a **LANGE** clinical manual

Family
Medicine

Ambulatory Care & Prevention

fourth edition

Edited by

Mark B. Mengel, MD, MPH
Professor and Chairman
Department of Community and Family Medicine
Saint Louis University School of Medicine
St. Louis, Missouri

L. Peter Schwiebert, MD
Professor and Director, Predoctoral Division
Department of Family and Preventive Medicine
University of Oklahoma College of Medicine
Oklahoma City, Oklahoma

Lange Medical Books/McGraw-Hill
Medical Publishing Division

New York   Chicago   San Francisco   Lisbon   London   Madrid   Mexico City   Milan
New Delhi   San Juan   Seoul   Singapore   Sydney   Toronto

Family Medicine: Ambulatory Care & Prevention, Fourth Edition

1234567890 DOC/DOC 0987654

ISBN: 0-07-142322-2

Notice

Medicine is an ever-changing science. As new research and clinical experience broaden our knowledge, changes in treatment and drug therapy are required. The authors and the publisher of this work have checked with sources believed to be reliable in their efforts to provide information that is complete and generally in accord with the standards accepted at the time of publication. However, in view of the possibility of human error or changes in medical sciences, neither the authors nor the publisher nor any other party who has been involved in the preparation or publication of this work warrants that the information contained herein is in every respect accurate or complete, and they disclaim all responsibility for any errors or omissions or for the results obtained from use of the information contained in this work. Readers are encouraged to confirm the information contained herein with other sources. For example and in particular, readers are advised to check the product information sheet included in the package of each drug they plan to administer to be certain that the information contained in this work is accurate and that changes have not been made in the recommended dose or in the contraindications for administration. This recommendation is of particular importance in connection with new or infrequently used drugs.

This book was set in Helvetica by Circle Graphics.
The editors were Janet Foltin, Harriet Lebowitz, and Penny Linskey.
The production supervisor was Catherine Saggese.
The index was prepared by Patricia Perrier.
R.R. Donnelley was printer and binder.

This book is printed on acid-free paper.

Contents

Contributors

Eve Ackerman, RN, MSN, ANP/CNP
Family Nurse Practitioner, College of Medicine at Rockford, Residency Program, Family Health Center, Rockford, Illinois

Alan M. Adelman, MD, MS
Professor, Department of Family and Community Medicine, Pennsylvania State University College of Medicine, Hershey, Pennsylvania

Kathleen C. Amyot, MD
Major USAFMC, Assistant Professor, Saint Louis University School of Medicine, Family Practice Residency Program, Belleville, Illinois

Joshua H. Barash, MD
Assistant Program Director, Department of Family Medicine, Thomas Jefferson University Hospital, Philadelphia, Pennsylvania

James R. Barrett, MD, CAQSM
Associate Professor, Department of Family Medicine, University of Oklahoma Health Sciences Center, Oklahoma City, Oklahoma

Heather Bartoli, PA-C
Clinical Assistant Professor, Department of Family and Preventative Medicine, University of Oklahoma Health Sciences Center, Oklahoma City, Oklahoma

Steven D. Bartz, MD, RPh
Assistant Professor of Family Medicine, University of Cincinnati, Cincinnati, Ohio

Frances Emily Biagioli, MD
Assistant Professor, OHSU Family Medicine, Oregon Health & Science University, Portland, Oregon

Richard B. Birrer, MD
Chief Executive Officer, St. Joseph Health Care System, Patterson, New Jersey, Professor of Medicine, Cornell Medical College, New York, New York

Shawn H. Blanchard, MD
Associate Predoctoral Director, Department of Family Medicine, Oregon Health & Science University, Portland, Oregon

Douglas G. Browning, MD, ATC-L
Assistant Professor and Director, Primary Care Sports Medicine Fellowship, Department of Family and Community Medicine, Wake Forest University School of Medicine, Winston-Salem, North Carolina

William E. Cayley, Jr., MD, MDiv
Assistant Professor, Eau Claire Family Medicine Residency, Department of Family Medicine, University of Wisconsin, Eau Claire, Wisconsin

Frank S. Celestino, MD
Associate Professor, Geriatrics Director, Wake Forest University School of Medicine, Health Promotion/Prevention, Winston-Salem, North Carolina

Isaac H. Cha, PharmD, BCPS, BC-ADM
Clinical Assistant Professor, Family and Community Medicine, University of Illinois
College of Medicine, Rockford, Illinois

Jason Chao, MD, MS
Professor of Family Medicine, Case Western Reserve University, University Hospitals
of Cleveland, Cleveland, Ohio

James C. Chesnutt, MD
Family Physician, Assistant Professor, Department of Family Medicine, Oregon Health
& Science University, Portland, Oregon

Leanne M. Chrisman-Khawam, MD, MEd
Assistant Professor, Department of Family Medicine, Case Western Reserve University,
University Hospitals of Cleveland, Cleveland, Ohio

Neal D. Clemenson, MD
Great Plains Family Practice Residency Program, Oklahoma City, Oklahoma

Stephen W. Cobb, MD
Residency Director, St. Joseph Hospital, Denver, Colorado

Jennifer Cocohoba, PharmD
Assistant Clinical Professor, Department of Clinical Pharmacy, School of Pharmacy,
University of California, San Francisco, San Francisco, California

Brian R. Coleman, MD
Assistant Professor, Department of Family and Preventive Medicine, University of
Oklahoma Health Sciences Center, Oklahoma City, Oklahoma

John L. Coulehan, MD, MPH
Professor, Preventive Medicine, SUNY at Stony Brook, Stony Brook, New York

Amy D. Crawford-Faucher, MD
Assistant Residency Director, Department of Family Medicine, Crozer-Keystone Family
Medicine Residency Program, Springfield, Pennsylvania

Michael A. Crouch, MD, MSPH
Associate Professor of Family and Community Medicine, Department of Family and
Community Medicine, Baylor College of Medicine, Houston, Texas

Mel P. Daly, MD
Director of Family Medicine, Subacute Unit, Greater Baltimore Medical Center,
Baltimore, Maryland

Janice E. Daugherty, MD
Associate Professor and Director of Predoctoral Education, Department of Family
Medicine, The Brody School of Medicine at East Carolina University, Greenville,
North Carolina

Kent W. Davidson, MD
Associate Professor, Department of Family and Community Medicine, University of
Arkansas College of Medicine, Little Rock, Arkansas

Pieter J. de Wet, MD
Formerly, Medical Director, Tyler Total Wellness Center, Associate Professor of Family
Practice, The University of Texas Health Center at Tyler, Tyler, Texas

Vanessa A. Diaz, MD, MS
Assistant Professor, Department of Family Medicine, Medical University of South
Carolina, Charleston, South Carolina

Victor Alejandro Diaz, Jr., MD
Assistant Professor, Department of Family Medicine, Jefferson Medical College, Thomas Jefferson University, Philadelphia, Pennsylvania

Larry L. Dickey, MD, MPH
Associate Adjunct Professor, Department of Family and Community Medicine, University of California, San Francisco, San Francisco, California

Philip M. Diller, MD, PhD
Associate Professor of Family Medicine, Department of Family Medicine, University of Cincinnati, Cincinnati, Ohio

Charles B. Eaton, MD, MS
Professor of Family Medicine, Director, Center for Primary Care and Prevention, Memorial Hospital of Rhode Island, Pawtucket, Rhode Island

Sarah R. Edmonson, MD
Primary Care Research Fellow, Department of Family and Community Medicine, Baylor College of Medicine, Houston, Texas

Mari Egan, MD, MHPE
Assistant Professor, Department of Family Medicine, Feinberg School of Medicine, Northwestern University, Chicago, Illinois

Ted D. Epperly, MD
Formerly, Chairman, Department of Family and Community Medicine, Eisenhower Army Medical Center, Fort Gordon, Georgia

David W. Euans, MD
Formerly, Clinical Associate Professor, Department of Family Medicine, Louisiana State University School of Medicine, Former Clinical Associate Professor, Department of Family and Community Medicine, Tulane University School of Medicine, New Orleans, Louisiana

Stephanie L. Evans, PharmD, BCPS
Assistant Professor, St. Louis College of Pharmacy, Clinical Pharmacist, Family Medicine of St. Louis, St. Louis, Missouri

Rhonda A. Faulkner, PhD
Assistant Professor, Department of Family Medicine, Northwestern University Feinberg School of Medicine, Chicago, Illinois

Jeanne M. Ferrante, MD
Associate Professor, Department of Family Medicine, UMDNJ-New Jersey Medical School, Newark, New Jersey

Scott A. Fields, MD
Professor and Vice Chair, Department of Family Medicine, Oregon Heath & Science University, Portland, Oregon

Brian J. Finley, MD
Assistant Professor, Department of Family Practice, University of Nebraska Medical Center, Omaha, Nebraska

Laura B. Frankenstein, MD
Formerly Family Physician, Lynn Community Health Center, Lynn, Massachusetts

Keith A. Frey, MD, MBA
Chair, Department of Family Medicine, Mayo Clinic Scottsdale, Associate Professor of Family Medicine, Mayo Clinic College of Medicine, Scottsdale, Arizona

Jennifer Gafford, PhD
Faculty Psychologist, Department of Family Medicine, Forest Park Hospital Family Medicine Residency Program, St. Louis, Missouri

Maria V. Gibson, MD, PhD
Medical Director of University Family Medicine, Assistant Professor, Department of
Family Medicine, Medical University of South Carolina, Charleston, South Carolina

Ronald H. Goldschmidt, MD
Director, Family Practice Inpatient Service, San Francisco General Hospital, Professor
and Vice Chair, Department of Family and Community Medicine, University of
California, San Francisco, San Francisco, California

Brian H. Halstater, MD
Assistant Clinical Professor, Department of Family Medicine Residency Program,
Department of Family and Community Medicine, Duke University School of Medicine,
Durham, North Carolina

John G. Halvorsen, MD, MS
Thomas and Ellen Foster Chair and Professor, Associate Dean for Community Health,
Department of Family and Community Medicine, University of Illinois College of
Medicine at Peoria, Peoria, Illinois

Richard J. Ham, MD
Director, Professor, Geriatric Medicine and Psychiatry, Center on Aging, Robert C. Byrd
Health Sciences Center at West Virginia University, Morgantown, West Virginia

Cynthia Haq, MD
Professor, Department of Family Medicine, The University of Wisconsin-Madison,
Madison, Wisconsin

D. Mike Hardin, Jr., MD
Faculty Member, Department of Family Medicine, McLennan County Medical Education
and Research Foundation, University of Texas Southwestern Medical School,
Waco, Texas

Radhika R. Hariharan, MD, MRCP (UK)
Assistant Professor, Department of Family and Community Medicine/Community Health
Program, Baylor College of Medicine, Houston, Texas

Shelly S. Harkins, MD
Assistant Professor, Department of Community and Family Medicine, Saint Louis
University School of Medicine, St. Louis, Missouri

John A. Heydt, MD
CEO, Drexel University Physicians, Chief Quality Officer, Chair, Department of Family,
Community and Preventive Medicine, Drexel University College of Medicine,
Philadelphia, Pennsylvania

Allen L. Hixon, MD
Assistant Professor, Department of Family Medicine, University of Connecticut School
of Medicine, Farmington, Connecticut

David Holmes, MD
Clinical Assistant Professor, Associate Vice Chair for Medical Student Education,
Family Medicine Clerkship Director, Department of Family Medicine, State University of
New York at Buffalo, Buffalo, New York

Felix Horng, MD, MBA
Assistant Clinical Professor, Department of Family Medicine, David Geffen School of
Medicine at UCLA, Los Angeles, California

May S. Jennings, MD
Assistant Professor, Department of Internal Medicine, University of Alabama School of
Medicine, Huntsville, Alabama

Andrew D. Jones, MD
Assistant Professor, Department of Family and Preventive Medicine, Associate Program
Director, Family Medicine Residency Program, University of Oklahoma Health Sciences
Center, Oklahoma City, Oklahoma

Cathy Kamens, MD
Assistant Professor, Department of Family Practice and Community Medicine,
University of Texas Southwestern Medical Center, Dallas, Texas

Mitchell A. Kaminski, MD, MBA
Chairman, Department of Family Medicine, Crozer-Chester Medical Center, Chester,
Pennsylvania

Nancy D. Kellogg, MD
Professor, Department of Pediatrics, The University of Texas Health Science Center at
San Antonio, San Antonio, Texas

Judith Anne Kerber, MD
Private Practice Physician, South Canadian Family Care Clinic, Mustang, Oklahoma

Sanford R. Kimmel, MD
Professor of Clinical Family Medicine, Department of Family Medicine, Medical College
of Ohio, Toledo, Ohio

Charles Kodner, MD
Associate Professor, Department of Family and Geriatric Medicine, University of
Louisville School of Medicine, Louisville, Kentucky

Geoffrey S. Kuhlman, MD, CAQSM
Primary Care Sports Medicine, Hinsdale Orthopaedic Associates, SC, Hinsdale, Illinois

David C. Lanier, MD
Associate Director, Center for Primary Care, Prevention and Clinical Partnerships,
Agency for Healthcare Research and Quality, Rockville, Maryland

Dennis P. Lewis, MD
Private Practice, Valencia, California, Formerly, Assistant Professor, Department of
Family Medicine, David Geffen School of Medicine at UCLA, Los Angeles, California

Martin S. Lipsky, MD
Regional Dean, University of Illinois-Chicago College of Medicine at Rockford,
Rockford, Illinois

Jonathan MacClements, MD, FAAFP
Director, Family Medicine Residency Program, Director of Medicine Education,
Assistant Professor of Family Medicine, Department of Family Medicine, The University
of Texas Health Center at Tyler, Tyler, Texas

Diane J. Madlon-Kay, MD, MS
Associate Professor, Institution Regions Family and Community Medicine Residency
Program, St. Paul, Minnesota

Arch G. Mainous III, PhD
Professor, Department of Family Medicine, Medical University of South Carolina,
Charleston, South Carolina

Robert Mallin, MD
Associate Professor, Department of Family Medicine, Medical University of South
Carolina, Charleston, South Carolina

Charles F. Margolis, MD
Professor of Clinical Family Medicine, Department of Family Medicine, University of
Cincinnati College of Medicine, Cincinnati, Ohio

James P. McKenna, MD
Director, Family Practice Residency, The Medical Center, Beaver, Pennsylvania

Anna L. Meenan, MD, FAAFP
Assistant Professor of Clinical Family Medicine, Department of Family and Community Medicine, University of Illinois-Chicago College of Medicine at Rockford, Rockford, Illinois

Mark B. Mengel, MD, MPH
Professor and Chairman, Department of Community and Family Medicine, Saint Louis University School of Medicine, St. Louis, Missouri

Angela D. Mickalide, PhD, CHES
Program Director, National SAFE KIDS Campaign, Washington, DC

Donald B. Middleton, MD
Vice President of Family Medicine Education, UPMC St. Margaret, Professor and Vice Chair, Department of Family Medicine, University of Pittsburgh School of Medicine, Pittsburgh, Pennsylvania

Leonard W. Morgan, MD, PhD*
Former Regional Chairman, Department of Family Medicine, Texas Tech University Health Sciences Center, Odessa, Texas

Karen D. Novielli, MD
Associate Professor of Family Medicine, Associate Dean for Faculty Affairs and Faculty Development, Jefferson Medical College, Thomas Jefferson University, Philadelphia, Pennsylvania

Jim Nuovo, MD
Professor and Assistant Dean for Graduate Medical Education, Department of Family and Community Medicine, University of California, Davis, Sacramento, California

Tomás P. Owens, Jr., MD
Chairman, Department of Family Medicine-Integris Baptist Medical Center, Associate Director, Great Plains Family Practice Residency Program, Clinical Associate Professor, Department of Internal Medicine, Geriatric Medicine, and Family and Preventive Medicine, University of Oklahoma Health Sciences Center, Oklahoma City, Oklahoma

Megeen Parker, MD
Clinical Assistant Professor, Department of Family Medicine, University of Wisconsin School of Medicine, Madison, Wisconsin

Ketan S. Patel, MD
Senior Associate Consultant, Department of Obstetrics and Gynecology, Mayo Clinic, Scottsdale, Arizona

Marjorie Shaw Phillips, MD, RPh, FASHP
Adjunct Clinical Associate Professor of Pharmacy Practice, University of Georgia College of Pharmacy and Pharmacist, Medical College of Georgia Hospital and Clinics, Augusta, Georgia

William G. Phillips, MD
Assistant Professor, Department of Family Medicine, Medical College of Georgia School of Medicine, Augusta, Georgia

Mark C. Potter, MD
Assistant Professor of Clinical Family Medicine, Department of Family Medicine, University of Illinois at Chicago, Chicago, Illinois

Brenda Powell, MD
Department of Family Medicine, Cleveland Clinic Foundation, Cleveland, Ohio

*Retired

Martin Quan, MD
Professor of Clinical Family Medicine, David Geffen School of Medicine at UCLA, Los Angeles, California

Kalyanakrishnan Ramakrishnan, MD
Associate Professor, Department of Family and Preventive Medicine, University of Oklahoma Health Sciences Center, Oklahoma City, Oklahoma

Goutham Rao, MD
Associate Professor, Departments of Family Medicine and Pediatrics, University of Pittsburgh School of Medicine and Children's Hospital of Pittsburgh, Pittsburgh, Pennsylvania

Brian C. Reed, MD
Assistant Professor, Department of Family and Community Medicine, Baylor College of Medicine, Houston, Texas

Steven E. Reissman, DO
Director of Adult Primary Care, Martin Army Community Hospital, Fort Benning, Georgia

John C. Rogers, MD, MPH
Professor and Vice Chair for Education, Department of Family and Community Medicine, Baylor College of Medicine, Houston, Texas

Michael P. Rowane, DO, MS, FAAFP, FAAO
Associate Professor, Family Medicine and Psychiatry, Case Western Reserve University, Residency Director, Case/University Hospitals of Cleveland, Family Medicine Residency Program, Co-Director, Case/University Hospitals of Cleveland, Family Medicine/Psychiatry Residency Program, Cleveland, Ohio

Robert C. Salinas, MD
Assistant Professor, Department of Family and Preventive Medicine, University of Oklahoma Health Sciences Center, Oklahoma City, Oklahoma

Ted C. Schaffer, MD
Director, Family Medicine Residency Program, UPMC St. Margaret, Pittsburgh, Pennsylvania

Richard O. Schamp, MD
Associate Professor, Department of Community and Family Medicine, Saint Louis University School of Medicine, St. Louis, Missouri

F. David Schneider, MD, MSPH
Associate Professor, Department of Family and Community Medicine, The University of Texas Health Science Center at San Antonio, San Antonio, Texas

L. Peter Schwiebert, MD
Professor and Director, Predoctoral Division, Department of Family and Preventive Medicine, University of Oklahoma College of Medicine, Oklahoma City, Oklahoma

H. Russell Searight, PhD, MPH
Director of Behavioral Medicine, Forest Park Hospital Family Medicine Residency Program, St. Louis, Missouri, Clinical Associate Professor of Community and Family Medicine, Saint Louis University School of Medicine, St. Louis, Missouri

Lowell G. Sensintaffar, MD
Assistant Professor, Department of Community and Family Medicine, Saint Louis University School of Medicine, St. Louis, Missouri

Aamir Siddiqi, MD
Associate Professor, Department of Family Medicine—Milwaukee Campus, St. Luke's Family Practice Residency, University of Wisconsin School of Medicine, Milwaukee, Wisconsin

Clark B. Smith, MD
Associate Professor and Vice Chairman for Clinical Affairs, Department of Family Medicine, University of Tennessee, Memphis, Tennessee

Jeannette E. South-Paul, MD
Professor and Chair, Department of Family Medicine, University of Pittsburgh School of Medicine, Pittsburgh, Pennsylvania

Rhonda A. Sparks, MD
Assistant Professor, Department of Family and Community Medicine, University of Oklahoma Health Sciences Center, Oklahoma City, Oklahoma

Nicole G. Stern, MD
Physician, Internal Medicine/Sports Medicine, Campus Health Service, University of Arizona, Tucson, Arizona

Carol Stewart, MD
Assistant Professor, Department of Family Medicine, David Geffen School of Medicine at UCLA, Los Angeles, California

Jeffrey L. Susman, MD
Professor and Chair, Department of Family Medicine, University of Cincinnati, Cincinnati, Ohio

Jay A. Swedberg, MD
Diplomate, American Board of Family Practice, Fellow, American Academy of Family Physicians, Casper, Wyoming

Melissa A. Talamantes, MS
Gerontologist, Department of Family and Community Medicine, The University of Texas Health Science Center, San Antonio, Texas

Patricia Taylor, MS, MPH, RN
ANP/CNP—Family Nurse Practitioner, Department of Family and Community Medicine, University of Illinois-Chicago College of Medicine at Rockford, Rockford, Illinois

Michael P. Temporal, MD
Associate Professor, Department of Community and Family Medicine, Saint Louis University, St. Louis, Missouri

William L. Toffler, MD
Professor and Director of Predoctoral Education, Department of Family Medicine, Oregon Health & Science University, Portland, Oregon

Terrence T. Truong, MD
Faculty, Great Plains Family Practice Residency Program, Oklahoma City, Oklahoma

Nancy Tyre, MD
Associate Physician Diplomat, Family Medicine, UCLA/Les Kelley, Santa Monica, California

Matthew E. Ulven, MD, MPH
Assistant Professor, Department of Community and Family Medicine, Saint Louis University School of Medicine, St. Louis, Missouri

Anthony F. Valdini, MD, MS, FACP, FAAFP
Clinical Associate Professor of Family and Community Medicine, Tufts University School of Medicine, Boston, Massachusetts, University of Massachusetts School of Medicine, Worcester, Massachusetts

Daniel A. Vogel, MD
Chief Fellow, Child and Adolescent Psychiatry, Cincinnati Children's Hospital Medical Center, Cincinnati, Ohio

H. Bruce Vogt, MD
Professor and Chair, Department of Family Medicine, University of South Dakota School of Medicine, Sioux Falls, South Dakota

Linda L. Walker, MD
Associate Director, Family Practice Residency Faculty, Columbus Regional Healthcare, Columbus, Georgia

Lara Carson Weinstein, MD
Instructor, Jefferson Family Medicine, Thomas Jefferson University, Philadelphia, Pennsylvania

Barry D. Weiss, MD
Professor of Clinical Family and Community Medicine, University of Arizona College of Medicine, Tucson, Arizona

Stephen F. Wheeler, MEng, MD
Associate Professor and Director of Residency Training, Department of Family and Geriatric Medicine, Associate Dean for Admissions, University of Louisville School of Medicine, Louisville, Kentucky

Lesley D. Wilkinson, MD
Associate Clinical Professor of Family Medicine, Department of Family Medicine, David Geffen School of Medicine at UCLA, Los Angeles, California

Deborah K. Witt, MD
Assistant Professor, Department of Family Medicine, Thomas Jefferson University, Jefferson Medical College, Philadelphia, Pennsylvania

Loyd J. Wollstadt, MD, MSc
Associate Professor of Medicine, Department of Family and Community Medicine, University of Illinois—Chicago College of Medicine at Rockford, Rockford, Illinois

Paul W. Wright, MD
Professor of Family Practice, Family Medicine Department, The University of Texas Health Center at Tyler, Tyler, Texas

Aleksandra Zgierska, MD, PhD
Family Medicine Resident, Department of Family Medicine, University of Wisconsin—Madison, Madison, Wisconsin

Preface

PURPOSE

This manual presents information on the most common complaints, problems, conditions, and diseases encountered by family physicians and other primary care providers who practice in the ambulatory setting. These common conditions, which have been selected from surveys taken in family practice, internal medicine, and pediatrics, are arranged alphabetically in five sections. Evidenced-based information is presented in such a way that busy practitioners can access it rapidly. Practical, specific treatment information, including starting doses of medications, is offered. This manual also addresses preventive interventions commonly used in the primary care setting.

ORGANIZATION AND SCOPE

Although most medical books are organized by organ system, we have structured this manual according to typical patient presentations in the primary care setting, for example, common symptoms and signs, follow-up needs for chronic physical or mental illnesses, and reproductive health concerns. In addition, we provide an evidence-based approach to preventive health care.

Section I contains information on the most commonly encountered acute problems in the primary care setting. Information is presented in such a way that a busy practitioner can quickly form a list of diagnostic possibilities, perform a cost-effective diagnostic work-up, and prescribe therapy for the most common causes of these complaints.

Section II offers information on the treatment of patients with common chronic illnesses. Each chapter provides practical follow-up strategies for such patients, integrating cost-effective clinical management with important psychosocial issues.

Section III is important because many patients who are seen in primary care clinics have either a primary psychiatric disorder or a psychiatric disorder complicating the management of co-existing medical conditions. Strategies that effectively identify and treat patients with psychiatric disorders are presented clearly and succinctly.

Section IV addresses reproductive health issues, including contraception, infertility, and prenatal and postpartum care.

Section V will assist primary care physicians in the prevention of important diseases in their patients. Authors recommend interventions that can be easily applied in primary care clinics; areas addressed include counseling, immunizations, screening tests, and chemoprophylaxis. New chapters on travel medicine and the preoperative evaluation are included.

In all chapters, authors have integrated principles of clinical decision-making and cost-effective clinical management and have considered psychosocial and contextual issues. When applicable, areas of controversy are identified. Where appropriate, alternative and complementary medicine interventions are discussed.

Other useful features of this manual include:

- A convenient outline format and selective use of boldface type to afford quick, easy access to key aspects of diagnosis and treatment.
- Flowcharts facilitating the diagnostic work-up or management of specific conditions.
- Emphasis on cost-effective, evidence-based strategies.
- Key Points that summarize main issues.
- Sidebars that highlight more than 70 special conditions.

- A streamlined organizational framework that makes it easier to find sections such as diagnoses, symptoms and signs, management strategies for chronic illnesses, treatment, and prognosis.

ACKNOWLEDGMENTS

First, we thank those of you who have used this manual. We received positive feedback from medical students and residents as well as from many practitioners who found the third edition to be a quick, practical reference text. We particularly appreciate those comments that have enabled us to strengthen many sections of the handbook and add new chapters and sections on topics that many readers considered important.

Second, we embarked on this fourth edition with some trepidation, as most of our authors are busy primary care physicians. We were pleasantly surprised to discover that many of these authors were eager to update their chapters and did so with great enthusiasm.

When time did not allow third edition authors to update their chapters, most were helpful in suggesting well-qualified authors willing to revise their work. We are delighted that all chapters have been updated and many have been totally rewritten, reflecting the rapid increase in information and changes in approach to therapy that have occurred in the mere 4 years since publication of the third edition.

Third, we thank the editors at McGraw-Hill for their encouragement and support. We had originally planned to revise this manual every 5 years; however, the editors were right in encouraging a shorter revision cycle. Also the outstanding editorial support of Linda Conheady, Janet Foltin, and Harriet Lebowitz has helped us express our ideas more clearly.

Last but far from least, we thank our spouses, Laura and Kathy, and our children, Sally, Kristin, and Matt, for their support and patience throughout this rapid editorial process. As we both had to take a great deal of work home, our families deserve special thanks and gratitude.

Mark B. Mengel, M.D., M.P.H.
L. Peter Schwiebert, M.D.
St. Louis, Missouri, and Oklahoma City, Oklahoma
November 2004

SECTION I. Common Complaints

1 Abdominal Pain

Kalyanakrishnan Ramakrishnan, MD

KEY POINTS

- Most patients presenting with abdominal pain have minor, nonsurgical causes. Nonspecific abdominal pain is most common and accounts for 90% of pain in children. Chronic abdominal pain is most often gastrointestinal in origin.
- Proper history taking and a stepwise physical examination enable a diagnosis to be made in most patients.
- Any woman of childbearing age presenting with abdominal pain should have a pregnancy test. Management in pregnancy should focus on both mother and fetus.
- Presentation in the elderly is modified by comorbid illness and medications. Classical history and physical findings are usually absent.

I. **Definition.** Abdominal pain is defined as a subjective feeling of discomfort in the abdomen. When the duration is less than 6 hours, it is referred to as acute. It may be caused by luminal obstruction (appendicitis, cholecystitis, renal or ureteral colic, diverticulitis), an inflamed organ (pancreatitis, hepatitis), ischemia (mesenteric ischemia, ischemic colitis), or bowel motility disorders/multifactorial causes (irritable bowel syndrome [IBS], nonspecific abdominal pain [NSAP]).

II. **Common Diagnoses.** Abdominal pain accounts for 2.5 million office visits and 8 million emergency-room visits every year in the United States and is the most frequent cause for gastroenterology consultation. Most patients have minor problems, such as dyspepsia, although 20–25% are found to have a serious condition requiring hospitalization. Table 1–1 lists the common causes of acute abdominal pain in adults and the elderly. In children, urinary tract disease, peptic ulcer, inflammatory bowel disease, and gastroesophageal reflux disease present acutely; constipation, lactose intolerance, midcycle pain, and psychological problems (secondary gain, sexual abuse, school phobia) are chronic.

A. **NSAP.** NSAP occurs in about one third (35%) of patients presenting with acute abdominal pain. Over 90% of children who have abdominal pain have NSAP. IBS rarely presents initially in the elderly.

B. **Appendicitis.** Appendicitis occurs in 7% of the US population (3% of women and 2% of men older than 50 years), with an incidence of 1.1/1000 people per year. It is the most common nonobstetric cause of surgical emergency during pregnancy and is more common in the second trimester. Perforation rates are higher in patients younger than 18 and older than 50 years.

C. **Gallstones.** About 10–20% of adults aged 20–50 years have gallstones; risk increases with aging, in Native Americans, and in younger women (where it is 2–6 times more frequent than in men). Other risk factors include pregnancy, oral contraceptive use, hormone replacement therapy, obesity, rapid weight loss, diabetes mellitus, liver cirrhosis, Crohn's disease, and sedentary lifestyle.

D. **Pancreatitis.** The incidence of acute pancreatitis in the United States is about 10 new cases per year per 100,000. The most common causes include cholelithiasis (40%), alcohol abuse (40%), drugs (steroids, azathioprine, estrogens, diuretics), trauma, viral infections, and hypercalcemia.

E. **Diverticular disease.** The prevalence of diverticular disease is age-dependent, increasing in the United States from <5% at age 40 to 65% by age 85; males and females are equally affected. Most cases (70%) are discovered incidentally, in 15–25% diverticulitis develops, and 5–15% bleed. Risk factors besides age include low fiber intake; increased consumption of red meat, fat, alcohol and caffeine; sedentary lifestyle; and obesity.

F. **Mesenteric vascular occlusion.** Risk factors for mesenteric vascular occlusion include age (>60 years) and atherosclerosis (embolic events in 50% and also thrombotic

TABLE 1-1. DISTRIBUTION OF ACUTE ABDOMINAL PATHOLOGY

Diagnosis	>50 years	<50 years
Intestinal obstruction	15–30%	2–6%
Biliary tract	15–30%	2–6%
Malignancy	4–13%	1%
Peptic ulcer	5–10%	2–8%
Diverticulitis	5–10%	<1%
Perforated viscus	4–6%	1%
Appendicitis	3–10%	15–30%
Hernia	3–4%	1–2%
Vascular emergencies	2–3%	<1%
Nonspecific abdominal pain	15–30%	40–50%

From Landry F: Evaluation of abdominal pain. In: *Emergency Clinical Guide.* Copyright Anisman SD. http://www.anisman.com/ecg/index.asp

or low-flow state with associated vasoconstriction). Hypercoagulable states, intra-abdominal sepsis, portal hypertension, and cancer increase risk for **mesenteric vein thrombosis,** although the cause in 5–10% of patients remains idiopathic. In the elderly, arteriosclerosis, shock, congestive heart failure, and aortoiliac surgery cause **ischemic colitis;** in younger patients, oral contraceptive use, vasculitis, and hypercoagulable states are risk factors.

   G. **Bowel obstruction.** Obstruction of the large or small bowel is a major health problem in the elderly, accounting for approximately 12% of cases of abdominal pain. Risk factors for small-bowel obstruction are adhesions due to previous abdominal surgery, neoplasms, or hernia. For large-bowel obstruction, risk factors include colon carcinoma, diverticulitis, and sigmoid volvulus.

   H. **Other causes.** Other common causes of abdominal pain not discussed here include dyspepsia (see Chapter 19), peptic ulcer disease (see Chapter 82), and pelvic inflammatory disease (see Chapter 51).

III. **Symptoms.** Proper history taking is the foundation for a correct diagnosis and should address a variety of features (Table 1–2). Knowing about a history of ulcer disease, biliary colic, or diverticulitis is helpful. Alcohol and drug use should be addressed. Alcohol abuse contributes to pancreatitis, hematemesis, esophageal rupture, and spontaneous bacterial peritonitis. Nonsteroidal anti-inflammatory drugs (NSAIDs), prednisone, and immunosuppressants cause bleeding and perforation; aspirin, NSAIDs, and anticoagulants increase risk of bleeding. Drugs in the elderly induce nausea, vomiting, anorexia, and constipation and affect vital signs. Menstrual history is also important; nausea, vomiting, constipation, frequency of urination, and pelvic or abdominal discomfort are experienced in normal pregnancy. Accuracy of history taking in the elderly may be affected by cognitive impairment, decreased auditory and visual acuity, and atypical symptoms.

   A. **NSAP and IBS.** Pain may be colicky or persistent, and aggravated by meals. Most patients have a long history of recurrent abdominal pain that is relieved with defecation, a change in the frequency or consistency of the stool, abdominal bloating, and passage of excessive mucus (Manning criteria). There is no weight loss, constitutional symptoms (fever, anorexia, nausea, arthralgia), or intestinal bleeding.

   B. **Appendicitis.** Anorexia and periumbilical pain followed by nausea, right lower quadrant (RLQ) pain, and vomiting occur in 50% of cases. Migration of pain has high sensitivity and specificity (approaching 80%). During pregnancy, the site of pain shifts progressively upward with increasing gestational age. Changes in bowel habits and hematuria/pyuria (pelvic appendicitis in 20%) may also be seen. Perforation results in generalized abdominal pain, fever, and tachycardia.

   C. **Cholelithiasis.** Over 50% of gallstones remain asymptomatic. Recurrent right upper quadrant or epigastric pain, radiating to the back or right shoulder blade, peaking over hours and resolving completely, suggests **biliary colic.** Upper abdominal pain in **cholecystitis** is severe, persistent, associated with constitutional symptoms and possibly jaundice. Perforation leading to **biliary peritonitis** causes spreading abdominal

TABLE 1–2. CORRELATION OF ABDOMINAL PAIN AND PATHOLOGY

Nature of Pain	Organ/Pathology
Acute or chronic (lasting weeks, months, years)	*Acute:* Biliary colic, renal colic, intestinal obstruction, perforated peptic ulcer, ruptured aneurysm, ruptured ectopic gestation *Chronic:* Peptic ulcer disease, chronic pancreatitis, diverticulosis
Onset of pain	*Sudden:* Sudden severe pain—perforated peptic ulcer, acute pancreatitis, ruptured aneurysm, ruptured ectopic gestation, renal/ureteric colic
Migration of pain	Appendicitis: Periumbilical, migrating to right iliac fossa Ureteric colic: From loin to groin
Referred pain	Biliary colic: Pain referred to the back and shoulder blades Pancreatitis: Referred to the back
Character of pain	*Burning pain:* Peptic ulcer *Colicky pain:* Biliary, renal, ureteric, intestinal colic (hollow organs) *Dull, continuous ache:* Solid organs (liver, spleen, kidneys)
Site of pain	*Epigastrium:* Stomach, liver, pancreas *Right hypochondrium:* Liver, biliary tree, hepatic flexure of colon *Left hypochondrium:* Spleen, tail of pancreas, splenic flexure of colon *Umbilicus:* Pancreas, transverse colon, small bowel *Right iliac fossa:* Appendix, cecum, ascending colon, terminal ileum, right tube, ovary, right ureter *Left iliac fossa:* Left tube and ovary, sigmoid colon, left ureter *Hypogastrium:* Urinary bladder, uterus *Back (renal angle):* Right/left kidney
Relieving factors	Antacids, food: Duodenal ulcer Sitting up, leaning forward: Pancreatitis Vomiting, antacids: Gastric ulcer
Associated symptoms	*Anorexia:* Gastric ulcer, appendicitis, peritonitis *Jaundice:* Biliary colic, cholecystitis, pancreatitis *Fever:* Appendicitis, cholecystitis *Vomiting:* Intestinal obstruction, pancreatitis, renal colic, ureteric colic, biliary colic, gastroenteritis *Hematemesis/melena:* Peptic ulcer disease *Diarrhea:* Gastroenteritis, colitis *Constipation:* Intestinal obstruction, appendicitis *Amenorrhea:* Pregnancy-related causes *Dysuria:* Urinary infection *Hematuria/smoky urine:* Renal/ureteric colic

pain and worsening constitutional symptoms. Stone in the common bile duct may cause deepening jaundice, associated with fever, chills, and pain—**Whipple's triad. Gallstone ileus** presents with pain, distention, and vomiting—features of small-bowel obstruction.
  D. **Mid-epigastric or diffuse abdominal pain,** relieved by bending forward, occurring 1–3 days after a binge or cessation of drinking, suggests **pancreatitis.** Nausea, vomiting, restlessness, and agitation accompany the pain. Chronic pancreatitis causes pain, malabsorption, diarrhea (steatorrhea), weight loss, or diabetes mellitus.
  E. **Diverticular disease.** Most diverticula are asymptomatic. **Diverticulitis** causes severe, abrupt worsening left lower abdominal pain, fever, anorexia, nausea, vomiting, and constipation.
  F. **Ischemic bowel disease** presents with severe localized or diffuse abdominal pain, unexplained abdominal distention, or gastrointestinal bleeding (bloody diarrhea, hematemesis) indicating bowel infarction. Elderly individuals with chronic mesenteric ischemia (**intestinal angina**) experience recurrent upper abdominal cramps 10–15 minutes after meals that subside over 1–3 hours. Bloating, flatulence, episodic vomiting, constipation,

or diarrhea and severe weight loss may occur. Steatorrhea develops in half of affected persons. A history of angina, claudication, or transient ischemic attacks may be present.

G. Bowel obstruction. Obstruction causes colicky pain, vomiting, abdominal distention, and constipation. In acute (small-bowel) obstruction, pain appears first followed by vomiting, distention, and constipation. In chronic (large-bowel) obstruction, constipation, followed by distention, pain, and vomiting, is seen.

IV. Signs (Table 1–3). The stability of the patient (pulse, respiration, blood pressure, level of consciousness) should be assessed initially. Shock, pallor, sweating, or fainting indicates serious abdominal pathologic findings. Rebound tenderness, guarding, and rigidity suggest a surgical cause. Operative scars suggest adhesions and bowel obstruction; abnormal orifices can be sites of hernias. Rectal and vaginal examinations assess pelvic or intraluminal pathologic findings. Guarding and rigidity are often absent during pregnancy, due to stretching of the abdominal wall and lack of direct contact with the parietal peritoneum of the underlying inflamed organ. To distinguish uterine from extrauterine tenderness, patients should be examined in the right or left decubitus position.

A. In **NSAP,** bowel sounds may be increased; a fecal mass may present in either iliac fossa.

B. Helpful findings in **appendicitis** include guarding, RLQ tenderness, rebound tenderness, pain on percussion, and rigidity. Nonspecific findings include Rovsing's sign (pain elicited by compression of the left iliac fossa), iliopsoas sign (pain precipitated by extension of the ipsilateral hip), and Cope's obturator test (pain on internal rotation of the right hip).

C. **Biliary colic** is characterized by right upper quadrant tenderness worse on deep inspiration (Murphy's sign), when the inflamed gallbladder comes in contact with the examiner's hand.

D. Patients with **pancreatitis** have epigastric or periumbilical guarding, abdominal distention, and ileus. In **hemorrhagic pancreatitis,** shock, coma, and signs of retroperitoneal bleeding may be present, as indicated by ecchymoses in the flanks (Grey Turner's sign) or around the umbilicus (Cullen's sign).

E. Localized peritonitis in **diverticulitis** may result in abdominal distention and ileus; rebound tenderness may be elicited in the left iliac fossa.

F. **Mesenteric ischemia** produces few significant abdominal signs in the early stages. A systolic upper abdominal bruit is heard in half of patients with intestinal angina. Mild tenderness and guarding in the left flank or iliac fossa is usual in ischemic colitis.

G. **Bowel obstruction** produces abdominal distention with hyperperistaltic bowel sounds. Guarding and rigidity suggest strangulation, as do the features of sepsis or shock. Hernial orifices and scars should be palpated for a mass, suggesting a hernia.

V. Laboratory Tests. The following approach relates to patients with **acute abdominal pain.** In **chronic abdominal pain** (see sidebars), testing must be individualized.

TABLE 1–3. PHYSICAL EXAMINATION IN ABDOMINAL PAIN

Inspection	Palpation	Percussion	Auscultation
Shape of the abdomen (scaphoid)	Guarding Rigidity	Tenderness Free fluid (ascites)	Bowel sounds
Whether all quadrants move equally with respiration	Of solid organs (liver, spleen, kidney, uterus, abdominal aorta, other palpable masses)	Organomegaly (liver, spleen, kidney, other masses)	Bruits (renal)
Engorged veins, visible abdominal pulsations, visible peristalsis	Testes, appendages (epididymis, spermatic cord)		
Hernial orifices (umbilical, inguinal, femoral)	Rectal/vaginal examination		
Scars of prior surgery			
Scrotum (testes, spermatic cord)			

ABDOMINAL WALL PAIN

Abdominal wall pain occurs in the young secondary to trauma, overexertion, or epigastric or incisional hernias. In the elderly it may be secondary to herpes zoster and postherpetic neuralgia, or soft tissue tumors (neurofibroma). The pain often has an insidious onset, being sharp initially and becoming dull over time. Straining, as in sneezing, coughing, or lifting heavy objects, aggravates it; changing positions or applying heat may relieve it. A positive Carnett's sign (tenderness reproduced by tensing the abdominal wall) may be present.

Useful measures include nonsteroidal anti-inflammatory drugs (eg, oral ibuprofen 400–600 mg three times daily), muscle relaxants (eg, cyclobenzaprine 10 mg three times daily, methocarbamol 1000 mg four times daily), antidepressants (eg, amitriptyline), local application of ethyl chloride or capsaicin cream 0.025%, and trigger point injections of bupivacaine hydrochloride 0.35% plus triamcinolone 10–40 mg (most effective).

INFLAMMATORY BOWEL DISEASE (IBD)

Chronic abdominal pain is more common in **Crohn's disease** than in **ulcerative colitis** and located in the right lower quadrant (RLQ). Fever, weight loss, arthralgia, and chronic diarrhea (with blood and mucus in stool) may be present, as are extraintestinal manifestations (arthralgias, skin ulcers, visual disturbances). Skin changes (pyoderma gangrenosum, erythema nodosum) and eye changes (iritis) may be present. A mass (thickened terminal ileum and cecum) may be palpable in the RLQ in **Crohn's disease.** Anemia, low serum albumin, elevated C-reactive protein level, and sedimentation rate are often present. Barium contrast studies and colonoscopy are diagnostic. Treatment involves long-term medications, including 5-aminosalicylic acid, steroids, and immunosuppressants such as azathioprine or 6-mercaptopurine. Ablative surgery (right hemicolectomy) may be necessary in the presence of obstruction, fistula formation, or non-response to medical management.

CHRONIC ABDOMINAL PAIN

Chronic pain implies persistence for 3–6 months and impact on the patient's activities of daily living. Evaluation begins with ruling out gastrointestinal causes. A blood count, sedimentation rate, chemistry, plain abdominal x-rays, abdominal ultrasound, and colonoscopy rule out most serious causes. When initial assessment suggests the possibility of a specific abnormality, specialized tests (eg, ERCP, angiography) can be considered. In children, sonography of the abdomen and pelvis is usually performed first to exclude nonintestinal pain.

Optimal treatment incorporates acknowledging the reality of the pain, reassuring the patient that an underlying serious abnormality is unlikely to be missed, setting appropriate goals to minimize the impact of the pain on daily patient functioning, minimizing testing, and treating pain early using a multidisciplinary approach. Psychological evaluation and treatment, biofeedback and relaxation therapy, use of oral antidepressants (eg, amitriptyline 25–50 mg at bedtime) as analgesic adjuncts, and referral to a pain management specialist may be indicated.

Recurrent abdominal pain syndrome in children is vague, unrelated to meals, activity, or stool pattern, and does not awaken patients. An epigastric location is sometimes reported. Pallor, nausea, dizziness, headache, and fatigue may be present. Family history is often positive for functional bowel disease. Indicators of serious disease in children include vomiting, localized pain away from midline, altered bowel habits, growth disturbance, nocturnal episodes, radiation of pain, incontinence, presence of systemic symptoms, and family history of peptic ulcer and IBD. Response to empiric intervention (trial of lactose elimination, reduction of excessive juice intake, addition of a fiber supplement in constipation) and behavior and psychological management are valuable, as is educating the child and parents about diagnosis and treatment options. A symptom diary allows the child to play an active role in the diagnostic process. It is important for the child to maintain a normal routine, including school activities and diet.

A. Hematologic tests. Initial lab tests in acute abdominal pain should include a complete blood count (CBC) with differential, serum chemistries (electrolytes, serum glucose, liver and kidney function tests, amylase and lipase), urinalysis, coagulation panel in the elderly or if the drug history indicates it, and a pregnancy test in women of childbearing age.

Investigations in children, other than a CBC, urinalysis, urine culture, and examination of the stool for blood, are selected based on clinical suspicion of specific pathologic findings (ultrasound in pelvic pain or appendicitis, endoscopic evaluation with pain suspected of gastrointestinal origin). Blood may need to be typed and crossmatched before surgery or with suspected bleeding. Blood cultures may be drawn if the patient is febrile. An electrocardiogram may be ordered in the elderly before surgery or if cardiac origin for the pain is considered.

  1. Blood count. Anemia is a feature of peptic ulcers, ruptured aneurysm, inflammatory bowel disease (IBD) (along with raised sedimentation rate), and malignancies. Thrombocytopenia (platelets <50,000) may be seen in Henoch-Schönlein purpura in children. Leukocytosis—white cell count >12,000—is seen in appendicitis (sensitivity 91%, specificity 21%), cholecystitis (sensitivity 78%, specificity 11%), diverticulitis, and bowel ischemia. Leukocytosis is typical in the second and third trimesters of pregnancy and in early labor.

  2. Serum chemistry.
    a. Hypocalcemia and elevations in serum amylase (sensitivity 74%, specificity 50%) and lipase may be seen in pancreatitis. Amylase is elevated early (within 24 hours) in pancreatitis and lipase within a few days after symptom onset.
    b. Metabolic acidosis (in 50% of patients) and elevations of serum and peritoneal fluid amylase, alkaline phosphatase, and inorganic phosphate are seen with mesenteric ischemia.
    c. C-reactive protein may be elevated in appendicitis; a normal test in patients symptomatic for 24 hours rules out appendicitis.

B. Radiologic tests
  1. X-rays in acute abdominal pain should include a flat plate and upright view of the abdomen, and an erect chest x-ray. X-rays have poor specificity (<15%), and in most instances do not change the clinical diagnosis.
    a. Chest x-ray is useful to visualize pneumoperitoneum and cardiopulmonary pathology.
    b. Abdominal films also identify subdiaphragmatic or retroperitoneal gas associated with perforation, features of bowel obstruction (distended bowel, air-fluid levels), air in the biliary tree (gallstone ileus), calcium deposits (eg, gallstones [10–20% sensitivity], renal or ureteral stones, appendicoliths, calcification in chronic pancreatitis, aortic aneurysm), foreign bodies, and pneumatosis (ie, air in the bowel wall suggesting possible ischemia).
  2. Ultrasound detects gallstones (sensitivity 85–90%), sludge, gallbladder wall thickening (>5 mm is diagnostic), pericholecystic fluid (in cholecystitis), and intrahepatic or extrahepatic bile duct dilatation, associated with biliary obstruction.
    a. Ultrasound can also identify pancreatitis, pseudocysts and tumors, ascites, chronic liver disease (eg, fatty liver or cirrhosis), gynecologic abnormalities, renal or adrenal pathologic findings, and acute appendicitis (sensitivity 85–90%, specificity 92–96%).
    b. Duplex ultrasonography is highly specific (92–100%) for mesenteric arterial stenosis or occlusion.
  3. Computerized tomography (CT) is the most sensitive study in evaluating patients with acute abdominal pain, particularly obese patients. It has high sensitivities (pancreatitis, 65–100%; appendicitis, 96–98%; pancreatic tumors, 95%; high-grade bowel obstruction, 86–100%). It detects smaller volumes of free air, as compared to plain x-rays, can detect loculated air, and is the diagnostic modality of choice in intraperitoneal and retroperitoneal abscess, in diverticulitis, and in determining the presence and extent of diverticular complications, such as fistulas or sinus tracts.

C. Radionuclide scanning
    a. In acute cholecystitis the cystic duct is obstructed; a technetium-labeled hepatic iminodiacetic acid scan (HIDA) shows nonvisualization of the gallbladder

and is 95% accurate. Poor fractional excretion of HIDA (<15%) is characteristic of biliary dyskinesia.

  b. In Meckel's diverticulum, there is a preferential uptake of sodium Tc-pertechnetate by ectopic gastric tissue in the diverticulum (sensitivity 85% and specificity 95% in children).

4. **Miscellaneous tests**
  a. **Magnetic resonance angiography,** with and without gadolinium, detects severe narrowing or occlusion of the celiac axis and superior mesenteric artery. **Mesenteric angiography** can show the presence and site of emboli and thrombi and mesenteric vasoconstriction as well as the adequacy of the splanchnic circulation. The angiographic catheter also provides a route for the administration of intra-arterial vasodilators or thrombolytic agents.
  b. **Barium enema or colonoscopy** is diagnostic in IBD and colonic ischemia, outlining ulcerations, thickened bowel, pseudopolyps, and strictures. **Water-soluble contrast medium** (meglumine diatrizoate [Gastrografin]) is preferred if contrast enema is to be performed in diverticulitis; it shows the diverticula and leakage and may outline a fistulous tract.
  c. **Endoscopic retrograde cholangiopancreatogram (ERCP)** is diagnostic in chronic pancreatitis, shows associated pseudocysts and glandular and ductal pathology (strictures, calculi), and helps rule out malignancy.

VI. **Treatment.** Once the patient's condition is stabilized, the physician can obtain a detailed history, perform a clinical examination and investigations, and formulate a treatment plan. Providing pain relief should not await a definitive diagnosis, because unrelieved acute pain produces adverse consequences and there is no evidence that immediate pain relief delays diagnosis or treatment.
  A. **NSAP.** Watchful waiting with close follow-up is recommended, because most patients have a benign, self-limited illness. Providing reassurance, having patients avoid foods that precipitate the pain, and prescribing oral antispasmodics such as dicyclomine hydrochloride (eg, Bentyl), 20 mg four times daily, or propantheline bromide (eg, Pro-Banthine), 15 mg before meals and at bedtime, are useful. Narcotic analgesics should be avoided.
  B. **IBS.** Treatment is directed at reducing anxiety and stress, increasing dietary fiber with bulk agents such as oral psyllium (eg, Metamucil), avoiding foods that exacerbate or trigger IBS, and using antispasmodics such as dicyclomine hydrochloride. Psychotherapy may be useful. In patients with diarrhea, oral loperamide hydrochloride (eg, Imodium) 2–4 mg, or diphenoxylate hydrochloride with atropine (eg, Lomotil), 10–20 mg four times a day, are useful. Frequent follow-up may be needed until symptoms stabilize.
  C. **Appendicitis.** Diagnostic scoring systems (Table 1–4) used to predict the likelihood of appendicitis offer sensitivity and specificity >90% and reduce rates of perforation and negative laparotomy by 50%. Appendectomy is the treatment of choice with early diagnosis, if an abscess develops, or in recurrent appendicitis. A laparoscopic approach is

TABLE 1–4. THE ALVARADO SCORING SYSTEM FOR LIKELIHOOD OF ACUTE APPENDICITIS

Features	Score
Migratory right iliac fossa pain	1
Nausea/vomiting	1
Anorexia	1
Right iliac fossa tenderness	2
Fever >37.3°C	1
Rebound tenderness in right iliac fossa	1
Leukocytosis >10,000/mm^3	2
Neutrophilic shift to the left >75%	1
Total score	**10**

Score <4: no appendicitis, 5 or 6 indicates compatible with acute appendicitis, 7 or 8 indicates probable acute appendicitis, 9 or 10 indicates very probable acute appendicitis.

less traumatic and has fewer complications (bleeding, wound infection, intra-abdominal sepsis) than open appendectomy. Other treatment measures include analgesics, intravenous (IV) fluids, and antibiotics. If an appendicular mass (inflamed appendix walled off by omentum) is noticed, nonoperative treatment (bowel rest, analgesics, IV fluids, and antibiotics) is continued until symptomatic improvement and resolution of the mass.

D. Biliary disease.
  1. Most patients with **biliary colic** respond to oral analgesics (eg, hydrocodone/acetaminophen 5–7.5/500 mg—eg, Lortab—every 4–6 hours) and clear liquids for 2–3 days.
  2. **Cholecystitis** responds to IV hydration, bowel rest, and broad-spectrum IV antibiotics (eg, cefotaxime 2 g three times daily) for 2–3 days. Interval elective laparoscopic cholecystectomy (6 weeks later) is curative.
  3. Chemical dissolution of gallstones using ursodiol 600 mg daily given in divided doses is reserved for patients refusing surgery or in whom it is contraindicated and is successful in 55% of patients over 12 months. An oral cholecystogram is performed initially to confirm normal gallbladder function, a prerequisite for dissolution.

E. Pancreatitis.
  1. Most patients improve on nothing by mouth, IV hydration, and pain relief for 2–3 days. Morphine sulfate 5–10 mg IV every 3 hours may be used in both biliary pathologic findings and pancreatitis; recent studies do not link morphine with causing or aggravating pancreatitis or cholecystitis.
  2. Once pancreatitis resolves, biliary stones should be removed and cholecystectomy performed. Alcohol intake should be avoided.
  3. Local complications include abscess formation, pseudocyst, bowel necrosis, pancreatic ascites, and splenic vein thrombosis. Shock or respiratory or renal failure is more likely in hemorrhagic pancreatitis. Initial leukocytosis (>16,000/mm^3), hyperglycemia (>200 mg%), elevated liver enzymes (lactate dehydrogenase >350 IU/L, aspartate aminotransferase >250 IU/L) and age >55 years are associated with a poorer prognosis (**Ranson's criteria**).
  4. Large pseudocysts may need surgical consultation for percutaneous or internal drainage. Medication intake (eg, steroids, azathioprine) may need to be modified, and metabolic abnormalities (eg, hypercalcemia) corrected to avoid recurrence and development of chronicity.
  5. Pain management in **chronic pancreatitis** is difficult and may require narcotics (despite the strong predilection in alcoholics for addiction), or celiac plexus block with phenol or alcohol by a radiologist. Steatorrhea should be treated with fat restriction (20 g/day) and Viokase (3 tablets with meals). Diabetes mellitus is treated appropriately (see Chapter 74 on diabetes mellitus).

F. Diverticulitis.
  1. Mild cases respond to a 7- to 10-day course of oral ciprofloxacin, 500 mg twice daily, and metronidazole (eg, Flagyl) 250 mg three times a day.
  2. Hospitalization for bowel rest, IV hydration, and antibiotics are required for vomiting, sepsis, or peritonitis. Laparotomy and bowel resection is indicated in bowel perforation or obstruction, fistula, suspected cancer, massive hematochezia, or failure of medical treatment. Percutaneous drainage of localized abdominal or pelvic abscesses by a radiologist under ultrasound or CT guidance is feasible.

G. Ischemic bowel disease requires hospitalization; patient stabilization; nasogastric aspiration; broad-spectrum antibiotics; interventional radiologist consultation for selective mesenteric arterial catheterization; possible vasodilator or thrombolytic infusion; and possible surgical consultation for embolectomy, bowel resection, or revascularization. Surgical resection is indicated in ischemic colitis if abdominal findings, fever, and leukocytosis suggest deterioration, or if the patient has diarrhea or bleeding for more than 2 weeks.

H. Patients with obstruction of the large or small bowel require hospitalization for IV hydration, correction of fluid and electrolyte imbalance, bowel rest, decompression through nasogastric aspiration, and administration of enemas to induce evacuation. Small-bowel obstruction due to adhesions and incomplete large-bowel obstructions respond to this treatment. Endoscopic decompression relieves a sigmoid volvulus. Surgical consultation is indicated in patients not responding to conservative treatment, with guarding and rigidity indicating bowel ischemia or irreducible hernia.

REFERENCES

Chan MYP, et al: Alvarado score: An admission criterion in patients with right iliac fossa pain. Surg J R Coll Surg Edinb Irel 2003;**1**:39.

Dominitz JA, Sekijima JH, Watts M: Abdominal pain. http://www.uwgi.org/cme/cmeCourseCD/ch_06/CH06TXT.HTM.

Fishman MB, Aronson MD: Approach to patient with abdominal pain. UpToDate 2002. http://www.uptodate.com/patient_info/topicpages/topics/Pri_Gast/2173.asp

Graff LG IV, Robinson D: Abdominal pain and emergency department evaluation. Emerg Med Clin North Am 2001;**19**:123.

Kizer KW, Vassar MJ: Emergency department diagnosis of abdominal disorders in the elderly. Am J Emerg Med 1998;**16**:357.

Perry R: Acute abdomen in pregnancy. eMedicine Journal, 2002, Volume 3, Number 5. http://www.emedicine.com/med/topic3522.htm

Portis AJ, Sundaram CP: Diagnosis and initial management of kidney stones. Am Fam Physician 2001;**63**:1329.

2   The Abnormal Pap Smear

Neal D. Clemenson, MD

KEY POINTS

- Human papilloma virus (HPV) infection causes most abnormal Pap smears and virtually all cervical dysplasia.
- Many abnormal Pap smears resolve spontaneously as the underlying HPV infection clears.
- HPV testing is now widely available and can assist with decision making in some situations.

I. **Definition.** The Pap smear, a cytologic examination of exfoliated cervical and endocervical cells, was developed in the 1930s by Papanicolaou and is currently used as a screening tool for cervical neoplasia and carcinoma. Largely because of the use of the Pap smear, deaths in the United States from cervical cancer fell 74% between 1955 and 1992; in 2003 we can expect 12,200 new cases of cervical cancer and 4100 deaths from it.

Advances in our understanding of cervical disease, new reporting systems, and new diagnostic and treatment modalities make a systematic approach to the abnormal Pap smear very important. Recommendations for the frequency and method of the Pap smear may be found in Chapter 102.

Several systems are used for reporting the results of the Pap smear. The Bethesda system provides the most complete information and has been widely adopted; its classification scheme, updated in 2001, is used in this chapter. Equivalent classifications in the World Health Organization (WHO) and cervical intraepithelial neoplasia (CIN) systems are provided. Since the systems are not interchangeable, it is essential that clinicians become familiar with the system used by their particular laboratory.

II. **Common Diagnoses.** Many types of cervical and vaginal abnormalities can be detected by the Pap smear, including the following.

A. **Atypical squamous cells (ASC).** These cells are further classified as "of uncertain significance" (ASC-US) or "cannot exclude HSIL" (ASC-H). (HSIL refers to high-grade squamous intraepithelial lesions.) ASC may be caused by infection (see section II,E), including HPV infection (section II,C) but may also occur in the absence of infection; the cause in this situation is not well understood.

B. **Low-grade squamous intraepithelial lesions** (LSIL, mild dysplasia, or CIN 1). These are generally caused by a transient **human papillomavirus (HPV)** infection. HPV is a small DNA virus that replicates in the nuclei of epithelial cells; some types may cause malignant transformation by incorporation into the host DNA, especially in chronic infections. The infection may be subclinical or may cause condylomata or other lesions on the vulva, vagina, or cervix. HPV infection is generally contracted by sexual contact with an infected partner, who may be asymptomatic, although infection from nongenital lesions may occur as well. As with other sexually transmitted diseases, the risk increases with the number and risk status of sexual partners and may be reduced by the use of barrier contraception (eg, condoms). HPV infection is common, especially in younger sexually active individuals; if the infection is cleared the Pap smear will often return to normal.

C. High-grade squamous intraepithelial lesions (HSIL). These include moderate and severe dysplasia (CIN 2 and 3) and carcinoma in situ (CIN 3). They often represent chronic HPV infection and are more likely to progress to more severe dysplasia or cancer.

D. Atypical glandular cells (AGC). These may be caused by inflammation or neoplasia in the endocervix, endometrium, or extrauterine sites such as the ovaries, breast, or gastrointestinal tract. They may be characterized as endocervical, endometrial, or not otherwise specified.

E. Frank cervical carcinomas. These include squamous cell carcinomas and adenocarcinomas, as well as noncervical carcinomas, including endocervical carcinoma and vaginal carcinoma. Cervical carcinomas are discussed in section V,E; the other carcinomas are beyond the scope of this chapter.

F. Organisms, including **bacteria** (eg, *Chlamydia* or *Gardnerella*), **fungi** (eg, *Candida*), or **protozoa** (eg, *Trichomonas*), can colonize or infect the vaginal or cervical epithelium. This may occur without altering the mucosa, or the infectious agent may elicit an inflammatory response and resultant cellular changes. *Chlamydia* and *Trichomonas* infections are sexually transmitted, and multiple sexually transmitted diseases may coexist. *Candida* infections are probably caused by alterations in the usual vaginal flora and may be triggered by antibiotics, altered host defenses, or other poorly understood causes. Frequent or severe *Candida* infections may occur in women with human immunodeficiency virus (HIV) infection or diabetes mellitus. Bacterial vaginosis is also caused by altered flora, but the cause of the alteration is not clear; it is generally believed not to be transmitted sexually.

III. Symptoms

A. ASC and **inflammation** are usually asymptomatic unless associated with an infection (see section II,F), although bleeding, especially after intercourse, may occur. Upon examination, the cervix may appear normal or may show redness, erosions, or friability, especially with some infections.

B. LSILs are usually asymptomatic. The cervix may appear normal or may show redness, erosions, friability, or gross lesions. Acetic acid application (see section IV,B,1) may identify lesions that are not grossly visible.

C. HSILs are usually asymptomatic but may be associated with bleeding; large lesions may cause vaginal discharge. The cervix may appear normal or may show redness, erosions, friability, or gross lesions. Acetic acid application (see section IV,B,1) may identify lesions that are not grossly visible.

D. AGC may be asymptomatic or may have symptoms related to the underlying disease (eg, irregular bleeding with endometrial neoplasia).

E. Carcinomas may be asymptomatic or may cause bleeding or vaginal discharge. Metastatic disease may be associated with abdominal fullness, weight loss, or other symptoms related to the sites and nature of the metastases.

F. Infections may be asymptomatic or may be associated with vaginal discharge, odor, or itching. Signs may include vaginal or cervical discharge or inflammation.

IV. Laboratory Tests

A. The **Pap smear** report should include the following information.

    1. Specimen adequacy. An unsatisfactory smear should be repeated; a less than optimal smear may warrant repeat, treatment, or follow-up, depending on the specific findings and clinical situation. Many authorities no longer consider the absence of endocervical cells alone to be an indication of an inadequate smear, and the need to repeat smears without endocervical cells is a clinical judgment.

    2. The report should specify any **epithelial cell abnormalities** using the terminology of the particular reporting system. Other findings may include organisms or other evidence of infection, reactive cellular changes (eg, inflammation), or endometrial cells.

    3. The report may include **educational notes and suggestions** regarding treatment, follow-up, or both. This information may be helpful, but the clinician should determine the plans for the patient, depending on the situation and his or her clinical judgment.

B. Additional tests

1. **Acetic acid application.** Applying 5% acetic acid solution to the cervix for 1 minute will cause many condylomata or dysplastic areas to turn white (acetowhite lesions). These lesions should be evaluated by colposcopy and biopsy (see section IV,B,3).

2. **Biopsy.** Prior to the widespread use of colposcopy, cervical biopsies of suspicious areas, or random biopsies of visually normal areas, were used to evaluate abnormal smears. With the availability of colposcopy, biopsy should be done only in conjunction with colposcopy.

3. **Colposcopy,** cervical examination under stereoscopic magnification by an experienced examiner, along with endometrial sampling and biopsy of abnormal areas, is the definitive procedure for assessing many Pap smear abnormalities.

4. **HPV testing** can be done to determine whether one of the types likely to cause malignancy is present. This technology is now widely available and is a useful option in the management of ASC-US (see section V,A,3). Many laboratories using fluid-based cytology can hold the sample for HPV testing after the Pap smear is reported.

5. **Cervicography** (photographing the cervix for interpretation by a specially trained technician) and **speculoscopy** (examining the cervix under chemiluminescent illumination) have been described as intermediate triage methods, but their role in clinical practice requires further study.

V. Treatment (Figure 2–1). Many strategies have been proposed for the treatment of abnormal Pap smears, especially ASC-US. The following strategies are based primarily on the

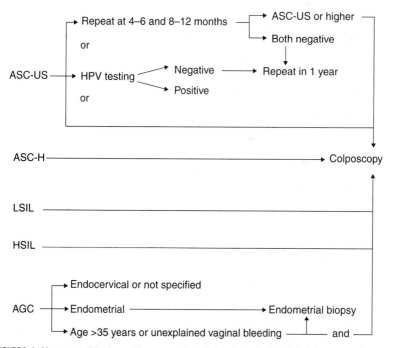

FIGURE 2–1. Management of the abnormal Pap smear. AGC, atypical glandular cells; ASC-H, atypical squamous cells, cannot exclude HSIL; ASC-US, atypical squamous cells of uncertain significance; HPV, human papilloma virus; HSIL, high-grade squamous intraepithelial lesions; LSIL, low-grade squamous intraepithelial lesions.

2001 Consensus Guidelines developed under the sponsorship of the American Society for Colposcopy and Cervical Pathology.
  A. ASC-US. Any of the following options is appropriate, depending on patient and clinician preferences and available resources.
   1. **Repeat cytologic testing.** Repeat Pap smears at 4- to 6-month intervals until 2 consecutive negative smears are obtained, after which the Pap smear should be repeated in 12 months. If a repeat smear shows ASC-US or a higher-grade abnormality, colposcopy should be performed. If the woman is postmenopausal and is not receiving estrogen replacement, the smear can be repeated 1 week after a course of vaginal estrogen (eg, conjugated estrogen cream, 2 g every other day for 4 weeks). If the smear remains abnormal, colposcopy should be considered.
   2. **Colposcopy.** Colposcopy is performed; if no CIN is found, the Pap smear should be repeated in 12 months.
   3. **HPV testing.** If negative for high-risk HPV, the Pap smear should be repeated in 12 months. If positive for high-risk HPV, colposcopy should be performed.
  B. ASC-H. Colposcopy should be performed on women with ASC-H results.
  C. LSIL. Colposcopy is currently recommended for most women with LSIL. In postmenopausal women, options also include repeat Pap smears at 6 and 12 months (with colposcopy if ASC-US or greater) or HPV testing at 12 months (with colposcopy if positive for high-risk types).
  D. HSIL. Colposcopy should be performed for HSIL.
  E. AGC. Colposcopy should be performed for AGC specified as endocervical or not otherwise specified. Endometrial sampling should be performed initially for AGC specified as endometrial cells. Women older than 35 years or with unexplained vaginal bleeding should have endometrial sampling and colposcopy.
  F. Carcinomas. The treatment of carcinomas is generally surgical; referral to a physician experienced in gynecologic oncology is indicated.
  G. Specific **vaginal infections,** with confirmation as clinically appropriate, should be treated as described in Chapters 31 and 64. If the infection was sexually transmitted, the patient's partner(s) should be treated in order to prevent reinfection. If reactive cellular changes, inflammation, or both are noted, reexamination of the patient may be appropriate to rule out infection. Empiric therapy with topical or systemic antimicrobial agents is not recommended.
  H. Endometrial cells may be found on a Pap smear taken during or shortly after menstruation, but if they are found in the second half of the menstrual cycle or in a postmenopausal woman, endometrial biopsy or other endometrial sampling should be considered.
  I. HIV. Since women with HIV are at higher risk for cervical neoplasia, some clinicians perform more frequent Pap smears. Annual colposcopy in place of Pap smears has also been recommended, but the practicality and cost-effectiveness of this approach are unclear.
  J. Pregnancy. The management of ASC-US in pregnancy is the same as discussed in section V,A, except that colposcopy should either be delayed until after delivery or performed without endocervical sampling. The recommendations for pregnant women with ASC-H, LSIL, or HSIL are complex and evolving; consultation with a gynecologic oncologist or other provider with experience in this situation should be considered.

REFERENCES

Apgar BS, Brotzman G: HPV testing in the evaluation of the minimally abnormal Papanicolaou smear. Am Fam Physician 1999;**59**:2794.

Kim JJ, et al: Cost effectiveness of alternative triage strategies for ASCUS. JAMA 2002;**287**:2382.

Melnikow J, et al: Management of the low-grade abnormal Pap smear: What are women's preferences? J Fam Pract 2002;**51**:849.

Nuovo J, et al: New tests for cervical cancer screening. Am Fam Physician 2001;**64**:780.

Solomon D, et al: The 2001 Bethesda system: Terminology for reporting results of cervical cytology. JAMA 2002;**287**:2114.

Wright TC, et al: 2001 Consensus guidelines for the management of women with cervical cytological abnormalities. JAMA 2002;**287**:2120.

3   Amenorrhea

Rhonda A. Sparks, MD, & Laura B. Frankenstein, MD

KEY POINTS

- Hypothalamic amenorrhea is the most common cause of secondary amenorrhea and is typically associated with stress, excessive strenuous exercise, chronic illness, or eating disorders.
- The **female athlete triad** is a commonly unrecognized disorder consisting of amenorrhea, eating disorder, and osteoporosis.
- Polycystic ovarian syndrome (PCOS) is a common endocrinopathy affecting 5–10% of premenopausal women.

I. **Definition.** Normal menstruation depends on integrated hypothalamic, pituitary, ovarian follicular and endometrial function, and a patent outflow tract. Hypothalamic gonadotropin releasing hormone (GnRH) stimulates release of pituitary gonadotropins luteinizing hormone (LH) and follicle-stimulating hormone (FSH), which stimulate ovarian production of 17-β estradiol and progesterone. Sequential cyclic endometrial stimulation by estradiol and progesterone thickens the endometrium, and cyclic withdrawal of these hormones causes endometrial sloughing (menstruation).

Amenorrhea is absence of menses for 3 months in a woman with previously normal menses, no menses by age 16 in an adolescent with normal sexual development, or no menses by age 14 in an adolescent without normal sexual development. **Primary amenorrhea** refers to women who have never menstruated, while **secondary amenorrhea** refers to cessation of menses in a previously menstruating female.

Causes of amenorrhea may be broadly considered in terms of anatomic or endocrine dysfunction at the hypothalamic, pituitary, or ovarian level. Amenorrhea may be due to **GnRH suppression from pituitary hyperprolactinemia** (eg, pregnancy/lactation, pituitary adenoma, medications, prolonged hypothyroidism), **low GnRH and pituitary gonadotropin levels** causing failed follicular development (hypothalamic amenorrhea), **high GnRH and FSH levels** associated with chronic anovulation (eg, PCOS), and **various anatomic defects** (eg, imperforate hymen, congenital absent uterus and vagina, or endometrial synechiae in Asherman's syndrome), which cause amenorrhea through outlet obstruction.

II. **Common Diagnoses.** Amenorrhea occurs in 5–10% of women.

A. **Pregnancy and lactation** interrupt menses predictably and are the most common cause of amenorrhea in women of childbearing age.

B. **Hyperprolactinemic amenorrhea** not associated with pregnancy or lactation may be secondary to **medications** that increase prolactin levels (Table 3–1) or to prolonged **hypothyroidism.** Prolactin-secreting tumors are less common but potentially more serious than the above causes of hyperprolactinemia.

C. **Hypogonadotropic amenorrhea (also known as hypothalamic amenorrhea)** is the most common cause of secondary amenorrhea and is typically associated with **stress, excessive strenuous exercise, chronic illness** such as chronic liver and renal disease, or **eating disorders.**

D. **Hypergonadotropic amenorrhea** is most commonly seen in POF, which can result from autoimmune disease, chemotherapy, or radiation therapy. POF may be inherited as an X-linked or autosomal condition; Turner's syndrome is the most common karyotype abnormality associated with amenorrhea.

E. **Polycystic ovarian syndrome (PCOS)** is the most common cause of **normogonadotropic amenorrhea,** an endocrinopathy affecting 10% of premenopausal women and associated with obesity in 50% of patients.

F. **Anatomic defects** may lead to amenorrhea via complete or partial outflow tract obstruction from **imperforate hymen** or **transverse vaginal septa.** The uterus or vagina may be absent. Rokitansky-Küster-Hauser syndrome is the most common anomaly

TABLE 3-1. MEDICATION CAUSES OF HYPERPROLACTINEMIA

1. Psychotropic drugs Benzodiazepines Selective serotonin reuptake inhibitors (SSRIs) Tricyclic antidepressants Phenothiazines Buspirone Monoamine oxidase (MAO) inhibitors	**4. Drugs that work on the gastrointestinal tract** H_2 blockers
	5. Cardiovascular drugs Atenolol Verapamil Reserpine Methyldopa
2. Neurologic drugs Sumatriptan Valproic acid Dihydroergotamine	**6. Herbal preparations** Fenugreek seed Fennel Anise
3. Hormonal medications Danazol Estrogen Depo-Provera Oral contraceptives	**7. Illicit drugs** Amphetamines Cannabis (marijuana)

resulting in absent uterus and vagina. **Asherman's syndrome** is obliteration of the endometrium caused by synechiae formation and is usually seen after D&C or other uterine surgery.

G. **Genetic disorders.** Turner's syndrome (XO karyotype) presents with primary amenorrhea due to failure of ovarian development; testicular feminization (46XY karyotype with androgen insensitivity) presents with primary amenorrhea due to absent outflow tract.

III. **Symptoms.** Symptoms other than missed menses may be few. A careful history elicits the cause of amenorrhea in 85% of cases and should always include the following:

A. A detailed **menstrual history,** including dates of last menstrual period (LMP).
   1. Age at **menarche** is important and separates **primary** (eg, outflow obstruction, genetic disorders) from **secondary amenorrhea.**
   2. **Oligomenorrhea progressing gradually to amenorrhea** characterizes PCOS, hypogonadotropic, or hyperprolactinemic amenorrhea.
   3. **Sudden missed menses** preceded by regular menses suggests pregnancy in reproductive-age women.

B. **Additional history**
   1. **Symptoms of pregnancy** including nausea, weight gain, breast tenderness, and urinary frequency.
   2. **Galactorrhea** (milky discharge from the breasts) indicating hyperprolactinemia.
   3. **Medication history** (Table 3-1) for medication-induced hyperprolactinemia. After discontinuation of oral contraceptives, amenorrhea may occur for several months.
   4. Symptoms of **hypoestrogenic state** such as hot flashes, vaginal dryness, or decreased libido, which may indicate POF or menopause, depending on age.
   5. **Hyperandrogenism** (acne, hirsutism) and infertility, which increase likelihood of PCOS.
   6. **Dietary history** and fluctuations in **weight** to look for evidence of eating disorders. A history of **excessive activity level** suggests the female athlete triad (see sidebar).

FEMALE ATHLETE TRIAD

The **female athlete triad** is a commonly unrecognized disorder consisting of amenorrhea, eating disorder, and osteoporosis. The prevalence of eating disorders and amenorrhea in athletes is reported as high as 66%. Athletic pursuits emphasizing low body weight (eg, gymnastics, figure skating, ballet, and distance running) increase the risk of the female athlete triad. Other risk factors include self-esteem focused on athletic pursuits solely, presence of stress fractures, and social isolation caused by intensive involvement in sports.

IV. Signs. In women presenting in primary care with amenorrhea, the physical examination is usually normal; focused examination should be guided by history and should address the following:

   A. Weight loss, signs of emotional distress (depression, agitation).
   B. **Hirsutism** (eg, acne, increased facial and body hair), which may be present in women with PCOS.
   C. **Virilization,** which is suggestive of ovarian or adrenal neoplasm. Manifestations include temporal balding, deepening voice, and clitoromegaly.
   D. **Galactorrhea** indicating **hyperprolactinemic** state.
   E. **Visual field defect** on confrontation suggesting pituitary adenoma.
   F. **Atrophic vaginal changes** and **vaginal dryness** suggesting a hypoestrogenic state.
   G. **Short stature, sexual infantilism, and neck webbing** characteristic of Turner's syndrome.
   H. Uterine or cervical anatomic defects.

V. Laboratory Tests. Unless the diagnosis is obvious from the history and physical examination, testing will be necessary. The work-up can be done in a stepwise fashion (Figure 3–1) to avoid unnecessary testing.

   A. A **pregnancy test** is always indicated.
   B. A test to determine the **level of thyroid-stimulating hormone (TSH)** is indicated because hypothyroidism, although rarely causing amenorrhea, cannot be ruled out by history and physical examination alone.
   C. **Serum prolactin level** should be tested, because 20% of cases of amenorrhea are associated with hyperprolactinemia. Levels of prolactin <100 ng/mL are usually related to medications, whereas levels >100 ng/mL suggest pituitary adenoma.
   D. Hyperprolactinemia warrants a **CT scan or MRI of the brain** to evaluate for pituitary adenoma.
   E. The **progestin challenge test** separates women with estrogen deficiency from those with normal or excess estrogen. Medroxyprogesterone acetate (Provera), 10 mg, is given orally once daily for 5–7 days. Any bleeding during the week following the final dose indicates that the patient has sufficient estrogen and that the amenorrhea is likely caused by anovulation. Absence of bleeding during the week after the final dosage indicates estrogen deficiency or possibly outflow tract obstruction.
   F. An **estrogen-progestin challenge** helps differentiate outflow obstruction from estrogen deficiency. Estrogen is given for 21–25 days and a progestational agent for the final 5–7 days of estrogen therapy to stimulate withdrawal bleeding. If no bleeding occurs, an outflow tract obstruction is present. If bleeding occurs, estrogen deficiency is present and further testing is necessary.
   G. **Gonadotropin levels.** An FSH level >40 mIU/mL suggests POF or menopause, depending on the patient's age. If FSH and LH levels are elevated, POF is the most likely explanation. An LH level is useful if PCOS is suspected, as the LH:FSH ratio will be >2:1.
   H. **Androgen testing** (testosterone, androstenedione, dehydroepiandrosterone sulfate [DHEA-S]) should be done in amenorrheic women with signs of androgen excess (virilization, hirsutism, acne). Testosterone levels >200 ng/dL and DHEA-S levels >7 mg/dL necessitate CT scan of the adrenals and ultrasound testing of the ovaries to rule out neoplasm.
   I. **Serum insulin levels** may be elevated in women with PCOS.
   J. **Karyotyping** should be performed in women with POF before age 30 or with stigmata of Turner's syndrome.
   K. Referral for **hysteroscopy** may be needed to evaluate the uterine lining if Asherman's syndrome is suspected.
   L. **Bone densitometry** is indicated in any women with amenorrhea >6–12 months.

VI. Treatment must be based on a firm diagnosis and must attempt to resolve **underlying problems** while restoring menses, treating symptoms associated with estrogen deficiency, and addressing fertility when applicable.

   A. **Hyperprolactinemic amenorrhea** is resolved when causative conditions are identified and corrected or when suppressive medication is used and menses return. If a pituitary

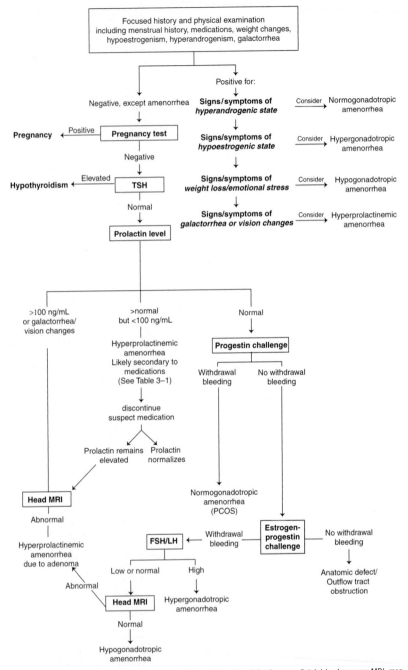

FIGURE 3–1. Evaluation of secondary amenorrhea. FSH/LH, follicle-stimulating hormone/luteinizing hormone; MRI, magnetic resonance imaging; PCOS, polycystic ovarian syndrome; TSH, thyroid-stimulating hormone.

adenoma is identified, the goals of treatment are to suppress prolactin, decrease tumor size, prevent recurrence, and induce ovulation.

1. **Bromocriptine** is the drug most often used for first-line therapy for hyperprolactinemia because it inhibits the secretion of prolactin and suppresses prolactin levels as long as it is taken. Bromocriptine shrinks prolactinomas, eliminates galactorrhea, and re-establishes menses and fertility. Menses usually return in 6–12 weeks once prolactin levels are normalized.

2. **Medroxyprogesterone acetate** (Provera), 10 mg/day taken for 10 days each month, is useful to induce menses if a women does not desire fertility, does not have galactorrhea, or cannot tolerate bromocriptine. Provera does not affect prolactinoma size or prolactin levels.

3. In the past, treatment of pituitary adenoma was commonly **transsphenoidal resection.** However, recurrence of these tumors is common and therefore bromocriptine is the usual first-line therapy for both microadenomas and macroadenomas. Microadenomas grow very slowly, and prolactin levels should be followed up yearly; neuroimaging should be done every 2–3 years.

B. **Hypogonadotropic amenorrhea (also known as hypothalamic amenorrhea)** is resolved when the stress causing the decreased GnRH secretion is lessened. In the meantime, other interventions are important.

1. **Dietary modifications** to increase caloric intake and maintain ideal body weight and a **decrease in activity level** to a point where menses resume are critical.

2. To protect the patient from bone loss, **estrogen supplementation** with oral contraceptives should be provided until normal menstruation is established.

3. **Smoking should be discouraged** and **adequate calcium intake** (1.5 g/day) and vitamin D (800 IU/day) encouraged to **prevent bone loss.** Antiresorptive therapy (eg, alendronate, 10 mg orally daily or 70 mg orally weekly) should be initiated if osteoporosis is identified.

C. **Hypergonadotropic amenorrhea** with diagnosed POF requires a hormone replacement therapy regimen that maintains bone mass. A higher **daily dose of estrogen** than what is generally administered in hormone replacement therapy is required in younger women with POF to prevent bone loss. **Calcium and vitamin D supplementation** should be initiated as above (VI,B,3.) and **osteoporosis treatment** (VI,B,3.) should be initiated.

D. **Normogonadotropic amenorrhea** manifested as PCOS may require multifaceted therapy including the following:

1. **Reduction of insulin resistance.** Insulin-sensitizing agents such as metformin have been shown to reduce hyperinsulinemia and restore ovulation. Oral metformin (500 mg three times a day) has been shown to enhance ovulation. Weight loss is recommended.

2. If pregnancy is desired, patients with PCOS are candidates for **induction of ovulation** with medications such as clomiphene citrate (Clomid).

3. If pregnancy is not desired, therapy should be directed at **interruption of the unopposed estrogen** and its effects. Use of oral contraceptives suppresses ovarian androgens and thus minimizes hirsutism, as well as providing a progestational agent to oppose estrogen.

4. Spironolactone, an aldosterone antagonist, is an androgen blocker used for the **treatment of hirsutism.** Oral doses of 100–200 mg/day are usually effective. Spironolactone works through a different mechanism than oral contraceptives and therefore using these agents concomitantly improves their effectiveness.

REFERENCES

Apgar B: Diagnosis and management of amenorrhea. Clinics in Family Practice 2002;**4**:3.
Hobart J, et al: The female athlete triad. Am Fam Physician 2000;**61**:3357–64, 3367.
Larsen PR: *Williams Textbook of Endocrinology,* 10th ed. Elsevier; 2003.
Moutos D: Amenorrhea. Rakel RE: *Conn's Current Therapy 2003,* 55th ed. Elsevier; 2003.
Richardson M: Current perspectives in polycystic ovary syndrome. Am Fam Physician 2003;**68**:697.
Speroff L, et al: *Clinical Gynecological Endocrinology and Infertility,* 6th ed. Williams & Wilkins; 1999.

4   Anemia

Andrew D. Jones, MD, & Mel P. Daly, MD

KEY POINTS

- Anemia is common in the primary care setting and iron deficiency anemia is the most common cause.
- Anemia is usually asymptomatic, although some syndromes are associated with specific signs and symptoms.
- Anemia can usually be diagnosed accurately with some simple laboratory tests such as red blood cell indices and reticulocyte count.

I. **Definition.** Anemia is an abnormally low hemoglobin (hgb) or hematocrit (hct) value of compared to age-matched norms (Table 4–1).

II. **Common Diagnoses**
   A. **Iron deficiency**
      1. **Nutritional/absorption.** Iron deficiency is the most common cause of nutritional anemia worldwide. However, iron deficiency anemia from nutritional deficiencies is uncommon in adults in developed countries, because such deficiencies must occur for at least 5 years to produce iron deficiency anemia in the presence of normal iron physiology. **Newborn infants** who are breast-fed or who are taking non–iron-enriched formulas are an exception and may become iron deficient in the first year of life. **Children aged 12–24 months** may also become iron deficient as they transition from iron-fortified formula to cow's milk and solid foods. (See the sidebar on anemia from cow's milk in children.) **Malabsorption** resulting from disease, resection of the small bowel, or partial gastric resection accounts for a small percentage of iron deficiency.

ANEMIA FROM COW'S MILK IN CHILDREN

One particular cause of anemia in children is iron deficiency anemia caused by early initiation of cow's milk feedings. To prevent this, the American Academy of Pediatrics recommends: (1) breast-feeding for 6–12 months, (2) using only iron-fortified formulas, (3) avoiding cow's milk during the first year of life, and (4) eating iron-enriched cereals with the initiation of solid foods.

TABLE 4–1. NORMAL VALUES FOR HEMOGLOBIN (g/dL) BY AGE, SEX, AND RACE

	Males		Females	
Age (yr)	Median	Range	Median	Range
1–2	12.3	10.7–13.8	12.3	10.7–13.8
3–8	12.5	10.9–14.3	12.5	10.9–14.4
9–11	13.2	11.4–14.8	13.2	11–14.8
12–14	14	12–16	13.4	11.5–15.0
15–17	14.8	12.3–16.6	13.5	11.7–15.3
18–44	15.3	13.2–17.3	13.5	11.7–15.5
45–64	15.2	13.1–17.2	13.7	11.7–16
65–74	14.9	12.6–17.4	13.9	11.7–16

In black children between 3 and 5 years of age, hemoglobin levels are a median of 0.4 g/dL lower than in white children of the same age.
In black men between 65 and 74 years of age, hemoglobin levels are a median of 1.1 g/dL lower than in white men of the same age.

2. **Blood loss.** In the absence of malnutrition or malabsorption, iron deficiency results from bleeding. **In young women,** most cases are caused by menstrual blood loss and increased iron requirements of pregnancy.

Gastrointestinal (GI) bleeding is another common source of blood loss; this is often due to the erosive effects of nonsteroidal anti-inflammatory drugs. In elderly patients, colonic carcinomas, diverticular disease, and vascular malformations are other major causes of GI bleeding. **Rare causes of blood loss** include chronic hemolysis, hemoptysis, and bleeding disorders. (Also see the sidebar on acute hemorrhage.)

ACUTE HEMORRHAGE

Acute hemorrhage is a potentially life-threatening cause of anemia. Acute severe blood loss is as much a problem of low circulating blood volume as it is of low Hgb or Hct. Acute blood loss may present with minimal to no reduction in hgb/hct yet still be clinically significant. Acute hemorrhage may be asymptomatic or may present with severe shock including fatigue, light-headedness, or alteration in level of consciousness, possibly accompanied by menorrhagia, melena, hematochezia, hematemesis, or hemoptysis. Acute hemorrhage is associated with a positive tilt test with orthostasis and is treated with hospitalization for fluid resuscitation, transfusion, and identification and management of underlying causes.

B. **Vitamin B_{12} deficiency** causes anemia in 5–10% of elderly patients. (See the sidebar on anemia in the elderly.)

ANEMIA IN THE ELDERLY

Anemia is common, present in 8–44% of those older than 65 years. Symptoms and signs of anemia may be difficult to detect in the elderly and may present as a worsening of underlying medical conditions. Therefore, a high index of suspicion is necessary in the evaluation of anemia in the elderly. Although the evaluation of anemia in the elderly is very similar to that described in this chapter, it must be remembered that low hgb or hct values are not a normal consequence of aging, and a cause for anemia must be sought.

1. **Malabsorption.** Vitamin B_{12} deficiency is almost always due to malabsorption related to atrophic gastritis. **Pernicious anemia (PA),** or failure to absorb vitamin B_{12} because of reduced production or secretion of intrinsic factor, occurs commonly; chronic histamine blockers, proton pump inhibitor treatment, and *Helicobacter pylori* gastritis may also play a role in development of PA. Other **less common causes of vitamin B_{12} malabsorption** include small-bowel overgrowth; ileal malfunction; acidification of the small intestine; pancreatic disease; and certain drugs (*p*-aminosalicylic acid, neomycin, and potassium chloride). Vitamin B_{12} deficiency increases the likelihood of subsequent development of gastric cancer or polyps, which is thought to be related to the gastritis associated with vitamin B_{12} malabsorption.
2. **Diet.** The only source of cobalamin is animal products; thus, vegans who eat no meat, eggs, or cheese for a number of years may develop a nutritional deficiency state.
C. **Folate deficiency** occurs because average dietary folic acid intake does not greatly exceed nutritional requirements and body folate reserves are relatively small, depleting in 4 months. Deficiency thus occurs in patients who either do not consume or absorb enough folic acid or who have some condition that depletes their body reserves.
1. **Decreased folate intake. Decreased intake** can occur when the diet is deficient in fresh green vegetables, nuts, yeast, and liver. Decreased intake may occur in the elderly, in alcoholics, and due to loss of food folate through excessive cooking.
2. **Decreased absorption/effectiveness. Folate malabsorption** can be caused by GI conditions such as jejunal atrophy from celiac disease and drugs such as phenytoin or sulfasalazine. **Folate antagonists** include certain chemotherapeutic agents;

antiviral drugs (eg, azidothymidine [AZT] and zidovudine); folate antagonists (eg, methotrexate); trimethoprim; nitrous oxide; primidone; and phenobarbital.
3. **Increased demand.** The increased nutritional demands of pregnancy and the increased requirements of chronic hemolytic anemia and exfoliative psoriasis may deplete folic acid reserves.

D. **Anemia of chronic disease (ACD)** is present in up to 6% of adults hospitalized by family physicians and is caused by reduced ability to incorporate stored iron into hemoglobin, despite adequate iron stores. ACD may also be exacerbated by features of the underlying disease, including blood loss, hemolysis, malabsorption, malnutrition, or bone marrow replacement or suppression by infection or drugs. (Also see the autoimmune hemolytic anemia sidebar.)

AUTOIMMUNE HEMOLYTIC ANEMIA

Autoimmune hemolytic anemia is rare and may occur idiopathically or secondary to other disorders, such as systemic lupus erythematosus, chronic lymphocytic leukemia, non-Hodgkin's lymphoma, Hodgkin's disease, and cancer. Drugs such as α-methyldopa, penicillin, rifampin, sulfonamides, quinidine, and chlorpropamide may induce an immune hemolysis, clinically indistinguishable from immune hemolytic anemia. Autoimmune hemolytic anemia may have a dramatic clinical presentation. The anemia may occur rapidly and be life-threatening, and patients may present with angina or congestive heart failure associated with jaundice developing over a 1- to 3-day period. Patients with thrombotic thrombocytopenic purpura, a type of autoimmune hemolytic anemia, may present with petechiae, fever, altered mental status, or focal neurologic findings.

E. **Hemolytic processes**
1. **Sickle cell disease** is inherited as an autosomal trait; it occurs in the heterozygous state as **sickle trait** in 8–10% of blacks in the United States. Sickle trait rarely occurs in Eastern Mediterranean people or people of Indian or Saudi Arabian ancestry. **Sickle cell disease** develops in persons who are homozygous for the sickle gene (*HbSS*) and affects about 2% of blacks in the United States. Other sickle syndromes, such as sickle-β-thalassemia and sickle C disease, are uncommon in the United States.
2. **Thalassemia** is most common in Mediterranean and Asian populations. Sporadic cases of thalassemia are found among Africans and American blacks.
3. **Hereditary elliptocytosis and spherocytosis** are autosomal dominant disorders affecting about 200–300 million people worldwide, although these conditions are uncommon in the United States. These membrane defects cause intravascular hemolysis of red blood cells (RBCs).
4. **Glucose-6-phosphate dehydrogenase (G6PD)** deficiency is one of the most common disorders causing hemolysis worldwide, affecting 10% of black males in the United States. The gene for G6PD is carried on the X chromosome, and female carriers are rarely affected.
5. **Pyruvate kinase deficiency** is another common RBC enzyme deficiency. The intravascular hemolysis caused by these conditions is particularly worsened by illness, stress, and, with G6PD, some medications.

F. **Bone marrow deficits**
1. **Aplastic anemia** occurs because of a marrow disturbance resulting in defective RBC synthesis. This may be due to marrow infiltration by tumor or fibrosis; dose-related, idiosyncratic, or hypersensitivity effects of drugs (eg, antithyroid medications, gold, chemotherapeutic agents, AZT, phenytoin, and phenylbutazone); radiation; autoimmune suppression (eg, with systemic lupus erythematosus); and infections such as tuberculosis, atypical mycobacterial infections, brucellosis, hepatitis A and B, and, rarely, mumps, rubella, infectious mononucleosis, influenza, human immunodeficiency virus, parvovirus, and fungal and parasitic infections.
2. **Myelodysplastic syndromes (MDSs)** are diagnosed in 1–10 per 100,000 people every year, and are more common in elderly males. MDSs are stem-cell disorders resulting in abnormal hematopoietic precursors causing disturbances of RBCs, white blood cells, and platelets. Previous treatment with radiation or mutagenic chemicals may result in MDSs.

III. Symptoms and Signs. In anemia, these may be nonexistent or may be vague. Some symptoms are more common in particular age groups and some syndromes do have characteristic symptoms and signs (Table 4–2).

IV. Laboratory Tests. One approach to the diagnosis of anemia using RBC indices and reticulocyte count is presented here (Figure 4–1).

A. Iron deficiency anemia. Essential diagnostic features include serum ferritin <20 ng/mL, low serum iron, and high iron-binding capacity; microcytic and hypochromic peripheral RBCs occur later with absent marrow iron stores. A normal red blood cell distribution width (RDW) effectively eliminates iron deficiency as a cause of microcytic anemia. Upper and lower GI endoscopy is indicated if laboratory studies suggest iron deficiency, especially if stool testing for occult blood is positive.

B. Vitamin B$_{12}$ and folate deficiencies. These deficiencies cause megaloblastic anemia (macrocytosis and hypersegmented granulocytes in the peripheral blood smear); mean corpuscular volume (MCV) elevation (frequently >110 fL but may be normal with co-existing thalassemia); indirect hyperbilirubinemia; elevated lactate dehydrogenase levels; normal mean corpuscular hemoglobin concentration (range, 31–35 g/dL); low reticulocyte count; and possibly decreased leukocyte and platelet counts. With macrocytosis, serum B$_{12}$ and folate levels should be obtained and, if these are normal, measuring levels of cobalamin metabolites (methylmalonic acid and homocysteine) should be considered. Normal levels rule out a vitamin B$_{12}$ or folate deficiency. In patients who are vitamin B$_{12}$ deficient, serum folate is usually normal or elevated unless there is a coexisting folate deficiency. Serum homocysteine levels are markedly increased in folate deficiency. **Bone marrow biopsy** may be necessary to rule out MDSs and malignancy if levels of vitamin B$_{12}$, folate, and metabolites are normal, since these disorders may present with peripheral megaloblastosis.

C. Anemia of chronic disease. ACD is usually mild in degree and not progressive, with the hct rarely falling below 25%, except in renal failure. Common findings in ACD are normochromic, normocytic red blood cells; low reticulocyte production; low or normal serum iron; low total iron-binding capacity; and usually normal RDW. Reticuloendothelial iron stores are usually adequate, serum ferritin levels are >50 ng/mL, and bone marrow iron is normal or increased. Serum erythropoietin levels are reduced in inflammatory disorders. The marrow is usually hypocellular, with decreased myeloid precursors.

D. Hemolytic anemia. The cardinal diagnostic feature of hemolytic anemia is significant reticulocytosis.

    1. Immunohemolysis is diagnosed based on Coombs' testing, with a positive direct Coombs' test indicating surface RBC antibodies and a positive indirect Coombs' test indicating circulating RBC antibodies. Cold agglutinins will be found in patients with immune hemolysis due to cold-reactive antibodies.

    2. In **extravascular hemolysis,** serum indirect bilirubin and lactate dehydrogenase levels rise, while haptoglobin decreases. In sustained and severe hemolytic anemia, nucleated RBCs may enter the circulation.

E. Hemoglobinopathies

    1. Sickle cell anemia

        a. Hemoglobin levels range between 5 and 10 g/dL, neutrophil and platelet counts are frequently elevated, and the blood smear shows sickle cells, Howell-Jolly bodies, reticulocytosis, and usually high white blood cell and platelet counts.

TABLE 4–2. FINDINGS IN COMMON ANEMIAS

Diagnosis	Abnormal Findings
Iron deficiency	Pica; esophageal webs (Plummer-Vinson syndrome); pallor of mucosa and nail beds; atrophic glossitis, angular stomatitis, cheilosis
B$_{12}$ deficiency	Tongue burning/soreness; numbness/paresthesias; yellow skin; vitiligo; glossitis; hepatomegaly; splenomegaly; mental status changes
Hemolytic anemia	Fever, pain; jaundice; hepatomegaly; cardiomegaly; murmur
Folate deficiency	Malnourishment; diarrhea, glossitis, cheilosis; no neurologic abnormalities but mild mental status changes
Thalassemia	Bony deformities; growth failure; hepatosplenomegaly

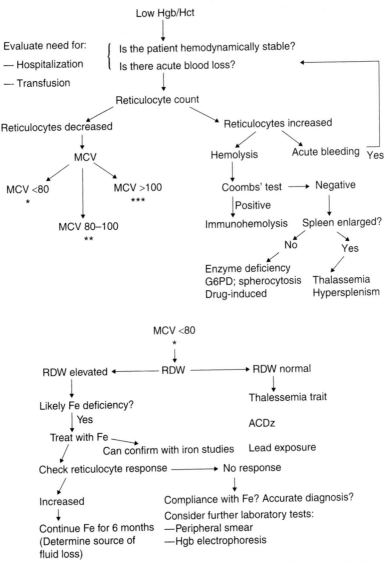

FIGURE 4–1. Diagnosis and treatment of anemia. ACD, anemia of chronic disease; G6PD, glucose-6-phosphate dehydrogenase; Hgb/hct, hemoglobin/hematocrit; MCV, mean corpuscular volume; MMA, methylmalonic acid; RDW, red blood cell distribution width.

    b. Hemoglobin electrophoresis shows RBCs containing 85–95% hgb S and, in homozygous S disease, no hemoglobin A. Elevated levels of hemoglobin A_2 on hemoglobin electrophoresis and a positive family history of thalassemia are characteristic of sickle-β-thalassemia.
  2. The peripheral smear in **thalassemias** shows hypochromia and microcytosis with basophilic stippling, potentially confusing them with iron deficiency anemia; however, findings with iron deficiency also include a reduced RBC count, an elevated

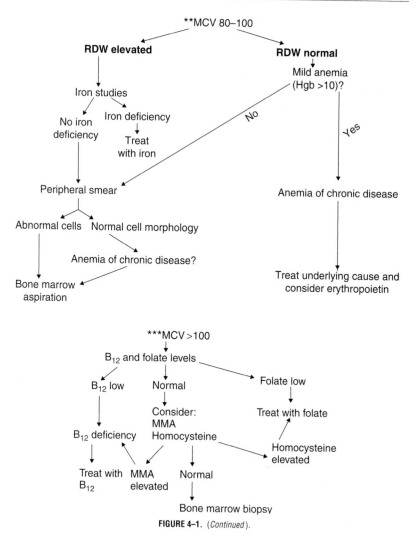

FIGURE 4–1. (*Continued*).

RDW, and reduced serum iron, whereas patients with β-thalassemia minor have normal or minimally reduced RBC counts, profound microcytosis, normal serum iron, and normal RDW. Hemoglobin electrophoreses in patients with β-thalassemia shows increased levels of hemoglobin A_2 and hemoglobin F.

V. Treatment. The treatment of anemia generally involves addressing underlying causes of anemia; options for most common conditions are discussed briefly here.

    A. Iron deficiency anemia. This form of anemia can usually be treated by correcting the cause of blood loss (see section IV,A).

        1. Iron preparations such as ferrous sulfate, ferrous gluconate, ferrous fumarate, or polysaccharide-iron complexes (ferric polymaltose) can replenish iron deficiency. The usual dose is 100–200 mg of elemental iron daily (eg, ferrous sulfate, 325 mg, three times a day). Reticulocytosis follows within a few days, and a rise in hemoglobin of 2 g/dL occurs within 3 weeks. Therapy should continue for 6 months to replenish iron stores.

2. **To minimize GI side effects,** iron therapy should begin with one tablet a day with meals, and the dose should be gradually increased. Ferrous gluconate, ferrous fumarate, and ferric polymaltose are less likely to cause GI side effects but are more expensive than ferrous sulfate.

3. **Nonresponse to iron therapy** is usually due to noncompliance, but may be caused by incorrect diagnosis (eg, anemia of chronic disease or thalassemia), ongoing GI blood loss, or, rarely, poor absorption.

B. **Vitamin B_{12} deficiency.** Patients with confirmed vitamin B_{12} deficiency from PA must receive vitamin B_{12} therapy for the duration of their lives. Intramuscular dosing is 1000 µg/day for the first week, then 1000 µg weekly until hematologic values normalize or for at least 6 months if neurologic complications exist, then 1000 µg monthly for life. Oral treatment with 1000–2000 µg daily is as effective but requires much greater patient compliance. Intranasal preparations also exist but are not first-line therapy.

C. **Folate deficiency.** This deficiency is treated with oral folic acid, 1 mg/day.

D. **ACD.** There is no specific treatment other than for the underlying illness. Recombinant erythropoietin should be considered for all patients with anemia of renal failure or patients undergoing chemotherapy. An additive deficiency state worsens the anemia; however, unless a specific deficiency exists, treatment with iron, vitamin B_{12}, and folic acid is useless.

E. **Hemolytic processes**

1. Patients with **sickle cell disease** should be immunized against *Streptococcus pneumoniae, Haemophilus influenzae,* hepatitis B, and influenza according to Centers for Disease Control and Prevention (CDC) recommendations. Infections should be treated early and aggressively. **Antibiotic prophylaxis** with penicillin should be given to children between the ages of 2 months and 5 years because of the high risk of pneumococcal infection. A typical regimen is oral penicillin, 125 mg twice daily until age 2–3, then 250 mg twice daily. **Regular ophthalmologic examination** should be done every 1–2 years beginning at age 10 years because of a high incidence of retinopathy. Patients should be maintained chronically on folic acid supplements.

2. The most common hemolytic condition requiring treatment is **sickle cell crisis.** Treatment of sickle cell crises consists of rest, hydration, and analgesia. Transfusions should be reserved for aplastic or hemolytic crises and for patients in the third trimester of pregnancy. No treatment is required for patients with sickle trait.

REFERENCES

Abramson SD, Abramson N: 'Common' uncommon anemias. Am Fam Physician 1999;**59**(4):851.
Bakerman S: *Bakerman's ABCs: Interpretive Laboratory Data,* 4th ed. 2002:53–59.
Brill JR, Baumgardner DJ: Normocytic anemia. Am Fam Physician 2000;**62**(10):2255.
Little DR: Ambulatory management of common forms of anemia. Am Fam Physician 1999;**59**(6):1598.
Sickle Cell Disease Care Consortium: Sickle cell disease in children and adolescents: Diagnosis, guidelines for comprehensive care, and care paths for management of acute and chronic complications. www.scinfo.org/protchildindex.htm
Smith DL: Anemia in the elderly. Am Fam Physician 2000;**62**(7):1565.
Walters MC, Abelson HT: Interpretation of the complete blood count. Pediatr Hematol 1996;**43**(3):599.

---

5   Ankle Injuries

Richard B. Birrer, MD

KEY POINTS

- Ankle sprains are among the most common injuries in sport and recreational activities.
- Forty percent of sprains have significant morbidity associated with them.
- Radiographic high-yield criteria can reliably identify fractures in the postpubertal patient.

I. Definition. An understanding of the major bones, ligaments, and tendons in the ankle is important to understanding ankle injuries (Figures 5–1 and 5–2A & B). Range of motion occurs in one plane: plantar flexion and dorsiflexion. Dorsiflexion is somewhat restricted due to the anterior widening of the talar dome. The subtalar joint of the foot allows for the full range of inversion, eversion, supination, and pronation. The medial malleolus (distal tibia) and the longer lateral malleolus (distal fibula) provide a significant amount of bony stability to the ankle joint through their downward extension along the talar dome.

    Ligaments provide medial and lateral stability (eversion and inversion). The tibiofibular ligament syndesmosis maintains cable mortise stability, and a variety of tendons traversing the joint serve as secondary stabilizers.

    Ankle injuries involve trauma to the bony or soft tissue structures of the ankle. **Sprains** involve tears to the ligaments, whereas **strains** involve tears of the muscle-tendon unit. They can be graded: 1—<30% of fibers; 2—30–70%, or 3—>70% of fibers. **Contusions** are bruises; **tenosynovitis** is the inflammation of the tendon and its sheath. Clues to the nature of ankle injuries are found in the mechanism of injury (Table 5–1).

II. Common Diagnoses. Ankle injuries account for 0.5% of visits in the primary care ambulatory setting.

    A. Sprains (85% of all ankle injuries). Sprains are particularly common in individuals who play basketball, volleyball, football, or racquetball. Between 10% and 15% of all ankle

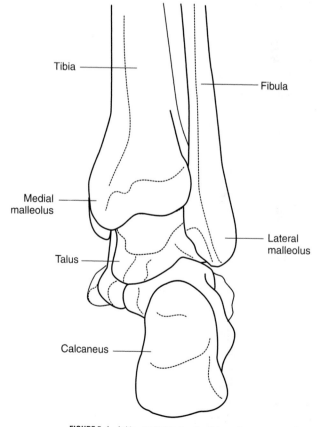

FIGURE 5–1. Ankle—posterior view showing mortise.

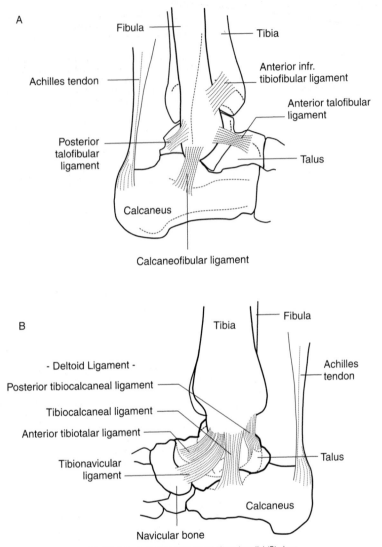

FIGURE 5–2. Ankle ligaments: lateral (**A**) and medial (**B**) views.

sprains involve the medial compartment, and this is usually a more serious injury than a lateral sprain.

B. Strains (5% of all ankle injuries). Strains are common in persons who engage in explosive activities, such as track and field events. These injuries result from overuse of the muscle-tendon unit, particularly in endurance running, dancing, or gymnastics.

C. Tenosynovitis (5% of all ankle injuries). Tenosynovitis most often occurs in individuals who are running, jumping, dancing, or cycling. This condition results from a direct blow or overuse with repetitive overloads and faulty technique.

TABLE 5-1. PATHOPHYSIOLOGY OF COMMON ANKLE INJURIES

Mechanism of Injury	Injury Examples
Lateral displacement	
Eversion with supinated ankle	Rupture of anterior inferior tibiofibular ligament, spiral oblique fracture of the fibula, posterior malleolar fracture, medial malleolar fracture, or deltoid ligament rupture
Eversion with pronated ankle	Rupture of deltoid ligament or fracture of medial malleolus, spiral fracture of fibula 2–3 inches above the top of the interosseus membrane, avulsion fracture of posterior malleolus, tear of interosseus membrane, in children (eg, type II or IV Salter fracture of tibia)
Adduction with pronated ankle	Fracture of medial malleolus or rupture of deltoid ligament, rupture of anterior inferior ligament, oblique fracture of distal fibula, posterior malleolar fracture
Adduction with dorsiflexed or plantar-flexed ankle	Medial malleolar fracture or tibiofibular diastases, medial or lateral osteochondral fractures
Medial displacement	
Inversion, plantar flexion, and adduction	Sequential tearing of the anchor talofibular, calcaneofibular, and posterior talofibular ligaments, avulsion fracture of the distal fibula, and transverse fracture of the medial malleolus
Adduction with supinated ankle	Avulsion of lateral malleolus or rupture of talofibular ligament, vertical fracture of the medial malleolus, in children (eg, type I or II Salter fracture of fibula, type III [Tilaux] or N of medial malleolus)
Axial compression of the talus	Impaction fracture, marginal fractures, tibiofibular diastases
Repetitive microtrauma	Medial osteochondral fractures or distal fibular stress fractures

    D. Contusions (<5% of all ankle injuries). Contusions involving the ankle are significantly underreported and occur in persons who participate in contact sports. Such injuries also result from faulty footwear and poor field conditions.

    E. Fractures (<5% of all ankle injuries). Fractures are more common than sprains in prepubertal children. They occur most frequently in persons who engage in high-velocity, high-impact sports (eg, football, soccer, skiing, hockey, or automobile racing).

        1. Stress fractures occur in running, gymnastics, or dancing.

        2. Salter type I and II fractures of the fibula are the most common ankle injuries in children. (For discussion of the Salter classification, see Chapter 29.)

III. Symptoms

    A. Painful injuries that affect weight-bearing ability may be sprains.

        1. Grade 1 sprains, which are microtears involving 20–30% of the ligament, cause minimal pain and disability. Weight bearing is not impaired.

        2. Grade 2 sprains, which are microtears involving 25–75% of the ligament, cause moderate pain and disability. Weight bearing is difficult in such cases.

        3. Grade 3 sprains, which are microtears involving >75% of the ligament, cause severe swelling, pain, and discoloration. Weight bearing is impossible.

    B. The **location of pain** provides a clue to the diagnosis of **strains.**

        1. Posterior pain on ambulation indicates a strain of the Achilles tendon.

        2. Pain at the posterior interior medial malleolus suggests a strain of the tibialis posterior tendon.

        3. A painful anterior tibia and ankle and medial foot indicate a strain of the tibialis anterior tendon.

        4. Posterior inferior lateral malleolar pain suggests a strain of the peroneal tendons.

    C. Pain and swelling over the affected tendon indicate tenosynovitis.

    D. A **painful lump** may be caused by a **contusion.**

    E. Abrupt moderate to severe pain and swelling. Immediate disability and discoloration and a patient report of an audible "pop" or crack indicate **acute fracture.** Patients with **chronic fracture** typically present with a history of a "sprained" ankle that resists all treatment, dull ache with slight swelling after excessive walking, increased pain with activity, and complete relief with rest.

IV. Signs
   A. Tenderness, swelling, and associated findings
   1. **Grade 1 sprains** of the lateral compartment result in slight tenderness and swelling over the ligaments and no laxity. Anterior drawer and talar tilt tests are negative. Medial compartment sprains cause tenderness and swelling over the deltoid ligament, no laxity, and slight pain with stress.
   2. **Grade 2 sprains** of the lateral compartment produce moderate tenderness and edema, hemarthrosis (40–50% of cases), and ecchymosis (30–40% of cases). Anterior drawer and talar tilt test results are positive. Medial compartment sprains cause tenderness and swelling over the ligament on eversion, as well as ecchymosis.
   3. **Grade 3 sprains** of the lateral compartment typically produce pronounced edema, loss of function, and severe pain, but may be painless. Hemarthrosis occurs in 80–90% of cases, and ecchymosis is present in 60–70% of cases. Anterior drawer and talar tilt test results are positive. Medial compartment grade 3 sprains cause diffuse swelling, tenderness, ecchymosis, and a positive talar tilt.
   4. **Sprains of the tibiofibular syndesmosis** are suggested by a positive compression test (squeezing the midthird of the calf).
   B. Crepitus ("packed snow" sensation) over the involved tendon indicates a **strain.** Additional specific findings include the following signs.
   1. Positive Thomas-Doherty squeeze test (Table 5–2) in Achilles tendon strain.
   2. Loss of medial longitudinal arch height and forefoot abduction in tibialis posterior tendon strain.
   3. Weakness or loss of foot elevation with tibialis anterior tendon strain.
   4. Weakness of eversion and dorsiflexion in strain of the peroneal tendons.
   C. Tenderness, thickening, erythema, crepitus, edema, weakness, and **nodule formation** are signs of tenosynovitis.
   D. Tenderness, ecchymosis, and **edema,** particularly over the malleolus, are evidence of contusions.
   E. Localized or point **tenderness, edema,** and possible **crepitus and ecchymosis** are signs of an acute fracture. Abnormal osteophony (ie, loss of sound transmission) may also occur. In chronic fractures, the physical examination findings are usually negative, except for point tenderness over the distal fibula (stress fracture) or on the talar dome with ankle plantar flexion (osteochondral fracture).
V. Laboratory Tests. Routine studies need not be performed if strains, tenosynovitis, and contusions are suspected.
   A. X-rays
   1. **X-rays** are indicated if there is **pain near the malleoli** and any of the following findings.
      a. **Bone tenderness** at the tip of either malleolus or at the posterior edge of the malleoli.
      b. **Inability to bear weight** both immediately and in the emergency department (four steps).

TABLE 5–2. MANEUVERS IMPORTANT IN EXAMINING THE INJURED ANKLE

Maneuver[1]	Findings
Anterior drawer test, which involves drawing the calcaneus and talus anteriorly while stabilizing the tibia	3–14 mm indicates grade 2 sprain; >15 mm indicates grade 3 sprain
Talar tilt test, which involves stressing the ankle laterally (inversion) and medially (eversion) while stabilizing the patient's leg	5- to 10-degree difference between ankles indicates grade 2 sprain; >10-degree difference indicates grade 3 sprain
Thomas-Doherty squeeze test, which involves squeezing the midthird of the calf with the knee flexed 90 degrees	Loss of plantar flexion with Achilles tendon rupture

[1] The anterior drawer, talar tilt, and stress tests can be facilitated by joint block. Lidocaine, 5–10 mL, is infiltrated into the joint opposite the side of injury and around the injured ligaments if necessary.

2. **Stress films** (ie, x-raying the ankle while applying varus or valgus stress) will be normal in grade 1 sprains. Such films will show a 5- to 10-degree tilt and 3- to 14-mm anterior displacement of the talus in grade 2 sprains and more than a 20-degree tilt with an anterior displacement of the talus of >15 mm in grade 3 sprains. Stress films should be performed to rule out associated ligamentous injury and joint instability if these findings are unclear from the physical examination.
3. Comparing anteroposterior, lateral, oblique, and mortise views between affected and uninjured ankles demonstrates fracture fragments. **Mortise** and **oblique views** are useful for detecting **osteochondral fragments.** Routine films will not show stress fractures for the first 2–3 weeks following injury.
B. **Arthrography**
  1. Arthrography is indicated in order to define the extent of damage. This technique is diagnostic for calcaneofibular tears (shown by extravasation of dye).
  2. **Disadvantages** of arthrography include expense, the need to schedule the procedure, allergic reactions to dye, and false-negative results several days after the injury. It should be used selectively in competitive athletes with significant disability.
C. **Computerized tomography (CT) and magnetic resonance imaging (MRI)** are >80% sensitive and specific in detecting soft tissue damage. These tests are recommended for locating fragments and determining the percentage of joint surface involved in osteochondral fractures. Compared to arthrography, CT and MRI have a greater predictive value and better patient acceptance.
D. **Bone scans** are helpful in detecting **stress fractures** in individuals with suggestive symptoms and normal plain films.

VI. **Treatment**
A. **Sprains**
  1. Management of **acute injuries**
    a. It is best to err on the conservative side when diagnosing the severity of a sprain and to be on the liberal side when treating and rehabilitating a sprain. Orthopedic consultation is recommended for grade 3 injuries and repeated sprains of any degree.
    b. **Rest, ice, compression, and elevation (RICE),** posterior splint or Aircast; and non–weight-bearing activities may be useful in treating sprains. Nonsteroidal anti–inflammatory drugs (NSAIDs) (eg, ibuprofen, 400–800 mg every 6–8 hours with food) and analgesics (eg, acetaminophen, 650 mg every 4–6 hours) should be given until edema and pain subside.
  2. **Long-term management**
    a. Grade 1: Weight-bearing brace or strapping for 2–3 weeks.
    b. Grade 2: Walking, well-padded dorsiflexion cast, Unna boot, weight-bearing brace, or air-stirrup for 2–4 weeks, followed by strapping at 90 degrees for 2–4 weeks. Severely swollen limbs shall not be placed in a cast.
    c. Grade 3: Dorsiflexion cast or weight-bearing brace for 3–6 weeks, followed by orthotic or strapping for 3–6 weeks; surgical repair. The best approach is unresolved, although age older than 40 years and athletic competition favor surgical repair.
    d. **Rehabilitation.** Isometric exercises while cast is on, then range of motion (ROM), progressive resistive exercises (PRE), and proprioceptive exercises (balance/wobble board), plus functional activity. Rehabilitation generally takes 2 weeks for grade 1 sprains, 4 weeks for grade 2, and 6 weeks for grade 3. Injection therapy can be used in a stable ankle that is chronically inflamed, preventing progression in a rehabilitative program. Ultrasound and cold packs have been found to offer no significant benefit over placebo, and the data on the benefit of diathermy over sham therapy are conflicting.
  3. **Prevention** of injury or reinjury involves the following measures.
    a. Using a **conditioning program** for the peroneal muscles that includes both isometric and isotonic exercises, emphasizing eversion and dorsiflexion.
    b. Teaching players to land with a relatively **wide-based stance.**
    c. **Taping, strapping, or bracing** previously injured ankles as well as uninjured ones.
    d. Using an **outer heel wedge** to avoid lateral sprains.
    e. Coordination training on a **balance board.**
    f. **Strengthening** of posteromedial muscles to prevent medial sprains.
    g. Using an **inner heel wedge** to avoid medial sprains.

B. Strains should be managed as described above for sprains (see section VI,A).

C. Tenosynovitis

1. **Initial treatment** includes **RICE, NSAIDs, and analgesics** as needed. **Injection of a corticosteroid** (eg, methylprednisolone acetate, 4 mg, with an equal volume of 1–2% lidocaine [Xylocaine]), may be helpful. This treatment is contraindicated in Achilles tendinitis, in the presence of infection, or if the patient has received a similar injection within the past 4 weeks or has a history of more than three such injections.

2. **Long-term management** includes application of a **short leg, non–weight-bearing cast, or protective strapping for 1–3 weeks.** ROM and PRE should be used for 1–3 weeks after cast removal (see section VI,A,2,d).

3. **Surgical consultation** is indicated in cases of refractory pain and disability that are unresponsive to conservative therapy. Tenolysis and debridement may prove helpful in such cases.

D. Contusions should be treated with **RICE and PRE.** Large hematomas should be aspirated and protected from further injury with foam and felt padding.

E. Fractures

1. **Initial management** of all fractures includes **RICE, NSAIDs, and analgesics** as needed. A **posterior splint** should be used, and no weight bearing should be permitted until pain and swelling subside. Consultation is advised for unstable, epiphyseal, and osteochondral fractures.

2. **Long-term management** of stable fractures includes a neutral, positioned **walking cast for 4–6 weeks. Rehabilitation** includes 2–4 weeks of ROM, PRE, and proprioceptive and functional exercises, as already described for ankle sprains (see section VI,A,2,d).

REFERENCES

Reisdorff EJ, Cowling KM: The injured ankle: New tests to a familiar problem. Emerg Med Reports 1995;**16**(5):39.

Safran MR, et al: Lateral ankle sprains: A comprehensive review. Med Sci Sports Exerc 1999; **31**(7S):429.

Stiell IG, et al: Implementation of the Ottawa ankle rules. JAMA 1994;**271:**827.

Struijs P, Kerkhoffs G: Ankle sprain. Clin Evid 2001;**6:**798.

Veenema KR: Ankle sprain: Primary care evaluation and rehabilitation. J Musculoskel Med 2000; **17:**563.

Wolfe MW, et al: Management of ankle sprains. Am Fam Physician 2001;**63**(1):93.

---

6   Arm & Shoulder Complaints

Brian R. Coleman, MD

KEY POINTS

- Knowledge of arm and shoulder anatomy is vital to proper diagnosis of arm and shoulder complaints.
- Overuse syndromes cause many shoulder complaints.
- Appropriate focused history and physical examination allows diagnosis of most arm and shoulder complaints and guides further testing.

I. **Definition.** The shoulder consists of four joints (glenohumeral, acromioclavicular, sternoclavicular, and scapulothoracic), which allow for movement in multiple planes. Unlike the hip, which is a stable joint having a deep acetabular socket, the shoulder is a mobile joint with a shallow glenoid fossa. The humerus has only minimal osseous support and is suspended from the glenoid by soft tissue, muscles, ligaments, and a joint capsule.

Glenohumeral stability is due to a combination of ligamentous and capsular constraints, musculature, and the glenoid labrum. **Static shoulder stability** is due to the joint surfaces and the capsulolabral complex. **Dynamic shoulder stability** results from rotator cuff muscles and the scapular rotators (trapezius, serratus anterior, rhomboids, and levator scapulae).

The **rotator cuff** is composed of four muscles, which assist in motion and depress the humeral head in the glenoid. The subscapularis assists internal rotation, the supraspinatus facilitates abduction, and the infraspinatus and teres minor assist in external rotation.

Arm and shoulder complaints comprise generalized or localized discomfort in the upper extremity. These may result from **direct trauma** (eg, acromioclavicular injuries, shoulder dislocation/subluxation, olecranon bursitis) or from **overuse** (eg, rotator cuff impingement/subacromial bursitis, olecranon bursitis, medial/lateral epicondylitis). Overuse of the musculotendinous unit evolves through several stages, beginning with inflammation (pain, swelling, erythema, warmth), followed by reparation (proliferative and maturation stages) and often, with continued overuse, fibrosis, which features histologically disorganized restructuring of the musculotendinous unit predisposing to degeneration, stenosing tenosynovitis, and even rupture. Aging also predisposes to these degenerative musculotendinous changes.

II. **Common Diagnoses** (Table 6–1). Arm and shoulder complaints are very common in family practice. Causes of these complaints are based on patient age and activity level. (See sidebars for information on burners/stingers, thoracic outlet syndrome, and acute brachial plexus neuritis.)

BURNERS/STINGERS

Burners/stingers are stretching/compression brachial plexus injuries caused by a blow to the patient's extended or flexed neck while in rotation. These injuries are most common in contact sports (eg, football, hockey, and lacrosse), are more common in males, and may also result from bicycling or motorcycle accidents.

Patients typically complain of burning/paresthesias of the arm and may experience some arm weakness hours to days after the injury, but should not have neck pain. Patients should have a thorough but brief neurologic examination of the affected extremity, as well as a cervical spine examination. Patients complaining of neck pain should be managed as if they have potential cervical spine injuries, with immobilization and emergency department evaluation. For uncomplicated stingers, radiographs are typically not required, and electromyography is required only if symptoms persist for 2–3 weeks (which occurs in <5–10% of patients). Stingers usually resolve on their own; in athletic play situations, the patient may return to play once burning resolves, provided there is no neck pain, weakness, or concussion.

THORACIC OUTLET SYNDROME

Thoracic outlet syndrome results from the compression of the neurovascular supply to the upper limb in the supraclavicular area and shoulder girdle. It tends to occur in young adults, particularly women, and has been associated with cervical ribs, diabetes, thyroid disease, alcoholism, and obesity. Patients may complain of pain in the neck or shoulder with numbness involving the entire upper extremity or forearm and hand; symptoms may be exacerbated by overhead activity. Nocturnal pain and paresthesias are common and should be distinguished from carpal tunnel syndrome. Thoracic outlet symptoms can often be reproduced and the condition diagnosed using the following maneuvers: Adson's maneuver (with the arm at the side and the neck hyperextended and turned to the affected side) and Wright's maneuver (with the arm abducted and externally rotated). Rib films will rule out cervical ribs or long transverse processes; if clinical evaluation is suggestive, cervical magnetic resonance imaging scan may help to rule out discogenic disease, and chest radiographs can evaluate for apical lung masses. Treatment for thoracic outlet syndrome involves management of underlying causes (eg, thoracic surgery consultation for cervical rib).

TABLE 6–1. DIFFERENTIAL DIAGNOSIS OF COMMON ARM/SHOULDER COMPLAINTS

Condition	Risk Factors	Symptoms	Signs	Testing
AC injuries	Male:female, 5:1, 16–30 yrs old Direct blow to tip of shoulder (eg, football, lacrosse, wrestling)	Pain with shoulder forward flexion/adduction	AC joint tenderness without gross deformity and with abnormal cross-arm test (Table 6–2) in Grade I or II dislocation; clavicular displacement (mildly and superiorly with Grade III and markedly superiorly or inferiorly or posteriorly accompanied by neurovascular or muscle compromise with Grades IV–VI)	Plain AP/lateral shoulder radiographs; stress radiographs are not recommended because they do not affect treatment
Glenohumeral instability	History of previous dislocation; adolescent female athletes; repetitive overhead activity (eg, gymnasts, swimmers, tennis, baseball pitching)	Vague pain referred to deltoid; feeling of impending dislocation or worse pain with overhead/abducted/extended rotated shoulder; "dead arm" after repetitive motion (eg, pitching)	Abnormal apprehension/sulcus tests (Table 6–1)	Results from AP/lateral shoulder radiographs are usually negative, but may show anteroinferior glenoid rim fracture (Bankart lesion)
Dislocation/subluxation	Contact sports (eg, football, lacrosse, rugby); fall on outstretched arm (eg, skaters, skiers, motorcyclists)	Pain: inability to abduct arm; possible arm paresthesias	Asymmetry compared to unaffected shoulder (prominent humeral head, sulcus between acromion and humerus)	Results from AP/transscapular lateral Y and axillary lateral views should be obtained; postreduction x-rays indicated to detect Bankart lesion
Impingement/bursitis continuum	Repetitive overhead motion (eg, throwing, racquet sports, swimming); overuse (eg, carpenters, painters, plumbers); >age 40	Pain with overhead activities, worse at night; anterolateral shoulder pain, possibly radiating to elbow	Abnormal Apley scratch, Neer's, Hawkin's, "empty can," or drop-arm tests (Table 6–2)	AP and transscapular lateral plain radiographs for degenerative changes; outlet or Alexander view visualizes subacromial space to grade acromial impingement; MRI 95% sensitive/specific detecting partial/complete tears, cuff degeneration, and chronic tendinitis

Adhesive capsulitis	Highest incidence in 40- to 50-year-olds; shoulder immobilization; involves nondominant arm more often and women > men	Painful loss of motion progressing to relatively pain-free restricted motion	Deltoid atrophy; decreased ROM, especially external rotation	AP/lateral radiographs useful to detect alternate diagnoses (fracture or calcification); arthrography may be helpful in diagnosis but is still controversial because of associated risks; MRI currently diagnostic test of choice
Olecranon bursitis	Direct contusion (eg, skaters, skateboarders, football players)	Swollen/fluctuant elbow extensor surface with or without pain	Fluctuant/tender or nontender mass over olecranon	Plain lateral radiograph may demonstrate bone spur or fracture with history of trauma or in recurrent, poorly responsive cases
Medial epicondylitis ("golfer's elbow")	Golfers; Little League pitchers	Pain medial elbow/forearm; decreased pitch control	Tender medial epicondyle	No testing, unless atypical presentation; plain radiographs can show fracture, OA, intra-articular loose bodies; EMG can document radiculopathy/neuropathy; MRI helpful in documenting soft tissue fraying or tear if surgical referral is considered.
Lateral epicondylitis ("tennis elbow")	Age 40–60; 7 times as common as medial epicondylitis, 75% involve dominant arm; found in carpenters/painters/tennis players or persons using poor equipment (wrong grip sizes, weight of racquet)	Pain lateral elbow/forearm (eg, holding a telephone, opening a door, or picking up a coffee cup); decreased grip	Tender lateral epicondyle, worse with resisted extension of middle digit	

AC, Acromioclavicular; AP, anteroposterior; EMG, electromyography; MRI, magnetic resonance imaging; OA, osteoarthritis; ROM, range of motion.

ACUTE BRACHIAL PLEXUS NEURITIS

Acute brachial plexus neuritis is an uncommon disorder, which can be confused with more common causes of shoulder pain. Brachial plexus neuritis most often affects those between ages 20 and 60 years, with a male-to-female ratio ranging from 2:1 to 11.5:1. A viral or other infectious cause has been suggested. Patients present with severe acute burning shoulder/upper arm pain without a known precipitant; the pain usually diminishes over days to weeks, replaced by upper arm weakness. Neck or arm movements typically do not affect pain. Brachial plexus neuritis must also be differentiated from cervical radiculopathy (Chapter 48), which radiates from the neck down the arm, may be related to trauma or exertion, and is exacerbated by neck movements. In brachial plexus neuritis, electromyography and nerve conduction studies 3–4 weeks after symptom onset reveal abnormalities in more than one nerve (ie, the brachial plexus); in contrast, cervical radiculopathy may feature osteophytes and interspace narrowing on cervical spine radiography and neuroforamenal disc impingement on magnetic resonance imaging scan. Treatment for acute brachial plexus neuritis is supportive, with physical therapy to maintain shoulder strength/mobility, analgesics as needed for pain, and reassurance that the condition generally will improve, albeit slowly.

    A. **Acromioclavicular (AC) injuries** are rare in skeletally immature individuals.
    B. **Glenohumeral instability** is an increase in translation of the glenohumeral joint and may occur in one or multiple directions. Generalized ligamentous laxity can also contribute to instability, especially in young athletic females and individuals with Marfan's syndrome.
    C. **Dislocations and subluxations** of the shoulder are common and account for 45% of all dislocations. Anterior dislocations account for approximately 90% of glenohumeral dislocations. Active patients younger than age 25 with a history of previous dislocation have an 85% risk of recurrence.
    D. **Rotator cuff impingement** and **subacromial bursitis** form a continuum, beginning with impingement with arm elevation, resulting in soft tissue edema/inflammation. **Under age 25,** ligamentous laxity predisposes to impingement; **beyond age 25,** impingement is usually related to overuse and frequently results in partial or full-thickness rotator cuff tears after age 40.
    E. **Adhesive capsulitis** is thickening and contraction of the capsule around the glenohumeral joint.
    F. **Olecranon bursitis** is inflammation of the superficial olecranon bursa caused by acute or chronic elbow trauma.
    G. **Medial epicondylitis** is inflammation of tendons and ligaments attaching to that structure.
    H. **Lateral epicondylitis** is pain over the lateral elbow precipitated by repetitive forearm dorsiflexion, supination, and radial deviation.

III. **Symptoms** (Table 6–1). Important elements include a careful history of the mechanism of acute injury, the patient's occupational/recreational activities, as well as location, precipitants, and any symptoms associated with the patient's shoulder/arm complaint.
    A. **Location**
        1. Vague pain radiating to the deltoid insertion occurs in patients with **glenohumeral instability.**
        2. Anterolateral shoulder pain possibly radiating to the elbow is consistent with **rotator cuff impingement/subacromial bursitis.**
        3. Lateral elbow pain characterizes **lateral epicondylitis;** medial elbow pain characterizes **medial epicondylitis.**
    B. **Precipitants**
        1. Pain with shoulder forward flexion/adduction characterizes AC **joint injury.**
        2. Pain with the shoulder overhead, abducted, and externally rotated occurs with **glenohumeral instability.**
        3. Shoulder pain with overhead activities and worsening at night is a clue to **rotator cuff impingement/subacromial bursitis.**
        4. Pain following a direct blow to the elbow may indicate **olecranon bursitis.**
    C. **Associated symptoms**
        1. A feeling of impending dislocation with the shoulder overhead, abducted, and externally rotated points toward **glenohumeral instability,** as does "dead arm" after repetitive shoulder motion.

   2. Painful decreased range of motion (ROM), developing over time into relatively pain-free restricted ROM, is consistent with **adhesive capsulitis.**
   3. Extensor elbow swelling indicates **olecranon bursitis.**
   4. Patients with lateral epicondylitis complain of decreased/weakened grip.
 IV. Signs (Table 6–1). Examination of the patient with arm/shoulder complaints should always include inspection (for asymmetry in AC or shoulder dislocations), palpation (for localized tenderness), and ROM/special maneuvers (Table 6–2).
 V. Laboratory Tests (Table 6–1). In most patients with arm and shoulder complaints, a careful history and physical examination should clarify the diagnosis. Further testing should be undertaken on a case-by-case basis.
 VI. Treatment of arm and shoulder complaints is directed at the underlying condition, which can be established through a careful focused history, examination, and selective testing.
   A. Grade I–III **AC joint injuries** are often treated with several days' rest and a shoulder sling for comfort. Ice and analgesics for pain and early range-of-motion exercises are important. Grade IV–VI (severe) AC sprains or dislocations warrant orthopedic consultation.
   B. Glenohumeral instability is treated primarily with physical therapy consultation for rotator cuff strengthening exercises. Nonsteroidal anti-inflammatory medications (NSAIDs) (eg, oral ibuprofen 600–800 mg three times daily with meals, or naproxen 550 mg twice daily with meals) may decrease pain and inflammation, but are not necessary. A history of recurrent dislocation warrants orthopedic consultation for consideration of surgical reconstruction.
   C. Rotator cuff injuries may be very difficult to treat. Initial therapy consists of rest, ice, and NSAIDs. Early physical therapy consultation is recommended for range-of-motion and strengthening exercises. A sling may provide some comfort, but could lead to

TABLE 6–2. MANEUVERS USED IN EVALUATING COMMON ARM/SHOULDER COMPLAINTS

Test Name	Description of Maneuver	Testing for . . .
Apley scratch test	Patient reaches (a) above/behind the head, then (b) behind the back, attempting to touch contralateral scapula	Rotator cuff (a) abduction/external rotation, (b) adduction/internal rotation
Neer's sign	Forced shoulder flexion with forearm extended/pronated (scapula stabilized)	Subacromid impingement
Hawkin's test	Forced shoulder internal rotation with arm forward elevated to 90 degrees	Subacromial impingement/rotator cuff tendinitis
"Empty can" test	With elbows extended, thumbs pointing downward and arms abducted to 90 degrees in forward flexion, patient attempts to elevate arms against examiner resistance	Rotator cuff (supraspinatus) weakness
Drop-arm test	After passive arm abduction, patient attempts to slowly lower arm to side	Rotator cuff tear/supraspinatus dysfunction (arm drops after 90 degrees)
Cross-arm test	Patient raises arm to 90 degrees, then actively abducts, attempting to touch opposite shoulder	AC joint dysfunction
Sulcus test	With arm extended and resting at patient side, examiner exerts downward traction on humerus, watching for sulcus or depression lateral/inferior to acromion	Glenohumeral instability
Anterior/posterior apprehension test	With patient's arm abducted to 90 degrees and elbow bent, examiner externally rotates arm and exerts (a) anterior or (b) posterior pressure on humeral head	(a) anterior (b) posterior glenohumeral instability
Yergason test	With patient's arm at side, elbow flexed to 90 degrees and thumb pointing up, examiner resists patient's attempts to supinate forearm and flex elbow	Biceps tendinitis (may be concomitant or confused with rotator cuff tendinitis)
Spurling's test	Patient extends neck; examiner axially compresses head and rotates it toward side of shoulder/arm complaint	Cervical nerve root compression

decreased ROM. **If a complete tear is noted,** then surgical intervention is necessary, but surgery is necessary in partial tears only after physical therapy has failed.

D. **Subacromial bursitis** is treated with relative rest, ice, range-of-motion exercises, and possible injection in the bursa (see sidebar).

SUBACROMIAL BURSA INJECTION

Informed consent should be obtained.

Equipment: 0.5–1 cc Aristocort 40 mg/mL and 3–4 cc lidocaine 1% combined in 5-cc syringe with 25G, 1½″ needle.

Technique: Injection can be done using either a posterolateral (just inferior to the posterior tip of the acromion into the space between the acromion and humeral head and directed anteriorly toward the coracoid process) or lateral approach; the lateral approach is described here. The patient should be seated with the arm hanging by the side to distract the humerus from the acromion. The edge of the acromion should be identified and marked. After cleansing the injection site with appropriate antiseptic rinse (eg, Betadine), the needle should be inserted with a slight upward angle at the midpoint of the acromion into the space between the humeral head and acromion. The needle is then slowly withdrawn while injecting the fluid in a bolus, ensuring there is no resistance. Occasionally the fluid will cause a visible swelling around the edge of the acromion. If needed, a "band-aid" dressing can be applied.

E. **Adhesive capsulitis** often resolves spontaneously, and treatment should focus on symptom relief. Gentle range-of-motion exercises, stretching, and **graded resistance training** have been shown effective. **Manipulation under anesthesia** requires orthopedic referral and is a very controversial treatment of capsulitis; it should be reserved for cases refractory to the foregoing measures. Corticosteroid injections (subacromial and intra-articular) may reduce pain but have not been shown to affect recovery.

F. **Olecranon bursitis** is treated with ice, NSAIDS, and close monitoring. Aspiration is performed only when swelling causes significant pain and loss of motion. Aspirated fluid should be analyzed for cell count, crystals, and Gram stain (see Chapter 39). Steroid injections have been used with mixed results and should only be performed if no infection is present.

G. **Medial epicondylitis** in youth is most easily treated conservatively with rest, ice, NSAIDs, and gradual increase in stretching-and-strengthening exercises. Local steroid injections (see section VI,H) should be considered if there is a poor response to 2–3 weeks' conservative therapy.

H. For **lateral epicondylitis,** conservative initial management involves NSAIDs, ice after activities or three times daily, emphasis on proper technique for work or sports activities, forearm or counterforce bracing, and physical therapy referral for stretching-and-strengthening exercises with a goal of pain-free ROM. Steroid injection (1 mL of betamethasone mixed with 3–5 mL bupivacaine into point of maximum tenderness in a spoke-and-wheel fashion) should be considered after poor response to 2–3 weeks' conservative management. Poor response to 6–12 months' treatment warrants consideration of orthopedic referral for possible debridement and tenotomy.

REFERENCES

Chumbly EM, O'Connor FG, Nirschl RP: Evaluation of overuse elbow injuries. Am Fam Physician 2000;**61**:691.

Miller JD, Pruitt S, McDonald TJ: Acute brachial plexus neuritis: An uncommon cause of shoulder pain. Am Fam Physician 2000;**62**:2067.

Tallia AF, Cardone DA: Diagnostic and therapeutic injection of the shoulder region. Am Fam Physician 2003;**67**:1271.

Woodward TW, Best TM: The painful shoulder: Part I. Clinical evaluation. Am Fam Physician 2000;**61**:3079.

Woodward TW, Best TM: The painful shoulder: Part II. Acute and chronic disorders. Am Fam Physician 2000;**61**:3291.

7   Bites & Stings

Brenda Powell, MD

KEY POINTS

- Mammalian bites cause morbidity from tissue destruction and introduction of pathogens.
- Insect and arachnid bites cause morbidity from hypersensitivity reactions, toxins, and introduction of pathogens.
- Treatment is based on the reaction type and the introduced infectious agent.

I. **Definition.** A **mammalian bite** is a skin wound caused by the teeth of a human or other mammal. Mammalian bites cause morbidity both from mechanical disruption and introduction of pathogens, which include oral aerobic and anaerobic flora and viruses such as hepatitis B and rabies, a fatal viral encephalitis.

    Insect and arachnid bites and stings involve penetration of the victim's skin by some part of the animal, with host reaction depending on the type of bite. Hypersensitivity to the organism occurs with lice, mosquito saliva, scabies, and hymenoptera stings. Spider bites can cause neurotoxicity and local necrosis with hemorrhage and thrombosis. Bites can transmit other diseases (eg, malaria and encephalitis from mosquitoes, Lyme disease and Rocky Mountain spotted fever from ticks, plague and typhus from fleas).

II. **Common Diagnoses.** About 1 million animal bites require medical attention each year in the United States. Lice and scabies are increasing in prevalence. Tick-borne diseases are the most common vector-borne illness in the United States. Hymenoptera stings cause more deaths than any other venomous animal (6 deaths per 100,000 people per year).

    The following animals cause most bites and stings that afflict humans in the United States.

A. **Mammals,** including humans and other mammals, both domestic and wild. About 90% of these bites are from dogs.

  1. **Bite injuries from humans** are common in fights; these involve primarily teenagers and alcohol-intoxicated males aged 30–35 years. Abused children, children who live in shelters for the homeless, and residents and staff of institutions for the mentally retarded are at especially high risk for human bites.

  2. Seventy-five percent of **animal bites** are considered "unprovoked." Sixty percent of dog bites involve neighborhood pets; 40% of these bites are superficial. Half of dog bite victims are children younger than 15 years. In the United States, rabies is found in unvaccinated domestic animals and wild animals such as skunks, raccoons, and bats.

B. **Insects,** including diptera (eg, mosquitoes, flies, and gnats); fleas and bedbugs; hymenoptera (eg, bees, wasps, hornets, yellow jackets, and ants); and pubic, head, and body lice. **Mosquitoes** breed in stagnant water during the warm season. **Fleas** can be found in grass, rugs, upholstery, floor cracks, and pet bedding, especially during warm, humid months; flea bites usually result from contact with dogs or cats. **Bedbugs,** which feed nocturnally on mammals and birds, may survive in clothing, furniture, and bedding for 6–8 weeks without a blood meal. **Bee and wasp stings** are common in suburbs and rural areas. The bites of **fire ants** are a significant problem in the southeastern United States. **Pubic lice** are usually transmitted by close body contact and are rarely spread by fomites. **Head lice,** which are commonly transmitted by the exchange of hats, combs, and brushes, may also be spread by close personal contact. Epidemics occur in schools. **Body lice,** associated with poor hygiene, are rare.

C. **Arachnids,** including mites that cause scabies, chiggers, hard and soft ticks, and brown recluse and black widow spiders. **Scabies** (adult mites or eggs) are readily transmitted by personal contact, especially within families or in crowded living situations. These parasitic mites burrow into the epidermis and lay eggs. **Chiggers (harvest mites)** are prevalent in brush in the southern and midwestern United States and bite gardeners, hikers, and campers. **Ticks** can be acquired by contact with pets, vegetation, or the burrows of host animals such as mice. Several human diseases are transmitted by ticks. Rocky Mountain spotted fever and tick-borne relapsing fever are endemic to the western mountain states. Tularemia from tick bites occurs mainly in western states. Lyme disease, which is endemic to semiwooded areas in New England, New York, and Wisconsin, occurs sporadically in the Midwest and the West. The bites of **brown recluse** and **black widow spiders** cause serious morbidity and result in about 5% of all deaths from venomous animals. **Brown recluse spiders** are endemic to the south central United States. These spiders, which are active nocturnally, hide both indoors and outdoors. They bite humans only when disturbed. **Black widow spiders** are found throughout the United States and Canada. They nest outdoors in crevices near the ground, especially where flies are present (eg, outhouses).

    D. Less common bites and stings not discussed in this chapter include **marine envenomations** and **snakebites.**

III. Symptoms and Signs

    A. Mammalian bite wounds. These bites may be **superficial abrasions; puncture wounds that are sometimes arcinate; lacerations, often with crushed and macerated edges,** or **wounds that may involve avulsion of tissue.** The wound should be examined for visible evidence of damage to underlying structures; diminished circulation or excessive bleeding; and decreased sensation, weakness, limited movement, or pain with movement. Signs of infection may become evident within hours of a bite. **Rabies** begins with pain and numbness in the area of the bite, followed by fever, dysphagia, pharyngeal spasms ("hydrophobia"), paralysis, convulsions, and death.

    B. Insect bite wounds. Itching is a symptom of **mosquito, flea, bedbug, lice, mite, and tick bites.**

        1. The bites of **mosquitoes** are **pruritic red papules or vesicles.**

        2. The bites of **fleas and bedbugs** are **pruritic red papules or vesicles.** They often occur in clusters or in a linear pattern on exposed areas, especially the wrists, ankles, and legs (fleas), and the hands, face, and neck (bedbugs).

        3. The normal local reaction to **hymenoptera venom** is heat, redness, and tenderness. A **local allergic reaction** consists of a red papule surrounded by a pale zone of edema, with varying amounts of local swelling. More severe **immediate hypersensitivity reactions** manifest the signs of generalized urticaria (see Chapter 62), redness, swelling, and anaphylaxis. A **delayed hypersensitivity reaction (serum sickness)** with fever, arthralgias, and malaise may occur 10–14 days after the sting. **Fire ants** cause multiple papules, which become necrotic pustules within several hours.

        4. The bites of **lice** are **pruritic red papules or vesicles.** The itching from lice begins about 21 days after infestation. **Pubic lice** live in pubic and axillary hair and skin, but move all over the body and may be found in eyelashes, eyebrows, and the hairline, especially in children. **Head lice** live on the scalp. The seams of clothing and folds of bedding should be searched for **body lice.** Nits of pubic and head lice attach to hairs at the skin level; since hairs grow 1 mm every 3 days, one can determine how recently nits were deposited by their distance from the skin on the hair shaft. This information is particularly helpful in deciding whether nits represent a new infestation following a course of treatment.

    C. Arachnid bite wounds

        1. Mites

            a. The female mite's burrow in **scabies** typically takes the form of a short, serpinginous lesion on wrists, elbows, or finger webs, or intertriginous areas. Myriad other skin lesions, including erythematous papules, nodules, scaly patches, excoriations, and secondary impetigo, can occur. Except in infants, scabies does not infest the scalp or the face.

            b. The bites of **chiggers** are **pruritic red papules or vesicles.** They often occur in clusters or in a linear pattern on exposed areas, especially the wrists, ankles, and legs. The bites of chiggers and flies have central puncta or vesicles, which may become hemorrhagic.

        2. After a **hard tick** has been attached for several days, its neurotoxin can cause an ascending progressive paralysis, similar to Guillain-Barré syndrome, with hyporeflexia.

            a. Lyme disease usually begins with a slowly spreading, annular skin lesion—erythema chronicum migrans—possibly accompanied by regional lymphadenopathy and minor constitutional symptoms. Early disseminated disease consists of multiple erythema chronicum migrans patches, lymphadenopathy, musculoskeletal pain, and attacks of arthritis. The nervous system may be involved and conduction abnormalities of the heart may be seen.

    b. The skin lesions of **Rocky Mountain spotted fever** are typically red macules on the peripheral extremities that may become purpuric and confluent.

    c. **Tularemia** is characterized by pain and ulceration at the bite site, with acutely inflamed, sometimes draining lymph nodes, or occasionally by severe pharyngeal inflammation with exudate, conjunctivitis, hepatosplenomegaly, or pneumonia.

3. Spiders

    a. A **brown recluse spider bite** is often unnoticed until local pain and itching begin; it becomes a hemorrhagic bulla surrounded by induration and erythema after 6–12 hours. The area of skin and subcutaneous necrosis may progress over a few days, forming an ulcer, which heals slowly over 2–4 months. Systemic symptoms include headache, fever, chills, malaise, weakness, nausea, vomiting, and joint pains. Signs of systemic intoxication, including morbilliform rash, tachycardia, hypotension, intravascular coagulopathy (petechiae, purpura, and bleeding diathesis), and hemolysis, may appear 1–3 days after the bite. Brown recluse spiders have a 3- to 5-cm leg span and a 1- to 2-cm brown, fuzzy body, with a violin-shaped dark band on the dorsum.

    b. The **black widow spider bite** is a mild prick, followed in 1–3 hours by severe, cramping pain at the bite site, spreading to adjacent parts of the body. Pain, cramps, anxiety, weakness, sweating, salivation, lacrimation, bronchorrhea, nausea, vomiting, and fever may subside in hours. The skin lesion develops a pale center with a red-blue border. Muscle rigidity, with tremor and fibrillations, develops in body parts near the bite. Signs of **cholinergic excess** (fever, lacrimation, rhinorrhea, and bradycardia) and **sympathetic activation** (hypertension and tachyarrhythmias), intensify over the next several hours, but may recur for up to 3 days. Black widow spiders have 1- to 2-cm shiny, black bodies, with a red hourglass mark on the underside.

IV. Laboratory Tests

  A. Mammalian bites

    1. Culture with sensitivity studies. More than one third of deeper human bite wounds and a smaller proportion of animal bites become infected; abrasions seldom reach that stage. Even apparently insignificant bites on the hand are prone to infection. Therefore, **culture with sensitivity studies** is recommended for the following types of mammalian bite wounds: deep puncture wounds, all bite wounds that are sutured, wounds that are clinically infected or require hospital treatment, and full-thickness bites on the hand.

    2. Radiograph. A plain radiograph should be obtained when osteomyelitis is suspected. Forceful injuries, such as a hand bite from a blow to a tooth, require an x-ray to look for fractures and embedded tooth fragments.

    3. Fluorescent antibody staining. An **animal suspected of being rabid** should be killed and its head sent to a health department laboratory, where the brain will be examined for rabies antigens by fluorescent antibody staining.

  B. Tests for possible scabies infestation. Scabies mites, eggs, or feces may be found by scraping open a pruritic lesion (especially the end of a burrow) with a No. 15 scalpel blade dipped in mineral oil, and then examining this material microscopically under a coverslip.

  C. Tests for suspected tick-borne diseases

    1. In the presence of **erythema chronicum migrans,** routine serologic testing for antibodies is not necessary and the patient should receive treatment with antibiotics. Otherwise, acute and convalescent titers of IgM and IgG to *Borrelia burgdorferi* can be drawn.

    2. Spirochetes can be seen in the blood smear in 70% of cases of **tick-borne relapsing fever.**

    3. Rocky Mountain spotted fever and **tularemia** are diagnosed by antibody titers to *Rickettsia rickettsii* and *Francisella tularensis,* respectively. Serology will be positive at 2 weeks. In **Rocky Mountain spotted fever,** the initial laboratory tests may often demonstrate normal or slightly depressed WBC, thrombocytopenia, elevated transaminases, and hyponatremia. In **tularemia,** the WBC and erythrocyte sedimentation rate may be normal or slightly elevated. The organism can be cultured, but this is not often done, due to the risk of transmission to laboratory workers.

  D. Tests for brown recluse spider bite with systemic involvement. If this kind of bite is suspected, order blood type and screen, coagulation studies, complete blood cell count, electrolytes, blood urea nitrogen, creatinine, and urinalysis.

V. Treatment
A. Mammalian bites
  1. Wound care is similar for human and other mammalian bites.
     a. **Thorough cleansing** is necessary. At home, this means repeatedly flushing the wound with soap and water, 3% hydrogen peroxide, or iodine solution. In the office, this involves pressure irrigation or scrubbing with gauze sponges (under local anesthesia if necessary) and 1% benzalkonium or povidone-iodine solution. The edges of a full-thickness wound should be debrided (see Chapter 41). Pressure irrigation should follow.
     b. **Closure**
        (1) **Primary closure** with sutures or wound tapes (Steri-Strips) may be considered for dog bites and for human and other animal bites on the face if the patient is treated within 3–6 hours after injury and if the wound appears to be uninfected. Subcutaneous sutures should be avoided. A pressure dressing should be applied for 24 hours, and the wound should be inspected for signs of infection after 48 hours.
        A single layer of skin sutures may be replaced with Steri-Strips after 5–7 days.
        (2) **Bite wounds on the hands should never be closed primarily.** A bitten hand should be immobilized, by splinting from the fingertips to the mid forearm, and elevated. Because of the risk of infection, the wound should be re-examined within 24 hours. After about 5 days, movement should be encouraged to minimize swelling and stiffness.
        (3) **Other bite wounds** should be packed with gauze impregnated with an antibacterial agent and seen 2 and 4–7 days later. Revision and delayed primary closure may be considered at that time.
     c. The **reporting of animal bites** (and of human bites in some locales) to the local health department is mandatory.
  2. **Antibiotic therapy**
     a. **Indications**
        (1) **Infected bite wounds** require antibiotic therapy. Patients with such bites on the hand should be hospitalized to receive intravenous antibiotics.
        (2) **Prophylactic antibiotics** should be considered for cat and human bites and for dog bites that are >8 hours old.
        (3) It is reasonable to treat with antibiotics bite wounds that have been sutured or followed up for possible delayed closure, all bites on the hand, bites causing deep puncture wounds, and all bites in diabetic patients or immunosuppressed persons.
     b. **Agents of choice and treatment regimens.** Animal bites (especially cat bites) may become infected with *Pasteurella multocida,* and human bites with *Eikenella corrodens* and *Bacteroides* spp, which are sensitive to penicillin and ampicillin but relatively resistant to clindamycin, first- and second-generation cephalosporins, and penicillinase-resistant penicillins. Staphylococci and other penicillinase-producing organisms are present in up to 41% of bite wound infections.
        (1) **Amoxicillin with clavulanic acid (Augmentin)** is the oral drug of choice for treatment (10-day course) or prevention (5-day course) of bite wound infection. The adult dose is 875 mg orally every 12 hours. Children should receive 30–50 mg/kg/day in three divided doses.
        (2) **Penicillin V,** 250 mg orally every 6 hours (30–50 mg/kg/day for children), may be adequate initial therapy for animal but not human bites. Infection developing within the first 24 hours suggests *Pasteurella* infection and constitutes an indication for penicillin.
        (3) Patients allergic to penicillin may receive the following antibiotics.
           (a) For adults and children aged 8 years or older: **erythromycin** (eg, **erythromycin ethylsuccinate,** 400 mg every 6–8 hours) *and* **tetracycline hydrochloride,** 250 mg orally every 6 hours, or **doxycycline,** 100 mg orally every 12 hours.
           (b) For children younger than 8 years, for whom tetracycline is contraindicated: **erythromycin** *alone,* 30–50 mg/kg/day in three divided doses.
  3. **Hospitalization** is indicated in the following situations:
     a. Bites to the hand, except those that are very superficial and do not appear to be infected.

     b. Bites involving tendon, joint capsule, bone, or facial cartilage.
     c. Signs of infection despite antibiotics or when treatment has been delayed.
     d. Severe disfigurement, or tissue loss that may require plastic surgery or grafting.
     e. Potential poor compliance with outpatient therapy.
  4. Rabies postexposure prophylaxis
     a. Indications (Table 7–1). Contact the local health department or the Rabies Investigation Unit, Centers for Disease Control and Prevention, Atlanta, Georgia, at (404) 639-3534 or (800) 311-3435 for additional information.
     b. Regimen. Human rabies immune globulin, 20 immunizing units per kilogram is given, half intramuscularly and half infiltrated around the wound, up to 8 days after exposure. Active immunization with human diploid cell rabies vaccine, 1 mL intramuscularly, is given on days 0, 3, 7, 14, and 28. Pregnancy is not a contraindication. Immunosuppressive drugs such as corticosteroids should be avoided if possible.
  5. Tetanus prophylaxis. Tetanus prophylaxis should be administered according to the indications outlined in Chapter 41.
B. Insect bites. Symptomatic relief is all that is needed for most bug bites, including those of mosquitoes, flies, fleas, and bedbugs. Topical lotions or creams such as **calamine** or **0.5% hydrocortisone** or applications of ice may relieve itching. Occasionally, an oral antihistamine, such as **diphenhydramine** (Benadryl), 25 mg three times a day for adults, ameliorates the urticarial reaction. Other, more specific treatments are discussed below.
  1. For flea and mite infestations, thorough **housecleaning,** including vacuuming, along with washing clothes and bedclothes, is indicated.
  2. Eradication of fleas and bedbugs is best performed by a professional exterminator. After **fumigation,** pets, children, and pregnant women should stay away for at least 4 hours.
  3. Pets with fleas should be treated with insecticide (eg, pyrethrum or malathion) after consultation with a veterinarian.
  4. Hymenoptera
     a. The **stinger** (if present) **should be removed** by scraping sideways so as not to squeeze the attached venom sac.
     b. Local pain and swelling may be controlled by applying ice and a protease (eg, a paste of meat tenderizer and water) to the site.
     c. Local allergic reactions should be treated with elevation to reduce swelling. **Antihistamines,** such as **diphenhydramine,** 25–50 mg (up to 1–2 mg/kg for children) orally every 6–8 hours, and **prednisone,** 1 mg/kg/day for 3 days, may also be effective.
     d. If **cellulitis** is present, an antibiotic, such as erythromycin, should be added to the above regimen (see Chapter 9).
     e. Immediate hypersensitivity reactions must be treated promptly with **epinephrine,** 1:1000, 0.01 mL/kg, up to 0.5 mL, injected subcutaneously, and repeated,

TABLE 7–1. RABIES POSTEXPOSURE PROPHYLAXIS

Animal	Animal Condition	Appropriate Treatment
Wild carnivores (eg, skunks, bats, or raccoons)	Available	Obtain fluorescent rabies antibody (FRA) test on animal. Begin HRIG[1] and HDCV.[2] Discontinue HDCV if FRA test is negative.
	Unknown	Assume rabid. Begin HRIG[1] and HDCV.[2]
Domestic dog or cat	Healthy/available	Observe animal for 10 days. If animal stays healthy, no treatment is necessary.
	Rabid/suspected rabid	Obtain FRA test on animal. Begin HRIG[1] and HDCV.[2] Discontinue HDCV if FRA test is negative.
	Unknown	Low risk of rabies in most areas. Consult local health department.
Rodents	Generally unknown	Prophylaxis rarely indicated. Consult local health department.

[1] Human rabies immune globulin, 20 U/kg intramuscularly on day 0. Before HRIG is given, serum should be drawn for measurement of rabies antibody titer.
[2] Human diploid cell vaccine, 1 mL intramuscularly on days 0, 3, 7, 14, and 28.
Adapted from the Centers for Disease Control and Prevention recommendations, 1991.

if necessary, in 5–10 minutes. A large-bore intravenous line should be started and the patient should be observed for at least 6–8 hours, since the vast majority of rebound or biphasic anaphylactic reactions will occur during this period. Additional measures for treatment of anaphylaxis should be available if necessary. Intravenous diphenhydramine, 50 mg, is given to block H_1 receptor sites. Aerosolized bronchodilators such as albuterol, 2.5 mg (0.5 mL of 5 mg/mL solution) in 3 mL of normal saline, should be used for bronchospasm. Simultaneous use of H_2 blockers (eg, ranitidine, 50 mg intravenously every 8 hours, or cimetidine, 300 mg intravenously every 6 hours) provides additional benefit.

   f. For **serum sickness** that occurs 10–14 days after hymenoptera stings, **prednisone,** 1–2 mg/kg/day orally in divided doses, should be tapered over 2 weeks.

   g. Prophylaxis. Any individual who has had *any* systemic allergic symptoms or progressively severe local reactions from hymenoptera stings should carry a kit with injectable epinephrine (eg, **Epi-Pen**), wear a medical identification bracelet, and avoid walking barefoot or wearing bright-colored clothing, flowers, or scent outdoors. Patients with allergic reactions may be evaluated by an allergist for desensitization treatment with venom extracts.

5. **Lice**
   a. Pediculosis capitis should be treated with a topical scabicide applied to dry hair and left on for 4 minutes before rinsing. (Permethrin 1% preferred, lindane 1% is an option, but not in children younger than 2 years or pregnant women.) After treatment, nits may be loosened by wrapping the hair for 30–60 minutes with a towel soaked in vinegar and may be combed out with a fine-tooth comb. Parents should check for treatment failure (new nits visible close to the skin) at 12 hours and every 2 days for 2 weeks; if failure occurs, a different medication should be used. Insecticides should be kept away from the eyes; on eyelashes, a thick coating of petroleum jelly should be applied twice a day for 8 days.
   b. Pediculosis corporis responds to a hot shower and laundering clothing/bed linens in hot water.
   c. Pediculosis pubis responds to the same measures as pediculosis capitis (ie, permethrin 1% as preferred agent, permethrin 5% a second option, and lindane 1% a third option).
6. **Scabies.** All household members should be treated simultaneously; bed linens and clothing should be washed in hot water.
   a. Permethrin 5% (Elimite cream), 1 oz per person, is massaged into the skin from the neck to the toes (and also on the head in infants) and left on for 8–14 hours, then thoroughly washed off.
   b. A less expensive and equally effective treatment is **1% gamma-benzene hexachloride** (lindane [Kwell or Scabene]) **lotion,** applied to cool skin from the neck down for 8–12 hours, then washed off with soap and water. Since systemic absorption and neurotoxicity can occur, it should not be used on children younger than 2 years, pregnant or lactating women, patients with seizures or other neurologic disease, or those with extensively inflamed skin.
   c. Despite elimination of live mites, pruritus and existing skin lesions may persist for several weeks. The itching may be treated with **hydrocortisone** or **0.1% triamcinolone cream, with or without oral antihistamines.**
   d. Oral ivermectin (Stromectol), 200 µg/kg in a single dose is effective in eradicating scabies, but is not approved by the US Food and Drug Administration for routine use. It should probably be reserved for scabies crustosa (Norwegian scabies).
7. **Ticks**
   a. Hard ticks should be removed. The tick should be grasped very close to the skin with blunt forceps, and pulled. If the tick is not completely removed, it should be excised (eg, using a skin biopsy punch). Sometimes a diligent search is required to locate an attached tick.
   b. Skin infections should be treated with antibiotics (see Chapter 9).
   c. For **Lyme disease** the length of treatment is dependent on the stage of the disease.
      (1) Early localized Lyme disease may be treated for 14–21 days with **doxycycline,** 100 mg twice a day, or **amoxicillin,** 250–500 mg three times a day (20–40 mg/kg/day for children).
      (2) Early disseminated disease is treated with intravenous therapy for 2–3 weeks. Options are ceftriaxone 2 g daily, cefotaxime 3 g twice a day,

and chloramphenicol 50 mg/kg/day in four divided doses. The risk of transmission of the disease is low, less than 5%, even in areas where the disease is hyperendemic; it is therefore probably not cost-effective to treat prophylactically with antibiotics after a tick bite.

d. For **Rocky Mountain spotted fever,** treatment should be started promptly with oral **tetracycline** (if the patient is older than 8 years), 25–30 mg/kg/day in four divided doses, or with one dose of **chloramphenicol,** 50 mg/kg, followed by 50 mg/kg/day in four divided doses. When the patient becomes afebrile, the dose should be halved, and then discontinued after 2–3 days.

e. Adults with **tularemia** can be treated with **streptomycin,** 0.5 g intramuscularly twice a day for 1 week.

f. **Tick-borne relapsing fever** in adults is treated with **tetracycline,** 500 mg orally four times daily for 10 days.

8. **Spider bites**

a. **Hospitalization** is indicated for patients with black widow spider bites who are symptomatic, elderly, or very young. Hospital treatment may also be necessary for patients with brown recluse spider bites if they have systemic symptoms or if laboratory evidence of intravascular coagulation and hemolysis exists.

b. For **local lesions caused by brown recluse spider bites,** good wound care is important. A bitten extremity should be splinted and elevated. Soaks and sterile dressings, and possibly topical antibacterial agents such as silver sulfadiazine, are applied to the necrotic ulcer. Systemic antibiotics such as **erythromycin ethylsuccinate,** 400 mg orally four times a day, have been used but are not routinely indicated. **Excision** of the bite wound is ineffective and **contraindicated.** Local and systemic corticosteroids are of no benefit. The following treatments are **experimental:** antivenom, hyperbaric oxygen, and dapsone, a polymorphonuclear cell inhibitor (dosage, 50–200 mg/day). The latter agent has potentially serious side effects.

c. Tetanus prophylaxis should be given (see Chapter 41).

d. Initial therapy for **black widow spider bites** consists of application of ice and extremity elevation. Calcium gluconate in a 10% solution (10 mL given by intravenous push over 5 minutes) may provide relief from muscle spasm. Narcotics and diazepam in standard doses can be initiated to relieve pain and muscle spasm.

e. Before administering **black widow spider antivenom,** testing for sensitivity to horse serum should be done. The test packaged with the antivenom can be used. One 2.5-mL ampule of black widow spider antivenom intramuscularly or intravenously in 10–15 mL of normal saline over 10–15 minutes can then be administered.

C. **Prevention**

1. **Hepatitis B.** Persons at occupational risk for human bites, including health and dental workers and employees of institutions for the mentally retarded, should receive hepatitis B vaccine.

2. **Rabies.** Veterinary workers occupationally exposed to animal bites and people traveling to areas where rabid dogs are common should be immunized with 1 mL of human diploid cell rabies vaccine intradermally on days 0, 7, and 21 or 28.

3. **Outdoor insect bites** can be prevented by avoiding their habitats, covering the skin with clothing, and using effective insect repellents that contain diethyltoluamide (DEET). Repeated applications to the skin can cause allergic and toxic effects. **Permethrin** (Permenone Tick Repellent) sprayed on clothing protects against mosquitoes and ticks.

REFERENCES

Bunzli W, et al: Current management of human bites. Pharmacotherapy 1998;**18:**227.

Dire DJ: Emergency management of dog and cat bite wounds. Emerg Med Clin North Am 1992;**10:**719.

Hogan DJ, Schachner L, Tanglertsampan C: Diagnosis and treatment of childhood scabies and pediculosis. Pediatr Clin North Am 1991;**38:**941.

Kelleher A, Gordon S: Management of bite wounds and infection in primary care. Cleve Clin J Med 1997;**54:**137.

Kemp E: Bites and stings of the arthropod kind. Postgrad Med 1998;**103:**88.

Norris R: Managing arthropod bites and stings. Physician Sports Med 1998;**26**(7):47.

Verdon M, Sigal L: Recognition and management of Lyme disease. Am Fam Physician 1997;**56:**2.

8   Breast Lumps & Other Breast Conditions

Diane J. Madlon-Kay, MD, MS

KEY POINTS
- Benign breast disease affects almost all women.
- Mammograms are not recommended for women younger than age 30.
- Family physicians can do needle aspirations of breast masses to determine whether they are cystic.

I. **Definition.** Breast lumps are any areas of the breast that feel different from surrounding breast tissue. The normal breast is lumpy due to its cystlike architecture.

II. **Common Diagnoses**
  A. **Fibrocystic changes** are the most common benign condition of the breast. The incidence of this disorder increases with age; approximately 25% of premenopausal women and up to 50% of postmenopausal women have this condition. Cysts may range in size from 1 mm to large macrocysts >1 cm.
  B. **Breast cancer** will eventually develop in one of every nine women. Risk factors include age, genetic factors, and hormonal factors.
  C. **Fibroadenomas** are most prevalent in women younger than age 25 and in black women.
  D. **Mastitis** is almost always associated with lactation. This condition results from the entrance of *Staphylococcus aureus* or streptococci into the breast tissue through abraded skin or a cracked nipple. Streptococcal infection usually leads to cellulitis, whereas staphylococcal infection may lead to abscess formation.

GYNECOMASTIA

Gynecomastia is a benign enlargement of the male breast. It may be asymptomatic or painful, unilateral or bilateral. It commonly occurs during puberty. It also occurs in adults, with the highest prevalence among 50- to-80-year-olds. Most patients seeing a physician for gynecomastia will have idiopathic gynecomastia (25%) or gynecomastia due to puberty (25%), drugs (10–20%), cirrhosis or malnutrition (8%), or primary hypogonadism (8%).

Gynecomastia appearing during mid-to-late puberty requires only a history and physical examination, including careful palpation of the testicles and, if the results are normal, reassurance and periodic follow-up. In most boys the condition resolves spontaneously within a year, and no further evaluation is necessary. Since gynecomastia is so common in men, the presence of nontender, palpable breast tissue on a routine examination should not lead to a major laboratory evaluation. In most instances taking a careful history is sufficient to uncover most of the conditions associated with gynecomastia. If no abnormalities are found on physical examination or after the assessment of hepatic, renal, and thyroid function by serum chemistry profiles, further specific evaluation is unlikely to be useful. The patient should be re-examined in 6 months. If a patient reports the recent onset of progressive breast enlargement and no underlying cause is apparent, measurements of serum chorionic gonadotropin, testosterone, estradiol, and luteinizing hormone may help elucidate the cause.

Most patients require no therapy other than the removal of any identified inciting cause. Specific treatment is indicated if the gynecomastia causes sufficient pain or embarrassment. Several medical regimens have been tried, including dihydrotestosterone, danazol, clomiphene citrate, tamoxifen, and testolactone. Surgical removal is also an option.

III. **Symptoms**
  A. One common symptom is **breast lumps.** In approximately 70–80% of women in whom breast cancer develops, the first and only symptom is the incidental discovery of a mass by the patient.

B. Breast pain is the most common symptom of fibrocystic changes. The pain is usually bilateral and often in the upper outer quadrants. Characteristically, the pain begins 1 week before menstruation and diminishes with the onset of menstrual flow. The pain is caused by breast swelling; breast volume may increase up to 15%.

C. Nipple discharge of a yellow or greenish-brown color occurs in up to one third of patients with mastitis. The second most frequent symptom of breast cancer, nipple discharge in women older than 50 years, is of more concern than it is in younger women. If the discharge is associated with a mass, the mass is the primary concern. Spontaneous, recurrent, or persistent discharge requires surgical exploration. The character of the discharge cannot be used to distinguish benign from malignant causes. However, bloody, serous, serosanguineous, or watery discharges should be regarded with suspicion.

MASTALGIA

Mastalgia is the most common breast symptom causing women to consult physicians. Although fibrocystic disease is often present in the biopsy specimens of women with breast pain, fibrocystic changes are also present in the breasts of 50–90% of asymptomatic women.

Most commonly, breast pain is associated with the menstrual cycle (cyclic), but it can be unrelated to the menstrual cycle or occur postmenopausally. Cyclic breast pain is usually bilateral and poorly localized. It is often described as a heaviness that radiates to the axilla and arm and is relieved with the onset of menses. Cyclic mastalgia occurs more often in younger women. Noncyclic mastalgia is most common in women 40–50 years of age. It is often unilateral and is described as a sharp, burning pain that appears to be localized in the breast.

In most women with breast pain, the physical examination and mammogram, if indicated, reveal no evidence of breast pathology. Patients can be reassured that breast pain has a spontaneous remission rate of 60–80%. Further treatment modalities are described in section VI,A.

IV. Signs

A. Breast lumps. Ideally, examination of the patient should take place 7–9 days after the onset of menstrual flow. In general, fibrocystic areas are slightly irregular, easily movable, bilateral, and in the upper outer quadrants. Compression often causes tenderness, especially premenstrually.

On palpation, a cancerous lesion is usually solitary, irregular or stellate, hard, nontender, fixed, and not clearly delineated from surrounding tissues.

Fibroadenomas are usually rubbery, smooth, well-circumscribed, nontender, and freely mobile.

B. Breast inflammation. Mastitis is characterized by inflamed, edematous, erythematous, indurated tender areas of the breast.

C. Surface of the breast

1. **Retraction.** Breast cancer frequently causes fibrosis. Contraction of this fibrotic tissue may produce dimpling of the skin, alteration of the breast contours, and flattening or deviation of the nipple.

2. **Edema of the skin.** Lymphatic blockage produces thickened skin with enlarged pores characteristic of the so-called pigskin or "orange peel" (*peau d'orange*) appearance in breast cancer.

3. **Venous pattern.** This may be prominent unilaterally in breast cancer.

V. Laboratory Tests. Diagnostic testing is unnecessary in women with multiple, bilateral, diffuse, symmetric breast lumps without dominant masses.

A. Mammography

1. **Indication.** A woman older than age 30 with a solitary or dominant mass or an area of asymmetric thickening in the breast should undergo mammography. A breast lump is described as a dominant mass when the breasts are diffusely nodular but one mass is clearly larger, firmer, or asymmetric in location.

2. **Contraindication.** Since breast tissue is very dense in young women, mammograms are *not* recommended in women younger than age 30. In older women, some fatty displacement of breast tissue has occurred, and mammograms are more worthwhile.

3. **Efficacy.** Although 85% of all breast cancers are documented by mammography, as many as 15% of women with breast cancers have a normal mammogram.

Therefore, a palpable mass is of concern even if a mammographic report shows no evidence of malignancy. **A biopsy is the only test that definitively excludes cancer.**

4. **Interpretation.** A mammogram is usually interpreted in one of three ways.
   a. **Normal.** No breast cancer is identified.
   b. **Indeterminate.** This usually means that an area of possible cancer or asymmetry is visible. It is not sufficiently suspicious to warrant immediate biopsy, however. A repeat mammogram in 3–6 months is often recommended.
   c. **Suspected breast cancer.** Mammogram findings suspicious for malignancy include a dominant or asymmetric mass, a typical microcalcification, a stellate pattern of denser tissue, an extension of streaks of denser tissue into the subcutaneous fat, retraction of the skin or nipple, and thickening of the skin.

B. **Other imaging techniques.** Although ultrasonography is not useful as a screening tool for breast cancer, it is useful for discriminating solid from cystic lesions. Other imaging techniques considered experimental or of no proven benefit for evaluation of breast conditions include thermography, diaphanography, computerized tomography, magnetic resonance imaging, and digital imaging.

C. **Aspiration of a suspected breast cyst.** Needle aspiration may be used to define the cystic nature of any breast mass.

   A 20- or 22-gauge needle attached to a 10- or 20-mL syringe should be used. After the skin is cleaned with alcohol, the cyst is fixed between the fingers of one hand while the needle is directed into the cyst with the other. The aspirated fluid is usually amber to green in color. If the fluid is bloody or if the mass is still palpable or reappears within 1 month of observation, a biopsy is necessary. The fluid is usually discarded.

D. **Breast biopsy.** The cytologic or histologic characteristics of a clearly dominant breast mass should be confirmed by biopsy, regardless of other clinical or mammographic findings.
   1. **Fine-needle aspiration biopsy** is used to determine the cytology of suspected breast cancer. Accurate interpretation requires proper smearing and fixation of the slides as well as an experienced pathologist. In expert hands, the false-negative rate is 1.4% and the false-positive rate is near 0%.
   2. **Excisional biopsy**
      a. Excisional biopsy is indicated if the results of the physical examination or mammogram suggest cancer even when the cytologic findings of aspiration are benign, or if a breast mass may be cancerous and fine-needle aspiration biopsy and cytologic evaluation are not available.
      b. The biopsy is usually performed as an outpatient procedure using local anesthesia. Removal of the entire mass is the objective.
   3. **Incisional biopsy** may be performed in the following circumstances.
      a. To confirm the diagnosis of advanced cancer. If the mass is strongly suspected of being malignant, a cutting-edge core needle can be used.
      b. To evaluate a breast mass that is too large to be excised easily and completely.

E. **Genetic testing for breast cancer.** Women at risk for genetic mutations should be identified by taking a thorough personal and family history for breast or ovarian cancer or both. Women at low risk for a genetic mutation should not undergo genetic testing because of the risk of indeterminate or false-positive results and the psychological and social risks associated with testing. A helpful tool to calculate breast cancer risk is the Breast Cancer Risk Assessment Tool developed by the National Cancer Institute, available by calling 1-800-4CANCER. For women in whom genetic testing is warranted, testing should be done only in the context of careful genetic counseling.

VI. **Treatment**
   A. **Fibrocystic changes**
      1. **General measures**
         a. **Supportive measures** that may be helpful include the use of loose, light clothing and a comfortable, supporting, well-padded bra.
         b. **Dietary changes**
            (1) **Caffeine intake.** Although studies of dietary restriction of **caffeine** and other methylxanthines are conflicting, some reports suggest that eliminating consumption of such substances may be efficacious.
            (2) **Vitamin E.** This vitamin has not been found to be beneficial in placebo-controlled studies.

(3) **Evening primrose oil** is often used by British physicians because of its significant response rate (60%), low incidence of side effects, and non-hormonal composition. The average dose is two 500-mg capsules three times a day for a minimum of 3–4 months. Evening primrose oil can be obtained without a prescription and costs about $1 a day.

2. **Pharmacologic therapy** (Table 8–1). Before beginning treatment, the woman's symptoms should be carefully evaluated. Minimal symptoms for only a few days of the month do not require drug therapy. It may take 3–4 months for evidence of improvement with any treatment regimen.

   Although other drugs can be used for this purpose, **danazol** is the only pharmacologic agent approved by the US Food and Drug Administration for use in the treatment of fibrocystic changes. Since danazol therapy is associated with significant side effects, however, this agent should be administered only by a physician familiar with its use.

3. **Surgery.** A subcutaneous mastectomy with implants or bilateral reduction mastectomies may be considered in the following patients.

   a. In women with an extremely high risk of breast cancer (eg, a history of breast cancer in a mother and a sister).

   b. In women with ductal or lobular atypical hyperplasia on biopsy. The risk of breast cancer is increased by a factor of approximately 5 in these women.

   c. In women with breast pain that is resistant to nonsurgical treatment.

B. **Breast cancer.** The objective of treatment is to provide the greatest chance for cure or long-term survival. Whether this objective can be met while preserving the major portion of the breast is controversial. Radical mastectomy is now performed rarely, since modified radical mastectomy results in comparable survival. Lumpectomy is an option for some women.

1. **Surgery.** The primary care physician is responsible for referring the patient to a surgeon, who should provide individualized counseling to the patient so that the appropriate option is selected. Breast cancers are staged at surgery, at which time tissue is obtained for estrogen and progesterone receptors.

   Most women can be fitted with a **prosthesis** within 3–6 weeks of surgery. The option of breast reconstruction should be discussed before surgery because it can often be performed at the same time.

2. **Chemotherapy, hormonal therapy, and radiation therapy** should be directed by an oncologist.

3. **Careful and frequent follow-up** is important. The history and the physical examination should be directed toward the breasts, bones, liver, chest wall, and nervous system. An annual mammogram of both breasts is recommended.

4. **Discussion of social and emotional issues is crucial.** The American Cancer Society's Reach to Recovery program is a valuable resource for patients.

C. **Fibroadenoma. Surgical excision,** preserving as much normal breast tissue as possible, is the preferred treatment. After excision, the patient should be reassured that she is at no increased risk of cancer.

TABLE 8–1. PHARMACOLOGIC THERAPY FOR FIBROCYSTIC CHANGES

Drug	Dosage	Effectiveness (%)	Significant Side Effects
Danazol[1]	100–400 mg by mouth daily for 4–6 months	60–90	Yes
Oral contraceptives (eg, Loestrin 1/20)	1 tablet by mouth daily for 1–2 years	70–90	Some
Medroxyprogesterone acetate	10 mg by mouth on days 15–25 of the menstrual cycle for 9–12 months	85	Some
Tamoxifen	10–20 mg by mouth daily for 4 months	70	Yes
Bromocriptine	1.25–5.0 mg by mouth daily for 2–4 months	50–80	Yes

[1] The only drug approved by the US Food and Drug Administration for the treatment of fibrocystic changes.

D. Mastitis. Lactating women should be encouraged to continue nursing.
   1. Ten days of an antibiotic effective against *S aureus* and streptococci should be sufficient.
      a. A penicillinase-resistant synthetic penicillin, such as dicloxacillin, 500 mg orally every 6 hours, should be used.
      b. For patients who are allergic to penicillin, erythromycin, 500 mg orally every 6 hours, is a reasonable alternative.
   2. Local heat is also of benefit.
   3. Failure of symptoms to respond to treatment in 48 hours or the development of a mass may indicate a breast abscess that requires incision and drainage. Inflammatory breast cancer must be considered in any mastitis that does not respond to treatment after 5 days or in nonnursing women with mastitis. A biopsy will establish the diagnosis.

REFERENCES

Morrow M: The evaluation of common breast problems. Am Fam Physician 2000;**61:**2371.
Neinstein LS: Breast disease in adolescents and young women. Pediatr Clin North Am 1999;**46:**607.
Pruthi S: Detection and evaluation of a palpable breast mass. Mayo Clin Proc 2001;**76:**641.
Rhodes DJ: Identifying and counseling women at increased risk for breast cancer. Mayo Clin Proc 2002;**77:**355.

---

9   Cellulitis & Other Bacterial Skin Infections

Donald B. Middleton, MD

KEY POINTS

- Most cellulitis and other skin infections are due to *Staphylococcus aureus* or *Streptococcus pyogenes,* which are sensitive to first-generation cephalosporins.
- Skin infection with certain organisms such as *Pseudomonas aeruginosa* suggests underlying bacteremia.
- Hospitalization is indicated for those who fail to respond to outpatient treatment, are toxic, or have high-risk medical conditions.

I. **Definition.** Infections of the skin follow bacterial invasion into the superficial or deep layers or specialized structures of the dermis. A breach of the skin's surface barrier allows bacteria to penetrate and produce infection, which may be a local process or reflect lymphatic or hematogenous spread from infection of another organ system. Factors facilitating infection include **primary skin diseases** (eg, eczema or psoriasis); **trauma** (eg, abrasions, burns, or bites); **immunologic defects** (eg, AIDS, alcoholism, multiple myeloma, or diabetes mellitus); **contaminated wounds** (eg, from dirty water, soil, or feces); concurrent or pre-existing **viral or fungal infections** (eg, herpes simplex cold sore or athlete's foot); **bacterial infection** in structures contiguous to the skin (eg, osteomyelitis, tooth abscess, or sinusitis); **circulatory dysfunction** (eg, edema or lymphedema); **bacteremia** (eg, sexually transmitted diseases or subacute bacterial endocarditis); **pruritus** (uremia); and **psychological distress** (neurodermatitis). Cytokines and lymphokines worsen the inflammatory warmth and erythema. Bacterial exotoxins enhance invasion. Although at least 100 different bacterial pathogens have been reported to produce skin infection, most are due to *S aureus* or *pyogenes.* The likelihood of other organisms depends on host factors (eg, age or immune status), source of inoculum (eg, human or animal bite), and lesion morphology (eg, erythema migrans in Lyme disease).

II. **Common Diagnoses.** In the primary care setting, bacterial skin infections account for 2% of ambulatory visits and are the 28th most common diagnosis in hospitalized persons. Common bacterial skin infections are:

A. Superficial infection (above or into the upper dermal papillae).
   1. **Impetigo** is endemic in children, especially preschoolers. At least 20% of children have one or more bouts of this infection. The incidence peaks in late summer and early fall, when minor trauma from insect bites or abrasions promotes infection. Close person-to-person contact or scratching from winter dryness, underlying chickenpox, scabies, pediculosis, or tinea can cause the infection and result in spread. Epidemics of impetigo occur occasionally, for example, infecting a whole wrestling team. Underlying chronic disorders like eczema or vascular stasis ulcers promote secondary infection.
   2. **Erysipelas** is common in alcoholics, diabetics, or immunocompromised hosts but occasionally arises spontaneously in preschool children or older adults. Roughly 30% of patients have recurrence bouts.
   3. **Erythrasma** affects young men. In tropical climates, 20% of men develop this infection.
B. Deep infection (epidermis and full dermal layer down into the subcutaneous fat).
   1. **Cellulitis** follows traumatic disruption of the skin's protective barrier or occurs spontaneously in the young, elderly, diabetic, alcoholic, edematous, or immunocompromised patient or in those with underlying dermatologic conditions. Cases occur throughout the year. Recurrent cellulitis is common in those with an underlying chronic process such as lymphedema or eczema. Many subtypes are recognized. For example, **necrotizing fasciitis** due to *S aureus* occurs most commonly in the elderly, a minority of whom have diabetes mellitus or myxedema. Intravenous drug abusers and those with malignancy, anal fissure, hemorrhoids, peripheral vascular disease, or penetrating trauma are also at risk for necrotizing fasciitis. In the young, *S pyogenes* fasciitis follows other illness such as chickenpox.
   2. A **furuncle (boil)** arises in an area prone to perspiration and friction and is most common in adults. Obesity, immunocompromise, and self-trauma, including squeezing a pimple, are important etiologic factors.
   3. A **carbuncle** usually develops in those with immunodeficiencies due to alcoholism or diabetes mellitus or who self-traumatize a furuncle.
   4. **Ecthyma** occurs in children or the neglected elderly, often after insect bites or skin excoriation.
C. Specialized skin structure infection (initially localized to a hair follicle, sebaceous cyst or sweat gland).
   1. **Folliculitis** usually follows water exposure such as immersion in a hot tub or with trauma such as shaving.
   2. **Sebaceous gland abscess** occurs in those with repetitive sebaceous cyst trauma from squeezing or rubbing.
   3. **Hidradenitis suppurativa**, a sweat gland infection, does not occur prepubertally and usually follows axillary or groin shaving, particularly in the obese. Men are more likely to have perianal infection, and women are more likely to have axillary disease. Some less common but important infections are listed in Table 9–1.

TABLE 9–1. DIAGNOSING AND TREATING LESS COMMON BACTERIAL SKIN INFECTIONS

Condition	Findings	Treatment
Anthrax (*Bacillus anthracis*)	Painless papule progressing to vesicle to ulcer over 3–5 days. Best diagnosed with punch biopsy of indurated plaque.	Penicillin, ciprofloxacin, or doxycycline ≥10 days
Gangrene (*Clostridium perfringens* or mixed)	Gas in wound.	Debride, oxygen, penicillin or clindamycin
Bacillary angiomatosis (*Rochalimaea henselae*)	Typically human immunodeficiency virus patient with cherry angiomatous or pyogenic granuloma–like lesions.	Erythromycin or doxycycline for 2 weeks
Chancriform lesions (venereal or mycobacterial)	Ulcerative lesions (syphilitic are painless; chancroid are painful).	Based on cause
Lyme disease (*Borrelia burgdorferi*)	Red ≥5 cm circinate macule or target lesion at site of tick bite; similar distant lesions occur with hematogenous spread.	Doxycycline or amoxicillin for 14–21 days

III. Symptoms. Most symptoms are common to all forms of infection.
   A. Pain at the site of infection occurs with most infections, except perhaps impetigo, Lyme disease, and erythrasma.
   B. Pruritus is common in impetigo, cellulitis, folliculitis, and erythrasma. Scratching often causes further trauma and promotes spread of infection.
   C. Feverishness, chills, and **malaise** can develop acutely. These symptoms often reflect invasion of deeper tissues or the bloodstream, especially when they occur with cellulitis, erysipelas, or carbuncles. Severely ill patients may become septic, slip into coma, or die. Erysipelas is especially prone to cause high fever.
IV. Signs (Table 9–2). The hallmarks of infection are pain, swelling, redness, and warmth. Most bacterial skin infections have a pathognomonic appearance. Nonetheless, bacterial infection must be distinguished from allergic conditions (eg, eczema), contact dermatitis (eg, poison ivy), insect stings, trauma, and viral or fungal infections. A red streak emanating from the rash suggests lymphangitic spread from an infectious cellulitis. Scattered purple or red skin papules or macules may reflect underlying bacteremia with agents such as *Pseudomonas* or gonorrhea.
   A. Superficial infection
      1. In **impetigo,** "kissing" lesions occur where two skin surfaces touch. Autoinoculation and multiple lesions are common, particularly around the face. Underlying viral or fungal infections can be distinguished from impetigo by the appearance of the primary lesions, such as the smaller vesicles of chickenpox or the circinate raised edge and central clearing of tinea corporis. Staphylococcal impetigo may mimic streptococcal disease.
      2. In **erysipelas,** the forehead, face, and abdomen are other sites of infection.
   B. Deep infection
      1. In **cellulitis,** propagation from a central traumatic lesion is centripetal and rapid, often resulting in lymphangitis or lymphadenopathy. An allergic reaction is seldom as warm, tender, or well demarcated. Infection is occasionally indolent and can spread to regional lymph nodes, blood, fascia, or muscle, creating a life-threatening situation.
         a. Cellulitis marked by a bluish discoloration and woody consistency of the cheeks indicates facial or buccal cellulitis, often secondary to *Haemophilus influenzae* type b or pneumococcus.
         b. Hand cellulitis often follows puncture wounds, such as animal bites or foreign body insertion. Cat or dog bites may often produce infection with *Pasteurella multocida.* **Cellulitis of the foot or the leg** often coexists with osteomyelitis in the immunocompromised or diabetic host.
         c. Cellulitis with a tense firm portion may indicate subcutaneous abscess formation.
         d. Infection in **necrotizing fasciitis** evolves over 1–3 days from cyanosis and edema into necrosis, sometimes accompanied by subcutaneous crepitans indicating gas-forming agents.
V. Laboratory Tests. Most skin infections, like impetigo or cellulitis, can be treated empirically based on morphology and likely causative agents. In these cases, cultures of the leading edge (10–15% positive), central abrasions (15–50% positive), or blood (a small percentage are positive) are minimally beneficial. Counterimmunoelectrophoresis on urine, tears, and other fluids; paired antibody titers; and cultures of skin biopsies also have marginal value.
   A. Cultures are warranted in certain situations.
      1. Blood cultures should be obtained from patients who are toxic or immunocompromised; who have preseptal or postseptal orbital cellulitis, necrotizing fasciitis, diabetes, facial cellulitis, or fever with scattered papules/macules; or who fail treatment. Blood cultures are positive in 80% of patients with *H influenzae* and in about 20% with pneumococcal cellulitis of the eye or face.
      2. Needle aspiration of unruptured bullae or pus from incised abscesses provides reliable culture data, especially with **paronychia** or a **boil.** However, cultures are unnecessary in most cases. **Gram stain** and **culture of pus** are often helpful, especially in severely ill patients.
      3. Conjunctival cultures may be useful in preseptal or postseptal cellulitis.
      4. Skin biopsy may help with atypical lesions. For example, anthrax is best diagnosed with a **punch biopsy** of the indurated plaque.
      5. Bone biopsy with culture is the definitive test to diagnose coexistent osteomyelitis. Orthopedic consultation is required for bone biopsy, although some neuropathic

TABLE 9–2. DIAGNOSIS AND TREATMENT FOR COMMON SKIN INFECTIONS

Class	Condition	Findings	Treatment (Table 9–3)
Superficial infections	Impetigo	Small vesicles, enlarging to 1–2 cm with red halo and central "honey" crust (strep) vs. bullous lesions with minimal surrounding erythema (staph).	Penicillinase-resistant penicillin, macrolide, or first-generation cephalosporin; topical agents for small areas or nasal carriage; good hygiene (avoid scrubbing)
	Erysipelas	Ill patient with well-demarcated erythema (70% involve lower extremity) with central peau d'orange appearance	Penicillin or erythromycin
	Erythrasma	Finely scaled red-brown lesions, especially in genital folds	Erythromycin for 14–21 days
Deep infections	Cellulitis	Typically poorly demarcated. Warmth/erythema/tenderness	Cephalosporin, fluoroquinolone, amoxicillin-clavulanate, azithromycin, clarithromycin, clindamycin; supportive care (limb elevation, warm soaks, and analgesics); hospitalization if severely ill, immunocompromised, or gram-negative or mixed aerobic/anaerobic cellulitis
	Preseptal orbital cellulitis	Red, swollen, tender eyelids	Hospitalization if ill-appearing
	Postseptal orbital cellulitis	Red, swollen, tender eyelids with proptosis, disconjugate gaze, painful eye movement	Hospitalization for parenteral antibiotics
	Necrotizing fasciitis	Abrupt, painful onset; ill patient with initially only mildly abnormal skin	Hospitalization for surgical debridement
	Furuncle	Hot/tender deep purulent boil. Typically neck, axilla, buttock, thigh	Moist heat, avoidance of squeezing, incision and drainage if fluctuant
	Ecthyma	Deep ulcerating lesions, especially in children or neglected elderly	Penicillin, cephalosporin; antipseudomonal if testing warrants
Special skin structure	Carbuncle	Conglomeration of boils, with multiple purulent sites	Hospitalization for parenteral antistaphylococcal antibiotics and possible incision and drainage (I and D)
	Folliculitis	Red dome-shaped pustule involving hair follicles	Antistaphylococcal antibiotics (antipseudomonal with warm compresses and avoidance of cosmetics if hot-tub folliculitis).
	Sebaceous cyst abscess	Painful, warm nodule with central black punctum	Office I and D, packing, 24-hr follow-up; possibly antistaph antibiotics for 3–7 days
	Hidradenitis suppurativa	Carbuncle in axilla or groin, varying from acute/tender to chronically draining lesions	**Acute:** Antistrep or antistaph antibiotics, warm compress, topical isotretinoin, avoidance of shaving or deodorants, surgical referral **Chronic:** May respond to ≥3 months of tetracycline

patients with open wounds may have protruding fractured bone fragments that can be removed for culture.
   B. Special procedures are sometimes helpful.
      1. Plain radiographs may detect tissue gas or foreign bodies, as well as bone, tooth socket, or sinus infection.

2. **Magnetic resonance imaging (MRI)** or **computerized tomography scans** can distinguish preseptal from postseptal cellulitis. MRI is useful to detect underlying osteomyelitis with severe cellulitis especially of the leg or foot in diabetics. Either technique can be used to identify complicating subcutaneous abscesses, which require drainage, common in diabetic or immunocompromised hosts.

3. **Bone scans** are beneficial in selected cases of cellulitis (diabetics with foot infection, cases of extremity cellulitis that fail to improve, or trauma victims with crush injury) to reveal concomitant osteomyelitis.

4. **Sonograms** of persistent cellulitis can reveal subcutaneous pus collections.

5. **Wood's lamp** illumination is useful in erythrasma because the infected skin fluoresces coral red.

VI. **Treatment** (Tables 9–2 and 9–3). A 7- to 10-day course of antibiotics is required for nearly all bacterial skin infections, most of which can be managed as outpatient therapy. Ordinarily, complete resolution is achievable, but recurrences are common. Therapeutic decisions include whether to hospitalize or seek consultation. Toxic patients or those with inadequate social supports are best hospitalized. Unfamiliar lesions are best handled through consultation.

A. **Superficial infection**

1. Although *S pyogenes* is the traditional cause of nonbullous **impetigo,** recent studies suggest that *S aureus,* usually phage group II, is also a major culprit. About 10% of all impetigo is bullous, a result of staphylococcal invasion. Therefore, **cephalexin** seems ideal for all cases of **impetigo,** but alternatives include any agent that eradicates streptococci and staphylococci, such as **clindamycin, azithromycin, clarithromycin,** or **amoxicillin-clavulanate.** Topical agents, especially **mupirocin** ointment (Bactroban) applied three times a day, are effective for small areas. Agents such as **hexachlorophene** are not highly efficacious. With treatment, impetigo responds rapidly in over 90% of cases, but the spontaneous resolution rate is 60% in 10 days. Glomerulonephritis or, rarely, toxic shock, may complicate streptococcal impetigo. Scalded skin syndrome, or, rarely, toxic shock may follow staphylococcal disease. Parents and patients should be warned to look for hematuria and peeling skin in the week following treatment.

2. **Erysipelas** (due to *S pyogenes*) usually defervesces within 24–48 hours of initiation of appropriate treatment, but may recur in up to 30% of cases.

3. **Erythrasma,** probably due to *Corynebacterium minutissimum,* can relapse into asymptomatic infection lasting for years.

B. **Deep infection. Cellulitis** is usually due to group A (rarely group C or G) *S pyogenes* and *S aureus.* Other bacteria capable of producing cellulitis include *H influenzae* type b (buccal cellulitis in young infants), *S pneumoniae* (preseptal or postseptal orbital cellulitis), mouth anaerobes such as peptostreptococcus (human bites), soil bacteria such as *Clostridia* (necrotizing fasciitis), *P multocida* (cat bites), and coliform organisms (decubitus ulcers).

1. In selecting an antibiotic for cellulitis, likely etiologic agents, cost, and side effect profile should be considered. In streptococcal disease, penicillin or cephalexin are the drugs of choice, whereas synthetic penicillins such as oxacillin are highly effective for both staphylococcus and streptococcus. Severely ill or immunocompromised patients should be broadly treated initially with an aminoglycoside and penicillin/β–lactam combination or a third-generation cephalosporin until culture results direct narrowing of the antibiotic regimen. Although no randomized controlled trials are available, a trial of intravenous **cefazolin** plus oral probenecid proved equal to intravenous **ceftriaxone** in adults with moderate to severe cellulitis.

2. Patients with underlying congestive heart failure, stasis ulceration, or diabetes mellitus frequently develop recurrent cellulitis of the legs. Support stockings or Unna boot therapy may help. Hyperbaric oxygen is of limited value for routine cellulitis but may benefit clostridial infections.

C. **Specialized skin structure infection**

1. Recurrent **folliculitis** may be treated prophylactically with chronic topical antibiotics. **Sycosis barbae,** a deep folliculitis of the beard, is treated with saline compresses, topical mupirocin or bacitracin and, if recalcitrant, with oral cephalosporins for 7–10 days.

2. In **sebaceous cyst abscess,** some advise antistaphylococcal antibiotics (eg, cephalexin) for 3–7 days to reduce chance of spread.

TABLE 9–3. ANTIBIOTICS FOR SKIN INFECTIONS (USUAL COURSE 7–14 DAYS)

Drug (Trade Name)	Route of Administration[1]	Pediatric Dose (mg/kg/day)[2,3]	Adult Dose (g/day)[2]	Interval (dose/day)
Penicillins				
Penicillin V	PO	25–50	1–2	4
Amoxicillin	PO	20–40	0.75–1.5	3
Ampicillin	PO, IV, IM	25–200	1–12	4
Ampicillin-clavulanate (Augmentin)	PO	20–40	0.75–1.5	3
Nafcillin	PO, IV, IM	50–200	1–12	4
Oxacillin	PO, IV, IM	50–200	1–12	4
Dicloxacillin	PO	12.5–25	1–2	4
Piperacillin	IV	Dose based on piperacillin content; 100–300; safety not established under age 12 years	6–24	4–6
Cephalosporins				
For use against gram-positive cocci and some gram-negative agents				
Cefadroxil (Duricef)	PO	30	1–2	1–2
Cephalexin (Keflex)	PO	25–100	1–4	4
For use against above plus *Haemophilus influenzae*				
Cefaclor (Ceclor)	PO	20–40	0.75–4	2–3
Cefprozil (Cefzil)	PO	15–30	0.5–2	1–2
Ceftibuten (Cedax)	PO	9	0.09–0.4	1
Cefuroxime axetil (Ceftin)	PO	20–30 or 125 or 250 mg/dose	0.5–1	2
Loracarbef (Lorabid)	PO	15–30	0.4–0.8	2
For use against primarily gram-negative agents and most gram-positive cocci				
Cefixime (Suprax)	PO	8	0.4	1
Cefpodoxime (Vantin)	PO	10	0.2–0.8	1–2
Ceftriaxone (Rocephin)	IV, IM	50–100	1–4	1–2
Other Antibiotics				
Erythromycin (many)	PO, IV	30–50	1–2	3–4
Clarithromycin (Biaxin)	PO	15	0.5–1	2
Azithromycin (Zithromax)	PO	5–10	0.5 initial, then 0.25	1
Doxycycline (many)	PO	Over age 8 yrs	200	2
Clindamycin (Cleocin)	PO, IV	10–40	0.6–2.7	3–4
Metronidazole (Flagyl)	PO, IV	15–30	0.75–2	3
Fluoroquinolones (over age 18 yrs only)				
Ciprofloxacin (Cipro)	PO, IV	Not used	0.5–1.5	2
Gatifloxacin (Tequin)	PO	Not used	0.4	1
Levofloxacin (Levaquin)	PO, IV	Not used	0.25–0.5	1
Lomefloxacin (Maxaquin)	PO	Not used	0.4	1
Moxifloxacin (Avelox)	PO, IV	Not used	0.4	1
Ofloxacin (Floxin)	PO, IV	Not used	0.4–0.8	2
Topical agents				
Mupirocin (Bactroban)	Topical			2–5 times/day
Bacitracin (many)	Topical			3–5 times/day

[1] PO, oral; IV, intravenous; IM, intramuscular.
[2] Dosage may require adjustment in renal failure.
[3] Not to exceed the adult dose.

3. In **hidradenitis suppurativa,** prednisone, 40–60 mg orally daily for 5–10 days, is sometimes used to diminish scarring. Chronic infection may respond to a tetracycline (eg, doxycycline) orally for ≥3 months.

REFERENCES

Bisno AL, Stevens DL: Streptococcal infections of skin and soft tissue. N Engl J Med 1996;**334**:240.
Cox NH: Management of lower leg cellulitis. Clin Med 2002;**2**:23.
Lowy FD: *Staphylococcus aureus* infections. N Engl J Med 1998;**339**:520.
Stevens DL: Infections of the skin, muscle, and soft tissues. In: Braunwald E, et al (editors): *Harrison's Principles of Internal Medicine,* 15th ed. McGraw-Hill; 2001:821.
Stulberg DL, et al: Common bacterial skin infections. Am Fam Physician 2002;**66**:119.
Swartz MN: Cellulitis and subcutaneous tissue infections. In: Mandell GL, et al (editors): *Principles and Practice of Infectious Diseases,* 5th ed. Churchill Livingstone; 1999:1037.
Swartz MN, Weinberg AN: Bacterial diseases with cutaneous involvement. In: Fitzpatrick TB, et al (editors): *Dermatology in General Medicine,* 6th ed. McGraw-Hill; 2003:1843.

---

10   Chest Pain

Leanne M. Chrisman-Khawam, MD, MEd

KEY POINTS

- Most chest pain encountered in ambulatory primary care is not life threatening and is chest wall or gastrointestinal in origin.
- A careful history and physical examination and focused testing uncover potentially deadly conditions, including coronary artery disease.
- Most causes of chest pain can be managed in the primary care ambulatory setting.

I. **Definition.** Chest pain is the sensory response to noxious stimuli caused by trauma or dysfunction of the chest wall, heart, lungs, pleura, diaphragm, esophagus, or stomach. Psychological disorders can cause chest pain in the absence of organic pathophysiology or may worsen the response to underlying organic disease.

II. **Common Diagnoses.** Chest pain is one of the most common and complicated symptoms for which patients seek medical attention. Most cases are due to myriad common and non-serious conditions; however, several deadly conditions including coronary artery disease, the number one cause of death in the United States, can easily be confused with more benign causes.

   A. Thirty-six to 38% of chest pain is **chest wall pain;** 20% is due to muscle pain; 13% to costochondritis; 2% to broken ribs; and <1% each to fibrocystic breast disease, sickle cell crisis, herpes zoster, and chest wall bruising or trauma. Chest wall pain is most common in active, young men and women, especially with a history of chest trauma or work/recreational activities involving repetitive upper extremity motion, lifting, or range of motion extremes.

   B. **Gastrointestinal (GI) sources** account for 20% of chest pain, including gastroesophageal reflux disease (GERD) and esophagitis (13%), achalasia and esophageal spasm (4%), dyspepsia (1–2%), peptic ulcer disease and gallbladder disease (1% each), and hiatal hernia and other esophageal motility disorders (<1% each). Factors increasing the likelihood of a gastrointestinal (GI) source of chest pain include past history of ulcers or dyspepsia, cigarette use, use of nonsteroidal anti-inflammatory drugs (NSAIDs), or use of other gastric irritants (eg, ethanol, aspirin, erythromycin, tetracycline, or alendronate).

   C. Twenty percent of chest pain is **cardiovascular,** including stable angina pectoris (10%); myocardial infarction (2–3%); mitral valve prolapse (2%); unstable angina (1.5%); cardiac arrhythmia (1%); and aortic dissection/aortic aneurysm, pericarditis, pericardial tamponade, and rare congenital defects (all <1% each). (Also see the sidebars on thoracic aortic dissection/aneurysm and pericarditis.) Risk factors for **coronary artery disease,** easily the most common cause of cardiovascular chest pain, include age (male 45 years or older, female 55 years or older); first-degree relative (male younger than 55 years or female younger than 65 years) with myocardial infarction (MI) or sudden cardiac death; diabetes mellitus; current cigarette use or use within 10 years; blood pressure ≥140/90 mm Hg or treatment with an antihypertensive drug, high-density lipoprotein cholesterol <45 mg/dL; low-density lipoprotein cholesterol >130 (mg/dL); left ventricular hypertrophy on electrocardiogram (ECG); or history of recent/chronic cocaine use. Minor risk factors include sedentary lifestyle and obesity (body mass index >28).

THORACIC AORTIC DISSECTION/ANEURYSM

Risk factors for this life-threatening condition include history of hypertension, congenital aortic valvular or ascending aortic disease, atherosclerotic inflammatory/collagen aortic disease, pregnancy, or tobacco abuse. Aortic dissection often presents suddenly with unremitting excruciating, tearing, knifelike chest pain, radiating through to the back. Less commonly, dissection presents as less severe, nagging mid-chest discomfort. Physical examination may reveal an anxious, dyspneic patient with hypo- or hypertension, differences between right and left arm blood pressures, absent arm or other pulses, a harsh/holosystolic heart murmur associated with aortic insufficiency, pulsus paradoxus, and less often, paralysis.

When dissection is suspected by clinical history, the patient should be hospitalized, with emergent cardiothoracic surgery consult and imaging studies (eg, chest computerized tomography) to confirm the diagnosis.

PERICARDITIS

Risk factors for pericarditis/myocarditis include infection (tuberculosis or viral infection); autoimmune disease (eg, lupus, acute rheumatic fever); recent MI or cardiac surgery; malignancy; mediastinal radiation therapy; uremia; and certain drugs (procainamide, hydralazine, isoniazid) or past history of pericarditis. Presentation is marked by constant substernal chest pain or pressure or left precordial chest pain consistent with angina. The pain of pericarditis often decreases with sitting and increases when supine or leaning forward. The classic feature of a two- or three-component friction rub may or may not be heard. Other findings include anxiety/dyspnea, tachycardia, fever, increased erythrocyte sedimentation rate, increased white blood cell count, pulsus paradoxus, and occasionally tamponade. Chest radiography may reveal cardiomegaly, a bottle-shaped heart in myocarditis, or be completely normal. Echocardiography detects wall motion abnormalities (myocarditis) or pericardial fluid (pericarditis). Treatment is supportive with serial monitoring and use of oral anti-inflammatory drugs; severely symptomatic patients, those whose initial studies are markedly abnormal, and those whose condition deteriorates during outpatient management should be hospitalized.

D. **Psychosocial sources** account for approximately 9% of chest pain; these include stress-related sources (8%) and panic disorder and somatization disorder (<1% each) Emotional stress may also exacerbate GERD, cardiac chest pain, and asthma.
E. Five to 10% of chest pain is **pulmonary,** including bronchitis (2%); pleurisy (1–2%); pneumonia (1%); and pneumonitis, sarcoidosis, obstructive lung mass, pulmonary embolus, pulmonary abscess, ruptured bullae, pneumothorax, asthma, or viral upper respiratory infection (<1% each). Risk factors for **bronchitis/pneumonia** include cigarette use and antecedent viral respiratory infection; additional risk factors for **pneumonia** include chronic lung disease, altered consciousness/impaired gag reflex, immunodeficiency, neuromuscular disease, and thoracic cage deformity. **Pneumonitis** tends to occur with occupational or other exposure to chemical irritants (eg, farming, factory/foundry work, cleaning). Teens who recreationally sniff chemicals and veterans of the last Gulf War are also at risk for pneumonitis. Risk factors for **deep venous thrombosis and pulmonary**

embolism (PE) (see sidebar) include prolonged immobilization, pregnancy or recent delivery, pelvic or lower extremity trauma, hypercoagulability, estrogen use, and malignancy. (See also Chapters 23 and 42.)

PULMONARY EMBOLISM (PE)

PE presents with sudden dyspnea, tachypnea, tachycardia, occasional hemoptysis, and hypo- or hypertension. Some patients present with few symptoms other than chest pain. Physical findings range from normal to tachypnea, isolated rales, and occasionally a pulmonary rub (an end-inspiratory rubbing sound). Pulmonary hypertension associated with PE may produce left heart failure (fine bibasilar lung rales) or be restricted to echocardiographic or angiographic abnormalities. Clinical scoring systems (Table 10–1) can be helpful in determining the risk for PE and the need for further testing, which should be done in the hospital setting.

    F. Although rare in the office setting, **major trauma** also produces chest pain (eg, cardiac tamponade, tension pneumothorax).

  III. Symptoms. A careful history can narrow the differential diagnosis of chest pain and should address location and quality of pain, risk factors, exacerbating/alleviating factors, and associated symptoms.

    A. Location/quality of pain

      1. Ischemic heart disease patients complain of substernal tightness, pressure, or both, which may radiate to either arm or to the jaw, the back, or both.

      2. Mitral valve prolapse (MVP) produces an often-sudden onset of chest discomfort, which may be less intense than angina, sharp, and in the left anterior chest. Often the pain can be fleeting and not usually relieved by nitrates.

      3. Pleuritic pain is often sharp and localized within the left or right hemithorax.

      4. Chest wall/muscle pain is also a sharp to dull ache and may be localized anywhere on the chest wall.

      5. GI pain may be substernal and burning (dyspepsia/GERD) or squeezing, substernal pressure (achalasia/esophageal spasm).

    B. Risk factors (see section II,A–E.)

    C. Exacerbating/alleviating factors

      1. Pain from ischemic heart disease is worsened with activity or stress and alleviated by rest or by oxygen, nitrates, or both.

TABLE 10–1. PREDICTION RULES FOR SUSPECTED PULMONARY EMBOLISM

Geneva Score	Points	Wells' Score	Points
Previous pulmonary embolism or deep vein thrombosis	+2	Previous pulmonary embolism or deep vein thrombosis	+1.5
Heart rate >100 beats per minute	+1	Heart rate >100 beats per minute	+1.5
Recent surgery	+3	Recent surgery or immobilization	+1.5
Age (years)		Clinical signs of deep vein thrombosis	+3
60–79	+1	Alternative diagnosis less likely than pulmonary embolism	+3
>80	+2	Hemoptysis	+1
P_aCO_2		Cancer	+1
<4.8 kPa (36 mm Hg)	+2		
4.8–5.19 kPa (36–38.9 mm Hg)	+1		
<6.5 kPa (48.7 mm Hg)	+4		
Clinical probability		Clinical probability	
Low	0–4	Low	0–1
Intermediate	5–8	Intermediate	2–6
High	>9	High	>7

2. **Chest wall/muscle strain pain** is worsened with arm movements or deep inspiration. **Pleuritic chest pain** may also be produced or exacerbated by deep inspiration or cough.
3. **GI pain** is exacerbated by meals (particularly by large meals) and supine position; antacids, protein pump inhibitors or histamine-2 (H_2) blockers typically alleviate this pain. In particular, **gallbladder pain** is classically brought on by high-fat meals.

D. **Associated symptoms**
   1. Nausea, dyspnea, diaphoresis, or sudden, severe overwhelming fatigue (particularly in women) may accompany **ischemic heart disease.**
   2. **MVP** may be associated with palpitations (especially when supine), lightheadedness, dyspnea, or anxiety or headaches.
   3. Cough frequently accompanies **pulmonary chest pain;** fever with productive or nonproductive cough occurs in **pneumonia;** insidious-onset cough with dyspnea and occasionally fever characterizes **pneumonitis.**
   4. **GI chest pain** is often associated with nocturnal/morning cough, flatus, belching, hoarseness, halitosis, dysphagia, or odynophagia.
   5. A sensation of dyspnea, an inability to breathe deeply, or frank hyperventilation often accompanies **psychogenic chest pain.** Such pain is frequently associated with other somatic pain (chronic headaches, abdominal or pelvic pain); panic disorder may feature the foregoing, along with paresthesias, dizziness, trembling, diaphoresis, and a sense of "impending doom."

IV. **Signs.** Important aspects of the focused physical examination in all patients with chest pain include general appearance and vital signs, palpation (chest wall and epigastrium), and cardiopulmonary auscultation.
   A. **General appearance/vital signs.** Those with **acute cardiac ischemia** (crescendo angina or MI) and those with **panic/anxiety** may appear anxious and dyspneic; **ischemic heart disease** may also cause hyper- or hypotension and diaphoresis; **panic/anxiety** may cause tremor.
   B. **Palpation**
      1. In **chest wall pain,** opposed movement or palpation of affected muscles or ligaments reproduces pain, while palpation of the costochondral junction (especially of the third and fourth ribs) reproduces **costochondral chest wall pain.**
      2. **GI pain** may be associated with mid-epigastric tenderness.
   C. **Auscultation**
      1. **Cardiac auscultation** in **ischemic heart disease** may be normal or may reveal a new murmur or S_3 or S_4 gallop; in **MVP,** auscultation classically reveals a mid to late systolic click and a late systolic murmur.
      2. **Pulmonary auscultation**
         a. **Pleuritic pain** may feature a friction rub, an end-inspiratory sound consistent with the rubbing of one's hand against rubber.
         b. Findings in **pneumonia** include localized rales, egophony ("e" to "a" changes), and expiratory sounds such as wheezes or more course rhonchi, which may decrease or be brought out by coughing.
         c. **Pneumonitis** may be accompanied by fine bibasilar rales.

V. **Laboratory Testing** (Figure 10–1). When a common cause of chest pain is highly probable based on focused history and examination (eg, chest wall pain or costochondritis), further testing is unnecessary and treatment can be initiated. Further testing is necessary when the etiology or severity of the chest pain remains unclear after focused history and examination, as is often the case with ischemic heart and pulmonary diseases.
   A. **Hematologic tests**
      1. **Complete blood count** may show leukocytosis and left shift with bacterial pneumonia and lymphocytosis with viral pneumonia.
      2. **Thyroid-stimulating hormone** levels may be low or undetectable in hyperthyroidism, which may contribute to anxiety states.
      3. Blood *Helicobacter pylori* testing can evaluate for this potential cause of refractory dyspepsia.
   B. **Chest radiograph** is helpful in both suspected cardiac and pulmonary causes of chest pain.
      1. **Cardiomegaly** may be seen in **dilated cardiomyopathy** due to chronic **ischemic heart disease (IHD).**

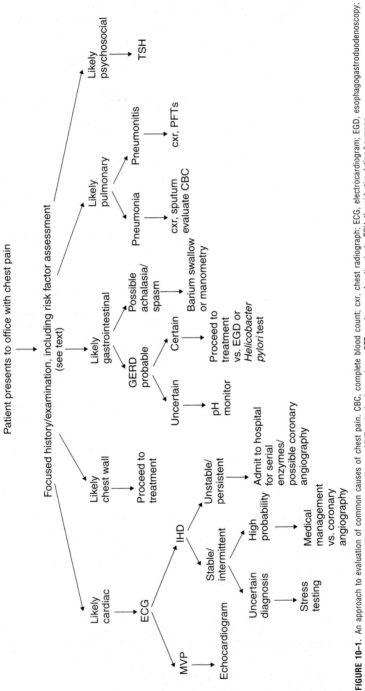

FIGURE 10–1. An approach to evaluation of common causes of chest pain. CBC, complete blood count; cxr, chest radiograph; ECG, electrocardiogram; EGD, esophagogastroduodenoscopy; GERD, gastroesophageal reflux disease; IHD, ischemic heart disease; MVP, mitral valve prolapse; PFTs, pulmonary function tests; TSH, thyroid-stimulating hormone.

2. **Infiltrates** may be apparent in pneumonia or pneumonitis.
   a. **Lobar consolidation** (bacterial pneumonia) or **diffuse infiltrates** (atypical or early pneumonia) may occur, but they generally lag behind clinical symptoms by hours to days and may be better visualized after rehydration.
   b. **Diffuse infiltrates** may also be seen in **pneumonitis**.
C. **Electrocardiogram (ECG)** is often normal in IHD; in a setting compatible with acute IHD, ST-segment elevation or depression can assist the decision to hospitalize.
D. **Stress testing**
   1. **Exercise stress electrocardiography** detects ECG changes occurring during exercise and absent on resting ECG. Dramatic ST-segment changes (>2 mm), particularly at low workloads (ie, <6 minutes on Bruce protocol or at <70% of age-predicted maximum heart rate) indicate severe IHD and the need for coronary angiography.
   2. **Exercise stress echocardiography** allows for similar evaluation as exercise stress ECG; however, echocardiography is preferred in certain patients, including women and those with obesity, pendulous breasts, left ventricular hypertrophy or previous ECG changes (such as a bundle branch block, pacemaker, or previous MI) precluding evaluation for ischemia using ECG alone. In addition to ECG changes, stress echocardiography can evaluate wall motion abnormalities and ventricular ejection fraction.
   3. **Pharmacologic stress testing** is preferred in individuals unable to achieve adequate heart rate through exercise; this inability may be due to severe arthritis, neurologic or vascular disease, or even severe deconditioning and morbid obesity. By increasing heart rate, a pharmacologic agent (eg, dobutamine) simulates exercise without the patient exercising.
   4. Intravenous administration of a **radioisotope** (eg, p-sestamibi) at the time of stress testing provides additional information about myocardial perfusion.
E. **Coronary angiography,** which delineates coronary artery anatomy, is the gold standard for confirming abnormal stress testing and guiding therapy (ie, medical vs. surgical management, including stenting and coronary artery bypass grafting).
F. **Pulmonary function tests (PFTs)** can be helpful in patients with pulmonary chest pain in clarifying obstructive vs. restrictive disease and its severity.
G. **GI studies**
   1. **Esophageal pH probe** can help confirm GERD in cases where symptoms are atypical or cardiac evaluation is normal.
   2. In known **GERD, esophagogastroduodenoscopy** can assess for complications or severity of disease (eg, Barrett's esophagus) and allow gastric biopsy to diagnose infection with *H pylori*.
   3. **Upper GI barium study** allows detection of fixed anatomic esophageal lesions (eg, Schatzki's ring, tumors) and may also help detect motility disorders and hiatal hernia; **manometry** increases sensitivity in detecting motility disorders.

VI. Treatment

A. **Chest wall pain/muscle strains**
   1. Treatment includes rest initially, avoidance if possible of precipitating activities, warm moist compresses, and local ice packs after activity.
   2. **Oral NSAIDs** (eg, ibuprofen, 600–800 mg with meals) may provide relief.
   3. Pain that is localized (eg, trigger point or costochondral), disabling, and resistant to the foregoing measures may be alleviated with an injection (eg, wheel-and-spoke administration of a local anesthetic, such as ½–1 cc of bupivacaine or 1–2% lidocaine, into a trigger point, or a mixture of ½–1 cc local anesthetic and ½ cc of Aristocort–40 into a costochondral joint). Particularly with intercostal trigger point injection, care must be taken to avoid pleural penetration.
B. **GI** (see Chapters 19 and 82).
C. **Cardiovascular**
   1. **Acute angina** or **escalating unstable or crescendo angina** or **suspected MI** is a medical emergency demanding immediate hospitalization for close monitoring, serial cardiac enzymes, oxygen, nitrates, pain management, and aspirin or other anticoagulation. Mortality has also been shown to be decreased through risk factor identification/modification (eg, lipid panel assessment and statin administration) and early beta blockade, if not contraindicated.
   2. **Chronic stable angina** (see Chapter 77).

3. MVP
  a. Explanation of the diagnosis and **reassurance** may be sufficient in those with minimal symptoms.
  b. **Those bothered with palpitations,** anxiety, or chest pain may be helped by counseling to minimize caffeine/ethanol intake and use of a beta blocker (eg, atenolol, 25–50 mg orally daily, with gradual upward titration of dose based on symptoms and heart rate).
  c. **Endocarditis prophylaxis** is indicated in MVP patients with auscultatory click-murmur or the following echocardiographic abnormalities: mitral valve thickening (>5 mm), elongated chordae, mitral regurgitation, or left atrial or ventricular enlargement. Prophylaxis is given an hour before dental, respiratory, or esophageal procedures; non–penicillin-allergic patients can take amoxicillin, 2.0 g (50 mg/kg in children). Penicillin-allergic patients can take cephalexin, 2.0 g (50 mg/kg in children).
D. Treatment of chest pain from **psychiatric disease** involves addressing underlying disorders (see Chapters 89, 92, and 94).
E. Pulmonary
  1. Pneumonia (see Chapter 13).
  2. Pleurisy may benefit from NSAIDs (see section VI,A,2). Incentive spirometry or deep breathing 10–20 times every few hours helps prevent atelectasis or secondary pneumonia from the splinting occurring with pleuritic pain.
  3. Pneumonitis
    a. With normal PFTs, pneumonitis requires avoidance of precipitants and periodic monitoring of symptoms/PFTs.
    b. Symptomatic pneumonitis with abnormal PFTs generally should be evaluated and initially managed by a pulmonologist, who may initiate oral steroids (eg, prednisone, 40–100 mg daily).

REFERENCES

American College of Emergency Physicians: Clinical policy for the initial approach to adults presenting with a chief complaint of chest pain, with no history of trauma. Ann Emerg Med 1995;**25**:274.

Chagnon I, et al: Comparison of two clinical prediction rules and implicit assessment among patients with suspected pulmonary embolism. Am J Med 2002;**113**(4):269.

Goyle KK: Diagnosing pericarditis. Am Fam Physician 2002;**66**(9):1695.

Heidelbaugh JJ: Management of gastroesophageal reflux disease. Am Fam Physician 2003;**68**(7):1311.

Kroenke K, Mangelsdorff AD: Common symptoms in ambulatory care: Incidence, evaluation, therapy and outcome. Am J Med 1989;**86**(3):262.

Mark DB: Risk stratification in patients with chest pain. Prim Care 2001;**28**(1):99.

Schmermund A: Assessment of clinically silent atherosclerotic disease and established and novel risk factors for predicting myocardial infarction and cardiac death in healthy middle-aged subjects: Rationale and design of the Heinz Nixdorf RECALL Study. Risk Factors, Evaluation of Coronary Calcium and Lifestyle. Am Heart J 2002;**144**(2):212.

11   Confusion

Robert C. Salinas, MD, & Heather Bartoli, PA-C

KEY POINTS

• Delirium is a syndrome for which a cause must be found; it represents a true medical emergency.
• Delirium may be due to a medical condition, drug of abuse, prescription medication, toxin, or a combination thereof.
• The elderly and those with underlying dementia are most susceptible to developing delirium.

TABLE 11–1. DSM-IV CRITERIA FOR DELIRIUM

- Disturbance of consciousness (ie, reduced clarity of awareness of the environment) with reduced ability to focus, sustain, or shift attention
- Change in cognition (such as memory deficit, disorientation, language disturbance) or the development of a perceptual disturbance that is not better accounted for by a pre-existing, established, or evolving dementia
- Disturbance that develops over a short period of time (usually hours to days) and tends to fluctuate over the course of the day
- Evidence from the history, physical examination, or laboratory findings that the disturbance is caused by the direct physiologic consequences of a specific medical condition, substance intoxication, substance withdrawal, multiple causes, causes not otherwise specified: insufficient evidence to establish a specific cause, or from other reasons such as sensory deprivation.

I. **Definition.** *Confusion* is a general term used to describe some aspect of global cognitive impairment, usually disorientation or inappropriate reaction to environmental stimuli. Confusion can develop suddenly (acute) or insidiously (chronic). Dementia and other chronic confusional states are discussed in Chapter 73. This chapter focuses on the evaluation and management of **delirium (acute confusional state),** which is a medical term used to describe a constellation of clinical symptoms characterized by acute onset, disturbance in consciousness, and impaired cognition and often precipitated by one or more underlying medical causes (Table 11–1).

II. **Common Diagnoses.** It is thought that up to 35% of elderly patients admitted to the hospital from the emergency department meet the criteria for delirium, as do over 50% of postoperative patients and 60% of nursing home patients older than 75 years. Delirium develops in a high percentage of hospitalized elderly patients, which increases morbidity and length of stay. Table 11–2 highlights risk factors for development of delirium; populations particularly at risk include (1) the **elderly,** due to sensory/cognitive impairment, underlying chronic illness, polypharmacy, and decreased synthesis of neurotransmitters (eg, acetylcholine) felt vital to attention, learning, and memory; (2) **abusers of ethanol and illicit**

TABLE 11–2. RISK FACTORS FOR DELIRIUM

Age	• Reduced capacity for homeostasis • Impairments in vision/hearing • Age-related changes in pharmacokinetics and pharmacodynamics • Chronic diseases • Psychosocial precipitants such as sleep loss, sensory deprivation, sensory overload, bereavement, or relocation • Structural brain disease
Pre-existing dementia	• Imbalance of noradrenergic/cholinergic neurotransmission • Inflammatory mechanisms • Hypothalamic pituitary axis abnormalities • Disrupted circadian rhythm
Hospitalization	• Relocation • Euthyroid sick syndrome • Severe illness • Disrupted sleep-wake cycle • Physical restraints • Bladder catheterization • Addition of new medications
Polypharmacy	• Drug interactions • Additive effects
Surgical factors	• Significant intraoperative blood loss • Hemodynamic instability • Emergent versus elective surgery • History of noncardiac thoracic surgery or abdominal aortic aneurysm repair
History of drug abuse	• Especially alcohol, cannabis, cocaine, hallucinogens

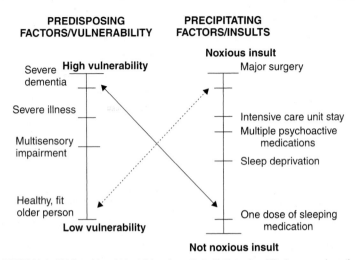

| PREDISPOSING FACTORS/VULNERABILITY | PRECIPITATING FACTORS/INSULTS |

FIGURE 11–1. Multifactorial model for delirium. In a patient with high vulnerability (eg, severe dementia, severe underlying illness, multisensory impairment), delirium may develop with a relatively benign insult (black arrow). Conversely, a patient with low vulnerability would be relatively resistant and require multiple noxious insults before delirium would develop (dotted arrow).

drugs (eg, cocaine and hallucinogens), due to drug-induced imbalances in neurotransmitters, such as acetylcholine, serotonin, and gamma-aminobutyric acid; (3) those with **underlying structural brain disease** (dementia, Parkinson's disease); and (4) the **terminally ill,** due to medications (eg, opiates) and anxiety/depression/sleep disturbance associated with disease progression. Figure 11–1 illustrates the complex interplay between patient and environmental risk factors causing delirium, particularly in the hospital setting.

A. Specific conditions predisposing to delirium
  1. **General medical conditions** (Table 11–3).
  2. **Substances**
     a. **Drug intoxication.** Drug intoxication, most often from cannabis, cocaine, or hallucinogens, is the most common cause of acute confusional state in older adolescents and young adults. **Substance withdrawal delirium** is most often caused by high doses of ethanol, sedative hypnotics, or anxiolytics. **Substance-induced delirium** is due to exposure to toxins (eg, carbon monoxide, insecticides, industrial solvents).
     b. **Prescription/herbal medications** (Table 11–4). Delirium from prescription medication should always be considered in the elderly, who consume approximately 36% of medication prescribed in the United States.

TABLE 11–3. GENERAL MEDICAL CONDITIONS OFTEN CAUSING DELIRIUM

Metabolic disturbances	Hyponatremia, hypo/hyperkalemia, hypo/hyperthyroidism, anemia, hypercarbia, hypo/hyperglycemia, dehydration, malnutrition, hypothermia, heat stroke
Neurologic	Head trauma, cerebrovascular accident, normal pressure hydrocephalus, subdural hematoma, meningitis, encephalitis, brain abscess, neurosyphilis, seizure disorders (ictal and post-ictal states)
Neoplastic	Primary intracranial neoplasm, metastatic disease to the brain
Cardiovascular	Myocardial infarction, congestive heart failure, arrhythmia, severe aortic stenosis, hypertensive encephalopathy
Pulmonary	Pneumonia, chronic obstructive pulmonary disease exacerbation, respiratory failure
Gastrointestinal	Fecal impaction, intra-abdominal infection, liver failure
Urinary	Urinary tract infection, urinary retention

TABLE 11-4. DRUGS WITH ANTICHOLINERGIC PROPERTIES

Classical anticholinergics Atropine Scopolamine	**Antipsychotics**
	Antispasmodics Gastrointestinal—ie, Bentyl, Levsin
Antidepressants Tricyclic—ie, Elavil, Sinequan	Urinary tract—ie, Ditropan
	Muscle relaxants
Antiemetics	**Prednisolone**
Antihistamines Benadryl	**Cimetidine**
Antiparkinsonian	

3. **Change in environment** (eg, transfer to hospital or a new place of residence).
4. **Structural brain disease** (Alzheimer's disease, vascular dementia, Lewy body dementia, Parkinson's disease).
5. **Depression.** Depression coexists in over one third of outpatients diagnosed with dementia and even more nursing home residents with dementia.
   B. **Conditions that often mimic delirium** include dementia (Chapter 73), depression (Chapter 92), other psychiatric disturbances, age-associated memory disorder (minimal cognitive impairment), malingering, and factitious disorder.
III. **Symptoms.** In delirium, obtaining a careful history from a caregiver may shed light on likely causes. History should include:
   A. **Onset and course** of the confusional state (Tables 11–5 and 11–6), which clarify whether delirium is present and its severity.
   B. **Other history**
   1. **Risk factors** (Table 11–2).
   2. **Chronic illnesses** (Table 11–3).
   3. **Drug use** (Table 11–4).
IV. **Signs.** A systematic examination often provides clues to underlying causes of delirium and should include:
   A. **Evaluation of mental status**
   1. The **Mini-Mental State Examination (MMSE)** (Table 11–7) has high sensitivity and specificity in evaluating memory loss and cognitive impairment; using a cutoff score of 23 or below, the MMSE has a sensitivity of 87%, a specificity of 82%, a

TABLE 11-5. THE CONFUSION ASSESSMENT METHOD (CAM) DIAGNOSTIC ALGORITHM[1]

Feature 1	**Acute Onset and Fluctuating Course** This feature is usually obtained from a family member or nurse and is shown by positive responses to the following questions: Is there evidence of an acute change in mental status from the patient's baseline? Did the (abnormal) behavior fluctuate during the day, that is, tend to come and go, or increase and decrease in severity?
Feature 2	**Inattention** This feature is shown by a positive response to the following questions: Did the patient have difficulty focusing attention, for example, being easily distractible, or having difficulty keeping track of what was being said?
Feature 3	**Disorganized Thinking** This feature is shown by a positive response to the following question: Was the patient's thinking disorganized or incoherent, such as rambling or irrelevant conversation, unclear or illogical flow of ideas, or unpredictable switching from subject to subject?
Feature 4	**Altered Level of Consciousness** This feature is shown by any answer other than "alert" to the following question: Overall, how would you rate this patient's level of consciousness? (alert [normal], vigilant [hyperalert], lethargic [drowsy, easily aroused], stupor [difficult to arouse], or coma [unarousable])

[1] The diagnosis of delirium by CAM requires the presence of features 1 and 2 and either 3 or 4.
Reprinted from Inouye SK, et al: Clarifying confusion: The confusion assessment method. Ann Intern Med 1990;**113**(12):947.

TABLE 11–6. FEATURES OF DELIRIUM AND DEMENTIA

Feature	Delirium	Dementia
Onset	Abrupt	Insidious
Duration	Acute illness, generally days to weeks	Chronic illness, characteristically progressing over years
Reversibility	Usually reversible	Usually irreversible, often chronically progressive
Orientation	Disorientation early	Disorientation later in the illness, often after months or years
Stability	Variability from moment to moment, hour to hour, throughout the day	Much more stable day to day (unless super-imposed delirium develops)
Physiological changes	Prominent physiological changes	Less prominent physiological changes
Consciousness	Clouded, altered, and changing level of consciousness	Consciousness not clouded until terminal
Attention span	Strikingly short attention span	Attention span not characteristically reduced
Sleep-wake cycle	Disturbed sleep-wake cycle with hour-to-hour variation	Disturbed sleep-wake cycle with day-night rever-sal, but not hour-to-hour variation
Psychomotor changes	Marked psychomotor changes (hyperactive or hypoactive)	Psychomotor changes characteristically late (unless superimposed depression)

TABLE 11–7. MINI-MENTAL STATE EXAMINATION (MMSE)

		Score	Points
Orientation			
1. What is the:	Year	_____	1
	Season	_____	1
	Date	_____	1
	Day	_____	1
	Month	_____	1
2. Where are we?	State	_____	1
	County	_____	1
	Town or city	_____	1
	Hospital	_____	1
	Floor	_____	1
Registration			
3. Name three objects, taking 1 second to say each. Then ask the patient to repeat all three after you have said them. Give 1 point for each correct answer. Repeat the answers until the patient learns all three.		_____	3
Attention and Calculation			
4. Serial sevens. Give 1 point for each correct answer. Stop after five answers. Alternate: spell the word *world* backwards.		_____	5
Recall			
5. Ask for names of three objects learned in question 3. Give 1 point for each correct answer.		_____	3
Language			
6. Point to a pencil and a watch. Have the patient name them as you point.		_____	2
7. Have the patient repeat, "No ifs, ands, or buts."		_____	1
8. Have the patient follow a three-stage command: "Take a paper in your right hand. Fold the paper in half. Put the paper on the floor."		_____	3
9. Have the patient read and obey the following: "Close your eyes." (Write it in large letters.)		_____	1
10. Have the patient write a sentence of his or her choice. (The sentence should contain a subject and an object and should make sense. Ignore spelling errors when scoring.)		_____	1
11. Have the patient copy a line drawing of intersecting pentagons. (Give one point if all sides and angles are preserved and if the intersecting sides form a quadrangle.)		_____	1
Add points for each correct response	**TOTAL**	_____	30

Adapted with permission from Folstein MF, Folstein SE, McHugh PR: "Mini Mental State: A Practical Method for Grading the Cognitive State of Patients for the Clinician." *Journal of Psychiatric Research*, 12(3):189–198, 1975. © 1998, MMLLC.

false-positive rate of 39.4%, and a false-negative rate of 4.7%. The MMSE cannot itself diagnose dementia or delirium, and results should be considered in the context of hearing, vision problems, physical disabilities, age, educational level, and cultural influences.

2. The "Confusion Assessment Method" (**CAM**) instrument (Table 11–5) has been used to evaluate hospitalized patients with suspected delirium.
3. **Hyperalert confusion** may result from alcohol withdrawal. A person who is excited, hyperalert, and hallucinating may be experiencing toxicity from amphetamine, lysergic acid diethylamide (LSD), cocaine, or phencyclidine (PCP).
4. An **agitated confusional state without focal signs** may occur following head trauma.

B. **Vital signs**
   1. If **diastolic blood pressure is >120 mm Hg,** hypertensive encephalopathy should be considered.
   2. If **systolic blood pressure is <90 mm Hg,** confusion may be from impaired cerebral perfusion secondary to shock. Drug overdose, adrenal insufficiency, and hyponatremia should also be considered.
   3. **Tachycardia** suggests sepsis, delirium tremens, hyperthyroidism, hypoglycemia, or an agitated, anxious patient.
   4. **Fever** may indicate infection, delirium tremens, cerebral vasculitis, or fat embolism syndrome. **Hypothermia** is defined as a core temperature (rectal or esophageal) below 35 °C (95 °F) and may cause confusion.
   5. **Tachypnea** suggests hypoxia. A patient with chronic obstructive lung disease receiving fractional inspiratory oxygen >0.28 may be confused from hypercarbia.

C. **Eye examination**
   1. **Papilledema** suggests hypertensive encephalopathy or an intracranial mass.
   2. **Dilated pupils** suggest sympathetic outflow, which is common with delirium tremens. **Pinpoint pupils** suggest narcotic excess or constricting eye drops.

D. **Other findings**
   1. **Bibasilar crackles** on lung auscultation indicate congestive heart failure with hypoxia. **Asymmetric crackles** suggest pneumonia with hypoxia.
   2. **Acute confusion, ataxia, bilateral sixth-nerve palsy, and diarrhea** suggest Wernicke-Korsakoff encephalitis.
   3. **Confusion, irritability, insomnia, and a photosensitive rash with diarrhea** suggest pellagra.

V. **Laboratory Tests.** Unless the cause of the confusional state is obvious from the history and physical examination, further diagnostic testing is important.

A. **Initial work-up** may include complete blood cell count with differential; erythrocyte sedimentation rate; serum chemistry profile, magnesium, and calcium; toxicologic screen of urine, blood, or both; urine analysis; chest x-ray; electrocardiogram; and serum drug levels of prescribed medication as indicated.
B. A **lumbar puncture** should be considered in any delirious patient with possible bacterial or viral meningitis. Relative contraindications include rapid improvement in the patient's clinical status and concerns about increased intracranial pressure from a mass lesion.
C. An **electroencephalogram** may identify partial complex seizures disorder, metabolic encephalopathy, or sedative use and should be considered in patients suspected of these disorders.
D. **Computerized tomography (CT)** of the head is the method of choice for the initial evaluation of confused obtunded patients to rule out subdural hematoma, epidural hematoma, stroke, cerebral abscess, or neoplasm. Repeat CT after 24–48 hours should be done if acute infarct is considered. Magnetic resonance imaging with magnetic resonance arteriography may be useful to rule out chronic subdural hematoma, regional blood flow abnormalities, or aneurysm.
E. **Additional tests** to be considered are arterial blood gas analysis, blood cultures, serum ammonia levels, liver function studies, thyroid function tests, cortisone levels, antinuclear antibodies, serum protein electrophoresis, serum B_{12} and folate levels, syphilis test (VDRL), serum and urine osmolality, HIV titer, and urine tests for heavy metals, porphyrins, and metanephrines.

VI. **Treatment**
A. **General principles.** Patients with delirium should usually be hospitalized for identification and management of underlying causes. Terminally ill hospice patients with delirium

may be managed at home or an inpatient hospice setting, depending on patient and family desires. Principles of management include:

1. **Supportive care.** Supportive care while work-up progresses includes a quiet private room with familiar objects, presence of a family member, and maintenance of a normal sleep-wake pattern.
2. **Drug therapy.** Agitation and behavioral problems posing harm to the patient or others may require neuroleptic agents for sedation. When considering such medication, the goal should be control of dangerous behavior, while avoiding excessive sedation.
   a. **Haloperidol** (0.25–2 mg) given intramuscularly may be helpful in the urgent setting. Occasionally, maintenance doses of haloperidol (2–5 mg orally two or three times daily) may be used until the underlying cause of delirium can be determined.
   b. Some of the newer atypical neuroleptic agents can also be used for maintenance purposes. **Risperidone** (0.5 mg orally twice daily up to 4–6 mg daily) has been shown to be effective in treating aggressive and violent patients with dementia.
   c. **Paradoxic physiologic reactions** can occur with all of these medications through anticholinergic properties and worsened extrapyramidal symptoms.
   d. **Benzodiazepines** may be useful in delirium from ethanol withdrawal. If a benzodiazepine is used, **lorazepam (Ativan)** is usually the drug of choice because of its relatively short half-life. However, this too can have a paradoxical effect in some patients and worsen the agitation.
   e. **In hospice patients,** the foregoing medications may benefit confusion; treatment of pain, anxiety, and depression may also be indicated.
3. **Open communication.** Open communication with family members about suspected causes and prognosis of the delirium is essential.
B. **Treatment of specific conditions.** (See Chapters 73, Dementia, and 92, Depression).
C. **Prevention.** The incidence of delirium may be decreased by limiting polypharmacy in the elderly, closely monitoring drug usage by the elderly, and recognizing prodromal symptoms of insomnia, nightmares, fleeting hallucinations, and anxiety.

REFERENCES

American Psychiatric Association: *Diagnostic and Statistical Manual of Mental Disorders,* 4th ed. American Psychiatric Association; 2000.

Chan D, Brennan NJ: Delirium: Making the diagnosis, improving the prognosis. Geriatrics 1999;**54**:28.

Eikelenboom P, Hoogendijk WJ: Do delirium and Alzheimer's dementia share specific pathogenetics mechanisms? In: Carlson LA, Gottfries CG, Winblad B, Robertson B (editors): *Dementia and Geriatric Cognitive Disorders.* Karger; 1999:319–324.

Inouye SK, et al: A multicomponent intervention to prevent delirium in hospitalized older patients. N Engl J Med 1999;**340**:669.

Inouye SK, et al: Clarifying confusion: The confusion assessment method. Ann Intern Med 1990; **113**:941.

Rummann TA, et al: Delirium in elderly patients: Evaluation and management. Mayo Clin Proc 1995; **70**:989.

---

12   Constipation

Steven D. Bartz, MD, RPh

KEY POINTS

- There is great variability in normal stool patterns. Individuals define constipation in many different ways.
- New-onset constipation in a geriatric population is a warning sign for cancer, especially if accompanied by rectal bleeding and weight loss.
- Dietary fiber, exercise, and hydration are all preferred treatment choices to laxatives.

I. Definition. The colon plays a vital role in water homeostasis. Water is absorbed through the osmotic gradient caused by the active transport of sodium ions across the large bowel's luminal surface. In a normally functioning colon, about 90% of the water entering the colon is absorbed. Colonic contents take approximately 24 hours to traverse the length of the colon, during which enteric bacteria digest foodstuffs, forming gas and feces. Bowel contents are stored in the distal colon and rectum until voluntarily expelled by relaxation of the external anal sphincter. Constipation occurs when either colonic transport time is delayed or evacuation is impaired due to a voluntary or involuntary problem. Most definitions of constipation use criteria of fewer than three bowel movements weekly. However, this frequency can be considered normal if it is not a change from past stooling frequency and is not bothersome to the patient.

II. Common Diagnoses. Constipation is a common medical condition afflicting all ages from the very young to the very old. It is one of the most common digestive complaints in primary care offices, accounting for more than 2.5 million office visits annually. Individuals spend $400 million yearly seeking symptomatic relief. Fortunately, in the vast majority of cases, the cause is benign and can be successfully treated. A variety of conditions can result in constipation.

    A. Functional causes are the most common etiologies. (See sidebars on fecal impaction and encopresis.)

        1. Willful suppression of the defecation reflex. Children are especially at risk from a previously painful or frightening experience (eg, aggressive toilet training, lack of toilets when needed). If not evacuated, large hard stools can accumulate in the rectum, resulting in a large, painful evacuation (eg, fecal impaction).

FECAL IMPACTIONS

Prolonged, severe constipation predisposes to a fecal impaction; 70% occur in the rectum, 20% occur in the sigmoid colon, and 10% occur in more proximal locations. Low-lying impactions should be manually removed using a scooping or scissoring motion with one's fingers. Inaccessible stool should be loosened with an enema. Occasionally endoscopy is needed to reach resistant or more proximal impactions. A cathartic agent should only be used after the bulk of the impaction has already been removed.

ENCOPRESIS

Encopresis is fecal soiling in a child with functional constipation. Stool accumulates in the rectum and becomes drier, harder, and more painful to pass. Stretching of the rectal wall can lead to hypercompliance and relative insensitivity to stool volume. When the mass is large enough, the anal sphincter loses competency and liquid stool seeps involuntarily. Encopresis is four times as common in boys than girls. Its prevalence is 3% at age 4 years and 1.6% at age 10. It is important to differentiate it from nonfunctional causes, especially Hirschsprung's disease (Table 12–1).

Treatment entails initial **disimpaction. Mineral oil** (up to 120 mL) or **milk and molasses enemas** (1:1 ratio) are both options. Mineral oil (30 mL per year of age) and **polyethylene glycol** solution of 25 mL/kg/hour are oral evacuants. Once the stool is disimpacted, a **routine oral laxative** can prevent reaccumulation of stool masses. **Sorbitol** (2 mL/kg/day), **Senna syrup** (5–10 mL twice daily), **Docusate liquid** (10–120 mg/day), or **bisacodyl** (5 mg) can be used to prevent reimpaction until regular toilet training is achieved.

        2. Dietary factors including insufficient dietary bulk/fiber and hydration. Individuals on low-fiber diets and patients taking diuretics are at particular risk.

        3. Physical inactivity (eg, hospitalized elderly).

        4. Motility disorders eg, irritable bowel syndrome (IBS), accounts for 59% of primary constipation.

    B. Pelvic floor dysfunction, loss of pelvic floor muscle strength, or paradoxical rectal sphincter hypertonicity, accounts for 25% of primary constipation cases. Risk factors include multiparity in women and years of straining while stooling.

TABLE 12-1. COMPARISON OF ENCOPRESIS AND HIRSCHSPRUNG'S DISEASE

Sign/Symptom	Encopresis	Hirschsprung's Disease
Age at onset	3 to 7 years	Typically first months of life
Constipation as newborn	Rare	Common
Meconium passage	No association	Typically delayed >48 hours
Fecal soiling	Common	Rare
Toilet avoidance	Common	Rare
Stool in rectal vault	Common	Rare
Stooling pattern	Intermittent large painful stools followed by resolution of symptoms	Small-diameter (ribbon) stools
Ganglia on rectal biopsy	Present	Absent

    C. Medications (see Table 12-2). Individuals taking numerous prescription and nonprescription medications frequently complain of constipation. Anticholinergic medications reduce bowel motility and are particularly problematic.

    D. Endocrine/metabolic disorders (eg, patients with hypothyroidism, diabetes mellitus, hypercalcemia, and hypokalemia).

    E. Anatomic lesions

        1. Individuals with **painful perianal lesions** such as rectal fissures or external hemorrhoids are prone to inhibit stooling.

        2. People with **prior abdominal surgeries** may form scars or strictures.

        3. **Obstructing lesions** (eg, tumors, large polyps, volvulus, rectoceles) can be a factor.

    F. Neuromuscular disorders (eg, Parkinson's disease, multiple sclerosis, Alzheimer's disease, muscular dystrophies, or scleroderma) may be associated with constipation. Infants with persistent constipation who fail to pass meconium within 48 hours of birth are at risk for Hirschsprung's disease.

III. Symptoms. A thorough history is essential to make a correct diagnosis. Many individuals have the misperception that they have constipation if they do not have daily bowel movements. However, lack of frequent bowel movements is not the most common symptom.

    A. Frequent complaints include **straining during stooling** (52%), **passage of hard stool** (44%), **inability to defecate at will** (34%), and **infrequent defecation** (33%).

    B. New-onset constipation in an older adult demands thorough evaluation. Additional clues to structural lesions, particularly cancers, include rectal bleeding, weight loss, and occasionally decreased stool caliber.

TABLE 12-2. MEDICATIONS ASSOCIATED WITH CONSTIPATION

Nonprescription Medications	Examples
Sympathomimetics	Ephedrine
Nonsteroidal anti-inflammatory drugs	Ibuprofen, naproxen
Antacids	Aluminum hydroxide, calcium carbonate
Calcium supplements	Calcium carbonate/citrate
Iron supplements	Ferrous sulfate/gluconate
Antidiarrheals	Loperamide, bismuth salicylate

Prescription Medications	Examples
Anticholinergics	Benztropine, trihexylphenidate
Antihistamines	Diphenhydramine
Antidepressants	Tricyclics, amitriptyline
Antiparkinson agents	Levodopa
Calcium channel blockers	Verapamil
Antispasmodics	Dicyclomine
Antipsychotics	Chlorpromazine
Diuretics	Furosemide
Narcotics	Codeine, morphine, oxycodone, hydrocodone

C. Neurologic disorders can have fecal leakage or urgency, urine or stool incontinence, and often a need for manual disimpaction.

D. Irritable bowel syndrome (IBS) can feature constipation, diarrhea, or often both. Abdominal pain or discomfort is common but is usually relieved by defecation. A feeling of bloating or abdominal distention and the passage of mucus can occur.

IV. Signs

A. Abdominal examination. Bowel sounds are typically normal or slightly hypoactive. Palpation usually causes either no discomfort or mild, diffuse discomfort. Diffuse mild pain is generally more characteristic of IBS. An abdominal mass may be a stool bolus, intussusception, or a carcinoma. Serial examinations are needed to rule out a fixed mass.

B. Rectal examination. Perianal inspection can identify hemorrhoids and anal fissures, both often painful to touch, or rectal prolapse. **Digital examination** should evaluate sphincter tone and presence of a firm, claylike mass indicating impaction.

V. Laboratory Tests (Figure 12–1). In most cases of constipation, further testing is not needed and is reserved for those presenting atypically or not improving with treatment, or when suspicion for systemic illness is present.

A. Reasonable initial **hematologic tests** for all patients include a **thyroid-stimulating hormone** test, serum **electrolytes**, serum **calcium**, and a **glucose test.**

B. Stool guaiac testing. In at-risk individuals, annual occult blood testing of three naturally expelled stools has been shown to be an effective, inexpensive screen for colon cancer (see Chapter 102). False-negative and false-positive results, however, are common. Hemorrhoids, anal fissures, and the digital rectal examination can give false-positive results.

C. Anoscopy allows visualization of local masses including internal hemorrhoids and the occasional rectal cancer.

D. Endoscopy (flexible sigmoidoscopy, colonoscopy) can visualize the colon and enable a biopsy specimen of suspicious lesions, verify internal hemorrhoids, and occasionally remove a high impaction.

E. Barium enema is less commonly used than in the past but can outline the luminal wall, visualizing polyps, diverticuli, and strictures.

F. Specialized tests including manometry, barium defecography, colonic transit studies, and balloon expulsion testing, are indicated in specific circumstances and are generally ordered in consultation with a gastroenterologist.

VI. Treatment should be directed by history, physical examination, and diagnostic testing. Most often, idiopathic constipation is the diagnosis. However, secondary causes should be identified and treated (eg, diabetes mellitus [Chapter 74]; thyroid disease [Chapter 87]).

A. Lifestyle modification is fundamental to effective management and should precede or accompany pharmacologic measures.

    1. Bowel retraining by establishing a regular stooling pattern is a useful first step. Patients can be instructed to attempt to move their bowels at the same time each day (ie, after breakfast) to utilize the postprandial gastrocolic reflex. Children can be encouraged to set a regular toileting time and be praised or rewarded with stickers for their efforts. It is important to avoid embarrassment or punishment in toilet training.

    2. Diet and exercise

        a. A **sedentary lifestyle** is thought to contribute to constipation. Regular exercise is always recommended.

        b. Adding **dietary bulk (Table 12–3) and hydration** is universally advised for constipation sufferers. Increases in indigestible fiber have been shown to increase gastric motility, shorten colonic transit time, and increase fecal volume. Adding dietary or supplemental fiber is easy and inexpensive.

        c. Large changes in the diet, including switching formulas in infants, can have a constipating effect.

B. Laxatives (Table 12–3). Although most are benign, some can have side effects and aggressive use can obscure underlying pathology.

    1. Bulk-forming agents including the fiber supplements **psyllium** (natural) and **methylcellulose/polycarbophil** (synthetic) are hydrophilic agents that promote water retention in the bowel lumen, resulting in softer, bulkier stools. These agents work slowly and will not produce results overnight. Synthetic agents are indigestible,

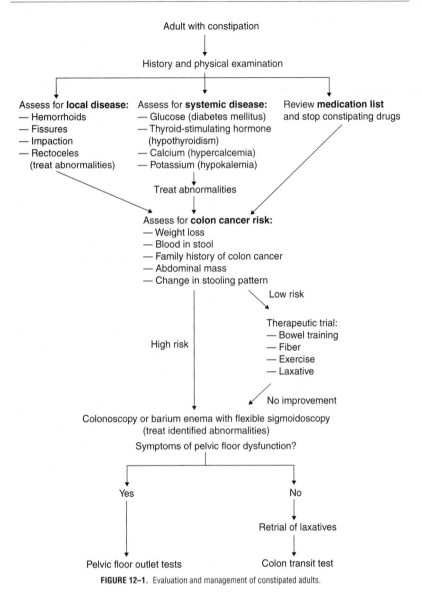

FIGURE 12–1. Evaluation and management of constipated adults.

so they have the advantage of producing less gas and bloating. Patients should be counseled to increase daily fluid intake (up to 2–3 quarts of water) to maintain adequate hydration.

2. **Surfactants** (stool softeners) act as detergents to reduce water/fat interface surface tension and soften the stool by increasing water penetration into it. These mostly benign agents are salts of docusate. As with bulk agents, they should be taken with plenty of water.

TABLE 12–3. COMMON LAXATIVES

Laxative	Generic Name	Brand Name	Adult Dosing	Onset (hrs)
Bulk forming	Bran	. . .	25 g/day	12–72
	Psyllium	Metamucil	12 g qd–tid	12–72
	Methylcellulose	Citrucel	19 g qd–tid	12–72
	Polycarbophil	FiberCon, Konsyl	500 mg/day	12–72
Stool softener	Docusate sodium	Colace	100–200 mg/day	24–72
	Docusate calcium	Surfak	240 mg/day	24–72
	Docusate potassium	Dialose Plus	100 mg qd–tid	24–72
Salines	Magnesium sulfate	Epsom salt	1–2 tsp qd–bid	0.5–3
	Magnesium hydroxide	Milk of Magnesia	30–60 mL/day	0.5–3
	Magnesium citrate	Citrate of Magnesia	200 mL/day	0.5–3
	Sodium phosphate	Fleets phospho–soda	up to 45 mL/day	0.5–3
Hyperosmolar agents	Sorbitol	. . .	30–60 mL/day	24–48
	Lactulose	Chronulac	30–60 g/day	24–48
	Polyethylene glycol	GoLYTELY, Miralax	17 g/day	0.5–4
Stimulants	Bisacodyl	Dulcolax, Correctol	5 mg qd–tid	6–10
	Senna	Senokot	8.6 mg qd–bid	6–10
Miscellaneous	Mineral oil	. . .	15–45 mL/day	6–8
	Castor oil	Purge	15–60 mL/day	2–6

3. **Saline laxatives** (salt formulations of sodium and magnesium) form an osmotic gradient, drawing water into the bowel lumen. Hypermagnesemia can result from chronic use of magnesium products, especially in patients with renal insufficiency.
4. **Hyperosmolar agents** are nonabsorbable sugars that have osmotic activity. **Lactulose** (prescription) and **sorbitol** (nonprescription) pass through the small bowel unchanged since humans lack enzymes to hydrolyze them. In the colon, bacteria metabolize the sugars to water and organic acids, providing an osmotic gradient keeping water in the lumen. **Polyethylene glycol** (PEG) solution also forms an osmotic gradient and in large doses is used to evacuate the bowel for endoscopy or surgery. **Glycerin suppositories** are locally active products when inserted in the rectum. They are usually used in young children with constipation. Insertion of the suppository also adds to its cathartic effect.
5. **Stimulants. Cascara, senna,** and **bisacodyl** are effective laxatives and are the most frequently used products for symptomatic relief. They work by both stimulating the colonic myenteric plexus and altering mucosal electron transport. Since they are fairly fast-acting, they are often taken at night for a morning bowel movement. Prolonged use can result in hyperpigmentation of the lumen (melanosis coli).
6. **Lubricants. Mineral** and **castor oil** are both older agents, which can cause a lipoid pneumonitis if aspirated. They are rather unpalatable and infrequently recommended.
7. **Enemas** are useful for evacuating the distal colon and rectum. Various agents are used, but plain warm water suffices in most cases. Enemas are usually the treatment of choice for fecal impactions.

REFERENCES

American Gastroenterological Association Clinical Practice and Practice Economics Committee. AGA Technical Review on Constipation. Gastroenterology 2000;**119**(6):1766.
Drug Facts and Comparisons, 57th ed. Lippincott Williams & Wilkins; 2003.
Felt B, et al: Guideline for the management of pediatric idiopathic constipation and soiling. Arch Ped Adolesc Med 1999;**153**:380.
Petticrew M, Watt I, Brand M: What's the "best buy" for treatment of constipation? Results of a systematic review of the efficacy and comparative efficacy of laxatives in the elderly. Br J Gen Practice 1999;**49**:387.
Physicians Desk Reference, 57th ed. Thomson; 2003.

13   Cough

David Holmes, MD

KEY POINTS

- The most common cause of acute cough is viral upper respiratory illness.
- The most common causes of chronic cough are postnasal drainage in nonsmokers and to-bacco irritants/chronic bronchitis in smokers. Other common causes are asthma and gastroesophageal reflux disease.
- Treatment of cough is directed at underlying disease. Antibiotics are not indicated for viral infections.

I. **Definition.** A **cough** is a sudden explosive forcing of air through the glottis, occurring immediately on opening the previously closed glottis. It is initiated by airway inflammation, mechanical/chemical irritation of airways, or pressure from adjacent structures.

Chronic cough has been thought of as any cough lasting more than 3 weeks. However, it takes 7 weeks for bronchial hyperreactivity to return to normal following viral upper respiratory illness (URI). Therefore, the following classification of cough will be used: **acute cough** lasts <3 weeks, **subacute cough** lasts 3–8 weeks, and **chronic cough** lasts >8 weeks.

II. **Common Diagnoses.** Cough is the fifth most common presenting complaint in primary care, accounting for about 30 million office visits each year in the United States. At any given time approximately 18% of people have a cough.

A. **Acute cough.** Common causes of acute cough are reflected in the mnemonic **AAA VIRUS**—that is, **A**sthma exacerbation, **A**cute Bronchitis (almost always viral), **A**spiration, **V**iral URI (most common cause), **I**rritants (ie, tobacco and marijuana smoke, allergens, air pollution, dust, sulfur dioxide, nitrogen oxide, ammonia, and ozone), **R**hinitis (allergic), **U**ncomplicated pneumonia, **S**inusitis/postnasal drainage (PND).

   1. **Asthma exacerbation.** Nine to 12 million people in the United States have asthma, and 4000–5000 die each year of it. Risk factors for asthma exacerbation include allergen exposure (ie, mold, pollen, dust, animal danders, cosmetics); respiratory infection; exposure to irritants (ie, smoke); certain medications (ie, beta blockers, aspirin); and psychological stress.

   2. **Acute bronchitis.** Acute bronchitis is one of the most common diagnoses in primary care. Up to 95% is viral—influenza (types A and B), respiratory syncytial virus, parainfluenza, coronavirus, and adenovirus; less common causes include *Mycobacterium pneumoniae, Bordetella pertussis,* and *Chlamydia pneumoniae.* Risk factors for acute bronchitis include exposure to viral URI, cigarette smoke and other irritants, and history of chronic obstructive pulmonary disease (COPD) or lupus.

   3. **Aspiration.** Virtually everyone aspirates what they are eating or drinking at some point in their lives, but subsequent cough reflex protects the airway. Risk factors for more serious aspiration include being very old or very young (younger than 3 years old) or having impaired gag or swallowing reflex.

   4. **Viral** upper respiratory illnesses (**URIs**). Viral URIs are the most frequent illnesses in humans, with a prevalence as high as 35% worldwide. Thirty to 50% of all common colds are due to rhinovirus; other causative organisms include echovirus, coxsackievirus, influenza virus, respiratory syncytial virus, parainfluenza virus, coronavirus, and adenovirus. Risk factors for development of URIs include exposure to URI, cigarette smoke, and other irritants.

   5. **Irritants.** Cigarette smoke is the most common offending irritant; the 20–25% of Americans who smoke and those breathing their smoke are at risk for this cause of coughing. Other irritants include pollutants and allergens.

   6. **Allergic rhinitis.** Allergies to dust mites, molds, animals, and pollen occur in 7% of North Americans, predominantly children and adolescents. Risk factors for allergic rhinitis include asthma, eczema, urticaria, and a family history of related symptoms.

7. **Uncomplicated pneumonia.** Each year there are 4 million cases of pneumonia in the United States, 600,000 hospitalizations, and 75,000 deaths, making pneumonia the sixth most common cause of death in the United States. Persons at highest risk for pneumonia include smokers; those with chronic lung disease; the elderly; the immunocompromised; those with renal or hepatic failure, diabetes, or malignancy; and those in nursing homes or hospitals. A patient's age helps determine likely causative organisms—ie, **<6 mo:** *Chlamydia trachomatis,* respiratory syncytial virus; **6 mo—5 yr:** *Haemophilus influenzae;* **young adults:** *Streptococcus pneumoniae, Mycoplasma pneumoniae,* and *C pneumoniae;* **elderly:** *S pneumoniae, H influenzae, Mycoplasma catarrhalis,* and *Legionella pneumophila.*
8. **Sinusitis/postnasal drainage (PND).** Sinusitis/PND is very common in the United States, resulting in 25 million office visits annually. Fifteen percent of sinusitis is viral; other identified organisms include *S pneumoniae* (most common bacterial etiology), *H influenzae, M catarrhalis,* Grp A streptococci, *Staphylococcus aureus,* and anaerobes. Risk factors for sinusitis include history of URI, allergic rhinitis, nasotracheal or nasogastric intubation, dental infections, barotrauma (deep-sea diving, air travel), cystic fibrosis, irritants, nasal polyps, and tumors (cause ostia obstruction).
B. **Subacute and chronic cough** (Table 13–1). Airway hyperresponsiveness following URI is a common cause of **subacute cough,** usually resolving by 7 weeks after the URI. The prevalence of **chronic cough** in the United States is 14–23% in nonsmoking adults and children and much higher in smokers. Chronic cough is more common in the elderly, school-aged children, and people exposed to air pollution in urban areas. In more than 90% of persons, chronic cough (>8 weeks) is caused by PND, asthma, smoking/chronic bronchitis, and gastroesophageal reflux disease (GERD). Often chronic cough is due to a combination of diagnoses. The differential diagnosis of subacute/chronic cough is incorporated in the mnemonic **GASP & HACK IT UP.**
  1. About 10 million people in the United States are infected with **tuberculosis (TB):** the risk of infection increases with history of travel to or immigration from countries where TB is prevalent (most countries in Latin America and the Caribbean, Africa, Asia, Eastern Europe, and Russia); African Americans and Hispanic Americans are also at increased risk.
  2. Other **uncommon** causes are reflected in the mnemonic: cough is "A CHEST BIZ"—Arnold's reflex (cerumen or hair on the tympanic membrane stimulating cough receptors), CHF (congestive heart failure), Cystic fibrosis (in children), Hyperthyroidism, Eosinophilic bronchitis, Sarcoidosis, Suture (retained), Tracheobronchial collapse, Bronchiectasis (irreversible dilation of bronchi/bronchioles due to inflammation or obstruction), Immunodeficiency and fungal disorders, and Zenker's (hypopharyngeal) diverticulum.
III. **Symptoms.** Diagnosis can be made by history alone in 70–80% of individuals with cough. Characteristics of cough, such as paroxysmal, barking, honking, brassy, self-propagating, and productiveness and timing during the day, have not proved reliable in determining diagnosis.
  A. **Acute cough**
    1. **Asthma exacerbation** (see Table 13–1).
    2. **Acute bronchitis/COPD exacerbation.** Following URI symptoms, in 90% of patients with bronchitis a nonproductive becoming productive cough develops that persists ≤3 weeks in 50% of patients, but over a month in 25%. Other symptoms include wheezing, fatigue, hemoptysis, and mild dyspnea.
    3. In **aspiration,** there is sudden intractable cough, which may be accompanied by choking, vomiting, wheezing, shortness of breath, dysphagia, and acute anxiety.
    4. **Viral URI.** Viral URI features coryza, malaise, chills, rhinorrhea, fever, sore throat, sneezing, and nasal congestion (see Chapter 55).
    5. With **irritants,** there may be few symptoms, other than cough. Chemical gas irritant exposure may in addition cause headache, lightheadedness, or confusion.
    6. **Rhinitis (allergic)** (see Table 13–1 under Postnasal drainage).
    7. **Uncomplicated pneumonia.** Symptoms include fever, chills, pleuritic chest pain, dyspnea, and myalgia; the elderly may also or predominantly present with confusion or delirium.
    8. **Sinusitis/PND.** Sinusitis/PND is suggested by URI symptoms lasting >10 days, nasal congestion, PND, maxillary or frontal headaches, purulent rhinorrhea, and poor response to over-the-counter antihistamines/decongestants. Fever is uncommon.

TABLE 13-1. DIFFERENTIAL DIAGNOSIS OF SUBACUTE AND CHRONIC COUGH: GASP & HACK IT UP

Differential Diagnosis	Etiology/Mechanism of Action	Risk Factors/History	Signs	Testing
Gastroesophageal reflux disease (GERD)	Transient loss of LES tone → increase in acid reflux and aspiration of gastric contents → irritation and airway inflammation	Cough is sole symptom in 43–75%; heartburn, sour taste in back of throat, sore throat, regurgitation, laryngitis, dysphonia, symptoms worse with lying down, exercise, caffeine, alcohol, acidic foods	Usually absent, possible epigastric tenderness	24-hr pH monitoring (consider if symptoms do not resolve after 3–6 mo of therapy); upper GI series and upper endoscopy in those chronically symptomatic to assess complications of GERD
Asthma	Inflammation and hyperresponsiveness of airways resulting in airflow obstruction	Nonproductive cough is only symptom in 50%; history of allergies and atopy, family history, wheezing, dyspnea, chest tightness, disturbed sleep. Symptoms exacerbated by exercise, cold air, nighttime, allergens, and respiratory infection.	Bilateral expiratory wheezing and prolonged expiratory phase; respiratory distress, dyspnea, tachypnea, use of accessory respiratory muscles	Sinus CT for concomitant sinusitis; PFTs (pre and post bronchodilator therapy); consider methacholine challenge test, pulse oximetry
Smoking and other environmental irritants	Irritation of airways	Smoker or exposure to secondhand smoke or other irritants, cough worse in specific environments such as work or home; cough >3 weeks occurs in 14–23% of nonsmokers	Often absent; may slow wheezing	CXR
Postnasal drainage (PND)	Rhinitis (allergic and nonallergic) and sinusitis cause PND, which is aspirated Bacterial causes of chronic sinusitis include *Haemophilus influenzae, Streptococcus pneumoniae,* and oral anaerobes	Most common cause of chronic cough in nonsmokers; persistent URI symptoms, history of seasonal allergies, feeling something dripping/tickling in back of throat, frequently clearing throat, hoarseness, facial pain, tooth pain **Allergic:** Red, itchy eyes, tearing, itching roof of mouth, otherwise unexplained cough, symptoms made worse by rhinitis or sinusitis, lying down, allergens, temperature changes, pregnancy	Erythematous and swollen nasal mucosa and turbinates, nasal polyps, deviated nasal septum, purulent nasal discharge, sinus tenderness; pharyngeal cobblestoning/postnasal drainage **Allergic:** Boggy nasal mucosa, conjunctivitis, tearing	Sinus CT
Hyperresponsiveness of airways after URI	URI → airway epithelial damage → hypersensitivity of the airway receptors to inhaled irritants	Recent URI; cough usually resolves in 3 weeks but may persist up to 7 weeks	Usually absent, possible wheeze	None
ACE inhibitors (ACEIs) and other medications	ACEI: unclear mechanism, but accumulation of bradykinin and prostaglandins that sensitize cough receptors is implicated. Beta blockers → bronchospasm Nitrofurantoin → pulmonary fibrosis	Five percent of those taking ACEI develop cough. Onset of cough is usually within 1 wk of starting suspect medication but may be delayed up to 6 mo.	Usually absent	None

Chronic bronchitis and COPD	Bronchial inflammation, excessive mucous production, and decreased ability of mucociliary system to clear secretions	Most common cause of chronic cough in smokers; history of smoking, ↑ sputum production, worse in morning, shortness of breath, dyspnea on exertion, wheezing. Chronic bronchitis is diagnosed with productive cough for at least 3 mo/yr for 2 consecutive years.	Scattered rhonchi, wheezes (especially forced expiration), crackles, prolonged expiration or distant breath sounds, thought lungs may be clear, no evidence of pulmonary consolidation	CXR, pulse oximetry, PFTs (pre and post bronchodilator therapy), ABG
Killer Kancer (primary pulmonary, Hodgkin's lymphoma, metastatic)	Mechanical compression of airways	Rarely presents solely with cough; weight loss, dyspnea, hemoptysis, history of smoking	Weight loss, cachexia, hemoptysis, fever	CXR, CT, MRI, bronchoscopy with biopsy, sputum cytology
Infants (aged <18 mo.) and children	Vascular anomalies most common in infants, asthma is most common in children	Wheezing, respiratory distress, persistent URI symptoms	Wheezing, dyspnea, tachypnea	CXR (all ages), barium swallow (infants) PFTs (children ≥5 yrs), consider sinus CT and pH probe
Tuberculosis (TB)	*Mycobacterium tuberculosis* infection transmitted by inhaling airborne bacilli from a person with active TB	History of TB exposure, HIV, immigration from countries with high prevalence, homelessness, substance abuse, in prison or nursing home; fatigue, fever, night sweats, weight loss, anorexia, dyspnea, hemoptysis, pleuritic chest pain	Fever, crackles near lung apices, septic appearing extrapulmonary TB may involve almost any organ and produce signs related to the specific site (such as recurrent UTIs, adenopathy, and meningitis)	PPD, CXR, acid-fast stain, and sputum culture (takes 2–6 wks to be positive) Testing for extrapulmonary TB as directed by history and examination.
Other Uncommon causes	"A CHEST BIZ" (See text)			One or more of the following (based on clinical suspicion): echocardiogram, BNP (CHF), sweat chloride (cystic fibrosis), HIV testing (AIDS), fungal antibody titers (suspected fungal infection)
Pertussis	Inflammation of larynx, trachea, and bronchi caused by *Bordetella pertussis*	Occurs in 5.5% of pts ≥16 years with persistent (average 6.5 weeks) cough: URI symptoms initially, then paroxysmal cough (not necessarily "whooping") develops 10–14 days after infected, posttussive vomiting	A febrile or slightly febrile, lung consolidation (in 20–25% of cases)	PCR testing of a nasopharyngeal specimen and serologic assays; WBC count (usually 15–20,000 and lymphocytosis >70%)
Psychogenic		Children ages 6–16 yrs, history of school phobia, cough is absent during sleep	Normal examination, or signs of anxiety/depression	No specific testing

ABG, arterial blood gases; BNP, B-type natriuretic peptide; CHF, congestive heart failure; COPD, chronic obstructive pulmonary disease; CT, computerized tomography; CXR, chest x-ray; GERD, gastroesophageal reflux disease; HIV, human immunodeficiency virus; LES, lower esophageal sphincter; MRI, magnetic resonance imaging; PCR, polymerase chain reaction; PFTs, pulmonary function tests; PPD, purified protein derivative; URI, upper respiratory infection; UTI, urinary tract infection.

B. Subacute/chronic cough (Table 13–1) may cause chest pain (chest wall, rib fracture), abdominal wall pain, insomnia, hemoptysis, urinary incontinence, syncope, bloodshot eyes (subconjunctival hemorrhage), shortness of breath (pneumothorax), headache, social isolation, anxiety, fatigue, myalgia, and dysphonia.

IV. Signs. The physical examination in patients with acute or chronic cough should focus on **temperature** (higher temperature tends to indicate bacterial infection); **ear canals** (for hairs/cerumen on tympanic membrane [Arnold's reflex]); **nares** (for edema, drainage, polyps, erythema); **sinuses** (for tenderness, possibly indicative of underlying sinusitis); **oropharynx** (for cobblestoning, indicative of PND); **neck** (for masses/lymphadenopathy, possibly indicative of infection or cancer); **lungs** (for localized inspiratory wheeze [foreign body or masses], diffuse expiratory wheeze [bronchospasm], basilar fine rales [pulmonary edema], percussion dullness, egophony, decreased breath sounds [pneumonia], or rhonchi [nonspecific], though absence of these findings does not exclude lung disease); **heart** (for S3 [CHF], or murmur [valvular disease]).

A. Acute cough
1. **Asthma exacerbation** (Table 13–1).
2. **Acute bronchitis/COPD** exacerbation may feature crackles, rhonchi, or wheezing (especially with forced expiration), but often lungs are clear. Fever, injected pharynx, or cervical lymphadenopathy may also occur.
3. Findings with **aspiration** may range from minimal to localized wheezing to severe dyspnea.
4. **Viral URI** often features normal examination, but may present with clear rhinorrhea, pharyngeal erythema, cervical adenopathy, low-grade fever, and clear lungs.
5. **Irritants** (see Smoking & other environmental irritants in Table 13–1).
6. **Rhinitis** (allergic) (see Postnasal drainage in Table 13–1).
7. **Uncomplicated pneumonia** may present with fever, tachypnea, hypoxia, cyanosis, and evidence of pulmonary consolidation, or localized rales or rhonchi. Atypical pneumonia may have minimal or no lung findings. The elderly may show mental status changes.
8. **Sinusitis/PND** (see Table 13–1).

B. Subacute/chronic cough (see Table 13–1).

V. Laboratory Tests. Tests are directed by history and examination findings (see Table 13–1). In patients with acute cough where a cause is clear, treatment can generally be initiated without further testing. However, even with a clear diagnosis of asthma, peak expiratory flow rate (PEFR) testing is wise, as is CXR in pneumonia or aspiration and complete blood count in pneumonia. Further testing in acute cough is generally reserved for the very ill, atypical presentations, or poor response to standard treatment (see below).

A. Hematologic tests
1. **White blood cell (WBC) count** assists in febrile patients to support a diagnosis of bacterial infection (increased neutrophils) or viral infection (increased lymphocytes).
2. **Antibody titers** may be helpful in suspected fungal infection (aspergillosis, histoplasmosis, or coccidioidomycosis).
3. **Arterial blood gases** can assist assessment of hypoxemia in patients with severe asthma, pneumonia, COPD, or other pulmonary disease.
4. **Serologic testing** (eg, enzyme-linked immunosorbent assay [ELISA]) helps confirm suspected human immunodeficiency virus (HIV) infection.
5. **B-type natriuretic peptide (BNP),** a cardiac neurohormone produced by the ventricles in response to ventricular volume expansion and pressure overload, may assist in differentiating a cardiac from a pulmonary origin of cough. Levels >100 pg/mL indicate CHF and those >480 pg/mL correlate with a nearly 30-fold increase in cardiac events over the next 6 months. Since samples remain viable <4 hours, this test is usually performed in the emergency room or inpatient setting.

B. Pulmonary function tests (PFTs) can differentiate obstructive from restrictive disease (respectively, asthma, COPD from sarcoid, pneumoconiosis, cystic fibrosis).
1. **Pre- and post-bronchodilator testing** clarifies fixed compared with reversible disease (eg, asthma).
2. **Bronchoprovocative testing** with methacholine inhalation uncovers subtle reversible airways obstruction in suspected asthmatic patients with normal or near-normal basic PFTs. Methacholine challenge is not widely available; its specificity approaches 100% in ruling out asthma, but its sensitivity is 60–80%, so positive testing does not conclusively rule asthma in.

3. PFTs are difficult to perform in children younger than 5 years old, so diagnosis in these patients is based on history, examination, and response to treatment.
4. **Peak expiratory flow rate (PEFR)** testing is an office procedure helpful in quantifying severity of airflow obstruction and response to treatment in acute asthma exacerbations.

C. **Radiography/special imaging**
1. **Chest x-ray (CXR)** is helpful in evaluating for pneumonia or complicated aspiration (localized infiltrates), bronchiectasis, COPD (hyperinflation/flat diaphragms), TB (fibronodular upper lobe infiltrates, cavitary lesions, hilar adenopathy, pleural effusion), sarcoid (hilar adenopathy), pulmonary edema/congestive heart failure (vascular congestion, Kerley B-lines, perihilar infiltrates, pleural effusion, cardiomegaly). This testing is readily available and, depending on clinical presentation/level of pretest diagnostic certainty, should be ordered early in the evaluation of cough.
2. **Barium swallow** is helpful in young children with chronic cough to assess for vascular anomalies, such as aberrant innominate artery.
3. **Upper GI series** assists in evaluating those with chronic cough and poorly responsive GERD (for hiatal hernia or complications, such as ulceration and stricture).
4. **Computerized tomographic (CT) or magnetic resonance imaging (MRI) scanning** of the chest assists in evaluating for mass lesions of sarcoid or neoplasms in patients whose clinical evaluation raises suspicion for these problems. CXR should precede CT or MRI imaging. **Sinus CT** is the gold standard for diagnosing chronic sinusitis and should be considered with chronic PND, recurrent episodes of sinusitis, or pediatric asthma. Approximately 50% of children with asthma have radiographic evidence of sinusitis, and studies have shown that treatment of sinusitis decreases bronchial hyperresponsiveness. Therefore, all children with asthma should be evaluated for concurrent sinusitis.
5. **2D echocardiogram** assesses left ventricular function and ejection fraction in suspected CHF. Multigated acquisition scan (**MUGA**) provides a more accurate ejection fraction than 2D Echo, but is more expensive and may not be as readily available.

D. **Endoscopy**
1. Referral for **bronchoscopy** is indicated in patients with (1) recurrent hemoptysis, (2) CT/MRI suggesting malignancy, or (3) chronic cough and negative results on basic clinical and testing evaluation.
2. **Nasopharyngoscopy** can be helpful in visualizing the turbinates/sinus ostia, pharynx, and larynx in individuals suspected of having cough originating in these structures (eg, those with chronic sinusitis).
3. **Esophagogastroduodenoscopy (EGD)** is used to evaluate for GERD complications (such as esophagitis, ulceration and stricture, Barrett's esophagus, and adenocarcinoma).

E. **Other tests**
1. **Sputum cytology** may be helpful if history or CT/MRI suggest malignancy.
2. **Sputum Gram stain, culture, and smears** may also be used. Gram stains of induced sputum may be useful in determining a likely cause of pneumonia. Although not useful in identifying gram-positive organisms, cultures are helpful in identifying gram-negative bacteria, penicillin-resistant *S pneumoniae, Mycobacterium* species (acid-fast stain), and fungi.
3. **24-hour esophageal pH monitoring** is 92% sensitive for GERD but is invasive. It should therefore be performed only after failure of empiric GERD treatment and a negative evaluation for asthma and sinusitis.
4. **Pulse oximetry** allows easy, noninvasive assessment of arterial oxygen saturation and is helpful in monitoring severity or response to therapy in patients with asthma or COPD.
5. **Purified protein derivative (PPD)** skin testing is a useful screen for pulmonary TB and should be considered in all patients with chronic cough, especially those at high risk. PPD needs to be read within 48–72 hours of placement. A test is considered positive if the diameter of the reaction measures ≥5 mm for HIV-infected and other immunocompromised individuals, ≥10 mm for those at high risk and ≥15 mm for all others. If a PPD test is positive, a CXR should be ordered. Symptomatic patients should be placed in respiratory isolation, pending results of a sputum smear with acid-fast stain and mycobacterium culture. The Centers for Disease Control and Prevention no longer recommends routine anergy testing in conjunction with PPD skin testing among HIV-infected individuals.

6. **Nasal smear** may be helpful in differentiating allergic from infectious rhinitis (showing eosinophils and white blood cells, respectively).
7. **Skin testing** for allergies may be helpful in clarifying the role of allergens in cough and in evaluating severe, poorly controlled perennial allergic symptoms for possible benefit from desensitization.
8. **Polymerase chain reaction** testing of a nasopharyngeal specimen is helpful in diagnosing pertussis in individuals with suggestive clinical findings.
9. **Sweat chloride testing** is necessary in evaluating children with cough and other features suggestive of cystic fibrosis (failure to thrive, gastrointestinal abnormalities, and recurrent infections).

VI. **Treatment** is directed at the underlying disease, which can be determined through methodical history taking, physical examination, and selective testing (Figure 13–1 and Table 13–1). For most conditions, management should include hydration, humidification, and rest. If the diagnosis is initially unclear, empiric treatment for the most likely cause may be preferable to extensive investigation, because such treatment may provide relief as well as diagnosis. Adequate treatment is important; in one study, many patients were correctly diagnosed by their primary care physician before pulmonology referral, but treatment was not aggressive enough to stop the cough.

Nonprescription medications for cough of presumed viral origin are no better than placebo and are associated with side effects, particularly in children younger than 6 years, where some adverse effects of over-the-counter medications may be life-threatening. Reported adverse reactions of common medications include hypertension, tachycardia, central nervous system (CNS) stimulation (agitation, psychosis, seizures, insomnia), dysrhythmias and myocardial infarction (**pseudoephedrine**); CNS depression and anticholinergic symptoms, tachycardia, blurred vision, agitation, hyperactivity, seizures, torsades de pointes (**chlorpheniramine and brompheniramine**); and lethargy, stupor, hyperexcitability, abnormal limb movements, and coma (**dextromethorphan**). One study showed a slight benefit using dextromethorphan for cough associated with acute upper respiratory tract infection. There are no randomized, controlled studies assessing the efficacy of prescription benzonatate (Tessalon Perles) compared with placebo.

If patients want to try an over-the-counter cough suppressant or expectorant (and are older than 6 years), they can, as there may be a beneficial placebo effect. Sucking on hard candies may have a similar effect.

Treatment of cough should always be directed at the underlying cause, but if the cough is severe and nonproductive, then a codeine antitussive should be considered as adjunct therapy, as there is solid evidence demonstrating the effectiveness of opioid antitussives, such as codeine, in controlling nonproductive cough. With less severe cough, benzonatate, dextromethorphan, or no treatment are options.

A. **Acute cough**
1. **Asthma exacerbation** (see Chapter 68).
2. **Acute bronchitis/COPD exacerbation** (see Chapter 70). Supportive treatment for acute bronchitis includes rest, fluids (3–4 liters per day, especially with fever), and albuterol inhaler if there is evidence of bronchospasm. Patients should expect to have a cough for 10–14 days. Due to their ineffectiveness and the risk of increasing resistance, Centers for Disease Control and Prevention guidelines state that antibiotics are not recommended for uncomplicated acute bronchitis regardless of the duration of the cough. Patient satisfaction with the office visit does not depend on receiving an antibiotic, but instead on effective doctor-patient communication. Patients should be advised that antibiotics are probably not going to be beneficial and that antibiotic treatment is associated with significant risks and side effects. To help patients understand the viral nature of their illness, it is helpful to refer to acute bronchitis as a "chest cold." Antibiotic prescription should be considered in patients with significant COPD, immunocompromised patients, patients with CHF, the elderly, and those appearing very ill or with high fever.
3. **Aspiration.** Most swallowed foreign bodies are coughed up or passed through the gastrointestinal tract without difficulty. Ten to 20% (especially swallowed button batteries) need intervention (laryngoscopy, bronchoscopy, esophagogastroscopy), and 1% need surgery. Surgical removal should be considered for a foreign body distal to the pylorus that serial abdominal plain films reveal to be unchanged in position over >5 days.
4. **Viral URI** (see Chapter 55).

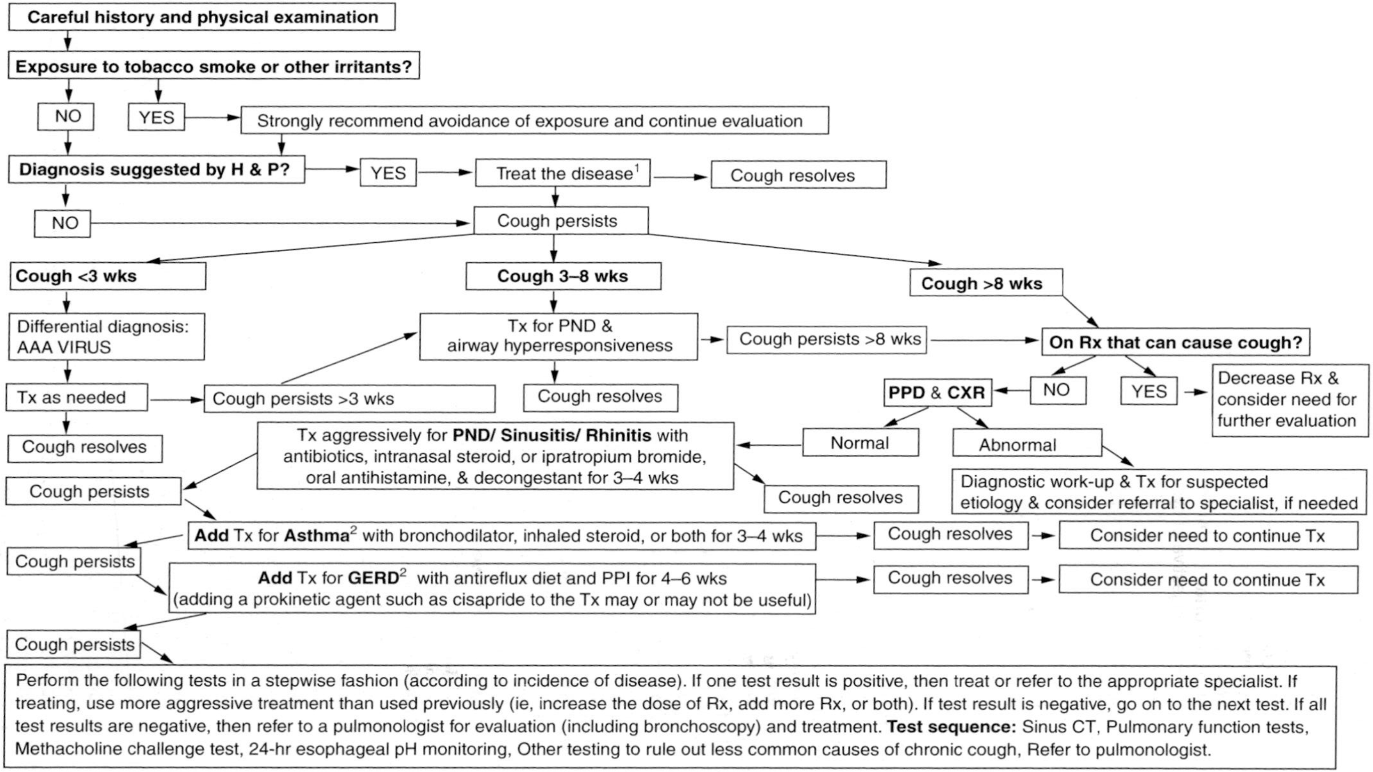

FIGURE 13–1. Cough management algorithm. [1]or discontinue medication, such as ACEI, if that is thought to be the cause of cough. [2]Tx for asthma and GERD are added, not substituted, based on the fairly high prevalence of patients having two (23–42%) or even three (3–15%) causes of chronic cough. ACEI, angiotensin converting enzyme inhibitor; CT, computerized tomography; CXR, chest x-ray; GERD, gastroesophageal reflux disease; PND, postnasal drainage; PPD, purified protein derivative; Rx, prescription; Tx, therapy.

Careful history and physical examination

Exposure to tobacco smoke or other irritants?
- NO
- YES → Strongly recommend avoidance of exposure and continue evaluation

Diagnosis suggested by H & P?
- YES → Treat the disease[1] → Cough resolves / Cough persists
- NO

Cough <3 wks
Differential diagnosis: AAA VIRUS
Tx as needed → Cough resolves / Cough persists

Cough persists >3 wks

Cough 3–8 wks
Tx for PND & airway hyperresponsiveness → Cough resolves / Cough persists >3 wks

Tx aggressively for PND/ Sinusitis/ Rhinitis with antibiotics, intranasal steroid, or ipratropium bromide, oral antihistamine, & decongestant for 3–4 wks → Cough resolves / Cough persists

Add Tx for Asthma[2] with bronchodilator, inhaled steroid, or both for 3–4 wks → Cough resolves / Cough persists

Add Tx for GERD[2] with antireflux diet and PPI for 4–6 wks (adding a prokinetic agent such as cisapride to the Tx may or may not be useful) → Cough resolves / Cough persists

Cough >8 wks
On Rx that can cause cough?
- YES → Decrease Rx & consider need for further evaluation
- NO → PPD & CXR
  - Normal → ... Cough resolves / Consider need to continue Tx
  - Abnormal → Diagnostic work-up & Tx for suspected etiology & consider referral to specialist, if needed

Cough persists >8 wks

Consider need to continue Tx

Perform the following tests in a stepwise fashion (according to incidence of disease). If one test result is positive, then treat or refer to the appropriate specialist. If treating, use more aggressive treatment than used previously (ie, increase the dose of Rx, add more Rx, or both). If test result is negative, go on to the next test. If all test results are negative, then refer to a pulmonologist for evaluation (including bronchoscopy) and treatment. **Test sequence:** Sinus CT, Pulmonary function tests, Methacholine challenge test, 24-hr esophageal pH monitoring. Other testing to rule out less common causes of chronic cough. Refer to pulmonologist.

5. **Irritant-related cough.** Avoidance of the offending agent and smoking cessation should be encouraged. Approximately 75% of people stop coughing within a month of eliminating offensive exposures. (See Chapter 100 for suggestions on effective smoking cessation techniques.)
6. **Rhinitis (allergic)** (see Chapter 55).
7. **Uncomplicated pneumonia**
   a. **Antibiotics** for outpatient treatment of community-acquired pneumonia include a macrolide (eg, erythromycin or azithromycin) for suspected *M pneumoniae* or trimethoprim-sulfamethoxazole or amoxicillin clavulanate for other causes. Treatment should generally continue for 10–14 days, and symptomatic improvement should occur within 2–3 days.
   b. **Supportive treatment** includes antipyretics/analgesia and hydration.
   c. **Hospitalization** may be necessary, depending on comorbidities, support at home, and severity of illness. Indicators of severe illness include age older than 65 years with multiple medical problems, altered mental status, hypoxia (O_2 saturation <90% or Pao_2 <60 mm Hg on room air), hypercapnia ($Paco_2$ >45 mm Hg), acidosis (arterial pH <7.35), hypotension, sepsis, multiorgan dysfunction, anemia (Hb <9 g/dL), significant leukopenia or leukocytosis (<4000 WBC/mm^3 or >30,000 WBC/mm^3, respectively), or multilobe densities or large pleural effusion on CXR.
8. **Sinusitis/PND** (see Chapter 55).
B. **Subacute/chronic cough**
   1. **Gastroesophageal reflux disease (GERD)** (see Chapter 19).
   2. **Asthma** (see Chapter 68).
   3. **Smoking and other environmental irritants** (see section VI,A,5).
   4. **Postnasal drainage (PND)** (see Chapter 55). Treatment with antihistamine and decongestant combination alone is successful in >50% of nonsmokers with PND and chronic cough.
   5. **Hyperresponsiveness of airways.** Hyperresponsiveness of airways persists for up to 8 weeks after URI and resolves without treatment. Significant cough warrants trial of a bronchodilator and an antihistamine, with addition of an inhaled steroid or oral steroid taper if cough persists using the bronchodilator or antihistamine. It is important not to misdiagnose "asthma" in this setting.
   6. **Angiotensin converting enzyme (ACE) inhibitors and other medicines.** ACE inhibitors and other medicines causing cough should be eliminated or changed (eg, substituting an angiotensin receptor blocker for an ACE). Cough should resolve within 4 weeks after these changes.
   7. **Chronic bronchitis/COPD** (see Chapter 70).
   8. **Killer Kancer.** Referral to an oncologist is indicated.
   9. In **infants and children,** underlying disease (usually asthma) should be treated; children with vascular anomalies should be referred to a vascular surgeon.
   10. **Tuberculosis**
       a. **Latent TB** (positive PPD and normal) is treated with oral isoniazid, 300 mg daily for 9 months, with addition of oral pyridoxine (Vitamin B_6), 25 mg daily to prevent neuropathy in those older than 35 years.
       b. **Active TB** (positive PPD test and abnormal CXR or positive acid-fast bacilli culture/smear) requires reporting to the local health department, respiratory isolation and multidrug therapy (eg, oral isoniazid combined with rifampin, pyrazinamide, streptomycin, or ethambutol). Because of variable resistance, consultation with an infectious disease specialist for assistance in drug selection and monitoring is prudent. During therapy, liver function tests should be monitored in those older than 35 years or with a history of drug/alcohol abuse or liver disease.
       c. To ensure compliance and effective treatment and to minimize the emergence of resistant strains, **directly observed therapy** should be implemented throughout treatment.
   11. **Other uncommon causes.** Treat according to etiology.
   12. **Pertussis**
       a. **Antibiotics.** Antibiotics do not alter the cause of the illness, unless initiated early in its course; however, antibiotics do prevent transmission and decrease the need for respiratory isolation from 4 weeks to 1 week.

    b. Suggested regimens
       (1) Macrolide antibiotics. Macrolide antibiotics are the treatment of choice; oral **erythromycin,** 500 mg four times a day in adults (40–50 mg/kg/day divided into four doses in pediatric patients, with maximum of 2 g/day) for 14 days, or oral **azithromycin,** 500 mg on day 1 and 250 g on days 2–5 for adults (10 mg/kg/day for 5 days in pediatric patients) are effective.
       (2) Alternative regimen. Oral **trimethoprim-sulfamethoxazole-DS** twice daily in adults (8 mg TMP + 40 mg SMX/kg/day divided into twice-daily doses in pediatric patients) for 14 days is also effective.
       (3) Hospitalization. Hospitalization is wise for seriously ill patients, especially infants.
    13. Psychogenic factors. Providing reassurance of normal test results (such as peak flow) can alleviate patient anxiety, increase patient acceptance of diagnosis, and decrease cough symptoms. Persistent psychogenic cough warrants consideration of a psychiatric consultation.

REFERENCES

D'Urzo A, Jugovic P: Chronic cough: Three most common causes. Can Fam Physician (August) 2002; **48:**1311.

Irwin RS, Madison JM: The diagnosis and treatment of cough. N Engl J Med (December 7) 2000; **343:**1715.

Poe RH, Kallay MC: Chronic cough and gastroesophageal reflux disease: Experience with specific therapy for diagnosis and treatment. Chest (March) 2003;**123:**679.

Schroeder K, Fahey T: Systematic review of randomized controlled trials of over the counter cough medicines for acute cough in adults. BMJ (February 9) 2002;**324:**329.

Tsao CH, et al: Concomitant chronic sinusitis treatment in children with mild asthma: The effect on bronchial hyperresponsiveness. Chest (March) 2003;**123:**757.

---

14   Dermatitis & Other Pruritic Dermatoses

Aleksandra Zgierska, MD, PhD, William G. Phillips, MD,
& Marjorie Shaw Phillips, MS, RPh, FASHP

KEY POINTS

- Generalized pruritus requires as specific a diagnosis and treatment plan as possible.
- Many serious systemic diseases produce generalized pruritus without skin manifestations.
- Chronic pruritus has a variety of psychological explanations and consequences.

  I. Definition. Pruritus is a sensation that causes one to itch, which is a peculiar irritating sensation in the skin that arouses the desire to scratch. **Dermatitis** is inflammation of the skin, whereas **dermatosis** is defined as any disease of the skin in which inflammation is not necessarily a feature.
    For the purposes of this chapter, dermatitis and pruritic dermatoses will be considered in terms of the following: (a) primary dermatoses, (b) symptoms of significant internal medical or surgical illness, and (c) primary psychological disturbances.
  II. Common Diagnoses. Approximately 15% of all patients presenting to generalist physicians do so for care of a skin disease or lesion, and pruritic dermatoses are a significant proportion of these. Severe and chronic pruritus may significantly affect quality of life, including causing insomnia/daytime drowsiness, anxiety, distraction from one's daily social functioning, and personal embarrassment.
    A. Pruritic dermatoses
      1. Atopic eczema is found in approximately 7–24 individuals per 1000 in the United States; it is more common in infancy and childhood. In 50% of affected children,

the condition persists into adulthood. Risk factors for persistent, more severe disease include positive family history, female gender, and coexisting allergic rhinitis/asthma.

2. Irritant **contact dermatitis** affects 1 in 1000 workers annually and accounts for 50% of occupational illness; those particularly at risk include workers in manufacturing, food production, construction, machine tool operation, printing, metal plating, and leather processing. Approximately three sevenths of occupational dermatosis is believed to be **allergic contact dermatitis.** Allergic contact dermatitis is uncommon in young children and less common in deeply pigmented individuals.

3. **Scabies,** caused by the mite *Sarcoptes scabiei,* is an extremely common pruritic infestation, which occurs in both genders and across the age range and is transmitted by close skin-to-skin contact. The development of an itchy rash in multiple family members at the same time is suspicious for scabies.

4. **Head lice (pediculosis capitis)** affect 6–12 million people in the United States annually, occur most frequently in school or day care settings, and require significant head-to-head contact for transmission. Head lice infest all levels of society and ethnic groups, although their incidence is lower in African American populations. **Pediculosis pubis** is transmitted sexually; it is frequently seen in the context of venereal disease clinics and student health services. **Body lice (pediculosis humanus)** are much less common than pediculosis pubis or capitis and are usually seen in a setting of poor hygiene, homelessness, and crowded conditions.

5. **Lichen simplex chronicus** is more common in adults than in children, particularly in middle-aged women, atopic individuals, and those suffering extreme stress.

6. **Lichen planus** typically begins in the fourth decade, is rare in children younger than 5 years, and is associated with an approximately 10% positive family history. It has been associated with liver disease (specifically, hepatitis C virus) as well as certain medications, including thiazides, Capoten, and antimalarials.

7. **Xerosis (dry skin)** is common in northern climates, particularly during the winter months, with low relative humidity and indoor heating. It is seen particularly in atopic individuals, at the extremes of age, with frequent bathing, with chemical or solvent exposure, as well as with hypothyroidism, or antiandrogen or diuretic therapy.

8. **Dyshidrosis** accounts for 5–20% of all hand dermatitis, is more common during spring and summer seasons in warmer climates, and may be associated with stressors.

9. **Pityriasis rosea** is seen more frequently in women than in men, and more than 75% of the patients are between ages 10 and 35 years. The incidence of the disease is higher during the colder months, and a small percentage of patients have a recent history of infection associated with fatigue, headache, sore throat, and fever.

10. **Psoriasis** affects more than 2% of people of European ancestry. It has a presumed autoimmune pathogenesis, and 40% of patients give a positive family history. Sunlight, relaxation, and the summer season are usually beneficial, but upper respiratory/streptococcal infections, trauma to the skin, stress, and medications (lithium, beta blockers, angiotensin converting enzyme inhibitors, indomethacin) can exacerbate psoriasis. In about 15% of patients with psoriasis, a seronegative inflammatory arthritis develops that has many clinical features of rheumatoid arthritis. **Guttate psoriasis** occurs in 2% of all patients with psoriasis, typically begins before age 30, and affects all races.

11. The estimated lifetime risk of acquiring a **dermatophyte infection** is between 10% and 20%. **Tinea capitis** is most common in 3- to 8-year-olds, particularly males. It may occur in epidemics. Farmers and children with pets are classically at risk for **tinea corporis.** Obesity, heat, humidity, perspiration, and chafing predispose individuals to **tinea cruris,** which occurs four times more common in young adults and males than in other population groups. Acquisition of **tinea pedis** appears to depend on a susceptibility factor. More males than females are affected with this condition, which is rare in children.

12. **Seborrhea** is often familial and most commonly occurs in adult males. It is associated with hyperandrogenicity (eg, polycystic ovarian disease, hirsutism), diabetes mellitus, sprue, Parkinson's disease, and epilepsy and may occur in patients affected with human immunodeficiency virus (HIV) infection before other more specific symptoms of this illness.

13. Nummular eczema typically occurs in young adults and, less commonly, in children. The cause is unknown, although the history is usually positive for asthma and hay fever. In the elderly, a history of a low-protein diet is often found.
   B. Pruritus in systemic disease. Pruritus can be a presentation of systemic disease in 10–50% of elderly patients. Systemic diseases associated with pruritus include hyperthyroidism, hypothyroidism, polycythemia vera, iron deficiency, obstructive biliary disease, multiple myeloma, and HIV. It is also a feature of lymphoma and Hodgkin's disease (up to 30% of Hodgkin's disease patients present with generalized pruritus). It is associated with end-stage renal failure (severe paroxysms of pruritus occur in 25% of patients with chronic renal failure).
   C. Pruritus with a prominent psychogenic component.
      1. Psychophysiologic disorders occur in individuals whose underlying dermatosis (acne, alopecia areata, atopic dermatitis, psoriasis, psychogenic purpura, rosacea, seborrhea, urticaria) is exacerbated by stressors (psychological, occupational, or social).
      2. Delusions of parasitosis, an example of a primary psychiatric disorder with dermatologic manifestations, occurs when persons carry the false belief of being infested by bugs, mites, worms, or other living creatures. These beliefs may be brought about by drug toxicity (alcohol, amphetamines, glucocorticoids, or cocaine withdrawal) or associated with vitamin B_{12} deficiency, cerebrovascular disease, neurosyphilis, multiple sclerosis, schizophrenia, psychotic depression, hypochondriasis, or an obsessional fear that parasites are present in the body.
      3. Localized psychogenic pruritus (localized scratching without identifiable physical pathology) occurs in 9% of patients with pruritus, typically begins between ages 30 and 45, and is more prevalent in women (52–92% of patients). Depression, anxiety, or both may play a significant role in the cause of the behavior.
 III. Symptoms. The intensity of pruritus in the pruritic dermatoses may vary from mild and annoying to intense. For all patients presenting with pruritus, especially when it is chronic and without characteristic lesions of common dermatoses (Table 14–1), symptoms of significant internal or psychiatric disease (eg, anxiety/depression, obsessive-compulsive disorder, and somatoform disorders) should be sought.
 IV. Signs (Table 14–1).
   A. Pruritic dermatoses. As with many dermatologic conditions, the diagnosis of most pruritic dermatoses is made on the basis of pattern recognition. **Pattern recognition** is the ability to identify a skin condition by its basic morphology, shape, size, color, distribution, and presence or absence of secondary features such as pruritus. At times, a particular feature of a lesion or the history of the lesion may be extremely helpful in achieving a diagnosis. Examples include (1) the presence of a "herald patch" in pityriasis rosea, (2) the classic distribution of lichen simplex chronicus on the back of the neck, (3) the presence of lice or nits in pediculosis, (4) the presence of eggs or feces in scabies, and (5) the linear vesicles or symmetric lesions of contact dermatitis.
      1. Lesions of **dyshydrosis** may resolve over 3–4 weeks and be replaced by 1- to 3-mm rings. Episodes may recur; chronic changes include lichenification and fissuring.
      2. Pityriasis rosea may take 6–8 weeks to spontaneously resolve. Instead of characteristic truncal lesions, African Americans may have facial or extremity lesions.
   B. Especially in elderly patients whose lesions lack the morphology of primary dermatoses (Table 14–1), signs of underlying systemic disease (eg, cholestasis, chronic renal failure, lymphoma, HIV, multiple myeloma) should be carefully sought.
   C. Primary psychiatric disorders. Patients with **delusions of parasitosis** have a positive "matchbox" sign, in which the patient brings in a matchbox or other container with bits of excoriated skin, debris, or insect parts as "proof" of infestation.
 V. Laboratory Tests
   A. The history and the physical examination are generally all that are necessary to diagnose common primary dermatoses. The tests listed below are also sometimes useful to confirm a particular diagnosis.
      1. Microscopic examination of burrow scrapings in mineral oil may reveal scabies mites, eggs, or feces.
      2. Potassium hydroxide (KOH) preparations are the classic tests for tinea. Skin scrapings are placed on a glass slide, one or two drops of 10–20% KOH are added, and the slide is heated gently to dissolve cellular material and reveal the hyphae and spores characteristic of tinea.

TABLE 14–1. DIFFERENTIAL DIAGNOSES OF COMMON PRURITIC DERMATOSES

Diagnosis	Locations(s) Affected	Usual Morphology
Atopic eczema	Symmetrical—cheeks/scalp/chest/ extensor (infants); lichenified flexural/ eyelids/perioral (children) flexural hands/ forearms/wrists/feet (teen/adult)	Thickened dry plaques
Contact dermatitis	At sites of irritant exposure; shape of irritant (eg, watchband)	Vesicles (acute) Crusty, lichenification (chronic)
Scabies	Web spaces of fingers, hands, wrists, axillae, buttocks, groin; facial/scalp (infants)	Linear vesicles, erythematous papules Lichenified, excoriated
Lice	Scalp, pelvic, pubic	Nits on hairs $1/4''$ from skin (capitis/pubis) Excoriation (body lice)
Lichen simplex chronicus	Back of neck, shoulders, forearms, lower legs, cheeks, perianal	Liner excoriations, scabs, scars
Lichen planus	Flexural wrists, scalp, trunk, ankles, genital, buccal mucosa	Violaceous flat-topped polygonal plaques White streaks on buccal mucosa (Wickham's striae)
Xerosis	Especially lower legs	Exaggerated skin lines, plaques with superficial fissures
Dyshydrosis	Palms/web spaces (80% of patients) Feet (10%) Feet and hands (10%)	Burning or itching, followed by deep ("tapioca-like") vesicles
Pityriasis rosea	Chest and trunk	Initially papulosquamous oval scaly 2- to 10-cm diameter pink "herald patch" followed by "Christmas tree" pink, scaly oval, salmon-colored macules on back
Psoriasis	Symmetrical—elbows/knees/ears/scalp/ umbilicus/gluteal cleft/genitalia/nails	Sharply demarcated erythematous plaque covered with grayish-white or silver-white scale; pitting/thickened nails 1- to 10-mm pink/red papules with fine scale (guttate)
Tinea corporis	Extremities, face, trunk	Flat scaly papules spreading radially into circinate lesion with raised scaly edge and central clearing
Tinea pedis	Interdigital; plantar	Interdigital scale/fissures Scaling plantar surface ("moccasin") Vesiculobullous
Tinea cruris	Groin folds	Radially expanding raised edge with central clearing, slight scale
Seborrhea	Scalp, nasolabial folds, upper chest, postauricular creases, brows, eyelashes	Occasional dry flakes to thick greasy scale Diffuse erythema to oozing cracks
Nummular eczema	Extremities	Coin-red plaques 1–5x cm diameter with minimal scaling
Primary psychological disorders	Face/scalp/trunk/arms/legs	Bitane excoriations due to scratching or self-inflicted damage from cigarettes, chemicals or sharp instruments without evidence of underlying skin disorder
Localized psychogenic pruritus	Localized lesions (neck, trunk, extremities)	Linear excoriations, scab, scar

3. **Wood's light examination** is useful in the differential diagnosis of tinea of the scalp, which fluoresces bright yellow-green, or of the skin (*Corynebacterium minutissimum*), which resembles tinea but fluoresces red.
4. **Patch testing** is the classic test for allergic contact dermatitis. Allergen is applied to the skin for 48 hours and then removed. The skin is observed 20 minutes later. Reactions may take place in one area of tissue but not in others.
5. **Biopsy**
   a. If lesions of atopic eczema involve the nipple and do not subside with simple treatment, Paget's disease must be excluded by biopsy. Unilateral eczema of the breast may be the only indication of a ductal adenocarcinoma.
   b. In cases of pityriasis, the physician should strongly consider a serologic test or a biopsy to rule out syphilis.
   c. In any case in which the diagnosis is in doubt, a biopsy should be considered.
B. In cases where a common primary pruritic dermatosis is in question and the above tests fail to confirm it, in the absence of reassuring historical risk factors (eg, localized lesions, recent travel, contacts with similar lesions, occupational exposure), in elderly patients, or in those with suspected underlying systemic disease, limited testing is indicated. Tests should include thyroid-stimulating hormone, bilirubin, alkaline phosphatase, blood urea nitrogen, creatinine, complete blood count, HIV testing, and chest radiographs.
VI. **Treatment.** Treatment goals include (1) appropriate management of diseases causing pruritus, (2) symptomatic relief, and (3) cosmetic improvement.
A. **General measures**
   1. **Nonmedication measures** include some or all of the following:
      a. **Bathing** no more frequently than daily for 5–10 minutes using warm (not hot) water.
      b. Using **mild soap** (eg, Alpha-Keri, Cetaphil, Dove, Nivea cream, Oilatum, Purpose, Basis) or soap-free cleansers (eg, Cetaphil lotion, Aquanil lotion, SFC lotion, Lowila, Aveeno cleansing) and soaping only vital areas (eg, axillae, genitals, feet).
      c. **Patting (not rubbing)** the skin during drying.
      d. **Applying emollients** within 3 minutes of bathing; emollients range from lotions (least occlusive) to creams (most cosmetically acceptable) to ointments (most occlusive, but leaves skin tacky). Additives such as urea (eg, Carmol, Aqua Care, Ureacin) or lactic acid (eg, Lac-Hydrin, Penecare) may further promote skin hydration.
      e. Using a **central humidifier** during cold months.
      f. **Soaking dry, pruritic areas** in cool solution of colloidal oatmeal (Aveeno) or baking soda.
      g. **Cutting fingernails** and wearing cotton gloves during sleep (for individuals who have difficulty controlling scratching).
      h. **Avoiding known irritants,** such as alcohol, caffeine, rubber shoes, dyed socks, cosmetics, hairspray, or jewelry.
   2. In individuals with more severe symptoms or lesions, or those refractory to nonmedication measures (section VI,A,1), one or a combination of the following **medications** may prove beneficial.
      a. **Topical medications**
         (1) **Corticosteroids** (Table 14–2).
             (a) The efficacy and risk of side effects depends on several factors, including **potency** (ranging from Group 1 to 7, where 1 is most potent), **vehicle** (ointment > cream > lotions), **anatomic area** (for a given agent, the greatest penetration occurs on the face and groin, the lowest on palms and soles), and **thickness of lesions** (thickened plaques are more resistant than thinner lesions).
             (b) As a general rule, the least potent effective medication/vehicle should be chosen to treat the lesion and the medication should be used for as short a time as necessary. For example, in pediatric patients or those with intertriginous lesions, a Group 6 or 7 corticosteroid should be prescribed; Group 1 or 2 agents are appropriate for thickened lesions on the palm or sole.
             (c) **Corticosteroid side effects** are mainly localized to the area of application and can include atrophy, telangiectasia, striae, hypopigmentation,

TABLE 14-2. TOPICAL STEROIDS FOR DERMATOSES

Generic Name of Product	Dosing[1]	Trade Name(s)	Cost[2]
Lowest potency			
Hydrocortisone (cream, ointment, lotion) 0.5–2.5%	qd–qid	Generic	$–$$
2.5% cream		Hytone, Synacort, etc	$$–$$$
0.5–1% available without prescription			
Dexamethasone (topical aerosol) 0.01%	bid–qid	Aeroseb-Dex[3]	$$$$
Low potency			
Betamethasone valerate (cream) 0.01%	qd–tid	Valisone Reduced Strength	$$$$
Fluocinolone acetonide (cream, ointment) 0.01%	bid–qid	Generic, Flurosyn	$–$$
		Synalar	$$
Flurandrenolide (cream,[3] ointment,[3] lotion) 0.025%	bid–tid	Cordran, Cordran SP	$$$$
Triamcinolone acetonide (cream, ointment,			
lotion, aerosol) 0.025%	tid–qid	Generic	$
		Aristocort, Aristocort A, Kenalog	$$$
High potency (for acute, self-limited dermatosis; avoid on face)			
Fluocinolone acetonide (cream) 0.2%	bid–qid	Synalar-HP	$$$$
Fluocinonide (cream, gel, ointment, solution) 0.05%	bid–qid	Generic	$$$
		Lidex, Lidex-E	$$$$
Halcinonide (cream, ointment, solution) 0.1%	qd, bid–tid	Halog, Halog-E	$$$$
Triamcinolone acetonide (cream, ointment) 0.5%	bid–qid	Generic	$
		Aristocort, Aristocort A, Kenalog	$$$$$

[1] Usual adult doses. Patients should be instructed to apply sparingly to skin in a light film and rub in gently.
[2] Average wholesale cost to the pharmacist for 15 g of ointment or cream: $, <$2; $$, $2–5; $$$, $5–10; $$$$, $10–20; $$$$$, >$20.
[3] Available as a 58-g spray.

rosacea, acne, or perioral dermatitis. The risk of systemic side effects (eg, cataracts, glaucoma, growth suppression in children, Cushing syndrome, hypothalamic-pituitary-adrenal suppression) increases with the percentage of body surface treated, duration of treatment, and potency of steroid.

    (2) Topical antihistamines (eg, diphenhydramine) and doxepin (eg, Zonalon) may relieve pruritus, but may also cause allergic contact dermatitis.

  b. Oral medications

    (1) Antihistamine medications

      (a) First-generation antihistamines include **hydroxyzine** (Vistaril or Atarax), 25–100 mg for adults, 12.5–25 mg for children over 6 years and 0.5 mg/kg up to 12.5 mg for children younger than 6 years, given three to four times a day; **diphenhydramine** (Benadryl), 50 mg at bedtime for adults and 12.5 mg every 4–6 hours for children aged 6–12 years. These medications are sedating and may help control pruritus.

      (b) Second-generation antihistamines (eg, Claritin 10 mg daily, Allegra 120–180 mg daily, or Zyrtec 10 mg daily) are less sedating but generally less effective in controlling pruritus than older agents.

      (c) Tricyclic antidepressants have antihistaminic effects and may be beneficial in inducing sleep and controlling pruritus. Examples include doxepin (Sinequan) or amitriptyline (Elavil) 10–75 mg at bedtime. These medications should be used with caution in the elderly, particularly those with cardiac conduction defects or prostatic hypertrophy.

    (2) Oral systemic steroids (eg, prednisone), given for a 4- to 7-day "burst" of 40–60 mg/day or starting with 60 mg a day and tapering over 10 days, may treat flare-ups or lesions uncontrolled with the foregoing measures. "Burst" therapy minimizes the side effects complicating long-term daily oral steroid therapy.

B. Therapies for specific dermatoses

1. **Atopic dermatitis (atopic eczema)**
   a. The foundation of treatment is conscientious **skin hydration** (see section VI,A,1).
   b. For mild breakthrough symptoms despite the foregoing treatment, a **low- to moderate-potency steroid** can be added; for persistent or more severe breakthrough symptoms, a higher potency topical steroid can be used (see Table 14–2).
   c. **Oral antihistamines** may be beneficial in relieving pruritus, in conjunction with topical measures and medications.
   d. Topical immunosuppressants **tacrolimus** and **pimecrolimus** are approximately as effective as medium-potency topical corticosteroids but do not cause skin atrophy and can be used when glucocorticoids are ineffective or contraindicated. Common side effects of tacrolimus ointment involve skin burning, erythema, and pruritus, but they are usually minor and resolve after a few days of therapy. **Tacrolimus (Prosopic)** should be applied twice daily and gently rubbed into dry skin. Improvement is seen within a week and treatment should continue for a week after lesions clear. In children aged 2–15 years the ointment should be used; adults can use either the 0.03% or 0.1% ointment. **Pimecrolimus** 1% cream (Elidel) should be used in the same manner as tacrolimus; it can be used for all patients older than age 2.
   e. Patients compliant with and responding poorly to the foregoing measures should generally be evaluated by a dermatologist for consideration of ultraviolet phototherapy or oral immunosuppressant therapy (eg, cyclosporin).
2. **Contact dermatitis** is best treated by identifying and removing the offending agent. **Acute** (weepy, edematous, vesicular) lesions are treated with cotton dressings soaked in Burow's solution (aluminum acetate diluted 1:40 with cool water), four to six times daily. **Chronic** (dry, scaly, thickened) lesions are treated with emollients (section VI,A,1) and topical corticosteroids (section VI,A,2,a,(1) and Table 14–2).
3. For treatment of **scabies** and **lice,** see Chapter 7, Bites & Stings.
4. Treatment of **lichen simplex chronicus (LSC)** involves treating underlying mood disorders (Chapters 89, 92, 94), and providing patient education regarding the itch-scratch cycle and efforts to control this cycle (see section VI,A).
5. **Lichen planus (LP)** should also be treated with general measures (section VI,A) and topical corticosteroids (section VI,A,2,a,(1) and Table 14–2); steroid gels (eg, fluocinonide, 0.05%) applied two to three times daily for flares are effective for intraoral lesions.
6. For **dry skin (xerosis, asteatosis)** elimination of medications and other aggravating factors is an essential aspect of treatment. Good skin hydration and lubrication as outlined in section VI,A,1 will alleviate symptoms.
7. For **dyshidrosis,** nonpharmacologic management includes using mild cleansers and soap substitutes, using protective gloves, and avoiding known hand irritants. Burow's solution (section VI,B,2) alleviates bullous lesions, medium- and high-potency topical corticosteroids can be used for flare-ups (section VI,A,2,a,(1) and Table 14–2), and an oral steroid taper (section VI,A,2,b,(2)) may benefit more severe or acute symptoms. Persistent or unresponsive cases should be referred to a dermatologist for psoralen plus ultraviolet A (PUVA) or low-dose methotrexate therapy.
8. There is no specific treatment for **pityriasis rosea.** Oral antihistamines as well as Aveeno baths may reduce pruritus. Patients need to be reassured that the condition may last for 6–8 weeks, but is benign.
9. **Psoriasis** treatment is related to reducing epidermal cell turnover.
   a. **Mild disease** can be treated with emollients (eg, **Desitin ointment,** applied three times a day to affected areas, or **A and D ointment,** applied three times a day) chronically to affected areas. Keratolytic agents, such as **salicylic acid** (eg, salicylic acid soap), applied daily, can bring limited improvement but can irritate inflamed skin. Mild to moderate corticosteroid ointments (see Table 14–2) are one of the mainstays of treatment but can cause localized skin atrophy.
   b. **Moderate disease** may respond to **ultraviolet (UV) light** or **tar preparations** (eg, Estar applied at bedtime to affected areas, allowing the gel to remain for 5 minutes and then removing any excess by patting with tissues) or a combination of UV light and tar preparation. **Calcipotriene** (Dovonex), a topical

treatment for psoriasis of mild to moderate severity, is a vitamin D derivative that inhibits epidermal cell proliferation in vitro. Calcipotriene should be applied twice daily to psoriatic plaques on the trunk, the extremities, or both, avoiding application with occlusive dressings; or to the face and the groin, where it may cause irritant dermatitis. Topical calcipotriene is about as effective as moderate- to high-potency topical steroids but may require 6–8 weeks of use before lesion improvement is noted. Absorption of calcipotriene is a problem only if large quantities (>100 g/week) are applied. It should not be used by patients with demonstrated hypercalcemia or evidence of vitamin D toxicity. It has a pregnancy category of C.

    c. Patients with **psoriatic arthritis** (5–8% of patients with psoriasis) or **more severe/unresponsive skin disease** should be referred to a dermatologist for consideration of ultraviolet phototherapy (PUVA or UVB), with or without oral methotrexate or retinoids (acitretin).

10. **Dermatophyte**
    a. **Tinea capitis** and **barbae** (see Chapter 32).
    b. **Tinea corporis.** Superficial and localized lesions respond well to topical agents applied once or twice daily for 1–2 weeks beyond when clinical response is first noted. These agents include clotrimazole (Lotrimin), econazole (Spectazole), ketoconazole (Nizoral), miconazole (Monistat derm), sulconazole (Exelderm), oxiconazole (Oxistat), terbinafine (Lamisil), butenafine (Mentax), or naftifine (Naftin). More extensive or topically unresponsive lesions should be treated for 2–4 weeks with an oral agent (eg, griseofulvin, 500 mg daily in adults or 7–10 mg/kg/day in children [ultramicrosize formulation]).
    c. **Tinea pedis.** Tinea pedis can be treated with a topical antifungal, although "moccasin" type may require 1 week's oral therapy—ie, griseofulvin, 500 mg/day in adults or 125–250 mg/day in children 30–50 lbs and 250–500 mg/day in children >50 lbs; terbinafine (Lamisil), 250 mg/day in adults or 3–5 mg/kg/day in children; or itraconazole (Sporanox), 200 mg/day in adults or 4–6 mg/kg/day in children.

11. **Seborrhea**
    a. In **adults,** conventional therapy for **seborrheic dermatitis** of the scalp is a shampoo containing one of the following compounds: **salicylic acid** (eg, X-Seb T or Sebulex), **selenium sulfide** (eg, Selsun or Excel), **coal tar** (eg, DHS Tar, Neutrogena T-Gel, or Polytar), or **pyrithione zinc** (eg, DHS Zinc, Danex, or Sebulon). Each of these shampoos can be used two or three times a week. After application, shampoos should be left on the hair and scalp for at least 5 minutes to ensure that the medication reaches the scalp skin. In more severe cases, adults may massage topical steroid lotions such as **2.5% hydrocortisone** (eg, Hytone) into the scalp once or twice daily.
    b. **Flares or more resistant cases** may respond to antifungals (eg, ketoconazole 2% shampoo) used daily on affected scalp or beard for at least a month. Scalp scale may be treated with 2% salicylic acid shampoo; a peanut oil/mineral oil/corticosteroid preparation (Derma Smoothe/FS) is helpful in individuals with dry scalps unable to tolerate daily shampooing with other products. Cases resistant to the foregoing treatments may respond to a 1- to 3-week course of oral ketoconazole, 200 mg/day.
    c. For **infantile seborrheic dermatitis,** the usual approach is conservative, with the use of a mild, nonmedicated shampoo (eg, baby shampoo used twice a week) first, followed by the use of a shampoo containing coal tar in resistant cases. Topical steroids should be avoided in infants if possible, because of significant percutaneous absorption.

12. **Nummular eczema** may respond to measures for **atopic dermatitis.**

REFERENCES

Cyr PR, Dreher GK: Neurotic excoriations. Am Fam Physician 2001;**64:**1981.
Hainer BL: Dermatophytic infections. Am Fam Physician 2003;**67:**101.
Koo J, Lebwohl A: Psychodermatology: The mind and skin connection. Am Fam Physician 2001;**64:**1873.
Moses S: Pruritus. Am Fam Physician 2003;**68:**1135.
Peate WF: Occupational skin disease. Am Fam Physician 2002;**66:**1025.
Russell JJ: Topical tacrolimus: A new therapy for atopic dermatitis. Am Fam Physician 2002;**66:**1899.

15   Dermatologic Neoplasms

Douglas G. Browning, MD, ATC-L

KEY POINTS

- The primary preventable cause of skin malignancies is chronic sun exposure.
- For any lesion exhibiting uncertain behavior, a biopsy should be done to rule out malignancy.
- A person with a history of a skin malignancy should have regular skin examinations to rule out any suspicious lesions.
- Early treatment or removal of actinic keratoses reduces a person's risk of developing squamous cell carcinoma.
- Melanoma is the skin malignancy with the poorest prognosis.

I. **Definition.** Neoplasm means new growth. A **dermatologic neoplasm** occurs when skin or subcutaneous cells begin to abnormally proliferate. Such new growths are extremely common and may be benign, premalignant, or malignant. They may arise in the **epidermis** (eg, acrochordon, keratoacanthoma, seborrheic keratoses, basal and squamous cell carcinomas, malignant melanoma, lentigines, nevi, verrucae, actinic keratoses), the **dermis** (eg, sebaceous hyperplasia, dermatofibromas, pyogenic granulomas, cherry angiomas, epidermoid cyst), or **subcutaneously** (eg, lipomas).

II. **Common Diagnoses.** Of patients who consult primary care physicians for skin problems, ~20% are diagnosed as having skin neoplasm or tumor. The skin is the most common cancer site, with over 1 million new cases of skin cancer diagnosed each year.

A. **Macular lesions**

1. All individuals develop **nevi** (moles), aberrant collections of melanocytes in the epidermis, dermis, or dermo-epidermal junction. Approximately 1% of infants have one or more nevi at birth. These nevi increase during adolescence to an average of 20–40 lesions by the third decade, and few remain by age 90. These lesions are more prevalent in whites, and sun exposure increases their number.

2. **Ephelides ("freckles") and lentigines** are hyperpigmented macular lesions found most commonly in children or young adults with light complexions. In elderly individuals, these lesions become more prevalent in sun-exposed areas, where they are recognized as age or liver spots.

3. **Giant congenital nevus** (bathing trunk nevus) is a large but rare nevus apparent at birth. Malignant melanoma occurs in 4–6% of patients; this transformation occurs in 50% before puberty.

4. **Mongolian patch** occurs in up to 80% of Asian, East Indian, and African American newborns, and 10% of whites.

5. **Atypical mole syndrome (dysplastic nevus syndrome)** is a familial autosomal dominant syndrome in which an individual may have >100 nevi (macular or papular). The risk for having cutaneous melanoma develop is 10–100 times that of the general population.

6. **Malignant melanomas** account for 2–3% of all skin cancers, but over two thirds of skin cancer mortality. Melanoma rates are highest in developed countries and areas closer to the equator. Greater ultraviolet light exposure through depletion of the ozone layer may contribute to the increasing incidence of melanoma; however, correlation with sun exposure is less frequent for melanoma than for basal and squamous cell cancers. Rather than duration, *intensity* of sun exposure (ie, a history of blistering sunburn before age 20) doubles the risk of melanoma. Precursors include atypical and congenital nevi, although most melanomas arise from apparently normal skin. A positive family history and a history of a previous (primary melanoma lesion) are also risk factors. Most individuals are diagnosed between the ages of 40 and 55; males and females are equally affected. The relative incidence of the four histologic subtypes of melanoma is:

    (1) **Superficial spreading** (70% of melanomas).
    (2) **Lentigo maligna** (12% of melanomas).

      (3) **Nodular** (10% of melanomas).
      (4) **Acral lentiginous** (8% of melanomas).
  B. Papular lesions
    1. Isolated lesions
      a. Nevi may be macular or papular.
      b. Cherry angiomas, dilated capillaries and postcapillary venules, occur in up to 50% of adults, beginning in young adulthood and increasing with age.
      c. Seborrheic keratoses (seborrheic or senile warts) are common in middle-aged and older individuals, occurring equally in men and women. They demonstrate autosomal dominant inheritance and are associated with oily-seborrheic skin.
      d. Verrucae (warts) can occur at any age, but are more common during the teenage years. Their incidence, severity, and prevalence are greater in the immunocompromised patient.
      e. Keratoacanthomas tend to occur in older individuals and may be related to sun exposure, human papillomavirus, or prolonged contact with coal tar derivatives.
      f. Pyogenic granulomas may be related to trauma or burns. They are most common in the first few years of life and incidence tends to decrease with age.
      g. Actinic keratoses are the most common premalignant skin lesions; they are found in middle-aged and older persons with light complexions and a history of chronic sun exposure. The lifetime risk of a cutaneous squamous cell carcinoma developing in an individual with actinic keratosis is approximately 20%.
      h. Basal cell carcinoma is the most common skin cancer. Two thirds of these neoplasms develop in sun-damaged areas of the body, and the remainder occur in covered areas where genetic disposition plays a role.
      i. Squamous cell carcinoma usually develops in sun-exposed areas of the body. The incidence of squamous cell cancer is higher in individuals with fair skin, immune disorders, outdoor occupations, and exposure to hydrocarbon fractions such as soot, coal tar, and lubricating oils.
    2. Eruptions of multiple lesions (**acrochordon, or skin tags**) are found in 25% of individuals and increase with age and obesity.
  C. Nodular lesions
    1. Lipomas, subcutaneous adipose cysts, occur in 1 of 1000 individuals. They are solitary in 80% of cases, but may be multiple, especially in young men.
    2. Dermatofibromas, subcutaneous scar tissue, may occur in reaction to trauma, insect sting, or folliculitis; multiple lesions may be associated with autoimmune disease.
    3. Epidermoid cysts are smooth, pearl-colored cysts that arise from the hair follicles.
    4. Sebaceous hyperplasia, enlarged sebaceous glands, are most common in middle-aged and older individuals; multiple sebaceous hyperplasia is associated with Gardner's syndrome.
III. Symptoms. Dermatologic neoplasms are often asymptomatic. When symptoms occur, they may include:
  A. Cosmetic change or disfigurement.
  B. Local irritation with friction from clothing (collars, bras, belts), jewelry, or skin folds, or trauma with shaving.
  C. Anxiety over changes in size or number of lesions, local discomfort, bleeding, discharge, or ulceration.
IV. Signs (Table 15–1).
  A. Common types of **verrucae (warts),** which can occur as single or grouped lesions, include:
    1. Flat warts (verruca plana), 1- to 3-mm lesions with smooth, flesh-colored surfaces, generally found on the face, neck, hands, and lower legs in a linear distribution.
    2. Periungual warts, rough-surfaced lesions found adjacent to and sometimes extending beneath the nails.
    3. Plantar warts, thick, coalescing lesions typically on the heels or balls of feet revealing pinpoint-sized bleeding points when pared.
    4. Genital warts (condylomata acuminata or venereal warts), velvety, moist, slightly raised, cauliflower-like lesions occurring singularly or in clusters genitally or perianally.

TABLE 15–1. DIFFERENTIAL DIAGNOSIS OF COMMON SKIN NEOPLASMS

Palpation	Lesion	Appearance	Location
Macule (flat skin discoloration)	Lentigines (B)	Tan to dark brown	Sun-exposed areas
	Ephelides ("freckles") (B)	Tan, darken with sun exposure	Sun-exposed, especially face
	Giant nevus (P)	Brown-black; macular at birth; plaquelike/hairy later	Lower torso or buttocks
	Mongolian patch (B)	Large, irregular gray to bluish-black	Sacrum-buttock
	Atypical mole (P)	Sudden onset multiple nevi in adolescent	Back, scalp, buttock, upper/lower limbs
Macule or papule	Nevi (B)	Tan to dark brown, well-demarcated macular (junctional) or domed (compound)	Ubiquitous, especially above waist; face/neck (intradermal)
	Malignant melanoma (M)	Nevus increasing in size, changing color (*ABCD*)	Interscapular (males), back and lower legs (females)
Papule (≤1 cm circumscribed solid superficial skin elevation) Such lesions >1 cm are plaques	Cherry angioma (B)	Pleomorphic/sessile (intradermal) round, bright red to dark red, nonblanching with pressure	Trunk, extremities
	Seborrheic keratosis (B)	Tan to brown, warty, domed "stuck-on"	Face/neck/trunk (not palms or soles)
	Verrucae (B)	Flesh-colored, papular or plaque, smooth or cauliflowerlike	Face, hands, feet, genital
	Keratoacanthoma (B)	Fast-growing (2–4 wk) papular growth becoming keratinized, often umbilicated	Face, upper extremities
	Pyogenic granuloma (B)	Rapid-growing solitary red/yellow moist papule, developing stalk	Head, neck, extremities mucous membranes
	Actinic keratoses (P)	Rough, "fine sandpaper," pink to tan plaques	Sun-exposed (face, head, neck, dorsa of hands/forearms)
	Basal cell carcinoma (M)	Papular/nodular, pearly with superficial telangiectasias, possible central ("rodent") ulcer	Sun-exposed areas
	Squamous cell carcinoma (M)	Thickened, indurated, scaly (often at site of actinic keratosis)	Sun-exposed areas
	Acrochordon (B)	1 mm–1 cm flesh-colored to brownish, pedunculated	Intertriginous/friction areas (neck/axillae, waist)
Nodule (≤1 cm solid lesion with depth); lesions >1 cm are tumors	Lipoma (B)	Firm, rubbery domed, flesh-colored, mobile, 2–10 cm	Especially shoulders, neck, trunk, arms
	Dermatofibroma (B)	Brown, yellow, pink 3- to 10-mm plaques or papule/nodules	Anterior surface lower legs
	Epidermoid cyst (B)	Round, mobile, skin-colored, with central keratin punctum	Back, face, chest
	Sebaceous hyperplasia (B)	Soft, skin-colored or yellow, domed	Forehead, cheeks, nose

B, benign; **P**, premalignant; **M**, malignant; *ABCD* (**A**symmetry, **B**order irregularity, **C**olor variation, and **D**iameter ≥5 mm).

B. **Epidermoid cysts** may become fluctuant and tender if inflamed.
C. **Atypical nevi (dysplastic nevus syndrome)** differ from common nevi in size (5–10 mm compared to <6 mm for common nevi), shape and contour (irregular borders with poor margination compared to symmetric, uniform borders for common nevi), and color (intra- and interlesional variations of brown, black, or red compared to more homogenous variations of tan, brown, or black for common nevi).
D. **Melanomas** classically show **a**symmetry, **b**order irregularity, **c**olor variation, and **d**iameter >5 mm (*ABCD*).

V. Laboratory Tests. In most cases, where physical examination clarifies the nature of a lesion, no further testing is necessary. Biopsies of suspicious lesions should be done. These lesions include:
  - **A. Newly discovered moles** in a patient older than 40 years.
  - **B. Mole >0.5 cm** accompanied by any tenderness, itching, bleeding, or ulceration.
  - **C. Lesions with recent growth, ulceration,** or characteristics suggestive of basal cell carcinoma, squamous cell carcinoma, or melanoma.
VI. Treatment
  - **A. Benign neoplasms** (Also see the sidebar on less common skin neoplasms.)
      1. **Nevi** usually require no treatment except for cosmetic or diagnostic purposes. Most are easily removed by shave, punch, or excisional biopsy.
          - a. **Shave excision** (Figure 15–1A) is useful for elevated lesions and those in which depth of excision is unimportant.
          - b. **Punch biopsy** (Figure 15–1B) is an easy way to obtain a full-thickness diagnostic specimen, although irregular, large, or cystic lesions may be better off excised.
          - c. **Excisional biopsy** (Figure 15–1C) allows for a complete, full-thickness excision of a worrisome skin lesion.

LESS COMMON SKIN NEOPLASMS

Neurofibromas are uncommon benign neoplasms arising from nerve sheath cells. They manifest as single or multiple submucosal nodules, sometimes with "café-au-lait" spots in the overlying skin. Surgical excision will cure single neurofibromas. The multiple form is inherited, causes disfigurement, and may lead to malignant change with a poor long-term prognosis.

---

   2. Removal of **seborrheic keratoses** may be achieved by cryosurgery or by shave excision after anesthetizing the skin with a local anesthetic.
   3. **Warts**
       - a. **Flat warts** may be treated with **cryosurgery** or **topical keratolytics (eg, cantharidin** (Cantharone), **bichloroacetic acid,** or **salicylic acid).** Alternatively, **tretinoin (retinoic acid)** cream or lotion (0.025%, 0.05%, or 0.1%) can be applied once or twice daily to produce mild inflammation and subsequent regression (may require several weeks). **Fluorouracil** (Efudex) cream, 5%, applied once or twice a day for 3–5 weeks, is also effective. Even weekly occlusion of the lesion with **duct tape,** with removal of the devitalized skin between applications, proved to be 85% effective in eradicating warts within 2 months according to one small study on a pediatric population.
       - b. **Periungual warts** should be treated cautiously because of the proximity of the nail bed. **Cryosurgery** can be done, taking care to avoid injury to the nail matrix and superficial nerves. Alternatively, **topical keratolytics** (section VI,A,3,a) may be applied weekly until the wart regresses. Occasionally, eradication can only be achieved by blunt dissection.
       - c. **Plantar warts** may cause foot pain. Topical keratolytic agents (section VI,A,3,a) may be used, but treatment usually requires several weeks. Application of **40% salicylic acid** under an occlusive pad to a wart that has been pared to its core has been successful. The pad should be reapplied every 24–48 hours, scraping away the devitalized skin between applications. Intralesional injection of a 1 U/mL solution of **bleomycin sulfate** is reported to have a cure rate of 48%. **Cryosurgery** or **excision** of these warts may be effective, but tends to temporarily cause pain and loss of mobility.
       - d. Treatment of **anogenital warts** (**condylomata acuminata** or venereal warts) is discussed in Chapter 31.
   4. **Lentigines** pose no health threat. Removal by topical or surgical techniques is unnecessary, and lesions tend to recur. Routine use of sunscreens or creams containing hydroquinone may make these lesions less noticeable.
   5. **Mongolian patch** generally fades during the first few months to the first year of life.

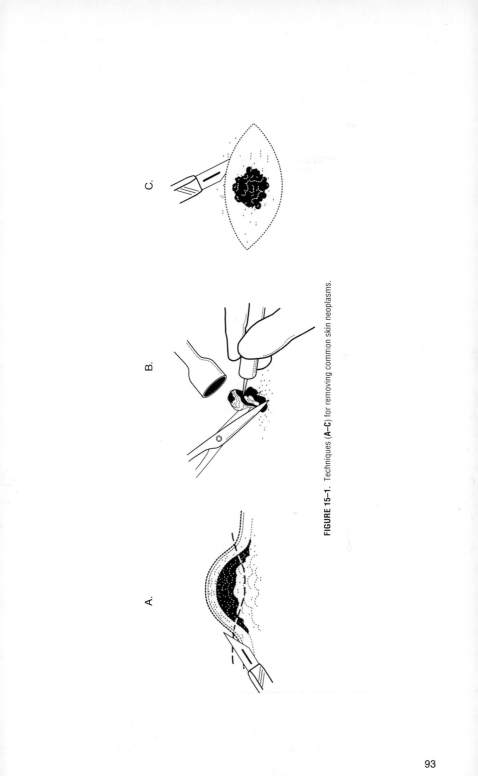

FIGURE 15–1. Techniques (**A–C**) for removing common skin neoplasms.

6. **Cherry angiomas** may be electrocauterized or removed by shave excision after local anesthesia, if necessary, but are usually left alone.

7. **Sebaceous hyperplasia** does not require treatment except for cosmetic purposes. Individual lesions may be removed by light cauterization. When they are severe, extensive, or disfiguring, oral isotretinoin (or in females, antiandrogens) may help improve their appearance.

8. **Acrochordon** ("skin tags") may be removed by cryosurgery with liquid nitrogen or by snip excision with sharp iris scissors.

9. **Dermatofibromas** require no treatment unless the lesion is symptomatic from repeated trauma, in which case partial removal with cryosurgery or shave excision may be indicated. For lesions that have recently changed in size or color, punch or elliptical excision with biopsy is indicated.

10. Although **keratoacanthoma** are benign, excision or destruction is recommended to prevent disfigurement from their aggressive expansion. Cryosurgery; topical 5-fluorouracil; intralesional 5-fluorouracil or methotrexate or interferon alfa 2a; or electrodesiccation can be used.

11. **For pyogenic granuloma,** shave excision is recommended to rule out amelanotic melanoma. If multiple lesions exist, local destruction may be accomplished by electrodesiccation or topical application of silver nitrate.

12. **Epidermoid (sebaceous) cysts** must be completely excised to prevent recurrence of the cyst. A small incision over the cyst will allow access; removal of the intact cyst and contents is desirable if possible. If the lesion is friable and intact removal is not possible, the cavity should be curetted to remove all parts of the cell wall and filled with an iodoform gauze wick. Antistaphylococcal antibiotics may be necessary if the cyst is infected.

13. **Lipomas** generally require no treatment, unless they interfere with the movement of adjacent muscles, in which case they may be removed by simple surgical excision or liposuction.

B. **Premalignant lesions** should be treated to prevent malignant degeneration. Patients with these lesions should be educated regarding **sun protection** (ie, covering exposed areas), **use of sunscreens** with a sun protection factor of 15 or more, **avoidance of sun exposure** between 10 AM and 4 PM, performance of regular **skin self-examination,** and avoidance of tanning salons.

   1. **Actinic keratoses.** Untreated actinic keratoses may progress to squamous cell carcinomas. **Electrodesiccation with curettage** or **excision** or **cryosurgery** is practical if lesions are few. For more extensive lesions, **topical 5-fluorouracil** (Efudex) is an effective alternative treatment available to primary care physicians.

      a. **For lesions on the face or lips,** a 1–2% solution or cream is applied twice daily. Over 2–4 weeks, lesions undergo inflammation, necrosis, and ulceration. With ulceration, treatment is discontinued and healing should begin to occur. Topical steroids may be used to decrease post-treatment inflammation as needed.

      b. **Actinic lesions on the scalp, neck, thorax, and extremities** are treated with a 5% concentration of 5-fluorouracil cream.

      c. **Tretinoin** (0.05% or 0.1%) **cream,** applied daily, may be used in patients with mild actinic damage.

      d. **Dermabrasion** and **chemical peel** are also effective, but should be performed only by physicians trained and experienced in these techniques.

   2. **Giant congenital nevi.** Most lesions are small and remain benign, but occasionally are extensive and cover a large area of the chest, back, shoulders, sacrum, or buttocks. They have a significant risk for malignant change. Patients with congenital nevi >20 cm in diameter should be referred to a plastic surgeon within the first decade of life for evaluation.

   3. **Atypical mole syndrome.** This syndrome should generally be referred to a dermatologist for frequent examinations, serial photographs, and early excision of any suspicious lesions.

C. **Malignant lesions** should be excised and submitted for pathologic examination.

   1. **Basal cell cancers.** Untreated basal cell carcinoma grows slowly, invading contiguous soft tissue, bone, and cartilage; metastasis is rare. The method of removal depends on lesion size, location, and physician preference. Treatment technique usually involves **excision,** although **electrodesiccation and curettage, cryosurgery,** and **radiation** have also been used. Punch or shave biopsy may be used

initially to confirm the diagnosis. **Basal cell cancers <2 cm** may be removed by a primary care physician using an elliptical excision to obtain clear margins around the lesion (Figure 15–1C). Clear margins surrounding the lesion in all directions should be verified by pathology. **Basal cell cancers >2 cm and those located on the nose, eye, or ear** should be referred for expert surgical removal. This might include excision by a dermatologist trained in **Mohs micrographic surgery,** or excision by a plastic surgeon.

2. **Squamous cell carcinomas.** Spread most commonly occurs by local extension and, less commonly, by metastasis. Management is similar to that of basal cell neoplasms, except that topical fluorouracil may be used for lesions arising from actinic keratoses. Squamous cell lesions arising within chronic ulcers, burns, or scar tissue or in mucous membranes have a high metastatic potential, and patients with such lesions should be referred to a specialist.

3. **Malignant melanomas.** Malignant melanomas have a tendency to spread rapidly and metastasize early. Thickness >1.70 mm or distal spread at diagnosis indicates a poor prognosis for survival. Patients with melanoma should be referred to an experienced surgeon for excision and need regular follow-up for recurrent disease.

REFERENCES

Champion RH, et al (editors): *Textbook of Dermatology,* 6th ed., vol. 2. Blackwell; 1998.
Habif TP: *Clinical Dermatology: A Color Guide to Diagnosis and Therapy,* 3rd ed. Mosby; 1995.
Jerant AF, et al: Early detection and treatment of skin cancer. Am Fam Physician 2000;**62:**357.
Luba MC, et al: Common benign skin tumors. Am Fam Physician 2003;**67:**729.
Rose LC: Recognizing neoplastic skin lesions: A photo guide. Am Fam Physician 1998;**58:**873.

---

16   Diarrhea

Jeanne M. Ferrante, MD

KEY POINTS

- Most episodes of acute diarrhea are self-limited.
- A thorough history is crucial to accurate patient assessment.
- Supportive care is usually the only required treatment.

I. **Definition. Diarrhea** is an increased number (three or more) or decreased consistency of stools (soft or liquid) during a 24-hour period.
   A. Duration of symptoms of 14 days or less is **acute diarrhea.** Causes include:
      1. **Viral infections** (eg, rotavirus, enteric adenovirus, Norwalk virus).
      2. **Bacterial infections** characterized as **enterotoxigenic** (*Escherichia coli/ Staphylococcus aureus/Bacillus cereus/Clostridium perfringens/Clostridium difficile*) or **inflammatory** (*Salmonella* spp/*Shigella* spp/*Campylobacter* spp/*Yersinia enterocolitica/Shiga toxin producing E coli* 0157:H7 [*STEC*]).
      3. **Parasitic infections** (eg, *Giardia lamblia, Cryptosporidium*).
      4. **Drugs** (eg, caffeine, alcohol, other prescription and over-the counter drugs).
      5. **Miscellaneous noninfectious causes** (eg, irritable bowel syndrome; fecal impaction with paradoxical diarrhea; inflammatory bowel disease; or ingestions of large amounts of lactose, fructose, or artificial sweeteners).
   B. Symptoms lasting more than 14 days define **persistent diarrhea,** and symptoms lasting more than 1 month constitute **chronic diarrhea.**
      1. **Chronic diarrhea** may be classified as:
         a. **Watery**—due to the following:
            (1) **Osmotic factors** (large volume decreased with fasting—eg, magnesium laxatives, lactase deficiency).

      (2) **Secretory factors** (endogenous—large volume not decreased with fasting, eg, carcinoid, gastrinoma; exogenous—large volume decreased with removal of offending agent, eg, stimulant laxatives, medications, toxins).

      (3) **Dysmotility** (eg, irritable bowel syndrome, diabetes, thyrotoxicosis).

  b. **Inflammatory**—due to **infections** (possibly with fever, eosinophilia—eg, parasitic, helminthic); **inflammatory bowel disease** (with fever, hematochezia—eg, ulcerative colitis); **neoplasia; ischemia;** or **radiation.**

  c. **Fatty**—due to **malabsorption** (eg, celiac disease) or **maldigestion** (eg, pancreatic insufficiency).

II. **Common Diagnoses.** Diarrhea is one of the most common symptoms for which patients visit their doctor. In the United States, there are an estimated 211 to 375 million annual episodes of diarrheal illnesses, resulting in 73 million physician visits, 1.8 million hospitalizations, and 3100 deaths. Approximately one third of travelers to less developed areas of the world (eg, Mexico, Latin America, Africa, the Middle East, and Asia) will have travelers' diarrhea, causing 40% of those affected to alter their travel plans, 20% to be bed-bound for at least 1 day, and 1% to require hospitalization. The prevalence of chronic diarrhea is estimated to be 5%, and the economic impact from medical care, disability, and lost productivity may exceed $350 million annually.

  For other causes of diarrhea, see the sidebars on sexually transmitted proctitis and colon ischemia.

A. **Acute diarrhea.** Most acute diarrhea is due to infections and usually occurs after the ingestion of contaminated food or water, or by direct person-to-person contact. **Underlying medical conditions** predisposing to infections include extremes of age, recent hospitalization, impaired immune system, human immunodeficiency virus, immunosuppressive therapy for organ transplant, long-term prednisone therapy, cancer chemotherapy, immunoglobulin A deficiency, or prior gastrectomy. **Other risk factors** include recent travel to developing countries, day care attendance, residence at an institution (nursing home, psychiatric facility, prison), and certain occupations (farmer, food handler, health care or day care provider). The common causes include:

  1. **Viral** (70–80% of acute infectious diarrhea). **Rotavirus,** the most frequent cause, typically presents in winter and may be transmitted by aerosol spread as well as through the fecal-oral route. Most cases occur between the ages of 3 months and 2 years. **Enteric adenoviruses** are the second most common type. Contaminated water, salads, and shellfish may transmit **Norwalk virus.**

  2. **Bacterial** (10–20% of acute cases). Risk factors include consumption of cooked foods that are later refrigerated, such as custard, pastries, and processed meats (*S aureus*); raw or undercooked meat (*Salmonella, Yersinia, STEC*) or seafood (*Vibrio, Plesiomonas*); improperly refrigerated foods (*B cereus, C perfringens*); or unpasteurized milk, juice, soft cheese, or unheated deli meats (*Listeria monocytogenes*). *Enterotoxigenic E coli* is the most common cause of travelers' diarrhea. *C difficile* causes approximately 20% of antibiotic-associated diarrhea. The most common antibiotics to cause *C difficile* infection are clindamycin, cephalosporins, and penicillin derivatives taken in the past 8 weeks.

  3. **Parasitic** (<10% of acute diarrhea). Parasitic infections (*G lamblia, Cryptosporidium, Entamoeba histolytica*) are uncommon in the general population but may be more prevalent in children in day-care centers, residents of mental institutions or nursing homes, immunocompromised persons, or persons exposed to untreated water from a lake or stream. *E histolytica* may be found in up to 30% of homosexual men.

  4. **Drugs.** Common causes include laxatives, anti-ulcer drugs, antibiotics, cardiovascular drugs, nonsteroidal anti-inflammatory drugs, antiparkinson drugs, colchicine, and excessive caffeine or alcohol. Any new drug or recent dosage change may result in diarrhea.

SEXUALLY TRANSMITTED PROCTITIS

Sexually transmitted proctitis can cause rectal pain, small-volume bloody diarrhea, and tenesmus. **Herpesvirus, gonorrhea, chlamydia,** and **syphilis** are likely causes. Those at risk are homosexual men and receptive partners during anal intercourse. Diagnosis is by sigmoidoscopy and cultures. Treatment consists of antiviral drugs or antibiotics for the sexually transmitted disease.

COLON ISCHEMIA

Colon ischemia is a rare cause of diarrhea, but it can be life-threatening. The diarrhea may be associated with mild to moderate abdominal pain or lower intestinal bleeding. Risk factors include recent aortic or cardiac bypass surgery, vasculitides (eg, systemic lupus erythematosus), infections (eg, *STEC*, **cytomegalovirus**), coagulopathies (eg, protein C and S deficiencies), medications (eg, oral contraceptives), drugs (eg, cocaine), long-distance running, preceding major cardiovascular episode with hypotension, and obstructing lesions of the colon (eg, carcinoma). Diagnosis is by colonoscopy or barium enema. Most cases resolve spontaneously and do not require specific therapy. Patients with severe or continuing symptoms should be hospitalized and placed on bowel rest (nothing by mouth for 48–72 hours), intravenous fluids, and antibiotics. Surgery is required for patients with peritoneal signs or those who are unresponsive to medical therapy.

    B. The differential diagnosis of **chronic diarrhea** is very extensive (Table 16–1).
        1. Most chronic diarrheas in **adults** are caused by:
            a. Irritable bowel syndrome (IBS), a complex of abnormal gastrointestinal motility, altered visceral sensation, and psychological factors, occurs in 20% of the US population, but only 10–20% of people with irritable bowel syndrome seek medical care. In more than 50% symptoms develop before age 35, and women are twice as likely to have irritable bowel syndrome develop as men.

TABLE 16–1. MAJOR CAUSES OF CHRONIC DIARRHEA

Osmotic diarrhea	**Secretory diarrhea**
Mg^{2+},PO_4^{-3},SO_4^{-2} ingestion	Addison's disease
Carbohydrate malabsorption	Bacterial toxins
Lactose intolerance	Disordered motility
Artificial sweeteners	Diabetic autonomic neuropathy
Excessive fructose	Irritable bowel syndrome
	Hyperthyroidism
Fatty diarrhea	Postsympathectomy
Malabsorption syndromes	Postvagotomy
Mucosal diseases	Drugs and poisons
Small bowel bacterial overgrowth	Idiopathic secretory diarrhea
Postresection diarrhea	Ileal bile acid malabsorption
Mesenteric ischemia	Inflammatory bowel disease
Maldigestion	Ulcerative colitis
Pancreatic insufficiency	Crohn's disease
Inadequate luminal bile acid (ileal resection)	Microscopic colitis
	Collagenous colitis
Inflammatory diarrhea	Diverticulitis
Inflammatory bowel disease	Neuroendocrine tumors
Ulcerative colitis	Carcinoid syndrome
Crohn's disease	Gastrinoma
Diverticulitis	Mastocytosis
Infections	Medullary carcinoma of thyroid
Pseudomembranous colitis	Somatostatinoma
Invasive bacteria	VIPoma
Yersinia, TB, others	Neoplasia
Ulcerating viral infections	Colon carcinoma
Cytomegalovirus	Lymphoma
Herpes simplex	Villous adenoma
Amebiasis/other invasive parasites	Vasculitis
Ischemic colitis	
Radiation colitis	
Neoplasia	
Colon cancer	
Lymphoma	

From Fine KD, Shiller LR: AGA technical review on the evaluation and management of chronic diarrhea. Gastroenterology 1999;**116**:1464–1486, with permission.

    b. Lactose intolerance, which is genetically controlled and due to a normal decline in the intestinal lactase activity after childhood. It is present in 75–90% of US blacks, Asians, American Indians, persons of Mediterranean origin, and Jews, compared to less than 5% of descendants of Northern and Central Europeans. Secondary lactose intolerance can develop from injury to the intestinal mucosa (eg, infectious diarrhea, celiac disease) or a decrease in mucosal surface (eg, resection), and is transient with successful treatment of the underlying disease.

    c. Idiopathic inflammatory bowel disease. Crohn's disease, characterized by transmural, focal, and asymmetric inflammation of any part of the gastrointestinal tract, occurs in 10–70 per 100,000 individuals and occurs most frequently in people of European descent, particularly Jews. The onset is usually in adolescence and young adulthood. **Ulcerative colitis** is a diffuse, continuous, superficial inflammation of the rectum and colon, occurring in 70–150 per 100,000 individuals. Its onset is between ages 15–35 years, with a second and smaller peak in the seventh decade. Ulcerative colitis is also more common in Jews, and there is a positive family history in approximately 10%. Occasionally, it develops after an acute infection.

    d. Malabsorption syndrome. Celiac disease, an autoimmune inflammatory disease of the small intestine precipitated by gluten ingestion, is more common than previously thought, at approximately 1 case per 250 persons. Approximately 75% of new adult cases are in women. Celiac disease should be considered in patients at genetic risk (ie, family history of celiac disease or personal history of type I diabetes) and in patients with unexplained chronic diarrhea, anemia, fatigue, or weight loss.

    e. Chronic infections (usually parasitic infections). Risk factors include travel to endemic areas, including Russia (*Giardia*), Nepal (*Cyclospora*), or any developing country (*E histolytica*), and drinking from lakes or streams (*Giardia*). Immunosuppressed individuals and the elderly may have persistent diarrhea from *Campylobacter* and *Salmonella*. Risk factors for relapse of *C difficile* infection (20% of patients) include intercurrent antibiotics, renal failure, and female sex. Other uncommon bacterial causes include *Aeromonas* (untreated water), *Plesiomonas* (foreign travel, raw shellfish, untreated water), *Yersinia* (contaminated stream and lake water, milk or ice cream), *Mycobacterium tuberculosis* (travel to undeveloped country).

 2. In **children,** most chronic diarrheas are due to the following factors:

    a. Postinfectious diarrhea. Postinfectious diarrhea is characterized by the persistence of diarrhea and failure to gain weight more than 7 days after hospital admission for gastroenteritis. Risk factors include being a neonate or very young; being nonwhite; using antibiotics or antidiarrheal agents before admission; or having a previous history of diarrhea, a longer duration of diarrhea before hospitalization, severe diarrhea during the initial enteritis, weight below the tenth percentile, low blood urea nitrogen, and bacterial etiology of the initial enteritis.

    b. Primary lactase deficiency. This deficiency starts between ages 3 and 5 years. Secondary lactose intolerance develops in 50% or more of infants with acute or chronic diarrhea (especially with rotavirus) and is also fairly common with giardiasis, inflammatory bowel disease, and the AIDS malabsorption syndrome.

    c. Cow's milk and soy protein hypersensitivity. Cow's milk hypersensitivity is the most common sensitivity in infancy, with an incidence between 0.3% and 7.0%. Thirty to 50% of infants with cow's milk protein sensitivity also may have soy protein hypersensitivity. Most patients achieve tolerance during their second year of life.

    d. Celiac disease (See section II,B,1,d).

    e. Chronic nonspecific diarrhea. Chronic nonspecific diarrhea (irritable bowel syndrome of children or toddler's diarrhea) appears between 6 months and 2 years of age. The cause is unknown but may follow an acute infection or gastroenteritis. It is self-limited, usually resolving spontaneously before age 4.

    Infrequent causes of chronic diarrhea in children include immune deficiencies, AIDS, endocrine disorders (eg, hyperthyroidism, adrenal insufficiency, diabetes), and anatomic lesions (eg, Hirschsprung's disease). Pseudomembranous enterocolitis with *C difficile* is rare, but it is severe and sometimes fatal. It is precipitated by antibiotics and causes profuse diarrhea, dehydration, abdominal pain, fever, electrolyte imbalance, hypoproteinemia, and leukocytosis.

III. Symptoms. A thorough history is key in guiding the evaluation and management of patients with diarrhea. Important questions include **when and how the illness began** (abrupt or gradual onset, duration of diarrhea), **stool characteristics** (frequency; quantity; watery, bloody, mucus-filled, purulent, greasy), symptoms of **dehydration** (thirst, lethargy, postural lightheadedness, decreased urination), presence of **dysentery** (fever; tenesmus; blood, pus, or both), and **associated symptoms** (nausea, vomiting, abdominal cramps, bloating, constipation, flatus or belching, headache, myalgias).

In **chronic diarrhea**, a history of **other medical conditions** may be helpful in diagnosis, such as seronegative spondyloarthropathies (inflammatory bowel disease), autoimmune diseases such as diabetes or thyroid disorders (chronic dysmotility diarrhea, celiac disease), and immune deficiencies (infections). Patients should be asked about **fecal incontinence,** especially with low-volume stools, because the evaluation for incontinence differs from that of diarrhea. **Previous surgery** to the gastrointestinal or biliary tracts may be the cause of chronic diarrhea. Use of all **current medications** including over-the-counter medicines, nutritional supplements, illicit drugs, and alcohol and caffeine should be elicited. Questions on antibiotic use in the past 8 weeks, a new or increased dose in medication, and laxative use should be specifically asked.

A. Viral diarrheas are usually self-limited, large volume, and watery, without blood, lasting from 1–2 days to 1 week. There may be nausea, vomiting, headache, low-grade fever, cramping, and malaise. Dehydration, especially in children, can occur.

B. Bacterial diarrhea
  1. **Food poisoning** by *S aureus* and *B cereus* cause symptoms within 1–6 hours of exposure. *C perfringens* causes symptoms within 8–16 hours. These symptoms are of sudden onset and generally last 2–12 hours. Nausea and vomiting are variable with some abdominal cramping. There is usually no fever, severe abdominal pain, headache, malaise, myalgia, or prolonged nausea and vomiting.
  2. Most **invasive bacterial diarrheas** are more gradual in onset, causing symptoms after 16 hours and lasting 1–7 days. Fever; tenesmus; and gross blood, pus, or both are usually present. *STEC* causes bloody diarrhea without high fever or leukocytes. Severe cases may lead to hemolytic-uremic syndrome (bloody diarrhea, thrombocytopenia, hemolytic anemia, and renal failure). Infection with *C difficile* can occur several days to 8 weeks after use of antibiotics. Watery diarrhea and abdominal cramps are typical. In severe cases, bloody diarrhea, fever, and abdominal pain can be present. There is usually no nausea or vomiting.

C. Parasitic diarrhea
  1. *G lamblia* causes watery diarrhea, sometimes with mucus. Nausea, anorexia, abdominal cramping, flatulence, steatorrhea, and weight loss may be present.
  2. *Cryptosporidium* causes prolonged diarrhea, associated with fatigue, flatulence, and abdominal pain. Fever is usually not present.
  3. Clinical symptoms of *E histolytica* vary from asymptomatic carriage to severe bloody diarrhea that can be indistinguishable from ulcerative colitis. Abdominal cramping, diarrhea with blood or mucus, and malaise are common. In severe cases, massive bleeding, obstruction, dilation, or perforation may occur. Liver abscesses may result from systemic spread.

D. Chronic diarrhea. Watery stools suggest osmotic or secretory diarrhea. **Gross blood in the stool** suggests inflammatory bowel or malignancy. The description of **foul-smelling,** light-colored, floating stool, or undigested foods in stool suggests malabsorption.
  1. The Manning criteria are helpful to differentiate **irritable bowel syndrome** from organic pathology. Four or more criteria make the diagnosis likely. The presence of less than two of the following excludes the diagnosis: pain relief with bowel movement, more frequent stools with onset of pain, looser stools with onset of pain, passage of mucus, sensation of incomplete evacuation, and abdominal distention as evidenced by tight clothing or visible appearance. In irritable bowel syndrome of children, the child may have 4–10 loose mucoid stools per day, mainly in the morning. The growth and development are normal, and there is no malabsorption.
  2. The severity of symptoms in **lactose intolerance** varies with the lactose load and other foods consumed at the same time, and may include diarrhea, bloating,

cramping, abdominal discomfort, flatulence, and rumbling (borborygmi). In children, vomiting is common and malnutrition can occur.

3. **Crohn's disease** typically presents with diarrhea, abdominal pain, and weight loss. The clinical picture of **ulcerative colitis** is variable, from occasional rectal bleeding to profuse watery and bloody diarrhea with crampy lower abdominal pain and weight loss.

4. **Celiac disease** may present with a range of symptoms including diarrhea, constipation, dyspepsia, gastroesophageal reflux, bloating, flatus, belching, fatigue, weight loss, depression, fibromyalgia-like symptoms, aphthous stomatitis, hair loss, and bone pain. Infants typically present with failure to thrive, diarrhea, abdominal distention, developmental delay, and occasionally, severe malnutrition. Older children may have constitutional short stature or dental enamel defects.

IV. **Signs.** The physical examination is most important in assessing volume status and nutrition. Other clinical signs may be important clues in differentiating chronic causes of diarrhea.

A. **Vital signs.** Fever greater than 101.3 °F suggests acute inflammatory diarrhea. Postural changes in systolic blood pressure (decrease of 10 mm Hg) and pulse rate (increase of 20 beats per minute) support dehydration. In children, acute body weight changes best assess dehydration; other helpful measurements include dry mucous membranes, decreased capillary refill time, absence of tears, and alteration in mental status. In chronic cases, weight loss and failure to thrive suggest malabsorption, inflammatory bowel disease, infection, and neoplasm.

B. **Skin.** Characteristic skin changes can be seen in less common causes of chronic diarrhea, such as carcinoid syndrome (flushing, telangiectasias), celiac disease (dermatitis herpetiformis), mastocytosis (urticaria, linear telangiectasias), and Addison's disease (hyperpigmentation).

C. **Oral.** Aphthous oral ulcers and stomatitis may be present in inflammatory bowel disease or celiac disease.

D. **Thyroid.** Nodules or mass may suggest medullary carcinoma of thyroid or thyroid adenoma.

E. **Cardiac.** Right-sided heart murmur may be present in carcinoid syndrome. Signs of severe atherosclerosis or peripheral vascular disease may be present with intestinal ischemia.

F. **Abdominal examination.** This examination should assess for distention (irritable bowel syndrome, infections), bruit (colon ischemia), tenderness (irritable bowel syndrome, inflammatory bowel disease, infections, ischemia), mass (neoplasia), and hepatosplenomegaly (amyloidosis).

G. **Rectal examination.** This examination should evaluate sphincter tone (fecal incontinence) and tenderness (proctitis). The presence of fistula, painless anal fissure, or a perirectal abscess may suggest Crohn's disease. Fecal impaction in pediatric or geriatric age groups may suggest overflow diarrhea.

H. **Extremities.** Edema and clubbing suggest malabsorption. Arthritis may be noted in inflammatory bowel disease, Whipple's disease, and some enteric infections.

I. **Lymphadenopathy.** Lymphadenopathy may suggest lymphoma or other neoplasm.

V. **Laboratory Tests**

A. **Acute diarrhea** (Figure 16–1). Testing is needed only in patients with dysentery, patients aged younger than 3 months or older than 70 years, immunocompromised patients, patients with persistent diarrhea, or those at risk of transmitting infections (eg, food handlers in food service establishments, health care workers, or attendees/residents or employees of day care or an institutional facility such as a psychiatric hospital, prison, or nursing home).

B. **Chronic diarrhea** (Figure 16–2). Findings from the history, examination, routine laboratory tests, and quantitative stool analysis should guide specific, confirmatory testing or a trial of empiric therapy.

1. The **complete blood count** may show anemia (blood loss, malabsorption) or leukocytosis (infection).

2. A **chemistry screen** may be helpful in assessing fluid/electrolyte balance and nutritional status (malabsorption).

3. A **48-hour quantitative stool collection** on a regular diet of moderately high fat (80–100 g fat/day) can help classify diarrhea as osmotic, secretory, inflammatory, or fatty. The fecal analysis should include weight, electrolytes, calculation of osmo-

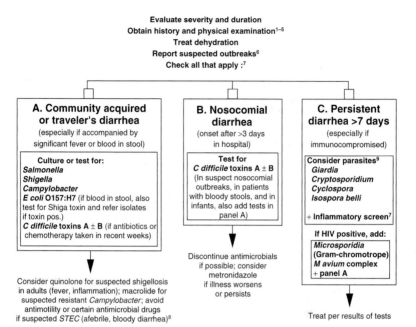

Evaluate severity and duration
Obtain history and physical examination[1-5]
Treat dehydration
Report suspected outbreaks[6]
Check all that apply :[7]

A. Community acquired or traveler's diarrhea
(especially if accompanied by significant fever or blood in stool)

Culture or test for:
Salmonella
Shigella
Campylobacter
E coli O157:H7 (if blood in stool, also test for Shiga toxin and refer isolates if toxin pos.)
C difficile toxins A ± B (if antibiotics or chemotherapy taken in recent weeks)

Consider quinolone for suspected shigellosis in adults (fever, inflammation); macrolide for suspected resistant Campylobacter; avoid antimotility or certain antimicrobial drugs if suspected STEC (afebrile, bloody diarrhea)[8]

B. Nosocomial diarrhea
(onset after >3 days in hospital)

Test for
C difficile toxins A ± B
(In suspect nosocomial outbreaks, in patients with bloody stools, and in infants, also add tests in panel A)

Discontinue antimicrobials if possible; consider metronidazole if illness worsens or persists

C. Persistent diarrhea >7 days
(especially if immunocompromised)

Consider parasites[9]
Giardia
Cryptosporidium
Cyclospora
Isospora belli
+ Inflammatory screen[7]

If HIV positive, add:
Microsporidia
(Gram-chromotrope)
M avium complex
+ panel A

Treat per results of tests

FIGURE 16–1. Diagnosis and management of acute diarrhea. [1]Seafood or seacoast exposure should prompt culture for *Vibrio* species. [2]Travelers' diarrheal illnesses that have not responded to empirical therapy should be managed with the above approach. [3]Persistent abdominal pain and fever should prompt culture for *Yersinia enterocolitica* and cold enrichment. Right-side abdominal pain without high fever but with bloody or nonbloody diarrhea should prompt culture for Shiga toxin producing *Escherichia coli* (*STEC*) O157. [4]Proctitis in symptomatic homosexual men can be diagnosed with sigmoidoscopy. Involvement in only the distal 15 cm suggests herpesvirus, gonococcal, chlamydial, or syphilitic infection; colitis extending more proximally suggests *Campylobacter, Shigella, Clostridium difficile*, or chlamydial (LGV serotype) infection, and noninflammatory diarrhea suggests giardiasis. [5]Postdiarrheal hemolytic uremic syndrome (HUS) should prompt testing of stools for *E coli* O157:H7 and for *Shiga* toxin (send isolates to reference laboratory if toxin-positive but *STEC*-negative). [6]Outbreaks should prompt reporting to health department. [7]Fecal lactoferrin testing or microscopy for leukocytes can help document inflammation. [8]Some experts recommend avoiding administration of antimicrobial agents to persons in the United States with bloody diarrhea. [9]Commonly used tests for parasitic causes of diarrhea include fluorescence and EIA for *Giardia* and *Cryptosporidium;* acid-fast stains for *Cryptosporidium, Cyclospora, Isospora,* or *Mycobacterium* species (as well as culture for *Mycobacterium avium* complex); and special chromotrope or other stains for *Microsporidia.* (Reproduced, with permission, from Guerrant RL, Van Gilder T, Steiner TS, et al: Practice guidelines for the management of infectious diarrhea. Clin Infect Dis 2001:**32**(3):331–351. University of Chicago Press.)

tic gap (290 – 2[Na$^+$ + K$^+$]), pH, occult blood, stool leukocytes (or lactoferrin), quantitative fecal fat and concentration, and analysis for laxatives.

VI. **Treatment** for acute and chronic diarrheas should include supportive measures as well as measures directed at underlying causes determined through careful history, examination, and appropriate laboratory evaluation (Figures 16–1 and 16–2).

A. **Maintenance of hydration and rehydration**

1. In the **healthy adult with mild to moderate acute diarrhea,** carbonated drinks, fruit juice, or sports drinks with saltine crackers are adequate. These should not be used in infants and young children because of excessive carbohydrate content and inadequate sodium and potassium.

2. For **children, the elderly, or those with moderate to severe diarrhea,** the World Health Organization formula or commercial oral rehydration solutions (ORS) such as Pedialyte, Rehydralyte, Infalyte, Naturalyte, or Resol are recommended and are superior to intravenous fluids in resolving diarrhea and gaining weight. **Homemade ORS** can be prepared using 8 oz apple, orange or other juice, ½ tsp corn syrup or

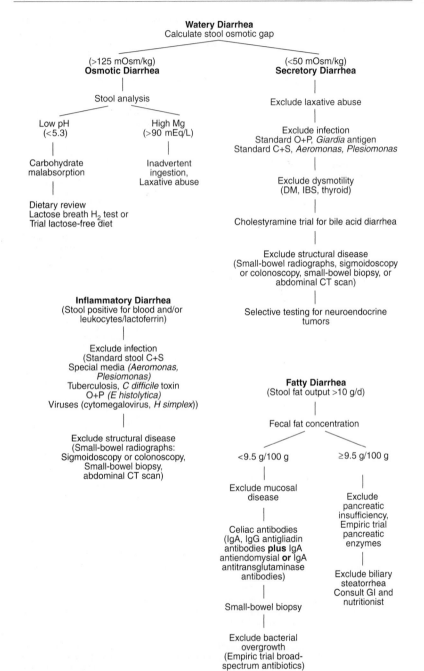

FIGURE 16–2. Further evaluation of chronic diarrhea. CT, computed tomography; DM, diabetes mellitus; GI, gastrointestinal; IBS, irritable bowel syndrome; O+P, ova and parasites test. Adapted from Fine KD, Shiller LR: AGA technical review on the evaluation and management of chronic diarrhea. Gastroenterology 1999;**116:**1464–1486, with permission.

honey, a pinch of salt, 8 oz water, and ¼ tsp of baking soda. **Rice-based ORS** decreases stool output compared to standard ORS and can be prepared by mixing ½ cup dry, precooked baby rice cereal with 2 cups water and ¼ tsp salt. Children should receive 30–60 mL ORS every 15 minutes with an additional 10 mL/kg for every stool or emesis.

3. In **severe dehydration** with obtunded mental status or when oral intake is not able to keep up with ongoing losses, intravenous fluids (0.9 N saline or Ringer's solution 20–40 mL/kg every hour for children, D5 Ringer's lactate or D5 0.9N saline 1 L every 1–2 hours for adults) should be given for 4–6 hours until adequate rehydration (determined by weight gain in children and clinical signs in adults) is established. The patient's usual diet supplemented with ORS can then be resumed.

B. Diet

1. **Children** should be continued on their preferred, usual, and age-appropriate diet. Frequent small feedings (every 10–60 minutes) of any tolerated foods or ORS may be helpful if vomiting occurs. Breast-feeding may be continued.

2. **Adults** should be encouraged to eat potatoes, rice, wheat, noodles, crackers, bananas, yogurt, boiled vegetables, and soup. Dairy products, caffeine, and alcohol should be avoided.

3. In **chronic diarrhea,** fasting can differentiate between osmotic diarrhea (which resolves with fasting) and some secretory diarrheas. Dietary measures beneficial in chronic diarrhea include eating a high-fiber diet for irritable bowel syndrome, avoiding lactose for lactose intolerance, and avoiding wheat, barley, and rye for celiac disease. In children with postinfectious diarrhea, management with a soy-based formula, lactose-free formula, or semielemental diet is indicated.

C. Symptomatic treatment

1. **Antimotility agents** may be considered in adult patients with watery, noninflammatory diarrhea. They should be avoided in young children and patients with dysentery. First-line therapies are usually opiate derivatives such as loperamide (Imodium) or diphenoxylate with atropine (Lomotil), used after each diarrheal movement, not to exceed 8 tablets per day.

2. In **chronic diarrhea,** bulk-forming agents (psyllium or methylcellulose) may be used to increase stool bulk and consistency, but they do not reduce stool weight. Opiates (eg, tincture of opium, 6 drops every 4–6 hours, or codeine, 15–30 mg every 4–6 hours) may be necessary.

D. Antibiotic treatment (See Table 16–2).

1. **Empiric treatment**

    a. Treatment for **travelers' diarrhea** without obtaining a stool specimen can reduce the duration from 3–5 days to less than 1–2 days.

    b. Patients with **persistent diarrhea** may be empirically treated for presumed giardiasis, especially if there was a history of travel or exposure to untreated water (eg, lake, stream, or well), and if other evaluations are negative.

    c. Empiric treatment can also be considered in those with **dysentery,** those who appear **septic or toxic,** and **high-risk patients** (infants younger than 3 months, persons older than 70 years, and immunocompromised patients) after a stool specimen is obtained.

    d. In **chronic diarrhea,** a therapeutic trial of broad-spectrum antibiotics may be considered for suspected small-bowel bacterial overgrowth (resulting from stasis of intestinal contents, eg, in diabetics with slowed intestinal motility, postgastrectomy, or persons with partial intestinal obstruction from Crohn's disease).

2. **Specific antibiotic treatment.** Other infections should be treated based on the specific causative organism. Antibiotics or antimotility agents should not be used in enterohemorrhagic shiga toxin producing *E coli* 0157:H7 (*STEC*), as they may enhance toxin release and increase the risk of hemolytic-uremic syndrome.

E. Probiotics

1. Probiotics containing *Lactobacillus species* or *Saccharomyces boulardii* can decrease the likelihood of **antibiotic-induced diarrhea** (from 23% to 13%) in children and adults. These products (eg, Culturelle) are sold over the counter and can be found in the vitamin or diarrhea section of the pharmacy. A typical dosage is 5–10 billion viable organisms three to four times a day in adults (half the dosage in children) for the duration of antibiotic use.

TABLE 16–2. ANTIBIOTIC TREATMENT FOR SPECIFIC PATHOGENS

Pathogen	Antibiotic of Choice	Alternative
Travelers' diarrhea	Fluoroquinolone[1] po bid × 3 d	TMP-SMZ[2] × 3 d, azithromycin 500 mg × 1, then 250 mg qd × 4 d (peds 5–10 mg/kg/d in 1 dose)
Shigella	Fluoroquinolone[1] po bid × 3 d	TMP-SMX[2] bid × 3 d, azithromycin 500 mg × 1 then 250 mg qd × 4 d, ceftriaxone 50–75 mg/kg/d × 2–5 d, nalidixic acid 1 g/d (children 55 mg/kg/d) × 5 d
Non-typhi species of *Salmonella*[3]	TMP-SMZ[2] bid × 5–7 d	Fluoroquinolone[1] po bid × 5–7 d, azithromycin 1 gm po once, then 500 mg qd × 6 d, ceftriaxone 100 mg/kg/d
Campylobacter species	Erythromycin 500 mg bid × 5 d	Fluoroquinolone[1] po bid × 7 d
Escherichia coli (except enterohemorrhagic)	TMP-SMZ[2] bid × 3 d	
Yersinia	Fluoroquinolone[1] po bid × 3 d, TMP-SMZ[2] bid × 3 d	Ceftriaxone 2 gm IV qd, doxycycline, aminoglycosides
Vibrio cholerae	Ciprofloxacin 1 gm po × 1	Doxycycline 300 mg single dose, TMP-SMZ[2] bid × 3 d
Aeromonas/Plesiomonas	TMP-SMZ[2] bid × 3 d	Fluoroquinolone[1] bid × 3 d
Clostridium difficile	Metronidazole 500 mg po tid × 10 d	Vancomycin 125–500 mg po qid × 10 d
Listeria monocytogenes	Ampicillin 200 mg/kg IV q6h	TMP-SMZ 20 mg/kg/d IV divided q6–8h
Giardia	Metronidazole 250 mg tid × 5 d	Furazolidone 100 mg qid × 7–10 d, paromomycin 500 mg qid × 7 d
Cryptosporidium species[3]	Paromomycin 1 gm po bid + azithromycin 600 mg po qd	
Isospora species	TMP-SMZ[2] bid × 10 d	Ciprofloxacin 500 mg bid × 7 d
Cyclospora species	TMP-SMZ[2] bid × 7–10 d	AIDS pt: TMP-SMZ[2] qid × 10 d, then 1 tab po 3×/week
Microsporidium species[3]	Albendazole 400 mg bid × 3 weeks	
Entamoeba histolytica	Metronidazole 500–750 mg tid × 5–10 d, followed by either iodoquinol 650 mg tid × 20 d or paromomycin 500 mg tid × 7 d	Tinidazole 1 gm po bid × 3 d or ornidazole 500 mg po bid × 5 d followed by either iodoquinol 650 mg tid × 20 d or paromomycin 500 mg tid × 7 d

[1] Ciprofloxacin 500 mg, ofloxacin 300 mg, or norfloxacin 400 mg.
[2] TMP-SMX: Bactrim DS or Septra DS, 160 mg/800 mg (pediatric dose, 5 mg/kg trimethoprim, 25 mg/kg sulfamethoxazole).
[3] Only for septic/toxic, extremes of age, or immunocompromised patients.

    2. In children, *Lactobacillus species* can reduce the duration of **acute diarrhea** (by 1–2 days) and duration of rotavirus shedding, but are most effective when given during the first 2.5 days of illness. The dosage is 10 billion colony-forming units twice daily for 5 days.

    F. Other agents for chronic diarrhea. Empiric trials of cholestyramine (for bile acid diarrheas, after ileal resection, vagotomy, or cholecystectomy) and pancreatic enzymes (for pancreatic insufficiency) may be diagnostic and therapeutic. Lactase capsules can be helpful in lactose intolerance.

REFERENCES

Acute Gastroenteritis Team: *Evidence Based Clinical Practice Guideline For Children With Acute Gastroenteritis.* Cincinnati Children's Hospital Medical Center; 2001:1–14.

Branski D, Lerner A, Lebenthal E: Chronic diarrhea and malabsorption. Ped Clin North Am 1996; **43**:307.

Fine KD, Schiller LR: AGA technical review on the evaluation and management of chronic diarrhea. Gastroenterology 1999;**116**:1464.

Guerrant RL, et al: Practice guidelines for the management of infectious diarrhea. Clin Infect Dis 2001;**32**:331.

Nelsen DA: Gluten-sensitive enteropathy (celiac disease): More common than you think. Am Fam Physician 2002;**66**:2259, 2269.

17 Dizziness

Diane J. Madlon-Kay, MD, MS

KEY POINTS

- Peripheral vestibular disorders are the most common cause of dizziness.
- A directed history and physical examination can usually rule out the few serious causes of dizziness.
- Treatment options are limited, although symptoms resolve spontaneously in most patients.

I. **Definition.** *Dizziness* is an imprecise term commonly used by patients to describe symptoms such as faintness, giddiness, lightheadedness, or unsteadiness.

II. **Common Diagnoses.** In up to 19% of cases, a definitive cause of dizziness cannot be found. The various diagnoses of dizziness can be divided into three main categories.

A. **Peripheral vestibular disorders,** which account for up to 44% of cases, include vestibular neuronitis, benign positional vertigo, Meniere's disease, acoustic neuroma (see sidebar), and otitis media. These patients have a disorder at some point along the course of the vestibular nerve other than at its origin in the brain stem. Most often, the problem is at the termination of the nerve in the inner ear, known as the labyrinth.

ACOUSTIC NEUROMA

Acoustic neuroma typically presents as unilateral tinnitus and hearing loss. Few patients have vertigo initially. Symptoms are slowly progressive, and continued growth of the tumor is associated with facial weakness and ataxia.

B. **Systemic diseases,** such as cardiac problems, diseases resulting from drug use, metabolic abnormalities, anemia, infection, and psychogenic causes, may result in dizziness. Twenty percent to 30% of all cases of dizziness are believed to be psychogenic. Disorders in almost any organ system can cause dizziness. Spatial orientation depends on the complex interaction of adequate sensation, central integration, and the proper motor response.

C. **Central nervous system diseases,** such as stroke, transient ischemic attack, or multiple sclerosis, are responsible for dizziness in 5% of patients (see sidebar). Any disease that disrupts the pathway between the vestibular apparatus and the brain may result in dizziness. Normally, impulses from this apparatus proceed through the eighth cranial nerve to the vestibular nuclei of the brain stem. From the brain stem, they are transmitted to the cerebellum and the cerebral cortex.

CENTRAL NERVOUS SYSTEM DISEASES

Central nervous system diseases, such as strokes, can cause vertigo. However, the vertigo is almost always accompanied by other central nervous system symptoms, such as facial numbness, hemiparesis, or diplopia. Dysarthria, facial numbness, hemiparesis, or diplopia may be found on examination.

III. **Symptoms.** Dizziness can be divided into four basic types: vertigo, presyncope, disequilibrium, and lightheadedness. The symptoms of each type are described in this section. Further details about the types of dizziness are shown in Table 17–1.

TABLE 17-1. TYPES OF DIZZINESS

	Vertigo	Presyncope	Disequilibrium	Lightheadedness
Sensation	Rotational; spinning or whirling .	Lightheaded, faint feeling	Unsteadiness; loss of balance on walking	Vague; may be floating sensation
Temporal characteristics	May be episodic or continuous	Typically episodes last seconds to hours	Usually present, although it may fluctuate in intensity	Usually present all or most of the time for days or weeks, sometimes years
Simulation tests	Dix-Hallpike maneuver	Orthostatic blood pressure measurement	Romberg test, tandem gait	Hyperventilation
Differential diagnosis	**Peripheral causes** • Vestibular neuronitis • Benign positional vertigo • Meniere's disease • Acoustic neuroma • Otitis media • Motion sickness • Drug use **Central causes** • Stroke • Transient ischemic attack • Multiple sclerosis • Basilar artery migraine • Temporal lobe seizure	• Arrhythmias • Vasovagal reflex • Orthostatic hypotension • Anemia • Aortic stenosis • Low cardiac output states • Carotid sinus hypersensitivity • Hypoglycemia • Hypoxemia	• Multiple sensory deficits • Altered visual input • Primary disequilibrium of aging • Parkinsonism • Cerebellar disease • Frontal lobe apraxia • Drug use	• Anxiety • Depression • Hyperventilation • Panic disorder

A. Complaints of **vertigo** (ie, a sensation of turning or spinning) accompanied by **nausea, vomiting, diaphoresis,** and **difficulty with balance** suggest peripheral vestibular disorders. Patients may also have **auditory symptoms** such as decreased hearing, tinnitus, or ear pain. Symptoms of particular disorders are described below.
  1. **Vestibular neuronitis or acute labyrinthitis.** After an acute onset of severe vertigo lasting several days, gradual improvement follows for several weeks. Symptoms frequently follow a viral illness.
  2. **Benign positional vertigo.** Instances of vertigo related to position are extremely brief, can be associated with nausea, and often will wake the patient from sleep when turning over in bed. Although the disorder is generally self-limited, its course is variable.
  3. **Meniere's disease.** Patients with this disease have discrete attacks of vertigo of abrupt onset. The attacks last for several hours, not days, and are often accompanied by nausea and vomiting. The interval between attacks may be weeks to months. Between attacks, the patient is asymptomatic. Fluctuating hearing loss, typically accompanied by tinnitus and a feeling of pressure in the ear, is usually present during attacks. Irreversible hearing loss and chronic tinnitus develop in the affected ear over time.
B. **Presyncope** is dizziness associated with the feeling of an impending faint. Actual loss of consciousness does not occur. It is episodic.
C. **Disequilibrium** is a problem with balance, usually associated with an unsteady gait. If patients are asked, "Is the dizziness in your head or in your feet?" those with disequilibrium respond with the latter choice.
D. **Lightheadedness** is a vague or floating sensation, often imprecisely described by the patient. Such dizziness is generally present much of the time. It is often accompanied by other somatic symptoms, such as headache and abdominal pain.

IV. Signs

A. The Dix-Hallpike (Nylen-Barany) maneuver can be helpful in distinguishing peripheral from central vestibulopathy. The patient should sit on the edge of the examining table and lie down suddenly, with the head hanging 45 degrees backward and turned 45 degrees to one side. Then repeat the test twice, once with the head turned to the other side and once with the head in the middle position. The patient's eyes should be kept open to observe (1) the development of vertigo and (2) the time of onset, duration, and direction of nystagmus. This maneuver will reveal a central or peripheral pattern of vertigo, as shown in Table 17–2.

B. Inspection of the eardrum may reveal otitis media or serous otitis.

C. Orthostatic blood pressure determinations are helpful when the history suggests dizziness due to hypovolemia from blood loss or dehydration. A drop in systolic blood pressure of as much as 20 mm Hg, a decline in diastolic pressure of up to 10 mm Hg, and a rise in pulse rate of up to 20 beats per minute can be normal findings with standing. If standing causes a greater blood pressure drop or pulse rise and reproduces the patient's symptoms, some form of hypovolemia is the most likely cause.

D. If the history suggests disequilibrium, gait and stationary testing should be done. Static balance can be tested with the Romberg test. The gait may be tested by asking the patient to rise from a chair, without using their arms, walk 10 feet, and then turn around. In addition, evaluation of muscle strength, coordination, reflexes, and proprioception should be conducted. The posture should be inspected. Often patients with postural instability stand bent over, with their knees and hips flexed. A gentle tap on the chest (the nudge test) while standing behind the patient can give an indication of the patient's likelihood of falling backward. Testing visual fields and acuity may uncover visual impairment.

E. If the history suggests a psychological cause, the patient should hyperventilate by blowing vigorously for 3 minutes on a paper towel held 6 inches from the mouth. This action may cause some circumoral and digital numbness, as well as reproduce the patient's dizziness.

V. Laboratory Tests

A. Few patients with suspected peripheral vestibular disorders require laboratory testing. Patients whose symptoms are progressive or recurrent should have an **audiologic evaluation** that includes a pure tone audiogram, speech discrimination testing, and tympanometry. Such patients should also undergo vestibular examination by **electronystagmography.**

Laboratory testing of patients whose dizziness may be caused by systemic diseases must be guided by the history and physical examination. Most "screening" laboratory tests, such as complete blood cell counts and electrolyte determinations, are rarely helpful.

B. Brain stem evoked response (BSER) testing is a useful screening in patients with suspected central causes of dizziness. A normal BSER safely excludes an acoustic neuroma. If the BSER is abnormal, an imaging procedure, such as magnetic resonance imaging, the most informative radiographic study, is indicated.

VI. Treatment

A. Peripheral vestibular disorders. The symptoms of vertigo are frightening to patients. The physician must be supportive and reassuring, since most causes of vertigo are not a serious health threat.

1. **Initial treatment** of acutely vertiginous patients usually involves having them lie still in a darkened room and avoid head movement. It is important to have patients mobilized as soon as the most severe nausea and vertigo subside, to avoid protracted disability.

TABLE 17–2. DISTINGUISHING PERIPHERAL FROM CENTRAL VERTIGO WITH POSITION TESTING

	Peripheral	Central
Latency (time to onset of vertigo or nystagmus)	3–10 s	None; begins immediately
Fatigability (lessening signs and symptoms with repetition)	Yes	No
Nystagmus direction	Fixed	Changing
Intensity of signs and symptoms	Severe	Mild

2. **Drug therapy** may provide symptomatic relief.
   a. **Antihistamines,** the most commonly prescribed drugs for vertigo, suppress the vestibular end organ receptors and inhibit activation of vagal responses. Patients should take the medication for a few weeks and then try discontinuing the drug. The major side effects are dry mouth and sedation. Commonly recommended drugs are meclizine, 25 mg orally every 4–6 hours, and diphenhydramine, 50 mg orally every 4–6 hours.
   b. **Antiemetics** can be tried when nausea and vomiting are pronounced. These agents suppress central vestibular pathways, which activate a vagal response. Their major side effect is sedation. Commonly recommended antiemetic drugs are prochlorperazine, 5–10 mg orally every 6 hours *or* 25-mg suppository by rectum twice daily, and trimethobenzamide, 250 mg orally every 6 hours *or* 200-mg suppository by rectum every 6 hours. Acute dystonic reactions may occur occasionally with prochlorperazine.
3. **Vestibular exercises** may be helpful, especially in cases of prolonged benign positional vertigo.
   a. The patient should be instructed to reproduce the vertigo by assuming the appropriate ear down, supine position and hold that position until the vertigo subsides. The vertigo usually returns upon resumption of sitting. The patient then repeats these maneuvers, usually five times, until the vertigo no longer recurs.
   b. Performing this exercise at least four times a day leads to longer symptom-free intervals and a reduction in the duration of symptoms.
4. The **canalith repositioning maneuver** eliminates symptoms of benign positional vertigo in up to 80% of patients after one treatment.
5. **Surgery** may be indicated if other medical therapies fail to adequately relieve severe vertigo. Surgical procedures include sectioning of the vestibular nerve, repair of an inner ear fistula, labyrinthectomy, or placement of a lymphatic shunt. Unilateral deafness may result.
B. **Systemic diseases.** Systemic diseases causing dizziness require treatment that is specific to the particular cause.
C. **Central nervous system diseases.** Symptomatic treatment of vertigo as described above may be helpful. Treatment of the underlying central nervous system condition is crucial.

REFERENCES

Baloh RW: Vestibular neuritis. N Engl J Med 2003;**348:**1027.
Froehling DA, et al: The canalith repositioning procedure for the treatment of benign paroxysmal positional vertigo: A randomized controlled trial. Mayo Clin Proc 2000;**75:**695.
Rubin AM, Zafar SS: The assessment and management of the dizzy patient. Otolaryngol Clin North Am 2002;**35:**255.
Sloane PD, et al: Dizziness: State of the science. Ann Intern Med 2001;**134:**823.

---

18   Dysmenorrhea

Rhonda A. Sparks, MD

KEY POINTS

- Primary dysmenorrhea is the most commonly reported gynecologic symptom in the United States, with an estimated 90% of all women being affected at one point in their life.
- If dysmenorrhea fails to respond to usual therapy with nonsteroidal anti-inflammatory drugs (NSAIDS), an underlying cause should be considered (ie, secondary dysmenorrhea).
- NSAIDs and oral contraceptive pills (OCPs) are the mainstay of treatment for dysmenorrhea. The newer COX-2 inhibitors provide pain relief with a better side effect profile.

I. Definition. Dysmenorrhea is pain with menstruation, usually cramping in nature, involving the lower abdomen and, in some women, the lower back and inner thighs. The distinction must be made between **primary dysmenorrhea,** in which no identifiable pelvic pathology is present, and **secondary dysmenorrhea** (pain secondary to organic pelvic pathology). Increased production of prostaglandin $F_{2\alpha}$ ($PGF_{2\alpha}$) and prostaglandin E_2 (PGE_2) or an inadequate $PGF_{2\alpha}$:PGE_2 ratio increases uterine resting tone, myometrial contractile pressure, frequency of uterine contractions, and dysrhythmic uterine contractions. These abnormalities lead to vasoconstriction, ischemia, and hypoxia of the uterus, all of which result in the pain of primary dysmenorrhea. Other possible factors contributing to primary dysmenorrhea include leukotrienes, platelet activating factor, and vasopressin. Psychosocial factors involving the patient, her family, or both may modulate the pain of primary dysmenorrhea.

Findings suggestive of secondary dysmenorrhea include pain during the first one or two menstrual cycles, pain onset after age 25 with no previous history of dysmenorrhea, abnormality on examination, and little or no response to usual therapy.

II. Common Diagnoses

A. Primary dysmenorrhea affects 40–70% of women of childbearing age. Cigarette smoking has been associated with an increased duration of dysmenorrhea with each cycle. Other risk factors for dysmenorrhea include obesity and frequent alcohol consumption. Studies have shown decreased prevalence and improvement of dysmenorrhea symptoms with exercise.

B. Secondary dysmenorrhea has several underlying causes:

1. **Endometriosis** occurs in 3–10% of women of reproductive age. Twenty-five percent to 35% of women with infertility have endometriosis.

2. **Leiomyomas (fibroids)** develop in 20% of women by age 40; most are asymptomatic. Black women have an increased incidence of uterine fibroids.

3. **Adenomyosis** is observed most frequently in women in the fifth and sixth decades. Fifteen percent of women with adenomyosis have associated endometriosis.

4. **Ovarian cysts** (see Chapter 51).

5. **Pelvic inflammatory disease (PID)** (see Chapter 51).

6. **Intrauterine devices (IUDs).**

7. **Miscellaneous causes.** Congenital abnormalities (bicornuate or septate uterus), cervical stenosis, imperforate hymen, uterine polyps, or uterine adhesions may cause secondary dysmenorrhea.

III. Symptoms

A. Primary dysmenorrhea is associated with ovulation and therefore usually presents 6–12 months after menarche when ovulation is established. Pain usually begins just prior to or 1–2 hours after menses and usually lasts <72 hours. Associated symptoms may include nausea and vomiting, fatigue, diarrhea, low back pain, inner or anterior thigh pain, and headache. Sixty percent of women with migraines have an increased incidence of headaches during menses.

B. The pain of **secondary dysmenorrhea** may be atypical or chronic and may vary in description and temporal relation to menses.

1. **Endometriosis** is usually a deep aching pain that begins several days prior to menses, may last throughout the cycle, and may be associated with dyspareunia, infertility, or menorrhagia.

2. Most **leiomyomas** (fibroids) are asymptomatic. Women may experience pelvic pressure, bloating, heaviness of the lower abdomen, menorrhagia, or metrorrhagia, depending on the location and size of the tumor.

3. **Adenomyosis** is usually associated with severe dysmenorrhea and menorrhagia. Thirty percent to 40% of patients are asymptomatic.

4. Pain associated with an **IUD** occurs after IUD placement.

IV. Signs

A. Primary dysmenorrhea. Most commonly, the physical examination will be normal. Tenderness on uterine palpation may be present.

B. Secondary dysmenorrhea

1. **Endometriosis** is classically associated with palpable nodules in the posterior cul-de-sac and a tender fixed uterus on bimanual examination, but may be present in a patient with a normal examination.

2. **Leiomyomata** are suspected if the uterus is irregularly enlarged or nodular.

3. **Adenomyosis** is associated with a symmetrically enlarged uterus.

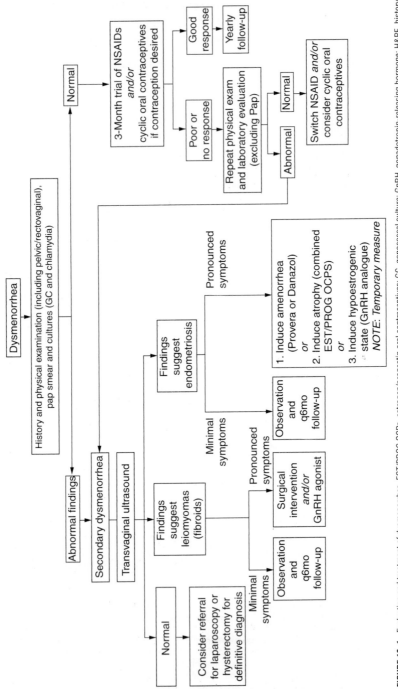

FIGURE 18–1. Evaluation and treatment of dysmenorrhea. EST/PROG OCPs, estrogen/progestin oral contraceptives; GC, gonococcal culture; GnRH, gonadotropin-releasing hormone; H&PE, history and physical examination; NSAIDs, nonsteroidal anti-inflammatory drugs.

TABLE 18–1. NONSTEROIDAL ANTI-INFLAMMATORY DRUGS MOST COMMONLY USED IN THE TREATMENT OF PRIMARY DYSMENORRHEA

Drug[1] (mg)	Initial Dose (mg)	Subsequent Dosage (mg)
Propionic acids		
Ibuprofen (Motrin, Advil)	400	400–600 qid
Ketoprofen (Orudis)	50	50 tid
Naproxen sodium (Anaprox)	550	275 q6h
Naproxen (Naprosyn)	500	250–375 bid
Acetic acids		
Sulindac (Clinoril)	200	200 bid
Diclofenac (Cataflam)	50	50 tid
Etodolac (Lodine)	400	300–400 bid

[1] Consult full prescribing information before administering any of these drugs.

    4. Ovarian cysts (see Chapter 51).
    5. PID (see Chapter 51).
V. Laboratory Tests
  A. Primary dysmenorrhea. With a suggestive history and a normal physical examination, no laboratory evaluation is indicated.
  B. For **secondary dysmenorrhea,** work-up may include:
    1. Gonococcal and chlamydia cultures if signs or symptoms suggest PID or the patient is at risk for sexually transmitted diseases.
    2. Pelvic ultrasound to diagnose fibroids, ovarian cysts, or mass lesions found on examination.
    3. Hysterosalpingography if a uterine anomaly is suspected.
    4. Laparoscopy for diagnosing endometriosis (visualize endometrial implants) and if other tests do not reveal the cause of secondary dysmenorrhea.
VI. Treatment (Figure 18–1)
  A. Prostaglandin synthetase inhibitors (ie, NSAIDs) (Table 18–1). Most NSAIDs are effective in relieving primary dysmenorrhea in 70–90% of cases. NSAIDs inhibit prostaglandin production without affecting endometrial development, can be started with the onset of pain associated with menses, and are rarely needed for >72 hours.
    If a patient is unresponsive to NSAIDs after 3 months and no new history or physical findings suggest secondary dysmenorrhea, another NSAID should be tried. If the patient remains unresponsive to NSAIDs, a work-up for underlying gynecologic pathology is warranted (Figure 18–1).
    Contraindications to NSAIDs include gastrointestinal ulcers and hypersensitivity. Side effects are mild and well tolerated and occur in <5% of patients (Table 18–2).
  B. Oral contraceptives (OCPs). OCPs suppress both menstrual fluid volume and prostaglandin release, but not synthesis. This is achieved by causing endometrial hypoplasia. OCPs are effective in 60–80% of patients and are an alternative to NSAIDs or an additional therapeutic option in patients desiring contraception. Combined OCPs with increased androgenic content (eg, Ovral and Loestrin) and progestin-only OCPs may be used. If OCPs and NSAIDs in combination do not provide relief after 3–6 months, reevaluation and work-up for underlying gynecologic pathology should be done (Figure 18–1).
  C. The **COX-2 inhibitors.** These are newer therapeutic options for both primary and secondary dysmenorrhea. The COX-2 inhibitors have an improved toxicity profile, particularly in the gastrointestinal tract and effect on renal function, over the conventional

TABLE 18–2. SIDE EFFECTS OF PROSTAGLANDIN SYNTHETASE INHIBITORS

Gastrointestinal symptoms	Indigestion, heartburn, nausea, abdominal pain, constipation, vomiting, diarrhea, melena
Central nervous system symptoms	Headache, dizziness, vertigo, visual disturbances, hearing disturbances, irritability, depression, drowsiness, sleepiness
Other symptoms	Allergic reaction, skin rash, edema, bronchospasm, hematologic abnormalities, eye effects, fluid retention, liver and kidney effects

NSAIDs. Available preparations include Vioxx, 50 mg every day for 5 days, Bextra 20 mg twice a day, and Celebrex, 400 mg at onset of pain and 200 mg every day thereafter.

D. Other treatments reported to improve pain associated with dysmenorrhea. These include the use of transcutaneous electrical nerve stimulation (TENS) units; acupuncture; and dietary supplementation, including calcium, magnesium, and thiamine.

E. Secondary dysmenorrhea treatment options. Endometriosis can be treated with OCPs, which induce endometrial atrophy and decrease symptoms. Danazol and progestin-only contraceptives can improve symptoms by inducing amenorrhea. Gonadotropin-reducing hormone (GnRH) agonists are sometimes used as a temporary measure or preoperatively to reduce endometrial implant size. Accepted regimens include (1) OCPs with high androgenic progesterone taken as a continuous 21-day pack for 6 months; (2) Depo-Provera 200 mg IM every month for 6 months; (3) Leuprolide (Lupron) 3.75 mg IM for 6 months. Other treatment options include surgical laparoscopy with lysis of lesions and, in extreme cases, hysterectomy.

REFERENCES

Coco AS: Primary dysmenorrhea. Am Fam Physician 1999;**60**:489.

Hacker NF, Moore JG: *Essentials of Obstetrics and Gynecology,* 3rd ed. Saunders; 1998.

Hayes EC, Osathanondh R: Dysmenorrhea. In: Bardin WC (editor): *Current Therapy in Endocrinology and Metabolism,* 5th ed. Saunders; 1997.

Rock JA: COX-2 inhibitors and their role in gynecology. Obstet Gynecol Surv 2002;**57**(11):768.

Shulman LP: Dysmenorrhea (Ch. 265). In: Rakel R: *Conn's Current Therapy,* 55th ed. Elsevier; 2003:1140–1142.

Sidani M, Campbell J: Gynecology: Select topics. Primar Care Clin Office Practice 2002;**29**:297.

Speroff L, Glass RH, Kase NG: *Clinical Gynecologic Endocrinology and Infertility,* 6th ed. Williams & Wilkins; 1999.

19 Dyspepsia

Alan M. Adelman, MD, MS

KEY POINTS

- Most patients with dyspepsia have no structural abnormality (nonulcer dyspepsia).
- Patients without alarm symptoms should be tested for *Helicobacter pylori* and, if test results are positive, treated with an appropriate antibiotic regimen ("test and treat" strategy).
- Patients with nonulcer dyspepsia may be treated with a proton pump inhibitor or histamine-2 blocking agent (H_2 blocker).

I. **Definition.** Dyspepsia is characterized by epigastric discomfort or pain and can be associated with epigastric heaviness or fullness, belching or regurgitation, bloating, early satiety, heartburn, food intolerance, nausea, or vomiting. Lower bowel function is usually not affected.

II. **Common Diagnoses.** Dyspepsia is a common complaint, occurring in 20–30% of the general population. It accounts for approximately 5–10% of all visits to general practitioners in England. Common causes include:

   A. **Medications.** Aspirin, nonsteroidal anti-inflammatory drugs (NSAIDS), erythromycin, tetracycline, alcohol, and potassium supplements can cause upper abdominal discomfort.

   B. **Nonulcer dyspepsia (NUD).** This disorder is found in 30–50% of patients with dyspepsia. The incidence of NUD is age dependent; approximately 70% of patients younger than age 40 have NUD, as opposed to only 40% of those older than age 60. The exact cause of NUD is unknown. No link between NUD and *H pylori* has been established.

   C. **Peptic ulcer disease (PUD).** PUD includes gastric and duodenal ulcers, gastritis, and duodenitis and is found in 20–30% of patients with dyspepsia. Together, NUD and PUD probably account for 50–80% of all cases of dyspepsia. PUD of the duodenum affects males twice as frequently as females. The peak incidence is between ages 45 and 64 in males and at age 55 in females. Gastric ulcer occurs much less frequently than duodenal ulcer and increases in incidence with advancing age. A past history of PUD, previous gastric surgery, male gender, and cigarette smoking all are associated with an increased chance of finding a structural abnormality (gastric or duodenal ulcers) on upper endoscopy.

D. Gastroesophageal reflux disease (GERD). GERD is found in 5–10% of patients with dyspepsia.

E. Gastric or pancreatic cancer. Fewer than 1% of patients with dyspepsia have cancer. The incidence of gastric cancer and pancreatic cancer increases with advancing age. Toxins (eg, nitrosamines or polycyclic hydrocarbons), genetic factors, pernicious anemia, and atrophic gastritis have been associated with gastric cancer.

F. Cholecystitis or cholelithiasis. (See Chapter 1). For irritable bowel syndrome, see Chapter 1.

G. Other causes of dyspepsia. Zollinger-Ellison syndrome, chronic pancreatitis, abdominal angina, and coronary artery disease are uncommon.

III. Symptoms. Although symptoms seem to be of little help in making a specific diagnosis in a patient with dyspepsia, they may be helpful in guiding the work-up (Figure 19–1).

A. Heartburn. Heartburn, regurgitation, and pyrosis are reliable symptoms of reflux.

B. Alarm symptoms. The presence of alarm symptoms including age older than 45 years, significant weight loss (>10–15 lbs), persistent vomiting, melena, hematemesis, or dysphagia should prompt immediate work-up, usually with endoscopy.

C. Symptoms that poorly discriminate between specific disease and NUD. These include relief with antacids or food, nocturnal pain, food intolerance (eg, fatty food intolerance), duration of pain, pain that occurs within 1 hour of eating, and anorexia.

D. Symptoms that may identify patients with complications of PUD. Symptoms that indicate complications of PUD or other specific causes of dyspepsia are:

    1. Hematemesis, melena, or both indicate gastrointestinal (GI) bleeding.

    2. Dizziness, especially upon sitting or standing, or syncope may indicate significant blood loss.

    3. Persistent vomiting is a symptom of gastric outlet obstruction.

    4. Pain that radiates straight through to the back may indicate a perforated ulcer, leaking abdominal aneurysm, pancreatitis, or pancreatic cancer.

    5. Pain radiating to the shoulder may result from diaphragmatic irritation due to pus, blood, or free air.

IV. Signs. In general, the physical examination is not helpful in determining the cause of dyspepsia. In uncomplicated cases, the examination usually reveals only mild to moderate epigastric tenderness. The following signs may be helpful in identifying patients with complications of PUD or serious systemic illness.

A. Unexplained tachycardia (pulse >120) or postural hypotension (orthostatic change in blood pressure >20 mm Hg) may indicate significant blood loss from GI bleeding.

B. Abdominal rebound or rigidity suggests peritoneal irritation. A perforated viscus, blood, or infection can cause peritoneal irritation.

C. Blood in the stool may indicate upper GI tract bleeding.

D. Jaundice may indicate biliary tract obstruction from pancreatic cancer or cholelithiasis.

V. Laboratory Tests. In general, the laboratory evaluation consists of testing for *H pylori* in those individuals without alarm symptoms. This is referred to as the "test and treat" strategy. (See Figure 19–1.)

A. Tests that may be useful include:

    1. Tests for *H pylori*. These can be either noninvasive (serology, or urea breath test) or invasive (rapid urease test, obtained at the time of upper endoscopy). Serology is the easiest and least costly.

    2. Upper GI series. The upper GI series is noninvasive and relatively inexpensive. The false-negative rate of this technique exceeds 18% the false-positive rate is between 13% and 35%. Even with double-contrast studies, the false-negative rate is still between 9% and 17%, and the false-positive rate is approximately 10%. In a patient with GERD, only severe esophagitis may be detected, although reflux and motility disorders of the esophagus can be seen. The presence of a hiatal hernia does not correlate with GERD.

    3. Upper endoscopy. Upper endoscopy is a relatively safe procedure, with a complication rate of 1.32 or less per 1000 cases. Over half of the complications

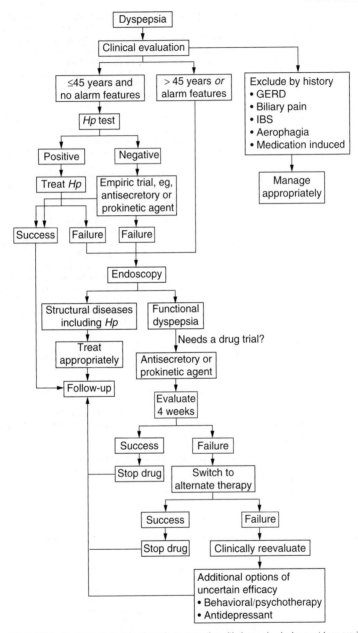

FIGURE 19–1. Management algorithm for patients presenting with dyspepsia who have not been previously investigated. GERD, gastroesophageal reflux disease; *Hp, Helicobacter pylori;* IBS, irritable bowel syndrome. (Adapted with permission from Clinical Practice and Practice Economics Committee, American Gastroenterological Association: American Gastroenterological Association medical position statement: Evaluation of dyspepsia. Gastroenterology 1998;**114:**579.)

(eg, hives and thrombophlebitis) in one study resulted from the medication used for sedation, with cardiopulmonary complications, perforation, bleeding, and infection representing the remainder of the complications. Upper endoscopy is preferred to upper GI barium study because lesions can be directly visualized and biopsy can be performed. In addition, testing for *H pylori* can be performed.

4. **Intraesophageal pH monitoring.** Most physicians consider this procedure to be the single best test for diagnosis for GERD. Coupled with a symptom diary, 24-hour monitoring has a sensitivity between 87% and 93% and a specificity of 92–97% for GERD.

5. **Scintigraphy.** Scintigraphy is best used to detect delayed gastric emptying. GERD and delayed gastric emptying can be detected using [^{99m}Tc] sulfur colloid, although intraesophageal pH monitoring is a better test for reflux.

B. **Indications for further testing.** A diagnostic investigation should be started promptly in patients with clinically obvious conditions, such as severe systemic illness, bleeding, perforation, symptoms of upper GI tract obstruction, or evidence of cancer.

1. **Persistence of symptoms** after empiric treatment in patients previously not evaluated with endoscopy or upper GI series requires further evaluation.

2. In patients who experience a **recurrence of dyspepsia** and who have previously been treated empirically for the condition, a specific diagnosis should be made.

VI. **Treatment.** Figure 19–1 presents the "test and treat" approach to a patient with dyspepsia.

A. A practical approach for patients with dyspepsia who are younger than 45 years and have no alarm symptoms, complications of PUD, or serious systemic illness is to treat empirically with an H$_2$ blocker or a proton pump inhibitor (see Table 19–1 for medications, dose, and frequency) and test for *H pylori.* If they test positive for *H pylori,* treat (see Chapter 82). Helidac (bismuth subsalicylate-metronidazole-tetracycline) plus a proton pump inhibitor or Prevpac (amoxicillin-clarithromycin-lansoprazole) are both effective in the treatment of *H pylori.* Both regimens are given for 14 days. Patients should also be encouraged to discontinue ulcerogenic medications (eg, alcohol or NSAIDS) and cigarette smoking.

B. For **individuals with dyspepsia who are older than 45 years,** empiric treatment should be followed by the establishment of a definitive diagnosis with upper endoscopy. If symptoms worsen or persist despite therapy, the patient should undergo further evaluation (see section V,B).

C. **When the cause of the patient's dyspepsia is known,** the following therapeutic measures may be helpful:

1. **NUD.** At present, the best therapy for NUD is unclear. Fortunately, in most individuals, abdominal discomfort resolves within several weeks. Treatment for *H pylori* is not appropriate.

2. **PUD.** (See Chapter 82).

3. **GERD.** Initial treatment of GERD includes antireflux measures and antiulcer agents (Table 19–1). Antireflux measures include losing weight, avoiding lying down or bending over after meals, consuming few large meals and bedtime snacks, elevating the head of the bed on 4- to 8-inch blocks, modifying the diet (such as avoiding

TABLE 19–1. H$_2$ BLOCKERS AND PROTON PUMP INHIBITORS USED IN THE TREATMENT OF DYSPEPSIA

Medication	Dose/Frequency
H$_2$ blockers	
Cimetidine	400 mg twice daily
Famotidine	20 mg once or twice daily
Nizatidine	150 mg twice daily
Ranitidine	150 mg twice daily
Proton pump inhibitors	
Esomeprazole	20–40 mg once daily
Lansoprazole	15–30 mg once daily
Omeprazole	20 mg twice daily
Pantoprazole	40 mg once daily
Rabeprazole	20 mg once daily

caffeine, chocolate, peppermint, and fatty foods), and discontinuing alcohol consumption and cigarette smoking. (See sidebar for pediatric GERD.)

   a. If symptoms persist or worsen, a **prokinetic agent** (eg, metoclopramide, 5–10 mg orally four times daily) may be helpful.

   b. **Antireflux surgery** should be considered if documented reflux persists despite full medical therapy.

PEDIATRIC GERD

Gastroesophageal reflux (GER) is fairly common in infants. It is marked by regurgitation with normal weight gain. The peak incidence is at 1–4 months and is usually resolved by age 1. "Happy spitters" can be treated conservatively by reassuring parents and using thickened feedings, hypoallergenic formula, and upright positioning after feedings. Although the supine position leads to less reflux, it is not recommended because of the increased incidence of sudden infant death syndrome in this position.

Infants who present with regurgitation and alarm symptoms such as respiratory problems (stridor, wheezing, cough), poor weight gain or growth, or irritability require further evaluation. Gastroesophageal reflux disease (GERD) should be considered in the differential diagnosis of these children. In older children and adolescents, GERD usually presents with heartburn, pyrosis, or lower chest pain. Infants or children with esophageal atresia with repair, neurologic impairment/delay, bronchopulmonary dysplasia, asthma, or cystic fibrosis have an increased risk of GERD. A pediatric gastroenterologist can help guide the work-up of GERD. Medical management includes H_2 blockers and proton pump inhibitors. Prokinetic agents may have a role.

   4. Gastric or pancreatic cancer. The primary treatment of gastric or pancreatic cancer is surgery. At present surgery offers the only chance for cure; chemotherapy and radiation therapy are experimental.

REFERENCES

Clinical Practice and Practice Economics Committee, American Gastroenterological Association: American Gastroenterological Association medical position statement: Evaluation of Dyspepsia. Gastroenterology 1998;**114:**579.

Institute for Clinical Systems Improvement. Health Care Guideline: Dyspepsia. Updated January, 2003. http://www.icsi.org/knowledge/detail.asp?catID=29&itemID=171

Jung AD: Gastroesophageal reflux in infants and children. Am Fam Physician 2001;**64:**1853.

Manes G, et al: Empirical prescribing for dyspepsia: Randomized controlled trial of test and treat versus omeprazole treatment. BMJ 2003;**326:**1118.

Rudolph CD, et al: Guidelines for evaluation and treatment of gastroesophageal reflux in infants and children: Recommendations of the North American Society for Pediatric Gastroenterology and Nutrition. J Pediatr Gastroenterol Nutr 2001;**32**(suppl 2):S1–S31.

Talley NJ, et al: AGA technical review: Evaluation of dyspepsia. Gastroenterology 1998;**114:**582.

---

20   Dyspnea

James C. Chesnutt, MD, Scott A. Fields, MD, & William L. Toffler, MD

KEY POINTS

- Dyspnea is mainly caused by cardiac or pulmonary disorders.
- The history and physical examination will reveal the cause in most cases.
- Quickly evaluate the ABCs to screen for life-threatening disorders, then proceed with diagnostic tests as needed.

I. **Definition.** Dyspnea is an unpleasant subjective sensation of difficult breathing (breathlessness). Respiratory physiology relies on sensory input from peripheral and central chemoreceptors (monitoring Po_2, Pco_2, and pH) and mechanoreceptors (located in the heart, lung, vessels, and chest wall) with central processing and control in the medulla, receiving additional input from higher brain centers, including the cerebral cortex. The sensation of dyspnea is related to a mismatch of sensory input, central respiratory drive, and peripheral ventilatory performance. Dyspnea can vary in quality and intensity and is affected not only by physiologic disturbances but also by psychological, social, and environmental factors.

II. **Common Diagnoses.** Dyspnea is an extremely common complaint of patients presenting for acute medical care. A chief complaint of shortness of breath accounts for 16–25% of nonsurgical admissions from the emergency room. Seventy percent of patients with advanced cancer have dyspnea, of which one quarter have moderate or severe symptoms. The most common causes of dyspnea relate to either cardiac or respiratory disorders. (See the sidebar for life-threatening causes of dyspnea.)

10 LIFE-THREATENING CAUSES OF DYSPNEA

1. Myocardial infarction
2. Ventricular tachycardia
3. Status asthmaticus
4. Anaphylactic laryngeal edema
5. Tension pneumothorax
6. Bacterial epiglottitis
7. Pulmonary embolism
8. Carbon monoxide poisoning
9. Guillain-Barré syndrome
10. Diabetic ketoacidosis

A. **Pulmonary disorders**
1. Those at risk for **obstructive lung disease** include pediatric patients (asthma, bronchiolitis, bronchitis), adults with asthma, and adults with a chronic cigarette smoking history (chronic bronchitis and emphysema).
2. Dyspnea due to **restrictive lung disease** is more likely with occupational exposure (asbestos, coal, beryllium, silica, uranium, cotton dust, grain dust, hay mold), those with severe scoliosis, the morbidly obese, and pregnant patients (due to uterine growth restricting lung expansion). Chest wall trauma and smoking are associated with pneumothorax.
3. Severe **pneumonia** also causes dyspnea; those at risk include immunocompromised patients (eg, *Pneumocystis carinii* pneumonia in HIV disease), the very young, the very old, and those at risk for aspiration (eg, alcoholics or individuals with stroke or history of swallowing disorders).
B. **Cardiac dyspnea.** Risk factors for cardiac dyspnea include known valvular heart disease, congestive heart failure, known ischemic cardiovascular disease (angina, myocardial infarction, claudication, or stroke), individuals with comorbid conditions (diabetes mellitus, hypercholesterolemia, or tobacco abuse), and those with a strong family history of premature coronary disease (ie, myocardial infarction in the 40s or 50s in first-degree relatives). Arrhythmias (eg, sick sinus syndrome, atrial fibrillation, and ventricular tachycardia) can cause dyspnea.
C. **Mixed cardiopulmonary dyspnea.** Risk factors for mixed cardiopulmonary dyspnea include hypercoagulable states, immobilization, major surgery or trauma, malignancy, and pregnancy and oral contraceptives (pulmonary embolism). Morbid obesity and a sedentary lifestyle contribute to deconditioning.
D. **Noncardiopulmonary causes**
1. Uncommonly, **neuromuscular diseases** (Parkinson's disease, amyotrophic lateral sclerosis, and Guillain-Barré syndrome) can cause dyspnea, due to respiratory muscle paralysis or dysfunction.

2. In the presence of clinical findings supporting them, the following **systemic diseases** can cause dyspnea: anemia, thyrotoxicosis, diabetic ketoacidosis, metabolic acidosis, and carbon monoxide poisoning.

3. A **psychogenic cause** for dyspnea should be considered in patients with a known history of psychiatric disease, multiple life stressors, and poor coping skills or a history of ill-defined somatic complaints. Extreme pain or hyperventilation can cause dyspnea.

4. **Upper airway causes** of dyspnea are more likely in children (tonsillar hypertrophy, croup, epiglottitis, or foreign body aspiration) and in alcoholics or individuals with a history of stroke or of swallowing disorders.

III. **Symptoms** (Table 20–1). Assessing the patient for dyspnea severity, onset (acute versus chronic), descriptive qualities, and associated symptoms and signs can be extremely helpful in identifying the underlying cause of the dyspnea.

Various studies show that different descriptive qualities of dyspnea are related to distinct physiologic abnormalities.

IV. **Signs** (Table 20–1). In order to quickly and accurately identify severe or life-threatening causes of dyspnea, special attention should be given to a rapid assessment of the patient's

TABLE 20–1. FINDINGS IN COMMON CAUSES OF DYSPNEA

Cause	Symptoms	Signs

Pulmonary
–OLD
–RLD
 	
–Pneumonia
	–"Chest tightness" (bronchospasm)
	–"Air hunger" (hypoxemia)
	–"Increased effort of breathing"
	   (COPD, RLD)
	–Exercise-induced coughing/wheezing
	   (asthma)
	–Daily sputum production (COPD)
	–Cough, purulent sputum (dark or rust)
	–"Air hunger" (hypoxemia)
	–Pleuritic chest pain
	–Chills, rigors
		–Tachypnea/tachycardia
		  Rales/rhonchi/wheezes
		–Nasal flaring, sternal retractions and
		  accessory muscle use (more severe)
		–Cyanosis or clubbing
		–Increased A-P chest diameter
		–Scoliosis, or chest wall deformity
		–Fever >38.5 °C (101°F)
		–Tachypnea, cyanosis
		–Coarse rales, dullness to percussion,
		  egophony

Cardiac	–Anginal chest pressure/pain, palpitations
	–Orthopnea, dyspnea on exertion, fatigue
		–Tachycardia, arrhythmia
		–Abnormal heart sounds (murmur,
		  rub, gallop)
		–Cardiomegaly, JVD
		–Dependent edema
		–Basilar fine rales and decreased
		  breath sounds

Mixed cardiopulmonary	–"Air hunger" (hypoxemia associated
	  with PE)
	–Pleuritic chest pain, syncope, unilateral
	  leg pain or swelling (PE)
	–"Heavy breathing" (deconditioning)
		–Tachypnea/tachycardia, cyanosis
		–Calf tenderness, edema, positive
		  Homan's sign (PE)
		–Obesity (deconditioning)

Noncardiopulmonary
–Neuromuscular
–Systemic disease
–Psychogenic
 	
–Upper airway obstruction
	–"Increased effort or work of breathing"
	  Fatigue, weakness, tremor, motor dysfunction (neuromuscular weakness)
	–Polyuria, polydipsia, polyphagia (DM)
	–Headache, confusion, dizziness (CO)
	–Anxiety, depression, pain (psychogenic)
	–Dysphagia, gagging, drooling, sore
	  throat, hoarseness (epiglottitis)
	–Allergic exposure: food, cat, drug, bee
	  sting (anaphylaxis/laryngeal/edema)
	–Snoring, sleep apnea, daytime fatigue
	  (OSAS)
		–Tachypnea/tachycardia
		–Abnormal muscle tone, strength, gait,
		  or reflexes (neuromuscular disease)
		–Pale (anemia)
		–Red skin CO poisoning
		–Hyperventilation
		–Tachypnea distress, inspiratory
		  stridor, high fever (epiglottitis)
		–Cyanosis, urticaria (angioedema)
		–Tonsil hypertrophy, nasal obstruction, obesity, large neck (OSAS)

A-P, anterior-posterior; CO, carbon monoxide; COPD, chronic obstructive pulmonary disease; DM, diabetes mellitus; JVD, jugular venous distention; OLD, obstructive lung disease; OSAS, obstructive sleep apnea syndrome; PE, pulmonary embolism; RLD, restrictive lung disease.

general level of distress and vital signs. In addition, cardiopulmonary examination is most helpful in identifying underlying causes of dyspnea.
  A. **Vital signs.** The patient's respiratory rate, temperature, pulse, and blood pressure should be determined. An increased respiratory rate (>20 respirations per minute) helps quantify dyspnea, but it is a nonspecific sign. Fever (>38.5 °C [101 °F]) is associated with respiratory infection. An increased pulse rate (>100 beats per minute) may be associated with pulmonary embolism, dysrhythmia, or metabolic disorder.
  B. **Focused examination**
    1. The **pulmonary examination** should consist of auscultation and percussion of the lungs to assess for the presence of rales, rhonchi, wheezing, decreased breath sounds, egophony, or dullness to percussion. Inspection of the oral/nasal cavities, chest wall, and extremities can reveal airway obstruction, an increased thoracic anterior-posterior diameter, chest wall deformity, or clubbing. Nasal flaring, sternal retractions, and accessory muscle use indicate more severe respiratory distress.
    2. The **cardiac examination** should include an evaluation for rhythm, abnormal heart sounds (S_3 and S_4), murmurs, rubs, increased jugular venous distention, peripheral edema and pulses, and pulmonary rales in the lower lung fields.
    3. The extent of additional **noncardiopulmonary examination** should be driven by the symptoms. If a dyspneic patient has weakness, tremor, gait problems, or other muscular or neurologic complaints, a screening neurologic examination should be performed, including testing gait; reflexes; sensation; and motor strength, tone, and coordination.
V. **Laboratory Tests.** The need for testing should be based on the patient's history and physical examination and ordered only if needed to help establish the cause or severity of the illness. A stepwise **"ABC and D"** approach to dyspnea diagnosis and testing may simplify the diagnostic process and decrease both cost and patient discomfort. When dyspnea is severe, a rapid assessment for life-threatening medical problems should focus on the ABCs (**A**irway, **B**reathing, and **C**irculation). Further diagnostic (**D**) testing can focus on evaluating the common causes of dyspnea.
  A. **Airway.** A **peak expiratory flow rate (PEFR)** of <150 L/min (normal value, 400–600 L/min) predicts a pulmonary cause for dyspnea, indicating significant obstructive airway disease that may require hospitalization. The PEFR is easily measured with a handheld peak flow meter and should be compared to the patient's baseline value and help guide a stepwise asthma/chronic obstructive pulmonary disease (COPD) treatment plan.
  B. **Breathing**
    1. **Pulse oximetry** can be used as a rapid and accurate assessment of oxygenation. For hypoxemia of <90% po_2 on pulse oximetry, an **arterial blood gas analysis (ABG)** profile should be considered, which provides precise levels of oxygenation, carbon dioxide, and pH (normal values: pH, 7.40; Pco_2, 40 mm Hg; Po_2, 90–100 mm Hg). An ABG can aid in the diagnosis of severe dyspnea or dyspnea of unclear origin.
    2. **Chest x-ray** is the next step. This can demonstrate an infiltrate, effusion, pneumothorax, or sign of congestive heart failure (eg, pulmonary vascular congestion or cardiomegaly) or lung disease (eg, fibrosis or tumor).
  C. **Circulation.** An **electrocardiogram (ECG)** is imperative for evaluation of cardiac arrhythmia or ischemia and can aid in the diagnosis of pulmonary embolism, pericarditis, or other cardiac problems. The ECG should be correlated with blood pressure and an assessment of perfusion.
  D. **Diagnostic testing.** Further testing can be based on likely disorders guided by the acuity and severity of symptoms, initial testing, and pertinent examination findings.
    1. **Cardiac tests**
       a. **BNP (brain or b-type natriuretic peptide)** is a validated test to evaluate for the presence of congestive heart failure (CHF) in patients with dyspnea. A low value (<80 pg/mL) has a high (99%) negative predictive value that helps to rule out CHF; a high value (>100 pg/mL) is nonspecific but is about 90% sensitive for CHF.
       b. **Other useful cardiac studies** may include **echocardiography, cardiac catheterization, cardiac event monitors, and exercise treadmill testing** but likely should be reserved to evaluate abnormal ECG or examination findings or suspicious unexplained symptoms. Exercise testing is helpful in the evaluation of cardiac abnormalities as well as in the diagnosis of exercise-induced asthma.

2. **Pulmonary tests.** These tests can tests evaluate possible lung disease. **Formal spirometry** is useful in the assessment of patients with lung disease. In **restrictive disease,** forced vital capacity (FVC) is low, and forced expiratory volume in 1 second (FEV_1) and the maximal mid-expiratory flow ($FEV_{25-75\%}$) may be low. The FEV-FVC ratio may be normal or even high. In **obstructive disease,** FVC, FEV, FEV_1-FVC ratio, or $FEV_{25-75\%}$, or all four, may be low. In mixed disease, all of these values are low.

3. **Mixed cardiopulmonary.** Pulmonary embolism can cause pleuritic chest pain, dyspnea, tachycardia, and hypoxemia. The following tests can help clarify the diagnosis.

   a. **D-dimer** is useful in determining risk for deep venous thrombosis (DVT) or pulmonary embolism (PE); a low result has a high negative predictive value for DVT and PE; a high result is nonspecific but requires further evaluation for presence of thrombosis.

   b. **Spiral CT of the chest** has become a standard, validated test for the evaluation of suspected PE.

   c. **Ventilation/perfusion (V/Q) scan** should be used in cases where computerized tomography is not available or is not conclusive for suspected PE. The result is often inconclusive, which may necessitate the use of **pulmonary angiogram** to clarify the diagnosis.

   d. **Doppler venous flow studies** are a noninvasive, accurate method to identify DVTs, which are correlated with PE (see Chapter 23).

4. **Noncardiopulmonary**

   a. **A complete blood cell count** can establish the presence of anemia or a possible underlying infection. Anemia leads to decreased oxygen-carrying capacity and therefore reduced oxygen delivery.

   b. **Blood glucose, basic metabolic test set, and thyroid-stimulating hormone** may be useful to assess metabolic status in unclear cases. Thyrotoxicosis results in increased oxygen demand. High levels of glucose can cause ketoacidosis. Renal or electrolyte abnormalities can cause dyspnea.

   c. A **carbon monoxide level** (normal value, <2%) may document a toxic exposure to smoke or exhaust from a furnace or other sources. Levels are elevated in active smokers (<10%), thereby decreasing oxygen-carrying capacity. Carbon monoxide binds to hemoglobin with 200 times the affinity of oxygen, severely compromising oxygen delivery to tissue. Lethal levels (>50%) can occur despite relatively normal arterial blood gas levels.

   d. Further neurologic testing or imaging should be guided by abnormal physical examination findings and is unlikely to be cost-effective if a screening neurologic examination is normal.

VI. **Treatment.** Once the underlying diagnosis has been made, treatment strategies should involve increasing oxygen delivery and correcting the underlying disease process, which usually relieves the sensation of dyspnea. For treatment of specific medical problems, please see the following chapters: asthma (Chapter 68), chronic obstructive pulmonary disease (Chapter 70), congestive heart failure (Chapter 72), cough (Chapter 13), ischemic heart disease (Chapter 77), and wheezing (Chapter 65).

Medical therapies aimed at alleviating the symptoms of dyspnea can be used while the disease process is being treated or in cases where the cause of dyspnea is uncertain or related to a terminal condition like cancer or end-stage COPD.

A. **Oxygen.** Oxygen delivered via nasal cannula at 1–4 liters per minute can provide good relief for mild or severe hypoxemia, at rest or with exercise, regardless of initial oxygen saturation; in COPD patients oxygen therapy can suppress respiratory drive and cause CO_2 retention, which can present as sedation.

B. **Bronchodilators.** Both beta-agonists and anticholinergics (better) alone or in combination (best) give good relief in COPD/asthma; longer-acting forms are most effective.

C. Intravenous **steroids** do not help dyspnea acutely; prolonged use of oral steroids can cause muscle weakness; inhaled steroids do show improved airway reactivity in asthma and COPD and are associated with decreased symptoms and hospitalizations.

D. **Pulmonary rehabilitation programs.** Education and structured exercise can reduce symptoms and increase exercise tolerance.

E. A Cochrane review found strong evidence that **opioids** relieve dyspnea and improve exercise tolerance in patients with cancer and severe COPD.

1. Immediate-release forms (eg, Roxicodone/oxycodone IR) are more effective than sustained-release forms (eg, OxyContin/oxycodone SR).
2. Constipation is a problem, but tolerance develops to other side effects.
3. Studies show opioids do not severely suppress respiration or cause early death in terminally ill patients.

F. Anxiolytics. In end-stage COPD and cancer, oral buspirone (eg, Buspar, 5–10 mg three times daily) or lorazepam (eg, Ativan, 0.5–2 mg every 4 hours as needed) may relieve anxiety associated with dyspnea rather than dyspnea itself.

G. Nonpharmacologic methods. Use of fans, open windows, cognitive therapy, stress management for patient and caregiver, and nutritional, spiritual, and emotional support have all proved useful in decreasing dyspnea.

REFERENCES

American Thoracic Society: Dyspnea mechanism, assessment, and management: A consensus statement. Am J Respir Crit Care Med 1999;**159:**321.
Collins SP, Ronan-Bentle S, Storrow AB: Diagnostic and prognostic usefulness of natriuretic peptides in emergency department patients with dyspnea. Ann Emerg Med 2003;**41:**532.
Legrand SB, et al: Opioids, respiratory function, and dyspnea. Am J Hospice Palliat Care 2003;**20:**57.
Morgan WC, Hodge HL: Diagnostic evaluation of dyspnea. Am Fam Physician 1998;**4:**711.
Runo JR, Ely EW: Treating dyspnea in a patient with advanced chronic obstructive pulmonary disease. West J Med 2001;**175:**197.

---

21   Dysuria in Women

L. Peter Schwiebert, MD

KEY POINTS

- In women with dysuria, consideration of historic risk factors should drive differential diagnosis and evaluation.
- Urinalysis or leukocyte esterase dipstick testing is the most important laboratory study in diagnosing urinary tract infection.
- Findings compatible with acute uncomplicated urinary tract infection warrant empiric treatment for *Escherichia coli.*

I. **Definition. Dysuria** is discomfort associated with micturition, commonly due to **bacterial urinary tract infection** (UTI). (Among uncomplicated UTIs, 75–90% are due to *E coli*, approximately 15% are due to *Staphylococcus saprophyticus*, and 5–10% are due to *Proteus mirabilis.*) The foregoing organisms may also cause recurrent or difficult to eradicate (ie, complicated) UTIs; such infections may also be due to *Serratia, Pseudomonas aeruginosa, Klebsiella,* enterococci, and Enterobacteriaceae species.

Other causes of dysuria include:

A. **Bladder or urethral irritation** (eg, interstitial cystitis [IC]).

B. **Urethral trauma, bubble baths, or dietary factors.**

C. **Vaginal atrophy** (postmenopausal or other hypoestrogenic state).

D. **Urethritis,** often due to sexually transmitted diseases (STDs), including *Chlamydia trachomatis, Neisseria gonorrhoeae, Trichomonas vaginalis,* or herpes simplex virus (HSV) virus infection.

E. **Psychogenic dysuria** (often a component of somatization disorder, depression, chronic pain, or sexual abuse).

II. **Common Diagnoses.** Clinical syndromes associated with dysuria account for 5–15% of visits to family physicians. Approximately 25% of American women report at least one bout of acute dysuria per year. UTI accounts for over 7 million visits and affects 50% of women at least once in their lifetime. Twenty percent of these women suffer recurrent UTIs.

A. Acute bacterial cystitis (25–35% of cases) is more likely with a past history of cystitis, sexual intercourse, diaphragm/spermicidal contraception, douching, or postponement of micturition. Risk factors for complicated UTIs include pregnancy, indwelling urinary catheter, urinary tract instrumentation within the past 2 weeks, urinary tract anomaly or stones, recent systemic antibiotic use, or immunosuppression (eg, poorly controlled diabetes mellitus).

B. Vulvovaginitis (21–38% of cases) is a more frequent cause of dysuria in college-aged women than are UTIs.

C. The likelihood of **acute or subclinical pyelonephritis** (up to 30% of cases) is increased in women who are symptomatic for more than 7 days before seeking medical attention, of lower socioeconomic status, presenting to an inner-city emergency room, are pregnant, or having recurrent UTIs (more than three in the past year), or in women with a history of first UTI before age 12, with recurrence of a UTI within 7 days of completion of appropriate antibiotic therapy, or with other risk factors for complicated UTI (see section II,A). Approximately one third of women with lower UTI symptoms will have unrecognized or subclinical pyelonephritis.

D. The likelihood of **dysuria without pyuria** (15–30% of cases) is increased with history of urethral trauma, in women in a postmenopausal state and not receiving estrogen replacement therapy, or with physical/chemical irritants (eg, douching, or consumption of citrus, ethanol, caffeinated carbonated beverages, sugar, or spicy foods). Ninety percent of patients with IC are women (up to 700,000 US women are affected); patients with this syndrome have a median age of 40 and tend to have a past history of childhood or adult UTIs.

E. Urethritis (3–10% of cases) should be considered in women with a recent new sex partner, multiple partners, or a partner with urethritis. Thirty to 50% of nongonococcal urethritis is due to *C trachomatis;* other organisms implicated include urea plasmids and *T vaginalis.*

III. Symptoms. The onset of symptoms is usually abrupt, and the patient may describe "internal" dysuria (ie, suprapubic pain), as opposed to stinging of the skin (ie, "external dysuria").

A. Dysuria

1. Dysuria is the cardinal symptom of acute bacterial cystitis. Other symptoms of this condition include urinary frequency, mild anorexia or nausea, nocturia, urgency, the voiding of small amounts, urinary incontinence, and suprapubic pain. A recent meta-analysis found that four factors significantly correlate with a diagnosis of UTI: frequency, hematuria, dysuria, and back pain. This same study found four factors (ie, absent dysuria or back pain, history of vaginal discharge or vaginal irritation) that decrease the likelihood of UTI; women with one or more symptoms of UTI have approximately a 50% likelihood of this diagnosis and combinations of the eight findings can raise the probability of UTI to >90%.

2. The dysuria accompanying urethritis often has a stuttering, gradual onset and is "internal." Increased frequency and urgency of urination may indicate dysuria without pyuria.

3. Patients who complain of external dysuria, or a burning sensation as the urine passes the inflamed labia, may have vulvovaginitis.

B. Vaginal discharge

1. Dysuria and an associated increase in vaginal discharge from concomitant cervicitis may indicate urethritis.

2. Patients with vulvovaginitis complain of vaginal discharge, odor, or itching.

C. Pain. Localized pain in the flank, low back, or abdomen and systemic symptoms, such as fever, rigors, sweats, headaches, nausea, vomiting, malaise, and prostration, can occur with UTI, particularly pyelonephritis.

D. Interstitial cystitis (IC) is characterized by persistent pelvic or perineal pain, temporarily relieved by voiding, and consistent urinary urgency and voiding 16–40 times daily, in the absence of a history of radiation, tuberculosis, or chemical cystitis.

IV. Signs

A. Acute bacterial cystitis

1. Fever almost never develops when a UTI is localized to the bladder.

2. Suprapubic tenderness is present in only about 10% of patients with cystitis. If this sign is present, however, it has a high predictive value for cystitis.

B. Vulvovaginitis. For signs of this condition, see Chapter 64.

C. **Pyelonephritis.** The patient often has a fever (temperature of 38–39 °C [101–102 °F]), costovertebral angle tenderness, and tachycardia.
D. **Dysuria without pyuria.** In this case, the physical findings just described are absent. The pelvic examination may show some periurethral or vulvar irritation, however.
E. **Urethritis.** Urethritis is frequently associated with mucopurulent cervicitis.
V. **Laboratory Tests** (Figure 21–1).
  A. A **clean-catch midstream urinalysis (UA)** is readily available in most offices and essential for evaluating patients with dysuria. Using the definition of significant bacteriuria as $>10^2$ of a single uropathogenic bacterial species per milliliter in a symptomatic patient, pyuria (>5 white blood cells [WBCs] per centrifuged high-power field) is found in up to 95% of patients with acute cystitis and $>10^5$ bacteria per milliliter and over 70% of patients with acute cystitis and 10^2–10^5 bacteria per milliliter. The **leukocyte esterase dipstick** test is 75–95% sensitive and specific in detecting pyuria and is a reasonable substitute if urine microscopy is unavailable. Microscopic hematuria is present in up to 60% of women with acute bacterial cystitis, but its absence does not rule out this diagnosis. Twenty percent of women with IC have gross hematuria without bacteriuria or WBCs.
  B. **Culture** (Figure 21–1).
    1. Urine culture is indicated in the following situations:
      a. If acute bacterial cystitis is suspected, but clinical findings and UA leave the diagnosis in question.
      b. If the patient has symptoms and signs of upper or complicated UTI (see section II,C).
      c. Two to four days after a patient completes treatment for a complicated UTI.
      d. After a patient self-administers antibiotics (see section VI,A,2).
    2. In women in whom **urethritis** is suspected, urethral and cervical cultures for N gonorrhoeae and C trachomatis should be performed.
  C. IC can be diagnosed with findings verifiable only with **cystoscopy** (ie, glomerulations or ulcers, absence of bladder tumor). **Urodynamic studies** will also demonstrate small bladder capacity—ie, <350 mL and urge to void at 150 mL.
VI. **Treatment** of women with dysuria is based on the clinical picture, supplemented by appropriate laboratory studies. In patients with findings compatible with acute uncomplicated bacterial cystitis, it is reasonable to initiate treatment for E coli based on UA findings alone.
A. **Acute, uncomplicated bacterial cystitis** (Table 21–1).
    1. **Short-course antibiotics**
      a. Trimethoprim-sulfamethoxazaole-double strength (TMP-SMX-DS), one tablet twice daily for 3 days, is the first-line treatment in non-sulfa-allergic women. However, up to 18% of E coli are resistant, and the likelihood of resistance increases with recent hospitalization, use of TMP-SMX during the previous 6 months, or recurrent UTIs during the past year.
      b. In patients with sulfa allergy, the following alternative regimens are effective: trimethoprim (TMP), 100 mg orally twice daily, nitrofurantoin, 100 mg orally four times daily, ciprofloxacin, 250 mg orally twice daily, ofloxacin, 200 mg orally twice daily, or fosfomycin, 3 g orally. All of these medications are taken for 3 days, except fosfomycin, which is taken as a single dose.
    2. **Recurrent UTIs.** Women with one to two uncomplicated UTIs per year can be given a prescription for an appropriate short-course antibiotic (see section VI,A,1,b). Women who experience three or more symptomatic UTIs over the preceding 12 months or two or more symptomatic UTIs over 6 months warrant prophylaxis.
      a. Measures shown to decrease the number of UTIs include frequent bladder emptying (especially following sexual intercourse), discontinuation of diaphragm use, and urine acidification using cranberry juice (>300 mL daily) or oral ascorbic acid.
      b. Since symptoms develop in 85% of women with recurring infections within 24 hours following sexual intercourse, postcoital antibiotics (one dose orally after sexual intercourse) may be helpful. Acceptable regimens include TMP-SMX, one single-strength tablet; nitrofurantoin, 50–100 mg; or sulfisoxazole, 500 mg.
      c. If a postcoital regimen is not effective, long-term prophylaxis is indicated. Recommended regimens include one of the following: TMP-SMX, one single-strength tablet taken at bedtime or three times weekly; TMP, 100 mg once daily at bedtime; norfloxacin, 200 mg once daily at bedtime; or nitrofurantoin,

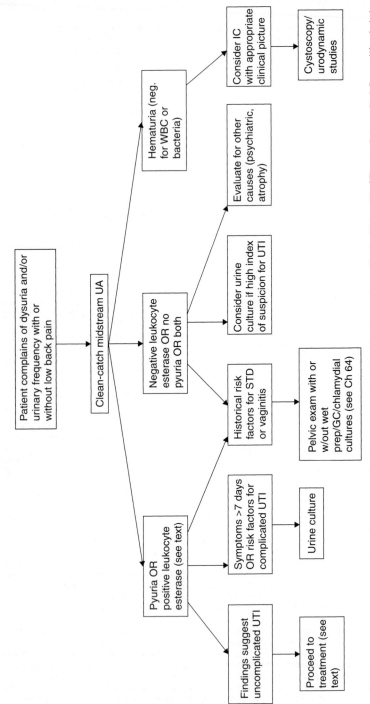

FIGURE 21-1. Approach to evaluation of ambulatory women with urinary tract symptoms. GC, *Neisseria gonorrhoeae*; IC, interstitial cystitis; STD, sexually transmitted disease; UA, urinalysis; UTI, urinary tract infection; WBC, white blood cells.

TABLE 21-1. ANTIBIOTICS RECOMMENDED FOR AMBULATORY MANAGEMENT OF UTIS IN WOMEN

Drug	Dosage (mg)
Trimethoprim-sulfamethoxazole (TMP-SMX)[1]	160/800 twice daily
Trimethoprim (TMP)[2]	100 twice daily or 200 daily
Nitrofurantoin[2]	100 four times daily
Ciprofloxacin[2,3,4]	250 twice daily
Ofloxacin[2,4]	200 twice daily
Fosfomycin[2,4]	3000 (single dose)

[1] Preferred agent in non–sulfa-allergic patients (3-day or 10- to 14-day regimen); in populations with low likelihood of resistance.
[2] Short-course (3-day) alternatives to TMP-SMX in sulfa-allergic patients.
[3] Preferred oral medication for ambulatory treatment of pyelonephritis (500 mg twice daily orally for 7 days).
[4] Relatively expensive.

50–100 mg once daily at bedtime. Antibiotics should be discontinued 3–6 months after initiating treatment to identify patients who will remain disease-free; women experiencing recurrences should receive extended (1- to 2-year) prophylaxis.

  d. Patients with one or two bouts of uncomplicated UTIs per year can be given an antibiotic prescription for a 3-day treatment course when symptoms occur.
 B. Vulvovaginitis (see Chapter 64).
 C. Pyelonephritis
  a. Febrile, ill-appearing patients should be hospitalized for treatment with parenteral antibiotics; those with mild symptoms (temperature <38.3 °C, no nausea or vomiting, good oral intake) in whom close follow-up is feasible can be treated as outpatients. A recent study found that 7 days of ciprofloxacin, 500 mg orally twice daily, resulted in greater bacterial and clinical cure rates than a standard 2-week course of TMP-SMX-DS.
  b. Patients with complicated UTI are at risk for subclinical pyelonephritis and should be treated with a standard 10- to 14-day regimen (Table 21-1).
 D. Dysuria without pyuria
  1. Offending agents identified through careful history should be eliminated.
  2. Postmenopausal women whose symptoms are believed due to estrogen deficiency may benefit from estrogen replacement (see Chapter 78).
  3. Other measures that may prove helpful include taking warm baths, avoiding acidic foods (eg, coffee, citrus fruits, tomato products, chocolate) and alcohol, artificial sweeteners, and carbonated beverages; increasing fluid intake (water is best) to dilute urine; drinking 8 oz water with 1 tbsp baking soda; or taking antispasmodics, such as phenazopyridine (eg, Pyridium) 100–200 mg orally three times daily, or hyoscyamine sulfate (eg, Levsin), 0.125–0.250 mg orally every 4 hours.
  4. For **IC**, a variety of agents have been used, without convincing evidence of efficacy in large, placebo-controlled trials (though there has been evidence of success in open-label trials). These agents include tricyclic antidepressants (eg, amitriptyline or imipramine, 25–75 mg orally at bedtime), antihistamines (eg, cimetidine, 300 mg orally twice daily, or hydroxyzine, 25–75 mg orally at bedtime).
  a. The only agent approved for IC by the US Food and Drug Administration is pentosan polysulfate (eg, Elmiron), 100 mg orally three times daily. Patients may take up to 6 months to respond and may experience side effects, including diarrhea, dyspepsia, headaches, rashes, or abdominal pain.
  b. Patients responding poorly to oral therapies and patients with severe symptoms may benefit from urologic referral for further management, such as intravesical dimethyl sulfoxide (DMSO).
 E. Urethritis. Empiric therapy for *C trachomatis* or *N gonorrhoeae* can be instituted in high-risk individuals while one is awaiting culture results. Because of the coprevalence of *N gonorrhoeae* and *C trachomatis* infection, patients should be treated with ceftriaxone (eg, Rocephin), 250 mg intramuscularly (one dose), and doxycycline, 100 mg orally twice a day for 7 days. Alternatives to ceftriaxone for *N gonorrhoeae* include cefixime (eg, Suprax), 400 mg, ciprofloxacin (eg, Cipro) 250 mg, or ofloxacin (eg, Floxin), 400 mg orally for one dose. Alternatives to doxycycline for *C trachomatis* include azithromycin, 1.0 g orally for one dose, or erythromycin base, 500 mg, or erythromycin ethylsuccinate,

800 mg orally four times daily for 7 days. **Pregnant or breast-feeding women should receive ceftriaxone plus erythromycin.** (Also see the sidebar on asymptomatic bacteriuria.)

ASYMPTOMATIC BACTERIURIA

Asymptomatic bacteriuria (ASB) is present in between 5% and 10% of pregnant women, with an increased likelihood in women who are sexually active or have diabetes, increased parity, or lower socioeconomic status. In 20–35% of women with ASB in pregnancy, overt UTI eventually develops. The American College of Obstetrics and Gynecologists recommends screening all pregnant patents with urine culture at the initial prenatal visit and in the third trimester.

Recommended antibiotics for treating UTI in pregnancy include nitrofurantoin (eg, Macrobid), 100 mg orally every 12 hours for 7 days, or a cephalosporin (eg, cephalexin), 250–500 mg orally four times daily for 7 days, with follow-up culture after treatment and monthly for the duration of the pregnancy, and consideration of prophylactic nitrofurantoin following a bout of pyelonephritis.

The evaluation and management of **elderly women with symptomatic UTI** is as described in the main text. In healthy **elderly women with asymptomatic bacteriuria,** there is no evidence that treatment reduces long-term renal problems; treatment increases cost, the likelihood of drug reactions (or drug-drug interactions), and the likelihood of drug-resistant microorganisms.

REFERENCES

Bent S, Saint S: The optimal use of diagnostic testing in women with acute uncomplicated cystitis. Am J Med 2002;**113**(1A):20S.

Bent S, et al: Does this woman have an acute uncomplicated urinary tract infection? JAMA 2002; **287**:2701.

Bremnor JD, Sadovsky R: Evaluation of dysuria in adults. Am Fam Physician 2002;**65**:1589.

Delzell JE, Lefevre ML: Urinary tract infections during pregnancy. Am Fam Physician 2000;**61**:713.

Metts JF: Interstitial cystitis: Urgency and frequency syndrome. Am Fam Physician 2001;**64**:1199.

---

22   Earache

Stephen W. Cobb, MD, & David W. Euans, MD

KEY POINTS

- Most causes of otalgia are benign and are easily diagnosed and managed in the office setting.
- The most important pathogen to consider when choosing an antibiotic in acute otitis media is *Streptococcus pneumoniae.*
- Otalgia not resolving with appropriate therapy should be evaluated by an otolaryngologist.

I. **Definition.** Earache (otalgia) is pain or discomfort perceived in the ear or surrounding structures. This pain may be due to middle ear pathology, including **eustachian tube dysfunction** (ETD) by itself or in combination with viral (influenza A, respiratory syncytial virus, or adenoviral) or bacterial (*Staphylococcus pneumoniae, Haemophilus–influenzae, Moraxella catarrhalis*) infection resulting in elevated middle ear pressure/inflammation (**acute otitis media** [AOM]). Earache can also be due to external auditory canal pathology, from canal trauma or water pooling and maceration, allowing infection with *Pseudomonas aeruginosa, Proteus vulgaris,* or fungi (**otitis externa** [OE]). Other sources of earache include pressure imbalance between the external and middle ear, possibly worsened by ETD (**barotrauma**); hematoma; tympanic membrane (TM) rupture; lacerations (**direct trauma**); or pain in surrounding structures perceived in the ear (**referred pain**).

II. **Common Diagnoses.** Earache most commonly originates from middle ear or external auditory canal pathology.

   A. **Acute otitis media (AOM)** occurs most frequently during the winter months, thus coinciding with the peak incidence of viral upper respiratory tract infections. The peak age incidence is 6 months to 7 years. Native Americans and Eskimos experience otitis media more frequently than do people of other races. Otitis media is also more prevalent in children with Down syndrome or cleft palate. Children who are in group day-care and whose parents smoke cigarettes are also at increased risk.

   B. **Otitis externa (OE)** is 10–20 times more common in the summer than in cooler months, particularly in individuals who swim in lakes or pools. This condition is more likely to affect diabetics, who are also more likely to develop invasive disease.

   C. **Barotrauma** most commonly occurs either after flying in an unpressurized aircraft or after scuba diving. Acute upper respiratory infections and allergies increase susceptibility to this condition.

   D. **Direct trauma** is seen more frequently in young males, resulting from fights or automobile accidents; in military personnel or miners, who may work near explosions; or in hikers, mountain climbers, or outdoor workers in cold climates, who may suffer frostbite.

   E. **Referred otalgia** occurs secondary to the complex innervation of the head and neck. The ear is innervated by sensory branches of the trigeminal, facial, vagus, and glossopharyngeal cranial nerves and by the lesser occipital and great auricular cervical nerves.

      1. **Temporomandibular joint (TMJ) dysfunction** tends to occur in patients with the following conditions: (1) dental malocclusion or poorly fitting dental prostheses, (2) bruxism (nocturnal tooth grinding), (3) trauma to the mandible, or (4) degenerative TMJ disease, especially in women in the third or fourth decade of life.

      2. Individuals with **poor oral hygiene** are likely to develop dental diseases, such as abscesses.

      3. Patients with a history of **heavy tobacco or alcohol use** or serous otitis (in adults), those of Chinese ancestry, and those with dysphagia or hemoptysis are at increased risk for cancers of the ear, nose, and throat region.

III. **Symptoms**

   A. **Pain**

      1. Severe deep pain or "up all night" ear pain may indicate **AOM,** but is nonspecific.

      2. Patients with **OE** may experience moderate pain, especially with lying on the affected side, or jaw movement.

      3. **Barotrauma** may progress from pressure to moderate to severe pain if unrelieved over a few hours.

      4. **Direct trauma** causes pain in the injured part of the ear; frostbite of the auricle usually causes burning pain lasting several hours.

      5. Pain in **referred otalgia** depends on the cause (Table 22–1).

   B. **Hearing impairment**

      1. Decreased hearing in the affected ear is common both in **ETD and AOM.**

      2. Hearing loss, along with tinnitus and vertigo, may occur with **barotrauma.**

      3. Complaints of impaired hearing are rare in **OE** unless the canal is so edematous it is partially or totally blocked.

   C. Patients with **OE** may present with itching.

   D. **Associated symptoms**

      1. Fever, dizziness, nausea, and vomiting may occur with **AOM.**

      2. Parents of infants and small children with **AOM** may observe irritability, decreased feeding, or pulling at the ears.

IV. **Signs.** Examination of patients with otalgia should be directed by the foregoing risk factors and symptoms and should include systematic evaluation of the auricle, auditory canals, and TMs, as well as sources of referred otalgia as indicated (Table 22–1).

   A. **Auricle**

      1. Erythema or crusting may occur if this portion of the ear is involved in **OE.**

      2. **OE** causes pain with movement of the auricle or pressure on the tragus.

TABLE 22–1. CAUSES OF REFERRED OTALGIA

Cause	Mechanism	Symptoms	Signs	Laboratory Tests	Treatment	Comments
TMJ dysfunction	Internal derangement of joint, malocclusion, poorly fitting dental prostheses, bruxism	Deep pain that becomes worse with eating	Pain on palpation, crepitus, asymmetry of motion	None	Ibuprofen, 200–400 mg tid–qid; moist heat; mechanical soft diet. Refer to dentist if not relieved in 3–4 weeks	
Dental disease	Inflammation or pressure on nerves by abscessed teeth, impacted third molars	Dull to lancinating pain that becomes worse with eating, tooth very sensitive to cold	Carious teeth, tender teeth, red or necrotic gingiva	None	Dental referral; codeine, 30–60 mg, and/or aspirin or acetaminophen, 325 mg q4h; penicillin V, 250–500 mg qid	
Head and neck tumors	Traction on or inflammation of nerves	Hoarseness, lump, dysphagia, slowly increasing pain or pressure	Tumor in nasopharynx or larynx	CT, MRI	Refer for excision or biopsy and possible radiation or chemotherapy	
Infection of sinuses, pharynx	Nerve irritation from infection	Retro-orbital or frontal pain, sore throat	Sinus tenderness, poor transillumination, exudative pharyngitis	Sinus x-rays, strep screen	See Chapters 55 and 57	
Carotodynia	Pain referred along same nerve pathways as the ear	Throat pain, dysphagia	Tender bifurcation of carotid artery	None	Aspirin, 650 mg qid, moist heat to affected side of neck	
Temporal arteritis	Collagen vascular disease with inflammation	Pain near affected arteries, weight loss, fever, jaw claudication	Tender, indurated temporal artery	Elevated ESR, temporal artery biopsy	Prednisone, 60 mg/day; taper by 10% weekly to 10 mg/day after 4–6 weeks; then taper 1 mg/week	Treat to prevent blindness. Use ESR to monitor therapy
Trigeminal, glossopharyngeal, or sphenopalatine neuralgia	Compression of nerves	Lancinating pain triggered by chewing or swallowing cold liquids	Trigger points in nasopharynx	None	Carbamazepine, 200 mg/day, up to 1600 mg/day; phenytoin, 300–400 mg/day; or baclofen, up to 20 mg tid. Surgical decompression, ablation for nonresponders	Aplastic anemia can occur with carbamazepine
GERD (gastroesophageal reflux disease)	Nerve irritation from acid stimulation	Worse at night or with stimulating foods	None	pH study, upper GI study	Diet and behavioral changes. Antacids H_2 blockers (see Chapters 19 and 82)	

ESR, erythrocyte sedimentation rate; CT, computerized tomography; GI, gastrointestinal; MRI, magnetic resonance imaging; TMJ, temporomandibular joint.

3. In **direct trauma,** injury to the auricle is evident from inspection; frostbite may initially present with auricular pallor, followed by erythema and sometimes, bullae.
   B. **External auditory canal**
   1. The canal in **OE** is red and edematous, usually with purulent drainage.
   2. Canal injuries with **direct trauma** include lacerations, abrasions, or hematomas.
   C. **Tympanic membrane (TM)**
   1. In diagnosing **AOM,** positive predictive values in the 90% range compared to myringotomy have been achieved with the following findings: an opaque TM, a bulging TM, and impaired TM mobility. The presence of a reddened TM alone, without pneumatic otoscopic evidence of immobility, is not sufficient to diagnose AOM, as an erythematous TM may also be due to increased intravascular pressure (eg, a crying infant or child).
   2. Vesicles may occur in **viral syndromes** or the Ramsay-Hunt syndrome; bullous myringitis was thought to be pathognomonic of *Mycoplasma* or other viruses, but the specificity of this finding has recently been questioned.
   3. Small yellow flecks behind the TM may be subtle findings of **cholesteatoma.**
   4. A purulent nonmalodorous discharge in the canal may be seen with TM rupture in **AOM;** perforation often occurs near the annulus, necessitating clear view of the entire TM.
   5. In **ETD,** the TM may appear normal, may have some hyperemia, or may be bulging (with positive middle ear pressure) or retracted (with negative middle ear pressure). Positive TM pressure is identified by exaggerated prominence of the umbo.
   6. In **barotrauma** the TM initially appears red, later becoming blue or yellow. With continued ET blockage, bubbles or air-fluid levels may be seen.
   D. Findings with **referred pain** are described in Table 22–1.
V. **Laboratory Tests.** The cause of otalgia is usually evident from the history and examination. Laboratory tests may be helpful in the following situations.
   A. If otitis media is suspected, **tympanometry** may be useful in equivocal cases. It may also be helpful for follow-up examination of patients treated for acute otitis media, especially those who are very young. The presence of significantly reduced pressure and poor TM movement helps diagnose a middle ear effusion. Tympanometry has not been found to be superior to pneumatic otoscopy when both are performed expertly.
   B. The **white blood cell count (WBC)** in cases of AOM is frequently elevated and shifted to the left, particularly in children. The complete blood count is not routinely done in nontoxic-appearing children with AOM.
   C. **Radiography** and **computerized tomography (CT)** are useful to determine the presence of other associated injury when occult fractures of the skull or intracerebral injury is suspected These techniques are usually not needed to diagnose ear injuries, however. If mastoiditis is suspected, CT is useful to rule out or confirm.
   D. **Referred pain** (see Table 22–1 for details).
VI. **Treatment**
   A. **Otitis media**
   1. **AOM** (see Table 22–2).
      a. **Antibiotic use** is controversial. In many countries, uncomplicated AOM is successfully treated without antibiotics. In selecting an antimicrobial, it is important to remember that the bacteria most commonly isolated with middle ear effusions are *S pneumoniae* (50%), *H influenzae* (30%), and *M catarrhalis* (25%). Of these, the most important pathogen is *S pneumoniae.* AOM caused by viruses, nontypeable *H influenzae,* or *M catarrhalis* is likely to resolve spontaneously and is unlikely to progress to more invasive disease. *S pneumoniae* is more likely to progress. Drug-resistant *S pneumoniae* is common and develops resistance by alterations in penicillin-binding proteins, not β-lactamase mechanisms. Therefore, in all but highly resistant organisms, resistance is overcome by higher doses of penicillin, not adding β-lactam stabilizers (eg, clavulanic acid).
      b. No studies have documented the efficacy of **decongestants or antihistamines** in the treatment of otitis media, but they are useful for symptomatic care (see Chapter 55 for dosage). **Analgesics** such as ibuprofen are also indicated for pain relief.
      c. The parents of young patients with acute otitis media should be **educated** concerning the importance of having the child finish the course of antibiotics as well as keeping follow-up appointments. They should also be made aware of

TABLE 22-2. ORAL DRUG THERAPY FOR ACUTE OTITIS MEDIA

Indication	Drug	Dosage		Comments
		Pediatric	Adult	
First-line therapy	Amoxicillin	50 mg/kg/day tid	500 mg tid	Least costly; treatment failures associated with resistant organisms
Second-line therapy	Amoxicillin[1]	80–90 g/kg/day		
Second-line therapy	Amoxicillin plus clavulanate	40 mg/kg/day tid	250–500 mg tid	Diarrhea common
Second-line therapy	Azithromycin	10 mg/kg/day, day 1; 5 mg/kg/day, days 2–5	500 mg, day 1; 250 mg, days 2–5	Long half-life allows short course of treatment
Second-line therapy	Cefaclor	40 mg/kg/day tid	500 mg tid	
Second-line therapy	Cefixime	8 mg/kg/day daily or bid	400–800 mg daily	Gastrointestinal side effects common
Second-line therapy	Cefpodoxime proxetil	10 mg/kg/day	200 mg bid	
Second-line therapy	Cefprozil	30 mg/kg/day	250–500 mg bid	Excellent antimicrobial spectrum
Second-line therapy	Cefuroxime axetil	30 mg/kg/day bid	250–500 mg bid	Diarrhea common; suspension may have unpleasant aftertaste
Second-line therapy	Erythromycin[2]	40 mg/kg/day qid	250–500 mg qid	For penicillin-allergic patients > age 4 years
Second-line therapy	Erythromycin (E) plus sulfamethoxazole (S)[2]	50 mg/kg/day qid (E) plus 150 mg/kg/day qid (S)		For penicillin-allergic patients between 2 months and 4 years of age
Second-line therapy	Loracarbef	30 mg/kg/day q12h	200 mg q12h	
Third-line therapy	Trimethoprim-sulfamethoxazole[2]	1 tsp/10 kg bid	1 double-strength tablet bid	Not effective against group A streptococci
	Ceftriaxone	50 mg/kg/day	One g IM for 1–3 days	

[1] Use higher dose with high rates of drug-resistant *Streptococcus pneumoniae* (DRSP). DRSP is more likely with day-care attendance, age older than 2 years, and antibiotic use within the preceding 3 months.
[2] Alternative drugs for penicillin-allergic patients.

        signs of possible invasive disease (ie, extreme irritability or somnolence, worsening pain, persistent fever). Risks, including tobacco smoke exposure and group day-care (6 or more households represented), should be reviewed.

  d. Follow-up

    (1) The patient should be **re-evaluated in 48–72 hours if fever or pain persists** at pretreatment levels. In this case, a 10-day course of a different antibiotic should be instituted. If the symptoms fail to improve after this intervention, the patient should be referred to a physician who can perform tympanocentesis for further evaluation, fluid culture, and management.

    (2) The patient should then **be re-evaluated at 2- to 4-week intervals** if an effusion has not resolved. An effusion may require up to 3 months to clear. Antibiotics are not indicated for persistent middle ear effusion in the absence of AOM. Effusions persisting beyond 3 months should be evaluated by an otolaryngologist.

(3) AOM is usually benign, but can be complicated by hearing loss, mastoiditis, and cholesteatoma. AOM that evolves into a chronically draining ear is highly suspicious for cholesteatoma. Severe complications include central nervous system infection and thrombosis.

e. **AOM in infants**

(1) Infants younger than age 2 months should be hospitalized for fever even if a source (eg, AOM) is identified. Children with fever and AOM between ages 2 and 6 months may be treated as outpatients after careful evaluation by a seasoned clinician. Children older than 6 months may be treated with an outpatient course of antibiotics if there is no complicating historical or physical finding (TM perforation, craniofacial abnormality, recurrent or chronic infection, or immunocompromise). A follow-up examination should take place in 3 weeks.

(2) A **polyvalent pneumococcal vaccine** is available for infants and has been shown to decrease the incidence of AOM and invasive pneumococcal disease.

2. **Recurrent AOM**

a. **Underlying conditions predisposing to recurrent disease** (defined as three episodes of AOM in a 6-month period or four or more episodes in a 12-month period) should be treated when associated with recurrence. Such disorders include enlarged adenoids, allergies, immunodeficiencies, nasal septal deviation, and sinusitis.

b. The insertion of **tympanostomy tubes,** which results in immediate improvement in hearing, has been advocated for the prevention of recurrent otitis media. However, surgical management has not been proved superior to antibiotic prophylaxis or interval treatment of recurrences for preserving hearing. The interpretation of these data is controversial.

c. Antibiotics used for prophylaxis of recurrent otitis media include **amoxicillin,** 25 mg/kg/day at bedtime; **sulfisoxazole,** 75 mg/kg/day at bedtime; and **trimethoprim-sulfamethoxazole,** 25 mg/kg/day at bedtime, based on the sulfamethoxazole component.

B. **Otitis externa**

1. First, the canal is gently and thoroughly cleansed of debris using a cotton-tipped applicator. Following this, an otic solution of polymyxin B, Neosporin, and hydrocortisone (eg, Cortisporin otic) should be instilled into the ear canal four times daily until symptoms are resolved. Adults should use four drops, and children, three drops, each application. An effective alternative is 2% acetic acid in propylene glycol (VoSol or VoSol HC) used in the same manner. Likewise, ofloxacin otic solution has been shown to be effective when used twice daily. With possible TM perforation, a suspension should be used instead of the solution, to minimize patient discomfort.

2. **If the auditory canal is very edematous,** the placement of a small absorptive wick in the canal will help to distribute the medication to the deeper parts of the canal. The wick may be removed once the edema has resolved.

3. **External otitis with cellulitis** of the auricle should be treated with systemic antibiotics effective against *Staphylococcus aureus* and β-hemolytic streptococci (see Chapter 9).

4. Patients with **necrotizing otitis externa,** a severe infection involving the deeper periauricular tissue, should be hospitalized and treated with parenteral antibiotics providing adequate pseudomonal coverage.

C. **Barotrauma**

1. The **acute episode** may be treated with decongestants (eg, **pseudoephedrine,** 30–60 mg every 4–6 hours) and analgesics (**acetaminophen,** 325–650 mg every 4–6 hours, or **codeine,** 30–60 mg every 4–6 hours).

2. **Patients with multiple episodes** of barotrauma should use a long-acting oral decongestant, such as timed-release **pseudoephedrine,** 120 mg once or twice daily, or a topical nasal decongestant such as **phenylephrine,** two sprays 5 minutes apart in each nostril 30 minutes prior to flying or diving. Individuals who use topical decongestants should be cautioned to apply them only intermittently to avoid

rhinitis medicamentosum. To prevent future recurrences, the diver or flier should be instructed in the proper methods of equalizing middle ear and ambient pressure, such as swallowing hard or exhaling against closed nostrils.

D. Direct trauma
   1. **Abrasions and small lacerations** of the auricle should be treated as are other minor skin injuries (see Chapter 41).
   2. **Hematomas** of the auricle should be aspirated, and a pressure dressing should be applied to prevent formation of a cauliflower ear.
   3. **Traumatic perforations** of the TM are treated by keeping the canal dry. If the perforations do not heal within several weeks, the patient should be referred to an otolaryngologist.

E. Referred otalgia (see Table 22–1).

REFERENCES

Dowell S, Schwartz B, Phillips W: Appropriate use of antibiotics for URIs in children: Part I. Otitis media and acute sinusitis. Am Fam Physician 1998;**58**:1113.

Dowell S, et al, and the Drug Resistant *Streptococcus pneumoniae* Therapeutic Working Group. Acute otitis media: Management and surveillance in an era of pneumococcal resistance—A report from the Drug Resistant *Streptococcus pneumoniae* Therapeutic Working Group. Pediatr Infect Dis J 1999;**18**:1.

Gilbert D, Moellering R, Sande M (editors): *The Sanford Guide to Antimicrobial Therapy*. Antimicrobial Therapy; 2003.

Jones R, Milazzo J, Seidlin M: Ofloxacin otic solution for treatment of otitis externa in children and adults. Arch Otolaryngol Head Neck Surg 1997;**123**:1193.

Karma P, et al: Pneumatic otoscopy and OM: The value of different TM findings and their combinations. In: Kim D, Bluestone C, Klein J, et al (editors): *Recent Advances in OM*. Proceedings of the Fifth International Symposium. Burlington, Ontario, December 1993, pp. 41–55.

---

23   Edema

Joshua H. Barash, MD

KEY POINTS

- Edema is a common complaint in primary care and often the manifestation of a serious underlying disease process.
- The underlying etiology causing a patient's edema is best determined based on the distribution of the accumulated fluid, in combination with a targeted history and carefully chosen diagnostic tests.
- Various nonpharmacologic measures are effective in controlling edema.

I. **Definition.** Edema is the excessive accumulation of fluid in the tissues. Responsible factors include (1) **increased capillary pressure**—(eg, congestive heart failure [CHF], deep vein thrombosis [DVT], venous insufficiency, pregnancy, or drugs); (2) **decreased plasma proteins** (eg, nephrotic syndrome, denuded skin areas [wounds], hepatocellular failure, or severe malnutrition); (3) **increased capillary permeability** (eg, allergic reactions, bacterial infections, burns, prolonged ischemia, or idiopathic edema); and (4) **lymphatic blockage** (eg, local lymphatic blockage from cancer or generalized lymphatic blockage [retroperitoneal]).

II. **Common Diagnoses.** Edema is a common complaint in primary care and often the manifestation of a serious underlying disease process.

   A. **Bilateral lower extremity edema**
      1. This condition **usually results from systemic conditions** (CHF, hepatocellular disease, or venous insufficiency). **Risk factors for CHF** include coronary artery disease or acute ischemia, valvular disease, alcohol excess (leading to alcoholic

cardiomyopathy), and hypertension. **Risk factors for hepatocellular disease** include a past history of alcoholism or hepatitis B or C infection. **Risk factors for chronic venous insufficiency** include a history of prior DVT, congenital valvular incompetence, or any process that destroys or damages deep venous valves.

2. Certain **drugs** (Table 23–1), as well as **hyperthyroidism and hypothyroidism,** can also cause bilateral lower extremity edema. **Lipedema** (leg swelling due to abnormal accumulation of fatty substances in the subcutaneous tissues) is commonly mistaken for lymphedema. This condition usually spares the feet and is found almost exclusively in young women.

B. **Unilateral lower extremity edema**
1. The most common causes are DVT (acutely) (see sidebar), or lymphedema (chronically). **DVT risk factors** include immobilization, malignancy, recent leg trauma, surgery, and hypercoagulable states. **Risk factors for lymphedema** include any process that results in obstruction of the lymphatic channels, such as malignancy, infection, surgery, trauma, or radiation exposure.
2. Other common causes of unilateral lower extremity edema include cellulitis, osteomyelitis, burns, and trauma (ruptured gastrocnemius, compartment syndrome, or soft tissue injury).

C. **Upper extremity edema** is rare and most commonly is due to the superior vena cava syndrome, usually from malignancy.

D. **Idiopathic edema** (hormone-related edema) is a diagnosis of exclusion. It is more common in women and may be hormonally mediated.

III. **Symptoms** (Figure 23–1).

A. In **bilateral swelling,** CHF is suggested by dyspnea on exertion, orthopnea, and paroxysmal dyspnea, whereas abdominal fullness in the absence of pulmonary symptoms is more common in patients with hepatocellular disease (cirrhosis).

B. In **unilateral swelling,** historical factors suggesting chronicity include old trauma, surgery, radiation, or old infection. Recent trauma suggests a ruptured gastrocnemius or compartment syndrome. Trauma (eg, puncture wound) followed by a focal area of erythema and pain suggests cellulitis. Recent inflammation may suggest a burn. Presence of risk factors may suggest an acute DVT.

C. In **idiopathic edema** (also referred to as **hormone-related edema**), the patient may gain several pounds during the day and exhibit significant edema of the hands, breasts, abdomen, and legs by evening. Upon lying down at night, the edema is mobilized, and nocturia often causes overnight loss of the excess weight.

IV. **Signs** (Figure 23–1).

A. **Bilateral pitting edema** with jugular venous distention, bibasilar fine rales, and wheezes points to CHF (see Chapter 72).

B. **Bilateral lower extremity edema** with ascites and absent pulmonary findings suggests hepatocellular disease.

C. **Chronic skin changes** (stasis dermatitis, brawny induration, ulcers) and absent pulmonary findings suggest chronic venous insufficiency.

D. **Unilateral edema associated with tenderness,** a palpable cord, or a Homan's sign (calf pain with passive dorsiflexion of the foot) suggests an acute DVT.

E. **Erythematous inflamed skin** may suggest an underlying cellulitis or osteomyelitis.

F. The **lack of involvement of the feet** characterizes lipedema and distinguishes it from lymphedema.

TABLE 23–1. MEDICATIONS KNOWN TO CAUSE PERIPHERAL EDEMA

Antidepressants	**Diabetic medications**
Monoamine oxidase inhibitors	Insulin sensitizers such as rosiglitazone
Antihypertensive medications	**Other medications**
Calcium channel blockers	Hormones
Direct vasodilators	Corticosteroids
Beta blockers	Estrogens/progesterones
Centrally acting agents	Testosterone
Antisympathetics	Nonsteroidal anti-inflammatory drugs (NSAIDs)

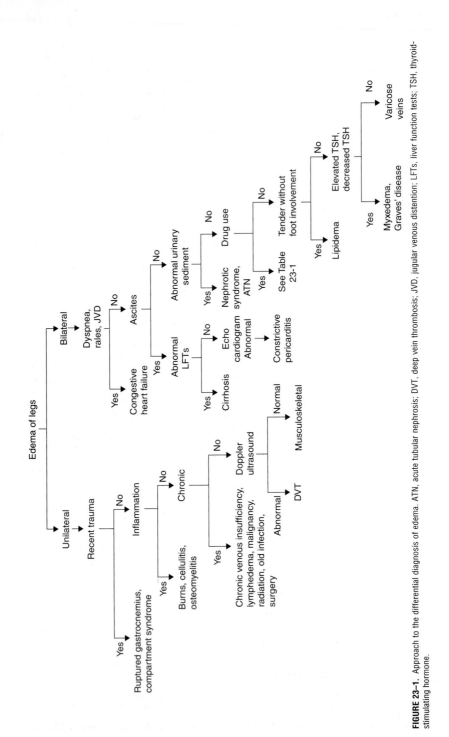

FIGURE 23–1. Approach to the differential diagnosis of edema. ATN, acute tubular nephrosis; DVT, deep vein thrombosis; JVD, jugular venous distention; LFTs, liver function tests; TSH, thyroid-stimulating hormone.

DEEP VEIN THROMBOSIS

Deep vein thrombosis. DVT can lead to significant morbidity and mortality if unrecognized and untreated. Although it is not possible to make a definitive diagnosis clinically, reasonable estimates of pretest probability for DVT can be made by ascertaining clinical features found to be independent predictors of DVT (see Table 23–2). Using an estimate of pretest probability in conjunction with results of noninvasive testing allows one to determine the need for anticoagulation, no anticoagulation, or further testing. For example, a person with a low pretest probability and a normal ultrasound test is effectively ruled out for DVT.

DVT below the knee carries a minimal risk of embolization (<1% per year) if the clot does not propagate into the thigh.

V. **Laboratory Tests** (Figure 23–1 and Table 23–3). After the physician does a targeted history and physical examination, a limited number of laboratory and diagnostic tests may be necessary to arrive at a diagnosis.
  A. In patients with **ascites in the absence of pulmonary signs,** abnormal liver function tests may suggest hepatocellular disease or cirrhosis.
  B. **Thyroid-stimulating hormone** can point to either hyperthyroidism or hypothyroidism in the absence of findings suggesting a cardiac or liver etiology, or in the absence of a drug side effect as a suspected cause of edema.
  C. A **urinalysis** demonstrating proteinuria may implicate the kidneys—for example, nephrotic syndrome or glomerulonephritis.
  D. Patients with unilateral lower extremity swelling and risk factors suggesting DVT may need the following tests.
    1. **Venous Doppler ultrasound** may be helpful in making a definitive diagnosis. The sensitivity and specificity of this test improve as pretest probability rises; in symptomatic patients sensitivity approaches 93% and specificity approaches 98%. In asymptomatic patients, the sensitivity falls to 59% while specificity remains at 98%.
    2. The **plasma D-Dimer test** is highly sensitive but not specific. It is useful in ruling out DVT in low-probability patients in conjunction with a normal Doppler ultrasound. Because of its low specificity, noninvasive testing is needed when a "positive" D-dimer test result is obtained.
    3. **Impedence plethysomography** detects changes in leg volumes using a thigh blood pressure cuff. In DVT, the normal pattern is altered and detected by plethysmography.
    4. **In questionable cases,** a venogram (nearly 100% sensitive and specific) usually provides a definitive diagnosis.

TABLE 23–2. MODEL FOR CLINICAL PREDICTION OF DVT[1]

Clinical Feature	Score
History	
Active cancer	1
Paralysis, recent plaster cast	1
Recent immobilization or major surgery	1
Physical examination	
Tenderness along deep veins	1
Swelling of entire leg	1
>3 cm difference in calf circumference	1
Pitting edema	1
Collateral superficial veins	1
Clinical assessment	
Alternative diagnosis likely	−2

[1] Pretest probability of deep vein thrombosis: high if score of 3 points or greater; intermediate if score of 1–2 points; and low if score of 0 or less.
From Wells PS, et al: Value of assessment of pretest probability of deep vein thrombosis in clinical management. Lancet 1997;**350:**1795.

TABLE 23–3. TESTS THAT MAY BE USEFUL IN EVALUATING THE CAUSE OF PERIPHERAL EDEMA

Test	Indication
Urinalysis	Glomerulonephritis, acute tubular necrosis, nephrotic syndrome
Thyroid-stimulating hormone	Hyperthyroidism, hypothyroidism
Liver function tests	Cirrhosis
Prealbumin	Malnutrition
D-dimer	Deep vein thrombosis
Chest x-ray	Congestive heart failure, lung cancer
Bone scan	Osteomyelitis
Ultrasound	Deep vein thrombosis, popliteal cyst
CAT scan	Malignancy, cirrhosis
Echocardiogram	Constrictive pericarditis, congestive heart failure

VI. Treatment. Specific diseases underlying edema should be treated (Chapter 72 for CHF, Chapter 84 for chronic renal failure). The following measures may be useful in managing other causes of edema discussed in this chapter.
  A. In patients with **varicose veins** and **venous insufficiency,** knee-length elastic stockings can aid venous return. In addition, periodic elevation throughout the day can help prevent edema; ideally, the leg should be above the level of the heart for this to be effective. Women should avoid the use of tight girdles, which can restrict superficial venous return at the thigh level. Finally, prolonged standing should be avoided if at all possible.
  B. Patients with **idiopathic edema (hormone-related edema)** should avoid diuretics because they can increase edema. Chronic diuretic use increases aldosterone secretion, exacerbating edema. Angiotensin converting enzyme (ACE) inhibitors have been used with success due to their suppression of aldosterone and salt and water retention. A common ACE inhibitor used for this purpose is captopril (Capoten), 25–50 mg by mouth two to three times each day. Sodium restriction may also benefit idiopathic edema.
  C. If an **offending medication** is implicated in edema, then a trial without the medicine should be instituted, substituting an alternative medication if necessary.
  D. Patients with **DVT** need initial clot stabilization with heparin followed by oral anticoagulation with coumadin.
    1. **Standard therapy** for acute DVT requires hospitalization and administration of intravenous *unfractionated* heparin, with concomitant initiation of oral coumadin. Heparin is continued until the patient achieves an international normalized ratio (INR) between 2.0 and 3.0, at which time heparin is discontinued and the patient is discharged home with continued oral coumadin.
    2. With the advent of **low-molecular-weight heparin,** inpatient hospitalization is not mandatory if close follow-up can be assured. Advantages of low-molecular-weight heparin include its efficacy, safety, and twice-daily dosing without the need for partial thromboplastin time (PTT) monitoring. A typical regimen is enoxaparin, 1 mg/kg twice daily by subcutaneous injection. Therapy is continued until an effective INR is achieved with oral coumadin.
    3. **Anticoagulation with oral coumadin** is usually continued for 3 months for a first-time DVT with known precipitant (eg, surgery or trauma). Recurrent DVTs or those without a clear etiology require treatment for at least 6 months and sometimes longer (eg, if serum lupus anticoagulant is identified).

REFERENCES

Andreoli TE: Edematous states: An overview. Kidney Int 1997;**51**(suppl 59):S2.
Blankfield RP, et al: Etiology and diagnosis of bilateral leg edema in primary care. Am J Med 1998;**105**:192.
Cho S, Atwood JE: Peripheral edema. Am J Med 2002;**113**:580.
Powell A, Armstrong M: Peripheral edema. Am Fam Physician 1997;**55**:1721.
Wells PS, et al: Value of assessment of pretest probability of deep vein thrombosis in clinical management. Lancet 1997;**350**:1795.

24   Enuresis

Patricia Taylor, MS, MPH, RN, Eve Ackerman, RN, MSN, ANP/CNP,
Isaac H. Cha, PharmD, BCPS, BC-ADM, Anna L. Meenan, MD, FAAFP,
& Loyd J. Wollstadt, MD, MSc

KEY POINTS

- Primary monosymptomatic nocturnal enuresis is the most common form of incontinence; there are usually no identifiable underlying pathologic findings.
- Diurnal enuresis suggests underlying bladder dysfunction.
- The most effective long-term treatment for primary monosymptomatic nocturnal enuresis is the alarm method.

I. **Definition. Enuresis** is involuntary urination after the age of expected urinary control. The International Children's Continence Society recommends the following terminology.
   A. **Nocturnal enuresis** should be considered in children 5–6 years old who have two or more bed-wetting episodes per month.
      1. **Primary monosymptomatic enuresis** is bed-wetting without a history of nocturnal continence and unassociated with other symptoms.
      2. **Secondary monosymptomatic enuresis** is recurrence of bed-wetting after at least 6 months of nocturnal continence.
      3. **Polysymptomatic nocturnal enuresis** is bed-wetting associated with urinary urgency, frequency, chronic constipation, or encopresis.
   B. **Diurnal enuresis** is diagnosed in children 5 years or older and is involuntary or intentional urination into clothing while awake or asleep.
II. **Common Diagnoses.** In the United States, it is estimated that 5–7 million children have primary enuresis, 80–85% are monosymptomatic, and no more than 5% will have an organic cause.
   A. Risk factors for **primary monosymptomatic nocturnal enuresis** include the following:
      1. **Family history.** The likelihood is 40% if one parent had nocturnal enuresis and there is a 70% risk if both parents had nocturnal enuresis.
      2. **Maturational delay.** Fifteen to 25% of 5-year-olds are enuretic, with this number decreasing by 15% per year, such that 5% of 10-year-olds and 1% of 15-year-olds are enuretic.
      3. **Male gender.** Fifty to 60% of bed-wetters and over 90% of nightly bed-wetters are male.
      4. **Deep sleep.** Most enuretic patients do not spontaneously awaken after wetting.
      5. **Bladder function.** Those with small capacity are at risk.
      6. **Lower nocturnal levels of antidiuretic hormone (ADH).**
   B. Twenty percent of enuretic children experience some daytime wetting. Risk factors for **diurnal** or **secondary enuresis** include constipation, urinary tract infection, psychological stress (dysfunctional home, abuse), and diabetes mellitus.
III. **Symptoms.** When evaluating a child with enuresis, responses to several key questions will assist in assessing causes and management for the problem. (See Table 24–1.)
IV. **Signs.** The child who presents in primary care with enuresis will generally have a normal examination. In most cases of enuresis presenting in primary care settings, relevant physical examination will be normal. However, the following focused evaluations are important in detecting underlying or contributing causes.
   A. **Blood pressure.**
   B. **Height/weight** plotted on a growth chart. Poor growth, elevated blood pressure, or both suggests renal disease.
   C. **Genitals.** Look for any anomalies.
   D. **Neurologic examination,** including gait/muscular strength and tone/deep tendon reflexes/sensory responses/rectal tone (for underlying neurologic disease).

TABLE 24-1. IMPORTANT HISTORY IN CHILDREN WITH ENURESIS

Question	Significance/Suggests
To distinguish primary from secondary enuresis:	
At what age was your child consistently dry at night?	"Never dry" suggests primary enuresis
To distinguish uncomplicated from complicated enuresis:	
Does your child wet his/her pants during the day?	Yes, complicated
	Nocturnal enuresis
Does your child appear to have pain with urination?	Urinary tract infection
How often does your child have bowel movements?	Infrequent stools: Constipation
Are bowel movements ever hard to pass?	Constipation
Does your child ever soil his/her pants?	Encopresis
To distinguish possible functional bladder disorder from nocturnal polyuria:	
How many times a day does your child void?	More than seven times a day: functional bladder disorder
Does your child have to run to the bathroom?	Positive response: functional bladder disorder
Does your child hold urine until the last minute?	Positive response: functional bladder disorder
How many nights a week does your child wet the bed?	Most nights: functional bladder disorder
	One or two nights: nocturnal polyuria
Does your child wet more than one time per night?	Positive response: functional bladder disorder
Does your child seem to wet large or small volumes?	Large volumes: nocturnal polyuria
	Small volumes: functional bladder disorder
To determine how parents have handled bed-wetting:	
How have you handled the nighttime accident?	Elicits information on interventions that have already been tried; be alert for responses suggesting that the child has been punished or shamed

Reprinted, with permission, from C. Thiedke.

    E. Observed voiding for stream/ability to initiate and interrupt in midstream (for neurologic disease or urethral strictures).

V. Laboratory Tests. Most children presenting in ambulatory primary care will have a **normal physical examination;** in these patients, the only testing indicated is **urinalysis (UA)** and **estimation of bladder capacity.** Bladder capacity is estimated by measuring the voided volume after the child reports an unbearable urge to void. The normal bladder capacity in ounces is the age plus 2. The normal adult bladder capacity is 12–16 oz.

    A. Children with normal examination, UA, and voided volume require no further laboratory evaluation.

    B. Children with abnormal examination, UA, or both may require further evaluation.

        1. Low specific gravity (<1.005) characterizes diabetes insipidus, acute tubular necrosis, and pyelonephritis. Specific gravity of 1.010 that remains unchanged despite fluid intake occurs in chronic glomerulonephritis with severe renal disease. High specific gravity (>1.035) occurs in nephritic syndrome, dehydration, acute glomerulonephritis, congestive heart failure, liver failure, and shock.

        2. Glycosuria commonly indicates diabetes mellitus or low renal glycemic threshold (eg, pregnancy).

        3. Proteinuria may be benign or indicate underlying disease (see Chapter 53).

        4. Hematuria can indicate cystitis or urinary tract calculi and warrants further evaluation (see Chapter 36).

        5. White blood cells suggest urinary tract infection, a cause of polysymptomatic enuresis with significant pyuria on a clean specimen (see Chapter 21); antibiotic treatment should be instituted. Children with urinary tract infection should be evaluated for vesicoureteral reflux; currently recommended testing includes voiding cystourethrogram and renal ultrasound.

VI. Treatment. Treatment for enuresis should not commence until the child is about 7 years old, unless enuresis causes severe emotional distress. The child must comprehend and perceive the condition as a problem and be a willing participant in therapy. Parental involvement is essential to the child's overall success. It is important to educate or reassure parents about rates of spontaneous resolution of enuresis (see section II,A).

A. Nonpharmacologic measures

   1. The following **lifestyle modifications** may be effective:

      a. Set a goal for **the child to get up at night and use the toilet** so that the child understands that he or she can solve the problem. Daytime and nighttime rehearsal can reinforce expectations. Alarm or parent-awakening approaches can be used.

      b. Improve **access to the toilet**—provide a bedside potty.

      c. Have the child consume 40% of fluids before noon, 40% in early afternoon, and only 20% in the evening. **Avoid giving excessive fluids** during the 2 hours before bedtime.

      d. Have the child avoid **caffeine-containing products.**

      e. **Encourage the child to empty the bladder** at bedtime.

      f. **Discontinue diapers** or pull-ups so that the sensation of wetness is recognized.

      g. **Include the child in morning cleanup** in a nonpunishing manner; criticism and punishment can cause secondary psychological problems.

      h. Provide a **diary or chart** to monitor progress.

      i. Use **positive reinforcement** (have the child place a favorite sticker on the calendar for dry days).

   2. **Behavioral conditioning** may be effective in children with frequent daytime voiding, few or no dry nights, or >1 enuretic episode per night; these children may have low functional bladder capacity and benefit from an alarm.

      a. **Enuresis alarm** (Table 24–2). Small transistorized mini-alarms are attached to the patient's bed or underwear and activate (via sound, vibration, or both) with the release of first few drops of urine. Eventually, a conditioned response occurs.

      b. **Nighttime alarm** (Table 24–2). An alarm clock is set for 3 hours after going to sleep to awaken the child to get up and void.

   3. **Self-hypnosis** with posthypnotic suggestion that the child will wake up and use the bathroom. The cure rate is reported at 77% for children 5 years and older.

B. Pharmacologic therapy (Table 24–2)

   1. The most common pharmacologic treatment is **desmopressin (DDAVP),** an effective and safe medication when used as directed. It is available in nasal spray and tablet. Dosage is not titrated to patient weight. This medication is best in children whose voiding pattern indicates likely arginine vasopressin (AVP) deficiency (ie, normal daytime voiding, and large nocturnal voids that are two times a week). Parents should be warned that the medication is to be used only as directed and that daytime use can result in water retention and dilutional hyponatremia.

   2. The tricyclic antidepressant **imipramine (Tofranil)** has been used to treat enuresis in the past. It is not commonly used today.

   3. The efficacy of **oxybutynin** is unclear from the medical literature. The drug has a high failure rate with discontinuation.

C. Follow-up. Regular follow-up visits are important to address issues or concerns, answer questions, and encourage the child and parents. In children receiving medications for enuresis, follow-up is recommended 2 weeks after initiation of therapy, then monthly for 3 months.

REFERENCES

Butler R, Stenberg A: Treatment of childhood nocturnal enuresis: An examination of clinically relevant principles. Br J Urol Int 2001;**88:**563.

Evans JHC: Evidence based management of nocturnal enuresis. BMJ (November 17) 2001; **323**(7322):1167.

Mikkelsen EJ: Enuresis and encopresis: Ten years of progress. J Am Acad Child Adolesc Psychiatry 2001;**40**(10):1146.

Schmitt BD: Nocturnal enuresis. Pediatr Rev 1997;**18:**183.

Thiedke CC: Nocturnal enuresis. Am Fam Physician 2003;**67:**1499.

TABLE 24–2. INTERVENTIONS FOR ENURESIS

Intervention	Mechanism	Dosage/Instructions	Side Effects/Comments	Efficacy	Cost
Parent-awakening with dry bed training program	Parent awakens child at timed interval	Parent awakens child 3 hrs after bedtime	Side effects: none Safe; does not require bed-wetting to initiate alarm	Initial cure rate: 92% Relapse rate: 20%	None
Enuresis alarm[1]	Alarm system activated by wetness that awakens child so child can get up to void	Worn nightly for 2–3 months	Side effects: none	Most effective intervention. Initial cure rate: 75–84% Relapse rate: 15–30% with discontinuance	$25.00
Desmopressin[1]	Synthetic analogue of vasopressin; reduces urine production by increasing water retention and urine concentration in the distal tubules	1 spray each nostril 20 µg (10 µg) nightly Oral: 0.2–0.6 mg qhs	Common side effects: headache, abdominal discomfort, nausea, and nasal discomfort. Comments: Contraindicated in patients who have habit polydipsia, hypertension, or heart disease.	Initial cure rates: 86% Relapse rate with discontinuation: 94%. Desmopressin plus anticholinergic may be appropriate for children where nocturnal enuresis pattern indicates arginine vasopressin deficiency and bladder instability.	Cost: $1.50 per spray $2.90 and up for 0.2-mg tablet
Imipramine	Mechanism of action combines anticholinergic effect that increases bladder capacity with a noradrenergic side effect that decreases bladder detrusor excitability	8–12 yr: 15–50 mg hs >12 yr: 50–75 mg hs	Common side effects: dry mouth, drowsiness, constipation, anxiety, nervousness, constipation, irritability **Comments: Most common causes of fatal poisoning in children 5 years old and younger.**	Initial cure rates: 10–60% Relapse rate with discontinuation: 90% Optimal treatment duration remains controversial. Should be used until the child has achieved (at minimum) 14–28 consecutive dry nights before it is gradually tapered.	Cost: $8–12 per 30 tablets
Oxybutynin[1]	Anticholinergic, antispasmodic effects that reduce uninhibited detrusor muscle contractions	6–12 yr: 5 mg hs >12 yr: 10 mg hs	Common side effects: dry mouth, flushing, drowsiness, constipation. Comments: Drug of choice for polysymptomatic enuresis.	Relapse rate with discontinuation: Anecdotal reports of benefit; prospective double-blind study showed no benefit vs. placebo.	Cost: 5 mg/5 mL (120 mL) $10–12

[1] Various studies indicate combination therapy will increase overall effectiveness.

25   Failure to Thrive

Cathy Kamens, MD

KEY POINTS

- Growth of children must be measured over time and plotted on a standardized growth chart at every visit.
- A thorough history and physical examination and selective laboratory tests are the foundation for accurate diagnosis and management of failure to thrive.
- Provision of calories and a multidisciplinary approach are keys to treating children with failure to thrive.

I. **Definition.** At each office visit, all infants and children should be accurately measured for weight, length (recumbent) or height (standing), and head circumference. These measurements should be plotted on standardized growth curves (see sidebar). Growth should be evaluated over time with attention to growth velocity and any change in growth percentiles. Weight should be compared to length (or height), as well as head circumference, to identify children with disproportionate growth.

  Failure to thrive (FTT) is a term used to describe children who are not growing adequately. It is a symptom or a sign of an underlying problem, but FTT itself is not a disease or disorder. There is no consensus on criteria for FTT, but investigation is appropriate in any child:

  A. Whose weight or height for age is below the fifth percentile.
  B. Whose growth slows to cross two major percentiles.
  C. Whose weight for height is less than the fifth percentile.

GROWTH CURVES

In May 2000, the Centers for Disease Control and Prevention (CDC) released revised growth curves, replacing the standard charts developed in 1977. These revised charts represent an ethnically diverse population from multiple sources, include breast-fed and bottle-fed infants, and exclude very low birth weight infants, who have different growth patterns. Two sets of growth charts are available: Set 1, from the 5th to the 95th percentile for average children, and Set 2, which includes the 3rd and the 97th percentiles, and are appropriate for evaluating children at the extremes of growth. These are available through the CDC or can be accessed at www.cdc.gov/growthcharts.

II. **Common Diagnoses.** FTT occurs in 3–10% of children, with the highest rates seen in urban and rural families living in poverty. FTT accounts for 1–5% of pediatric hospital admissions. FTT is usually identified in the infant or young child—more than 80% of cases are identified before age 18 months. It is important for health care providers to consider FTT, because many parents will not recognize the subtle slowing of growth that characterizes most FTT. The differential diagnosis for FTT is long (see Table 25–1). FTT can be approached as one of three types.

  A. Nonorganic FTT is due to a psychosocial or behavioral problem. This type accounts for 60–80% of cases of FTT.

  B. Organic FTT results from an underlying medical illness. It can be attributed to inadequate intake of calories, inadequate absorption, or increased loss or increased utilization of calories. In one study of hospitalized infants, gastroesophageal reflux or diarrhea were identified in 66% of infants with an organic cause of FTT. Other organic causes for FTT include renal, cardiac, respiratory, or endocrine illnesses.

TABLE 25–1. DIFFERENTIAL DIAGNOSIS, PRESENTATION, AND LABORATORY EVALUATION OF FAILURE TO THRIVE (FTT)

Cause	History	Signs	Laboratory Tests
Psychosocial			
Breast-feeding problems	Sore nipples, lack of engorgement or milk let-down	Asymmetric FTT (see section IV,B,1), cracked nipples	None
Feeding errors	Insufficient quantity offered, formula preparation error, excessive juice intake	Asymmetric FTT	None
Infant behavior/bonding	Refusal of bottle, irritability, ignorance of infant cues	Apathetic, withdrawn behavior, minimal smiling, decreased vocalizations	None
Abuse or neglect	Maternal depression or mental illness, parental drug use, "chaotic" family style, spousal abuse	Poor hygiene, bruises in different stages of healing, characteristic patterns of injury	None
Economic deprivation	Homelessness, public assistance, "rationing" food supplies	Asymmetric FTT, poor hygiene	None
Gastrointestinal			
Gastroesophageal reflux	Very frequent "wet burps"	Emesis, cough, wheezing	Esophageal pH probe
Craniofacial abnormalities Cleft lip/palate Choanal atresia Micrognathia	Nasal regurgitation, choking, unilateral rhinorrhea	Cleft or small jaw seen on examination, unable to pass catheter through nose	None
Malabsorption Celiac disease Lactose intolerance Milk protein intolerance Pancreatic insufficiency	Diarrhea, abdominal pain, foul-smelling stools	Abdominal distention, dehydration, fatty stools	Lactose tolerance test, stool pH, electrolytes, sweat test, fecal fat, jejunal biopsy, anti-endomysial antibodies
Inflammatory bowel disease	Abdominal pain, diarrhea, melena	Heme-positive stool, fever	Stool Hematest, ESR, barium enema
Biliary disease Atresia Cirrhosis	Pale stools	Jaundice, hepatomegaly	LFTs, abdominal ultrasound, liver biopsy
Obstruction Pyloric stenosis Malrotation Hirschsprung's disease	Vomiting, may be projectile vomiting after meals	Abdominal distention, palpable mass (olive), dehydration	Electrolytes, KUB, abdominal ultrasound
Renal			
Renal tubular acidosis	Polyuria, vomiting	Tachypnea, muscular weakness	US, electrolytes, blood gas
Chronic renal failure	Listlessness, pruritus	Pallor, edema	Serum, BUN, creatinine, US
Diabetes insipidus	Polyuria, thirst	Dehydration, irritability	US, electrolytes

Cardiopulmonary			
Congenital heart defects	Shortness of breath, blue lips	Cyanosis, murmur	CXR, ECG, echocardiogram
Congestive heart failure	Shortness of breath, swelling, blue lips	Cyanosis, rales, edema	CXR, echocardiogram
Asthma	Cough, shortness of breath	Tachypnea, wheezing	Pulmonary function tests
Bronchopulmonary dysplasia	History of prematurity or respiratory disease	Tachypnea, retractions	Pulse oximetry, pulmonary function tests
Cystic fibrosis	Frequent respiratory infections	Tachypnea, wheezing	Sweat test
Anatomic upper airway abnormalities	Slow feeding, coughing and choking, history of pneumonia	Stridor, inability to pass a catheter into the stomach	CXR, barium esophagram
Tracheoesophageal fistula			
Vascular slings			
Endocrine			
Thyroid disease	Dry or moist skin, cold or heat intolerance	Irritability or slow movements, warm or cold skin	Serum thyroxine, TSH
Diabetes mellitus	Polydipsia, polyphagia, polyuria	Lethargy, Kussmaul respirations	US, serum glucose, pH
Adrenal disorder	Obesity, poor sleeping	Hypertension or hypotension, diabetes mellitus	Urine-free cortisol, plasma, ACTH
Parathyroid disorders	Muscle pain and cramps, abdominal pain	Tetany, cataracts	Calcium, PTH
Pituitary disorders	May have none	Prominent forehead, large abdomen	"Provocative" growth hormone test
Growth hormone deficiency			
Neurologic			
Developmental disorder	History of developmental delay	May be normal or with dysmorphic features	None
Hydrocephalus	Irritability, lethargy, vomiting	Increased head circumference, wide bulging fontanelle, dilated scalp veins	Head CT or MRI
Neuromuscular disorder	History of developmental motor delay	Spasticity or hypotonia, microcephaly	Head CT or MRI
Cerebral palsy			
Hypotonia			
Myopathy			
Cerebral hemorrhages	Headache, vomiting, history of trauma	Nuchal rigidity, hemiparesis	Head CT or MRI
Infectious			
UTI	Fever, irritability	Fever, suprapubic tenderness	UA and culture
Infectious diarrhea	Diarrhea, melena	Abdominal distention, pain, fever	Stool culture, ova & parasites
Thrush	Refuses bottle	White plaque on oral mucosa	None
Recurrent tonsillitis	Sore throat, bad breath, mouth breathing	Tonsillar hypertrophy, cervical lymphadenopathy	Throat culture
Tuberculosis	Travel in high-risk area or exposure to high-risk persons	Lymphadenopathy	PPD, CXR
Human immunodeficiency virus	Maternal history of high-risk behaviors	Fever, lymphadenopathy	HIV antibody test
Hepatitis	Maternal history or risk factors for hepatitis	Jaundice, hepatomegaly	LFTs, hepatitis serology
Immunologic deficiency	Frequent infections	Lymphadenopathy	CBC, quantitative serum IgG, IgM, IgA

(continued)

TABLE 25–1. (*Continued*)

Cause	History	Signs	Laboratory Tests
Metabolic			
Inborn errors of metabolism	Lethargy	May be normal	Newborn screen
Congenital			
Chromosomal abnormalities Turner's syndrome Down syndrome	Advanced maternal age, loose neck skin and hand puffiness	Dysmorphic features such as short/webbed neck, cubitus valgus, epicanthal folds, simian crease	Chromosomes
Skeletal dysplasias	Positive family history	Short extremities, trident hands	Pelvic, lumbar, extremity x-rays
Congenital syndromes Fetal alcohol syndrome	Maternal history of alcohol ingestion or drug use, delayed development	Symmetric FTT, short palpebral fissures, epicanthal folds, maxillary hypoplasia, micrognathia	None
Miscellaneous			
Malignancy	Fever, fatigue	Lymphadenopathy, tumors	CBC, ESR
Drugs or toxins Lead poisoning Accidental intake	Exposure to lead paint, medication errors	May be normal	Lead levels, toxicology screen
Nutritional deficiencies Iron deficiency Zinc deficiency	Exclusive breast-feeding, unsupplemented formula	Pallor, dermatitis	CBC
Vitamin D deficiency (rickets)	Exclusive breast-feeding, no exposure to sunlight	Large fontanelle, bony deformities	X-rays, calcium, alkaline phosphatase
Connective tissue disease	Fever, arthralgia, myalgia	Arthritis, rash, myositis	ESR, CBC, ANA
Normal Variants			
Familial short stature	Short members of family	Symmetric FTT (see section IV,B,2), normal examination	Bone age x-rays
Constitutional delay of growth	Family history of late puberty	Symmetric FTT, normal examination, delayed puberty	Bone age x-rays
Intrauterine growth retardation	Small for gestational age at birth	Hepatosplenomegaly, chorioretinitis	Viral antibody titers, urine for CMV

ACTH, adrenocorticotropic hormone; ANA, antinuclear antibody; BUN, blood urea nitrogen; CBC, complete blood count; CMV, cytomegalovirus; CT, computerized tomographic test; CXR, chest radiograph; ECG, electrocardiogram; ESR, erythrocyte sedimentation rate; FTT, failure to thrive; HIV, human immunodeficiency virus; KUB, kidney/ureter/bladder (abdominal plain radiograph); LFTs, liver function tests; MRI, magnetic resonance imaging; PTH, parathyroid hormone; PPD, purified protein derivative (TB test); TSH, thyroid-stimulating hormone; UA, urinalysis; US, ultrasound; UTI, urinary tract infection.

C. Mixed organic and nonorganic FTT is most common. This accounts for the coexistence of the biological, psychosocial, and behavioral problems that contribute to poor growth.
D. FTT must be distinguished from the following normal variants:
   1. **Familial short stature,** in which growth deceleration represents a physiologic adjustment for the child's growth potential. About 30% of normal babies have a downward shift in growth between 3 and 18 months. Calculation of the midparental height (see sidebar) can be helpful in establishing a child's growth potential. Familial short stature can be diagnosed when:

MIDPARENTAL HEIGHT

Girls:
(Father's height – 13 cm [5 in] + Mother's height ÷ 2
Boys:
(Mother's height + 13 cm [5 in]) + Father's height ÷ 2

---

   a. There is a proportional decrease in weight and length (symmetric FTT).
   b. Bone age is consistent with chronological age.
   c. There is a family history of short stature.
   d. The child maintains a normal annual growth rate without further deceleration.
   2. **Constitutional growth delay** occurs when growth decelerates in the first 2 years of life, followed by stabilization on a new growth curve until adolescence, when a growth spurt occurs.
      Constitutional growth delay is suspected when:
   a. Weight and height are proportionally decreased (**symmetric FTT**).
   b. Bone age is less than chronological age. There may be a 2- to 4-year delay in skeletal maturation.
   c. There is a family history of a parent or sibling with a similar growth pattern.
   d. A work-up does not reveal inadequate intake, or any other cause of growth delay.
   3. **Intrauterine growth retardation** is failure of intrauterine growth due to prenatal factors and not genetic predisposition.
   a. These infants are easily identified by their birth weight below the fifth percentile.
   b. Many of these infants catch up to their peers within the first 6 months, but growth may be slow for the first several years.
   c. Careful monitoring over time should show an improvement in growth. Low birth weight infants should double their birth weight by age 4 months and triple it by 1 year.
   d. Very low birth weight (VLBW) infants (weighing less than 1500 g), due to prematurity, should be followed up on a specific VLBW graph, with postnatal age adjusted for gestational age.
   4. **Breast-feeding infants** may show a decrease in growth around 6–8 months. There are no growth charts specific to breast-fed babies, so it is not clear how to interpret this decrease.
III. Symptoms. A thorough history should be elicited in poorly growing children, including the following specific areas (see Table 25-1):
   A. Feeding history. Query method, breast-feeding patterns, engorgement and let-down, frequency, quantity, formula preparation, length and quality of feeding time, feeding techniques, and personal and cultural beliefs about food and feeding.
   B. Dietary history. Query 24-hour recall or 72-hour food diary.
   C. Past medical history. Query birth weight, prenatal and birth history, illnesses, and hospitalizations.
   D. Developmental history. Query gross and fine motor milestones, language milestones, behavior, and temperament.
   E. Social history. Query living situation, financial constraints, family stressors, parental employment, parental substance abuse, and domestic violence or abuse.
   F. Family history. Query mental illness in the family (especially maternal depression), childhood illnesses, mental retardation, genetic abnormalities, history of growth delays in parents or siblings, and midparental height.

    G. Review of systems. Query vomiting, spitting up, choking, diarrhea, dyspnea, and tachypnea.

IV. Signs (Table 25–1)

    A. A careful examination may identify physical findings that provide clues to the cause of FTT in children and should include:

        1. Accurate measurements and plotting of weight, height, and head circumference. Measurement or plotting errors can give the appearance of FTT, and therefore, the first step in the diagnosis should be to recheck the child's measurements and re-plot them on the growth curve.

        2. General appearance and vital signs.

        3. Dysmorphic features or structural anomalies.

        4. Signs of abuse or neglect.

        5. Cardiac, respiratory, and gastrointestinal findings and checking of the oropharynx and lymph nodes.

        6. Neurologic examination.

    B. Patterns of growth may provide helpful clues to diagnosis.

        1. Asymmetric FTT, in which the head circumference is preserved, is generally due to psychosocial factors or a systemic illness. In severe FTT, the height may also be decreased.

        2. Symmetric FTT, in which weight, height, and head circumference are proportional, may represent a normal variant or a primary central nervous system disorder.

        3. Isolated short stature, where the weight is preserved, is likely to represent an endocrine or genetic disorder.

V. Laboratory Tests (Table 25–1). No routine laboratory tests are indicated in the child with FTT, and less than 1% of all laboratory tests ordered in a typical FTT work-up provide useful information. Evaluation of the poorly growing child should be completed in a timely manner, usually over 2–3 weeks, and should be conducted concurrently with efforts to improve the child's feeding and growth.

VI. Treatment. Treatment must be individualized for each child according to the medical, family, social, and psychological risk factors identified.

    A. Treatment goals must be clearly established:

        1. Identify and treat any underlying disorder.

        2. Achieve catch-up growth.

            a. An increase in calories of 1.5 to 2 times expected intake is required for catch-up growth (see sidebar).

CALORIE REQUIREMENTS FOR CATCH-UP GROWTH

Median weight for age (kg) ÷ Current weight (kg) × 120 kcal/kg

---

            (1) High-calorie concentrated formula is the mainstay of intervention for the infant.

            (2) Glucose polymers or extra lipids may be added to increase calories.

            (3) Prescribe a multivitamin with iron and zinc for all children with FTT.

        b. Growth should be monitored closely and follow-up should be scheduled based on the child's age and severity of growth failure.

            (1) The child may require 1–2 weeks of refeeding to demonstrate weight gain.

            (2) Several months may be needed for return to baseline growth curve.

        3. Parental education.

            a. Success is dependent on establishing a longitudinal alliance with the child and the caretakers. A nonjudgmental attitude and ongoing support are vital.

            b. Education should focus on the nutritional needs of the child, in addition to any behavioral and psychosocial problems identified.

    B. Hospitalization allows for improvement in growth, as well as a controlled environment to assess caloric needs, feeding techniques, and parent-child interaction.

        1. Hospitalization may be indicated when:

            a. There is evidence of, or high risk for, physical abuse or severe neglect.

    b. The child is severely malnourished or medically unstable.

    c. Outpatient management has failed to demonstrate any appreciable improvement.

  2. A 10- to 14-day hospitalization may be necessary to demonstrate weight gain.

  3. An inpatient multidisciplinary team should be available to address all aspects of the child's and parent's needs.

  4. Enteral feeds or gastrostomy are required only in children who are unable to achieve the required caloric intake under controlled circumstances, and is usually indicated only in children with a significant developmental or neurologic diagnosis.

VII. Prognosis

  A. There is consistent evidence of a long-term impact on growth in many children diagnosed with FTT. These children remain small at follow-up, as far out as age 9 years, and this may be due to a persistent impact on eating behaviors or chronic undereating.

  B. Some studies show long-term cognitive impairment and developmental delay, but others demonstrate no appreciable difference in these outcomes. It is possible that the timing or the length of growth failure may affect outcomes.

  C. The effect of environmental and socioeconomic factors, even after establishment of appropriate feeding, may influence outcomes for these children.

REFERENCES

Boddy J, Skuse D, Andrews B: The developmental sequelae of non-organic failure to thrive. J Child Psychiatry 2000;**41**(8):1003.

Gahagan S, Holmes R: A stepwise approach to evaluation of undernutrition and failure to thrive. Pediatr Clin North Am 1998;**45**(1):169.

Maggioni A, Lifshitz F: Nutritional management of failure to thrive. Pediatr Clin North Am 1995; **42**(4):791.

Rudolph CD, et al: Failure to thrive. In: *Rudolph's Pediatrics,* 21st ed. McGraw-Hill; 2003:7–12.

Samuels RC, Cohen LE: Understanding growth patterns in short stature. Contemporary Pediatrics 2001;**18**(6):94.

Schwartz ID: Failure to thrive: An old nemesis in the new millennium. Pediatr Rev 2000;**21**(8):257.

---

26   Fatigue

Anthony F. Valdini, MD, MS, FACP, FAAFP

KEY POINTS

- The longer a person is fatigued, the more likely a psychological problem is present.
- The history and physical examination are much more likely to reveal the cause of fatigue than blind laboratory testing.
- Most patients complaining of fatigue are depressed.
- Fatigue can be caused by physical, psychological, physiologic (appropriate, as in lack of sleep), or mixed etiologies. The mixed category is more common than once thought and may explain the difficulty in resolving the symptom. Just because an abnormality is discovered does not mean that the problem of fatigue is "solved." First, there is often more that one etiology to the complaint. Second, the abnormality discovered may be treated and resolved without changing the patient's complaint of fatigue.

  I. Definition. Fatigue is a subjective complaint of tiredness, weariness, or lack of energy.

 II. Common Diagnoses. Fatigue is the seventh most common symptom in primary care and accounts for more than 10 million office visits every year. Various studies have found the prevalence of fatigue in primary care at between 10% and 20%. One group of investigators found that 6.7% of patients presenting to a family medicine clinic had a primary complaint of fatigue. Patients identified as fatigued visit the physician and are admitted to the hospital more often, incur greater charges for prescription medications, have more new diagnoses, and have a greater proportion of their diagnoses containing a psychological component than do their nonfatigued counterparts. Fatigue may result from virtually every physical and psychological illness. Four major classes of fatigue useful in evaluating the tired patient are listed below.

A. Physiologic fatigue is due to overwork, lack of sleep, or a defined physical stress, such as pregnancy. It can normally be expected in a mentally and physically healthy individual experiencing such a stress. Females, as a group, work more hours in a day and more years in their lives than males, and this may partially account for women visiting physicians more often for fatigue than men. Individuals with irregular or inadequate sleep patterns (including parents of young children), those on reducing diets, or those getting excessive or minimal exercise or spending long hours commuting and working are at increased risk for physiologic fatigue.

B. Physical fatigue is due to infections, endocrine imbalances, cardiovascular disease, anemia, and medications (prescription or over-the-counter drugs, alcohol, or other drugs of abuse); less commonly, cancer, connective tissue diseases, and other ailments cause physical fatigue.

C. Psychological illness, including depression, anxiety, stress, and adjustment reaction, can cause fatigue. Children of alcoholics have an increased incidence of fatigue and depression.

D. "Mixed" fatigue, which is often overlooked, involves any of the above categories occurring in combination.

III. Symptoms (Figure 26–1).

A. Duration. Fatigue lasting 1 month or less is commonly a result of physical causes; fatigue lasting 3 months or more is likely to be caused by psychological factors.

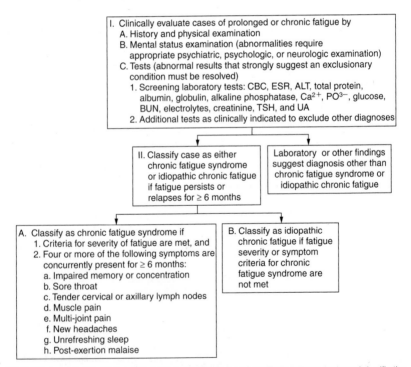

FIGURE 26–1. International Chronic Fatigue Syndrome Study Group recommendations for evaluation and classification of unexplained chronic fatigue. ALT, alanine aminotransferase; BUN, blood urea nitrogen; CBC, complete blood cell count; ESR, erythrocyte sedimentation rate; PO$_4$, phosphorus; TSH, thyroid-stimulating hormone; UA, urinalysis. (Adapted with permission from Fukada K, et al, and the International Chronic Fatigue Syndrome Study Group: The chronic fatigue syndrome: A comprehensive approach to its definition and study. Ann Intern Med 1994;**121**:955.)

B. Fever, chills, sweats, and **significant weight loss** are associated with infection and carcinoma.

C. Specific historical features (see Table 26–1) including endocrine and cardiovascular review of systems may indicate psychological, physical, or mixed origins of fatigue. Review of sleep patterns and work and travel history, in addition to physical functional capacity, can help elucidate the cause of fatigue. The feature most solidly linked with physical versus psychological causes is the chronicity of fatigue; that is, acute fatigue is likely to be caused by physical or physiologic events, whereas chronic fatigue is associated with psychological and mixed causes. Fatigue should be distinguished from weakness and hypersomnolence, which indicate a different origin, such as neuromuscular (eg, myasthenia) or sleep disorder (obstructive sleep apnea, narcolepsy).

D. Chronic fatigue syndrome (CFS) is a distinct diagnostic category. The International Chronic Fatigue Syndrome Study Group has revised the case definition. It includes a duration of 6 months or longer, absence of an identified cause, and the presence of at least four specific symptoms (see Figure 26–1). Among the symptoms and signs associated with CFS, Komaroff and Buchwald (1991) found the following frequencies: low-grade fever (60–95%), myalgias (20–95%), sleep disorder (15–90%), impaired cognition (50–85%), depression (70–85%), headaches (35–85%), pharyngitis (50–75%), anxiety (50–70%), weakness (40–70%), postexertional malaise (50–60%), arthralgias (40–50%), and painful lymph nodes (30–40%). Despite the findings of "subtle and diffuse" immunologic abnormalities and associated viruses—Epstein-Barr virus, enteroviruses, herpesvirus type 6, retroviruses, and others—the syndrome remains enigmatic.

   1. Chronic idiopathic fatigue. Not all patients with chronic fatigue symptoms meet the criteria for CFS. Persons tired for 6 months or longer for no apparent cause who do not meet CFS criteria for severity or specific symptoms are classified as having "chronic idiopathic fatigue."

   2. Most patients who are tired for more than 1 year have significant psychological problems.

   Because depression is the most common psychological cause of fatigue, and not all providers feel comfortable making the diagnosis, an instrument to measure depression (such as Beck's) may be useful. (See Chapter 92.)

IV. Signs

A. The **physical causes** of acute fatigue (eg, rales, edema, and gallops of congestive heart failure) may be obvious.

B. Subtle signs of infections (eg, lymphadenopathy or temperature elevation), connective tissue disease (eg, extra-articular manifestations), and cancer should not be overlooked.

V. Laboratory Tests (Figure 26–2). The patient often needs the reassurance of a laboratory investigation. The clinician should bear in mind, however, that laboratory investigations of persons fatigued for more than 1 year have been remarkably unproductive. Laboratory investigation based on signs will be more productive than screening based on the complaint of

TABLE 26–1. CHARACTERISTICS PROPOSED TO DISTINGUISH PSYCHOLOGICAL FATIGUE FROM PHYSICAL FATIGUE

Characteristic	Psychological	Physical
Duration	Chronic	Acute
Primary deficit	Desire	Ability
Onset	Stress related	Unrelated to stress
Diurnal pattern	Worse in morning	Worse in evening
Course	Fluctuates	Progressive
Effect of activity	Relieves	Worsens
Associated symptoms	Multiple and nonspecific	Few and specific
Previous problems	Functional	Organic
Family	Stressful	Supportive
Appearance	Anxious/depressed	Ill
Family history	Psychological/alcoholism	None
Placebo effect	Present	Absent
Effect of sleep	Unaffected/worsened	Relieved
Decreased activity to cope	No	Yes

Adapted with permission from Katerndahl DA: Differentiation of physical and psychological fatigue. Fam Pract Res J 1993;**13**:82.

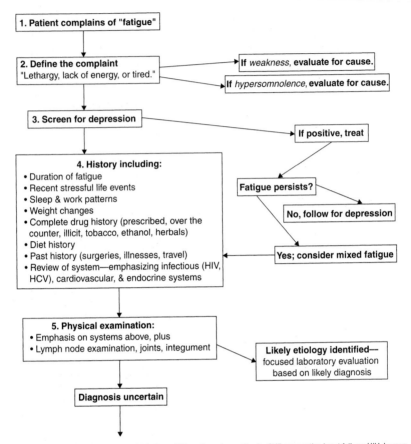

FIGURE 26–2. Evaluation of patient with fatigue. ANA, anti-nuclear antibody; CHF, congestive heart failure; HIV, human immunodeficiency virus; HCV, hepatitis C virus; PPD, purified protein derivative; VDRL, venereal disease research laboratory test.

fatigue alone. The most common physical causes of fatigue are infectious (especially viral infections), endocrine (thyroid disease and diabetes mellitus predominate), and cardiovascular.

   A. Level 1, 2, and 3 laboratory evaluations consist of tests outlined in Figure 26–2.

   B. **Abnormal laboratory findings.** Treatment of the underlying condition until the laboratory abnormality resolves is necessary to determine whether it represented the cause of the fatigue. One should be prepared to resume the search if a particular laboratory value returns to normal but the patient's condition does not.

VI. **Treatment**

   A. **Etiology identified.** Specific treatments for defined physical and psychological causes should be administered when possible.

   B. **Etiology undetermined**

      1. **Behavioral treatment.** Despite intensive investigation and follow-up, the cause of chronic fatigue often remains undetermined. In such a case, cognitive behavioral therapy and graded exercise programs have been shown to be effective. Additionally, group therapy may provide some solace. These modalities should be offered to all fatigued patients whose problems do not resolve with more specific treatment.

      2. **Drug therapy.** A host of medications have been advocated for fatigue of unknown origin. A partial list includes vitamins, thyroid supplementation (for subclinical hypo-

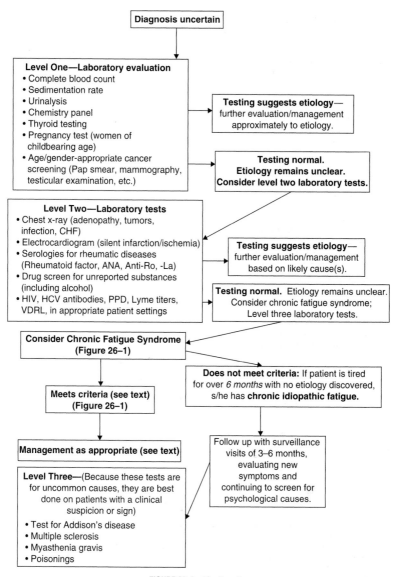

FIGURE 26–2. *(Continued)*.

thyroidism), growth hormone, amphetamines, pemoline, and hydrocortisone. The use of any medication for treatment of a symptom without a specific, identified cause is problematic. However, the likelihood of depression or fibromyalgia causing fatigue in persons with no obvious cause probably warrants a 2-month therapeutic trial of antidepressants.

3. **Diet therapy.** Several unproven diets have been proposed. Although fatigue has been associated with a body mass index of 45 or greater, it is not certain that weight loss will alleviate fatigue in greatly obese persons. Nevertheless, achieving

and maintaining ideal body weight through balanced nutrition is recommended for general health and may be helpful in fatigued patients.

4. **Complementary/alternative medical therapy (CAM).** While studies of CAM therapies have not, as yet, provided significant positive benefit, there have been no reports of adverse effects on fatigued patients using CAM. The use of CAM for fatigued patients is empirical.

VII. Patient Follow-up. It is not known exactly how often the fatigued patient should return to the physician. A few bimonthly visits early in the investigation of the complaint will serve to cement the patient-doctor relationship and establish good faith. If no identifiable cause of fatigue is determined, the physician should avoid the inclination to stop seeing the patient for the problem. Regularly scheduled visits, even as seldom as twice a year, remind the patient that he or she is not adrift and that the reported changes in the patient's condition will receive serious consideration.

At each visit, a review of physical, environmental, and psychological symptoms and signs should be conducted. Physician support, reassurance, and follow-up are important for the patient whose fatigue appears to have no clear cause.

VIII. Natural History. In one series, in which 73 fatigued and 72 nonfatigued subjects were reevaluated after 1 year, 41% of the fatigued patients were no longer fatigued, based on Rand Index of Vitality scores. Fifteen of the 72 nonfatigued subjects became fatigued after 1 year. The difference in improvement between fatigued patients with physical diagnoses and those with psychological diagnoses was not significant.

REFERENCES

Fukada K, et al, and the International Chronic Fatigue Syndrome Study Group: The chronic fatigue syndrome: A comprehensive approach to its definition and study. Ann Intern Med 1994;**121**:953.

Katerndahl DA: Differentiation of physical and psychological fatigue. Fam Pract Res J 1993;**13**:81.

Komaroff AL, Buchwald D: Symptoms and signs of chronic fatigue syndrome. Rev Infect Dis 1991; **13**(suppl 1):S8.

Kroenke K, et al: Chronic fatigue in primary care: Prevalence, patient characteristics and outcome. JAMA 1988;**260**:929.

National Center for Infectious Diseases. Chronic Fatigue Syndrome. www.cdc.gov/ncidod/diseases/cfs

Valdini AF, et al: A one year follow-up of fatigued patients. J Fam Pract 1988;**26**:33.

Whiting P, et al: Interventions for the treatment and management of the Chronic Fatigue Syndrome. JAMA 2001;**286**:1360.

---

27   Fluid, Electrolyte, & Acid-Base Disturbances

Lara Carson Weinstein, MD

KEY POINTS

- In the ambulatory care setting, fluid, electrolyte, and acid-base disturbances often present initially as abnormal chemical screening panels in patients with known chronic disease, new medications, previously undiagnosed endocrine disorders, or acute gastrointestinal illnesses.
- Disorders of salt and water balance are exceedingly common in geriatric patients.
- Primary hyperparathyroidism is the most common cause of outpatient hypercalcemia and is often diagnosed through incidental hypercalcemia noted on routine screening.

I. **Definition and Common Diagnoses**
   A. **Decreases in effective circulating volume** commonly occur from **gastrointestinal (GI) losses** (vomiting, diarrhea); **loss through skin** (sweating, fever); **renal losses** (diuretics, interstitial renal disease); and **third-space accumulations** (pharmaceutical excess vasodilatation, pancreatitis). **Expansion of interstitial volume** causes edema. The most common edematous conditions seen in the outpatient setting result from con-

gestive heart failure. Edema is also seen in cirrhosis, renal failure, and the nephrotic syndrome.

1. **Hyponatremia,** serum sodium <135 mmol/L, uncommonly occurs with hyper- or iso-osmolar states (hyperglycemia or severe hyperlipidemia or hyperproteinemia. Most commonly, hyponatremia is hypo-osmolar and due to decreased renal water excretion or increased water intake.

   a. Hypervolemic hypo-osmolar hyponatremia occurs in patients with congestive heart failure, liver disease, chronic renal failure, or pregnancy.

   b. Euvolemic hypo-osmolar hyponatremia occurs with hypothyroidism, primary polydipsia, or syndrome of inappropriate secretion of antidiuretic hormone (SIADH). SIADH is most commonly associated with central nervous system (trauma, infection, tumors) or pulmonary (tuberculosis, pneumonia, bronchogenic carcinoma) pathology; other causes include a variety of neoplasms (pancreatic/prostatic/bladder carcinomas, lymphomas, thymoma) and drugs (eg, nonsteroidal anti-inflammatory drugs, clofibrate, carbamazepine).

   c. Hypovolemic hypo-osmolar hyponatremia, from decreased real or effective circulating volume, occurs most commonly with GI losses (diarrhea, vomiting); renal losses (diuretic use, osmotic diuresis, diabetes insipidus); or sequestration without actual loss (eg, intestinal obstruction, pancreatitis, peritonitis).

2. **Hypernatremia** is serum sodium >145 mmol/L. Hypernatremia results from a relative water deficit or, less commonly, from a primary sodium gain. Elderly individuals with decreased fluid intake, infants fed overly concentrated formula, individuals with untreated severe hyperglycemia, and those with diabetes insipidus are at risk for hypernatremia.

3. **Hypokalemia,** plasma potassium <3.5 mmol/L, most commonly occurs with diuretic use, eating disorders (with laxative use and vomiting), and less commonly, with primary or secondary hyperaldosteronism.

4. **Hyperkalemia,** plasma potassium >5 mmol/L, occurs with ingestion of potassium supplements or, in chronic renal insufficiency, with medications (eg, potassium-sparing diuretics, angiotensin-converting enzyme inhibitors, nonsteroidal anti-inflammatory drugs) interfering with potassium excretion. Pseudohyperkalemia occurs with blood sample hemolysis.

5. **Hypocalcemia,** serum calcium of <8 mg/dL, is seen in chronic renal insufficiency, hypoparathyroidism following thyroid surgery, and premature/low birth weight infants.

6. **Hypercalcemia** is serum calcium >10 mg/dL. Primary hyperparathyroidism or malignancy cause more than 90% of hypercalcemia. Primary hyperparathyroidism occurs in 1/500 elderly women. Rare causes of hypercalcemia include sarcoidosis, hyperthyroidism, lithium use, and the milk-alkali syndrome.

B. Common causes and mechanisms of **primary acid-base disorders** are outlined in Figure 27–1.

II. **Symptoms** associated with fluid, electrolyte, and acid-base disorders are subtle, nonspecific, and less sensitive than laboratory testing in detecting these disorders. Symptoms are more likely with large shifts in fluid, electrolyte, or acid-base status. The most common symptoms include lethargy, fatigue/weakness, or irritability.

A. **Seizures** can occur with severe hypernatremia or hypocalcemia.

B. **Palpitations** can occur with hyperkalemia.

C. **Hypercalcemia** is associated with a symptom complex including anorexia/nausea/vomiting, constipation, nephrolithiasis, confusion, and polyuria.

D. **Respiratory alkalosis/hyperventilation** is associated with irritability, paresthesias, muscle cramps, and lightheadedness.

E. **Vomiting** suggests metabolic alkalosis.

III. **Signs** of common fluid, electrolyte, and acid-base disorders are also less sensitive/specific in diagnosis than laboratory testing; findings associated with particular disorders include the following:

A. Spasticity, muscle twitching, and hyperreflexia are seen in **hypernatremia.**

B. **Chvostek's sign** (facial muscle twitching when the facial nerve is tapped anterior to the ear) occurs with **hypocalcemia.**

C. **Ectopic soft tissue calcifications** may be seen with hypercalcemia.

D. Anxiety and tachypnea may be seen in **respiratory alkalosis** or **acidosis.**

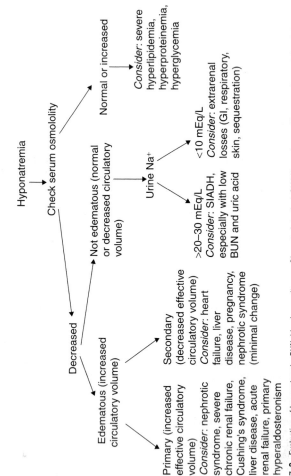

FIGURE 27–2. Evaluation of hyponatremia. BUN, blood urea nitrogen; GI, gastrointestinal; SIADH, syndrome of inappropriate antidiuretic hormone release.

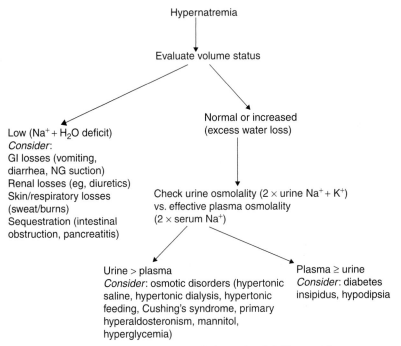

FIGURE 27–3. Evaluation of hypernatremia. GI, gastrointestinal; NG, nasogastric.

   2. **Severe hyperkalemia (>6 mEq/L)** requires hospitalization for possible administration of calcium gluconate, insulin, sodium bicarbonate, and other therapies.

 E. **Hypocalcemia.** Treatment in the office of mild hypocalcemia (ionized calcium of 3.2–3.9 mg/dL) includes oral calcium supplementation (eg, calcium carbonate, 1–2 g of elemental calcium per day).

   1. **Vitamin D supplementation** with ergocalciferol or vitamin D analogue (eg, Calcitrol) is indicated, with dose depending on the underlying cause.

     a. Patients without associated absorptive or metabolic problems can receive **ergocalciferol,** 50,000 IU weekly for 2 months; with normalization of 25 **hydroxy vitamin D** level (25–45 ng/mL), maintenance can be with a daily multivitamin containing 400 IU of vitamin D.

     b. Patients with impaired vitamin D metabolism (eg, chronic renal insufficiency and hypoparathyroidism) should receive **Calcitrol,** 0.25–1 μg twice daily, generally in consultation with an endocrinologist, nephrologist, or both, with close monitoring to avoid hypercalcemia.

   2. **Vitamin D therapy** requires close laboratory monitoring to avoid hypercalciuria, hypercalcemia, and renal toxicity.

   3. **Hospitalization should be considered** for management of ionized calcium levels <3.2 mg/dL or with signs of neuromuscular irritability (Chvostek's sign or carpopedal spasm).

 F. **Hypercalcemia**

   1. Patients with **serum calcium levels >13 mg/dL or severe symptoms** require hospitalization for evaluation and treatment. Hydration with normal saline, initially to replace volume and then to promote calcium excretion, is the most important initial aspect of therapy.

   2. Patients with mild hypercalcemia (<13 mg/dL) of known etiology (ie, known cancer diagnosis) may be treated as outpatients with oral rehydration.

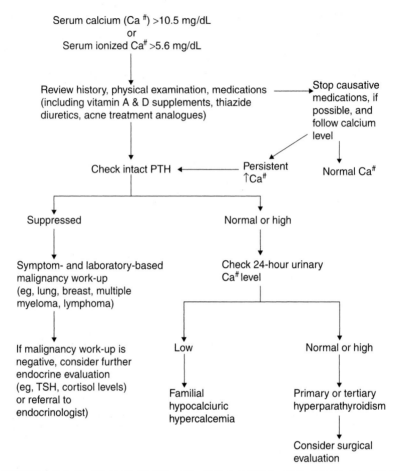

FIGURE 27–4. Evaluation of hypercalcemia. PTH, parathyroid hormone; TSH, thyroid-stimulating hormone. (Adapted from Carroll MF: A practical approach to hypercalcemia. Am Fam Physician 2003;**67**:1959.

   3. Malignancy-related hypercalcemia may be controlled with intermittent pamidronate (eg, 60 mg pamidronate every other week) following hospital discharge.
   4. Referral to a neck surgeon for consideration of parathyroidectomy is appropriate for normo- or hypercalciuric hyperparathyroidism.
G. **Metabolic acidosis and alkalosis**
   1. **Metabolic acidosis** is managed by providing nutrition and rehydration for alcoholic or starvation ketosis (often in a hospital setting), eliminating suspect drugs, or treating underlying diabetes mellitus (Chapter 74), diarrhea (Chapter 16), or causes of lactic acidosis. Renal tubular acidosis should initially be evaluated and managed in consultation with a nephrologist.
   2. **Metabolic alkalosis** management likewise depends on its cause. Suspected causative medications (eg, diuretics) should be eliminated if possible, vomiting or nasogastric losses should be replaced (often in the inpatient setting), renal failure should be managed in consultation with nephrology, and mineralocorticoid excess

(Cushing's syndrome, primary aldosteronism) should be managed by treating the underlying disease.
H. Respiratory acidosis is managed by correcting or stabilizing underlying disorders and improving ventilation. This may include controlling bronchospasm (Chapter 68) and congestive heart failure (Chapter 72).
I. Respiratory alkalosis treatment also focuses on underlying disorders. For example, patients with symptomatic, anxiety-related hyperventilation may respond to rebreathing (eg, breathing into a paper bag) when symptoms develop.

REFERENCES

Adelman RD, Solhaug MJ: Pathophysiology of body fluids and fluid therapy. In: Behrman RE, Kliegman RM, Jenson HB (editors): *Nelson Textbook of Pediatrics,* 16th ed. Saunders; 2000.
Carroll MF: A practical approach to hypercalcemia. Am Fam Physician 2003;**67:**1959.
Don H: Metabolic acidosis, metabolic alkalosis. In: Greene HL, Johnson WP, Maricic MJ (editors): *Decision Making in Medicine.* Mosby–Year Book; 1993.
Klahr S: Acid-base and fluid and electrolyte disorders. In: Noble J (editor): *Textbook of Primary Care Medicine,* 3rd ed. Mosby; 2001.
Kraut JA, Madias NE: Approach to patient with acid-base disorders. Respir Care 2001;**46:**392.
Kugler JP, Hustead T: Hyponatremia and hypernatremia in the elderly. Am Fam Physician 2000; **61:**3623.

---

28 Foot Complaints

James R. Barrett, MD, CAQSM, & Kent W. Davidson, MD

KEY POINTS

- One should look for contributing factors, such as improper footwear, when evaluating foot pain since correcting these will decrease the chance of pain recurrence.
- Stress fractures are a common cause of foot pain and may have no initial x-ray findings. A high index of suspicion should be maintained.
- Four injuries need to be identified early to reduce morbidity and improve successful treatment: Achilles tendon rupture, Lisfranc injury, and fractures of the fifth metatarsal and navicular bones.

I. Definition. The foot, which has 26 bones and 55 articulations, acts as a platform and shock absorber to support the weight of the body as well as a powerful lever to propel the body. Foot complaints are usually related to overuse, trauma, or degenerative changes. Contributing factors include foot type—such as high arch (pes cavus) and flatfoot (pes planus)—foot deformities (ie, hallux valgus); improper footwear; excessive weight; and underlying systemic diseases (ie, diabetes or osteoporosis). The foot and ankle can have numerous accessory ossicles that can be confused with a possible fracture.

II. Common Diagnoses. Due to the amount of weight that the foot carries every day, it is little wonder that 18% of the population each year will have foot problems, an incidence that increases with age. Diagnosis can be facilitated by considering three distinct regions of the foot: the forefoot, the midfoot, and the hindfoot (Figure 28–1).

A. Forefoot. The forefoot, comprising the toes and metatarsals, is the most common site of foot complaints, with a prevalence of 2–10%. Most forefoot conditions are caused by poor shoe selection (tight toe boxes, high-heeled shoes); foot deformities (hallux valgus, hammer toes); overuse; or degenerative changes. Common conditions affecting the toes (followed by their prevalence) include calluses/corns (4.5%), plantar warts (2%), onychomycosis (10%), ingrown toenails (3–5%), phalangeal fractures, and peripheral neuropathy. Common conditions affecting the metatarsals include bunions (hallux valgus) (1.8%), hallux limitus (2%), metatarsalgia, Morton's (interdigital) neuromas, fractures (stress and fifth metatarsal), and sesamoiditis.

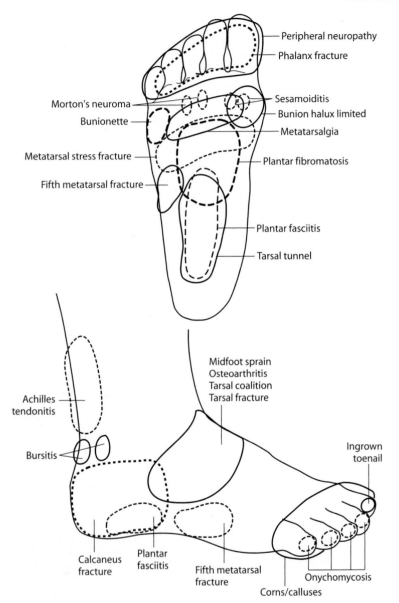

FIGURE 28–1. Foot complaints by location.

B. Midfoot. Midfoot complaints, caused by degenerative changes, trauma, or foot deformity, are relatively uncommon but can lead to significant disability. Common conditions affecting the midfoot, which comprises the cuneiforms, cuboid, and navicular bones of the foot, include midfoot sprain, osteoarthritis, tarsal fractures, plantar fibromatosis, posterior tibialis dysfunction, and tarsal coalition. (Also see the sidebars for Lisfranc injury and tarsal navicular bone fractures.)

LISFRANC INJURY

Lisfranc injury is a severe form of midfoot sprain to the tarsometatarsal articulation and is frequently missed. Pain and swelling over the tarsometatarsal articulation and inability to bear weight on tiptoes are clues to the injury. Weight-bearing x-rays of the foot may show avulsed bone between the first and second metatarsals and loss of congruity between the first metatarsal and the first cuneiform, second metatarsal, or both and the second cuneiform. Computerized tomography of the foot may be necessary for diagnosis. Patients with this injury should be placed in a non–weight-bearing cast and referred to orthopedics.

TARSAL NAVICULAR BONE FRACTURES

Tarsal navicular bone fractures are easily missed, because patients may have minimal pain over the midfoot and medial arch; these fractures are important to diagnose early because navicular fractures have a high rate of nonunion. Examination reveals tenderness over the navicular bone and increased pain with hopping on the foot. Plain x-rays of the foot are often inconclusive; therefore, bone scan, computerized tomography, or magnetic resonance imaging may be necessary for diagnosis. Treatment of nondisplaced fractures involves a non–weight-bearing cast for 6–8 weeks. Displaced fractures require orthopedic consultation.

C. **Hindfoot.** Hindfoot conditions are the second most common type of foot complaint, with a prevalence of 1%. Common conditions affecting the hindfoot, which comprises the calcaneus and talus, include plantar fasciitis (0.4% prevalence), calcaneal stress fractures, Achilles tendinosis, and bursitis. Most hindfoot conditions are caused by overuse or excessive weight. (Also see the sidebar on Achilles tendon rupture.)

ACHILLES TENDON RUPTURE

Achilles tendon rupture usually causes acute pain in the posterior heel. Examination will often reveal swelling and ecchymosis over the posterior heel, a palpable defect of the Achilles tendon, inability to walk normally, and a positive Thompson test (no plantar flexion when the calf is squeezed). Treatment is usually surgical and warrants an urgent referral to orthopedics.

III. **Symptoms** (see Tables 28–1 to 28–3 and Figure 28–1).
IV. **Signs** (see Tables 28–1 to 28–3 and Figure 28–1).
V. **Laboratory Tests** (see Tables 28–1 to 28–3).
   A. Laboratory tests are generally not necessary in evaluating foot complaints. Atraumatic symmetric foot swelling and pain can be caused by systemic arthritis (such as rheumatoid arthritis and systemic lupus erythematosus) and should be evaluated with tests for sedimentation rate, complete blood count (CBC), rheumatoid factor, antinuclear antibody, and uric acid. Pain due to a peripheral neuropathy is evaluated with a CBC (pernicious anemia, lead poisoning), complete metabolic profile (diabetes, renal disease, liver disease), thyroid-stimulating hormone (TSH), tests for vitamin B_{12}, and, depending on the history, urine heavy metal screen and serum protein electrophoresis (multiple myeloma).
   B. **Radiography.** X-rays of the foot should be performed on initial presentation in four instances: (1) when bony deformity is present, (2) when fracture is suspected, (3) when trauma to the foot has occurred, or (4) when the diagnosis is in question. Typically, standing anterior-posterior, oblique, and lateral views are obtained. **Technetium bone scan** can be used for identifying stress fractures if plain x-ray does not show any abnormality. Bone scan is very sensitive but not very specific in identifying stress fractures. **Magnetic resonance imaging (MRI)** is useful in identifying stress fractures and soft tissue abnormalities (eg, ligament/tendon pathology). It is very sensitive and specific but is more costly than a bone scan. Local expertise and procedure availability may

TABLE 28–1. EVALUATION AND MANAGEMENT OF COMMON FOREFOOT COMPLAINTS

Diagnosis	Symptoms	Findings	Testing	Treatment
Corn/callus	Pain with pressure on lesion	Skin thickening under bony prominence (calluses) or between toes (corns); tenderness with pressure directly over lesion	None	Paring of calluses[1] Padding[4] Shoes with wide toe box
Plantar wart	Pain with pressure on lesion	Skin thickening or papules that interrupt skin lines and have blood vessels within core; tenderness on squeezing lesion	No routine testing but can do a biopsy for diagnosis	Observation (some spontaneously resolve within 6–12 months) Wart removal[5]
Onychomycosis (fungal toenail infection)	Thickened nail, occasionally painful	Thickened discolored nail, occasionally crumbles	Fungal culture from scraping	Trimming/thinning of nail Shoes with wide toe box Oral antifungals Nail removal
Ingrown toenail (Onychocryptosis)	Pain, swelling, and discharge along border of nail	Nail border swollen, erythematous, occasional discharge	None	Ingrown toenail removal[2] If surrounding cellulitis, use antibiotic
Phalanx fracture	Acute pain and swelling of digit usually after trauma	Bony tenderness, swelling, ecchymosis, pain with toe motion	X-ray	**Nondisplaced fracture:** Buddy taping to adjacent toe, hard-soled shoe **Displaced fracture:** Referral to foot specialist
Peripheral neuropathy	Tingling, burning and/or pain initially in toes, then later in a stocking distribution, usually bilateral	May have decreased light touch, vibratory, and temperature sensation over toes. Sensation abnormalities tend to progress to involve entire foot with associated loss of motor strength in foot and loss of Achilles tendon reflex	Electromyography and nerve conduction velocity; laboratory tests to rule out underlying condition	Identify and treat underlying condition if present. Amitriptyline or gabapentin
Bunion or bunionette	Painful bony protuberance of first or fifth metatarsophalangeal joint (MTP)	Tender bony MTP prominence with valgus first MTP deformity (bunion) or varus fifth MTP deformity (bunionette)	X-ray reveals bony angular deformity (angle between first and second metatarsals >15°, angle between fourth and fifth metatarsals >10°)	Shoes with wide toe box Bunion shield Acetaminophen or NSAID Arch support orthotic Surgical removal if continued pain despite conservative treatment for 6–12 months

Condition	Symptoms	Signs	Diagnosis	Treatment
Hallux limitus or hallux rigiditus	Pain and swelling with movement, especially at toe off stage of gait	Loss of motion of first metatarsal, pain with extension of first metatarsal	X-ray may show degenerative spurs and loss of joint space of first MTP	Padding[4] Acetaminophen or NSAID Hard-soled shoes Surgery if severe pain despite conservative measures for 6–12 months
Metatarsalgia	Pain at metatarsal heads	Tenderness on palpation of metatarsal heads	X-ray to rule out fracture, arthritis	Relative rest Padding[4] Acetaminophen or NSAID
Morton's neuroma (interdigital)	Pain between metatarsal heads, numbness and tingling into toes, cramping of toes	Tenderness with squeezing metatarsal heads—occasionally accompanied by a click, fullness, or occasional soft tissue mass between metatarsal heads	None	Shoes with wide toe box; Morton's neuroma injection[3] If continued pain referral to foot specialist for excision
Metatarsal stress fracture	Pain and swelling over foot with activity, particularly during toe off stage of gait	Exquisite tenderness over metatarsal, occasional swelling and/or ecchymosis	X-ray findings may be absent; periosteal reaction, fracture line, or bony callous formation may be present. Bone scan or MRI if negative x-ray result.	Short leg removable cast-brace, hard-soled shoe or short leg walking cast for 4–8 weeks Orthopedic referral for fifth metatarsal stress fractures as healing is often delayed
Fifth metatarsal fracture	Pain over lateral foot	Tenderness to palpation of fifth metatarsal Swelling over lateral foot	X-ray to evaluate for avulsion fracture vs. Jones fracture (Figure 28–2)	**Avulsion fracture:** Short leg walking cast or air stirrup for 4–6 weeks; **Jones fracture:** Non–weight-bearing short leg cast until callous formation (3–6 weeks) then short leg walking cast for 3–6 weeks Orthopedic referral if non–union after 3 months, displaced fracture, stress fracture, or patient preference

(continued)

TABLE 28-1. *(Continued)*

Diagnosis	Symptoms	Findings	Testing	Treatment
Sesamoiditis	Pain in ball of foot (first MTP) with toe off stage of gait	Tenderness and swelling over plantar first MTP and just proximal to joint	X-ray to rule out sesamoid fracture	Padding[4] Relative rest NSAID

[1] For **paring of calluses**, soak the feet in lukewarm soapy water for 10–15 minutes. Dry the feet. Using a No. 15 blade scalpel, shave the callus shallowly with the blade parallel to the skin using an up-to-down motion repeatedly. Apply counterpressure with the back of the hand on the patient's foot to prevent slipping and shakiness. Continue until skin lines are apparent or until the callus has been completely removed. Make sure to remove the rim around the callus, not just the center portion. Diabetic patients, in particular, may have an ulcer beneath the callus. If the callus has a boggy feel to it or a bruised appearance underneath, it must be removed to prevent ulcer progression and possible infection.

[2] For **ingrown toenail removal**, materials needed are a 10-cc syringe with 25-gauge 11/2-inch needle; 10 cc lidocaine without epinephrine; alcohol swabs; Betadine; Penrose drain; 2 hemostats; nail lifter; nail separator (can use Beaver blade, sharp scissors, nail nipper, or #15 blade scalpel); cotton tip; triple antibiotic cream; 4 × 4 pad; and tape (alternatively, can also use tube gauze, cling, or Coban wrap).
Obtain informed consent from the patient. Perform a digital toe block with 10 cc of lidocaine without epinephrine, evenly distributing anesthetic laterally, medially, inferiorly, and superiorly (Figure 28–3). Sterilely clean the area with Betadine and drape. Apply tourniquet (Penrose drain and hemostat) to the proximal aspect of the toe to reduce the amount of blood in the field; remove as soon as the procedure is finished. Lift section of toenail to be removed (usually 1/4 to 1/3 of nail) with lifter or hemostat blade (blunt end down) all the way to the base of the nail (Figure 28–4). Separate nail to be removed with Beaver blade (#61), sharp scissors, nail nipper, or scalpel (#15 blade) all the way to the nail bed. Avulse the nail by clamping it with a hemostat, and roll the nail starting at the cut side until the section of the nail is removed, including the ingrown portion. Use a cotton tip to sweep under the fleshy part of the nail–skin border to ensure that the nail has been completely removed. Remove any remaining nail fragments with the hemostat. Dress with antibiotic cream and folded 4 × 4. Hold the dressing in place with tape, tube gauze, cling, or Coban dressing. Advise the patient to change the dressing in 24 hours using an adhesive bandage or 4 × 4 until the nail is healed and no longer drains or bleeds. The area may be washed after 24 hours. Schedule a follow-up examination of the area in 3–5 days to evaluate healing.

[3] For **Morton's neuroma injection**, materials needed are a 1-cc syringe; 1/2 cc lidocaine without epinephrine; 1/2 cc triamcinolone acetate (40 mg/mL); alcohol swabs, Betadine swabs, or both; and an adhesive bandage.
Obtain informed consent. Place the patient in a seated position. Localize the area to be injected using the metatarsal heads on either side of the neuroma as landmarks. The injection site is 1/2 cm proximal to the space between the metatarsal heads on the dorsal side of the foot. Draw up into a 1-cc syringe a mixture of 1/2 cc lidocaine and 1/2 cc of triamcinolone acetate (20 mg). Thoroughly clean the area to be injected with alcohol or Betadine. To provide local anesthesia, apply topical refrigerant (such as ethyl chloride) over the area where the needle will penetrate the skin. Inject using a dorsal approach perpendicular to the skin. Completely inject the mixture within the soft tissue space. Remove the needle. Clean the area and apply the adhesive bandage. Have the patient limit weight-bearing activities for 2 weeks.

[4] For **padding**, materials needed are high-density adhesive foam or felt (or moleskin) and scissors.
Padding takes weight off pressure points or inflamed areas. As a general rule, padding is placed just proximal to the area of irritation to take pressure off that site; the adhesive side is attached to the insole of the shoe. Calluses can be padded by cutting a doughnut-shaped pad and placing the hole of the pad over the callus. Corns need padding cut to a size that separates the two surfaces that are causing friction without being overly bulky.

[5] For **wart removal**, this procedure can be performed by two main methods: salicylic acid application or liquid nitrogen. All methods require debridement of the overlying thickened warty tissue with a #15 blade scalpel until there is slight bleeding (at surface of capillary bed) prior to the procedure.
50% salicylic acid paste method: In a 2″ × 2″ piece of 1/8″ adhesive foam, cut a hole slightly larger than the diameter of the wart (alternative—use a nonmedicated corn pad). Place adhesive foam (adhesive side on foot) with the hole centered over the wart. Fill the hole with salicylic acid paste and cover the top with an adhesive bandage. Secure the foam and bandage circumferentially around the foot with tape or Coban dressing, making sure the tape is not restricting circulation. Leave in place for 3–5 days. Remove the bandage and debride the dead skin. The procedure can be repeated in 1–2 weeks if the wart is not completely removed.
Liquid nitrogen method: Apply liquid nitrogen with cotton tip applicator or with spray applicator to the wart surface until white coloration of the wart extends past the wart's diameter by approximately 1/8″ and the lesion takes 15 seconds to return to normal color. Repeat this process three times in one session. Warn the patient that the lesion will itch and may form a blister at the base. The skin normally sloughs in 5–7 days. The procedure may be repeated at 1- to 2-week intervals until the wart is completely removed.
MRI, Magnetic resonance imaging; NSAID, nonsteroidal anti-inflammatory drug.

TABLE 28–2. EVALUATION AND MANAGEMENT OF COMMON MIDFOOT COMPLAINTS

Diagnosis	Symptoms	Findings	Testing	Treatment
Midfoot sprain	Swelling and pain diffusely over midfoot with hyperflexion	Tender midfoot diffusely	X-ray to rule out Lisfranc injury	Relative rest Acetaminophen and/or NSAID Shoes with supportive arch cushions Surgical referral if Lisfranc injury
Osteoarthritis	Midfoot pain and stiffness	Diffuse tenderness, occasional diffuse swelling, bony prominence	X-ray may show spurring, loss of joint space; laboratory tests to rule out other types of arthritis	Acetaminophen and/or NSAID Shoes with supportive arch cushions
Plantar fibromatosis	Painful bumps on bottom of foot	Nodules on plantar aspect of foot	Usually none but can do biopsy for diagnosis	No treatment, as there is high recurrence with excision; scars from excision can cause pain
Posterior tibialis dysfunction	History of twisting injury, sudden loss of arch, pain posterior and inferior to medial malleolus	Medial ankle swelling, asymmetric pes planus, inability to walk on toes, poor internal rotation and inversion, tenderness posterior and inferior to medial malleolus	MRI if rupture suspected (no strength with inversion and internal rotation, tendon not palpable)	Relative rest Arch support (OTC or custom) Surgery if continued pain despite conservative treatment for 6–12 months
Tarsal coalition	Vague midfoot pain, frequent ankle sprains, lower leg pain with activity	Limited inversion and eversion of foot, tenderness of midfoot and ankle	X-ray may show bony bridge between talus-navicular or talus-calcaneus, CT if suspicion but no x-ray findings	Custom arch support Surgery if continued pain despite conservative treatment for 6–12 months
Tarsal tunnel syndrome	Numbness or burning pain over bottom of foot, worse with walking and sometimes awakens patient from sleep	Positive Tinel's sign (tingling over bottom of foot) on tapping over posterior tibial nerve inferior-lateral to medial malleolus	Laboratory tests for peripheral neuropathy EMG/NCV	NSAID Arch support (OTC or custom) Physical therapy referral if no improvement in 1–2 months Referral to foot specialist in cases of severe pain not responsive to conservative management in 2–6 months

CT, computerized tomography; EMG, electromyography; MRI, magnetic resonance imaging; NCV, nerve conduction velocity; NSAID, nonsteroidal anti-inflammatory drug; OTC, over the counter.

TABLE 28-3. EVALUATION AND MANAGEMENT OF COMMON HINDFOOT COMPLAINTS

Diagnosis	Symptoms	Findings	Testing	Treatment
Plantar fasciitis	Dull, achy pain in inferior heel, especially upon awakening	Tender calcaneal tubercle and arch	X-ray to rule out stress fracture of calcaneus; calcaneal spurs do not correlate with pain (10–27% of asymptomatic patients have spurs)	Stretching and strengthening of plantar fascia and Achilles tendon NSAID Heel cup, arch support Night splint Physical therapy referral if no improvement after 2–3 months Plantar fascia injection[1] Referral to foot specialist if no improvement in 6–12 months of conservative treatment
Calcaneus stress fracture	Heel pain and swelling with walking, ecchymosis	Squeeze tenderness of calcaneus	X-ray may reveal stress reaction Bone scan or MRI	Relative rest Short leg removable cast-brace or short leg walking cast for 4–8 weeks
Achilles tendinosis	Activity-related pain and swelling behind heel	Swelling, tenderness over Achilles tendon (2–6 cm proximal to insertion), weak plantar-flexion	None	Relative rest NSAID Heel lift Stretching of Achilles tendon Physical therapy if no improvement after 1 month of above measures
Bursitis (superficial calcaneal or retrocalcaneal)	Pain and swelling localized on posterior ankle near Achilles tendon insertion	Tender posterior ankle, localized swelling/erythema, Haglund's deformity (prominent bony deformity of posterior calcaneus)	None	See Achilles tendinosis treatment

[1] For **plantar fascia injection**, materials needed are a 3-cc syringe, 1 cc lidocaine (optional); 1 cc triamcinolone acetate (40 mg/mL); topical refrigerant (optional); alcohol swabs, Betadine swabs, or both; and adhesive bandage.

Obtain informed consent from the patient, which should mention the risk of steroid flare and plantar fascial rupture. Ask the patient to lie down. Localize the area to be injected using the calcaneal tubercle as the main landmark. Normally the tubercle is the area of maximal tenderness on examination and can be palpated readily over the plantar aspect of the heel. Draw up into a 3-cc syringe a mixture of 1 cc lidocaine, 1 cc bupivacaine (optional), and 1 cc triamcinolone acetate (40 mg). Thoroughly clean the skin over the medial calcaneus with alcohol or Betadine. To provide local anesthesia, apply topical refrigerant (such as ethyl chloride) over the area where the needle will penetrate the skin. Inject using a medial approach approximately 1 cm up from the plantar aspect of the heel and 3 cm from the rear aspect of the heel using the calcaneal tubercle as a landmark (injection is just distal to the tubercle). Fan the mixture across the area of the fascial insertion. Remove the needle. Clean the area and apply an adhesive bandage. Have the patient limit weight-bearing activities for 2 weeks.

MRI, magnetic resonance imaging; NSAID, nonsteroidal anti-inflammatory drugs.

influence the decision between having an MRI or a bone scan. Computerized tomography is useful in evaluating bony pathology such as tarsal fractures if initial x-ray results are negative and there is strong clinical suspicion of fracture.

C. **Electromyography and nerve conduction velocity** are frequently ordered to evaluate neurogenic pain when an obvious source is not identifiable or for confirmation of clinical diagnosis. These tests are usually performed by a neurologist or physiatrist and help to anatomically localize the nerve involved or distinguish between mononeuropathies and polyneuropathies.

VI. **General Treatment Principles.** (Also see Tables 28–1 through 28–3 and Figures 28–1 through 28–4.)

A. **Appropriate footwear** can prevent and, in some cases, resolve many problems related to the foot. Characteristics of good footwear include roomy wide toe box, supportive arch, and low heel with a firm cushioned heel counter at the back of the shoe.

B. **Treatment of pain and inflammation** involves the use of relative rest, ice, and medications. **Relative rest** means decreasing pain-provoking activity to the point where there is no pain with that activity and substituting alternative minimal weight-bearing activities (ie, swimming, biking) during healing. Acetaminophen (Tylenol) (500–1000 mg orally four times a day) can be used for pain. Nonsteroidal anti-inflammatory medications (eg, ibuprofen, 400–800 mg orally three times daily, or naproxen, 250–500 mg orally

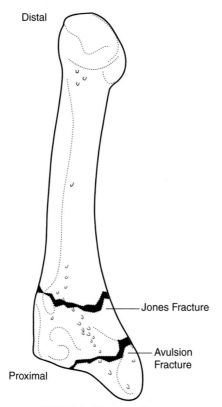

FIGURE 28–2. Fifth metatarsal fractures.

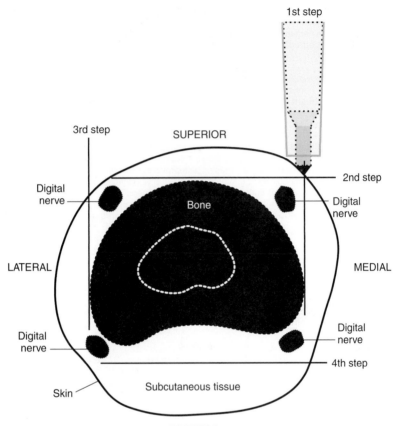

FIGURE 28–3. Digital nerve block. Cross-section through proximal phalanx. **Procedure:** Apply ethyl chloride for topical anesthesia. Insert 25-gauge 1½ needle into the skin at the medial base of the proximal phalanx until bone is touched, aspirating, then injecting a small amount above the bone. Advance the needle along the medial side. While withdrawing the needle, fan 1–2 cc of lidocaine evenly along the side. Repeat this step superiorly, laterally, and inferiorly. Allow at least 5 minutes for the block to become effective.

twice daily) can be used for pain, inflammation, or both. Chronic neurogenic pain can be treated with amitriptyline, 10–100 mg orally at bedtime, or gabapentin (Neurontin), 300–800 mg orally two to four times daily, starting with low doses, slowly titrating the doses higher to obtain pain relief and minimize side effects.

C. **Stretching exercises** are commonly used for foot complaints (especially plantar fasciitis and Achilles tendinosis) and involve stretching the plantar fascia and posterior heel cord muscles (gastrocnemius and soleus). Stretching for the plantar fascia is accomplished in a seated position by grasping the forefoot, dorsiflexing it for 10 seconds, then releasing and repeating this three to five times a day. The posterior heel cord is stretched by standing facing a wall with one foot placed approximately 24 inches from the wall and the other foot placed 48–60 inches from the wall. The patient leans toward the wall with hands on the wall in a "pushing fashion," keeping both heels on the ground. The knee of the leg in back is extended, while the front knee is slightly flexed. This position is held for 10–20 seconds, repeated three to five times, alternating which foot is forward.

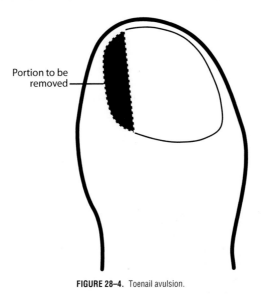

FIGURE 28–4. Toenail avulsion.

D. Orthotics are used for a wide variety of foot conditions.
  1. Over-the-counter (OTC) **arch cushion insoles** can be used initially for plantar fasciitis, bunions, and posterior tibialis dysfunction. OTC bunion shields, made of felt or silicone, can be used to protect the medial aspect of a bunion.
  2. **Heel lifts,** made of cork, felt, or visco-elastic material, are commonly used for Achilles tendinosis and bursitis.
  3. A **tension night splint for plantar fasciitis** can be commercially obtained or made with fiberglass splinting material, placing the ankle in an 80- to 90-degree angle, with the splint over the plantar aspect of the foot and posterior ankle and calf. ACE bandages secure the posterior splint.
  4. If these items are not helpful, referral to a foot specialist or orthotist for custom-made arch supports is appropriate.
  5. A short leg removable cast brace (cam walker boot) can be used for most stress fractures of the foot.
E. Systemic antifungal drugs may be used for onychomycosis. They are expensive, require treatment for 3 months, have a high rate of recurrence of infection (complete cure in <50%), and require monitoring of liver function tests (and CBC for terbinafine) at baseline, 6 weeks, and 3 months. Common systemic antifungal drugs given orally include terbinafine (Lamisil), 250 mg daily (for 3 months), and itraconazole (Sporanox), 200 mg twice daily for 1 week, repeated monthly for a total of 3 consecutive months. Topical ciclopirox 8% nail lacquer may also be used for onychomycosis. It is applied daily to the nail for 48 weeks but is seldom effective, as only 5–8% of patients have a complete cure.
F. Systemic antibiotics are used for foot infections such as cellulitis. (See Chapter 9.)

REFERENCES

Amundsen G, et al: *Office Surgery*. FP Essentials, edition no. 290, AAFP Home Study. Leawood, Kansas: American Academy of Family Physicians, July 2003.
Burroughs KE, Reimer CD, Fields KB: Lisfranc injury of the foot: A commonly missed diagnosis. Am Fam Physician 1998;**58**(1):118.
Corris EE, Lombardo JA: Tarsal navicular stress fractures. Am Fam Physician 2003;**67**(1):85.

Greene WB (editor): *Essentials of Musculoskeletal Care,* 2nd ed. American Academy of Orthopaedic Surgeons; 2001:407–515.
Noble J (editor): *Textbook of Primary Care Medicine,* 3rd ed. Mosby; 2001;1207–1226.
Young CC, Rutherford DS, Niedfeldt MW: Treatment of plantar fasciitis. Am Fam Physician 2001; **63:**467.

29   Fractures

Ted C. Schaffer, MD

KEY POINTS

- After trauma, one should assume a fracture has occurred and immobilize the affected region until x-rays have been obtained.
- The hallmark symptom of a new fracture is pain. Although the amount of pain correlates poorly with fracture severity, the absence of pain with an abnormal x-ray result makes it unlikely that a fracture has occurred.
- When x-ray results are negative but clinical suspicion for fracture is high, a magnetic resonance imaging scan (high cost with high sensitivity/specificity) or bone scan (lower cost but lower specificity) can provide supplemental information.

I. **Definition.** A fracture is a complete or incomplete break in the continuity of a bone. Fractures can be caused by direct trauma to the bone, repetitive forces to a bone (stress fracture), or abnormal bone architecture (osteoporosis or bone tumors).

II. **Common Diagnoses.** Evaluation of musculoskeletal injuries that are potential fractures accounts for 3–5% of all office visits. A fracture should be differentiated from a **sprain** (joint injury to ligaments attaching to bone), a **strain** (injury to the musculotendinous unit that attaches to bone) and a **contusion** (injury to the soft tissue surrounding the bone). Conditions associated with fractures include **dislocations** (complete loss of continuity between two articular surfaces) and **subluxations** (partial loss of continuity).

During **infancy,** as many as 1% of newborns may sustain a fractured clavicle at the time of delivery. In **childhood,** the incidence of long bone fractures increases, with common areas including buckle fractures of the arm, clavicle fractures, and growth plate injuries. Common **adult** trauma includes finger, metacarpal, and wrist fractures, as well as fractures of the ankle, metatarsals, and toes. The **elderly** are at greater risk for osteoporotic fractures such as vertebral, pelvic, and wrist fractures.

III. **Symptoms**
   A. **Pain** is the hallmark of new fracture occurrence. Often, however, the amount of pain experienced by the patient correlates poorly with the amount of bone damage. In children, pain at an epiphyseal plate is usually a fracture, not a joint sprain, since the growth plate is often the weakest area when a joint is stressed.
   B. **Loss of motion** can occur with fractures, especially when the fracture is located near a joint surface.
   C. **Loss of function** may be noted by the patient, either because of the pain involved or because of soft tissue swelling.

IV. **Signs**
   A. **Tenderness** to palpation should be present over a new fracture site. If there appears to be radiographic evidence of a fracture but the area is not tender on examination, the diagnosis of a fracture is suspect.
   B. **Swelling and deformity** may be apparent when the area of injury is inspected. The deformity may appear either as an obvious angulation at the bone or as an abnormal manner in which the extremity is being held.
   C. **Crepitus** can sometimes be noted with a displaced fracture.
   D. **Abnormal mobility** may be observed. Motion of the joint above and the joint below the injured area should always be tested to ensure that these adjacent regions are not also affected by the injury.

V. Laboratory Tests

A. An **x-ray** of any suspected fracture must be performed, since this is the method by which most fractures are confirmed. At least two views directed 90 degrees apart are required, since a nondisplaced fracture may not be visible if only a single view is obtained. Comparison x-rays of the opposite limb should be obtained in children to aid the physician in distinguishing a fracture line from a normal epiphyseal growth plate.

B. When clinical suspicion for fracture is great but initial x-ray results are negative, the area can be immobilized and x-rays repeated in 7–14 days to look for a new fracture line. If a fracture diagnosis is more urgent, then a **bone scan** or **magnetic resonance imaging (MRI)** scan can be obtained. The MRI is more costly than a bone scan, but its high degree of sensitivity and specificity has made it the diagnostic test of choice for many physicians when initial x-ray results are negative and an early diagnosis is important for management. A bone scan has a high degree of sensitivity but lacks the specificity of an MRI.

VI. Treatment

A. **General principles** for the management of a potential fracture are as follows:
1. **The physician should assume a fracture** has occurred until an x-ray examination has proved otherwise.
2. A **splint** should be applied to the injured area in order to decrease bone motion and hold the bone in place. This procedure will alleviate pain and prevent further tissue damage.
3. **Ice applied immediately** for 20–30 minutes will curtail swelling and provide pain relief. The ice should not directly touch the skin. Ice therapy may be repeated at 90-minute intervals.
4. Most **dislocations** should not be reduced until x-rays have been taken. Reduction before x-ray is advisable when there is evidence of vascular compromise to an extremity that may be relieved by immediate reduction of the dislocation or fracture. Immediate post-traumatic reduction of a dislocation is also permissible when the patient is having substantial pain and the reduction is easily accomplished, such as in an anterior shoulder or finger dislocation.

B. The following **specific fractures** can be managed in an ambulatory setting:
1. **Finger fractures**
   a. **Distal phalangeal fractures** are usually crush injuries, which can be managed by immobilization and protection. If the extensor tendon has been involved, then a mallet finger injury has occurred (see Chapter 33).
   b. **Middle and proximal phalangeal** fractures can be managed if the injury is nondisplaced, without angulation or rotation. Fracture angulation is evident on x-ray and is caused by the pull of intrinsic hand muscles as they attach to the bone. Rotation is evaluated by having the patient flex their fingers into the palm and observing that the fingers remain parallel and do not overlap. Nondisplaced fractures should be treated with a finger splint on the flexor surface for 2–4 weeks, keeping the PIP (proximal interphalangeal) joint at 30–50 degrees flexion and the DIP (distal interphalangeal) joint at 10–20 degrees flexion.
   c. **PIP joint** dislocations often occur with a hyperextension injury, causing a dorsal dislocation of the middle phalanx on the proximal phalanx ("a coach's finger"). These are usually easily reduced by **gentle** traction and **gentle** hyperextension, followed by a flexor surface splint for 2–4 weeks.
2. **Metacarpal fractures**
   a. **Fractures of the neck of the fifth metacarpal** ("Boxer's fracture") commonly occur after punching a person or wall. An ulnar gutter splint extending from midforearm to the fingertip can be applied for 3–6 weeks, keeping the MCP (metacarpal phalangeal) joint in 90 degrees of flexion.
   b. **Fracture of the shaft of the fourth and fifth metacarpal** can be treated with an ulnar gutter splint if there is angulation less than 30 degrees and no rotational injury (see section VI,B,2,a).
   c. **Fractures of the first, second, and third metacarpals** generally require orthopedic referral because of functional problems related to residual angulation.
3. **Wrist and arm fractures**
   a. The **scaphoid** is the most common wrist fracture. Those that involve the distal scaphoid (5% of fractures) or middle scaphoid (80% of fractures) have a good blood supply and can be immobilized for 8–12 weeks with a long arm (ex-

tending above the elbow) or a short arm cast (extending to the proximal forearm); the thumb must be immobilized to the level of the IP (interphalangeal) joint. Fractures of the proximal scaphoid have a poor blood supply and a high risk of nonunion and are therefore referred to an orthopedic surgeon.

   b. **Nondisplaced distal radial fractures** can be treated with short arm cast immobilization for 6 weeks in adults. The cast should extend from the metacarpals to the proximal forearm, with the thumb allowed free mobility.

   c. Children more commonly sustain a nondisplaced fracture of the radius above the growth plate, which is known as a **buckle fracture.** The patient should wear a short arm cast for 3–4 weeks. Casting should extend from the metacarpal to the proximal forearm.

   d. **Proximal radial head** fractures near the elbow can also occur with a fall on an outstretched hand. Unless there is x-ray evidence of a displaced radial head, these fractures can be managed with a long arm splint extending along the ulnar surface from the metacarpals to the proximal humerus, with the elbow at 90 degrees flexion. The splint should be maintained for 3–4 weeks with early mobilization to maintain elbow motion, especially in the elderly.

   e. **Humeral head fractures** are common in elderly individuals after falling on an outstretched arm or sustaining a blow to the lateral arm. Eighty percent of proximal humerus fractures are minimally displaced. Treatment, even if the shaft of the humerus is impacted, consists of providing the patient with a shoulder sling for 1–2 weeks and, after the sling is removed, providing the patient with range-of-motion exercises. The major risk involved in humeral head fractures is loss of shoulder motion after immobilization. Orthopedic referral is needed if there is >1 cm fracture displacement between the proximal and distal components.

4. **Clavicle fractures**
   a. **Middle third (midclavicular) fractures** account for 80% of clavicle fractures and are easily managed. A "figure-of-8" or clavicular strap is worn for 3–6 weeks by children and for 6 weeks by adults. A residual callus is often left, but the fracture usually heals well.

   b. **Distal fractures,** which are present in 15% of fractures, can be more complicated than midclavicular fractures. The initial management is the same and can be performed by a family physician. However, a painful acromioclavicular joint arthritis may develop, necessitating orthopedic resection of the distal clavicle.

   c. **Proximal fractures** occur in 5% of these cases and should be evaluated carefully. The physician should look for signs of vascular injury due to the close proximity of the great vessels of the neck. Orthopedic consultation should be strongly considered.

5. **Simple torso fractures**
   a. **Rib fractures** are common in the elderly with only minor trauma. In young adults and children, they are usually the result of greater traumatic force. A chest x-ray should be obtained to exclude pneumothorax or pulmonary contusion. Rib fractures are easily managed if the bones are not displaced.

      (1) **Pain relief** is the main focus of treatment. Oral systemic narcotics (eg, codeine, 30 mg four times daily), and **nonsteroidal agents** (eg, ibuprofen, 600 mg three times daily) are usually adequate, but **intercostal nerve blocks** (usually done by an anesthesiologist) can be considered if a patient is in severe pain. Rib belts should be avoided, since they cause substantial atelectasis and increase the incidence of pneumonia.

      (2) **Hospitalization** should be considered for multiple rib fractures (three or more) because of the increased risk of pulmonary contusion and atelectasis. In the elderly, even a single rib fracture can occasionally lead to pulmonary compromise.

   b. **Lumbar compression fractures** are common in elderly patients with osteoporosis and can occur with minimal trauma. They can be seen from the T-4 through L-5 vertebrae, and neurologic compromise is extremely rare. Treatment is aimed at pain relief, with immobilization for a few days followed by **ambulation** with a support such as a lumbosacral garment.

   c. **Undisplaced pelvic fractures** are another problem in the elderly, occasionally complicated by blood loss, even with minor fractures. Treatment is aimed at pain relief (see above) and **ambulatory support** with devices such as a walker or cane until pain resolves.

6. **Ankle fractures**

   a. **Fibular fractures below the tibial dome** are avulsion fractures caused by ligamentous pulling during sudden inversion of the foot. Treatment is a posterior leg splint for 5–7 days until the swelling has subsided, followed by a short leg walking cast for 3–6 weeks. A pneumatic ankle support (eg, Aircast) may be considered as an alternative to casting since ankle inversion/eversion will be protected. In children, tenderness over the epiphyseal plate of the distal fibula should be regarded as a Salter I fracture (see Figure 29–1), not an ankle sprain. Treatment consists of a short leg walking cast for 3–4 weeks.

   b. When fibular fractures are **at or above the tibial dome,** greater ligamentous instability occurs, because the syndesmotic ligaments and interosseous membrane are involved. Referral is indicated in these cases, since surgery may be required.

7. **Foot and toe fractures**

   a. **Second, third, and fourth metatarsal** fractures often occur as stress fractures from overuse. Frequently initial x-ray results are negative, but repeat films in 2–4 weeks show healing callus. The treatment is relative rest and use of a hard-soled shoe for 2–4 weeks until pain subsides. Patient education is important to prevent recurrent injury.

   b. **Fifth metatarsal** fractures can be treated if they are within 1.5 cm of the proximal styloid tip. These are avulsion injuries, which respond to relative rest and a hard-soled shoe. More distal fifth metatarsal fractures have a high incidence of nonunion, often require operative intervention, and are best referred to someone with management experience.

   c. **Toe fractures** are common, and generally require just buddy-taping to an adjacent toe for symptomatic relief of 1–2 weeks. A small piece of gauze or tissue should be placed between toes to prevent skin maceration.

C. Special features of **pediatric fractures** are described below.

   1. The time needed for **cast or splint immobilization** for fractures in children is generally one half to one third the time needed for immobilization of an adult fracture, since bone healing occurs much faster in children than in adults.

   2. The Salter-Harris classification of pediatric fractures should be understood (see Figure 29–1).

      a. Salter I fractures through the epiphyseal plate are a clinical diagnosis, often with normal x-ray findings. The prognosis is excellent. Salter II fractures through the metaphysis are also stable injuries. Salter I and II fractures are treated like any other fracture with cast or splint immobilization for several weeks.

      b. Salter III and IV fractures, which involve the epiphysis, and Salter V fractures, which are crush injuries to the growth plates, are more serious problems, especially when they involve long bones of the body.

      c. Parents of children with growth plate injuries should be advised of the possibility of growth abnormalities. These abnormalities are quite rare with Salter I and II fractures, except when the fractures are in the distal femur or tibia.

      d. In children, tenderness at the growth plate is assumed to be a bony injury rather than a ligamentous sprain, since the ligaments are stronger than the bone at this age. Immobilization often with casting is indicated, depending on the bone involved. Common growth plate fractures include the ankle and wrist.

D. **Fractures requiring referral.** In an ambulatory setting, the physician must know which injuries should be managed by an orthopedist because of the increased risk of complication. The following list serves as a guideline for situations in which consultation is advisable.

   1. **Open fractures** increase the risk of infection, especially osteomyelitis, and fracture nonunion.

   2. **Neurovascular compromise** is an orthopedic emergency necessitating immediate care by a qualified surgeon.

   3. **Unstable fractures,** where bone alignment cannot be maintained without external forces, usually require open reduction and internal fixation.

   4. **Intra-articular fractures** create a high risk for the development of long-term traumatic arthritis. Open surgical reduction is often required in order to achieve the best possible bone alignment.

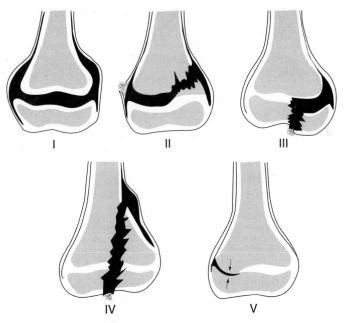

FIGURE 29–1. Salter-Harris classification of epiphyseal injuries in children. (Reproduced, with permission, from Way LW [editor]: *Current Surgical Diagnosis & Treatment*, 9th ed. Originally published by Appleton & Lange; 1991. Copyright © 1991 by the McGraw-Hill Companies, Inc.)

     5. Growth plate injuries of long bones that involve the epiphysis (Salter III, IV, or V fractures) create a high risk of complications, and therefore the patient may require long-term orthopedic management.

REFERENCES

Greene WE (editor): *Essentials of Musculoskeletal Care,* 2nd ed. American Academy of Orthopaedic Surgeons; 2001.
Greenspan A: *Orthopedic Radiology: A Practical Approach.* Lippincott Williams & Wilkins; 1999.
Johnson R (editor): *Sports Medicine in Primary Care.* Saunders; 2000.
Simon RR, Koenigsknecht SJ: *Emergency Orthopedics: The Extremities,* 4th ed. McGraw-Hill; 2001.

---

30   Gastrointestinal Bleeding

May S. Jennings, MD

KEY POINTS

- Initial assessment of hemodynamic status and appropriate triage of patients with gastrointestinal bleeding are strongly linked to patient outcomes.
- 80% of gastrointestinal bleeds will resolve spontaneously with appropriate supportive care.
- The risk of further upper gastrointestinal bleeding can be minimized by changes in lifestyle and use of medications.

I. **Definition.** Gastrointestinal (GI) bleeding is blood loss from any part of the GI tract, including both symptomatic and occult blood loss.

II. **Common Diagnoses.** The estimated incidence in the United States is 1 per every 1000 people. GI bleeding accounts for 300,000 hospitalizations annually in the United States. The mortality rate for GI bleeding remains around 10% despite modern technological advances.

  A. **Upper GI (UGI) bleeding** is defined as any GI bleeding proximal to the ligament of Treitz.

   1. **Peptic ulcer disease** makes up 50% of significant UGI bleeding. Risk factors include nonsteroidal anti-inflammatory drugs (NSAIDS), alcohol, *Helicobacter pylori* infection, and excess acid production.

   2. **Gastritis** is the presence of subepithelial hemorrhages and erosions in the mucosa. It is associated with NSAIDS, alcohol, and stress.

   3. **Esophagitis** is especially common in geriatric patients and can be associated with drug-induced injury.

   4. **Mallory-Weiss tear** is frequently associated with alcohol ingestion and represents 5–15% of UGI bleeds.

   5. **Esophageal and gastric varices** are associated with portal hypertension, generally as a result of cirrhosis. The overall mortality rate from bleeding varices is 30%.

  B. **Lower GI (LGI) bleeding** is defined as any GI bleeding distal to the ligament of Treitz.

   1. **Diverticulosis** is the most common cause of significant LGI bleeding in the older adult population. It is estimated that half of all US adults older than 60 years have diverticuli.

   2. **Vascular ectasias** are the second most common cause of LGI bleeding in the older adult population. Twenty-five percent of geriatric patients have vascular ectasias in the cecum and right colon.

   3. **Colitis** can cause GI bleeding and may be due to infection, inflammation, radiation, or ischemia.

   4. **Neoplasms and polyps** generally cause occult GI bleeding.

   5. **Hemorrhoids,** both external and internal, can be associated with bleeding after excessive straining and hard stools. They are rarely associated with significant LGI bleeding.

   6. **Anal fissure** is associated with blood around the stool after a painful bowel movement. It is associated with minor LGI bleeding.

  C. **LGI bleeding in children.** UGI bleeding in children is extremely rare in the outpatient setting. Significant LGI bleeding is not common.

   1. **Meckel's diverticulum** is the most common cause of significant GI bleeding in children. It is a congenital abnormality that is generally located in the small intestine. It can present as UGI or LGI bleeding.

   2. **Intussusception** is the second most common cause of significant LGI bleeding. It is caused by the involution of one segment of bowel into another segment of bowel.

   3. **Juvenile polyps** are generally benign, but can be associated with familial polyposis syndromes.

   4. **Colitis** is due to infection, inflammation, or allergic etiologies. Inflammatory bowel disease often presents in childhood and young adulthood.

   5. **Anal fissure or rectal foreign bodies** are frequently associated with minor rectal bleeding in children.

III. **Symptoms.** (Also see the sidebar on rare but serious conditions.)

  A. **Bleeding history**

   1. **Hematemesis** is vomiting blood. A careful history must be taken to exclude nasopharyngeal bleeding and hemoptysis.

   2. **Melena** is black, tarry stools. It is generally indicative of UGI bleeding.

   3. **Hematochezia** is passing blood through the rectum. It is indicative of LGI bleeding 85% of the time. If it originates from an UGI source, it denotes a very brisk bleed.

   4. **Currant jelly stool** is blood, mucus, and stool in combination. It is generally seen in intussusception or acute colitis.

  B. **General history.** The history is frequently not helpful in identifying the source of the GI bleed, especially in UGI bleeding. In fact, the clinical judgment of physicians is only correct 40% of the time. Important features of the history are listed below.

1. **Confusion, dizziness, or syncope.** Any recent history represents a hemodynamically unstable patient who requires urgent attention.
2. **Abdominal pain.** In UGI bleeding, pain would be more consistent with peptic ulcer disease and gastritis. In LGI bleeding, pain would be most consistent with colitis in adults or Meckel's diverticulum in children. Bowel perforation should always be considered in patients with severe pain.
3. **Coughing, vomiting, or retching.** These symptoms suggest Mallory-Weiss tear.
4. **Number of stools.** Knowing the number of stools in the last 24–48 hours may be helpful in determining the rate of the bleeding.
5. **History of prior GI bleed.** This knowledge may or may not be helpful, since 30% of patients with known varices will bleed from other sites.
6. **Atherosclerotic disease.** Atherosclerotic disease such as coronary artery disease or peripheral vascular disease raises the possibility for ischemic colitis. Historical features that go along with this diagnosis include abdominal pain after meals and abdominal pain followed by LGI bleeding.
7. **NSAIDS, warfarin, and alcohol.** NSAID use increases the risk of UGI bleeding by threefold in adults, fivefold in the elderly.
8. **Weight loss** suggests carcinoma. Colon carcinoma is suggested by weight loss plus change in bowel habits.

RARE BUT SERIOUS CONDITIONS

1. **Vomiting, pain and blood in the stool** of a young child are suggestive of intussusception.
2. **History of an aortic aneurysm repair or aortic bypass** suggests a potentially life-threatening aortoenteric fistula, usually to the duodenum, as the cause of GI bleeding.

IV. **Signs.** Like the history, the examination may not be very helpful in terms of pinpointing the etiology of the GI bleed.
  A. **Vital signs.** Orthostasis (rise in pulse by 20 beats per minute and a fall in systolic blood pressure by 20 mm Hg when standing) indicates hemodynamic instability and rapid bleeding. The presence of orthostasis represents a 20% blood loss and a clinical emergency. Other signs of hypovolemic shock, such as a drop in the patient's usual systolic blood pressure by 40 mm Hg, should be considered an emergency. Beta blockers may mask the tachycardia normally associated with hemodynamic instability.
  B. **Altered mental status.** Altered mental status is an ominous finding and should be considered a sign of hypovolemic shock until proved otherwise.
  C. **Abdominal examination**
    1. **Peritoneal signs or severe tenderness** raise suspicion for bowel perforation.
    2. **Pain that is disproportional to the abdominal examination** suggests ischemic colitis.
  D. **Rectal examination.** Rectal examination is mandatory in all patients with GI bleed. This includes:
    1. **Inspection and digital examination for masses,** hemorrhoids, and anal fissures.
    2. **Examination of retrieved stool** for melena and hematochezia. If no obvious bleeding is noted, stool guaiac testing is indicated.
      a. Stools will appear black (not tarry) after ingestion of iron or bismuth subsalicylate.
      b. Tomatoes, rare meat, and cherries may cause a false-positive stool guaiac study.
      c. Guaiac-positive stools may continue for up to 3 weeks after an acute bleeding episode.
  E. Any **sequelae of chronic liver disease** including spider angiomas, ascites, caput medusa, palmar erythema, jaundice, or splenomegaly suggest variceal bleeding.
  F. A **nasogastric (NG) tube** should be placed to try to differentiate UGI from LGI bleeding, regardless of history. Bright red blood or "coffee ground" material in the NG tube suggests a UGI source. There is no contraindication to NG tube placement in patients

with known or suspected esophageal varices. Guaiac testing of the nasogastric aspirate is not recommended.

V. Laboratory Tests

A. Endoscopy (esophagogastroduodenoscopy [EGD], or colonoscopy) is the first step in further evaluation of most patients with GI bleeding. In addition to localizing the source of bleeding, endoscopy allows therapeutic interventions, including banding of varices and mucosal biopsy to diagnose *H pylori* (EGD) and sclerotherapy, cauterization, and snaring of polyps (colonoscopy).

   1. In patients with hematochezia and hemodynamic instability, EGD should precede colonoscopy.
   2. In patients older than 40 years with occult GI bleeding (guaiac-positive stool with minimal or no symptoms), colonoscopy is indicated; with negative colonoscopy result further work-up may not be productive, unless iron deficiency anemia is present (see Chapter 4).
   3. In patients younger than 40 years with minor rectal bleeding, anoscopy (Chapter 52) or sigmoidoscopy that reveals a likely cause is often a sufficient work-up.
   4. Data suggest improved outcomes when EGD is performed within 24 hours of upper GI bleed onset, likely because this allows early interventions for the 20% of bleeds not resolving spontaneously.

B. Hematologic studies
   1. **Hemoglobin and hematocrit** should be done, though they will be normal early in acute bleeding. A low hematocrit and mean corpuscular volume without hemodynamic compromise suggests slow, chronic bleeding.
   2. A **blood urea nitrogen to creatine ratio** ≥ 36 suggests UGI bleeding.
   3. **Prothrombin time, partial thromboplastin time, and platelet count** assess possible contribution of coagulopathy or thrombocytopenia to the bleed.

C. An electrocardiogram is recommended in adults, especially those with known coronary artery disease.

D. Barium studies and **gastric lavage** (see section IV,F) are generally not as helpful as endoscopy in evaluating GI bleeding.

E. Technetium red cell scan can locate LGI bleeding sources, but results are not highly reliable. However, the scan is the procedure of choice in confirming Meckel's diverticulum.

F. Angiography is highly sensitive and allows therapeutic intervention during the procedure, but it carries procedure-related risks and cannot locate very slow bleeds.

VI. Treatment. GI bleeding is an emergency until proved otherwise.

A. Hospitalization is always indicated for those with signs or symptoms of hemodynamic instability and those with melena or comorbid disease. Hospitalization is also recommended for elderly patients, due to poor functional reserves and frequent comorbidities. The inpatient setting allows for aggressive intravenous fluid resuscitation; transfusion (packed red blood cells, fresh frozen plasma, or platelets as indicated); efficient localization of bleeding source (see section V); and initiation of specific therapy (eg, octreotide for acute variceal bleeding). **Surgery** is a last resort for bleeding uncontrolled with other interventions.

TABLE 30–1. INITIAL PREDICTORS OF POOR CLINICAL OUTCOME IN GI BLEEDING[1]

Age >60 years	**Laboratory tests**
	Elevated liver function tests
Comorbidities	Elevated prothrombin time
Presence of 3 or more	Hypoalbuminemia
Cardiac, pulmonary, renal, or liver disease	Thrombocytopenia
	Leukocytosis
Medications	Elevated creatinine
Warfarin	Hemoglobin <10 mg/dL
Corticosteroids	Electrocardiographic changes
Melena	
Hemodynamic instability	
Bloody nasogastric aspirate	

[1] Poor clinical outcome is defined as risk of rebleeding and risk of death.

B. Outpatient management is appropriate for patients not meeting criteria for hospital management (eg, individuals with occult bleeding).
C. Preventive measures are often effective in minimizing recurrences, once the bleeding source has been identified and controlled. (See Chapters 1, 19, and 52.)
D. Prognosis. In all types of GI bleeding, 80% resolve spontaneously with supportive care. Even 60% of variceal bleeds resolve spontaneously without aggressive intervention. Seventy percent of mortality from GI bleeding is attributed to comorbid diseases (Table 30–1).

REFERENCES

Bono MJ: Lower gastrointestinal tract bleeding. Emerg Med Clin North Am 1996;**14**(3):547.
Fox VL: Gastrointestinal bleeding in infancy and childhood. Gastroenterology Clinics 2000;**29**(1):37.
Hussain H, Lapin S, Cappell MS: Clinical scoring systems for determining the prognosis of gastrointestinal bleeding. Gastroenterology Clinics 2000;**29**(2):445.
McQuirk TD, Coyle WJ: Upper gastrointestinal tract bleeding. Emerg Med Clin North Am 1996;**14**(3):523.
Pianka JD, Affronti J: Management principles of gastrointestinal bleeding. Primary Care; Clinics in Office Practice 2001;**28**(3):557.
Rosen AM: Gastrointestinal bleeding in the elderly. Clin Geriatr Med 1999;**15**(3):511.

---

31   Genital Lesions

Tomás P. Owens, Jr., MD

KEY POINTS

- In evaluating patients with genital lesions, a history of sexual preferences/practices is important.
- Most genital lesions can be diagnosed by a careful history and examination, with minimal laboratory testing.
- Human immunodeficiency virus testing should always be considered in patients with genital lesions believed to be sexually transmitted.

I. Definition. Genital lesions are any acquired abnormality of the external genitalia.
II. Common Diagnoses. The 2001 National Ambulatory Medical Care Survey describes diseases of the skin and subcutaneous tissue as being the principal diagnosis in 5.3% of all office visits and diseases of the genitourinary system as 3.3% of all office visits.
  A. Ulcerative lesions
   1. **Herpes simplex virus types 1 and 2** (HSV-1 and -2). The presence of antibodies to **HSV-2** varies from 3% in nuns to 70–80% in prostitutes and seems to be directly proportional to sexual activity. **HSV-1,** which is present in 90% of the population, can cause genital herpes, although less frequently.
   2. **Primary syphilis** (chancre). The United States showed a 90% decline in the number of cases reported from 1991 to 2000, but a 9.1% increase was noted from 2000 to 2002, with the highest incidence among non-Hispanic blacks and in the South. During the last year there has been an upsurge in cases of men who have sex with men (MSM).
  B. Verrucoid/papillomatous lesions
   1. **Condylomata acuminata** due to human papillomavirus, most commonly serotypes 6 and 11, are the most common sexually transmitted entity, although this condition can also be transmitted nonsexually. Condylomata are most common during the reproductive years, are commonly associated with other sexually transmitted

- diseases (STDs), and may grow dramatically with pregnancy, human immunodeficiency virus (HIV), or corticosteroid use.
    2. **Secondary syphilis** condyloma latum (see section II,A,2).
    3. Genital lesions of **molluscum contagiosum** are associated with, but not always due to, sexual transmission. HIV infection is associated with an increased number and size of lesions.
    4. **Pearly penile papules** are present in up to 30% of men. There are no known predisposing risk factors.
  C. **Pruritic lesions**
    1. **Balanitis,** irritation of the glans penis, occurs most commonly in uncircumcised diabetic patients, and those with poor hygiene. It can be precipitated by smegma and exogenous contact irritants.
    2. **Erythrasma** is a chronic bacterial infection that occurs more often in obese dark-skinned men.
    3. **Phthirus pubis** (pubic lice) occurs only in humans, most commonly in young adults, is very contagious, and is transmitted sexually or by sharing clothing, towels, or bed linens. It prefers moist environments, seldom goes into neighboring skin, and has been described rarely on facial hair.
    4. **Vulvar dystrophy/lichen sclerosus et atrophicus (LSA)** is a common process of unknown etiology in postmenopausal women but is seen in all age groups. In men, it is very rare and is called balanitis xerotica obliterans (**BXO**). It is more common in middle-aged diabetic patients but can be seen in all age groups.
  D. **Cystic lesions**
    1. **Bartholin's gland cysts or inflammation** occurs on either side of the lower vaginal vestibule. They account for 2% of all new patients in a gynecological practice, are more common after menarche and before menopause, and are unrelated to STDs. Other causes of genital lesions discussed elsewhere include psoriasis, seborrheic dermatitis, scabies, tinea cruris, allergic/contact dermatitis (see Chapter 14); testicular torsion, epididymo-orchitis, spermatocele/epididymal cyst/varicocele (see Chapter 56); folliculitis (see Chapter 9); urethritis (see Chapter 61); and vaginitis, cervicitis, and chlamydia (see Chapters 51 and 64). Causes of genital lesions not discussed here because of their relative rarity include penile cancer, bowenoid papulosis of the penis/vulvar epithelial neoplasia, testicular cancer, lymphogranuloma venereum, granuloma inguinale, lichen planus, fixed drug eruption, erythroplasia of Queyrat, Peyronie's disease, penile/vulvar trauma, penile prostheses, and priapism.
III. **Symptoms**
  A. **Ulcerative lesions**
    1. **HSV-1 or -2**
      a. The incubation period is 2–14 days. Primary infection, which is associated with viremia, may manifest as fever, generalized myalgia, malaise, headaches, and weakness, peaking 3–4 days after the onset of lesions. Painful inguinal or deep pelvic lymphadenopathy arises 2–3 weeks later. Burning pain and pruritus along with vaginal or urethral discharge and dysuria are common.
      b. There is a prodrome of burning, lancinating pain 1–2 days before eruption. Direct local inflammatory changes and cytolysis account for most of the syndrome in recurrences, which rarely cause systemic symptoms.
    2. **Chancres** are painless, unless secondarily infected. Patients present for evaluation of the lesion or for accompanying lymphadenopathy.
  B. **Verrucoid/papillomatous lesions**
    1. **Condylomata acuminata** have an incubation period from weeks to years, are painless, and commonly recur during the first few years. Rarely, a patient may complain of hematuria from a urethral condyloma.
    2. **Condyloma lata** are painless lesions, although generalized myalgia, fever, chills, and arthralgia may occur in the early phase of eruption, which occurs 6–24 weeks after untreated primary syphilis or, rarely, synchronously with the chancre.
    3. The lesions of **molluscum contagiosum** develop slowly over a 2- to 3-month period and rarely are pruritic.
    4. **Pearly penile papules** are asymptomatic but worrisome to some patients.

C. **Pruritic lesions**
   1. **Balanitis** is associated with pruritus and burning pain during or after sexual intercourse or with excessive smegma production. Dysuria and more severe pain occur with more severe disease.
   2. Pruritus and long-standing rash persisting after fungicidal therapy are common presentations for **erythrasma.**
   3. **Phthirus pubis** infestation manifests as pruritus, rarely severe. Some patients describe nits on their pubic hair.
   4. Patients with **vulvar dystrophy/LSA** and **BXO** present with varying degrees of pruritus and concerns about the lesion's appearance.
D. **Cystic lesions**
   1. Small **Bartholin's gland cysts** are usually asymptomatic. Larger lesions cause discomfort, pruritus, and sometimes dyspareunia. As the lesions become infected, there is at times very severe pain, external dysuria, and vulvar discharge. Systemic symptoms are rare.

IV. **Signs**
A. **Ulcerative lesions**
   1. **HSV-1 or -2** initially is an erythematous papule, which is followed hours to a few days later by small, grouped vesicles on the glans, on the distal and sometimes proximal shaft of the penis, or on the scrotum in males. The entire vulva can be involved. Pustules, erosions, or ulceration occur, which heal by crusting in 2–4 weeks, leaving some hypomelanosis or hypermelanosis. Scarring occurs only with manipulation or secondary infection. **Primary infection** produces larger numbers of lesions than **recurrent infection.**
   2. Primary infection with *Treponema pallidum* produces a **chancre** at the site of inoculation 10–90 days after direct contact with secretions of an infected person. The **chancre** is a papule that erodes into a single, round, beefy-red ulcer with hard, raised borders and yellow-green exudative material on its base. Chancres occur in the inside penile foreskin, coronal sulcus, shaft, or base, or on the cervix and vagina (where patients seldom detect it), vulva, or clitoris. Extragenital sites for chancres are the mouth, lips, breast, fingers, and thighs. Multiple chancres can be seen in HIV infection.
B. **Verrucoid/papillomatous lesions**
   1. **Condylomata acuminata** are skin-colored or pink-red tumors, which are localized, fleshy, soft, moist, elongated, and dome-shaped with filiform or conical vegetating projections in grape- to cauliflower-like clusters on moist surfaces. They can be keratotic and smooth papular warts in dry surfaces or subclinical "flat" warts. Large lesions occur perianally in immunosuppressed persons.
   2. **Condylomata lata** are soft, flat-topped, moist, skin-colored or pale pink papules, warts, nodules, or plaques, which may become confluent. These lesions occur in any body surface, but have a preference for the anogenital area and intertriginous sites.
   3. **Molluscum contagiosum** presents as pearly white papules or nodules 2–8 mm in diameter, which are mostly round or oval with a classic umbilicated top. The papules are localized in clusters, with preference for the genital area, neck, and trunk and may evolve to pustules and small crusts or plaques. Large size or large number of lesions, particularly in the face, suggests HIV.
   4. **Pearly penile papules** histologically are angiofibromas that first appear around puberty. They are thin, conical, white, or pale pink uniformly sized groups of papules, forming multiple parallel lines mostly on the corona, but also in the balanopreputial sulcus.
C. **Pruritic lesions**
   1. Erythema, excess amounts of smegma, and flat white-gray "empty" or erythematous papules suggest **balanitis;** erosions and fine scaling sometimes associated with marked edema of the prepuce suggest **balanoposthitis. Phimosis** (a contraction of the distal foreskin) may be present, revealing only edema and obstructing the view of the glans. In uncircumcised males, phimosis can be a cause or a complication of balanitis (or both). Paraphimosis can occur if the foreskin has been retracted, constricting the glans or the shaft just proximal to the glans and causing ischemia, which presents as swelling and acute pain. Any papule, plaque, or white discoloration that is not resolved by therapy (see section VI,C,1,c) is a clue to possible malignancy.

2. An erythematous to brownish-red plaque with sharp borders and minimal scaling located on the inner thigh extending into the scrotum or vulva suggests **erythrasma**.

3. Minuscule white-gray nits are seen attached to hair shafts, and brownish-gray lice of similar size (1–2 mm) are seen on the perifollicular skin in *Phthirus pubis* infestation. Papules, lichenification, and excoriations from scratching can be seen.

4. **Vulvar dystrophy/LSA** varies from nonspecific thinned skin, to multiple flat, irregular pearly/ivory white or pink/reddish (less common) papules or macules in multiple sites. They may eventually coalesce into white plaques involving the entire perineum. Hyperplastic dystrophy and leukoplakia are less common and considered premalignant; vulvar carcinoma is uncommon. In **BXO** there is a ring of white sclerotic tissue at the tip of the foreskin (which causes phimosis) or meatus but is not accompanied by inflammatory changes. Kraurosis vulvae (atrophy and shriveling of the skin or mucous membranes) with hypomelanosis, telangiectasias, and a "keyhole" vaginal opening is an old, now abandoned gynecologic term for end-stage atrophy not necessarily due to sclerosis.

D. **Cystic lesions**
   1. A rubbery, soft, renitent bulge in the inner aspect of the lower vaginal vestibule (outside of the introitus) suggests **Bartholin's gland cyst;** if infected, the cyst is red and extremely tender.

V. **Laboratory Tests**
   A. **Ulcerative lesions.** Testing for chlamydia, gonorrhea, and HIV (with adequate counseling) should be considered in persons with primary HSV-1 or -2, syphilis, or chancroid (see sidebar), with retesting in 3–6 months. In addition, testing for syphilis is recommended in those with primary HSV-1 or -2.

CHANCROID

Chancroid is a highly contagious disease that has declined steadily since 1987 to just 38 cases in 2001. It is caused by *Haemophilus ducreyi,* a gram-negative coccobacillary organism. Occasional discrete outbreaks occur, commonly associated with the influx of Central American, Caribbean, and Southeast Asian immigrants. Underreporting is common because of difficulty in diagnosis. As many as 10% of patients with chancroid may be coinfected with *T pallidum* or HSV. The disease may have an important role in the transmission of HIV, primarily among heterosexuals. Chancroid is a tender genital papule that erodes into single or multiple round, oval, or serpiginous painful ulcers with sharp, flat, nonindurated borders. Ulcers can become confluent and large. Regional lymphadenopathy is typical. The diagnosis of **chancroid** is **clinical** and based on excluding other ulcerative processes such as syphilis and herpes. Rapid plasma reagin (RPR) test performed 1 week after identification of the lesion is more reliable than initial RPR in ruling out syphilis. **Gram stain** for coccobacillary clusters is unreliable, and **culture** is difficult and expensive. Commercially available polymerase chain reaction tests can be used but none is approved by the US Food and Drug Administration. Persons with **chancroid** should be treated with azithromycin, 1 g orally in a single dose, *or* ceftriaxone, 250 mg intramuscularly in a single dose, *or* erythromycin base, 500 mg orally four times daily for 7 days, *or* ciprofloxacin, 500 mg orally twice daily for 3 days. Ciprofloxacin should not be given to children or pregnant/lactating patients. There has been intermediate resistance to ciprofloxacin and erythromycin worldwide. Uncircumcised males and HIV patients are more resistant to therapy and may require retreatment or longer courses if the condition is not resolved in 7 days.

---

1. Laboratory studies are rarely necessary in HSV-1 or -2; they are reserved for situations in which the diagnosis is not clear and certainty is imperative, such as a primary infection soon before parturition or when strict confirmation is necessary for medicolegal cases.
   a. In the **Tzanck test,** a vesicle is unroofed and its fluid is smeared on a slide, dried, and stained with Giemsa or Wright's stain. Presence of giant multi-

nucleated acanthocytes is considered a positive test result for **Herpesviridae** (simplex or zoster).
   b. **Viral culture** is expensive and must incubate 7 days before being read. Positive cultures can occur in persons with nonherpetic lesions who shed the herpesvirus regularly.
   c. **Microscopic pathology** and **electron microscopy** can be used, although this is rarely necessary.
2. **Primary syphilis**
   a. **Dark-field microscopic examination** of the lesion's secretions is diagnostic but rarely available to the clinician. It reveals treponemes contracting and kinking, but these may not be seen if the chancre has been treated with topical antibiotics.
   b. **Rapid plasma reagin (RPR) and VDRL tests,** the nontreponemal tests, turn positive 1 week after the appearance of the chancre. These tests become negative up to 1 year after treatment, but may remain positive for life at a low titer in a small percentage of patients.
   c. Confirmatory treponemal tests such as the **fluorescent treponemal antibody-absorption** (FTA-ABS) or *T pallidum* **hemagglutination assay** (TPHA) may take 2 weeks to become positive. Treponemal tests remain weakly positive for life.
B. **Verrucoid/papillomatous lesions.** Testing for chlamydia, gonorrhea, and HIV (with adequate counseling, including safe-sex information) should be considered in persons with condylomata acuminata, condyloma lata, or molluscum contagiosum. In addition, testing for syphilis is recommended in those with condylomata acuminata.
   1. The diagnosis of **condylomata acuminata** is clinical.
      a. Occasionally, a **biopsy** confirms the diagnosis.
      b. Subclinical lesions can be soaked with **5% acetic acid** (white vinegar) for 5 minutes, resulting in white epithelium that can be observed with a colposcope or magnifying glass of 4–10× magnification. White papules may be noted, although other changes such as mosaicism and punctation are possible.
   2. RPR and VDRL tests are always positive when **condyloma lata** are present. FTA confirmation is warranted.
   3. Sticking a needle through a lesion releases the semisolid core of **molluscum contagiosum,** which is considered diagnostic. Microscopic observation, rarely necessary, reveals inclusion "molluscum" bodies or Lipschütz cells.
   4. No laboratory is necessary to diagnose **pearly penile papules.** A biopsy reveals an angiofibroma.
C. **Pruritic lesions**
   1. **Balanitis** is a clinical diagnosis; however, biopsy of any associated glanular mass is needed. Biopsy can be done under local anesthesia using a shallow punch at the office.
   2. Wood's lamp examination shows a classic coral-red fluorescence in **erythrasma.** Scraping of the lesions may show gram-positive rods and do not show hyphae.
   3. Lice and nits can be observed microscopically in *Phthirus pubis* infestation. Testing for chlamydia, gonorrhea, syphilis, and HIV (with adequate counseling) should be considered in those who were infested by direct sexual contact.
   4. Biopsy is necessary in **vulvar dystrophy** to distinguish **LSA/BXO** from leukoplakia, vitiligo, lichen planus, or carcinoma. This can be accomplished in the office under local anesthesia using a punch biopsy of the leading edge or a full excision if the lesion is less than 1 cm in diameter.
D. **Cystic lesions.** Diagnosis of **Bartholin's gland cyst** is clinical. Cultures should be considered only when cellulitis is present.
VI. **Treatment**
A. **Ulcerative lesions**
   1. Maximal viral shedding in HSV-1 or -2 occurs within 24 hours of the appearance of lesions and diminishes by the fifth day; nevertheless, viral shedding occurs intermittently in the absence of any signs in many persons. Herpes is generally self-limited, with recurrences decreasing over the years. Therapy does not eradicate **HSV-1 or -2,** nor does it affect the severity or rate of recurrences after discontinuation. Significant clinical improvement is seen when therapy is started promptly after onset of symptoms.

    a. For primary infection, oral drugs of choice include acyclovir, 400 mg, or famciclovir, 250 mg three times per day, *or* valacyclovir 1 g twice a day for 7—10 days. It is unclear whether higher doses (eg, acyclovir, 400 mg five times per day) are warranted for stomatitis, pharyngitis, or proctitis.

    b. For recurrent infection

       (1) At onset, oral acyclovir, 200 mg five times per day, or 400 mg three times daily, or 800 mg twice daily for 5 days, *or* famciclovir 125 mg or valacyclovir 500 mg twice daily or 1000 mg every day for 5 days, may be prescribed.

       (2) Oral suppressive therapy options include acyclovir, 400 mg, or famciclovir, 250 mg twice daily, *or* valacyclovir, 500 mg or 1 g once a day for 1 year, with consideration of a drug-free period at that point to assess the need for continued therapy.

    c. Counseling regarding potential for recurrence, amelioration of symptoms over the years, transmission through viral shedding in the absence of lesions, and the need for condom use is important.

  2. Primary syphilis is treated with benzathine penicillin G, 2.4 million U intramuscularly in a single dose. Some experts recommend 2 extra doses, a week apart, in patients with HIV. Persons who are allergic to penicillin should receive doxycycline, 100 mg orally twice daily for 2 weeks. If compliance is an issue, penicillin desensitization should be considered. Dosages and effectiveness of azithromycin and ceftriaxone have not been defined.

B. Verrucoid/papillomatous lesions

  1. Condylomata acuminata resolve spontaneously in 6–15 months, except in immunocompromised persons. Most clinicians treat to avoid persistent growth. Treatment removes only the wart and does not eliminate the virus, which could remain for months to years. Recurrences are common during the first year, even after adequate removal. An additional Papanicolaou smear is recommended in women at the time of diagnosis with warts.

    a. Most effective therapies include the following.

       (1) For **cryotherapy** with liquid nitrogen, the cryotherapy probe, spray "gun," or cotton-tipped applicator is applied until blanching occurs no more than 1 mm around the perimeter of the lesions, which fall off in 24–72 hours, leaving a shallow ulcer.

       (2) **Trichloroacetic acid** or **bichloroacetic acid** 80–90% can be applied, only to warts, and turns them white in seconds. Lesions should be powdered with talc or sodium bicarbonate immediately to remove unreacted acid. Treatment can be repeated weekly as necessary.

       (3) **Imiquimod** (Aldara) 5% cream is applied by the patient's finger on each lesion at bedtime and washed off in the morning, three times a week for as long as 16 weeks.

       (4) **Podophyllin,** 10–25%, in compound tincture of benzoin, is applied to warts. The total amount applied per session should be limited to 0.5 mL or less than 10 cm^2 to avoid systemic toxicity; medication should be washed off in 4 hours. Treatment may be repeated weekly and is contraindicated in pregnancy.

       (5) **Podofilox** (Condylox), 0.5% solution, for self-treatment, is applied twice daily for 3 days followed by 4 days of no therapy. Treatment can be repeated up to four cycles and is contraindicated in pregnancy. The health care provider should teach the patient which lesions to treat and how to apply the drug.

       (6) **Electrodesiccation** or **electrocautery** is contraindicated in patients with anal lesions or with a pacemaker.

       (7) **Surgical tangential shave/scissor excision** or **curettage.**

    b. Alternative therapies include the following.

       (1) **Carbon dioxide laser** is necessary only with warts that are very extensive or very resistant to other therapies.

       (2) **Interferon alpha-2b** (Intron-A) can be injected on the base of lesions three times per week for 3 weeks and repeated as needed. This drug is extremely expensive, and its use should be restricted to recalcitrant cases.

  2. Treatment for **secondary syphilis,** which is extremely contagious, is the same as for primary syphilis.

3. Spontaneous remission of **molluscum contagiosum** occurs in weeks to several months. **Cryotherapy, curettage,** or **electrocautery** can be done (see section VI,B,1,a).
4. Reassurance is all that is necessary for **pearly penile papules.**

C. **Pruritic lesions**
1. **Balanitis**
   a. The foreskin should be kept retracted as much as possible.
   b. The glans should be dried thoroughly after showering and micturition.
   c. Candidiasis superinfection should be treated with an **imidazole** cream (ketoconazole, butoconazole, clotrimazole, econazole, miconazole, isoconazole, tioconazole, or terconazole), ciclopirox, or **nystatin** cream, topically twice daily, or fluconazole, 150 mg orally in a single dose. Ketoconazole and itraconazole might be as effective but have a higher potential for toxicity. Terbinafine should not be used as a primary agent for *Candida*.
   d. The glans and prepuce should be washed with soap and water and dried thoroughly after sexual intercourse.
   e. **Circumcision** may be needed if phimosis develops or in resistant cases, since chronic balanitis is a potential precursor of premalignant penile glanular changes.
2. Povidone-iodine soap cleansing can be sufficient for **erythrasma. Econazole** cream twice daily for 7–10 days or **erythromycin base** 250 mg orally four times daily for 14 days is also effective against the causative agent (*Corynebacterium minutissimum*).
3. **Lindane** 1% shampoo applied for 4 minutes or **permethrin** 1% creme rinse or **pyrethrins with piperonyl butoxide** applied for 10 minutes and then thoroughly washed off are effective treatments for **pubic lice.** Lindane should be avoided in children and during gestation and lactation. **Permethrin** has less potential for toxicity than lindane.
4. **Vulvar dystrophy/LSA and BXO**
   a. When biopsy reveals intraepithelial neoplasia, either **laser therapy** or conventional **surgical excision** is indicated.
   b. In **LSA/BXO topical testosterone** is no longer recommended. Highly potent **topical steroids** (eg, clobetasol 0.05%) should be carefully rubbed on the lesion twice daily for 1 month and then once daily for 2–3 weeks) followed by lower-potency steroids (triamcinolone acetonide 0.1% or betamethasone valerate 0.1%) twice daily for a few weeks. Tacrolimus ointment 0.1% and pimecrolimus cream 1% twice daily are also effective (off-label use). Leukoplakia requires close follow-up; 5-fluorouracil topically is often used instead.

D. **Cystic lesions**
1. **Bartholin's gland cysts/inflammation**
   a. Hot, wet dressings or sitz baths may promote spontaneous drainage of cysts.
   b. Incision and drainage are effective in most abscesses.
   c. Marsupialization is recommended for recurrences.
   d. **Antibiotic therapy** is not necessary unless there is associated cellulitis, generally due to staphylococci, streptococci, coliforms, or anaerobes.

REFERENCES

Fitzpatrick TB, et al: *Color Atlas and Synopsis of Clinical Dermatology,* 4th ed. McGraw-Hill; 2001.
Gilbert DN, Moellering RC, Sande MA: *The Sanford Guide to Antimicrobial Therapy,* 33rd ed. Antimicrobial Therapy; 2003.
MMWR 2002 Guidelines for Treatment of Sexually Transmitted Diseases MMWR (May 10) 2002; **51:**RR-6. http://www.cdc.gov/std/treatment/TOC2002TG.htm
National Ambulatory Medical Care Survey (NAMCS): *2001 Summary. Advance Data from Vital and Health Statistics No. 337.* National Center for Health Statistics, Centers for Disease Control and Prevention; (August 11) 2003.
Pickering LK (editor): *Red Book: 2003 Report of the Committee on Infectious Diseases,* 26th ed. American Academy of Pediatrics; 2003.

32   Hair & Nail Disorders

Amy D. Crawford-Faucher, MD, & Frank S. Celestino, MD

KEY POINTS

- Ninety-five percent of alopecia cases presenting to primary care physicians are potentially treatable.
- Hirsutism associated with virilization requires hormonal evaluation.
- Only 50% of dystrophic nails are onychomycotic; accurate diagnosis is key to appropriate therapy.
- Melanoma and metastatic cancers sometimes present as nail disorders.

   I. **Definition.** Hair follicles produce one of two types of human hair: **vellus hair** is fine, hypopigmented, and barely visible; and **terminal hair,** which is coarse and usually pigmented. Follicles cycle through three stages: anagen (hair growth), catagen (transition), and telogen (rest). Hair shafts mature and are shed after the telogen phase. Scalp hair follicles normally stay in anagen for 2–8 years, producing potentially long hairs, then "rest" in telogen for 2–3 months. Follicles cycle at different rates; while only 5–15% of scalp hairs are in telogen phase at any given time, 40–50% of hair follicles on the trunk are in telogen phase. Abnormal hair growth or loss is usually not medically serious, but can indicate systemic disease, and may cause significant emotional distress.

   Alopecia (hair loss) may be localized, patchy, diffuse, or total. It usually occurs when hair follicles are damaged by chemical or physical agents, or by infectious or immunologically mediated inflammation. Slowing or disrupting the normal hair growth cycle can also result in alopecia, as from metabolic diseases, many medications, and physiologic stresses. When hair follicles (and potential for regrowth) are retained, alopecia is **noncicatricial (nonscarring)**. When hair follicles are lost, alopecia is **cicatricial (scarring)**.

   Hirsutism is excess hair growth in a typically male distribution and is due to excess androgen (testosterone and its precursors dehydroepiandrosterone sulfate [DHEA-S] and 17 alpha hydroxyprogesterone [17-OHP]) originating in the ovaries, adrenals, or exogenously from medications. These androgens act on a woman's androgen-sensitive follicles (located primarily on the face, chest, upper back, lower abdomen, and inner thighs) to produce terminal instead of vellus-type hair. Hirsutism may be an isolated condition or occur in conjunction with other virilizing symptoms and signs that indicate androgen excess. **Hypertrichosis** refers to excess hair growth that may be diffuse and is not sensitive to androgens.

   Normal nail anatomy includes a vascular and highly innervated nail bed that underlies the nail, which is composed of dead keratin. The proximal end of the nail bed comprises the matrix, from which new nail grows. The perionychium folds around the nail edge proximally and laterally, producing the nail folds. Abnormal nails result from trauma, infection, systemic disease, or congenital conditions or may be variants of normal. Damage to the matrix can cause permanent nail growth abnormalities. Accurate diagnosis of nail disorders is necessary for effective treatment and for prompt evaluation of potentially serious systemic disease.

  II. **Common Diagnoses**
   A. **Alopecias.** (Table 32–1). Before the era of approved medical therapy for common male pattern baldness, approximately 1 of every 2000 office visits to family physicians was for some form of hair loss; this figure is likely higher today. Nonscarring alopecias account for >95% of the hair loss seen by primary care physicians. The six causes listed below are the most common and important.
      1. **Androgenetic alopecia,** including male and female pattern baldness, is more common than all other causes of alopecia combined. It affects nearly three quarters of men to some degree, and less than one fifth of women. More than half of men show signs of this hair loss by age 50. In genetically susceptible people, androgens gradually transform terminal follicles on the scalp to vellus-like follicles, which eventually atrophy. Androgenetic alopecia is controlled by one dominant,

TABLE 32–1. DIAGNOSES AND ETIOLOGIC CLASSIFICATIONS OF ALOPECIA

Cicatricial (scarring) alopecias
1. **Neoplastic:** localized or metastatic
2. **Nevoid:** nevus sebaceous, epidermal nevus
3. **Physical or chemical:** burns, freezing, trauma, radiation, acids, alkalis
4. **Infectious:** bacterial, fungal, protozoal, viral, mycobacterial
5. **Congenital or developmental:** aplasia cutis, Darier's disease, recessive X-linked ichthyosis, keratosis pilaris atrophicans
6. **Dermatosis-related:** lichen planus, necrobiosis lipoidica diabeticorum, cicatricial pemphigoid, folliculitis decalvans
7. **Systemic disease:** lupus erythematosus, sarcoidosis, scleroderma, dermatomyositis, amyloidosis

Noncicatricial (nonscarring) alopecias
1. **Drug-induced:** antimetabolites, anticoagulants, beta blockers, antidepressants, lithium, levodopa
2. **Congenital:** ectodermal dysplasias, hair shaft disorders
3. **Infectious:** secondary syphilis, tinea capitis, human immunodeficiency virus infection
4. **Toxic:** arsenic, boric acid, thallium, vitamin A
5. **Nutritional:** anorexia nervosa, marasmus, kwashiorkor, "crash" diets, iron or zinc deficiency
6. **Traumatic:** trichotillomania, traction, friction, chemical, thermal
7. **Endocrine:** hyper- or hypothyroidism, hypopituitarism, hyper- or hypoparathyroidism
8. **Immunologic:** alopecia areata
9. **Genetic or developmental:** male and female pattern baldness (androgenetic alopecia)
10. **Radiation-induced:** x-ray epilation
11. **Physiologic:** telogen effluvium (postpartum, postsurgical, febrile illness, severe psychological stress, puberty)

sex-limited, autosomal gene that may be incompletely expressed because of polygenic modifying factors.

2. **Traumatic alopecia** is relatively common on the occiput of infants who sleep on their backs, and in persons with hairstyles (tight braids, curlers) that put continuous traction on the follicle. Recurrent, compulsive hair plucking (trichotillomania) can also lead to traumatic alopecia.

3. **Infectious alopecia,** mainly related to **tinea capitis,** most commonly affects children and young adults. Intense inflammation injures the hair follicles.

4. **Physiologic alopecia,** called **telogen effluvium,** results in diffuse hair loss and most often occurs 2–3 months postpartum, following the cessation of oral contraception or corticosteroids, or after serious illness or stress. This hair loss occurs when an unusually large number of follicles (25–45%) abruptly end anagen and move through catagen and into telogen (rest) phase. Large numbers of telogen hairs then synchronously fall out.

5. **Alopecia areata** occurs in approximately 0.1% of the general population, affecting men and women equally. More than half the cases arise by age 40, and there is a familial tendency. Alopecia areata tends to occur in those with other presumed autoimmune disease, such as pernicious anemia, vitiligo, Hashimoto's thyroiditis, and atopic dermatitis, and in Down syndrome. While most cases eventually resolve spontaneously, cases that present before puberty, are recurrent, or do not respond to treatment carry a poor prognosis for hair regrowth.

6. **Hair loss caused by systemic processes** including thyroid disease, other endocrinopathies, and malnutrition, either slow the rate of hair growth or alter the balance between the anagen and telogen phases in the hair follicles.

B. **Hirsutism** (Table 32–2) affects up to 10% of all women.

1. **Idiopathic hirsutism** is most common in women of Mediterranean ancestry and is thought to represent increased follicle sensitivity to normal levels of circulating androgens. Idiopathic hirsutism is a diagnosis of exclusion.

2. **Polycystic ovarian syndrome (PCOS)** is the most common androgen-excess condition causing hirsutism and affects about 6% of reproductive-age women.

3. Prevalence of **adult-onset congenital adrenal hyperplasia (CAH)** is unclear but clearly varies with ethnic background. The disorder is uncommon in women of Northern European ancestry and occurs with greater frequency in Ashkenazi Jews, Hispanics, and Central Europeans.

4. **Cushing's syndrome** is a rare cause of hirsutism.

TABLE 32-2. CAUSES OF HYPERTRICHOSIS AND HIRSUTISM

Hypertrichosis	Hirsutism
Idiopathic	Polycystic ovarian syndrome (PCOS)
Familial	Congenital adrenal hyperplasia
Puberty	Adrenal or ovarian neoplasm
Pregnancy	Cushing's syndrome
Menopause	
Hypothyroidism	
Acromegaly	
Hurler's syndrome	
Porphyria cutaneous tarda	
Multiple sclerosis	
Encephalitis	

5. **Ovarian or adrenal tumors** are rare causes of hirsutism.
6. **Medications** can cause both hirsutism and hypertrichosis (Table 32–3).

C. **Nail disorders.** The most common nail disorders are listed below.

1. **Onychomycosis,** a fungal infection of the nails, comprises one half of nail diagnoses, affecting up to 20% of adults, and a much smaller percentage of children. Toenails are more commonly involved than fingernails and prolonged or repeated foot dampness and locker room exposure may predispose to infection.
2. **Paronychia,** infection of the proximal or lateral nail folds, is due acutely to local trauma, such as a "hangnail," and chronically to repeated exposure to moisture, as in dishwashers or swimmers.
3. Direct trauma to the nail and fingertip can cause a **subungual hematoma,** blood from ruptured nail bed vessels collecting in the potential space between the nail bed and plate.
4. **Ingrown nails** are also common, occurring most commonly on the medial edge of the great toenail. Ill-fitting shoes, nail dystrophies, and onychomycosis can all predispose to the condition.
5. **Discolored nails** can be due to a wide variety of conditions (Table 32–4).
6. **Systemic diseases** can manifest as nail disorders. Alopecia areata, chronic hypoxia, iron deficiency anemia, zinc deficiency, and hypocalcemia can cause nail abnormalities.

III. **Symptoms.** Evaluation of patients with **alopecia** should include duration and location of hair loss, major life changes, physical trauma, drug intake, and hair care habits. For **hirsutism,** the onset, associated signs and symptoms, medication use, ethnic origin, and affected family members are important.

A. The vast majority of processes leading to alopecia, hirsutism, and hypertrichosis are remarkably symptom-free locally. Trauma or infectious processes such as tinea capitis may cause itching and pain. Women with **hirsutism from androgen excess** commonly

TABLE 32-3. MEDICATIONS CAUSING HYPERTRICHOSIS OR HIRSUTISM

Hypertrichosis	Hirsutism
Minoxidil (forearms and legs in women)	Anabolic steroids
Cyclosporine	Danazol
Corticosteroids	Reglan
Diazoxide	Aldomet
Streptomycin	Progestins
Interferon	Reserpine
Acetazolamide	Phenothiazines
Phenothiazines	Testosterone
Phenytoin	
Psoralens	

TABLE 32–4. CAUSES OF DISCOLORED NAILS

White (Leukonychia)
Fungus
Physical stress/mild trauma (transverse lines or spots that grow out with the nail)
Nail bed injury (transverse lines that do not move with the nail)
Heavy metal poisoning (eg, arsenic) (transverse lines)
Liver disease (all-white nails)
Renal failure and uremia (half white, half pink nails)
Idiopathic (spots and lines)
Congenital

Brown/Black
Lines common in dark-skinned persons
Nevus (confined to nail)
Melanoma (may "run over" onto nail fold)
Fungus
Psoriasis or alopecia areata
Chloroquine (bluish)
Quinacrine (bluish)
Several chemotherapeutic agents
Heavy metal poisoning

Yellow
Fungus
Non-pseudomonal bacteria
Psoriasis (usually not uniform)
Alopecia areata (usually not uniform)
Lymphedema
AIDS
Addison's disease

Green
Pseudomonal infection

Blue
Minocycline
Doxorubicin (brownish)
Wilson's disease
Ochronosis (gray-blue)

Red
Darier's disease (longitudinal streaks)

report rapid onset of postpubertal virilization and irregular menses. Those with **idiopathic hirsutism** report gradual onset of mild hirsutism, normal menses, and no virilizing signs. Women with hirsutism and *PCOS* often give a history of oligomenorrhea and infertility. Many patients experience psychological distress over their hair loss or excess growth.

   B. **Pain** is a common complaint with ingrown nails from any cause, and from acute or chronic paronychia. Onychomycosis and other nail infections may be painless. Significant throbbing pain at the nail is the hallmark of subungual hematoma, occurring within hours to a day of a crush injury to the fingertip and nail.

IV. **Signs.** With **hirsutism,** signs of virilization should be sought; including varying degrees of clitoromegaly, cystic acne, decreased breast size, deepened voice, increased libido, increased muscle mass, malodorous perspiration, oligomenorrhea, and temporal hair recession and balding. With **alopecia** a helpful clinical clue is the presence of follicular orifices, which implies a noncicatricial (potentially reversible) process. The following local signs will rapidly narrow the differential diagnosis in alopecia, hirsutism, and nail abnormalities.

   A. **Androgenetic alopecia**
      1. **Male pattern baldness** is most often characterized by frontotemporal hairline recession with variable hair loss at the scalp vertex.
      2. **Female pattern baldness** shows a predominance of diffuse or vertex hair loss with sparing of the hair along the frontal hairline.

   B. **Traumatic alopecia** usually shows patchy hair loss but may also be diffuse. Localized breakage with variously shortened hairs suggests mechanical damage.

   C. **Infectious alopecia** due to tinea capitis exhibits discrete patches of partial hair loss and breakage overlying scaly, inflamed skin. Less commonly, a **kerion** induced by the dermatophyte *Trichophyton tonsurans* causes a deep, purulent folliculitis. With severe fungal infections or marked cellulitis, inflammation and suppuration can cause destruction and scarring. Secondary syphilis, in contrast, leads to a diffuse, moth-eaten appearance of the scalp.

   D. **Physiologic alopecia** is suggested by acute, diffuse, yet reversible hair thinning. When present, transverse nail depressions (Beau's lines) imply a subacute physiologic injury.

   E. **Alopecia areata** is characterized by abrupt, patchy, but very well-demarcated hair loss. This process leaves discrete areas of smooth, hairless, noninflamed skin that is surrounded by easily plucked hairs. Another helpful (and some say pathognomonic) finding is that of "exclamation point" hairs, which are short, heavily pigmented shafts with wide, brushlike distal ends that taper at the skin surface. There can be complete loss of scalp hair (**alopecia totalis**) or of all body hair (**alopecia universalis**), although this is less common than other types of hair loss. Pitted nails are seen in up to one third of patients.

  F. **Systemic diseases,** such as thyroid disease, exhibit their specific associated signs in addition to diffuse hair loss and thinning.

  G. **PCOS** is associated with obesity.

  H. **Adrenal or ovarian neoplasms** are associated with rapid onset of significant hair growth many years after puberty and with other virilizing signs. (See sidebar for other neoplasms.)

MELANOMA/CARCINOMA AND NAILS

Malignant melanoma can present as a new hyperpigmented longitudinal line on a nail, especially if it "runs over" onto the proximal nail fold or takes over the entire nail.

  Squamous cell carcinoma, melanoma or, rarely, **metastatic cancer** can manifest as a paronychia that does not respond to usual treatments. Biopsy of the nail bed is necessary to diagnose these cancers.

  I. **Onychomycosis**
    1. **Distal onychomycosis** causes nails to become white, yellow, or brownish. The nail thickens and subungual debris collects at the distal tip.
    2. **White superficial onychomycosis** causes soft, rough nails that crumble.
    3. **Proximal onychomycosis** is least common and occurs when *Trichophyton rubrum* invades the proximal nail fold, infects the newly formed nail plate, and moves distally.
  J. **Acute paronychia** presents with significant erythema, tenderness, and fluctuance along the proximal or lateral nail border. **Chronic paronychia** often involves many nails and is less erythematous. Affected nails become tender intermittently, especially after water exposure. The proximal nail folds become edematous but are rarely fluctuant.
  K. **Subungual hematoma** causes an exquisitely tender nail that may appear partially or completely red-blue, purple, or black due to accumulated blood. If significant portions of the bed are affected, the nail may separate partially or completely (onycholysis).
  L. **Ingrown nails** act as a foreign body to cause inflammation and sometimes infection at the site where the corner of the nail grows into the adjacent lateral nail bed. With chronic inflammation, granulation tissue grows over the affected portion of nail. The area is extremely tender to touch and may be fluctuant.
  M. **Systemic diseases** can manifest specific nail abnormalities. **Psoriasis** most commonly causes deep pits in the nails, but also can cause separation (onycholysis), discoloration, and subungual thickening with nail debris accumulation. These findings may be confused with onychomycosis. Usually the nail involvement occurs in conjunction with typical skin symptoms, but it may be the sole sign of the disease. **Alopecia areata** causes shallow pitting with progressive opacification. Clubbing from **chronic hypoxemia** is a chronic and permanent convex nail curvature and swelling of the skin around the proximal nail fold. Occasionally clubbing occurs as a normal variant. Spoon-shaped (concave) nails in adults can occur with **iron deficiency anemia,** transverse depressions (Beau's lines) may indicate **zinc deficiency** or **physiologic stress,** whereas whitish nails may occur in hypocalcemia.
  N. **Nail curvature, hypertrophy, or splitting** may result from repeated nail trauma, such as from constricting shoes, although the etiology is not always clear.
  V. **Laboratory Tests**
    A. Most cases of **alopecia** can be diagnosed by a thorough personal history and a careful physical examination. Ancillary tests may be helpful in certain situations.
      1. The **hair pull or pluck test** involves a moderately firm pull of 10–20 closely grouped hairs. Normally, less than 20% of the shafts will be removed, but in telogen effluvium and active androgenetic alopecia, over 40% of the shafts will be uprooted.
      2. **Wood's light examination, potassium hydroxide (KOH) preparation,** and more rarely, **fungal cultures of hair shafts** aid in diagnosing fungal infection.
      3. A **trichogram** involves the microscopic analysis of at least 50 plucked hairs to determine hair structure and the proportion of telogen follicles. These hairs are removed

from one area using a hemostat. Telogen hairs have small, unpigmented, ovoid bulbs and no internal root sheath. Anagen hairs have larger, elongated, pigmented bulbs shaped like the end of a broom, with a narrow internal root sheath. In telogen effluvium, between 20% and 60% of the patient's hair will be telogen hairs. Anagen hairs that show atrophied bulbs are typical in patients with androgenetic alopecia.

4. A **hair count** is the actual count of all hairs lost over several days. Up to 100 hairs per day is considered normal. Elevated counts are typical of telogen effluvium.

5. **Scalp biopsy** is usually reserved for cases of uncertain origin but may be helpful in determining the prognosis of patients with alopecia areata and lupus erythematosus based on the degree of perifollicular lymphocytic infiltration and antibody deposition, respectively.

6. **Assessment of endocrine dysfunction** may include thyroid tests (eg, thyroid-stimulating hormone). Women with androgenetic hair loss should undergo the same evaluation as hirsute women (see section V,B).

7. **Hematologic, serologic, rheumatologic,** and **blood chemistry tests** should be performed only when systemic disease is suspected, except for balding women, in whom a complete blood cell count, antinuclear antibody test, and ferritin level are routinely indicated.

B. Women with **hirsutism** associated with mild hair growth, normal menses, and no other virilizing signs do not need extensive laboratory evaluation. With more significant symptoms/signs, laboratory tests can help detect serious systemic disease; a sequential approach is best (Figure 32–1).

1. With **irregular menses,** thyroid function, prolactin, 17-OHP, and testosterone should be measured; if these are normal, PCOS and anovulation are likely. For suspected PCOS, blood glucose and lipid screening should be done, and measurement of serum insulin levels considered.

2. With **virilization, testosterone, DHEA-S,** and **17-OHP levels** are used in initial screening for ovarian or adrenal tumors. These hormones can be normal or mildly increased in PCOS; marked elevations suggest ovarian or adrenal tumors, respectively. Virilization also requires imaging (computerized tomography or magnetic resonance imaging) of the adrenal glands or ovaries.

C. Many **nail conditions** can be adequately diagnosed by careful history and physical, including search for other signs of systemic illness. Testing primarily confirms the diagnosis of onychomycosis.

1. **KOH stain and fungal cultures** are necessary to diagnose onychomycosis, because only 50% of dystrophic nails are actually mycotic. Although office-based tests exist, the standard remains KOH stain, culture, or both. Affected nail and nail bed should be sampled, using a #15 blade or sharp curette to obtain debris from different locations on multiple affected nails. Testing for specific species is generally not warranted, as current treatments are effective against most fungi.

2. **Biopsy** is indicated to diagnose tumors, inflammatory disease, and infections when the diagnosis is unclear. The nail bed, perionychium, or matrix can be biopsied. As nail matrix biopsy can cause permanent nail dystrophy, referral to a dermatologist is usually warranted.

VI. **Treatment**

A. The goals of **alopecia** treatment are slowing hair loss and maximizing hair regrowth. No "magic pill" exists, and any gains may be subtle. Treatment may be required indefinitely to prevent further hair loss.

1. **Androgenetic alopecia**

a. **Minoxidil (Rogaine)** solution is a topical agent with unclear mechanism of action that can increase the number of new hairs in thinning scalp. One milliliter is applied to affected areas morning and night.

(1) Minoxidil is not effective on receding temporal baldness, and is most successful in those with hair loss of <5 years, vertex baldness <10 cm, and with the presence of many indeterminate (between vellus and terminal) hairs.

(2) Approximately 40% of men report acceptable hair regrowth after 1 year of treatment.

(3) Minoxidil comes as 2% and 5% solutions. The stronger concentration is recommended for men; the 2% solution is recommended for women. The main side effect in women is hypertrichosis of the face and arms that generally resolves over a year of continued use.

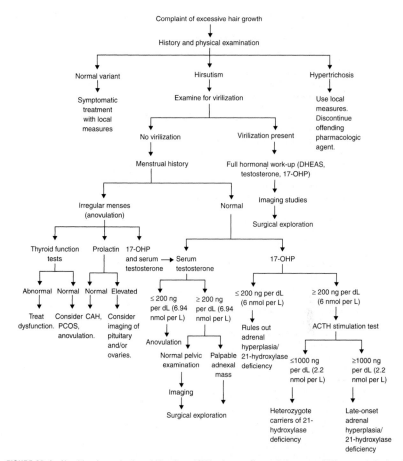

FIGURE 32–1. Algorithm for evaluation of hirsutism. ACTH, adrenocorticotropic hormone; CAH, congenital adrenal hyperplasia; DHEAS, dehydroepiandrosterone sulfate; PCOS, polycystic ovary syndrome; 17-OHP, 17α-hydroxyprogesterone. (Reproduced, with permission, from Hunter MH, Carek PJ: Evaluation and treatment of women with hirsutism. Am Fam Physician 2003;**67**:2565–72.)

   b. Finasteride (Propecia) is the only oral medication approved for baldness. Dosed at 1 mg daily, it inhibits 5 α-reductase in the follicle to reduce the effects of testosterone. Results can be slow; a 12-month trial is usually needed before declaring the drug ineffective. Side effects are uncommon.
   (1) After 3–4 months of treatment, 88% of trial participants reported that their hair loss stabilized, and 60% realized hair regrowth. Recent studies support the safety and efficacy of long-term (ie, 5-year) therapy.
   (2) Propecia is not effective for alopecia in postmenopausal women.
   c. Oral contraceptives do not treat androgenetic baldness in women, but progesterones with low androgen effects (eg, norgestimate, norethindrone, desogestrel, and ethynodiol diacetate) can help prevent worsening of alopecia.
   d. Other medical therapies may improve androgenetic alopecia. Oral spironolactone, 50–200 mg/day, may be helpful as adjunctive treatment in women,

and combination therapy (eg, minoxidil with tretinoin) shows promise in men and women.

   e. **Surgical methods,** including hair transplantation, remain options for men, but results are generally less satisfactory in women whose hair loss is usually more diffuse.

  2. **Traumatic alopecia** is treated by avoidance of the causative action. Trichotillomania can be difficult to treat; a combination of psychological counseling and antidepressant medication may be effective.

  3. Treatment of **tinea capitis** continues to move from griseofulvin to the newer oral antifungals, which seem to be safe, at least as effective, and allow shorter courses of therapy. While not approved by the US Food and Drug Administration (FDA) in children, terbinafine (Lamisil), itraconazole (Sporanox), and fluconazole (Diflucan) are being used in children and adults. The following dosages seem to produce equivalent results after a 3-week course: **terbinafine,** 250 mg daily (125 mg/day if weight 20–40 kg; 62.5 mg/day if <20 kg), **fluconazole,** 6 mg/kg/day, or itraconazole, 5 mg/kg/day. (In children, **itraconazole** can be dosed at 100 mg every other day for weight 10–20 kg, 100 mg alternating with 200 mg daily for weight 30–50 kg, and 200 mg/day for children >50 kg.)

  4. **Telogen effluvium** requires recognition of the inciting event and reassurance that hair growth will normalize.

  5. **Alopecia areata** remains challenging to treat.

    a. **Intralesional steroid injection** is the treatment of choice for less severe cases (<50% of the scalp affected). **Triamcinolone (Kenalog)** 5 mg/mL is used: 0.1 mL is injected intradermally into multiple sites of each patch up to a monthly maximum of 15–20 mg. Applying **minoxidil,** a mid-potency topical steroid, or both in between injections may hasten resolution.

    b. **Strategies for more severe cases** (affecting >50% of the scalp) can be complex and include topical immunotherapy, anthralin, and topical or systemic steroids. Therapy for severe alopecia areata is best managed by practitioners experienced with the disorder.

B. Hirsutism can be controlled either through hair removal processes, suppression of androgens, or a combination of both.

  1. **Hair removal**

    a. **Mechanical hair removal** includes shaving, plucking, and waxing. These techniques are relatively inexpensive, but the results are variably short (2–3 days for shaving, 2 weeks for plucking, up to 8 weeks for waxing), can be painful, and often are unacceptable to women.

    b. Over-the-counter **chemical depilatories** can provide a 2-week hair-free interval. Local skin irritation is common.

    c. **Electrolysis** is performed by specially trained technicians. While considered effective for permanent hair removal, the results are operator- and technique-dependent. Electrolysis is time-consuming, requiring multiple sessions.

    d. **Laser therapy** is becoming more popular for hair removal. Usually performed by dermatologists, lasers are directed at the follicles; the absorbed energy damages and sometimes destroys the follicle. Lasers work best on dark hair, because the pigment best absorbs the heat. Because dark tones absorb more heat, darker skinned or even tanned individuals may not be candidates for laser therapy. Multiple treatments are needed but may produce permanent results.

    e. **Eflornithine HCl (Vaniqa)** is a topical hair growth modulator that can be effective against unwanted facial hair in women. Eflornithine is applied twice daily to the affected areas of the face; results are usually apparent after 4–8 weeks of regular use. Often prescribed by primary care physicians, eflornithine may be used indefinitely, and is most effective when used in conjunction with other modalities of hair removal (such as laser therapy or hormonal treatment).

  2. Several **hormonal therapies** have proved effective in suppressing androgens. These medications are not approved by the FDA for hirsutism, and are labeled pregnancy category D or X; reliable contraception is an important component of therapy.

    a. **Oral contraceptives (OCs) with low-androgen effects** (see section VI,A,1,c) can decrease hair growth by 50–75%. They confer other benefits to patients with PCOS and are frequently used in conjunction with other medications.

b. Spironolactone (see section VI,A,1,d) suppresses testosterone production and inhibits uptake through 5α-reductase in the follicle.

c. Flutamide (Eulexin) is an antiandrogen dosed at 250 mg orally two to three times a day. Monthly liver function testing (for 4 months, then periodic monitoring) is necessary.

d. Finasteride (Proscar) is an antiandrogen; daily dose is 5 mg orally. Results are slow, because effects may be delayed >1 year.

e. Metformin (Glucophage) is an insulin-sensitizing agent that results in decreased amounts of free testosterone and moderate hair reduction in women with PCOS. Dosing regimens include 500–1000 mg orally twice daily, or 850 mg three times daily.

f. Gonadotropin-releasing hormone (GnRH) antagonists are potent therapies usually prescribed by endocrinologists or gynecologists experienced with their use. **Leuprolide (Lupron)** is given as an intramuscular injection dosed at 3.75 mg monthly up to 6 months. It may be used with severe or resistant hirsutism, but its side effect profile demands careful risk-benefit analysis. **Cyproterone** is a progestin that acts as a GnRH blocker. It is not available in the United States but is commonly used in other countries as a combination OC (**Diane**) for maintenance therapy.

g. Dexamethasone (0.5 mg nightly) or prednisone (5–10 mg daily) may be helpful in CAH, but its significant side effect profile may restrict its use by experienced practitioners for resistant or severe hirsutism.

C. Treatment of **nail disorders** is specific to the underlying cause.

1. Oral antifungal therapy is the mainstay of treatment for **onychomycosis,** because local agents cannot penetrate the nail. Terbinafine (Lamisil), itraconazole (Sporanox), and fluconazole (Diflucan) can be used. The treatment regimens are compared in Table 32–5.

2. Subungual hematomas respond best to immediate drainage to relieve pressure. Any heated probe, such as an electrocautery probe or even the tip of a paper clip (heated until red hot), is pressed against the nail over the hematoma to make a small puncture. The blood is expressed with gentle pressure, affording almost immediate pain relief.

3. Ingrown nails with mild inflammation can be treated conservatively with warm soaks, elevating the nail corner with cotton to avoid the inflamed tissue as it grows out, and oral antibiotics if there is a superinfection. Patients should be counseled to trim the nails straight across, which prevents cutting the corners of the nail too short, and to avoid shoes with a narrow toe box. If the ingrown nail does not resolve with these methods, the medial third of the nail should be removed (see Chapter 28).

4. Acute paronychia usually requires incision and drainage of any fluid collections. The most fluctuant area along the nail fold can be drained by incising with a small

TABLE 32–5. ANTIFUNGAL THERAPY FOR ONYCHOMYCOSIS

Continuous Therapy	Dose	Monitoring
Terbinafine (Lamisil)	250 mg/day for 6 weeks (fingernails); 12 weeks (toenails)	CBC, AST, ALT at baseline, then every 4–6 weeks
Itraconazole (Sporanox)	200 mg/day for 6 weeks (fingernails); 12 weeks (toenails)	AST and ALT at baseline, then every 4–6 weeks
Pulse therapy		
Itraconazole (Sporanox)	200 mg twice daily for 7 consecutive days per month; repeat for 2–3 months (fingernails) and 3–4 months (toenails)	None recommended
Fluconazole (Diflucan)	150 mg once weekly for 6–9 months (until nail is improved)	None recommended

CBC, complete blood count; ALT, alanine aminotransferase; AST, aspartate aminotransferase.
From Rogers P, Bassler M: Treating onychomycosis. Am Fam Physician 2001;**63:**663–672, 677–678.

blade (either a #11 or #15 blade), or by gently separating the nail fold from the nail plate to facilitate drainage without cutting the skin. The incision is irrigated and followed up with frequent warm soaks to keep the wound open. Antibiotics are usually not necessary, but clindamycin (Cleocin) or amoxicillin-clavulanate (Augmentin) is appropriate if local drainage and soaks do not resolve the paronychia.

5. **Chronic paronychia** is more difficult to treat, because several nails are affected and incision and drainage is usually not an option. Treatments include avoiding chronic exposure to moisture (or wearing cotton-lined rubber gloves when unable to prevent exposure) and using 1:1 vinegar-water soaks and topical steroids. In addition, areas of inflammation or discharge should be cultured to allow specific treatment. Chronic candidal infection responds to topical or oral antifungal therapy. *Staphylococcus* species and *Pseudomonas* have also been implicated and require oral antibiotics. Treatment failures should prompt a search for underlying systemic disease, such as psoriasis.

6. **Nail changes of underlying systemic disorders,** such as psoriasis and alopecia areata, may improve with treatment of the disease, but nail-specific treatment has not been overly successful. Clubbing is usually a permanent change.

REFERENCES

Behrman RE, et al: Cutaneous fungal infections. In: *Nelson Textbook of Pediatrics,* 17th ed. Saunders; 2004:2230.

Gupta AK, et al: Treatment of tinea capitis caused by *Trichophyton* species: Griseofulvin versus the new oral antifungal agents, terbinafine, itraconazole, and fluconazole. Pediatr Dermatol 2001;**18**(5):433.

Habif TP: Hair diseases. In: Habif TP (editor): *Clinical Dermatology,* 3rd ed. Mosby; 1996:739.

Habif TP: Nail diseases. In: Habif TP (editor): *Clinical Dermatology,* 3rd ed. Mosby; 1996:758.

Hunter MH, Carek PJ: Evaluation and treatment of women with hirsutism. Am Fam Physician 2003; **67**:2565.

Rogers P, Bassler M: Treating onychomycosis. Am Fam Physician 2001;**63**:663–72,677–8.

Sinclair R: Male pattern androgenetic alopecia. Br Med J 1998;**317**:865.

Thiedke CC: Alopecia in women. Am Fam Physician 2003;**67**:1007.

---

33   Hand & Wrist Complaints

Nicole G. Stern, MD

KEY POINTS

- Overuse injuries are common.
- Fractures and tendon injuries should not be missed.
- A normal neurovascular examination should always be documented.
- The contralateral side should be examined for comparison.

I. **Definition.** The hand and wrist consist of 28 bones, numerous articulations, and 19 intrinsic and 20 extrinsic muscles. The surface anatomy can be separated into dorsal, volar (palmar), radial, and ulnar sides. The palm is divided into thenar, midpalm, and hypothenar areas; the **thenar eminence,** containing the small thumb muscles, represents the area just proximal to the thumb, and the opposite side of the palm is the **hypothenar eminence.** Overall, the unique anatomy of the hand and wrist, with closely situated and interrelated structures, allows for extensive variability of movement necessary in functional and recreational activities. Whether occurring acutely or chronically, injuries to the hand or wrist can be debilitating. **Common complaints involving the hand and wrist** include pain, numbness, tingling, instability, weakness, skin discoloration, coldness, swelling, and bony deformity. These are most often due to overuse, trauma, nerve compression, and underlying systemic diseases such as diabetes mellitus, hypothyroidism, and rheumatoid arthritis. This chapter provides an approach to the differential diagnosis and management of common hand and wrist disorders.

II. **Common Diagnoses.** Hand and wrist injuries are particularly common in certain occupations, hobbies, and sports. Incidence is difficult to assess; however, a study from the University of Rochester Sports Medicine Center reported a 5% incidence of hand injuries in 3431 cases of sports medicine consultations. Knowing which special tests to perform in the clinical setting can assist the examiner in adequately diagnosing the condition of an injured patient. By understanding the functional anatomy of the hand and wrist (Figure 33–1), a careful diagnosis and specific treatment plan can be achieved by the primary care provider.

A. **Tendon injuries,** including tendon ruptures or tendinitis, are common especially in sports and in industrial workers.

1. **Boutonnière deformity** (Figure 33–2) can be seen in athletes, especially those involved in contact or ball sports.

2. **Mallet deformity** (Figure 33–3) occurs in athletes, especially those who hit or catch a ball, and results from an axial blow to the terminal phalanx causing forced flexion of the distal interphalangeal joint (DIP), often rupturing the terminal extensor tendon and causing distal phalangeal avulsion fracture.

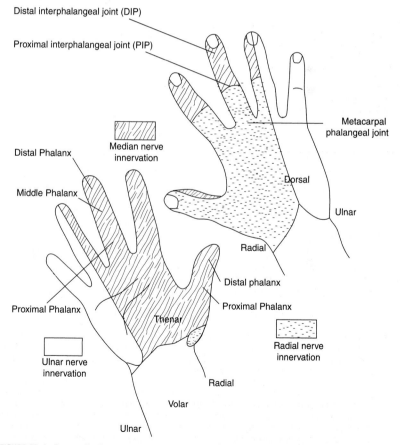

FIGURE 33–1. Sensory distribution of the hand. (Reprinted with permission from Snider RK (editor): *Essentials of Musculoskeletal Care.* American Academy of Orthopaedic Surgeons; 1997:256.)

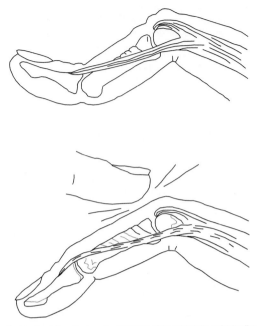

FIGURE 33–2. Boutonnière deformity caused by disruption of the central slip and volar displacement of the lateral bands. The point tenderness test elicits tenderness over the base of the middle phalanx.

   3. **Jersey finger** occurs when an athlete attempts to tackle an opponent who is pulling away. In one study, 75% of cases of jersey finger in football and rugby players involved the ring finger.
   4. **Trigger finger** (Figure 33–4) (stenosing tenosynovitis) usually occurs from continuous direct pressure over the distal palm or metacarpophalangeal (MCP) flexion crease in athletes holding a racquet, golf club, or bat.
   5. **de Quervain's tenosynovitis** occurs in athletes and industrial workers who engage in repetitive wrist motion, which includes radial and ulnar deviation as well as flexion and extension. Sports and activities most commonly associated with de Quervain's include racquet sports, golf, and fishing.
B. **Sprains and contusions** represent the most common injuries seen in sporting events (especially basketball, football, and skiing) and likely comprise a majority (incidence unknown) of the hand, finger, and wrist injuries that account for 3–9% of all sports-related injuries reported in the literature.
   1. **Swan-neck deformity** (Figure 33–5) occasionally occurs in athletes playing either contact or noncontact sports. Chronically, swan-neck deformities can also occur in patients with inflammatory arthritis, such as rheumatoid arthritis or gout.
   2. **Ulnar collateral ligament injury of the thumb metacarpophalangeal (MCP) joint** commonly occurs in football players, skiers, and wrestlers when athletes attempt to break their fall with their hand.
   3. **Triangular fibrocartilage complex (TFCC) tears,** often seen in sports such as baseball and gymnastics, result when the athlete suddenly, or repetitively, loads all their weight on their wrist with or without simultaneous, excessive torque.
C. **Bennett's** and **scaphoid fractures** are among the most commonly seen in a primary care provider's office. In addition, scapholunate dissociation should not be missed.
   1. **Bennett's fracture** occurs most often in football players and athletes requiring a strong pinch-grip mechanism in their sport, such as in racquet sports, hockey, or bull-riding.

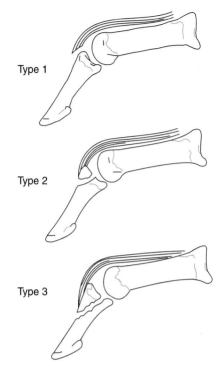

Type 1

Type 2

Type 3

FIGURE 33–3. The three types of mallet finger.

    2. Scaphoid fractures may represent two thirds of all carpal fractures. They are usually due to a fall onto an outstretched hand with the wrist in hyperextension.

    3. Scapholunate dissociation (Figures 33–6 and 33–7) also occurs commonly in those sustaining a fall onto an outstretched hand.

D. Among **ganglia injuries,** dorsal and volar wrist ganglion cysts are the most common soft tissue masses of the hand and wrist. The incidence is unknown, but there may be a predilection in those with carpal tunnel syndrome, previous wrist impaction injury, or in athletes such as gymnasts.

E. Arthritis. The hands, notably the base of the thumb, are susceptible to osteoarthritis; carpometacarpal (CMC) arthritis is very common in women, especially those doing repetitive activities (eg, professional seamstresses). CMC arthritis also occurs idiopathically in women and following trauma in men.

F. Entrapment neuropathies are commonly seen in the workplace or other situations requiring repetitive hand movement.

    1. Carpal tunnel syndrome is considered the most common entrapment neuropathy and is seen in occupations requiring continuous typing and in athletes, but it may also occur spontaneously in pregnant women or in diabetic, hypothyroid, or acromegalic patients. About 50% of patients have bilateral carpal tunnel syndrome.

    2. Ulnar neuropathy, also called Guyon's canal syndrome, can be seen in cyclists and racquet sport athletes where repetitive power gripping is required. Injury to the ulnar nerve occurs when there is continuous pressure on the nerve, causing inflammation, and from traumatic fractures of the hamate or pisiform.

    3. Radial nerve compression, also known as "handcuff neuropathy," is commonly seen in tennis and other racquet sports in which the athlete performs repetitive ulnar flexion, pronation, and supination.

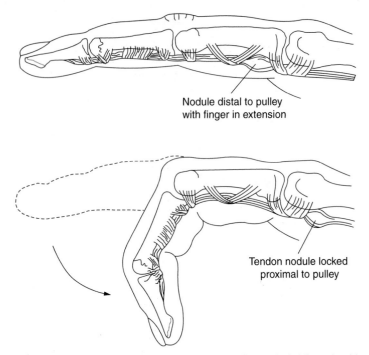

Nodule distal to pulley
with finger in extension

Tendon nodule locked
proximal to pulley

FIGURE 33–4. Trigger finger results from nodular constriction of the flexor tendon by inflammation of the fibrous sheath at the metacarpophalangeal joint. (Reprinted with permission from Snider RK [editor]: *Essentials of Musculoskeletal Care.* American Academy of Orthopedics; 1997:249.)

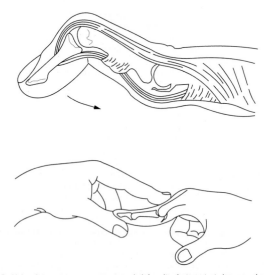

FIGURE 33–5. Volar plate rupture causes swan-neck deformity. A stress test shows an abnormal increase in extension.

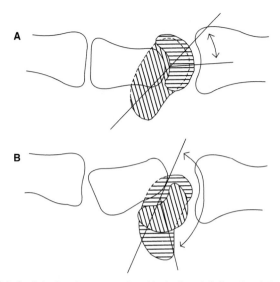

FIGURE 33–6. Scapholunate angle measurements on lateral radiograph. **A:** Normal scapholunate angle is 30–60 degrees. **B:** Vertical scaphoid and lunate subluxated palmarward in an abnormal scapholunate angle measured greater than 65 degrees.

III. **Symptoms** (Table 33–1). An accurate history, including occupation, activities, and mechanism of injury for acute injuries, is critical in diagnosing hand and wrist complaints. In addition, localizing symptoms to specific areas, such as dorsal, volar, radial, or ulnar, can assist in narrowing the differential diagnosis.

IV. **Signs** (Table 33–1). Examination of individuals with hand and wrist complaints is facilitated by knowledge of relevant anatomy and a systematic approach, beginning with inspection (deformity, skin color changes, and edema), followed by palpation (tenderness), range of motion (active, passive, instability check), neurovascular examination (Figures 33–1 to 33–7), and specific provocative testing.

   A. **Special tests**
      1. **Finkelstein's test.** This test is used to diagnose de Quervain's tenosynovitis, which is inflammation of the extensor pollicis longus, extensor pollicis brevis, and

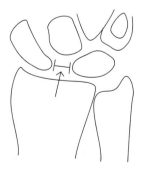

FIGURE 33–7. Distance between the scaphoid and lunate is greater than 3 mm, sometimes called the "Terry Thomas" or "David Letterman" sign.

TABLE 33-1. DIFFERENTIAL DIAGNOSIS AND MANAGEMENT OF COMMON HAND AND WRIST COMPLAINTS

Diagnosis	Symptoms	Signs	Testing	Treatment
Boutonnière deformity	Pain after sudden forced flexion of PIP	Swelling Flexion of PIP and hyperextension of DIP (Figure 33–2) Tenderness with pressure directly over base of middle phalanx	X-ray anteroposterior and lateral, rule out avulsion fracture	Splint PIP full extension/Leave DIP free Immobilize 6–8 weeks and athletes for 4–6 weeks more Surgery if fracture
Mallet deformity	Pain after forceful axial blow causing forced flexion of the DIP	Tenderness on DIP Cannot actively extend distal phalanx (Figure 33–3)	X-ray to rule out fracture	Splint DIP in extension for 6–8 weeks, nighttime splint for 3–4 weeks, then wean depending on severity of injury
Jersey finger (flexor digitorum profundus tendon rupture or avulsion)	Pain on flexor side from forced extension of the DIP during maximum contracture	Patient cannot flex at DIP PIP swelling or palm tenderness from FDP retraction in these areas	X-ray to rule out fracture	Early surgical repair of tendon insertion Conservative therapy if chronic injury
Trigger finger (digital flexor tenosynovitis)	Nodule on distal palm, "catching" or "triggering" of finger	Nodular thickening of flexor tendon within distal palm resulting in loss of smooth extension or flexion of the finger (Figure 33–4)	X-ray not necessary unless concern for tumor	Corticosteroid injection into sheath (Table 33–2) Surgical decompression of the A-1 pulley
de Quervain's tenosynovitis	Pain, swelling near or over radial styloid	Tenderness, swelling over radial styloid (inflammation in first dorsal extensor compartment); positive Finkelstein's test (see section IV,A,1)	X-ray to rule out bony pathology	Thumb/wrist immobilization in thumb spica splint NSAIDs Steroid injection (Table 33–2) and/or surgical decompression if conservative therapy fails

	Signs and Symptoms	Physical Examination	Diagnosis	Treatment
SPRAINS				
Swan-neck deformity	Pain at PIP, deformity often chronic and seen in RA	Tender at PIP, deformity with hyperextension at PIP, and flexion at DIP (Figure 33–5)	X-ray shows deformity	Open repair of volar plate if acute, and if deformity causes disability in chronic cases
Ulnar collateral ligament (UCL) sprain of thumb MCP (gamekeeper's or skier's thumb)	Pain at MCP of thumb from abduction force across the joint	Tender at MCP of thumb and a positive gamekeeper's test (see section IV.A.2)	X-ray to rule out avulsion fracture MRI if plain films negative	Grade I/II immobilize in thumb spica cast 2–4 weeks, then thumb spica splint 2–4 weeks or more Grade III often treated surgically
Triangular fibrocartilage complex (TFCC) tears	Dorsal ulnar-sided pain during ulnar deviation with pronation and supination	Pain with forced passive pronation and supination of the wrist; dorsal subluxation of the ulna often with a painful "clunk"	X-ray to rule out radioulnar arthritis or other bony pathology; magnetic resonance arthrogram	Neutral splint NSAIDs, rest; surgical referral for refractory symptoms
FRACTURES				
Bennett's fracture	Pain after blow to distal thumb while flexed, swelling base of thumb	Base of thumb metacarpal displaced up and back, while tip of thumb is held into the palm	X-ray to demonstrate oblique fracture of base of thumb metacarpal and dislocation (if present)	Nondisplaced thumb spica (TS) cast 3–4 weeks, then splint; dislocation/displaced fracture requires surgery
Scaphoid fracture	Radial-sided pain after fall onto outstretched hand	Tender in anatomic snuffbox or volar side of radiocarpal area	X-ray: need longitudinal view of scaphoid. Bone scan/MRI often needed for definitive diagnosis	*Nondisplaced fracture:* Short arm TS cast or splint 4–6 weeks *Middle/proximal fractures:* Long arm TS cast 6 weeks, then short arm TS cast 4–14 weeks until x-ray union *Displaced fractures:* Long arm TS cast or splint, refer to hand surgeon
Scapholunate dissociation	Dorsal radial wrist pain, decreased grip strength, and "clicking"	Tender in anatomic snuffbox or dorsal wrist at the scapholunate joint	X-ray (AP and lateral): scapholunate angle >60 degrees (Figure 33–6) or scapholunate space >3 mm ("Terry Thomas or David Letterman" sign) (Figure 33–7)	Immobilize and refer to hand surgeon

(continued)

TABLE 33–1. *(Continued)*

	Diagnosis	Symptoms	Signs	Testing	Treatment
GAN-GLIA	Ganglion cysts	Often originate on tendon sheath; pain or "bump"	Tender or nontender mobile soft tissue mass over radial or dorsal wrist or over flexor/extensor tendon sheath	X-ray to rule out bony pathology; arteriogram as needed to rule out radial artery aneurysm or traumatic pseudo-aneurysm	Observation if asymptomatic; neutral wrist splint, aspiration, injection (Table 33–2) or excision
ARTH-RITIS	Carpometacarpal (CMC) of thumb arthritis	Pain at base of thumb with pinching and gripping activities; pain can radiate up arm with "clicking" or "catching" sensation in thumb	Tender over volar or radial sides of CMC joint; positive grind test (see section IV,A,3)	X-ray shows loss of joint space, subchondral sclerosis, bone spurs, subluxation or dislocation at the CMC joint	Immobilize in TS splint 3–6 weeks; injection (Table 33–2); referral to hand surgeon if failed conservative treatment
N E U R O P A T H I E S	Carpal tunnel syndrome	Numbness, tingling, pain in palmar wrist and hand; worse in morning, after repetitive use, and cold sensitivity, color changes	Swelling, weakness, sensation loss in nerve distribution (Figure 33–1); positive Tinel's test; negative Spurling's test (see section IV,A,7)	X-ray to rule out bony pathology; nerve conduction studies (NCVs) show delayed terminal sensory latency; c-spine x-ray if indicated to rule out cervical neuroforaminal encroachment	Ergonomic correction, night neutral wrist splints, NSAIDs; injection (Table 33–2) and/or surgery for carpal tunnel release if conservative treatment fails
	Ulnar neuropathy	Numbness and tingling in 4th and 5th digits, pain and weakness (Figure 33–1)	Swelling, weakness, sensation loss; positive ulnar Tinel's test (see section IV,A,4)	X-ray to rule out bony pathology (eg, hamate fracture); NCVs and Allen's test (see section IV,A,6)	Immobilize, cryotherapy, NSAIDs; surgical decompression for refractory cases
	Radial nerve compression	Pain/numbness/tingling over dorso-radial aspect of wrist and thumb (Figure 33–1)	Swelling, weakness, sensation loss; positive radial Tinel's test	X-ray to rule out bony pathology; NCVs, two-point discrimination test (see section IV,A,8)	Immobilize, NSAIDs, molded or-thoses; surgical decompression and nerve transfer for refractory cases

DIP, distal interphalangeal joint; FDP, flexor digitorum profundus; MCP, metacarpalphalangeal joint; MRI, magnetic resonance imaging study; NSAIDs, nonsteroidal anti-inflammatory drugs; PIP, tendon proximal interphalangeal joint; RA, rheumatoid arthritis.

abductor pollicis longus. It is considered positive if the test reproduces a patient's pain when the patient fully flexes the thumb into the palm, followed by passive ulnar deviation of the wrist by the examiner.

2. **Gamekeeper's test.** This test is used to diagnose ulnar collateral ligament (UCL) injury at the thumb MCP joint. With one hand, the examiner holds the patient's thumb metacarpal, and the other hand holds the patient's thumb proximal phalanx. A gentle radial deviation is applied to the thumb tip MCP joint to stress the UCL. A UCL sprain will show laxity, while a complete rupture (called a **Stener lesion**) can be diagnosed on clinical examination by not feeling an end point during stress testing in either full extension or 30 degrees of MCP flexion. A Stenar lesion should not be missed and involves the interposition of the adductor aponeurosis between the torn UCL and its insertion site, preventing ligament healing.

3. **Grind test.** This test is helpful in diagnosing thumb CMC arthritis. The examiner holds the patient's wrist with one hand and the other hand holds the patient's thumb metacarpal. The examiner then provides an axial load to the thumb and gently rotates it side-to-side. A positive test reproduces pain and crepitus and sometimes shows instability.

4. **Tinel's test.** This test is provocative for carpal tunnel syndrome and is positive if it reproduces the patient's paresthesias (in a median nerve distribution) when the examiner percusses over and just distal to the distal palmar crease midline on the volar wrist. Percussing the distal crease over the radial or ulnar nerve may also assist in diagnosing ulnar or radial neuropathy.

5. **Phalen's test.** This is another test for carpal tunnel syndrome that is positive if paresthesias occur within 1–2 minutes of holding the wrists in maximum flexion.

6. **Allen's test.** This test is useful to rule out vascular disorders such as hypothenar hammer syndrome (ulnar artery injury) or Raynaud's disease (seen in collagen vascular diseases). The patient rests a hand on the knee or a table while the examiner compresses the radial artery with one thumb and the ulnar artery with the other thumb. Next, the patient clenches and opens the fist three times. Then the patient opens the palm and the radial artery is released to see how fast color returns to the palm. The test is then repeated, this time releasing the ulnar artery.

7. **Spurling's test** creates neural foraminal narrowing that may or may not reproduce radicular arm pain, numbness, or tingling. With the patient sitting upright on the examination table, the examiner provides gentle axial loading on top of the head while passively extending the neck, then tilting the head to the side. A positive test may represent cervical disk herniation or cervical spondylosis (osteoarthritis).

8. **Two-point discrimination.** Use two sterile pins to simultaneously prick the skin on the hand in the area of numbness. The pins are separated at different distances in order to determine when the patient perceives the pins as two points versus one. Fingertip two-point discrimination is normally 2–8 mm.

V. **Laboratory Tests** (Table 33–1). When diagnosing hand and wrist complaints, initial evaluation often includes obtaining a plain radiograph following physical examination. In tendon injuries, it is essential to rule out an avulsion fracture while reviewing a plain x-ray.

VI. **Treatment** (Table 33–1).

A. The cornerstone of treatment of most hand and wrist injuries often involves one or more of the following: **nonsteroidal anti-inflammatory drugs (NSAIDS)** (eg, oral ibuprofen, 600–800 mg with food three times daily, or naproxen, 500 mg with food twice daily), for 2 weeks or longer depending on the condition, with precautions for **renal and gastrointestinal toxicity, immobilization, injection** (Table 33–2), or **surgery.**

B. Due to the risk of avascular necrosis, patients with **suspected scaphoid fractures** should be aggressively treated. Patients with a negative x-ray result and scaphoid pain should be placed in a cast until a follow-up x-ray result is obtained in 2–3 weeks or should have further evaluation with bone scan or magnetic resonance imaging.

C. Treatment of **carpal tunnel syndrome** should be conservative if symptoms are mild and of short duration. Patients should first be educated about ergonomic corrections at work or home to prevent further injury. Nighttime neutral wrist splints are usually used to decrease nighttime and morning symptoms. Sometimes NSAIDS help relieve pain, but often patients require local corticosteroid injection if they fail conservative treatment. In refractory cases, carpal tunnel release, either arthroscopic or open, is required.

TABLE 33–2. HAND AND WRIST INJECTIONS

Diagnosis	Equipment	Anesthetic	Corticosteroid	Injection Technique
Carpal tunnel syndrome	25–30 gauge, 1.5-inch needle with a 5-mL syringe	2–3 mL 1% lidocaine or 0.25–0.5% bupivacaine	1 mL betamethasone (Celestone) or 40 mg per mL methylprednisolone	Insert needle at 30-degree angle on volar wrist at proximal wrist crease just ulnar to the palmaris longus tendon aiming at the fourth digit
1st CMC arthritis	25–30 gauge, 1-inch needle with a 3-mL syringe	0.5 mL 1% lidocaine or 0.25–0.5% bupivacaine	0.25–0.5 mL Celestone or methyl-prednisolone	Insert needle on ulnar side of extensor pollicis brevis just proximal to first metacarpal on extensor surface
de Quervain's teno-synovitis	25–27 gauge, 1.5-inch needle with a 5-mL syringe	2 mL 1% lidocaine or 0.25–0.5% bupivacaine	1 mL Celestone or methylprednisolone	Insert needle into first extensor compartment, direct proximally toward radial styloid (not into tendon)
Ganglion cysts	18 gauge, 1- to 1.5-inch needle with a 20- to 30-mL syringe	1–2 mL 1% lidocaine or 0.25–0.5% bupivacaine	1 mL Celestone or methylprednisolone	Insert needle into cyst, aspirate. Use hemostat to stabilize needle, change syringe, then inject
Trigger finger	25–30 gauge, 1- to 1.5-inch needle with a 3-mL syringe	0.5–1 mL 1% lidocaine or 0.25–0.5% bupivacaine	0.5 mL Celestone or methylprednisolone	Insert needle at 30-degree angle over palmar aspect distal to the metacarpal head, then direct needle proximally, almost parallel to the skin, toward the nodule

CMC, carpometacarpal joint.

REFERENCES

Eiff MP, Hatch RL, Calmbach WL: *Fracture Management for Primary Care*. Elsevier Science; 2003.

Nguyen DT, McCue III FC, Urch SE: Evaluation of the injured wrist on the field and in the office. Clin Sports Med 1998;**17**:421.

Nicholas JA, Hershman EB: *The Upper Extremity in Sports Medicine*. Mosby; 1990.

Rettig AC: Tests and treatments of hand, wrist, and elbow overuse syndromes: 20 Clinical pearls. J Musculoskel Med 2003;**20**:136.

Rettig AC: Wrist and hand overuse syndrome. Clin Sports Med 2001;**20**(3):591.

Snider RK (editor): *Essentials of Musculoskeletal Care*. American Academy of Orthopaedic Surgeons; 1997.

Tallia AF, Cardone DA: Diagnostic and therapeutic injection of the wrist and hand region. Am Fam Physician 2003;**67**:745.

---

34 Headaches

Stephen W. Cobb, MD

KEY POINTS

- Most headaches are benign and treatable in the primary care office setting.
- Careful attention to a focused set of symptoms and signs will alert the clinician to more serious causes of headache.
- Neuroimaging is not usually necessary in the evaluation of headache when the history clearly suggests a primary headache disorder and a careful neurologic examination is normal.

I. **Definition.** Headache, or **cephalgia,** is pain or discomfort perceived in the head, neck, or both. **Primary headache disorders** are recurrent benign headaches whose causes are multifactorial; trigeminal serotonin receptors are felt to play a significant role in the inflammation and vasodilation contributing to pain in migraine headaches. **Secondary headaches** result from an underlying pathology caused by a distinct condition (eg, aneurysm, infection, inflammation, or neoplasm).

II. **Common Diagnoses.** Most people will experience an episodic headache during their lifetime. The annual prevalence may be as high as 90%, with a minority of those sufferers pursuing medical evaluation. Still, headache is the second most common pain syndrome in primary care ambulatory practice. There are many headache classification systems. Using the International Headache Society system, **the most common primary headaches in primary care are episodic migraine, tension-type headache, cluster, and medicine-associated headache.** Secondary headaches comprise fewer than 10% of headaches in primary care, but include some important treatable and life-threatening entities.

A. **Episodic migraine.** Migraine affects 18.2% of US women and 6.5% of men each year. Prevalence in the United States was reported for 1999 to be 27.9 million sufferers. The onset of symptoms is usually between adolescence and young adulthood. The peak prevalence is between 30–39 years of age, where it affects about one in four women and 1 in 10 men. A strong correlation with family history of migraine has been observed in migraineurs. It is estimated that only 51% of women and 41% of men who experience migraine have actually been diagnosed. Over 60% of migraineurs are treated only by their primary care physicians for headache.

B. **Tension-type headache (TTH),** also called muscle contraction headache. Onset varies widely, and can be at any age. Fewer than half of these patients have a positive family history of headache; there is a positive association between chronic TTH and mood disorders. Once felt to be the most common headache diagnosed in the primary care office, a refined definition of migraine has identified migraines that were previously considered tension type. "Mixed headache," another common syndrome consisting of migraine and TTH in the same headache, may actually be a migraine variant or two distinct headache types.

C. **Cluster.** Although not common in the primary care office, cluster headaches are recognized as one of the more common primary headache disorders in the general population (lifetime prevalence about 0.1%). Males are affected more commonly than females, with onset between ages 30 and 50 years. There is a positive association with smoking.
D. **Medication-associated headache.** There are very little data on the incidence of medication-associated headaches in primary care. Anecdotally, medicines commonly contribute to headache syndromes, particularly in the setting of long-standing **chronic daily headache** and chronic analgesic use. All currently available abortive medications have been associated with overuse or rebound headache. Drugs most commonly associated with rebound headache include acetaminophen, ergot alkaloids, opioids, butalbital, nonsteroidal anti-inflammatory drugs, and Midrin.
E. **Secondary headaches.** Fewer than 0.4% of headaches in primary care are from serious intracranial disease. Headaches seen with regularity in primary care include those associated with neoplasm, infections (eg, meningitis, purulent sinusitis, abscess), temporal arteritis, acute glaucoma, and cerebral aneurysm.
III. **Symptoms.** Differentiation among types of headaches is usually based on the patient's history. Emphasis should be placed on the history of onset, quality and intensity of pain, frequency, provoking influences, and associated symptoms. Patients frequently experience more than one headache type; to avoid misdiagnosis, it is important to define each type carefully. A headache diary can help with ongoing evaluation of episodic headaches.
A. **Migraine.** Episodic migraine is classified as migraine with aura (classic) or without (common) (see sidebar). Associated symptoms may include a prodrome (vague symptoms such as smells or emotions), an aura (visual or hemisensory symptoms), or even focal neurologic deficits (complicated migraine). The aura is usually stereotypical, with visual scotomata being the most common. Ninety percent of migraineurs do not exhibit aura or prodrome. Nausea and vomiting may be prominent symptoms.

DIAGNOSTIC CRITERIA: EPISODIC MIGRAINE WITHOUT AURA

At least five attacks that include:
• Headache lasting 4–72 hours
• At least two of the following:
  – Unilateral location
  – Pulsating quality (throbbing)
  – Moderate to severe intensity (inhibits or prohibits daily activity)
  – Aggravated by climbing stairs or similar activity
• At least one of the following:
  – Nausea, vomiting, or both
  – Photophobia, phonophobia, or both

B. **TTH** (see sidebar) originates with pain in the occipital or vertex regions of the skull, evolving into a "band-like" distribution. Though primarily bilateral, unilateral tension headaches also occur. The pain is usually not throbbing, but dull. Nausea is an occasional associated symptom. The duration may be hours to days.

DIAGNOSTIC CRITERIA: EPISODIC TTH

A. At least 10 previous headache episodes fulfilling B–D below. Fewer than 180 headache days/month. (If >180 days, and B–D are present, then it is chronic TTH)
B. Headache lasting 30 minutes to 7 days
C. At least two of the following pain characteristics:
   1. No-pulsating quality: pressing or tightening
   2. Mild or moderate intensity. Not activity prohibiting
   3. Bilateral location
   4. No aggravation by routine physical activity
D. Both of the following
   1. No nausea or vomiting
   2. Either photophobia or phonophobia is absent

C. **Cluster headache.** These headaches peak very quickly after onset and are "clustered" temporally over weeks to months. Pain-free intervals are variable in length. The pain is sharp, excruciating in intensity, lasting 15–180 minutes. The location is usually unilateral and in the orbital, supraorbital, or temporal region. Parasympathetic overactivity (lacrimation and ipsilateral rhinorrhea) is common.

D. **Medication-associated headache** (see sidebar). Since headaches may be caused by medications or medication withdrawal, taking a careful headache and medication history may reveal an association.

DIAGNOSTIC CRITERIA: MEDICATION-ASSOCIATED HEADACHE

1. Headache >15 days each month
2. Onset after the intake of ergotamines or general analgesics used more than 15 times each month for more than 3 months
3. Disappears after withdrawal therapy

E. **Secondary headaches.** Symptoms of a "worrisome" headache that should elicit a search for an underlying cause include the following. (See sidebar on "SNOOP" mnemonic for worrisome headache.)

1. **Headache, new in onset, that is constant, prevents sleep, or progressively worsens over several weeks** (indicative of possible intracranial mass lesion or infection). The new headache occurring later in life is less likely to be migraine or tension.

2. **Headache that is abrupt, explosive, and extremely severe** (eg, "the worst headache of my life"), suggestive of intracranial hemorrhage.

3. **Headache beginning with exertion** (consider leaking aneurysm, increased intracranial pressure, or arterial dissection). Exertional headache also may be a primary headache type.

4. **Headache in a drowsy or confused patient** (consider sepsis, trauma, etc).

5. **New headache in the elderly** (consider temporal arteritis, glaucoma, cerebrovascular accident, etc).

6. **Unremitting moderate or severe headache in obese females** (consider pseudotumor cerebri).

"SNOOP" MNEMONIC FOR WORRISOME HEADACHE

S—Systemic symptoms or signs (fever, weight loss). Systemic disease (cancer, autoimmune).
N—Neurologic symptoms or signs.
O—Onset sudden.
O—Onset late in life.
P—Pattern change.

IV. **Signs.** A complete physical examination including careful neurologic, otologic, ophthalmologic, and head and neck evaluation is essential. Vital signs may reveal fever or hypertension. Although there are a few physical examination findings that are common in primary headaches, the examination is most often normal.

A. **Migraine.** There may only be evidence of pain behavior (eg, avoidance of bright light and sound), or there may be focal neurologic deficits, such as hemiparesis or a visual field disturbance.

B. **Tension.** A physical examination may reveal muscle tightness, or "trigger points," over the posterior cervical and occipital regions. The neck examination may provide clues to underlying causes of tension headache, such as cervical arthritis (eg, stiffness, decreased range of motion, or crepitus with movement), inflammatory processes (eg, trigger points or nodules), or infectious causes (eg, lymphadenopathy).

C. **Cluster headaches.** Photophobia, tearing, nasal stuffiness, or Horner's syndrome may be present. The patient may be unable to sit still during the interview.

D. Secondary headaches. Signs of a "worrisome" headache are listed below.
1. **Fever** may indicate meningitis, purulent sinusitis, otitis, dental abscess, etc.
2. A **stiff neck** may indicate infection or blood in the cerebrospinal fluid.
3. **Focal neurologic deficits** or **elevated blood pressure** [>200 mm Hg systolic or >120 mm Hg diastolic] may indicate increased intracranial pressure from mass effect, bleed, or accelerated hypertension.
4. A **palpable, tender temporal artery** suggests temporal arteritis.
5. **Papilledema** suggests increased intracranial pressure.

V. Laboratory Tests. Diagnostic testing is unnecessary for most patients with chronic, recurring headaches and for low-risk patients (ie, young patients who [1] have prior or family history of headache, [2] are improving during their evaluation, [3] have none of the abovementioned "worrisome" symptoms or signs, [4] are alert and oriented, and [5] have no focal neurologic signs). For these individuals, repeated history taking and physical examinations over time, in addition to observations of response to treatment, are the best diagnostic tools. The following tests should be considered in patients not meeting low-risk criteria.

A. Radiologic evaluation
1. **Plain skull films** are rarely useful in the evaluation of headache.
2. **Computerized tomography (CT)** may assist in evaluating for sinusitis or diagnosing subarachnoid or intraparenchymal hemorrhage in the patient with a severe and acute headache. The acutely ill patient who requires monitoring will be most easily evaluated by CT, although a normal CT scan does not rule out an acute bleed. If the clinical suspicion remains high, a lumbar puncture (LP) should be performed.
3. **Magnetic resonance imaging (MRI)** is generally more informative than CT in patients with chronic headaches. Characteristic MRI findings have been described in patients with migraine, trigeminal neuralgia, and temporomandibular joint dysfunction. This procedure is also superior to CT in demonstrating subacute subdural hematoma in patients with a history of trauma and is useful in further characterizing lesions detected by CT. MRI has excellent resolution in the posterior fossa. Most patients with primary headache disorders will have an unremarkable study.

B. The purposes of **LP** are (1) to establish the presence or absence of blood or inflammatory cells in the cerebrospinal fluid, (2) to detect hemorrhage or infection in the patient with a stiff neck, and (3) to determine the organism responsible for infection by fluid culture. Although LP is easy to perform and readily available, it is an invasive, uncomfortable procedure that has no role in routine headache evaluation. LP should *not* be performed when increased intracranial pressure is suspected, until mass effect is ruled out. LP opening pressure also may be elevated in pseudotumor cerebri.

C. Blood analysis. A complete blood cell count is rarely useful or definitive in the evaluation of headache and has no place except in the febrile patient. The erythrocyte sedimentation rate is indicated in the older patient with a new headache to support a diagnosis of temporal arteritis.

D. Other studies. Radionucleotide imaging and **angiography,** which are usually less helpful than CT scans for identifying or ruling out significant intracranial disease, should be reserved for the few patients with normal CT scans and cerebrospinal fluid findings whose evaluations strongly suggest an intracranial lesion. MRI has largely replaced these studies. **Magnetic resonance angiography (MRA)** is useful to demonstrate small aneurysms. Temporal arteritis should be confirmed by **arterial biopsy;** this procedure should not delay treatment when clinical suspicion is strong. **Electroencephalography (EEG)** is not routinely helpful for the patient with a new headache, although it may be useful in ruling out seizure disorder in the chronic headache patient responding poorly to therapy.

VI. Treatment
A. Episodic migraine (with or without aura)
1. **General measures** include patient education and avoidance of precipitating factors, such as alcohol, certain foods (eg, foods containing tyramine or monosodium glutamate), fatigue, and life stressors. Alternative therapies are frequently prescribed for migraine sufferers and include aerobic exercise, biofeedback, progressive self-relaxation, meditation, massage therapy, or acupuncture. The most widely researched botanical for migraine headache is a wildflower called feverfew (*Tanacetum parthenium*), which is modestly efficacious for either acute treatment or prophylaxis (Table 34–1).
2. **Acute therapy** is appropriate when migraine attacks occur less than two to four times a month. The most effective approach is individualized and stratified, based on a given drug's ability to preserve normal function. An abortive medication with

TABLE 34–1. PROPHYLAXIS FOR RECURRENT MIGRAINE HEADACHES

Class	Medication	Tablet Dose (mg)	Oral Dosing/Max	Notes
Beta blockers	Propranolol (Inderal)	10/20/40/80; 80/120/160—LA	20–40 mg tid–qid	Beta blockers are first-line preventive drugs; caution with asthma/COPD/bradycardia
	Nadolol (Corgard)	20 mg	20–160 mg	
Tricyclic antidepressants	Amitriptyline (Elavil)	25/50/75/100/125	25–150 mg, HS	Sedating/serotonergic/anticholinergic
	Nortriptyline (Norpramin)	25/50/75/100	25–75 mg, HS	
	Imiprimere (Tofranil)	25/50/75/100	25–150 HS	
Calcium channel blockers	Verapamil (Calan)	120, 180, 240, 360 SR	40–160 mg bid–qid	Agents of choice if beta blocker intolerant or contraindicated (asthma/CHF/bradycardia)
	Diltiazem (Tiazac)	30, 60, 90, 120 (60, 90, 120 SR)	30–90 mg bid–tid	
Antiepileptic drugs (AEDs)	Divalproex (Depakote)	125, 250, 500	25–500 mg bid	
	Topiramate (Topamax)	25, 100, 200	50–200 mg bid	
	Carbamazepine (Tegretol)	200	200–400 mg bid	
	Tiagabine (Gabitril)	2, 4, 12, 16, 20	4–16 mg qd	
Ergot	Methysergide (Sansert)	2; tid–qid	tid–qid; 16 max	Not commonly used due to reported adverse effects, including retroperitoneal and cardiopulmonary fibrosis
Herbal	Feverfew	125	1 tablet bid	Effective, but concerns with product reliability
Antihistamine	Cyproheptadine (Periactin)	4, 2 mg/5 cc	2–4 mg tid	Useful in childhood migraine
Miscellaneous agents	Fluoxetine (Prozac)	20	20 mg daily	SSRI—modestly effective
	Clonidine (Catapres)	.1, .2 mg	1–.2 mg bid–tid	Central alpha blocker; sedation; possibly effective

CHF, congestive heart failure; COPD, chronic obstructive pulmonary disease, HS, hour's sleep (bedtime); SSRI, selective serotonin reuptake inhibitor.

(continued)

TABLE 34–1. (Continued)

Class	Medication	Tablet Dose (mg)	Formulations	Dosing (tablets unless specified otherwise)	Notes
Combination products	Acetamin/butalb/caffeine (Fioricet)	325/50/40	T	T 1–2 po q 4 hours. Max 6 tabs/day	Also available with 30 mg codeine
	Acetamin/dichloralphea/ isometheptine (Midrin)	325/100/65	T	2 at onset, 1 q 30 min. Max 5/day	Effective for mild to moderately intense migraines
Simple analgesics/NSAIDs	Aspirin	325	T	1–2 po q 4 hours. Max 4 g/day	Gastrointestinal upset, gastritis, ulcers
	Ibuprofen (Motrin)	200–800	T	1 po q 8 hours	
Antiemetics	Chlorpromazine	10, 25	T, RS, IM	25 po q 4–6 hours po	Use 50–100 q 6–8 pr
	Promethazine (Phenergan)	12.5, 25	T, RS, IM, IV	12.5–25 q 4–6 hours	
	Prochlorperazine	5, 10, 25	T, RS, IM, IV	5–10 mg q 6 hours	25 PR q 12 hours, 5–10 mg IV
Narcotic analgesics	Codeine (Tylenol #3)	300/30	T	1–2 q 4 hours	
	Oxycodone ± acetaminophen (Lortab)	5 g or 7.5 mg/500 mg	T	1–2 q 6 hours	
	Butorphanol tartrate (Stadol NS)	1 mg	IN	1 mg IN, repeated in 1 hour, then q 3–4 hours	
Sedative hypnotics	Secobarbital (Seconal)	100 mg	T, IM	100 single dose	Sedate—"sleep off" headache
	Triazolam (Halcion)	.125, .25	T	1–2 single dose	Data on efficacy lacking

DHE, dihydroergotamine; DT, dissolving tablet; IM, intramuscular; IN, intranasal; NSAIDs, nonsteroidal anti-inflammatory drugs; RS, rectal suppository; SC, subcutaneous; T, tablet.

receptor-specific therapy (**eg, a triptan**) should be prescribed initially and administered at migraine onset, or in the prodromal/aural phase if possible. Ergot alkaloids are a good alternative to triptans; these drug classes share contraindications. If triptans or ergotamines fail or are contraindicated, **rescue medications,** such as simple analgesics, may be tried. Rescue medications also include combination products, sedatives, antiemetics, and narcotics. These are often effective, but seldom allow the patient to function normally.

The following specific agents are commonly used (Table 34–2).

   a. **Triptans** are selective serotonin receptor agonists affecting primarily 5-HT 1B/1D receptors. They have proved to be very effective in the treatment of migraines, with success rates approaching 70%. There are many triptans available, with important differences in route of administration (oral tablet, dissolving oral tablet, injectable, intranasal); onset of action; and duration of action. Triptans should be used with caution in patients with suspected coronary artery, cerebrovascular, or peripheral vascular disease, since they have been associated with vasospasm. They should not be used in basilar or complicated migraine. Patients should be limited to two administrations each week, and triptans should not be taken within 24 hours of an ergot alkaloid.

   b. **Ergot alkaloids** also target serotonin receptors, but are less selective. These drugs are estimated to be effective within 2 hours in >90% of cases when administered parenterally, 80% when given rectally, and up to 50% when given orally. They are also available in sublingual and intranasal forms. Since ergotamine preparations may result in dependency and rebound headaches, they should not be used more often than 2 days/week.

   c. **Combination products.** A combination of acetaminophen, butalbital, and caffeine (Fioricet) is commonly used for migraine; however, no studies have addressed the efficacy of butalbital.

   d. **Simple analgesics** are effective. The best evidence exists for aspirin, ibuprofen, naproxen sodium, and tolfenamic acid. There are little data supporting use of acetaminophen alone. There is no strong evidence for the use of injectable ketorolac.

TABLE 34–2. MEDICATIONS FOR ACUTE MIGRAINE HEADACHES

Class	Medication	Tablet Dose (mg)	Formulations	Dosing (tablets unless specified otherwise)	Notes
Triptans	Zolmitriptan (Zomig)	2.5, 5.0	T/DT	1 po × 1. May repeat in 2 hours	
	Sumatriptan (Imitrex)	25, 50, 100	T/SC/IN	1 po × 1. May repeat in 2 hours	May repeat SC (6 mg) in 1 hour. SC and IN good for early morning migraine
	Rizatriptan (Maxalt)	5, 10	T/DT	1 po × 1. May repeat in 2 hours	Caution with propranolol, use 5-mg dose
	Naratriptan (Amerge)	2.5	T	1 po × 1. May repeat in 4 hours.	Long half-life
	Almotriptan (Axert)	6.25, 12.5	T	1 po × 1. May repeat in 2 hours.	
	Frovatriptan (Frova)	2.5	T	1 po × 1. May repeat in 2 hours.	Long half-life, indicated for menstrual migraine
	Eletriptan (Relpax)	20, 40	T	1 po × 1. May repeat in 2 hours	40-mg dose preferred
Ergot alkaloids	D.H.E. 45	1	IV/IM	1 mg IM/IV × 1. May repeat in 1 hour × 1.	
	Ergotamine/ caffeine	1/100 tab, 2/100 supp	T/RS	1–2 po or pr. May repeat after 30 minutes	

    e. Antiemetics administered either by mouth, intramuscularly (IM), or by rectal suppository may be useful to offset the nausea and gastric stasis associated with migraine. They may be used alone or as adjunctive therapy with narcotics.

    f. Narcotic analgesics such as **codeine** or **oxycodone** are effective during an acute attack, but their use must be carefully balanced with the risks of habituation and rebound headache. The potential for abuse is less with agonist-antagonist opioids (eg, **butorphanol tartrate**) than with receptor agonists.

    g. Sedative hypnotics such as **secobarbital** or **triazolam** may be helpful in allowing the patient to "sleep off" the headache. There are not strong data to support or refute this practice.

  3. Prophylactic therapy (Table 34–1) is indicated for more than three or four attacks per month or for headaches occurring on a predictable schedule (eg, with menses). Effective medications include the following:

    a. Beta blockers are the most important drugs for migraine prevention. Once- or twice-daily dosing improves compliance.

    b. Tricyclic antidepressants have also proved useful, probably because of serotonin effects. The full dosages normally used for depression are unnecessary.

    c. Calcium channel blockers are not as effective as beta blockers for prophylaxis. Nifedipine may actually increase headaches.

    d. Reflecting the changing perception of migraine as a neurologic phenomenon perhaps propagated centrally, **antiepileptic drugs (AEDs)** have been used more frequently to suppress migraines. Experience with **divalproex sodium** has been most encouraging. **Topiramate carbamazepine,** and **tiagabine** may also be effective. AEDs are generally more expensive than other agents and require monitoring for adverse effects (eg, abnormalities in liver function).

    e. Other agents. Clonidine or carbamazepine may also be effective; selective serotonin reuptake inhibitors like fluoxetine have been only modestly effective.

    f. Follow-up and education. Patient education during an acute headache is not very effective. The mutually cooperative, understanding relationship critical to long-term success can be established with frequent visits during medicine trials and titration. Communicating therapeutic goals clearly is essential to success. Follow-up visits to assess response to therapy, patient understanding, and frequency of attacks can be therapeutic.

B. TTH

  1. General measures. A supportive cooperative physician-patient relationship is essential. Education, insight into family and life events, consideration of environmental and emotional triggers, and counseling may help both decrease headache frequency and increase coping skills. Headache diaries, biofeedback, stress management, muscle relaxation techniques, exercise programs, and dietary changes may also help. Addressing psychiatric comorbidities (see Chapters 89, 92, and 94) contributes to successful treatment of headaches.

    Individuals with **chronic tension headaches** may benefit from a multidisciplinary approach using both drug and nondrug treatments, including individual/family therapy and physical therapy.

  2. Used sparingly, **muscle relaxants** (eg, cyclobenzaprine, 10 mg three times daily for up to 21 days; chlorzoxazone, 500–750 mg three times daily; methocarbamol, 1000–1500 mg four times daily; or diazepam, 5 mg two to three times daily) can be helpful adjunctive therapy. Narcotic analgesics generally should be avoided.

  3. Preventive therapy. Medications used for migraine prophylaxis (specifically, beta blockers and tricyclic antidepressants, alone or in combination) have also proved useful in patients with frequent, recurrent, and chronic TTH.

  4. Follow-up

    a. Most **acute headache patients** will see their primary physician only once for this complaint. Early follow-up is recommended **with new headaches** to gauge response to therapy and reconfirm history and physical findings. Review of headache diaries, precipitating factors, and life stressors may help patients identify/avoid precipitants, thereby reducing the number of headache days.

    b. Clinicians tend to underestimate the therapeutic value of **regularly scheduled follow-up,** often monthly, for **chronic pain complaints like chronic TTH.**

C. Cluster headaches

  1. Acute therapy during an attack includes (1) **inhalation of 100% oxygen** by mask at a rate of 7–10 L/min; (2) **inhaled ergotamine,** one puff every 5 minutes for a maximum of five puffs per day; or (3) **sublingual nifedipine,** 10–20 mg, repeated every 6–8 hours (not to be used with ergotamine).

2. **Prevention** is preferable once clusters begin. Effective oral medications, alone or in combination, include (1) **methysergide,** 2–8 mg/day; (2) **lithium,** 300 mg three times per day (monitoring blood levels weekly to avoid toxicity); (3) **prednisone,** 40–60 mg/day for 5 days, followed by tapering over 10–14 days; and (4) **calcium channel blockers,** such as nifedipine, 10–20 mg three times daily. **Indomethacin,** 25 mg orally three times a day, is very effective for benign paroxysmal hemicrania, an entity similar to cluster headache.

D. **Chronic daily headaches** probably represent a heterogeneous collection of chronic migraine and tension- and medication-associated headaches, rather than a distinct entity. If there has been a long history of poorly controlled episodic migraines that evolve into chronic daily headaches, chronic migraine should be considered.

1. Those taking narcotic medication chronically may require inpatient detoxification both to treat the headache and the medication dependence. This is largely a successful enterprise.

2. **Severe chronic migraine** and **medication-associated headache requiring detoxification** are problems best managed in collaboration with a headache expert.

3. **Continuity of care** with a single knowledgeable physician remains essential for these patients.

E. **Secondary headaches.** Treatment of the underlying disease, whether medical or neurosurgical, is the best approach.

REFERENCES

Bigal ME, et al: Chronic daily headache: Identification of factors associated with induction and transformation. Headache 2002;**42**(7):575.

Lipton RB, et al: Prevalence and burden of migraine in the United States: Data from the American Migraine Study II. Headache 2001;**41**:646.

Maizels M: The clinician's approach to the management of headache. West J Med 1998;**168**:203.

Matthew NT: Serotonin 1D (5HT1D) agonists and other agents in migraine. Neurol Clin 1997;**15**:61.

Saper JR: Diagnosis and treatment of migraine. Headache 1997;**37**(suppl 1):S1.

Silberstein SD, Lipton RB: Overview of diagnosis and treatment of migraine. Neurology 1994; **44**(suppl 7):S6.

Tepper SJ, Rapoport A, Sheftell F: The pathophysiology of migraine. Neurolog (September) 2001; **7**(5):279.

---

35   Hearing Loss

Robert C. Salinas, MD, & Heather Bartoli, PA-C

KEY POINTS

- Hearing loss is classified as sensorineural, conductive, or mixed type.
- Sudden deafness is a medical emergency and warrants prompt referral to an otolaryngologist.
- The treatment of hearing loss is dependent on its etiology and involves environmental alteration, assistive listening devices, active medical/surgical intervention, and hearing aids.

I. **Definition.** Hearing loss may be defined as a reduction in an individual's ability to perceive sound. The intensity of sound is measured with the decibel (dB), a logarithmic unit whose reference is 0 on the audiogram. Normal hearing is from 0 to 20 dB. Thresholds in the 20- to 40-dB region constitute a mild hearing loss, 40- to 60-dB thresholds are moderate hearing loss, and thresholds greater than 60 dB are considered severe hearing loss.

Hearing loss is a very common problem encountered in primary care and may be classified as **sensorineural** (due to deterioration of the cochlea or lesions to the eighth cranial nerve); **conductive** (due to lesions of the external or middle ear that impede passage of sound waves to the inner ear); **mixed** (sensorineural and conductive); or **central** (due to lesions of the auditory pathways proximal to the cochlea). Hearing loss may further be described as congenital or acquired. A more complete listing of etiologies of hearing loss may be found in Table 35–1. (Also see the sidebars on acoustic neuroma and sudden deafness.)

ACOUSTIC NEUROMA

Ninety-five percent of acoustic neuromas are idiopathic; 5% occur in patients with neurofibromatosis, in which cases tumors are more aggressive and more likely to undergo malignant transformation. The most common presenting symptoms are tinnitus and progressive hearing loss. About 50% of patients also have disequilibrium.

Audiometric findings include loss of discrimination that is disproportionate to pure-tone results, and high-frequency sensorineural loss. About 5% have normal audiograms. Thin-section magnetic resonance imaging with gadolinium can detect temporal bony acoustic neuromas measuring just a few millimeters. Treatment for acoustic neuroma is surgical excision; however, since acoustic neuromas are usually very slow-growing, the elderly or those with multiple medical problems may choose observation.

SUDDEN DEAFNESS

Sudden deafness is a sensorineural deafness that occurs instantly or is noticed over hours or days. The degree of hearing loss may range from mild to complete and is typically unilateral. Potential causes include **localized lesions** of the temporal bone (ie, acoustic neuroma, aneurysm of the anterior inferior cerebellar artery), **systemic diseases** (ie, macroglobulinemia, leukemia, polycythemia, sickle cell disease, syphilis, bacterial infection, ototoxic drugs, mumps, multiple sclerosis), **barotrauma,** or **head trauma.** Sudden deafness should be thought of as a medical emergency, requiring prompt referral to an otolaryngologist. Prognosis is dependent on the timeliness of therapy, which may include treatment of identified causes or supportive/empiric therapies (eg, corticosteroids, vasodilators, anticoagulants, bed rest, sedation, or a low-sodium diet).

TABLE 35–1. COMMON ETIOLOGIES OF HEARING LOSS ENCOUNTERED IN PRIMARY CARE

Conductive	Sensorineural
Cerumen impaction	Genetic[1]
Cholesteatoma	Alport's syndrome
Cysts	Usher's syndrome
Exostosis	Waardenburg's syndrome
Eustachian tube dysfunction	Meniere's disease
Foreign body	Multiple sclerosis
Hemotympanum	Noise-induced
Ossicular malformations	Ototoxicity
Ossicular discontinuity	Presbycusis
Otitis externa	Sarcoidosis
Otitis media	Sudden idiopathic hearing loss
Otosclerosis	Syphilis
Previous ear surgery	Trauma
Trauma	Vascular
Perforated tympanic membrane	Migraine
Temporal bone fracture	
Tumors	
Tympanic membrane perforation	
Tympanic membrane retraction	
Tympanosclerosis	

[1] Many genetic syndromes causing hearing loss have been identified; some of the more common examples are listed above.

II. Common Diagnoses (Table 35–1). Approximately 15 million people in the United States are hearing impaired, and approximately 2 million Americans are functionally deaf. Hearing loss is also the third most prevalent chronic condition in older Americans, after hypertension and arthritis. Approximately 90% of Americans older than 65 years have some degree of hearing impairment, and approximately 15% of school-aged children have a 16–dB hearing loss. One of every 2000 individuals is deaf or severely hearing impaired. At least 90% of these hearing problems are secondary to middle ear disorders that are potentially treatable.

   A. Sensorineural loss. More than 90% of hearing loss is sensorineural. Some common etiologies of sensorineural loss include presbycusis, acoustic damage, ototoxicity, and Meniere's disease.

   1. **Presbycusis** is the most common type of hearing loss in the United States, is associated with aging, and may begin in middle age.

   2. **Acoustic damage** (noise-induced hearing loss) may be caused by chronic exposure to excessive noise levels or from more acute acoustic trauma (ie, shotgun blast or firecracker explosion).

      a. **As many as 30 million Americans are exposed to excessive noise levels at work,** and as many as 17% of these workers have hearing loss.

      b. **Males are affected more frequently than females** presumably due to occupational noise exposure, military service, and recreational shooting.

      c. **Noise exposure is not limited to the workplace.** Noise-induced hearing loss has been demonstrated in children and adolescents.

   3. **Ototoxicity** is caused primarily by exposure to drugs and is the most common cause of deafness in children. The correlation between ototoxicity and plasma drug levels is poor. An increased risk of ototoxicity is associated with decreased creatinine clearance, advanced age, certain drugs (especially if administered parenterally), and drug treatment longer than 14 days. Environmental exposure and workplace exposure are less common causal agents. Cigarette smokers are 1.69 times as likely to have hearing loss as nonsmokers.

   4. **Meniere's disease** is the most common type of hearing loss that occurs between the fourth and sixth decades but may occur at any age.

   5. **Congenital sensorineural hearing loss,** a form of significant hearing loss, is one of the most common major abnormalities present at birth. One in 200 children is born with some degree of congenital hearing loss, and one third to three fourths of these losses have a genetic component. More than 70 syndromes have been identified that involve a genetic basis for hearing loss. Increased risk of congenital hearing loss is associated with a family history of congenital hearing loss; low birth weight; craniofacial abnormalities; syndromes known to cause hearing loss (Usher's syndrome, Waardenburg's syndrome, etc); intrauterine infections (ie, toxoplasmosis, syphilis, cytomegalovirus, rubella); hyperbilirubinemia; prolonged stay in the neonatal intensive care unit; and low Apgar score.

   B. Conductive loss. This type usually involves abnormalities of the middle and external ear, and generally has a mechanical cause (eg, perforated eardrum, fluid in the middle ear, disarticulation of the ossicular chain, cerumen impaction).

   1. **Obstruction.** Hearing loss often results from obstruction of the external ear canal by cerumen or foreign bodies, such as crayons, food, or toys. Cerumen sometimes accumulates in the auditory canal of individuals with either excessive production of cerumen or ineffective self-cleaning mechanisms. In the third and fourth decades of life, the hairs found in ear canals become coarser and longer, which secondarily reduces natural clearance of cerumen. Edema associated with otitis externa may also obstruct the canal.

   2. **Otosclerosis,** a progressive sclerotic fixation of the stapes in the round window dampening sound conduction to the cochlea, causes deafness in 50% of affected adults. Otosclerosis is transmitted through autosomal dominant inheritance with variable expression, typically occurs in women during the second or third decades of life, and is 10 times more common among whites than blacks.

   3. **Otitis media** (suppurative or serous), a collection of fluid behind the tympanic membrane, most commonly causes hearing loss in children younger than age 5 with a history of recurrent ear infections.

   C. Central hearing loss. This may be caused by demyelinating disease, ischemia, neoplasm, or hematoma.

III. Symptoms
A. Reduced hearing acuity
1. **Presbycusis** may not cause reduced hearing acuity until late in the disease process and may manifest as difficulty understanding conversation when ambient noise levels are relatively high, as in crowded or large areas or on the telephone. Some patients complain of sensitivity to loud noises or that people mumble.
2. Patients with **noise-induced hearing loss** first notice some muffling of sound, but they usually consult a physician only when they begin to experience difficulties hearing speech, which is a late finding.
3. With **conductive hearing loss,** patients tend to hear conversation better in noisy rooms than in quiet rooms. Reduced hearing acuity is common in patients with impacted cerumen.
B. Timing/onset of symptoms may suggest particular etiologies.
1. **Noise-induced hearing loss** may be most pronounced shortly after the patient leaves the workplace, and the patient's hearing may improve while away from work.
2. A temporal relationship between the **use of a toxic agent** and the symptomatology is generally present in patients with ototoxicity.
3. Symptoms of hearing loss from **impacted cerumen** frequently begin suddenly following bathing or swimming, when a drop of water closes the passageway.
4. Hearing loss associated with **presbycusis** is typically of gradual onset and bilateral.
C. Associated symptoms
1. **Vertigo, imbalance, nausea, and disequilibrium** may occur in patients with ototoxicity.
2. **High-pitched tinnitus** may occur in individuals with presbycusis, noise-induced hearing loss, and otosclerosis.
3. **Pain, discomfort, or itching** can occur in patients with hearing loss from impacted cerumen, otitis media, or otitis externa.
4. **Chronic cough** may be present in patients with impacted cerumen if the impaction abuts the tympanic membrane. The cough should disappear with removal of the impaction.
5. In **Meniere's disease,** fluctuating, unilateral hearing loss is classically associated with vertigo and tinnitus.
6. **Behavioral changes** resulting from isolation and depression caused by hearing loss may include fear, anger, depression, frustration, embarrassment, or anxiety. Elderly people with hearing loss suffer depression twice as often as the general population.

IV. Signs. Physical findings may be limited.
A. Otoscopic examination
1. **Impacted cerumen or a foreign body** may be evident.
2. Findings consistent with **otitis externa or otitis media** (see Chapter 22) may be seen.
3. The medial wall of the middle ear promontory may appear reddish in patients with **otosclerosis.**
B. Tuning fork tests
1. **The Weber test** is performed by placing the handle of a vibrating tuning fork (512 cycles/s) against the midline of the patient's forehead. A patient with normal sensorineural function and no conductive hearing loss hears the sound equally in both ears. Lateralization of the Weber test to one side means either a conductive loss on that side or a sensorineural loss on the opposite side.
2. The **Rinne test** assesses air and bone conduction. The handle of a vibrating 512-cycles/s tuning fork is placed against the mastoid until the patient can no longer hear it and then the tines are held near the ear canal to assess whether the patient can still hear it. Air conduction persists longer than bone conduction in a patient with no hearing loss. Equal hearing levels at both positions are consistent with hearing loss of mixed cause. If air conduction is louder, either normal hearing or sensorineural loss may exist. If bone conduction is louder, conductive loss exists.
C. Developmental milestones. The primary care practitioner should be familiar with milestones associated with normal speech and hearing. Any deviation from these norms should alert the clinician to consider audiologic testing.
1. From **birth to 3 months** infants should have a startle reflex to loud sounds. At this age they are generally comforted by familiar voices.

2. The **ability to localize sound usually develops at around 6 months of age,** while responding to their name and mimicking environmental sounds usually takes place around 9 months.
3. Infants usually learn to say **their first meaningful word around 12 months,** and by 24 months usually have a vocabulary of about 20 words.

V. Laboratory Tests

A. **Audiometry** measures the threshold levels (ie, the intensity at which the patient is able to perceive sound correctly 50% of the time). This level is usually measured by presenting pure tones to the individual at preset frequencies through air conduction and occasionally through bone conduction.

1. **Indications**
   a. **Audiometry is indicated in all patients with hearing loss,** except those patients with a foreign body or acute infection whose hearing normalizes following treatment.
   b. **Baseline audiometry should be performed within 3 days of institution of therapy with ototoxic agents** for patients who are alert enough to cooperate with the examination. Serial audiometry on an individual basis should be considered.
   c. **Follow-up should be performed annually** after treatment, if indicated by the patient's condition.

2. **Findings**
   a. **Sensorineural loss** causes lower thresholds in low frequencies than in higher frequencies.
      (1) Individuals with **presbycusis** display a pattern with a greater high frequency loss at 8000 than at 4000 cycles, often described as a smooth, ski slope–shaped curve, and the loss is generally bilateral. It is not always possible to distinguish, from an audiogram alone, whether the hearing loss is the effect of presbycusis, noise exposure, or ototoxic agents.
      (2) The classic **noise-induced pattern** on the audiogram shows high frequency loss, greatest at 4000 cycle, with improvement at 8000 cycles. The audiogram should be measured at least 14 hours after the last significant noise exposure in order to minimize the confusion of temporary versus permanent threshold shifts.
   b. **Conductive loss** causes low-frequency (ie, 125–500 cycles) loss rather than high-frequency loss. Bone conduction testing in patients with conductive hearing loss reveals normal hearing thresholds.
   c. **Mixed loss** causes audiometric patterns with features of both sensorineural and conductive hearing loss.

B. **Tympanometry.** Tympanometry is a simple, reliable test that may be rapidly performed in the clinic setting. This test assesses function of the tympanic membrane and Eustachian tube. A small probe is inserted into the external auditory canal and a tone of fixed characteristics is presented via the probe. The compliance of the tympanic membrane is measured electronically while the external canal pressure is artificially varied.

1. **Indications.** Tympanogram is useful to confirm an otoscopic diagnosis, aid in diagnosis when otoscopy is equivocal or difficult (especially in children), and as a screening test for ear disease.
2. **Findings** (Figure 35–1). In general, tympanograms may be described as Type A, Type B, or Type C. Compliance is greatest when pressures are equal on both sides of the tympanic membrane. A peak will be present when the compliance is normal. **Type A tympanogram** describes normal compliance of the tympanic membrane. **Type B tympanogram** looks flat, because no impedence peak may be identified. There is little or no mobility, often due to fluid in the middle ear. Type B may also be seen with patent pressure equalization tubes and perforations. **Type C tympanogram** shows a peak in the negative range, which is consistent with a retracted tympanic membrane and Eustachian tube dysfunction.

C. **Otoacoustic emission (OAE).** Without screening, congenital hearing loss is often not diagnosed until as late as 2½ years of age, and therefore results in impaired speech, language, and cognitive development. Over 30 states have mandated newborn screening with OAE testing.

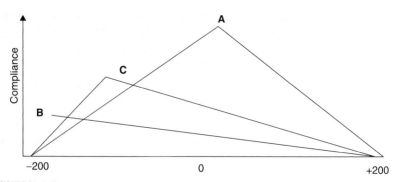

FIGURE 35–1. Tympanogram patterns. **A:** Type A tympanogram, with normal compliance of the tympanic membrane. **B:** Type B tympanogram, with no impedance peak. **C:** Type C tympanogram, with a peak in the negative range.

VI. Treatment

A. General points/preventive measures. Effective measures to prevent or minimize hearing loss are described below.

   1. **The treatment of hearing loss is dependent upon its etiology** and involves environmental alteration, assistive listening devices, active medical/surgical intervention, and hearing aids.
   2. **Both conductive and sensorineural hearing loss may benefit from environmental alteration** and usage of assistive listening devices. Perhaps the most important way the listening environment may be altered is by minimizing the amount of background noise.
   3. Physicians should **minimize the use of ototoxic drugs** and carefully monitor patients taking these drugs.
   4. **Individuals with exposure to noise at home or work** should receive education concerning the use of ear protection during noise exposure and should be fitted for proper ear protective devices.

B. Sensorineural loss

   1. **Presbycusis.** Patients with a presumptive diagnosis of presbycusis should be referred to an audiologist for further testing to confirm the diagnosis and for rehabilitation. Patients may increase the effectiveness of communication by cupping the hand behind the ear, reducing distractions and background noise levels, using good lighting to see the speaker and understand gestures, and learning lipreading. Hearing aids or other assistive devices may be beneficial. Psychological support, particularly for elderly patients, is very helpful. Left untreated, presbycusis can lead to social isolation and depression.
   2. **Noise-induced loss.** Patients with this type of loss should be referred to an otolaryngologist for assessment of asymmetric hearing loss, rapid and progressive hearing loss, permanent threshold shift, or an occasional finding of low-frequency loss. All patients with losses presenting at threshold >25 dB are candidates for hearing aids.
   3. **Ototoxicity.** For patients with ototoxicity, early removal of the offending agent will reduce the likelihood of permanent hearing loss. Hearing impairment may be either permanent (eg, when caused by drugs such as mercury, arsenic, lead, or aminoglycosides) or temporary (eg, when caused by drugs such as aspirin, quinine, or certain diuretics). Actual recovery may be delayed and is often incomplete. Thus, follow-up with an audiologist may be necessary to evaluate for ototoxic sequelae.

C. Conductive hearing loss

   1. **Foreign bodies or cerumen** in the external auditory canal can almost always be removed by irrigation, forceps, or earloops. Patients with objects wedged in place should be referred to an otolaryngologist because of potential risks of damage to the tympanic membrane or bony structures by attempted removal.

    a. **Hard cerumen can be softened** fairly quickly prior to irrigation with a few drops of over-the-counter cerumen softener. The ear can be irrigated with water approximately 20 minutes after the softening agent is applied. The use of water at a temperature of 35–37.8 °C (95–100 °F) will prevent vertigo.

    b. **Water irrigation is contraindicated** with vegetable foreign bodies (ie, dry beans) because it can cause swelling. Alcohol solutions should be used in such cases. A perforation in the tympanic membrane is an absolute contraindication to irrigation.

  2. **Otitis externa** or **otitis media** should be treated with appropriate medication (see Chapter 22); hearing should normalize following treatment of infection and resolution of middle ear effusion, which may take up to 3 months.

  3. Patients with **otosclerosis** can be successfully treated with stapedectomy and should be referred to an otolaryngologist.

REFERENCES

Bogardus ST Jr, Yueh B, Shekelle PG: Screening and management of adult hearing loss in primary care: Clinical applications. JAMA 2003;**289**(15):1986.

Cohn ES: Hearing loss with aging. Clin Geriatr Med 1999;**15**(1):145.

Isaacson JE, Vora NM: Differential diagnosis and treatment of hearing loss. Am Fam Physician 2003; **68**:1125.

Lee KJ: *Essential Otolaryngology—Head & Neck Surgery,* 7th ed. McGraw-Hill; 1999.

Rabinowitz PM: Noise-induced hearing loss. Am Fam Physician 2000;**61**:2749, 2759.

Yueh B, et al: Screening and management of adult hearing loss in primary care: Scientific review. JAMA 2003;**289**(15):1976.

---

36   Hematuria

Brian H. Halstater, MD, Felix Horng, MD, Dennis P. Lewis, MD, & Leonard W. Morgan, MD, PhD

KEY POINTS

- Hematuria occurs with common urinary tract diseases (eg, urinary tract infection, prostatic disease, urinary stones), but may herald neoplasm.
- Careful urinalysis is an important first step in laboratory evaluation of hematuria and may guide further evaluation.
- Most common causes of hematuria can be managed by primary care physicians.

I. Definition. Hematuria is the presence of red blood cells (RBCs) in urine. It can be classified as either gross or microscopic. Significant hematuria is three or more RBCs per high-power field in a centrifuged specimen.

II. Common Diagnoses. Microscopic hematuria occurs in 3–4% of the adult population.

  A. **Urinary tract infections (UTIs),** such as cystitis and pyelonephritis (34% of all cases of gross hematuria, 28% of all cases of microscopic hematuria). Cystitis is more common in females than in males.

  B. **Prostatic diseases,** such as benign prostatic hypertrophy (BPH) and prostatitis (18% of all cases of gross hematuria, 13.2% of all cases of microscopic hematuria).

    1. **BPH.** Clinically significant BPH affects an average of 23% of males by age 45 and 88% of males by age 90.

    2. **Prostatitis.** This disease occurs with equal frequency in postpubertal males of all ages.

  C. **Neoplasms** resulting from renal, bladder, and prostatic cancer (22.5% of all cases of gross hematuria, 3–10% of all cases of microscopic hematuria).

    1. **Carcinoma of the bladder,** which accounts for two thirds of neoplasms associated with hematuria, occurs mainly after the sixth decade. This cancer is more common

TABLE 36–1. DRUGS THAT MAY CAUSE HEMATURIA

Drug	Induced Condition
Aspirin-phenacetin combination	Papillary necrosis, analgesic nephropathy, uroepithelial tumors
Penicillins	Allergic interstitial nephritis
Cephalosporins	
Sulfonamides	
Phenytoin (Dilantin)	
Cyclophosphamide (Cytoxan)	Chemical hemorrhagic cystitis, uroepithelial tumors
Mitotane (Lysodren)	
Anticoagulants	Spontaneous urinary tract bleeding, bleeding from occult urinary tract neoplasm
Primaquine	Hemoglobinuria resulting from hemolysis in individuals with
Nitrofurantoin (Furadantin, Macrodantin)	glucose-6-phosphate dehydrogenase deficiency

in males than females (3:1 ratio). Risk factors include work in the printing/leather/ dye industries and smoking.

2. **Renal cell carcinoma** accounts for up to 90% of all renal tumors. Risk factors include smoking, male gender, and age greater than 50 years.
3. **Carcinoma of the prostate** is a common disease affecting 10% of all men in the fifth decade and up to 50% of all men older than age 80.
4. **Wilms' tumor,** the most common malignancy in children, occurs most often in children younger than 6 years old.

D. **Urinary stones** (5.3% of all cases of gross hematuria, 0.4% of all cases of microscopic hematuria). These stones occur in 2–3% of the general population and are the third most common urinary system disease. Those at risk include white males (estimated lifetime risk of 1%); residents of the southeastern United States; and individuals who consume inadequate fluids, have gout or leukemia (receiving chemotherapy), or have a positive family history of nephrolithiasis.

E. **Trauma** (2% of all cases of gross hematuria), which may either be direct (ie, blunt trauma) or indirect (prolonged physical exertion in a marathon runner).

F. **Intrinsic renal diseases,** such as glomerulonephritis, which are rare in adults. However, post-streptococcal glomerulonephritis is responsible for 50% of pediatric hematuria.

G. **Drugs.** See Table 36–1.

H. **Pseudohematuria** (Table 36–2), when the urine is red or contains non–urinary tract RBCs. This condition is common in women late in the luteal phase of their menstrual cycle.

III. **Symptoms**

A. Hematuria associated with **suprapubic pain, dysuria, urgency, frequency,** and **nocturia,** especially in women, makes cystitis a likely diagnosis (see Chapter 21).

TABLE 36–2. CAUSES OF "RED URINE" (PSEUDOHEMATURIA)

Endogenous substances	Exogenous substances
Red blood cells (hematuria)	*Dyes*
Free hemoglobin	Beets
Myoglobin	Blackberries
Bilirubin	Rhubarb
Urobilinogen	*Drugs*
Porphyrins	Anthraquinone-containing laxatives
	Chloroquine (Aralen)
	Deferoxamine (Desferal)
	Doxorubicin (Adriamycin)
	Metronidazole (Flagyl)
	Phenothiazines
	Phenytoin (Dilantin)
	Rifampin (Rifadin, Rimactane)
	Sulfasalazine (Azulfidine)

B. **Acute prostatitis** presents with **dysuria, fever, suprapubic or back pain, urinary frequency/urgency,** and occasionally hematuria; **chronic prostatitis** usually presents with isolated back pain, dysuria, or posterior urethral discomfort upon ejaculation. **Prostatism** is commonly associated with obstructive symptoms, such as dribbling, incomplete voiding, urgency, and hesitancy. Nocturia is also common and is probably related to incomplete voiding (see Chapter 61).

C. **Hematuria,** usually **without other symptoms,** is the most common presentation of **bladder carcinoma** (85% of such patients). Urgency, frequency, and difficult micturition may also be present. **Hematuria occurs in 90% of renal cell carcinomas;** constitutional symptoms, such as fever, malaise, weakness, and weight loss are generally associated with metastatic disease. The classic triad of pain, hematuria, and abdominal mass is rare.

D. **Sudden onset of excruciating unilateral flank pain** and gross or microscopic hematuria unassociated with a precipitating event characterizes **urinary stones.** As a stone progresses, pain migrates medially and caudally.

E. Patients with **primary renal diseases** (such as glomerulonephritis) may present with **gross or microscopic hematuria, with or without flank pain.** In contrast, secondary conditions (eg, systemic lupus erythematosus or endocarditis) are more likely to be silent or present with systemic symptoms.

F. **Gross hematuria** may be induced by exercise. **Blunt trauma** may result in pain at the site of injury.

IV. **Signs**

A. **Pyelonephritis** can usually be differentiated from cystitis by the presence of fever, costovertebral angle tenderness, and a "toxic" appearance (see Chapter 21).

B. **Digital rectal examination (DRE)** in **BPH** may reveal enlarged but firm lateral lobes. The degree of obstruction generally correlates with median lobe hypertrophy, which cannot be evaluated by rectal examination. In **acute prostatitis,** DRE reveals an enlarged, boggy prostate gland, occasionally with increased warmth to the touch. There are no specific physical findings in **chronic prostatitis.**

C. The utility of physical examination is limited in **urologic malignancies.** Weight loss, muscle weakness, and an abdominal mass are late findings in **renal carcinoma,** generally associated with metastatic disease. DRE commonly reveals a stony-hard or nodular prostate in **prostatic carcinoma.** An abdominal mass is the most frequent and consistent physical finding of **Wilms' tumor.**

D. **Hematuria from vigorous exercise** usually has no associated clinical signs. However, blunt trauma may cause tenderness, ecchymoses, or abrasions at the point of impact.

E. Patients with **glomerulonephritis** commonly present with hypertension and edema, but they may also lack signs of disease. Secondary glomerulonephritis may be characterized by fever, rash, joint tenderness, heart murmur, or splinter hemorrhages of the nail beds.

V. **Laboratory Tests** (Figure 36–1).

A. **Urinalysis (UA).** Dipstick and microscopic evaluation of a centrifuged urine specimen should be the initial step in the diagnostic work-up of patients with hematuria. A midstream specimen improves the chances of a good sample for analysis and culture.

1. **True hematuria** should be differentiated from **pseudohematuria.** Pseudohematuria can be derived from at least two sources: chemical agents (Table 36–2), or cervical or vaginal bleeding in females.

2. **Initial hematuria** (hematuria with initiation of micturition) suggests a lesion in the urethra, whereas **terminal hematuria** (hematuria at the end of micturition) suggests a bladder neck or a prostatic urethral lesion. **Total hematuria** (hematuria occurring throughout micturition) occurs with bladder, ureteral, or renal lesions.

3. **Associated findings** narrowing the differential diagnosis include **crystals** in nephrolithiasis, **bacteria** in infections, and >2+ (100 mg of protein per deciliter) **proteinuria or RBC casts** in glomerular disease. **Dysmorphic RBCs** with a wide range of alterations in the urinary sediment also suggest glomerular disease. **White blood cell casts** may be seen in pyelonephritis. **Pyuria with hematuria** may be from infection, stones, tumors, or glomerulonephritis.

4. Some urine dipsticks can test for nitrates, which suggest UTI. **Because dipstick testing often gives false-positive results, it is important to corroborate dipstick findings with microscopic examination.**

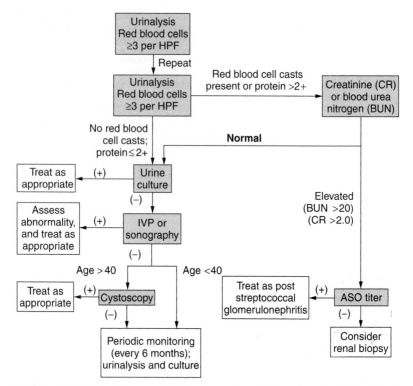

FIGURE 36–1. Algorithm for laboratory and radiologic work-up of hematuria. ASO, antistreptolysin O; HPF, high-power field; IVP, intravenous pyelography.

- **B. Urine culture.** Regardless of UA results, urine culture is a reasonable next step in hematuria evaluation. The patient's history, physical examination, and urine culture results can establish the diagnosis of pyelonephritis, cystitis, or prostatitis. A positive culture result in patients older than 40 years does not rule out malignancy, and further evaluation is indicated (see sections V,G and J).
- **C. Phase contrast microscopy.** Evaluation of urine RBC morphology to determine the site of bleeding has been used extensively over the last few years. Phase contrast microscopy is the technique most often used and has a high sensitivity (90–95%) and specificity (95–100%) in differentiating glomerular from lower tract bleeding. This test should be used early in evaluation of hematuria (after excluding a UTI).
- **D. Multichemistry profile.** In patients with suspected glomerular disease, blood urea nitrogen (BUN), creatinine (Cr), serum protein, and serum lipid determinations can be helpful. For example, elevated BUN and Cr, a decreased albumin level, and hyperlipidemia may occur in glomerulonephritis.
- **E. Complete blood cell count.** This test can document the degree of blood loss and indicate the presence of systemic involvement (eg, pyelonephritis or cystitis). Target cells or sickle cells suggest hemoglobinopathy as a possible cause of hematuria.
- **F. Erythrocyte sedimentation rate.** Because of its non-specificity, this test should be considered only if a secondary glomerular disease is suspected.
- **G. Intravenous pyelography (IVP).** This technique is the most effective method for evaluating upper urinary tract anatomy; addition of a cystourethrogram allows visualization of the lower urinary tract. IVP has demonstrated utility in the evaluation of urolithiasis, renal tumors, renal trauma, carcinoma of the bladder, and BPH is indicated if UA confirms hematuria on two separate specimens with negative urine culture results.

1. **Bladder tumors 1 cm** or larger can be visualized only 75% of the time. Therefore, absence of a radiolucent bladder lesion does not exclude a bladder tumor.
2. All patients with a history of **renal trauma and hematuria** should undergo an IVP or radiographic evaluation.
3. Conditions that may preclude IVP are allergy to the dye and diminished renal function.
H. **Nephrotomography.** This radiographic test, combined with an IVP, improves detection of small renal carcinomas.
I. **Ultrasonography.** This technique has some limitations. It is not as sensitive as IVP in detecting urolithiasis and carcinoma of the bladder. Ultrasonography can be quite helpful if the patient is allergic to IVP dye, has diminished renal function, or if a cystic renal lesion is suspected.
J. **Cystoscopy.** This technique allows direct visualization and biopsy of lesions and sampling of lesions for cytologic analysis. Cystoscopy is indicated in all patients older than age 40 with gross hematuria; patients older than 40 years who have microscopic hematuria and negative urine culture, IVP, or sonogram results; and patients suspected of having bladder carcinoma even with negative IVP and cystourethrogram results.
K. **Computerized tomography (CT).** This technique is used to evaluate small lesions of the kidney and for staging bladder carcinoma. **Noncontrast helical CT** is 95–100% sensitive and 94–96% specific for all types of urinary stones.
L. **Angiography.** This procedure is rarely needed in the evaluation of hematuria because CT scans, ultrasonography, and other diagnostic tools can provide the similar information more safely and cost-effectively.
M. **Renal biopsy.** Renal biopsy is indicated in two instances: (1) when other diagnostic tests have yielded little information and hematuria persists, and (2) if history and laboratory data suggest glomerulonephritis as the cause of hematuria.

VI. **Treatment**
A. **Urinary tract infections.** See Chapter 21.
B. **Prostatic diseases.** See Chapter 61.
C. **Neoplasms.** Surgery, chemotherapy, and radiation are possible modalities. Details of therapeutic interventions are beyond the scope of this chapter.
D. **Urinary stones**
1. In general, stones ≤4 mm have an 80% chance of spontaneous passage, those 4–5 mm a 40–50% chance of passage, and those >6 mm a <5% chance of spontaneous passage.
2. **Stones likely to pass** can be managed expectantly with hydration, analgesia (eg, oral acetaminophen with codeine or oxycodone), and follow-up within a week or two.
3. **Urologic consultation** is indicated for obstructive hydronephrosis, sepsis, or stones >5 mm diameter. Urologic referral for lithotripsy may benefit individuals with renal calculi.
4. **Prophylactic therapy** should be instituted after resolution of the acute episode. Reasonable prophylaxis against recurrent stones is achieved by maintaining a urine flow rate of 3–4 L/day. A low-purine diet and uricosuric agents (eg, oral allopurinol, 200–600 mg daily, adjusted based on urinary urate levels) may prevent recurrence of uric acid stones.
E. **Trauma.** Exercise-induced hematuria is self-limited. Urologic trauma is best managed with the assistance of a urologist.
F. **Renal diseases.** Therapy for post-streptococcal glomerulonephritis is generally limited to treating associated hypertension. Rapid or continued deterioration of renal indices (increasing BUN and Cr) requires nephrology consultation.

REFERENCES

Brendler CB: *History, Physical Examination, and Urinalysis: Campbell's Urology,* vol. 1, 7th ed. Saunders; 1998:146.
Crompton CH, Ward PB, Hewitt IK: The use of urinary red cell morphology to determine the source of hematuria in children. Clin Nephrol 1993;**39**:44.
Grossfeld GD, et al: Asymptomatic microscopic hematuria in adults: Summary of the AUA best practice policy recommendations. Am Fam Physician 2001;**63**(6):1145.
Mohammad KS, et al: Phase contrast microscopic examination of urinary erythrocytes to localize source of bleeding: An overlooked technique? Clin Pathol 1993;**46**:642.

37   Insomnia

Jeffrey L. Susman, MD, & Daniel A. Vogel, MD

KEY POINTS

- When assessing sleep problems, explore the role of underlying medical and psychiatric illnesses, medication use, and current sleep habits.
- Implement good sleep hygiene for all sleep disorders and consider nonpharmacologic approaches to treatment whenever possible.
- The accurate diagnosis of many primary sleep disorders requires full polysomnography in an accredited sleep laboratory; currently, actigraphy and home polysomnography are inadequate substitutes for such an evaluation.

I. **Definition.** Adequate sleep is essential for healthy tissue growth and repair, regulation of immune function, and memory integration. Normal sleep may be divided into five stages. **Non–rapid eye movement (non-REM) sleep** includes the transition period from wakefulness to sleep or light sleep (stages 1 and 2) and deep sleep (stages 3 and 4). Deep sleep is characterized by decreased muscle tone, blood pressure, and respiratory rate. **REM sleep,** or "dream sleep" (stage 5), is associated with skeletal muscle atonia, variability of vital signs, and dreaming. A person normally goes from wakefulness through stages 1–4 followed by the first REM period after approximately 90 minutes of sleep. Cycles of REM and non-REM sleep occur at 1- to 3-hour intervals, with decreasing amounts of deep sleep in later cycles. Most adults require 6–8 hours of sleep each day. Approximately 2% require less than 5 hours, and another 2% require more than 9 hours each day. **Insomnia** is the inability to fall asleep (long sleep latency) or stay asleep (excessive or prolonged awakenings), and sleep disorders may be associated with disruption of the quality, quantity, or timing of one or more stages of sleep.

II. **Common Diagnoses.** A National Sleep Foundation poll reported in 2003 that over two thirds of Americans older than 55 years reported sleep problems, but only 1 in 8 had their problem diagnosed. One third of children and adolescents may experience sleep problems. While the relative incidence of sleep disorders in primary care populations is less clear, almost all individuals suffer from occasional sleep disturbance. The major categories of insomnia include:

A. **Transient conditions** due to situational stress or conflict; environmental factors, such as excessive noise, bright light, and improper temperature; travel problems, including jet lag and adjustment to new sleeping environments; hospitalization or institutionalization; and shift work.

B. **Psychiatric diseases** including alcohol and drug abuse (see Table 37–1); depression (Chapter 92); bipolar disorder, mania, or dementia (Chapter 73); delirium (Chapter 11); post-traumatic stress disorder or other anxiety disorders (Chapter 89); and patients with excessive neurotic symptoms or the inability to deal effectively with anger and emotions.

C. **Physiologic, age-, or gender-related insomnia.** More than 50% of elderly people will admit to sleep problems, and females are more likely to complain of insomnia than males.

D. **Medical disorders** such as symptomatic prostatic hypertrophy, congestive heart failure, and gastroesophageal reflux.

E. **Primary sleep disorders**

   1. **Disturbances of the sleep-wake cycle or circadian rhythm sleep disorders** are common in people who are hospitalized, institutionalized, do night or changing shift work, or have jet lag.

   2. **Sleep-related movement disorders** include restless legs syndrome and nocturnal myoclonus. One third of patients with **restless legs syndrome** have a family history of this disorder. This problem is sometimes associated with iron deficiency, motor neuron disease, renal disease, or circulatory problems. **Nocturnal myoclonus** is more common in older individuals.

TABLE 37-1. MEDICATIONS ASSOCIATED WITH SLEEP DISTURBANCE

Excessive wakefulness
Theophylline
Amphetamines
Caffeine
Anticonvulsants
Antidepressants (eg, many of the selective
  serotonin reuptake inhibitors)
Alcohol
Nicotine
Triazolam (rebound phenomena)
Thyroid hormone
Methylphenidate
Sympathomimetics including herbals
  (eg, ma huang, ephedra)

Nightmares
Beta blockers (especially lipophilic agents
  such as propranolol)
Tricyclics
Antiparkinsonian agents
Quinidine
Buspirone
Selective serotonin reuptake inhibitors (SSRIs)

Excessive somnolence
Benzodiazepines
Antihistamines
Anticonvulsants
Antidepressants
Antipsychotics (both typical and atypical)
Tricyclics (especially amitriptyline, doxepin, and trazodone)
Monoamine oxidase inhibitors
Antihypertensives (especially clonidine)

Other symptoms
Diuretics (nocturia)
Levodopa and tricyclics (sleep-related myoclonus)
Caffeine (nonrepetitive muscle contractions at sleep onset
  or hypnic jerks)

3. **Parasomnias** include nightmares, sleep terrors, sleepwalking, REM sleep behavior, and sleep paralysis. The first three are more common in the pediatric population.
   a. **Nightmares** occur in REM sleep and may be associated with post-traumatic stress disorder.
   b. **Night terrors** are a non-REM phenomenon; in adults, night terrors may be associated with neurologic or psychiatric disorders.
   c. **Sleepwalking** is a non-REM phenomenon, is seen most frequently in children, and new-onset somnambulism in an adult may suggest a central nervous system or psychiatric disorder.
4. **Disorders of excessive somnolence**
   a. **Sleep apnea syndrome.** Central sleep apnea usually has a readily apparent cause such as stroke, brain stem infarction, or neoplasia. Obstructive sleep apnea (OSAS) is associated with an upper airway abnormality and with medical conditions such as thyroid dysfunction, hypertension, cor pulmonale, obesity, and severe pulmonary dysfunction. Obstructive sleep apnea is most common in men and in older individuals.
   b. **Narcolepsy.** Narcolepsy is most likely to occur in young to middle-aged males.
F. **Conditioned or learned insomnia.** These conditions often occurs as patients develop poor sleep habits and come to associate bedtime with a frustrating experience trying to fall asleep or maintain sleep.
G. **Drug/alcohol-related** (Table 37-1).
III. **Symptoms.** Patients with insomnia may present with unusual or nonspecific symptoms, such as headache and irritability, in addition to complaints of difficulty in initiating or maintaining sleep. A sleep diary for a week (see Table 37-2), a tape recording of the patient's sounds while sleeping, and a history of the patient's sleep patterns provided by the patient's bed partner are useful tools in diagnosing the causes of insomnia.
A. **Snoring** is common in the general population and becomes more common as the patient increases in age. Over 60% of men and 45% of women older than the age of 60 snore. Unusually loud or disruptive snoring (especially when accompanied by periods of apnea), however, may be a symptom of a more serious problem such as sleep apnea syndrome.
B. **Pain, paresthesias, cramps, cough,** and **breathlessness** may indicate that the insomnia is caused by illness or disease.
C. **Sleep phase disorders**
   1. **Delayed sleep phase.** Patients with this problem have difficulty falling asleep, have no problems once asleep, and awaken later than usual.

TABLE 37–2. SLEEP DIARY

Date and day of the week
Habits prior to sleep, including food, drink (especially alcohol and caffeine), and medication
Activities prior to bedtime, including reading, television, telephone, sex, work, exercise, and socializing
Bedtime
Time it takes to fall asleep
Quality of sleep, including awakenings and nightmares
Dreams, snoring, or unusual movements
Time awake
Total sleep time
Symptoms and alertness upon awakening
Daytime sleepiness and naps
Other unusual or important factors

    2. Advanced sleep phase. Patients cannot stay awake in the evening, have no difficulty once asleep, and awaken early in the morning.
    3. Irregular sleep phase. Patients complain of frequent drowsiness and naps and excessive time in bed.
  D. Difficulty maintaining sleep, periodic hypersomnolence, headache, impotence, enuresis, personality changes, unusual movements, and **loud sounds or snoring** during sleep may indicate sleep apnea syndrome.
  E. Excessive daytime sleepiness and **"sleep attacks," hypnagogic or bizarre hallucinations,** and **cataplexy** (sudden muscle weakness, especially at times of extreme emotion) are common symptoms of narcolepsy. The symptoms usually begin before age 30.
    1. Cataplexy is pathognomonic; however, episodes of cataplexy may be very short, infrequent, and easily overlooked.
    2. Periodic amnesia or **accidents** may be the presenting symptoms because of the patient's "sleep attacks" and cataplexy.
  F. Restless legs syndrome is characterized by a "creepy" or "crawling" sensation and an irresistible urge to move one's legs, particularly when just retiring and frequently during the day when in confined spaces (such as at a movie theatre). **Nocturnal myoclonus** is associated with repetitive stereotypic spasms of the legs in non-REM sleep and with muscle aches and daytime fatigue. These disorders are often coexistent.
  G. Parasomnias include **nightmares,** which are associated with limited vocalization, vivid recall, and easy arousal; and **night terrors,** which are associated with blood-curdling screams, little recall, and more difficult arousal. There is also minimal recall associated with **somnambulism.**
IV. Signs of the psychiatric disorders and medical diseases mentioned previously should be sought, as discussed in detail elsewhere (see Chapters 11, 73, 88, 89, and 92). A large neck, large tongue, or abnormalities in the ear-nose-throat examination may be associated with obstructive sleep apnea.
V. Laboratory Tests. In most cases, a careful history and physical examination will obviate the need for laboratory evaluation and will point to underlying medical conditions.
    Iron studies (eg, ferritin) should be ordered in patients with restless legs syndrome; consideration should also be given to renal (blood urea nitrogen, creatinine), folate, and thyroid (TSH) assessment. A thyroid-stimulating hormone (TSH) level should be ordered in patients with sleep apnea. A **sleep study** is indicated in the following situations.
  A. The diagnosis remains obscure or the problem persists or worsens.
  B. There is suspicion of sleep apnea, especially in patients with hypertension, signs of cardiopulmonary difficulties and respiratory symptoms, or daytime somnolence.
  C. Periodic hypersomnia is present. A sleep study is particularly important when this is associated with functional impairment.
  D. Serious disorders of the sleep-wake cycle occur that are not associated with transient changes in work or travel.
  E. The patient feels that the problem is becoming more severe and interfering with daily activities.

The accurate diagnosis of many primary sleep disorders requires full polysomnography in an accredited sleep laboratory; currently, actigraphy and home polysomnography are inadequate substitutes for such an evaluation.

VI. Treatment. Psychiatric and medical disorders associated with sleep disturbance should always be treated optimally, and instituting good sleep hygiene (see Table 37–3) is useful for most sleep disturbances.

A. Transient insomnia

1. **Environmental factors** such as proper light, noise levels, and temperature should be optimized. **Drug and alcohol use** should be carefully assessed. **Good sleep hygiene** (Table 37–3) should be instituted.

2. **Adjustments to new sleeping environments, shift work,** and **jet lag** should be addressed. Small delays in the sleep-wake cycle (ie, staying up longer and going to bed later before westbound travel) are more easily accommodated prior to travel than in the opposite situation (ie, going to bed earlier before eastbound travel). Adjustment to shift work is difficult if the schedule rotates irregularly. If possible, a routine of sleep-wake periods should be established. Melatonin (5 mg of the immediate-release formulation at the desired bedtime) is effective in patients with jet lag. Exposure to bright light during the day is also helpful.

3. **Pharmacologic agents** may be used in select cases of transient sleep disorders unassociated with more serious problems (see Table 37–4). The drug of choice for sleep onset problems is usually zolpidem (Ambien) and for sleep maintenance difficulty, zaleplon (Sonata), with benzodiazepines reserved for nonresponders. Guidelines for hypnotic therapy include:

    a. Making a presumptive diagnosis and ruling out primary sleep disorders or underlying medical problems that pharmacologic therapy might aggravate.

    b. Determining the goals of therapy.

    c. Educating the patient on the use of medication.

    d. Beginning with a low dose of medication and increasing as needed based on improved sleep and daytime functioning.

    e. Following up in 1 week to reassess the patient's condition. Telephone contact is reasonable for reliable patients.

    f. Limiting medication use to no more than 3–4 weeks (especially if using a benzodiazepine) or using medications three or four times per week when longer therapy is warranted.

    g. Educating the patient about the possibility of withdrawal symptoms, especially with benzodiazepines.

B. Physiologic or age-related insomnia

1. The patient should be reassured.

2. **Good sleep hygiene** should be recommended.

TABLE 37–3. SLEEP HYGIENE

Awaken at a regular hour
Exercise daily on a regular basis (not close to bedtime)
Control the sleep environment (proper temperature, decreased noise and light)
Eat a light snack before bedtime (if not contraindicated)
Limit or eliminate alcohol, caffeine, and nicotine
Use hypnotics on a short-term basis only
Wind down prior to bedtime
Have a "worry time" early in the evening
Go to bed when sleepy
Avoid excessive sleep on weekends or extremes of sleep
Use relaxation and behavioral modification techniques
Use bed for sleeping only
Eliminate naps unless part of the schedule
Get up if you cannot get to sleep in 15–30 minutes
Sleep where you sleep best
Recognize the adaptation effect in new environments

TABLE 37–4. PHARMACOLOGIC THERAPY FOR TRANSIENT INSOMNIA

Class and Selected Agents	Initial Dose (mg)	Comments
Nonprescription		
Aspirin or acetaminophen (Tylenol)	325–650	May relieve troublesome aches or pains and thus enhance sleep
Antihistamines		
Diphenhydramine citrate (Excedrin PM)		May be effective transiently but have potential
Diphenhydramine hydrochloride (Benadryl, Nytol)		for carry-over, anticholinergic side effects, and can induce paradoxical wakefulness
Doxylamine succinate (Unisom)		
Hydroxyzine (Atarax, Vistaril)		
Prescription		
Chloral hydrate	500–1000	May cause nausea and displace warfarin and phenytoin from albumin
Trazodone (Desyrel)	50–150	Sedating; may be associated with priapism, particularly with higher doses
Gabapentin (Neurontin)	100–400	Particularly useful with neuropathic pain syndromes
Benzodiazepines		Recommended for 1 month or less of continuous therapy
		Decreases sleep latency and nocturnal awakenings. May be associated with withdrawal.
Triazolam (Halcion)	0.125–0.25	Intermediate onset and rapid elimination; may cause rebound insomnia
Alprazolam (Xanax)	0.25	Intermediate onset of action and elimination;
Lorazepam (Ativan)	1	give at least 1 hour prior to bedtime
Temazepam (Restoril)	15	Slower onset of action; give several hours
Oxazepam (Serax)	15	prior to bedtime
		Intermediate half-life
Estazolam (ProSom)	0.5–2.0	Should be used cautiously because of long
Flurazepam (Dalmane)	15	half-lives and potential for accumulation,
Chlordiazepoxide (Librium)	5–10	especially in elders. Associated with falls
Diazepam (Valium)	1–5	and hip fractures.
Non-benzodiazepines		
Zolpidem (Ambien)	5–10	Agent of choice for sleep onset problems; less potential for withdrawal and is more specific for sedative properties alone
Zaleplon (Sonata)	5–10	Best agent for sleep maintenance difficulty; very short elimination half-life
Alternatives		
Melatonin	5 immediate release at time of desired sleep	Effective for jet lag
Valerian	300–600 of root extract	Conflicting data about efficacy but appears to have few substantial side effects; may potentiate other psychoactive drugs
Kava-kava		May be associated with fatal liver failure even after one dose; contraindicated

3. **Medications** should be avoided.
4. In the absence of underlying disease, patients who **snore** should be advised to consider:
   a. Exercise during the day or early evening.
   b. Avoidance of sedatives and alcohol.
   c. Sleeping on the side, not on the back. Sewing a tennis ball in the back of the pajamas may make this position easier to maintain.
   d. Raising the head of the bed 6 inches.
   e. Using a soft collar.
   f. Drinking a cup of coffee before going to bed.

C. Underlying **medical disorders** should be treated whenever possible. Certain problems may be associated with underlying primary sleep disorders (eg, hypertension and obesity with sleep apnea syndrome). In the absence of contraindications, short-term pharmacologic therapy is often useful for hospitalized patients.

D. Primary sleep disorders

1. **Disturbances of the sleep-wake cycle.** Slow advancement or delay of the patient's bedtime, usually in conjunction with a sleep laboratory, is the therapy for this disorder. The irregular sleep phase disturbance will respond to strict structuring of a patient's waking and sleeping hours.

2. **Sleep-related movement disorders.** These disorders may respond to the treatment of underlying medical conditions such as iron deficiency or uremia; the avoidance of stimulants, including caffeine; and the judicious use of **benzodiazepines or dopaminergic agents. Oral clonazepam,** 1–4 mg, or **carbidopa-levodopa,** 25/100 mg at bedtime; **pergolide,** 0.1–0.5 mg three times daily; or **pramipexole,** 0.125–1 mg three times daily, are useful for restless legs syndrome. A trial of iron supplementation is occasionally effective for restless legs syndrome even when iron studies are normal. Opioid analgesics, gabapentin, and a host of other agents are also occasionally used for restless legs syndrome.

3. **Disorders of excessive somnolence**

   a. **Sleep apnea syndrome. Central sleep apnea** usually requires treatment by a pulmonary or neurologic specialist and is usually directed at the underlying disorder. For patients with **OSAS,** consultation with pulmonary and otorhinolaryngology (ORL) specialists is often indicated. Upper airway abnormalities may be amenable to ear, nose, and throat surgery, especially adenotonsillectomy for children, or oral appliances specifically fitted to the patient. Obesity and underlying medical conditions should be treated aggressively. Even a small amount of weight loss can translate into a significant reduction in apneas. Patients should sleep on the side and should avoid depressants that affect the central nervous system. Nasal continuous positive airway pressure (CPAP) is the treatment of choice for most patients. Unfortunately, long-term adherence to CPAP is less than 50%. Many problems can be corrected with refitting of the mask, trial of alternative delivery systems (such as nasal pillows) or the use of BIPAP, and appropriate humidification. Occasionally, uvulopalatopharyngoplasty (UPP) or tracheostomy is necessary if more conservative measures fail. Consultation with a skilled sleep specialist and ORL are important.

   b. **Narcolepsy** should be managed by a specialist skilled in the evaluation and control of this disorder. Multiple newer medications (eg, modafinil) are available to help maintain wakefulness and combat cataplexy.

4. **Conditioned insomnia** will usually respond to strict sleep hygiene, cognitive behavioral measures, and other counseling approaches such as sleep restriction therapy.

5. **Psychiatric and medical disorders** exacerbating insomnia should be treated (see Chapters 11, 73, 89, and 92).

6. **Alcohol use** should be limited, and alternatives should be sought for drugs felt to be exacerbating insomnia (Table 37–1).

VII. Follow-up of sleep disorders and insomnia should be dictated by the severity of the problem. For serious sleep disorders, close supervision and careful follow-up are necessary. On the other hand, when more serious problems have been ruled out, a 2- to 4-week trial of good sleep hygiene is indicated. The identification of hidden medical or psychophysiologic causes of sleep disturbance should be pursued.

REFERENCES

Early CJ: Restless legs syndrome. N Engl J Med 2003;**384:**2103.

Estivill E, et al: Consensus on drug treatment, definition and diagnosis of insomnia. Clin Drug Invest 2003;**23:**351.

Howard BJ, Wong J: Sleep disorders. Pediatr Rev 2001;**22:**327.

Morin CM: Contributions of cognitive-behavioral approaches to the clinical management of insomnia. Prim Care Comp J Clin Psych 2002;**4**(suppl 1):21.

Schenck CH, Mahowald MW, Sack RL: Assessment and management of insomnia. JAMA 2003; **289:**2475.

White DP: Tragedy and insomnia. N Engl J Med 2001;**345:**1846.

38   Jaundice

Brian J Finley, MD, & L. Peter Schwiebert, MD

KEY POINTS

- Most jaundice is due to one of three underlying mechanisms: liver disease, isolated disorders of bilirubin, and biliary obstruction.
- Jaundice has many causes but can be effectively evaluated based on age, risk factors, physical examination, and limited laboratory testing.
- Jaundice is very common in newborns and can usually be managed at home, if treatment is required.

I. **Definition.** The major source of bilirubin is degradation of hemoglobin from senescent red blood cells. Bilirubin from the periphery is tightly bound to albumin during transport in the blood to the hepatocyte. Inside the hepatocyte, nonpolar bilirubin is enzymatically conjugated by uridine diphosphoglucuronyl transferase (UDPGT) to form water-soluble bilirubin glucuronides. UDPGT activity is physiologically decreased in neonates, increasing unconjugated bilirubin levels. (In white and African American neonates, bilirubin levels rise steadily, peaking at 5–6 mg/dL between the second and fourth days of life, then slowly declining to adult levels by days 10–12. In Asians and Native Americans, bilirubin levels rise more rapidly, peaking at 8–12 mg/dL by days 4–5, then declining more slowly than in white or African American neonates.) After conjugation, bilirubin is excreted in the bile and transported in the biliary system to the gastrointestinal tract.

Jaundice is the yellow discoloration of the skin and mucous membranes caused by an elevated serum bilirubin. In adults, jaundice is visible at bilirubin levels of 2–3 mg/dL. In newborns, the threshold for visible jaundice is 5–6 mg/dL. Based on bilirubin physiology just described, jaundice can be categorized as being due to (1) **excessive hemoglobin degradation/bilirubin overproduction,** as in immune hemolysis (eg, ABO incompatibility or Rh isoimmunization); nonimmune hemolysis (eg, glucose-6-phosphate-dehydrogenase [G6PD] deficiency or spherocytosis); extravascular hemolysis (eg, cephalohematomas in newborns); or intramarrow hemolysis (eg, "ineffective erythropoiesis" in thalassemia or pernicious anemia); (2) **defective hepatic uptake/conjugation,** as in Gilbert's or Crigler-Najjar syndrome or hepatitis; or (3) **impaired excretion,** as in hepatocellular disease, drug effects, primary biliary cirrhosis, or bile duct obstruction.

II. **Common Diagnoses.** Jaundice is very common in newborns, affecting 60% of full-term and 80% of preterm infants; after the neonatal period, jaundice is less prevalent, but still significant, accounting for up to 4% of admissions to acute care hospitals annually. Jaundice has myriad causes; while recognizing that more than one pathophysiologic process can be present in a single patient, it is helpful to approach jaundice based on age of onset, risk factors, and the test by which jaundice is initially assessed—ie, **unconjugated** (indirect fraction of bilirubin exceeding 80% of total) vs. **conjugated** (indirect fraction of bilirubin ranges from 20% to 60% of total bilirubin).

A. **Childhood jaundice**

1. **Unconjugated hyperbilirubinemia**

a. **Neonatal onset**

(1) **Physiologic jaundice** is present in as many as 50% of newborns.

(2) **Jaundice in breast-fed infants. Breast-feeding jaundice** occurs in 5–10% of breast-fed infants and is due to decreased caloric intake and subsequent weight loss; dietary supplementation with formula is an additional risk factor. **Breast milk jaundice** occurs in less than 1% of breast-fed infants and is believed to be due to some substance in the breast milk that causes the baby's intestine to reabsorb excessive amounts of bilirubin.

(3) **Hemolytic anemia** is the most common pathologic cause of jaundice, usually resulting from ABO incompatibility or, less commonly, Rh incompatibility, spherocytosis, enzyme deficiency, or a hemoglobinopathy.

African Americans are prone to certain types of hemolytic anemias (eg, sickle cell disease and G6PD deficiency). Patients of Mediterranean descent and Asians are at increased risk for the thalassemias.

   (4) Other causes of unconjugated neonatal jaundice include polycythemia, hematoma reabsorption, pyloric stenosis, and congenital hypothyroidism.
   b. Infancy and childhood onset. Jaundice may result from hemolytic diseases (eg, G6PD deficiency and spherocytosis), Gilbert's syndrome, and Crigler-Najjar syndrome.
  2. Conjugated hyperbilirubinemia
   a. Neonatal onset. Sepsis, neonatal hepatitis, TORCHS infections (**t**oxoplasmosis, **r**ubella, **c**ytomegalovirus [CMV], **h**erpes, and **s**yphilis), extrahepatic obstruction in biliary atresia or choledocholithiasis, and metabolic diseases, such as galactosemia, α_1-antitrypsin deficiency, or tyrosinemia may result in jaundice.
   b. Infancy and childhood onset. Viral hepatitis (see section II,B,2,a,(1)) is the most common cause of jaundice in a previously healthy child. Less common causes include Wilson's disease and milder forms of galactosemia.
B. Adult onset
  1. Unconjugated hyperbilirubinemia may occur with **hemolytic anemia, ineffective erythropoiesis** (eg, thalassemias, sideroblastic anemias, and pernicious anemia), and **impaired uptake and conjugation of bilirubin** (eg, Gilbert's syndrome, which occurs in 3–7% of the US population, and Crigler-Najjar syndrome type II, an uncommon disorder). In addition to risk factors already mentioned for hemolytic anemia, a positive family history may be associated with Gilbert's syndrome or hemolytic anemia.
  2. Conjugated hyperbilirubinemia
   a. Impaired intrahepatic excretion
    (1) Viral hepatitis accounts for 75% of jaundice in patients younger than 30 years but only 5% in patients older than 60 years. Risk factors for **hepatitis A** include ingestion of raw shellfish, travel to countries with unsanitary water supplies, household contact with infected persons, and exposure to diapered infants in day care. Risk factors for **hepatitis B** include living in a country where the virus is endemic (eg, sub-Saharan Africa or Asia), birth canal exposure of the infant to an infected mother, and sexual contact with an infected patient. A history of blood transfusions (especially before 1992), intravenous drug abuse, multiple sexual partners, hemodialysis, and health care occupations are risk factors for both **hepatitis B and hepatitis C.**
    (2) Cirrhosis causes about one third of jaundice in 30- to 60-year-old patients. Females have a higher incidence of primary biliary cirrhosis; males have a higher risk for alcoholic liver disease.
    (3) Congestive heart failure (CHF) accounts for 10% of jaundice after age 60. Risk factors include a history of hypertension and atherosclerotic cardiovascular disease (see Chapter 72).
    (4) Metastatic disease causes 13% of jaundice after age 60.
    (5) Other causes include drugs (erythromycin, nonsteroidal anti-inflammatory drugs, anabolic and contraceptive steroids, phenothiazines and sulfonylureas), pregnancy, primary biliary cirrhosis, primary hepatocellular carcinoma, and Dubin-Johnson and Rotor's syndromes.
   b. Extrahepatic obstruction (eg, gallstones, strictures, and tumors, especially pancreatic cancer) accounts for 60% of jaundice in patients older than 60 years. Gallstones are more common in females than males.
III. Symptoms
 A. Onset of jaundice
  1. A rapid onset suggests infection, drug reaction, hemolytic anemia, or acute choledocholithiasis.
  2. Intermittent or fluctuating jaundice occurs in Gilbert's syndrome (typically with fasting or intercurrent illness), Crigler-Najjar syndrome, Dubin-Johnson or Rotor's syndrome, recurrent common bile duct stones, and congestive heart failure.
  3. A gradual onset occurs in cirrhosis, intrahepatic metastases, pregnancy, or primary biliary cirrhosis.
 B. Pruritus. Severe pruritus and excoriations suggest extrahepatic obstruction.

C. **Abdominal pain** occurs more often with obstructive jaundice than with hepatocellular disease. Colicky, right upper quadrant pain prior to the onset of jaundice suggests choledocholithiasis, especially in middle-aged to older patients.

D. **Fever with chills** suggests biliary obstruction and cholangitis. **Flulike symptoms** suggest viral or drug-induced hepatitis.

E. Additional clues to **obstructive jaundice** include a >2-week history of acholic stools or severe jaundice without systemic symptoms.

F. Sixty percent to 70% of patients with **acute hepatitis C** are asymptomatic, 20–30% have jaundice, and 10–20% complain only of fatigue, anorexia, or abdominal pain.

G. **In neonates,** historical clues include history of premature rupture of membranes (sepsis), delay in clamping the cord (polycythemia), and history of jaundice in a sibling (metabolic disorders or anemias). In **breast-feeding** infants, both **breast milk** and **breast-feeding jaundice** develop in the first week of life.

IV. **Signs**
   A. **Urticaria** suggests hepatitis B infection.

   B. **Cutaneous xanthomas** suggest hypercholesterolemia seen in patients with chronic cholestasis (eg, primary biliary cirrhosis).

   C. **Spider angiomata,** palmar erythema, white nails, gynecomastia, testicular atrophy, ascites, and signs of portal hypertension are signs of chronic hepatocellular disease or cirrhosis.

   D. **Kayser-Fleischer ring** of the cornea is pathognomonic of Wilson's disease.

   E. A **palpable (Courvoisier's) gallbladder** suggests malignant common duct obstruction (eg, cancer of the head of the pancreas) or, more commonly, an obstructing stone in the cystic duct.

   F. **Large nodules** in the liver suggest a metastatic cancer.

   G. **Splenomegaly** is found in many patients with cirrhosis, chronic active hepatitis, and acute alcoholic liver disease. However, splenomegaly is present in less than 5% of patients with acute viral hepatitis, gallstones, or malignant biliary obstruction. Hepatomegaly, especially if the liver span is ≥15 cm and tender, suggests alcoholic hepatitis or malignancy.

   H. **In newborns,** jaundice can be detected by examining the child in a well-lighted room and blanching the skin with digital pressure, revealing skin and subcutaneous tissue color. Icterus is first seen in the face and progresses to the trunk and the extremities; the degree of cephalocaudad progression correlates roughly with the bilirubin level (ie, the face, approximately 5 mg/dL; midabdomen, approximately 15 mg/dL; and the soles of the feet, approximately 20 mg/dL).

   I. **Infants** should be examined for signs of infection, increased hemoglobin load, a metabolic disorder, or biliary obstruction.

V. **Laboratory Tests** (Figures 38–1 and 38–2). Most causes of jaundice can be determined with a history, physical examination, and simple laboratory evaluation.

   A. **Basic tests.** In all jaundiced patients, total and direct bilirubin levels and complete blood count should be done.

      1. In **neonates** (Figure 38–1), Coombs' testing, peripheral smear, and reticulocyte count should also be done; ill or premature infants with jaundice also should be evaluated for infection (chest x-ray, blood/urine cultures).

      2. In jaundiced **nonneonates** (Figure 38–2), liver function tests are required in all patients, with further testing based on clinical findings.

         a. **Liver profile**
            (1) In classic hepatocellular disease, the **alkaline phosphatase** value is less than three times the upper limit of normal; in obstructive disease, values are greater than three times normal.
            (2) **Transaminase values** (alanine aminotransferase [ALT] and aspartate aminotransferase [AST]) generally reflect the degree of hepatocellular disease. With typical **obstructive jaundice,** transaminases are typically two to three times the upper limit of normal, whereas values generally are at least five times normal with hepatocellular disease.

         b. **A peripheral smear, reticulocyte count,** and **Coombs' testing** should be done in all jaundiced patients with unconjugated hyperbilirubinemia or anemia.

         c. **A prothrombin time (PT)** should be done with suspicion of obstruction or severe liver dysfunction. In **obstructive disease,** a prolonged PT may respond

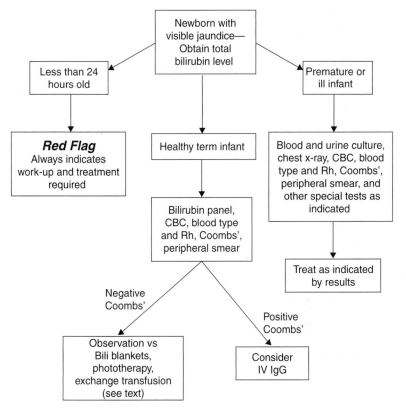

FIGURE 38–1. Evaluation of the newborn with jaundice. CBC, complete blood count; IV, IgG, intravenous.

dramatically to 10 mg subcutaneous vitamin K, whereas minimal improvement with vitamin K implies hepatocellular disease.

    d. Urinalysis for bilirubin and urobilinogen can be helpful, because it is inexpensive and detects only conjugated bilirubin.

B. Additional special testing (Figure 38–2).

    1. Imaging studies

        a. In patients with suspected extrahepatic obstruction, **ultrasonography** is indicated to detect dilated biliary ducts. Dilated biliary ducts indicate obstruction; ultrasound is over 90% specific, and, with jaundice greater than a week, is close to 90% sensitive in detecting obstruction.

        Computerized tomography (CT) is similar in sensitivity and specificity to ultrasound, but is more expensive. CT is indicated when ultrasonography is unsatisfactory because of equivocal findings or technical limitations (eg, overlying bowel gas).

        b. Endoscopic retrograde cholangiopancreatography (ERCP), percutaneous transhepatic cholangiography (PTC), or **magnetic resonance cholangiopancreatography (MRCP)** is indicated if extrahepatic obstruction is strongly suspected on clinical grounds (even if ultrasound results are negative) or if additional anatomic information is required for diagnosis. The choice of ERCP vs. PTC vs. MRCP depends mainly on local expertise and availability. ERCP is often preferred if planned therapy includes papillotomy, stenting, pancreatic stone removal, or biopsy. MRCP is becoming the preferred test for evaluating anatomy because of no risk for inducing post-procedure pancreatitis.

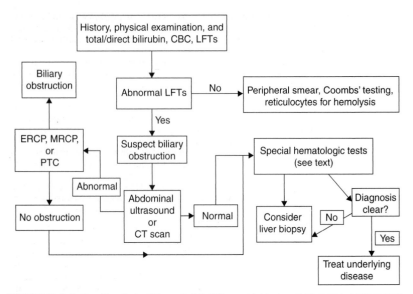

FIGURE 38–2. Evaluation of jaundice in children and adults. CBC, complete blood count; CT, computerized tomography; ERCP, endoscopic retrograde cholangiopancreatography; LFTs, liver function tests; MRCP, magnetic resonance cholangiopancreatography; PTC, percutaneous transhepatic cholangiography.

2. **Hematologic testing**
   a. **Viral hepatitis studies**
      (1) **Immunoglobulin M (IgM) hepatitis A antibody** appears at the onset of symptoms of hepatitis A infection and clears within 6 months during convalescence.
      (2) **Hepatitis B surface antigen (HBsAg)** is the first serologic marker to appear in hepatitis B infection, starting 2–6 weeks before symptoms. The antigen generally clears within 6 months, but persists in patients with chronic active or persistent infection.
      (3) **Hepatitis B core antibody (anti-HBc)** is present in virtually all patients with active hepatitis B infection. Since anti-HBc appears later than HBsAg but often before clinical symptoms develop, it serves to confirm hepatitis B infection when HBsAg is present. Anti-HBc persists for life.
      (4) **Hepatitis C antibody** becomes detectable by **enzyme immunoassay (EIA)** in 90% of patients by 12 weeks after infection. Because of possible acquired maternal antibody, EIA testing in neonates at risk is not considered reliable until 12 weeks of age. Although EIA is >97% sensitive in detecting hepatitis C, it cannot differentiate acute, chronic, or resolved infection and should be confirmed by **recombinant immunoblot assay (RIBA)** testing.
         (a) Negative EIA test or positive EIA coupled with negative RIBA rules out hepatitis C; an indeterminate RIBA should be followed with reverse transcriptase–polymerase chain reaction (RT-PCR) for hepatitis C RNA.
         (b) Indeterminate RIBA coupled with negative RT-PCR and normal ALT rules out hepatitis C.
      (5) **IgM antibody to Epstein-Barr virus and CMV** should also be considered in the appropriate clinical setting, although screening for hepatitis A and B should usually be done first.
   b. **Antimitochondrial antibody** to screen for primary biliary cirrhosis should be considered in patients aged 30–60 years (especially females) with evidence of chronic cholestasis. Antibodies are positive in 85–90% of patients with primary biliary cirrhosis.

    c. Antinuclear and smooth muscle antibodies are positive in about two thirds of patients with lupoid hepatitis (autoimmune hepatitis) and should be considered in patients (especially females) who have chronic liver disease without a clear cause.

    d. Serum iron, transferrin saturation, and ferritin to screen for hemochromatosis should also be considered in patients whose chronic liver disease lacks a defined cause. In hemochromatosis, the plasma iron exceeds 200 U/dL and transferrin saturation exceeds 70%.

    e. Serum protein electrophoresis is useful to screen for α_1-antitrypsin deficiency.

    f. Serum ceruloplasmin and urine copper levels to screen for Wilson's disease should be considered in patients younger than 30 years of age or in patients with hepatitis and neurologic dysfunction.

    g. One study indicated that **serum secretory component** is more reliable than alkaline phosphatase in differentiating mechanical from hepatocellular cholestasis.

    3. Liver biopsy may be useful in the following situations: (1) to differentiate chronic active from chronic persistent hepatitis, (2) to diagnose malignant involvement of the liver, and (3) to document or diagnose hepatocellular disease when the diagnosis is not otherwise possible on clinical grounds.

VI. Treatment of jaundice is directed at its underlying cause, and this should be revealed through careful history, examination and, particularly, appropriate selective laboratory evaluations.

    A. Therapy for **neonatal jaundice** is directed at treatment of underlying causes and prevention of kernicterus, a form of unconjugated hyperbilirubinemia-induced neurotoxic basal ganglial/hippocampal damage. At least three factors affect risk in neonatal hyperbilirubinemia: (1) **gestational age**—in healthy term infants, risk is low even with total serum bilirubin (TSB) as high as 23 mg/dL, whereas tolerable level is lower in premature infants; (2) **age at which jaundice is evident**—clinical jaundice at ≤24 hours of life is always nonphysiologic; and (3) **maternal/infant symptoms or signs of significant underlying disease.**

    1. With **physiologic jaundice,** which begins between the second and fourth days of life, TSB levels are <15 mg/dL, direct bilirubin is ≤1.5 mg/dL, and bilirubin rises <5 mg/dL in 24 hours and resolves by 1 week (term infants) or 2 weeks (preterm infants).

    2. Treatment of the hyperbilirubinemia of **breast-feeding jaundice,** which begins on or after the fourth day of life and peaks by day 10–15, is more frequent breast-feeding and possible involvement of a lactation consultant.

    3. Breast milk jaundice, beginning on the fourth through seventh day of life and lasting 3–10 weeks, can be treated by alternating breast and formula feeding for 2–3 days. Breast pumping should be done at formula feedings; full-time breast-feeding can be resumed when hyperbilirubinemia improves.

    4. Phototherapy exposes infants to blue-range lights, producing photoisomers of unconjugated bilirubin that are water soluble and may be excreted in bile or urine without conjugation.

        a. Phototherapy should be considered at TSB >15 mg/dL at 25–48 hours of age, >18 mg/dL at 49–72 hours of age, or >20 mg/dL past 72 hours of age. A favorable response to phototherapy is a decrease of 1–2 mg/dL within 4–6 hours, with subsequent continued decreases. Discontinuation of phototherapy should be considered once the TSB is 2 mg/dL below the threshold for initiation of therapy.

        b. The eyes of the newborn must be covered during phototherapy to prevent retinal damage if using bili-lights in the hospital. Bili-blankets are now being used more and more to allow babies to go home with their mother. Adequate fluid intake promotes the elimination of bilirubin and counteracts the dehydration associated with phototherapy.

    5. Exchange transfusion is traditionally performed when the TSB exceeds the threshold for phototherapy by 5 mg/dL or if phototherapy fails. The threshold for exchange transfusion should be lowered by 1–2 mg/dL when additional risk factors for kernicterus are present, such as perinatal asphyxia; respiratory distress; hypoglycemia; metabolic acidosis (pH ≤7.25); hypothermia (temperature, <35 °C [95 °F]); hypoproteinemia (protein, ≤5 g/dL); and signs of clinical or central nervous system deterioration.

    6. Neonates with hemolytic jaundice (Rh or ABO incompatibilities) can now be treated with high-dose intravenous immunoglobulins (IgG) to prevent both the anemia and the hyperbilirubinemia that can develop. Those infants identified with these conditions should have their hemoglobin, hematocrit, and bilirubin levels and signs of hemolysis monitored serially.

B. **Viral hepatitis.** Most patients can be treated symptomatically as outpatients. Hospital admission is indicated for inability to maintain hydration or for evidence of severe hepatocellular failure or ascites.
  1. If liver enzymes fail to return to normal within 6 months, liver biopsy is indicated.
  2. Alfa-interferon can induce sustained remissions in some patients with chronic hepatitis B, C, and D. Consultation should be sought with a gastroenterologist familiar with its use.

C. **Extrahepatic obstruction**
  1. Surgical therapy is generally required for extrahepatic biliary obstruction.
  2. If fever and chills develop, suggestive of cholangitis, prompt hospitalization for intravenous antibiotics and surgical consultation is necessary. Nonoperative biliary drainage can be performed in selected patients via ERCP on transhepatically placed stents.

D. **Unconjugated hyperbilirubinemia**
  1. **Hemolytic anemia,** particularly if associated with marked hyperbilirubinemia, should be managed with appropriate specialty consultation (eg, perinatology for neonates, hematology for others).
  2. Mild unconjugated hyperbilirubinemia (eg, Gilbert's, Dubin-Johnson, Rotor's syndrome) rarely requires treatment to lower bilirubin levels.

E. **Cholestatic jaundice**
  1. **Ursodeoxycholate** (usual dose, 10–12 mg/kg/day) improves both biochemical abnormalities and symptoms in primary biliary cirrhosis and other forms of chronic cholestasis.
  2. Since **pruritus** may be disabling for some patients, leading to depression and even suicide, early treatment is advisable. Oral agents used to treat pruritus include **cholestyramine,** one packet or scoop in juice or applesauce three times a day; and antihistamines (eg, **diphenhydramine,** 25–50 mg three or four times a day).

F. **Underlying diseases** contributing to jaundice should be treated (see Chapter 71—Cirrhosis; Chapter 72—Congestive Heart Failure; Chapter 87—Thyroid Disease; Chapter 50—Pediatric Fever); drugs contributing to jaundice should be eliminated or substituted.

G. **Other hepatocellular disease.** Periodic monitoring of patients is necessary with clinical examination and liver function tests (see Chapter 43). When the disease is progressive, liver biopsy may be indicated for definitive diagnosis.

REFERENCES

Dennery PA, Seidman DS, Stevenson DK: Neonatal hyperbilirubinemia. N Engl J Med 2001;**344:**581.
Feldman M: *Sleisenger and Fordtran's Gastrointestinal and Liver Disease,* 7th ed. Saunders; 2002.
Goldman L: *Cecil Textbook of Medicine,* 21st ed. Saunders; 2000.
Pashanker D, Schreiber RA: Jaundice in older children and adolescents. Pediatr Rev 2001;**22**(7):219.

---

39   Joint Pain

L. Peter Schwiebert, MD

KEY POINTS

- In evaluating the complaint of joint pain, it is helpful to differentiate intra-articular from periarticular processes.
- A careful focused history, physical examination, and selective testing allow accurate diagnosis of most common causes of joint pain.
- Physicians should always consider bacterial arthritis in acute monarthritis, because delayed treatment of septic arthritis risks severe joint damage.

I. Definition. Joint pain (arthralgia) is discomfort in one or more joints, with or without evidence of joint effusion, swelling, erythema, or tenderness. Joint pain can be due to **intra-articular** or **periarticular** processes. **Intra-articular** processes include **synovitis** (viral or bacterial infection, transient synovitis, gout/pseudogout, rheumatoid arthritis [RA], rheumatic fever [RF], idiopathic) or **degenerative disease** (osteoarthritis [OA], post-traumatic). **Periarticular processes** include **soft tissue diseases** (fibromyalgia, hypermobility syndromes, viremia, primary Lyme disease) and **idiopathic diseases** (growing pains, psychogenic rheumatism).

II. Common Diagnoses. Surveys reveal 11% of patients visiting general and family physicians in the United States have complaints related to the back and the upper or lower extremities. Unspecified arthritis is the 14th most common principal diagnosis seen by these physicians.

A. Intra-articular processes
   1. Synovitis
      a. Bacterial/viral
         (1) Transient synovitis occurs in children 3–10 years old, related to recent (within the past week) viral infection. Males are affected more frequently than females.
         (2) Viral synovitis can occur with a variety of infections, especially hepatitis B, mumps, and rubella.
         (3) Over 50% of adult **bacterial arthritis** is due to *Neisseria gonorrhoeae;* risk factors include past history of gonorrheal infection, multiple sex partners, and non-use of barrier contraceptives. Other causes of adult **bacterial arthritis** (*Staphylococcus aureus,* group A and B streptococci, gram-negative bacteria) tend to occur with immune compromise (diabetes mellitus, malignancy, human immunodeficiency virus disease); chronic liver disease; periarticular cellulitis or skin ulceration; intravenous drug use; or history of a damaged joint (eg, with chronic severe RA). Ninety-six percent of bacterial arthritis in children younger than 6 years old is due to *Haemophilus influenzae;* children with sickle cell disease are at risk for infection with salmonella species.
      b. Crystal-induced
         (1) Gouty arthritis, intra-articular uric acid crystal deposition caused by enzyme deficiency/overproduction/underexcretion, occurs most commonly in men older than 40 years and postmenopausal women, especially with a positive family history of gout. Medications (eg, thiazide diuretics, aspirin, niacin); myeloproliferative disorders; multiple myeloma; hypothyroidism; chronic renal disease; and alcohol ingestion are also associated with gouty attacks.
         (2) Pseudogout, calcium pyrophosphate dihydrate (CPPD) deposition disease, most commonly occurs in those older than age 60 and can be associated with a variety of metabolic diseases (eg, hyperparathyroidism, hypothyroidism, diabetes mellitus, Wilson's disease, gout).
      c. Immune-complex
         (1) Rheumatoid arthritis (RA), one of a family of autoimmune inflammatory disorders (including systemic lupus erythematosus [SLE], polymyalgia rheumatica, and polymyositis/dermatomyositis) mainly affects synovial membranes. One to 2% of the US population has RA, with a female:male prevalence of 3:1 and usual age of onset between 20 and 40 years. A positive family history is a risk factor. Eighty-five percent of patients with SLE are women, blacks are affected four times as frequently as whites, and positive family history also plays a role. A variety of drugs can cause a lupus-like syndrome; the most common offenders include chlorpromazine, hydralazine, isoniazid, methyldopa, procainamide, and quinidine.
         (2) Lyme disease, transmitted by a bite from a tick carrying the spirochete, *Borrelia burgdorferi,* can manifest as autoimmune synovitis in stage 3 (late) disease. Incidence of Lyme disease is highest in summer months, particularly in the Northeastern United States, Wisconsin, Minnesota, and California.
         (3) Rheumatic fever (RF), due to group A β-hemolytic streptococcal (GABHS)–induced immune complex synovitis, is rare (<1:10,000), and its

overall incidence is progressively declining. RF is most common in 5- to 15-year-olds, with slight male predominance.

2. **Degenerative disease**
   a. **Osteoarthritis (OA)** is the most common joint disease, affecting at least 20 million US adults; radiologic evidence of OA is present in weight-bearing joints of 90% of individuals by age 40. Age increases the likelihood of symptomatic disease.
   b. **Traumatic arthritis** is more likely with a history of recent or remote trauma to affected joint(s) (eg, falls, motor vehicle accidents, sports injuries, and overuse).

B. **Periarticular processes**
   1. **Soft tissue**
      a. **Viremia** can occur at any age; in winter months in the Northern hemisphere, influenza is commonly implicated.
      b. **Hypermobility syndromes** cause arthralgias most commonly in 10- to 15-year-olds, especially but not exclusively associated with Ehlers-Danlos or Down syndromes.
      c. **Fibromyalgia** is most common in 20- to 50-year-old women, affecting 3–10% of the general population; it may be associated with sleep disorders, depression, heightened perception of normal stimuli, and hypothyroidism.
   2. **Idiopathic**
      a. **Growing pains** occur in up to 18% of school-aged children, peaking at age 11 years and continuing through adolescence. This problem is more common in females than males and with a family history of similar symptoms.
      b. **Psychogenic pain** is more common with depression or school phobia (eg, separation anxiety or overly dependent parent-child interaction).

III. **Symptoms.** A systematic history often assists in narrowing the joint pain differential diagnosis; in addition to evaluating for risk factors, history includes:
   A. **Location/number of joints involved**
      1. **Monarticular arthralgia**
         a. **Septic arthritis** typically affects the knee, but may involve the hip, wrist, shoulder, or ankle.
         b. **Gout** classically presents with first metatarsophalangeal (MTP) arthritis, though it also commonly involves the foot, ankle, or knee.
         c. **Transient synovitis** typically affects the hip.
         d. **Lyme disease** is typically monarticular, characteristically targeting the knee.
         e. **OA** affects large joints (eg, knee, hip) and the first carpometacarpal (CMC) and distal interphalangeal (DIP) hand joints.
         f. **Pseudogout** also commonly affects large joints (eg, knees, wrists) and may also affect metacarpophalangeals (MCPs), hips, shoulders, elbows, or ankles.
      2. **Polyarticular arthralgia**
         a. **Viremia** and **growing pains** cause polyarticular arthralgia.
         b. **Rheumatologic/autoimmune** diseases (eg, RA) typically present with symmetrical multiple joint involvement, often of smaller, non–weight-bearing joints (eg, hand proximal interphalangeals [PIPs], MCPs, wrists, toes, ankles).
         c. One criterion for **RF** is polyarticular involvement, especially ankles, knees, hips, wrists, elbows, and shoulders.
   B. **Chronology**
      1. The pain of **trauma, gout, pseudogout,** and **septic arthritis** is typically **acute** onset.
      2. Arthralgias associated with growing pains, fibromyalgia, hypermobility, OA, and collagen diseases (eg, RA) tend to follow an **insidious/chronic/recurrent** pattern.
   C. **Exacerbating/alleviating factors**
      1. Osteoarthritis, traumatic arthritis, overuse injuries, and growing pains tend to **worsen with activity.**
      2. **Psychogenic pain** associated with school phobia worsens before school and improves on weekends.
      3. **Nocturnal worsening** is associated with growing pains; an **acute gout attack** may begin at night.
   D. **Associated symptoms**
      1. Complaint of a **red, very tender joint** and feverishness/chills are associated with septic arthritis, gout, and RF.

2. **Stiffness** following immobilization is associated with **osteoarthritis** and **autoimmune arthritis** (eg, RA); OA stiffness ("gelling") typically abates within 15 minutes of activity, whereas RA stiffness persists at least an hour.
3. Depending on specific underlying disease, **autoimmune arthritis** may be associated with rashes (eg, butterfly malar rash, sun sensitivity, alopecia, or discoid lesions with SLE).
4. **RF** may be associated with a macular, circinate erythematous truncal rash; Sydenham's chorea (choreoathetoid facial, tongue, or upper extremity movements); and subcutaneous nodules of tendon sheaths (especially in children) (see Table 39–1).
5. **Psychogenic arthralgia** may be associated with symptoms of anxiety, depression, or other psychiatric disease.
6. **Fibromyalgia** frequently is associated with fatigue, sleep disorders, chronic headaches, and irritable bowel symptoms.

IV. **Signs.** A careful, focused physical examination is crucial in differentiating articular from periarticular processes and, together with symptoms and risk factors, guides testing strategies.
  A. **Vital signs/general appearance**
     1. **Fever** is associated with septic arthritis, viral arthralgias, gout, and RF.
     2. **Ill or toxic appearance** (or both) raises suspicion of septic arthritis.
     3. **Integument/mucous membranes**
        a. **Erythema migrans (EM)** occurs in 90% of patients with early Lyme disease 3–30 days following a tick bite. EM begins as a red papule at the site of the bite, enlarging circumferentially over days to a month with central clearing and typical resolution over 3–4 weeks.
        b. A generalized evanescent, pinkish maculopapular exanthem makes **viremia** a likely cause of arthralgias.
        c. **SLE** lesions include malar erythema ("butterfly rash"), discoid macular plaquelike lesions, alopecia, or oral ulcers.
  B. **Joint findings. Intra-articular processes** have abnormal findings of affected joints, ranging from heat/erythema, to firm or boggy swelling, to synovial or joint line tenderness, to restricted range of motion (ROM). In **periarticular processes,** by contrast, the joint examination is often normal or minimally abnormal.
     1. **Intra-articular processes**
        a. In **transient synovitis,** there is decreased hip ROM, especially internal rotation.
        b. **Bacterial synovitis/septic joint** presents dramatically with a warm/erythematous joint, joint effusion, and restricted ROM.
        c. **Viral synovitis** may show tenderness and synovial involvement, but no deformity.
        d. **Gouty arthritis** presents with swollen, red, tender-to-the touch joint or less dramatically with swollen joint, restricted ROM, and painful weight-bearing. Following multiple attacks, tophaceous invasion may grossly deform affected joints.

TABLE 39–1. JONES CRITERIA FOR RHEUMATIC FEVER

Major Manifestations	Minor Manifestations	Supporting Evidence of Antecedent Group A Streptococcal Infection
Carditis	Clinical findings	Positive throat culture or rapid
Polyarthritis	Arthralgia	streptococcal antigen test
Chorea	Fever	Elevated or rising ASO or antiDNAse B titer
Erythema marginatum	Laboratory findings	
Subcutaneous nodules	Elevated acute phase reactants	
	Erythrocyte sedimentation rate	
	C-reactive protein	
	Prolonged PR interval on ECG	

If supported by evidence of preceding group A streptococcal infection, the presence of two major manifestations or one major and two minor manifestations indicates a high probability of acute rheumatic fever.
ASO, antistreptolysin-O; ECG, electrocardiogram.
From Adnans D: Guidelines for the diagnosis of rheumatic fever: Jones criteria, updated 1992. Circulation 1993;**87**:302.

     e. Pseudogout shows less dramatic inflammation than gout; one may note firm hypertrophy due to chronic chondrocalcinosis.

     f. OA findings typically include crepitus, tender joint line, firm swelling (bony hypertrophy and osteophytes, rather than synovitis), and restricted extremes of ROM.

     g. Traumatic arthritis findings are similar to OA; there may be deformity at the site of previous trauma or surgery.

     h. RA findings include symmetric, swollen, warm, tender boggy joints; chronic active disease produces deformities, including ulnar deviation of digits, and Boutonnière/"swan-neck" digit deformities.

     i. A tender joint, with or without synovitis, occurs with stage 3 **Lyme disease** (late persistent infection).

     j. RF may produce tender joints/synovium (large joints); RF may be monarticular in adults.

  2. Periarticular

     a. Five criteria establish a diagnosis of **hypermobility;** these include (1) passive opposition of thumb to flexor forearm, (2) passive finger hyperextension parallel to forearm, (3) elbow hyperextension, (4) knee hyperextension, and (5) palms on floor with knees extended.

     b. Fibromyalgia is diagnosed by reproducing >11 of 18 mainly axial designated tender sites (occiputs, supraspinati, glutei, greater trochanters, upper trapezius borders, anterior cervical 5–7 interspaces, second anterior rib lateral to the costochondral junction, lateral epicondyles, and medial fat pads of knees).

     c. There are no characteristic articular or periarticular findings with **growing pains** or **psychogenic arthralgias.**

V. Laboratory Tests (Figure 39–1) can be selective and based on careful history and focused physical examination as described. Because some diagnoses become apparent only over time, serial evaluation and testing may be necessary to arrive at a correct diagnosis. No further testing is necessary if hypermobility syndrome is suspected or for findings consistent with growing pains in absence of articular inflammation. If joint effusion is present and diagnosis is uncertain, or if septic arthritis is suspected, arthrocentesis is indicated (Table 39–2).

  A. Hematologic tests

     1. In **acute RF,** erythrocyte sedimentation rate (ESR) and antistreptolysin-O (ASO) are elevated, though these are normal in 10% of patients with other findings compatible with RF.

     2. In 75% of patients with **RA, rheumatoid factor** is positive; false-positive results occur with syphilis, sarcoidosis, endocarditis, advanced age, or asymptomatic relatives of patients with autoimmune diseases. Twenty percent of **RA patients** have a positive antinuclear antibody (ANA) test.

     3. Hematologic abnormalities associated with **SLE** include positive ANA (in 95–100%), anti-native DNA (in 50%), anti-smooth muscle (in 20%), anemia (in 60%), leukopenia (in 45%), and thrombocytopenia (in 30%).

     4. In acute **gouty** attack, uric level is increased (>7.5 mg/dL) at some point during the attack, though a single level is normal in up to 25% of acute gouty patients. Commonly, the white blood cell count and ESR are elevated during an acute gouty attack.

     5. In **Lyme disease** up to 50% of patients can be enzyme-linked immunosorbent assay (ELISA)-antibody negative during the first several weeks of illness. Repeat titers should be obtained in these cases; a fourfold rise in titer is diagnostic of recent infection. All positive or equivocal ELISA *B burgdorferi* tests should be confirmed with Western immunoblot testing.

  B. Joint fluid examination (Table 39–2). **Gouty arthritis** is definitively diagnosed by finding urate crystals (needlelike, negatively birefringent); pseudogout crystals are rhomboid-shaped.

  C. Radiology

     1. In **OA,** plain radiographs show joint space narrowing and irregularity, periarticular spurring, and juxta-articular sclerosis.

     2. In **RA,** no radiographic abnormalities may be evident during the first 6 months of disease. The earliest changes are evident in the wrists and feet and include soft tissue swelling and juxta-articular demineralization. Later changes include joint space narrowing and periarticular erosions.

     3. Pseudogout manifests with changes similar to those in OA, along with cartilage calcification.

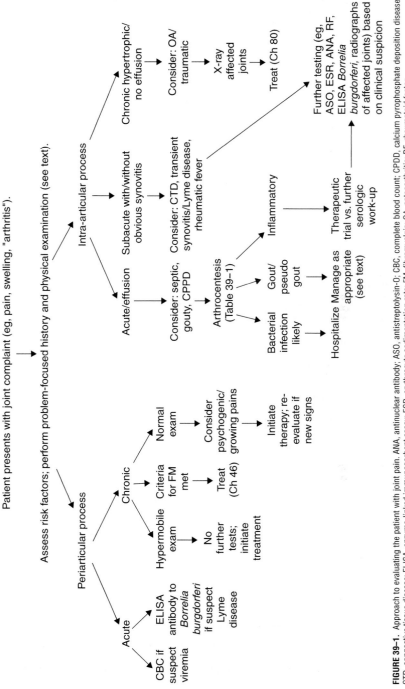

FIGURE 39–1. Approach to evaluating the patient with joint pain. ANA, antinuclear antibody; ASO, antistreptolysin-O; CBC, complete blood count; CPDD, calcium pyrophosphate deposition disease; CTD, connective tissue disease; ELISA, enzyme-linked immunosorbent assay; ESR, erythrocyte sedimentation rate; FM, fibromyalgia; OA, osteoarthritis; RF, rheumatoid factor.

TABLE 39–2. JOINT FLUID FINDINGS

	Normal	Trauma	Infection	Crystalline Disease	Inflammatory
Color	Clear to yellow	Bloody to xanthrochromic	Yellow to cloudy	Yellow to cloudy	Yellow to cloudy
Cell count (cells/µL) WBC/RBC	<200/0	<1000/many	1000–200,000/few	1000–2000/few	1000–20,000/few
Crystals	Negative	Negative	Negative	Yes; pseudogout and gout	Negative
Culture	Negative	Negative	Positive	Negative	Negative

RBC, red blood cell count; WBC, white blood cell count.

    4. In **transient synovitis,** soft tissue periarticular swelling may be evident, but is a nonspecific finding.

    5. In **RF,** one manifestation of carditis may be cardiomegaly and other signs of congestive heart failure on plain chest radiographs.

  D. Other testing

    1. Proteinuria occurs in 30% of **SLE** patients.

    2. Echocardiography in RF may confirm valvular disease or dilated cardiomyopathy with decreased ejection fraction.

VI. Treatment is directed at the underlying cause of joint pain, which can accurately be arrived at via appropriate history, focused examination, and selective testing.

  A. Intra-articular diseases

    1. Transient synovitis usually resolves on its own over a few days. Bed rest, traction with slight hip flexion, with or without age-appropriate oral nonsteroidal anti-inflammatory drugs (NSAIDs) may increase comfort. Follow-up plain hip radiographs at 1 and 3 months can detect avascular femoral head necrosis, a possible complication of transient synovitis.

    2. Septic arthritis requires treatment with systemic antibiotics and possible orthopedic consultation, which should occur in a hospital setting.

    3. Gouty arthritis

      a. Acute attack

        (1) NSAIDs (eg, oral indomethacin, 25–50 mg every 8 hours for 5–10 days or until symptoms are controlled) are the first-line treatment.

        (2) Alternately, **colchicine** (0.5–0.6 mg orally hourly until symptoms are controlled or diarrhea develops, with maximum of 8 mg) is effective but limited by gastrointestinal (GI) toxicity. GI symptoms can be limited using intravenous colchicine, 2 mg in 25–50 mL normal saline, with additional 1-mg doses every 6 hours for 2 doses (maximum: 4 mg total). Colchicine should not be used in those with hepatic and renal impairment.

        (3) Intra-articular steroids (eg, 10–40 mg of triamcinolone) can be effective for monarticular gout; an oral steroid (eg, prednisone, 40–60 mg initially and tapered over 7 days) may be effective for polyarticular acute gout.

        (4) Analgesics (other than aspirin, which may precipitate gout) may be necessary for pain control.

        (5) Bed rest during the acute attack is also helpful.

      b. Chronic management

        (1) Patient education

          (a) Patients should be advised to avoid or limit their intake of high-purine foods, including meats, seafood, meat extracts and gravies, yeast and yeast extracts, alcoholic beverages, beans, peas, lentils, oatmeal, spinach, asparagus, cauliflower, and mushrooms.

          (b) The following medications can precipitate gouty attacks and should be avoided: thiazide and loop diuretics, low-dose aspirin (<3 g/day), and niacin.

        (2) The decision to initiate **preventive medication** depends on the individual patient's risk of recurrent gouty arthritis; for example, an individual who had a single attack and is willing to avoid alcohol and lose weight is low risk, while an older individual with multiple attacks or mild chronic renal insufficiency, or requiring a diuretic, is considered high risk.

    (a) **Oral colchicine,** 0.6 mg twice daily, may be effective prophylaxis in individuals with mild hyperuricemia and few acute attacks; colchicine therapy also decreases the risk of an acute attack when initiating uricosurics.

    (b) **Urate-lowering** therapy is indicated for patients with frequent acute attacks, those not controlled on colchicine, or those with tophi or renal disease. The goal of therapy is to keep serum uric acid <6 mg/dL, and medication choice is guided by results of a 24-hour urine collection for uric acid (if <800 mg/24 hr, a uricosuric should be used; if >800 mg/24 hr, allopurinol should be used).

        (i) **Uricosurics,** which block tubular reabsorption of urate, include oral probenecid, 500 mg initially with gradual increase to 1–2 g, or **sulfinpyrazone,** 50–100 mg twice daily, increasing as needed to 200–400 mg twice daily. Uricosurics should not be used in patients with chronic renal failure (serum creatinine >2 mg/dL), and patients should consume sufficient fluids to assure at least 2 L urine output daily.

        (ii) **Allopurinol,** a xanthine oxidase inhibitor that lowers plasma urate concentrations and can mobilize tophi, is indicated in patients with tophi, who overproduce uric acid, who have failed uricosuric therapy, or who have a history of renal urate stones. Dosing should begin at 100 mg orally daily for the first week, with dose increases depending on serum uric acid response. Most people require 200–300 mg/day. With tophaceous gout, the goal is to maintain uric acid at <5 mg/dL, and this may require combined allopurinol and uricosuric therapy.

  (3) Prognosis depends on age at first attack and number of attacks; destructive arthropathy is rare in those having their first attack after age 50.

4. Pseudogout treatment is directed at underlying disease. Acute symptoms may be helped with oral NSAIDs, oral colchicine (0.6 mg twice daily may benefit prophylaxis), and joint aspiration followed by intra-articular steroid injection (eg, triamcinolone, 10–40 mg, depending on joint size), as with monarticular gout.

5. RA, like other autoimmune diseases, follows a variable course, with prognosis depending on disease severity; severe disease demands early aggressive treatment with disease-modifying antirheumatic drugs (DMARDs).

  a. Supportive therapy

    (1) Patients should be educated about the disease, its variable course, and their role in self-monitoring and management.

    (2) Rest in bed is important for a severe disease flare; 2 hours' rest per day is sufficient for milder inflammation. Activity should be liberalized as tolerated by symptoms.

    (3) Exercise depends on disease activity and should start with passive ROM/hydrotherapy when pain or stiffness is worse, progressing to active then resisted ROM as symptoms abate. Joint stretching may help prevent contractures. Activities producing pain for greater than an hour after concluding the activity should be avoided.

    (4) Heat, cold therapy, and assistive devices can also control symptoms and improve quality of life.

  b. Response to **medications** can be gauged, based on the patient's stiffness, fatigue, and degree of joint swelling.

    (1) NSAIDs (eg, oral ibuprofen, 600–800 mg three to four times daily, or naproxen, 550 mg twice daily) are first-line anti-inflammatory/analgesic therapy; therapy should be carefully monitored for GI toxicity.

    (2) Poor response to NSAIDs warrants consideration of DMARDs (eg, methotrexate, gold, tumor necrosis factor inhibitors) and possible rheumatology consultation for drug selection and monitoring.

6. Lyme disease/EM (see Chapter 7).

7. RF

    a. Bed rest is indicated until the patient is afebrile without antipyretics and has a normal pulse rate, ESR, and electrocardiogram.

    b. Acute medications

       (1) Salicylates (eg, oral aspirin, 600–900 mg every 4 hours in adults) can markedly improve fever and joint symptoms.

       (2) An **oral steroid** (eg, prednisone, 40–60 mg, initially and tapered over 7 days) may relieve joint symptoms poorly controlled by salicylates.

       (3) Benzathine penicillin, 1.2 million units intramuscularly (IM) in a single dose, or **procaine penicillin,** 600,000 units IM daily for 10 days, will eradicate streptococcal infection in nonallergic patients.

    c. Endocarditis prophylaxis is indicated in children (20% have recurrent RF within 5 years) or others with RF carditis.

       (1) Benzathine penicillin, 1.2 million units IM, should be given monthly.

       (2) Prophylaxis can be discontinued after 5 years of treatment or in patients older than 25 years.

  8. Traumatic arthritis/OA (see Chapter 80).

B. Periarticular diseases

  1. Viremia-induced arthralgias should be treated symptomatically and supportively (see Chapter 55).

  2. Hypermobility enjoys a good functional prognosis with graded conditioning to provide muscle support of affected joints.

  3. Fibromyalgia (see Chapter 46).

  4. Treatment of **growing pains** involves reassurance, symptomatic analgesics, and instructions to follow up if the symptom pattern worsens.

  5. In **psychogenic arthralgia,** underlying stress or abnormal family dynamics should be identified and treated.

REFERENCES

Harris MD, Siegel LB, Allowa JA: Gout and hyperuricemia. Am Fam Physician 1999;**59**:925.

Johnson MW: Acute knee effusion: A systematic approach to diagnosis. Am Fam Physician 2000; **61**:2391.

Lane S, Gravel JW: Clinical utility of common serum rheumatologic tests. Am Fam Physician 2002; **65**:1073.

Richie AM, Francis ML: Diagnostic approach to polyarticular joint pain. Am Fam Physician 2003;**68**:1151.

Siva C, et al: Diagnosis of acute monarthritis in adults: A practical approach for the family physician. Am Fam Physician 2003;**68**:83.

---

40   Knee Complaints

Mitchell A. Kaminski, MD, MBA

KEY POINTS

- A careful history of the complaint coupled with knowledge of knee anatomy and a focused physical examination lead to accurate diagnosis.
- Evidence-based application of tests (x-ray, magnetic resonance imaging, blood work, and joint aspiration) can cost-effectively enhance diagnosis.
- Knowledge of when to refer to an orthopedist is critical in acute injuries; medication and an appropriate exercise program often benefit the patient with chronic complaints.

I. Definition. The knee is a complex, weight-bearing hinge joint comprising ligaments, cartilage, bone, and bursae (Figures 40–1 and 40–2). Knee complaints can be **acute,** most often reflecting medial or lateral external force (collateral ligament tears), excessive anterior or posterior forces with torsion (cruciate ligament injuries), or direct trauma (fractures). Immediate pain and swelling suggest hemarthrosis and more serious injury. **Chronic complaints**

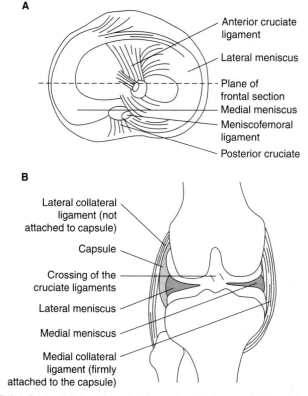

A

Anterior cruciate ligament

Lateral meniscus

Plane of frontal section

Medial meniscus

Meniscofemoral ligament

Posterior cruciate

B

Lateral collateral ligament (not attached to capsule)

Capsule

Crossing of the cruciate ligaments

Lateral meniscus

Medial meniscus

Medial collateral ligament (firmly attached to the capsule)

FIGURE 40–1. Relationship between the menisci, the capsule, and the ligaments of the knee. **A:** A superior view of the menisci and cruciate ligaments. **B:** A posterior view of a frontal section of the knee through the middle third. (Modified with permission from Steinberg GG, Akins CM, Baran DT, et al [editors]: *Ramamurti's Orthopaedics in Primary Care,* 2nd ed. Williams & Wilkins; 1992.)

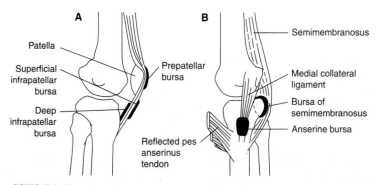

A

Patella

Superficial infrapatellar bursa

Deep infrapatellar bursa

Prepatellar bursa

B

Semimembranosus

Medial collateral ligament

Bursa of semimembranosus

Anserine bursa

Reflected pes anserinus tendon

FIGURE 40–2. Bursae about the knee. **A:** The lateral view. **B:** The medial view. (Modified with permission from Steinberg GG, Akins CM, Baran DT, et al [editors]: *Ramamurti's Orthopaedics in Primary Care,* 2nd ed. Williams & Wilkins; 1992.)

reflect overuse, inflammation such as friction between the iliotibial band and the lateral femoral condyle (iliotibial band syndrome) (or both); patellofemoral tracking abnormalities (patellofemoral arthralgia, chondromalacia, and subluxation); or traction trauma (of the calcifying tibial apophysis in Osgood-Schlatter disease, or of the distal pole of the patella in Sinding-Larsen-Johansson syndrome). **Bursitis** results from acute bursal contusion (prepatellar or superficial infrapatellar), overuse (deep infrapatellar or anserine bursa), or intraarticular inflammation (Baker's cyst.) The symptoms of **rheumatoid arthritis and osteoarthritis** are chronic, unlike the arthritis of **gout or pseudogout,** which flares acutely.

II. **Common Diagnoses.** The knee joint is a frequent source of complaints in primary care practice. Each year, 1 of every 10 persons in the United States suffers an injury to the leg warranting medical care or activity restriction. The knee, after the back, ankle, and foot, is the most common site for arthritis.

   A. **Acute ligamentous** (collateral, cruciate, or iliotibial band) **and cartilaginous (meniscal) injuries** are more likely in young and active patients. Collateral and cruciate ligament injuries are more common in sports involving contact or torsion of the lower extremity (eg, football, soccer, and skiing). The medial collateral ligament is more often injured. Cruciate ligament tears are often accompanied by other injuries due to the severe trauma involved.

   B. **Patellofemoral dysfunction** is an overuse syndrome occurring most often in jumping sports (eg, basketball). It is most frequent in tall, adolescent females with an abnormal "Q" angle (Figure 40–3). Abnormal patellar tracking in the femoral condylar groove with chronic stresses, recurrent dislocation, or both leads to degeneration of the patellar cartilage (chondromalacia patellae).

   C. The **iliotibial band syndrome** occurs most frequently in runners and can be precipitated by a change in footwear, an increase in a running schedule, or prolonged downhill running.

   D. **Bursitis** (prepatellar, infrapatellar, or anserine; Baker's cyst) can reflect acute or chronic injury.

   E. **Fractures** of the patella or femoral condyles follow acute trauma; compressive, rotational, or lateral stresses can result in tibial plateau fracture. Bone that is pathologically weaker (eg, osteoporosis) than ligaments will fracture before the ligaments will tear. Dis-

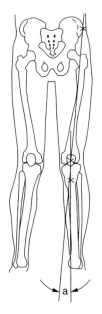

FIGURE 40–3. "Q" angle. A normal "Q" angle is <14–15 degrees.

tal femoral Salter type I fractures in adolescents may initially mask as a "ligament tear."
- **F. Osgood-Schlatter disease** (traumatic apophysitis of the tibial tubercle) and **osteochondritis dissecans** occur in adolescents. Osgood-Schlatter disease is more common in males than females; the additional risk factors for osteochondritis dissecans are unknown.
- **G. Arthritis** (rheumatoid or osteoarthritis, gout, or pseudogout) often underlies chronic knee complaints; increasing patient age makes those disorders more likely. Arthritis of the knee is associated with obesity and repetitive trauma, both occupational and recreational. Illnesses such as diabetes mellitus, sickle cell anemia, and recurrent infections often underlie septic arthritis. (See also Chapters 39 and 80.)
- **H. Pain referred from the hip** should be considered especially in pediatric patients, and in older patients at risk for metastatic disease and fracture of the hip (Chapter 42).
- **III. Symptoms.** In approaching the patient with knee complaints, taking a careful history is vital to arriving at the diagnosis. The history should include the mechanism of injury, precipitating factors, or both; chronology; location of symptoms; and exacerbating and alleviating factors. The site of pain and swelling often helps localize the abnormality. Some symptoms are suggestive of specific disorders.
  - **A. Pain**
    1. **Mild pain** over the lateral side of the knee suggests iliotibial band syndrome or collateral ligament strain. **Moderate to severe pain** usually occurs with fractures.
    2. **Localized pain** and **effusion** occur with incomplete disruption of ligaments. **Diffuse pain,** especially with climbing stairs or getting up from a squatting position, is a hallmark of chondromalacia patellae.
    3. **Pain with weight bearing** often occurs with meniscal tears and with osteochondritis dissecans. Inability to bear weight is common with fractures.
    4. **Pain with resisted knee extension** (eg, from running, climbing, jumping, or kicking) occurs with Osgood-Schlatter disease, Sinding-Larsen-Johansson syndrome, and chondromalacia patellae.
    5. **Aching pain** in the knee, even at rest, may indicate osteochondritis dissecans. Knee pain from rheumatoid arthritis is worse after inactivity, while activity tends to precipitate pain in osteoarthritis.
    6. **Pain limited to the knee** is common with septic arthritis. Knee pain referred from the hip may be the only symptom of hip disease.
  - **B. Mechanical symptoms**
    1. A **"pop" followed by knee instability** may occur with complete ligament disruption, particularly of the cruciate ligaments, and with patellar or quadriceps tendon rupture.
    2. **"Locking"** or **"giveway"** suggests a bucket handle meniscal tear.
    3. A loose joint body may cause **locking or restricted range of motion** in advanced cases of osteochondritis dissecans.
  - **C. Swelling**
    1. **Rapid swelling** is usual with hemarthrosis.
    2. **Swelling behind the knee** with variable to no pain is seen with Baker's cyst.
    3. **Swelling with pain over the tibial tubercle** is seen with Osgood-Schlatter disease. **Swelling and pain over the respective bursa** is seen in prepatellar, infrapatellar, and anserine bursitis (Figure 40–2).
    4. **Joint swelling** is more common with rheumatoid arthritis than with osteoarthritis (see Chapter 80).
  - **D. Stiffness**
    1. A patient may feel **"something out of place"** and be unable to flex or extend the knee with patellar dislocation.
    2. **Stiffness that is worse after inactivity** is common with rheumatoid arthritis.
  - **E.** A **limp** may be noticed in patients who have knee pain referred from the hip.
  - **F. Systemic symptoms**
    1. Rheumatoid arthritis is accompanied by systemic symptoms more often than is osteoarthritis.
    2. **Fever and chills** are common with septic arthritis.
- **IV. Signs.** *A careful history combined with a systematic knee examination leads to a more accurate diagnosis.* Examination after an acute injury is often limited by pain and swelling and may require orthopedic referral for examination under anesthesia. Knee examination involves ***inspection, palpation, and special maneuvers.***
  - **A. Inspection. Tense effusion** is seen in patellar fracture, and a tense, hot effusion is common with septic arthritis. Varying amounts of joint effusion are seen with rheumatoid

arthritis, osteoarthritis, and the arthritis of gout and pseudogout. **Shortening** and **deformity** may occur with femoral condylar fractures and to varying degrees with rheumatoid arthritis, osteoarthritis, and the arthritis of gout and pseudogout. **Patella alta** (high position) or **patella baja** (low position) are seen with knee flexion in patellar tendon or quadriceps tendon rupture, respectively. **Erythema** may appear in patients with femoral condylar fractures, and it is present to varying degrees in patients with rheumatoid arthritis, osteoarthritis, and the arthritis of gout and pseudogout. **Hemarthrosis** may occur with femoral condylar fractures.

B. **Palpation.** Localization of tenderness by palpation provides valuable diagnostic clues (Figure 40–4). **Localized swelling and tenderness** over the affected bursa will be found in bursitis. Tenderness is also common with femoral condylar fractures. Hip or groin tenderness and pain with rocking of the hip are the primary clues to knee pain referred from the hip. **Crepitance** is palpable with patellar fracture.

C. **Special maneuvers.** Special maneuvers (Table 40–1) may reveal signs of ligamentous or meniscal injury or patellar instability. **Limitation in range of motion** is common with septic arthritis, effusion, and muscle spasm. Irritation with range-of-motion testing, and possibly a restriction of range of motion caused by a loose body, are seen with osteochondritis dissecans and meniscal tear. **Neural compromise** (altered sensation or loss of motor ability) and **vascular compromise** (loss of peripheral pulse) may occur with femoral condylar fractures. **Increased pain with compression** of the affected side of the joint occurs with tibial plateau fractures.

V. **Laboratory Tests.** In most patients, a careful history and focused examination will allow for accurate diagnosis without additional testing. Additional studies can be ordered if a diagnosis is in doubt, or if findings will affect decisions on additional surgical or medical treatment.

A. **Imaging studies**

1. **Plain radiographs** should be ordered whenever the severity of injury or physical signs suggests a fracture. The Ottawa Knee Rule (Figure 40–5) is a highly validated, sensitive, and specific guideline for accurately determining the need for x-ray in acute knee injury.

   a. **Anteroposterior, lateral,** and **30-degree sunrise views** are standard.

   b. **A lateral x-ray of the tibial tubercle** will show fragmentation of the apophysis of the tibial tubercle in Osgood-Schlatter disease, but is usually not required.

   c. The **intercondylar notch or tunnel x-ray** view is helpful in searching for loose bodies, such as those that may be found in osteochondritis dissecans.

2. **Magnetic resonance imaging (MRI)** has not been proven superior to clinical evaluation by an experienced examiner in acute knee injuries, but is extremely helpful

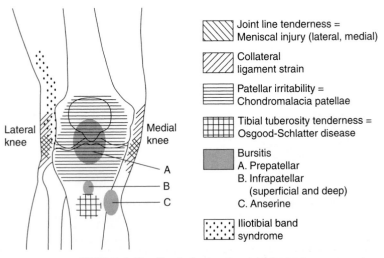

FIGURE 40–4. Sites of knee tenderness and suggested diagnoses.

TABLE 40–1. SPECIAL MANEUVERS IN THE KNEE EXAMINATION

Test	Method	Significance
McMurray's	Extend axially compressed knee with internal tibial rotation and then with external tibial rotation	Locking or popping suggests meniscal injury
Drawer sign	Pull/push tibia anteriorly and posteriorly with 90-degree flexion and foot planted	Laxity found with cruciate ligament tear
Lachman's maneuver	With knee flexed 20 degrees and femur supported, pull tibia anteriorly	Step-up from lower patella to tibial tuberosity indicates anterior cruciate ligament instability
Collateral ligament stressing	Valgus varus stress of knee in full knee extension then 30-degree flexion	Laxity with full extension suggests collateral and cruciate ligament injury. Laxity only at 30-degree flexion suggests collateral ligament tear
Apprehension sign	Valgus varus stress on patella with quadriceps relaxed, knee extended	Extreme guarding suggests patellar subluxation
Patellar irritability	Compress patella against femoral condyles	Tenderness indicates chondromalacia patellae
Thigh circumference measurement	Measure thigh circumference at an equal distance above both midpatellae	Decreased circumference of thigh above affected knee suggests subacute or chronic disorder with quadriceps atrophy

in accurately assessing torn meniscus or cruciate ligaments. MRI may also be useful in assessing bone pathology underlying chronic knee pain.

3. **Arthrography** or MRI definitively diagnose a **Baker's cyst.**

B. **Aspiration of effusion** may be done for diagnostic purposes; aspiration of tense effusion will also provide some pain relief.

A knee x-ray series is only required for knee injury patients with any of these findings:
1. Age 55 years or older
   or
2. Isolated tenderness of patella*
   or
3. Tenderness at head of fibula
   or
4. Inability to flex to 90 degrees
   or
5. Inability to bear weight both immediately and in the emergency department (4 steps)†

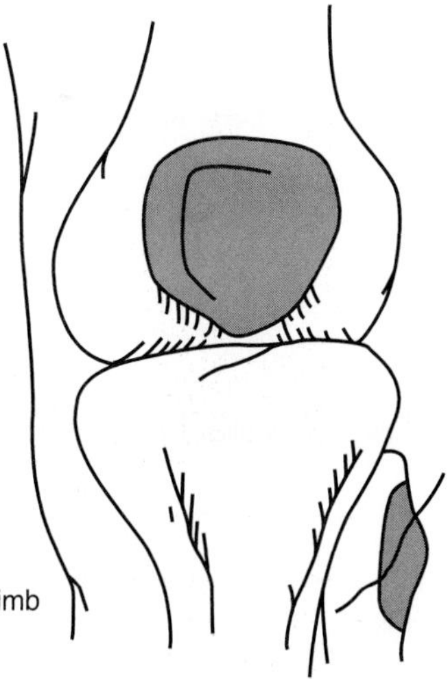

* No bone tenderness of knee other than patella.
†Unable to transfer weight twice onto each lower limb regardless of limping.

FIGURE 40–5. The Ottawa Knee Rule for the use of radiography in acute knee injuries. (From Stiell IG, et al: Validity of the "real" Ottawa Knee Rule. Ann Emerg Med 1999;**33**(2):241.)

1. The anterior knee is prepared with Betadine and covered with a sterile drape. A small area just medial or lateral to the patella is anesthetized with intradermal 1% Xylocaine hydrochloride. A large-bore (16- or 18-gauge) needle is inserted through the anesthetized area, and the syringe plunger is withdrawn until fluid is obtained. Bloody fluid should be sent to the laboratory in a heparinized test tube if cell counts are desired. The aspiration site is then covered with an adhesive bandage or similar dressing.

2. See Chapter 39 for information on joint fluid analysis.

C. See Chapter 39 for the laboratory evaluation of arthritis.

VI. **Treatment.** Focused history/examination and testing should differentiate those patients likely to improve with conservative care from those in whom urgent or eventual orthopedic referral is likely. Indications for urgent orthopedic referral are included in Table 40–2.

A. **Ligamentous and cartilaginous injuries**

1. **Collateral and cruciate injuries** with little or no laxity on testing should be managed as follows.

   a. **Immobilization** is accomplished with a compression dressing (cotton batting wrap with firm Ace wrap application), knee immobilizer (Velcro or strap type with lateral stays), or cylindrical cast. The length of immobilization depends on the extent of injury; protected early range of motion is an option after several days for mild sprains.

   b. **Weight bearing** is allowed as tolerated. Crutches for aid in ambulation are often initially helpful. **Isometric quadriceps exercises** (tensing of the quadriceps, 10 contractions every few hours while awake) are recommended during immobilization to minimize atrophy.

   c. **Cold application** with an ice pack through the immobilization apparatus is recommended for 24–48 hours after an acute injury. Elevation of the knee above heart level is helpful in decreasing swelling during this period.

   d. **Oral nonsteroidal anti-inflammatory drugs (NSAIDs)** such as aspirin, 600–1000 mg four times a day, or ibuprofen, 400–800 mg three times a day, with gastrointestinal precautions, are beneficial for treatment of pain and inflammation.

   e. After immobilization, **gradual rehabilitation** to full activity is necessary. The rehabilitation interval should be twice as long as the period of immobilization. For most knee injuries, strengthening of the quadriceps muscle with straight leg lifting, 10 repetitions three times daily, will promote knee stability and decrease the likelihood of reinjury. The use of ankle weights, with progressive increases in 2- to 4-lb increments, will maximize the benefit of this exercise. Many knee injuries will improve with low-impact activities and exercises to improve muscular strength and flexibility.

      If the initial examination is limited by pain and swelling, the foregoing regimen can still be followed. An adequate examination will often be possible after 1 week.

2. **Iliotibial band syndrome**

   a. **Ice** should be applied for 24 hours. NSAIDs can also be used (see section VI,A,1,d).

   b. **Rest** and avoidance of aggravating activities usually for 1–2 weeks until pain and inflammation subside will facilitate the healing process. Resumption of full activity should be gradual. Rehabilitation is recommended (see section VI,A,1,e).

TABLE 40–2. INDICATIONS FOR URGENT ORTHOPEDIC REFERRAL

Neurovascular compromise
Suspected complete ligamentous disruption
Locked knee—unable to be manipulated into place
Fractures
    Patellar (complete)
    Femoral condylar
    Tibial plateau
    Any compound fracture
Severe injury with limited examination (examination under anesthesia may be indicated)

3. **Meniscal tears** are treated acutely the same as ligamentous injuries. After the acute injury, if the knee is persistently locked or if locking or clicking in the knee recurs, orthopedic referral is indicated.

B. **Patellofemoral dysfunction**
   1. **Patellar subluxation** is treated like an acute ligamentous injury (see section VI,A). If the patella is still dislocated, it can be reduced by hyperextending the knee and pushing the patella back into place. Follow-up referral to an orthopedic surgeon within 1 week is necessary.
   2. Acute pain in **chondromalacia patellae** is treated with ice, elevation, and NSAIDs, as for ligamentous injuries (see section VI,A). The knee should be immobilized for 1 week if pain is severe. Climbing, jumping, running, and squatting should be limited until pain subsides, usually for 2–4 weeks. Quadriceps strengthening exercises (see section VI,A,1,b) are also beneficial.
   3. **Patellar or quadriceps tendon rupture.** Complete ruptures require surgical repair; partial tears are treated as ligamentous injuries (see section VI,A,1).

C. **Bursitis**
   1. For **prepatellar, infrapatellar, and anserine bursitis,** ice should be applied for 24 hours and NSAIDs may be used (see section VI,A,1,d). Aggravating activities should be avoided until pain and inflammation subside (usually several days to several weeks). A tense, inflamed, noninfected bursa can be aspirated (see section V,B,1), and corticosteroid solution (eg, triamcinolone acetonide, 20–40 mg, depending on bursa size) is then injected.
   2. A **Baker's cyst** may be aspirated to relieve pressure and pain. The cyst will re-form unless underlying irritation is corrected.

D. **Fractures.** Most fractures of the patella, femoral condyles, and tibial plateaus require prompt referral to an orthopedic specialist, as noted in Table 40–2.
   1. **Patellar fractures** without complete disruption of the patella can be immobilized (see section VI,A,1,a), with orthopedic follow-up in 1 week. Cylindrical casting is usually required for 6 weeks.
   2. **Tibial plateau fractures** require immobilization and no weight bearing. Surgical reduction is usually required for fracture displacement >3 mm.
   3. **Femoral condylar fractures** should be stabilized with a splint until a specialist can attend. If a neurovascular deficit is found, a vascular surgeon should be consulted.

E. **Osgood-Schlatter disease** and **Sinding-Larsen-Johansson syndrome.** These conditions are treated symptomatically by avoidance of resisted knee extension (running, climbing, jumping, and kicking) until symptoms subside. Immobilization of the affected knee should be considered for 1–2 weeks, if walking aggravates pain. **Osteochondritis dissecans** requires limited weight bearing. NSAIDs can be prescribed (see section VI,A,1,d). Because of the potential for chronic knee pain and the occasional need for removal or fixation of fracture fragments, orthopedic follow-up should be arranged.

F. For the management of **osteoarthritis,** see Chapter 80. Patients with septic arthritis should be hospitalized for parenteral antibiotic therapy to minimize morbidity.

G. **Pain referred from the hip.** (See Chapter 42.)

REFERENCES

Kiningham R, et al: Knee pain or swelling: Acute or chronic. University of Michigan Health System; 2002. Available at cme.med.umich.edu/pdf/guideline/knee.pdf.

Smith BW, Green GA: Acute knee injuries: Part I. History and physical examination. Am Fam Physician 1995;**51**:615.

Smith BW, Green GA: Acute knee injuries: Part II. Diagnosis and management. Am Fam Physician 1995;**51**:799.

Solomon DH, et al: Does this patient have a torn meniscus or ligament of the knee?: Value of the physical examination. JAMA 2001;**256**:1610.

Stiell IG, et al: Validity of the "real" Ottawa Knee Rule. Ann Emerg Med Feb 1999;**33**(2):241.

Tandeter HB, et al: Acute knee injuries: Use of decision rules for selective radiograph ordering. Am Fam Physician 1999;**60**:2599.

Zuber TJ: Knee joint aspiration and injection. Am Fam Physician 2002;**66**:1497–500, 1503–4, 1507, 1511–2.

41   Lacerations & Skin Biopsy

Jason Chao, MD, MS

KEY POINTS

- The goals of laceration repair are to gently appose tissue so that normal healing may take place, and to minimize complications, especially infection and unsightly scars.
- Anesthesia may be accomplished using topical anesthetic or injection.
- Wound closure options include sutures, cyanoacrylate adhesive, staples, and adhesive tape.

I. **Definition.** A laceration is a cut or tear in the skin or mucosa that extends through the epidermis into deeper, underlying tissues. Lacerations may result in two ways: (1) from a **shearing force** that slices through the skin or (2) from **blunt trauma** that compresses or stretches the skin. Blunt trauma requires greater energy and results in more extensive tissue damage. This creates an increased inflammatory response and contributes to additional scarring and greater risk of infection.

Tensile strength of the healing wound increases most rapidly during the first 3 weeks. Unfortunately, sutures must be removed by 2 weeks to minimize suture scars, and dehiscence may occur at this time. Local factors that increase infection rates include poor local blood supply and the presence of any necrotic tissue, foreign bodies, hematoma, or dead space.

II. **Common Diagnoses.** Lacerations and open wound injuries occur in 5–10 of every 100 persons each year in the United States. These wounds constitute one quarter of all injuries in this country, occurring mostly in the home environment. Lacerations are more common among males and happen more frequently during the summer. There is a bimodal age distribution, with one peak of lacerations occurring in persons younger than 5 years and a second peak occurring in persons between 18 and 24 years of age.

A. In **superficial wounds,** the surface epidermis is left intact by contusions or bruises or is abraded, leaving underlying tissue intact.

B. In **puncture wounds,** a small surface opening may hide a deeper, serious injury. An electrical or chemical wound with a break in the skin requires special attention, since the patient may have severe soft tissue injury that is not apparent initially.

C. **Clean lacerations**

D. **Wounds with extensive tissue loss or injury,** including dirty lacerations, compound lacerations, and electrical wounds.

III. **Symptoms.** Lacerations cause **pain, bleeding,** and **swelling.**

IV. **Signs**

A. **Tissue damage**

1. A partial or complete severing of bones, muscles, tendons, ligaments, major blood vessels, or nerves may occur in **compound lacerations.**

    a. Loss of a pulse or slow capillary refill after the application of pressure distal to wounds may indicate a vascular injury that must be treated.

    b. Sensorineural function distal to wounds should be assessed before anesthesia is administered. Loss of sensation or movement suggests a nerve injury that must be investigated. Poor finger flexion or extension indicative of a tendon injury is common in hand lacerations because the hand lacks subcutaneous fat.

2. **Dirty lacerations** are contaminated with foreign matter. The depth and degree of contamination of lacerations and the surrounding tissue must be assessed. Full exploration of wounds is best performed after the administration of anesthesia.

3. Inflammatory reaction with surrounding erythema begins several hours after the patient sustains a laceration. Marked erythema or pus signifies wounds that are not recent and are probably infected.

V. **Laboratory Tests**

A. A **deep wound culture** is usually indicated if the laceration is dirty, more than 24 hours old, or obviously infected. The culture results are helpful as a guide in the treatment of the wound if it does not improve with initial therapy.

   B. X-rays may be appropriate for patients with compound or deep lacerations to check for a fracture, subcutaneous air, or a foreign body that might be associated with the laceration. Most glass is visible on x-ray.

VI. Treatment. The goals of treatment are to assist the healing process by approximating the wound when possible and to minimize complications, including infection and unsightly scars.

   A. Wound preparation. Most bleeding can be stopped by the application of direct pressure for 10–15 minutes. Hemostasis of active bleeders can be obtained using ligation, electrocautery, or Gelfoam.

   1. Thorough cleansing of the wound is performed to ensure that no foreign body is left in the wound.

      a. Gentle rinsing with saline solution is an adequate cleanser for many lacerations. An antiseptic solution such as Betadine or Hibiclens is often used, but laboratory studies have shown that these disinfectants inhibit the wound repair process.

      b. Dirty lacerations should be forcefully irrigated with copious amounts of sterile saline. A 20- to 50-mL syringe and a 19-gauge needle should be used. Sharp debridement with a scalpel or scissors is sometimes necessary to remove the most contaminated tissue. Scrubbing the wound should be avoided if possible in order to prevent additional trauma to the wound.

      c. Areas such as the face or the neck that have a rich blood supply require less debridement than other areas.

   2. If hair removal is required, clipping with scissors is preferable to using a straight razor, to reduce tissue trauma. Eyebrows should not be shaved, since they grow slowly and a defect in the eyebrows is very noticeable.

   3. Wound edges should be perpendicular to the skin surface. If they are beveled, skin should be removed to produce a sharp perpendicular edge that will approximate with the other side. Small skin flaps with inadequate blood supply should be excised to ensure that the skin at the margins of the laceration is vascularized.

   4. If tissue is missing, so that easy closure of the wound is precluded, the physician may undermine the subcutaneous layers to free the overlying skin, which in turn will allow approximation of the skin margins.

   B. Anesthesia. Anesthesia is used for pain relief and to aid in adequate examination, debridement, and repair. Landmarks that need to be approximated should be identified and marked before local anesthesia is administered in order to prevent distortion.

   1. **Local infiltration** of the wound with anesthesia is often sufficient. A slow injection (ie, for more than 10 seconds) of 1% **lidocaine hydrochloride** through a 27-gauge needle is commonly used. Mixing the lidocaine with **sodium bicarbonate** in a ratio of 9:1 will reduce the pain of injection. This procedure provides adequate anesthesia for as long as 2 hours.

   2. **Epinephrine, a vasoconstrictor,** may be included in an injection with lidocaine except in an area with reduced circulation, such as the fingers, toes, tip of the nose, penis, or earlobes. Contaminated wounds should not be injected with epinephrine because these wounds become easily infected when their blood supply is reduced.

   3. **Topical anesthetic** avoids painful injection, and does not distort local landmarks. LAT (4% lidocaine, 1:2000 adrenaline, and 0.5% tetracaine) or TAC (0.5% tetracaine, 1:2000 adrenaline, and 11.8% cocaine) can be used, especially in children. However, serious complications including seizures and death have been reported with improper use. Anesthesia using lidocaine and prilocaine (EMLA) cream is more effective but may take up to an hour to become effective, compared with a half hour using LAT or TAC.

   4. A **regional block** may be suitable for wounds that are very large or involve the distal fingers or toes.

   C. Biopsy

   1. For a diffuse skin eruption, a new or fresh lesion should be chosen. In blistering disorders, a rim of normal tissue should be included. Complete removal of a small to moderate-sized lesion can serve both diagnostic and therapeutic purposes. If malignancy is a concern, adequate margins around the lesion should be obtained.

   2. **Shave biopsy** is indicated for benign exophytic lesions such as warts, seborrheic keratoses and skin tags, and superficial nodulo-ulcerative processes. After cleansing the skin and adequate anesthesia, a scalpel blade is positioned almost parallel to the skin surface and the skin specimen is obtained in a single gentle scoop under

the lesion, leaving a shallow defect with smooth borders. This wound is left to heal by secondary intention.

3. **Punch biopsy** is indicated for diagnosis in diffuse eruptions, deeper lesions, suspected vasculitis, or other inflammatory lesions requiring direct immunofluorescence. After cleansing the skin and adequate anesthesia, the skin should be stretched perpendicular to skin tension lines. The other hand is used to twist the punch into the skin down to the plastic hub of the punch. The plug of skin is gently removed and cut at the base with scissors or blade. A 4-mm punch is generally adequate. Smaller punches may be useful in cosmetically important areas, but have a lower diagnostic yield. Larger lesions may require up to a 6-mm punch. The wound is closed with sutures as described below.

4. **Excisional or incisional biopsy** is indicated for most pigmented lesions, suspected malignancies, and deep or subcutaneous lesions. After cleansing the skin and adequate anesthesia, a fusiform-shaped cut is made around the lesion. The length of the biopsy should be three times its width.

D. **Wound repair**

1. **Wound closure.** When clean lacerations present within 12–24 hours, they can be closed primarily. Lacerations closed during this "golden period" are likely to heal without infection. Evidence suggests that head wounds with good blood supply may be closed even after 24 hours and still heal well.

   Lacerations with extensive devitalized tissue or evidence of infection require thorough debriding but should not be closed primarily. Delayed closure, 3–4 days later, may be performed if the wound appears free of infection and is adequately supplied with blood. The following techniques may also be used to close clean surgical wounds.

2. **Equipment.** The equipment required to repair a laceration includes a needle holder, smooth and toothed small forceps, scissors, small hemostats, a scalpel, sterile gauze, suture material, gloves, and drapes. Skin hooks are optional; they allow less traumatic handling of the skin. A disposable skin hook may be created by gently bending a needle with a hemostat. Adequate lighting is essential.

   The choice of suture material depends on the location and purpose of the suture (Table 41–1).

   a. **Absorbable sutures** should be used for dermal or fascial layer repair or for ligation of vessels. They lose their tensile strength by gradual degradation over days to weeks. Synthetic absorbable polymers (eg, Dexon, Vicryl, PDS, or Maxon) retain their tensile strength longer than does plain or chromic gut.

   b. **Nonabsorbable sutures** should be used for epidermal repair. Nonabsorbable sutures include silk, cotton, synthetic monofilament nylon or polypropylene (eg, Ethilon, Dermalon, Prolene, Surgilene, or Deklene), and braided polyester. Nonabsorbable sutures remain strong but induce a cellular reaction and increase the likelihood of infection in dirty wounds. Synthetic monofilament is the most commonly used material for the final epidermal closure.

3. **Placement of sutures.** Tissue should be handled gently to minimize additional trauma to the wound.

   a. **Dermal sutures** are used to approximate larger wounds, close dead space, and provide hemostasis and tensile strength. Sutures in fat lead to infection and should be avoided. An inverted suture will bury the knot deep in the wound.

   b. **Skin sutures** should approximate the wound edges and not be tied too tightly. Excessive tightness of sutures restricts blood flow and produces a depressed scar that is more noticeable.

TABLE 41–1. WOUND CLOSURE

Site of Wound	Size of Subcutaneous Suture (Absorbable)	Size of Surface Suture (Nonabsorbable)	Time to Removal (Days)
Scalp	#4-0 or #5-0	#3-0 or #4-0	5–7
Face	#5-0 or #6-0	#6-0 or #7-0	3–5
Trunk and extremities	#3-0 or #4-0	#4-0 or #5-0	7–10
Hands, feet, and skin over joints	None	#3-0 or #4-0	7–14

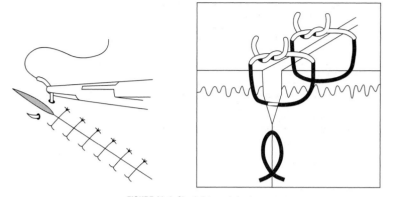

FIGURE 41–1. Simple interrupted suture.

c. **Simple interrupted sutures** (Figure 41–1) are the most commonly used epidermal suture and provide good cosmetic repair. The deep portion of the suture should be wider than the surface to help evert the skin edges and prevent
a depressed scar. **Vertical mattress sutures** (Figure 41–2) evert skin edges
more than do simple sutures, but they are time-consuming and may lead to increased inflammatory reaction. **Half-buried horizontal mattress sutures**
(Figure 41–3) are useful when the patient has skin flaps that appear viable.
These sutures are least likely to compromise vascular supply to the flap.

d. **Running simple sutures** (Figure 41–4) provide the fastest repair; however,
they are generally not used in cosmetically important areas. **Locked running
sutures** (Figure 41–5) are particularly useful when the laceration is in mucosal
surfaces, such as the vagina or the rectum. Absorbable suture material should
be used. **Subcuticular (buried running) sutures** (Figure 41–6) are time-
consuming but produce good cosmetic results without suture marks when used
to close small, clean lacerations. Absorbable sutures may be used. If nonabsorbable sutures are used, the ends should be left on the outside of the skin
so the suture can be easily removed.

e. In patients with facial lacerations, slight misalignments in repair of the eyebrows and the vermilion border of the lips become very noticeable even at a
distance. The first sutures that are placed should align the edges of these structures. Lacerations inside the mouth do not need to be closed primarily. For
through-and-through wounds, the skin and muscle should be closed, and the
oral mucosa should be left alone to heal by secondary intention.

f. For patients with scalp lacerations, choosing a suture of a color different from that
of the patient's hair helps the physician in repairing the laceration and during
suture removal.

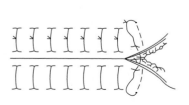

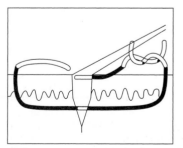

FIGURE 41–2. Vertical mattress suture.

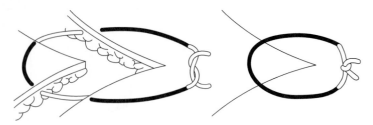

FIGURE 41–3. Half-buried horizontal mattress suture.

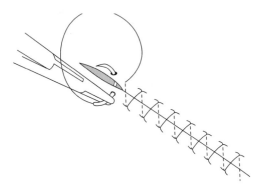

FIGURE 41–4. Running, or continuous, simple suture.

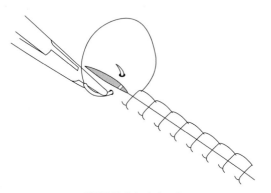

FIGURE 41–5. Locked running suture.

    g. Discussion of Z-plasty and other plastic techniques is beyond the scope of this chapter. These techniques may be used on patients with long lacerations that do not follow the natural contours of the body or with lacerations over joints that are likely to involve excessive motion during the healing process.

E. Tissue adhesive for closure

    1. Octylcyanoacrylate (Dermabond) tissue adhesive has been shown to have **comparable cosmetic outcome to suturing** in repair of selected traumatic lacerations. Tissue adhesive closure is **faster** and **less painful** than suturing. Skin moisture is the catalyst for the adhesive to polyermize, generating heat.

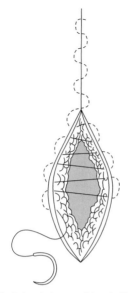

FIGURE 41–6. Subcuticular (buried running) suture. (Adapted with permission from Stillman RM [editor]: *Surgery: Diagnosis & Therapy*. Appleton & Lange; 1989.)

    2. Most **facial and selected trunk and extremity lacerations** are suitable for tissue adhesive closure. It should not be used on hands or over joints.

    3. When using topical tissue adhesive, care should be taken to **keep adhesive out of the wound,** which would act as a foreign body and inhibit wound healing (Figure 41–7).

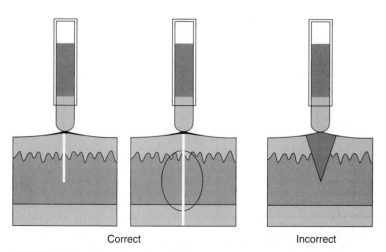

Correct   Incorrect

FIGURE 41–7. Proper tissue adhesive closure (**left, center**); improper use (**right**). (Adapted with permission from Quinn J, Wells G, Sutcliffe T, et al: Randomized trial comparing octylcyanoacrylate tissue adhesive sutures. JAMA 1997;**277**:1529. © 1997, American Medical Association.)

TABLE 41–2. GUIDE TO TETANUS PROPHYLAXIS

Type of Wound	Immunization Status (Doses of Tetanus Toxoid Received)	
	Uncertain, Less Than 3, or None Within the Last 5 Years	3 or More (Booster Within 5 Years)
Clean wound	Td[1]	No prophylaxis necessary
Dirty wound[2]	Td,[1] and human tetanus immune globulin, at different site	Consider human tetanus immune globulin

[1] Adult tetanus and diphtheria toxoids, 0.5 mL intramuscularly. If the patient is younger than 7 years old, diphtheria-tetanus or diphtheria-tetanus-pertussis is given intramuscularly.
[2] A wound that is grossly contaminated, is more than 8 hours old, contains devitalized tissue, or is of a form that prevents adequate irrigation.
Modified with permission from Chesnutt MS, Dewar TN, Locksley RM: *Office & Bedside Procedures.* Appleton & Lange; 1992.

4. Wound edges should be apposed when applying the first layer of adhesive, and the adhesive should dry 3 minutes between layers. A minimum of **three layers** of adhesive should be applied.
5. The patient should be instructed to **avoid washing or soaking** the wound, but may get it wet, as in a shower.
F. **Staples.** Staples can be applied quickly, but accurate placement may be difficult and they are more painful to remove than sutures. Infection rates are comparable to those of sutures.
G. **Prevention of infection**
1. The physician should provide **tetanus immunization** if it is indicated (Table 41–2).
2. Prophylactic antibiotics are not necessary except in selected cases, such as in patients with dirty compound lacerations or with lacerations that involve significant tissue ischemia because of blunt trauma. Most patients with bite wounds should receive antibiotics.
H. **Patient education.** Patients should be given the following advice.
1. **Keep the wound clean and dry** for the first 24 hours, after which the dressing should be removed, and the wound should be cleaned daily.
2. **Contact a physician** if redness, excessive swelling, tenderness, or increased warmth of the skin around the wound occurs; if pus or watery discharge occurs; if there are tender bumps or swelling in an armpit or groin area; if red streaks appear in the skin near the wound; if there is a foul smell from the wound; or if generalized body chills or fever develop.
3. **Elevate an extremity** with a laceration to reduce swelling.
4. **Limit activity** somewhat for 1 week after the sutures are removed to avoid reopening the wound. Wound healing takes several weeks.
5. **Use sunscreen** to protect the scar from sunlight in order to avoid marked pigment changes that occur in lighter-skinned patients. A scar normally appears red and slightly raised or thickened for several months after an injury.
VII. **Patient Follow-up.** See Table 41–1 concerning the timing of suture removal.
A. The physician should see patients with contaminated or deep lacerations 48 hours after the sutures are placed in cases in which infection is likely to present.
B. When lacerations are in areas of tension, every other suture may be removed initially and replaced by adhesive bandages, with tincture of benzoin applied to the normal skin to prolong bandage adhesion. The remaining sutures should be removed several days later.

REFERENCES

Bruns TB, Worthington JM: Using tissue adhesive for wound repair: A practical guide to Dermabond. Am Fam Physician 2000;**61**:1383.
Hollander JE, Singer AJ: Laceration management. Ann Emerg Med 1999;**34**:356.
Leach J: Proper handling of soft tissue in the acute phase. Facial Plast Surg 2001;**17**:227.
Wilson JL, Kocurek K, Doty BJ: A systematic approach to laceration repair: Tricks to ensure the desired cosmetic result. Postgrad Med 2000;**107**:77.
Zuber TJ: The mattress sutures: Vertical, horizontal, and corner stitch. Am Fam Physician 2002; **66**:2231.

42   Leg & Hip Complaints

Geoffrey S. Kuhlman, MD, CAQSM

KEY POINTS

- Leg and hip complaints in children and adolescents often reflect serious conditions and should be treated as such until proved otherwise.
- Leg pain in athletic individuals is usually due to overuse injuries, including stress fracture or medial tibial stress syndrome.
- The history and physical examination should guide appropriate diagnostic testing in the evaluation of hip and leg complaints.

I. **Definition. Hip complaints** arise from processes in the hip joint (eg, transient synovitis, bacterial infection, avascular necrosis of the femoral head, slipped capital femoral epiphysis [SCFE], osteoarthritis, rheumatoid arthritis); other soft tissues (eg, bursitis); or neurovascular structures (eg, meralgia paresthetica). **Leg complaints** arise in the lower extremity proximal to the ankle from infection (eg, osteomyelitis of the long bones); joints (eg, osteoarthritis); muscle (eg, nocturnal leg cramps); vasculature (eg, arterial insufficiency, deep vein thrombosis [DVT], or varicose veins); neuropathy; overuse (eg, stress fracture, medial tibial stress syndrome, or chronic compartment syndrome); or idiopathic etiologies (eg, growing pains).

II. **Common Diagnoses** (Table 42–1 and Figures 42–1 to 42–4). Hip and leg complaints are common in family medicine. Some causes demand urgent attention, such as osteomyelitis, septic arthritis, and SCFE. Many of the less urgent diagnoses are quite debilitating for patients, causing significant pain, inability to work or exercise, or difficulty sleeping. Likely causes of hip and leg complaints depend on age and activity.

   A. Hip complaints in **children and adolescents** include transient synovitis, septic arthritis, Perthes disease, and SCFE.

   1. **Transient synovitis** is acute nonspecific inflammation in the hip joint and is the most common atraumatic cause of hip pain in childhood. Risk factors include antecedent upper respiratory infection, recurrent microtrauma, or allergic hypersensitivity.

   2. **Septic arthritis** of the hip joint can occur at any age but is most common in infants and toddlers.

   3. **Perthes disease,** avascular necrosis of the femoral head (see sidebar), is bilateral 12% of the time. Low birth weight and family history are risk factors, but the cause is undetermined, and no consistent hereditary pattern exists.

   4. **SCFE** is bilateral in 25–40% of cases.

AVASCULAR NECROSIS

Atraumatic **avascular necrosis of the femoral head** begins between ages 25 and 45 years. Predisposing factors in 75% of cases include systemic corticosteroid therapy, alcoholism, sickle cell disease, or dysbaric trauma (underground or undersea work). Avascular necrosis presents with abrupt hip pain followed by progressive, intermittent episodes in 85% of patients, worsened by movement. Rest pain is present in two thirds of patients and night pain in 40%. Findings on examination include limp and limited abduction/internal rotation.

Plain radiographs have a 19% false-negative rate early in avascular necrosis. Initial plain radiographic findings include a crescent sign (Figure 42–3), with bone collapse and degenerative arthritic changes occurring later.

Radioisotope bone scans increase sensitivity in detecting avascular necrosis, and magnetic resonance imaging scanning is the most sensitive, specific and low-risk means of making this diagnosis.

Management of avascular necrosis involves orthopedic consultation for possible core decompression or, for more advanced disease, hip arthroplasty.

TABLE 42–1. EVALUATION OF COMMON HIP AND LEG COMPLAINTS

Diagnosis	Risk Factors	Symptoms	Signs	Testing
Transient synovitis	3- to 10-yr-olds; M:F, 2:1; recent upper respiratory infection	Insidious or acute painful limp	Afebrile, voluntary limited hip range of motion	Hip US
Septic hip arthritis	Infants/toddlers	Rapid-onset, constant hip thigh/knee pain, worse with movement, failure to thrive	Febrile/ill, thigh edema Flexed/abducted/externally rotated hip	Elevated WBC; plain x-rays show lateral displacement of femoral head; ESR; hip US guides needle aspiration
Perthes disease	4- to 10-yr-olds; M:F, 5:1	Insidious pain/stiffness of groin/ lateral hip/medial knee, then limp	Antalgic gait, decreased hip range of motion, occasional flexion contracture	Crescent sign on x-ray (Figure 42–3), followed by progressive changes in femoral epiphysis/femoral head
SCFE	Obese early adolescence; M:F, 3:2	Groin/buttock/lateral hip or knee pain, simultaneous pain + limp in 50%	Antalgic gait, hip externally rotated	X-ray (Figures 42–3, 42–4)
OA/RA	90% of adult hip pain	Stiffness after rest, insidious pain referred to groin/thigh/knee	Limp, decreased hip range of motion, especially internal rotation/abduction	X-ray—spurring, narrowed joint space, periarticular sclerosis (OA)
Trochanteric bursitis	40- to 60-yr-old females	Thigh, posterolateral hip pain	Tender grt. Trochanter. Increased with resisted abduction (Figure 42–1)	
Ischial bursitis	Prolonged sitting on hard surfaces	Buttock pain, worse with sitting	Tender ischial tuberosity (Figure 42–1), painful SLR	
Iliopsoas bursitis	Sports (eg, soccer) requiring repetitive hip flexion/adduction	Deep groin pain, worse with hip extension	Tender and cystic mass (30%) over bursa (Figure 42–1), limited hip extension	Hip US detects enlarged bursa; CT confirms

Meralgia paresthetica	Abdominal obesity, middle-aged men, pregnancy	Anterolateral thigh pain, paresthesia	Reproduced by pressing lateral femoral cut. N. Against anterior Superior iliac spine (Figure 42–2)	None, NCV if diagnosis in question
Growing pains	15% of children 4- to 14-yr-old	Intermittent bilateral nocturnal thigh and lower leg pain	Normal examination	None
Medial tibial stress syndrome	Adolescent/early adult runners, sudden increased training	Achy posteromedial distal tibia, initially during exercise, progressing to rest pain	Tender medial edge, distal third of tibia	None
Stress fractures	Late teen to early adult athletes, increase in physical activity; oligoamenorrhea/weight loss	Insidious local pain: tibia (34%), fibula (24%), metatarsal (20%), femur (14%), pelvic (6%)	Focal bony tenderness, poorly resolving soft tissue symptoms	X-ray shows periosteal reaction, then fracture (2–4 wk after symptom onset) MRI or radioisotope bone scan more sensitive
Chronic compartment syndromes	Late teen to early 20s, distance runners/sprinters/basketball players/soccer players	Gradual exercise-associated achiness: anterolaterally (anterior tibial compartment) calf pain/plantar paresthesia (posterior compartment), lateral lower leg achiness: lateral compartment)	Involved muscle groups tender during/shortly after exercise; normal examination after adequate rest	Compartment pressure measurement (by orthopedist or physiatrist)
DVT	Immobility, leg trauma, hypercoagulable state, major surgery, history of DVT or cancer, estrogen therapy, CHF, pregnancy, atrial arrhythmias	Variable, nonspecific unilateral swelling, pain, erythema	Edema/red/warm (>50% of DVTs not clinically detectable)	Duplex US (proximal DVT), D-Dimer assay, contrast venography
Nocturnal leg cramps	All ages (especially elderly), occasionally associated with denervation or electrolyte disorders	Abrupt nocturnal calf, plantar cramps	Tender affected muscles	Serum electrolytes if abnormality suspected

CHF, congestive heart failure; CT, computerized tomogram; DVT, deep vein thrombosis; ESR, erythrocyte sedimentation rate; M:F, male:female ratio; MRI, magnetic resonance imaging; NCV, nerve conduction velocity; OA, osteoarthritis; RA, rheumatoid arthritis; SCFE, slipped capital femoral epiphysis; SLR, straight leg raise (seated or supine); US, ultrasound; WBC, white blood cell count.

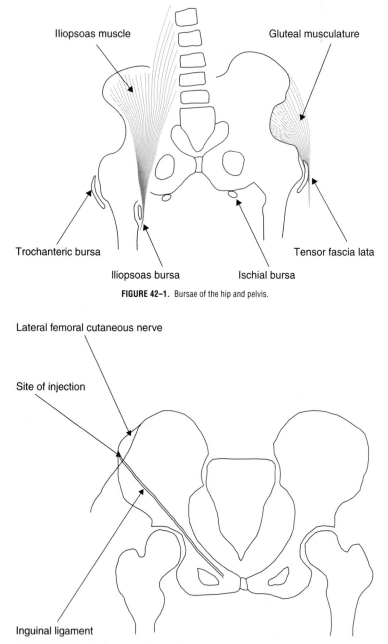

FIGURE 42–1. Bursae of the hip and pelvis.

FIGURE 42–2. Meralgia paresthetica. The lateral femoral cutaneous nerve is compressed under the inguinal ligament medial to the anterior superior iliac spine (ASIS). Therapeutic injection is performed 1 cm medial to the ASIS (see text).

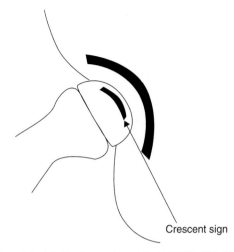

FIGURE 42–3. Crescent sign. In Perthes disease or in avascular necrosis of the hip in an adult, a radiographic finding is the crescent sign, a curvilinear lucency along the articular surface of the head of the femur.

B. Hip complaints in **adults** include osteoarthritis and rheumatoid arthritis, bursitis, meralgia paresthetica, referred pain, avascular necrosis, and malignancy. Hip bursitis is usually associated with trauma or overuse.

C. Leg complaints in infants and toddlers (0–3 years) include septic arthritis of the hip, osteomyelitis (see sidebar), and fracture.

D. Leg complaints in children (4–14 years) include transient synovitis of the hip, Perthes disease, SCFE, growing pains, and a variety of injuries. Growing pains are idiopathic.

E. Common leg complaints in adolescents (11–16 years) are SCFE, growing pains, and knee disorders such as Osgood-Schlatter disease and Sindig-Larsen-Johansson syndrome (see Chapter 40), risk factors for which include jumping activities and tight quadriceps muscles.

F. Leg complaints in athletic adolescents and adults
  1. Medial tibial stress syndrome, periostitis of the origin of the soleus muscle on the distal posteromedial aspect of the tibia, typically develops from repetitive dorsiflexion, as in running.

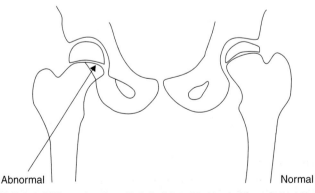

FIGURE 42–4. In SCFE, an early radiographic finding is loss of the triangle of Caper. On the right side of the picture, the entire ischium is seen (normal view). On the left side of the picture, slippage of the femoral epiphysis causes the femur metaphysis to shift medially, obscuring part of the ischium (abnormal view).

OSTEOMYELITIS

Risk factors for osteomyelitis in children include male gender (male:female, 2:1), lower socioeconomic status, immunocompromise, and the autumn season. Osteomyelitis presents with rapid-onset leg pain and refusal to walk in children. Findings include fever >38 °C (100.4 °F), ill appearance, and redness/warmth/tenderness of the involved region with limited motion of adjacent joints. Early in osteomyelitis, plain radiographs show loss of normal fascial planes and fat shadows, due to edema. Bony changes appear 7–10 days after symptoms and include (1) destruction, with or without periosteal elevation, (2) fading cortical margins, and (3) absence of adjacent reactive new bone. Radioisotope bone scanning detects osteomyelitis before plain radiographs, and magnetic resonance imaging is the most sensitive, specific, low-risk means of diagnosing osteomyelitis. Suspected osteomyelitis requires hospitalization for blood cultures and prolonged parenteral antibiotics.

2. Chronic compartment syndrome is ischemic or neuropathic pain resulting from increased muscle mass within an unyielding compartment. **Posterior compartment syndromes** are common in cyclists; **lateral compartment syndromes** are common in football and soccer players.
3. Other causes include patellofemoral pain, iliotibial band syndrome, and muscle strain.
G. **Leg complaints in adults**
1. **Deep vein thrombosis (DVT)** occurs in the setting of venous stasis, venous injury, or increased blood coagulability.
2. **Nocturnal leg cramps** are sudden contraction of the plantar flexor muscles causing painful cramps during sleep.
3. Other causes include patellofemoral pain (see Chapter 40), iliotibial band syndrome (see Chapter 40), peripheral neuropathy (see sidebar), peripheral arterial disease (see sidebar), acquired spinal stenosis (see sidebar), cancer (see sidebar), osteoarthritis (see Chapter 80), gout and other crystal arthropathies, and rheumatoid arthritis.

PERIPHERAL NEUROPATHIES

Peripheral neuropathies can be classified as **mononeuropathy** (a single nerve affected, usually due to trauma, compression, or entrapment [eg, common peroneal neuropathy at the fibular head causing dorsal foot/lateral calf sensory loss and weakened foot dorsiflexion and eversion]) or **polyneuropathy** (affecting multiple nerves simultaneously). Polyneuropathy can be classified as axonal or demyelinating. The **axonal** type involves distal sensory, burning, or tingling progressing proximally in a stocking/glove distribution and initially affecting fine touch and temperature—eg, diabetes, vitamin B_{12} deficiency, Lyme disease, uremia, drugs, toxins, or human immunodeficiency virus. The **demyelinating** type manifests early with diffuse loss of reflexes and strength—eg, Guillain-Barré syndrome, multiple myeloma, or chronic inflammatory demyelinating polyneuropathy.

In approaching a patient with peripheral neuropathy, it is important to assess risk factors (eg, history of recent viral illness, chronic systemic disease, new medications, and occupational or other exposure to toxins, such as alcohol/pesticides/heavy metals); distribution (ie, likely mono- vs. polyneuropathy); and rapidity of onset. (With regard to rapidity of onset, massive intoxications or Guillain-Barré syndrome develop over days to weeks; many toxins will develop over weeks to months; and diabetic, hereditary, or dysproteinemic neuropathies evolve over months to years.) Examination confirms/localizes deficits (ie, sensation, reflexes, strength, or proprioception). Further testing is based on the foregoing clinical evaluation; helpful basic testing when the cause is not clear includes blood glucose, sedimentation rate, vitamin B_{12} or methylmalonic acid levels, serum blood urea nitrogen and creatinine, and serum protein/immunoelectrophoresis. Electrodiagnostic studies (eg, nerve conduction velocity) are also helpful in clarifying the type and location of neuropathy. Treatment of neuropathy depends on its causes (eg, controlling diabetes or renal failure, eliminating inciting drugs or toxins, treating vitamin B_{12} deficiency) and may involve neurologic consultation in puzzling cases.

PERIPHERAL ARTERIAL DISEASE (PAD)

PAD results from endothelial injury, lipid deposits, vasoconstriction, and plaque disruption, which reduce arterial blood flow and oxygen delivery to affected muscles, causing exertional calf or leg angina or nocturnal leg pain improved with walking. (This should be distinguished from neurogenic claudication due to lumbar nerve root compression from spinal stenosis.) PAD shares risk factors (eg, hypercholesterolemia, tobacco abuse) with coronary artery disease (CAD), and significant CAD coexists in 60% of patients with PAD. The best screen for leg claudication is the ankle-brachial index (ABI), the ratio of systolic blood pressure in the posterior tibial artery/systolic blood pressure in the brachial artery, and is performed supine using a Doppler ultrasound. Since ankle pressure normally is higher, a normal ABI is >1. Severity of PAD correlates with ABI values, such that ≤0.90 diagnoses PAD, 0.70—0.89 indicates mild disease, 0.5—0.69 indicates moderate disease, and <0.5, severe disease. Treatment for PAD starts with lifestyle modifications (exercise to develop collateral blood flow, smoking cessation, dietary reduction in cholesterol) and extends to pharmacologic intervention (lipid-lowering drugs, antiplatelet agents—eg, aspirin, cilostazol, clopidogrel, ticlopidine, and red-cell morphology-altering agents—eg, pentoxifylline). Vascular surgical referral should be considered in cases: refractory to medical management, for rest pain, tissue loss, persistent ulcers, or gangrene.

SPINAL STENOSIS

Spinal stenosis can be congenital or acquired; 75% of cases are acquired, and risk factors include old age (men > women) and history of degenerative arthritis, although up to 20% of adults with spinal stenosis on imaging studies are asymptomatic. Degenerative spinal stenosis can be **central** (circumferential spinal cord compression) or **lateral** (narrowing of neuroforamina).

In differentiating spinal stenosis from disk disease and vasculogenic claudication, it is helpful to know that sciatica caused by spinal stenosis is more commonly bilateral (vs. unilateral with lumbar disk disease) and that the cramping calf pain in patients with spinal stenosis is relieved with sitting, lying, or leaning forward (vs. vascular claudication, which is relieved by decreased muscular activity, without the need to sit or lean forward). In those suspected of having degenerative spinal stenosis, an enhanced magnetic resonance imaging scan is the preferred imaging study; a dural sac with <10 mm anterior-posterior diameter is consistent with this diagnosis. Initial management of spinal stenosis is symptomatic, using NSAIDs and proper positioning; surgical decompression is reserved for those with significant pain despite medical therapy, whose spinal stenosis significantly impacts daily activities, or with focal neurologic findings. Surgery is 65–80% successful in providing relief, although approximately 25% of patients develop recurrent spinal stenosis within 5 years.

CANCER

Cancer, most commonly metastatic from breast, prostate, lung, kidney, or thyroid tumors, but also from multiple myeloma in the elderly, causes pain through osteoclastic bone resorption and resulting osteopenia and pathologic fractures. Cancer pain is often nocturnal and described as a deep ache, is exacerbated by movement, and may cause acute disability with pathologic fracture. Typically, physical findings may initially be minimal; later palpable swelling and pain over bony prominences may develop. Pathologic fracture may cause immediate inability to bear weight, though occult fracture may manifest with normal motion, except at extremes of internal or external rotation.

Plain radiographs may show punched-out osteolytic lesions. Cancer patients with osteolytic lesions and increasing pain unresponsive to analgesics (including combination opioids and acetaminophen or NSAIDS) or palliative radiotherapy, in whom radiographs show destruction of >50% of bone cortex or lesions >3 cm in diameter, should be considered for prophylactic internal fixation, in consultation with an orthopedic surgeon.

III. Symptoms (Table 42–1)

- **A. Transient synovitis** pain occasionally will awaken children at night.
- **B. In Perthes disease,** knee pain alone occurs in 15%. The patient usually tolerates symptoms for 1–12 months before seeing a physician.
- **C. In SCFE,** about 20% of patients present acutely with a history of a sudden twisting or falling injury.
- **D. Osteoarthritis** and **rheumatoid arthritis** (see Chapters 39 and 80).
- **E. Bursitis**
    1. In **trochanteric bursitis,** running or lying on the affected side worsens the pain.
    2. **Iliopsoas bursitis** causes pain with hip extension, as when rising from a chair or lying in bed, and patients often limp with the hip flexed and externally rotated.
- **F.** In **meralgia paresthetica,** prolonged standing and walking may worsen the pain; sitting may relieve it.
- **G. Chronic compartment syndrome** gradually develops over 1 year or longer, and how far the patient can walk or run before symptoms occur is usually constant, but discomfort may worsen over time.
    1. In **anterior tibial compartment syndrome,** numbness in the web space between the first and second toes and dorsiflexion weakness may occur.
    2. Complaints of ankle instability are common with **lateral compartment syndrome.**
- **H.** In **stress fractures,** pain initially occurs toward the end of exercise, and usually increases over days to weeks; the pain eventually develops early in activity and finally occurs at rest if training is not decreased.

IV. Signs (Table 42–1). Physical examination of hip and leg complaints begins with taking vital signs and observing the patient's general appearance. The hips and legs are inspected for asymmetry, deformity, discoloration, and edema. Gait is observed for symmetry, antalgia (quick soft steps to favor a painful area), hip circumduction (swinging one thigh outward to reduce ipsilateral hip pain), and Trendelenburg sign (dropping one side of the pelvis due to contralateral hip weakness). Palpation of bony landmarks and soft tissue should be done with precision to localize tenderness. Particularly in patients with suspected vascular or neurologic disease, quality of pulses (femoral, popliteal, posterior tibial, and dorsal pedal) and of sensation (light touch, sharp, vibration, temperature) are assessed. Range of motion (ROM) testing should include passive, active, and resisted. Hip (flexion, extension, abduction, adduction, and internal and external rotation) and knee (flexion and extension) ROM are best performed with the patient supine, whereas ankle motion (dorsiflexion, plantar flexion, inversion, and eversion) and Homan's sign (rapid passive dorsiflexion to elicit pain from DVT) are done seated. Tendon reflexes should be tested. If the examination does not clearly localize the problem, then sources of referred symptoms should be examined (eg, pelvis, lumbar spine).

- **A.** In **Perthes disease,** thigh and calf circumferences are diminished; late in the process, leg length may decrease.
- **B.** In **SCFE,** passive hip flexion elicits external rotation and abduction of the hip; half of the patients will have thigh atrophy, and half will have shortening of the extremity up to 1 inch.
- **C. Osteoarthritis** and **rheumatoid arthritis** (see Chapters 39 and 80).

V. Laboratory Tests (Table 42–1).

- **A.** In **evaluating hip complaints, plain x-rays** of the involved hip in adults (anterior and lateral views) and both hips in children (often including a frog leg lateral view) are the single most cost-effective adjunctive test. When combined with age-adjusted history and thoughtful interpretation of physical signs, radiography approaches 90% sensitivity and 90% specificity.
    1. **Perthes disease** shows the following sequence: crescent sign (Figure 42–3), lateral displacement of the femoral head, widening and increased density of the femoral epiphysis, flattening of the femoral head and widening of the femoral neck, demineralization and fragmentation of the femoral head, and finally, re-ossification of the femoral head.
    2. The **SCFE** appears widened with irregular margins. The femoral head is displaced posteriorly and medially (Figure 42–4).

VI. Treatment

- **A. The pain of transient synovitis is relieved with bed rest** at home for 7–10 days and **nonsteroidal anti-inflammatory agents (NSAIDs)** such as **ibuprofen** (5–10 mg/kg three times daily) as needed. Patients may use crutches to resume weight bearing. Most children have only a single attack of transient synovitis, but it may recur. Because 6–15% of patients with transient synovitis develop Perthes disease, patients and their parents should be instructed to seek care if hip or leg complaints occur.

B. Losing weight and avoiding constrictive garments are key to treating **meralgia paresthetica.** Abdominal muscle strengthening is also helpful. Local corticosteroid injection at the site of lateral femoral cutaneous nerve compression may provide relief in refractory cases (eg, triamcinolone, 10–20 mg with 1 mL lidocaine via a 27-gauge 1¼-inch needle, Figure 42–2). Patients should be reassured that this condition is benign and self-limited.

C. **Stretching** overlying muscle to reduce friction on a bursa is the key to treating **bursitis.** Oral analgesics might be helpful (eg, ibuprofen, 200–800 mg three times daily or naproxen, 375–500 mg twice daily as needed for adults). If pain persists or function is limited, the affected bursa should be injected with 20–40 mg of **triamcinolone** or **methylprednisolone** added to 1–2 mL of 1% lidocaine. No more than three injections should be given each year.

D. **Osteoarthritis** is managed with lifestyle modification (weight reduction, moderate exercise as tolerated), topical and oral analgesia, and assistive devices (see Chapter 80).

E. **Surgical intervention**
1. A patient with **bacterial infection** of the hip must be hospitalized for **arthrotomy** to drain all purulent material and for intravenous antibiotics. Poor prognosis is correlated with delayed action. Results of ultrasound-guided aspiration may allow selection of a smaller high-risk group for operative drainage and may also shorten operative time.
2. Perthes disease requires the orthopedic use of **braces, casts,** or **surgery** in order to retain the normal spherical shape of the femoral head during the natural repair process. Under the best of circumstances (eg, younger age or earlier diagnosis), minimal deformity and normal function will result. Premature osteoarthritis of the hip can develop.
3. SCFE is best treated with immediate cessation of weight bearing and **surgical stabilization.** Premature osteoarthritis of the hip is common.
4. Under ultrasound or computerized tomography guidance, diagnostic and therapeutic **aspiration and drainage** of an enlarged **iliopsoas bursa** refractory to previously described measures can be accomplished. Prophylactic intravenous antibiotics will lessen the need for repeat aspiration.

F. Because the cause of **growing pains** is unknown, treatment consists of supportive measures including heat, ice, massage, and acetaminophen or NSAIDs. If symptoms persist despite a negative work-up, referral to a rheumatologist or pediatric orthopedic surgeon should be considered.

G. **Chronic compartment syndrome** often requires surgical decompression of the affected fascial compartment. Reducing or changing sports participation is another option. Some cases might respond to a few weeks of stretching the lower extremity musculature two to four times daily, which might improve compliance of fascia enclosing compartments.

H. **Stress fractures**
1. Weight-bearing exercise should be discontinued until x-ray evidence of healing is seen and there is no tenderness, after which gradual resumption of activity may proceed.
2. Use of analgesics is discouraged because of the possibility of masking pain, which reflects ongoing bone stress.
3. Stress fractures of the pelvis, femur, and anterior tibia have high risk for complications and are best managed by a subspecialist.

I. **Medial tibial stress syndrome**
1. The initial treatment includes rest for 5–7 days, ice, and wrapping or taping the leg.
2. Once symptoms resolve, soleus muscle stretching should be initiated, and the patient may gradually return to running. Patients whose feet pronate excessively might benefit from arch support and heel control, such as with off-the-shelf or custommade orthotics.
3. In rare instances surgical release of the involved fascia is necessary.

J. DVT (see Chapter 23).
K. Nocturnal leg cramps
   1. When cramping occurs, the calf muscles should be stretched by dorsiflexion. Calf stretching at bedtime can prevent symptoms.
   2. Quinine sulfate, 200–300 mg orally at bedtime, may be helpful. Side effects include nausea, vomiting, headache, tinnitus, hearing loss, vertigo, and vision disturbance.

REFERENCES

Anand SS, et al: Does this patient have deep vein thrombosis? JAMA 1998;**279:**1094.
Bradshaw C: Hip and groin pain. In: Brukner P, Khan K (editors): *Clinical Sports Medicine.* McGraw-Hill; 2001:375–394.
Bradshaw C: Shin pain and calf pain. In: Brukner P, Khan K (editors): *Clinical Sports Medicine.* McGraw-Hill; 2001:508–534.
Hart JJ: Transient synovitis of the hip in children. Am Fam Physician 1996;**54:**1587.
Leet AI, Skaggs DL: Evaluation of the acutely limping child. Am Fam Physician 2000;**61:**1011.
Loder RT: Slipped capital femoral epiphysis. Am Fam Physician 1998;**57:**2135.

---

43   Liver Function Test Abnormalities

James P. McKenna, MD

KEY POINTS

- An AST:ALT >2:1 is highly suggestive of alcoholic hepatitis.
- Persistent elevations of liver function tests for >6 months suggest chronic liver disease; patients should be evaluated for treatable causes and referred for liver biopsy.
- Alcohol liver disease, hepatitis C, and nonalcoholic steatohepatitis are the most common causes of persistently abnormal liver function tests.

I. **Definition.** Abnormalities in liver function tests (LFTs) are elevated levels of static biochemical tests, including aspartate aminotransferase (AST) (formerly serum glutamic-oxaloacetic transaminase [SGOT]), alanine aminotransferase (ALT) (formerly serum glutamate pyruvate transaminase [SGPT]), alkaline phosphatase, bilirubin, and albumin. The tests are most frequently obtained as part of LFT panels. Tests other than those mentioned are often included in LFT panels but are less useful in evaluating the spectrum of liver disease, and therefore are not discussed here. Cellular injury in the liver causes release of AST and ALT. ALT is a more specific indication of liver disease, whereas AST elevations may be secondary to damage of other organs (heart, kidney, brain, intestine, placenta). **Alkaline phosphatase** is associated with cellular membranes, and elevated levels may be caused by injury to the liver, bone, kidneys, intestines, placenta, or leukocytes. In the liver, the enzyme is located in the bile canaliculi. Biliary obstruction induces increased synthesis of alkaline phosphatase and spillage into the circulation. **Hyperbilirubinemia** may be caused by increased production (hemolysis, ineffective erythropoiesis); extravasation of blood (hematoma); decreased metabolism (hereditary disease, Gilbert's syndrome, or acquired defects in bilirubin conjugation); or reduced bilirubin excretion due to bile duct obstruction.

   Hepatic clearance tests measuring liver metabolism of lidocaine or caffeine may be used by hepatologists to assess liver function in patients with chronic compensated liver disease.

II. **Common Diagnoses.** In asymptomatic populations, the frequency of abnormal LFTs on routine screening ranges from 1% to 6%. The prevalence of liver disease is approximately 1%.
   A. **Elevated aminotransferases** are found to some degree in almost all patients with liver disease and represent hepatocellular dysfunction (Table 43–1).

TABLE 43-1. CAUSES OF ELEVATED AMINOTRANSFERASES

Alcoholic hepatitis	Drug-induced hepatitis[1]
Viral hepatitis	Autoimmune hepatitis[1]
Hepatitis A	Toxic hepatitis
Hepatitis B[1]	Nonalcoholic steatohepatitis (NASH)[1]
Hepatitis C[1]	Metabolic hepatitis[1]
Hepatitis D[1]	Hemochromatosis
Hepatitis E	α_1-Antitrypsin deficiency
Hepatitis G[1]	Wilson's disease
Cytomegalovirus	
Epstein-Barr virus	

[1] These conditions may cause chronic active hepatitis.

    1. In asymptomatic populations, as many as 6% of patients have abnormal values of AST.

    2. Alcohol liver damage, hepatitis C, and nonalcoholic steatohepatitis (NASH) are the most common causes of aminotransferase abnormalities in adults.

    3. Hepatitis A virus is the most common cause of aminotransferase abnormality in children.

  B. **Elevated alkaline phosphatase** is secondary to intrahepatic or extrahepatic obstruction, cholestasis from medication, or infiltrative disease (eg, cancer or granulomas). It has been found in as many as 4% of asymptomatic patients.

  C. **Hyperbilirubinemia** may signify hepatobiliary disease or hemolysis.

    1. Mild degrees of indirect hyperbilirubinemia may be found in as many as 10% of asymptomatic patients with Gilbert's syndrome.

    2. Prior to age 30, hepatitis causes 75% of hyperbilirubinemia.

    3. After age 60, extrahepatic obstruction causes 50% of hyperbilirubinemia (eg, gallstones or pancreatic cancer).

III. Symptoms

  A. Abnormal LFTs in asymptomatic patients may indicate very mild hepatic dysfunction or may represent a more serious illness in its presymptomatic phase. Subsequent testing and follow-up are usually necessary to determine which abnormality exists.

  B. Fatigue, nausea, malaise, pruritus, jaundice, anorexia, or right upper quadrant discomfort are common complaints of patients with compensated liver disease and abnormal LFTs. The severity of the complaints is often related to the acuteness and extent of the illness.

  C. Fatigue, anorexia, weight loss, abdominal distention, hematemesis, hematochezia, confusion, jaundice, and abdominal discomfort are symptoms of hepatic decompensation in patients with decompensated liver disease and abnormal LFTs.

IV. Signs

  A. Hepatomegaly or an unusually firm liver may be present in asymptomatic patients.

  B. Fever, jaundice, splenomegaly, and a tender, enlarged liver may indicate compensated liver disease.

  C. Ascites, edema, jaundice, vascular spiders, esophageal varices, splenomegaly, hepatic encephalopathy, testicular atrophy, gynecomastia, or loss of pubic and axillary hair may indicate decompensated liver disease.

V. Laboratory Tests

  A. A **stepwise approach to evaluating LFT abnormalities** is recommended (Figure 43–1).

    1. **LFTs should be repeated** to confirm any abnormalities in asymptomatic patients. Any offending agents (Table 43–2) should be discontinued, and the test should be repeated in 1–3 months.

      If abnormal LFTs persist for more than 6 months, treatable causes of chronic hepatitis should be ruled out. Such causes include hemochromatosis; autoimmune hepatitis; α_1-antitrypsin deficiency; hepatitis B, C, and D; NASH, and Wilson's disease (see Chapters 38 and 71).

    2. A **γ-glutamyltransferase (GGT) test** should be ordered in patients with abnormal alkaline phosphatase levels to confirm the hepatic origin of the enzyme.

    3. Direct and indirect **bilirubin fractions** should be obtained if total bilirubin levels are increased. If the indirect (unconjugated) fraction is elevated (>80% of total),

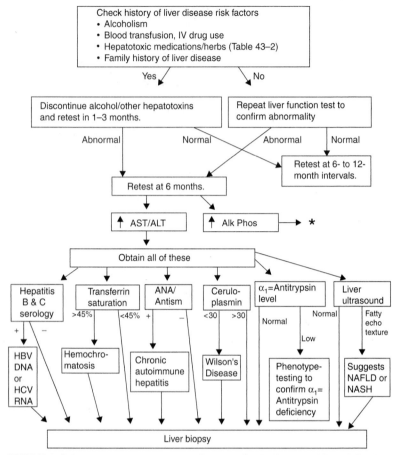

FIGURE 43–1. Evaluation of the asymptomatic patient with abnormal liver function tests. Alk Phos, alkaline phosphatase; ALT, alanine aminotransferase; ANA, antinuclear antibody; AntiSm, anti–smooth muscle antibody; AST, aspartate aminotransferase; ERCP, endoscopic retrograde cholangiopancreatography; GGT, gamma glutamyltransferase; HBV DNA, hepatitis B virus deoxyribonucleic acid; HCV RNA, hepatitis C virus ribonucleic acid; IV, intravenous; NAFLD, nonalcoholic fatty liver disease; NASH, nonalcoholic steatohepatitis; ULN, upper limit of normal; US, ultrasound.

a reticulocyte count and a peripheral blood smear should be obtained (see Chapter 4).

4. **Serum albumin** determinations are indicated in any symptomatic patient. Decreased levels reflect decreased synthesis (from poor nutrition or hepatic dysfunction) or increased loss (from the kidneys or the intestines). Serum levels correlate poorly with prognosis in acute liver disease, although patients with decompensated liver disease routinely have low levels.

5. **Prothrombin time (PT)** reflects hepatic synthesis of vitamin K–dependent clotting factors (II, VII, IX, and X) and should be ordered for patients with acute or chronic liver disease or coagulopathy.

   a. Improvement by 30% after a 10-mg subcutaneous injection of vitamin K suggests intact hepatocellular function and makes biliary obstruction the likely cause of the abnormal PT.

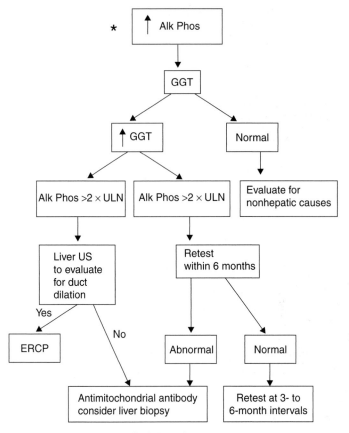

FIGURE 43–1. (*Continued*).

   b. If the PT fails to improve after administration of vitamin K, significant loss of
      hepatocellular function exists and the prognosis is poor.
 6. If evidence suggests hepatitis, further serologic testing is indicated to confirm the
      diagnosis (see Chapter 38).
         Liver biopsy should be considered for any patient with abnormal LFTs for
      6 months. A biopsy sample should be obtained before the end of the 6-month pe-
      riod if the patient's condition deteriorates. Liver biopsy is the only definitive
      means of establishing a diagnosis of chronic hepatitis.
B. Interpretation of particular abnormal LFT patterns
   1. Alcoholic liver disease results in modest elevations of the transaminases. An
      elevation of ALT >300 IU is not consistent with alcoholic liver damage. The ratio of
      AST to ALT is useful diagnostically, since a ratio of 2:1 or greater suggests a high
      probability of alcoholic liver disease. Elevated mean corpuscular volume and GGT
      suggest alcoholic liver disease.
   2. Viral hepatitis often causes significant elevations of the transaminases, with lev-
      els exceeding 1000 IU. ALT is typically elevated more than AST; the AST-ALT ratio
      is <1.
   3. Medications causing cholestasis (Table 43–2) may result in transaminase and
      alkaline phosphatase elevations that are as much as 10 times the normal levels.

TABLE 43–2. MEDICATIONS THAT MAY ADVERSELY AFFECT LIVER FUNCTION TESTS

Cholestatic pattern	Cytotoxic pattern
Amoxicillin/clavulanic acid	Acetaminophen
Anabolic steroids	Amiodarone
Chlorambucil	L-Asparaginase
Chlorpromazine	Aspirin and nonsteroidal anti-inflammatory drugs
Chlorpropamide	Carbamazepine
Erythromycin estolate	Etretinate
Estrogen (oral contraceptives)	Halothane
Methimazole	Hydralazine
Phenobarbital	Imipramine
Tolbutamide	Isoniazid
	Ketoconazole
	Lovastatin
	6-Mercaptopurine
	Methotrexate
	Methyldopa
	Nicotinic acid (especially sustained-release)
	Nitrofurantoin
	Phenytoin
	Propylthiouracil
	Rifampin
	"Statins"
	Sulfonamides
	Tetracycline
	Valproic acid

   4. **Cytotoxic reactions** from medications may cause severe injuries resembling viral hepatitis, with transaminase values as high as 500 times the normal levels.
   5. **Intrahepatic or extrahepatic obstruction** cause values of alkaline phosphatase to be five or more times higher than normal. The highest values are found in primary biliary cirrhosis.
   6. **Infiltrative diseases** such as neoplasm, granulomas, or amyloidosis may cause moderate to marked elevations of alkaline phosphatase. Bilirubin is minimally elevated, however.
   7. **Hemolysis** causes an elevated reticulocyte count and an abnormal peripheral smear, with the bilirubin level generally <5 mg/dL.
   8. **Gilbert's syndrome** is characterized by indirect bilirubin levels of 2–3 mg/dL, normal LFTs, and no evidence of hemolysis.
 VI. **Treatment.** For information on the management of the following causes of abnormal LFTs, refer to the chapters indicated.
   A. **Cholelithiasis** (see Chapter 1).
   B. **Hemolysis** (see Chapter 4).
   C. **Hepatitis** (see Chapter 38).
   D. **Cirrhosis** (see Chapter 71).
   E. **Alcohol and drug abuse** (see Chapter 88).

REFERENCES

Harrison SA, et al: Nonalcoholic steatohepatitis: What we know in the new millennium. Am J Gastro-enterol 2002;**97:**2714.

Moodie SJ, et al: Testing for haemochromatosis in a liver clinic population: Relationship between ethnic origin, HFE gene mutations, liver histology and serum iron markers. Eur J Gastroenterol Hepatol 2002;**14:**223.

Pratt DS, Kaplan MM: Evaluation of abnormal liver-enzyme results in asymptomatic patients. N Engl J Med 2000;**342:**1266.

Riley TR, Bhatti AM: Preventive strategies in chronic liver disease. Am Fam Physician 2001;**64:**1555.

Sherwood P, et al: How are abnormal results for liver function tests dealt with in primary care? Br Med J 2001;**322:**276.

Skelly MM, James PD, Ryder SD: Findings on liver biopsy to investigate abnormal liver function tests in the absence of diagnostic serology. J Hepatol 2001;**35:**195.

44   Low Back Pain

David C. Lanier, MD

KEY POINTS

- Up to 95% of patients seen in primary care settings for acute low back pain have no evidence of serious underlying spinal pathology, and diagnostic testing should not be a routine part of their initial evaluation.
- The clinical history and physical examination are generally effective in identifying the few patients who potentially have serious causes of LBP and need further evaluation immediately. A patient's failure to improve with conservative treatment is also an indication for further evaluation.
- The treatment goal for acute or chronic LBP is for the patient to be active as soon as possible. Prolonged bed rest should be avoided.

I. **Definition.** Low back pain (LBP) is pain, muscle tension, or stiffness below the costal margin and above the inferior gluteal folds, with or without pain or neuromotor deficits in the leg (sciatica). Most back pain symptoms are **nonspecific** and result from overuse or injury of the ligaments and muscles that hold together the lumbosacral (LS) vertebrae or from degenerative osteoarthritis of the articular processes of the facet joints. **Specific** mechanisms resulting in LBP include:

    A. Herniation of an intervertebral disk, causing inflammation or direct pressure on nerve roots exiting from the LS spinal cord.

    B. Fracture of a vertebra, which may be traumatic or pathologic.

    C. Malignant neoplasm of the spine.

    D. Spinal stenosis, mechanical pressure on neural structures resulting from a degenerative narrowing of the bony spinal canal.

    E. A defect of the vertebral arch (spondylolysis) leading to slippage of all or part of a vertebra on another (spondylolisthesis).

    F. Spinal infection.

    G. Inflammatory diseases.

    H. Referred visceral pain from vascular, genitourinary, or gastrointestinal diseases.

II. **Common Diagnoses.** LBP is a common condition that affects >80% of individuals at some time during their active life and accounts for about 4% of adult primary care visits.

    A. **Back strain** tends to affect men at an earlier age (30–50 years) than women, who are more likely to report symptoms after age 60. Risk factors include repetitive lifting (especially in a twisted position), exposure to mechanical vibrations, static work postures (eg, prolonged sitting), cigarette smoking, and a sedentary lifestyle.

    B. Degenerative **osteoarthritis** of the LS spine, the prevalence of which increases with age, can almost universally be detected in individuals older than 75 years of age.

    C. **Lumbar disk herniation** occurs most frequently in individuals between the ages of 30 and 55 years, but can occur at any age. Only about 35% of individuals with disk herniation develop leg symptoms (sciatica), a condition seen in <2% of all patients with acute LBP. **Cauda equina syndrome,** a massive central disk herniation compressing the spinal cord, is even rarer, with a prevalence among all patients with LBP estimated at 0.0004.

    D. **Compression fracture.** Older patients with osteoporosis, especially postmenopausal women, are at greatest risk, with African American and Mexican-American women having 25% fewer compression fractures than white women. Only about 30% of patients with fractures have a history of identifiable trauma.

    E. **Spondylolysis** is found in 5% of people older than age 7. **Spondylolisthesis** is the most common cause of LBP in patients younger than age 26, especially athletes, but is rarely the sole cause of LBP after age 40. (Also see the sidebar on idiopathic scoliosis.)

    F. **Malignant neoplasms** are the cause of LBP in <1% of episodes. Metastatic lesions (eg, from breast, prostate, or lung) are 25 times more common than primary bone tumor.

G. **Visceral pain** referred to the back (eg, from abdominal aortic aneurysm or gastro-intestinal cancer) is observed primarily in adults older than 50 years.

H. **Inflammatory diseases** (eg, rheumatoid arthritis, ankylosing spondylitis, Reiter's syndrome) account for about 0.3% of episodes of LBP.

I. **Lumbosacral infections** (LS spine osteomyelitis, diskitis, or epidural abscess) are even rarer, occurring most often in individuals who have diabetes mellitus, use intravenous drugs, or have a history of septicemia, sickle cell disease, or recent spinal or urinary tract infection.

J. **Anxiety, depression,** and **social/psychological distress** may amplify or prolong back pain and often play an important role in the transition from acute to chronic LBP. Occupational risk factors include job dissatisfaction, monotonous tasks, and poor relationships with coworkers.

IDIOPATHIC SCOLIOSIS

Idiopathic scoliosis of the spine, most commonly found in young females, rarely causes back pain unless the spinal curvature is severe (>40 degrees). However, since the condition is present in 2–4% of children between 10 and 16 years of age, less severe scoliosis may be a coincidental x-ray finding in patients with back pain. The initial evaluation of the adolescent found to have scoliosis should focus on the severity of the curvature noted on x-ray (eg, Cobb angle), associated warning signs, and the potential for progression. Since 90% of thoracic curves are to the right, a left thoracic curve deserves further evaluation with a magnetic resonance imaging scan to rule out spondylolisthesis, tumors, or syringomyelia. Unusual pain or abnormal neurologic findings should also prompt further evaluation. Greater potential for curve progression is associated with gender (females have a 10 times higher risk than males of curve progression) and future growth potential. An estimate of remaining skeletal growth can be determined by radiographic assessment of bony fusion of the iliac apophysis (Risser grades).

Adolescents with curvatures of less than 20 degrees and no evidence of an underlying etiology can be safely followed up for progression with x-rays every 6 months. Patients with curvatures on diagnosis of greater than 20 degrees and patients with curves that demonstrate progression should be referred to an orthopedic subspecialist. Surgery is not a consideration until spinal curvature of 40 degrees or greater is observed. Bracing has been shown to halt progression of less severe curvatures.

The principal screening test for scoliosis is the forward bend test on examination to detect a rotational deformity (rib hump) as the patient bends over. However, since the positive predictive value of this test varies with the degree of curvature, the prevalence of scoliosis in the screened population, and the skills of the examiner, the US Preventive Services Task Force has found insufficient evidence for or against routine screening of asymptomatic adolescents. When examining adolescents, clinicians should remain alert for large spinal curvatures.

III. Symptoms

A. **Onset.** Back strain typically has an acute, sudden onset, as may the pain from a compression fracture. Pain caused by medical conditions (eg, inflammation, cancer, or referred visceral pain) generally has a more gradual or insidious onset.

B. **Frequency and duration.** Most mechanical LBP occurs in intermittent episodes that last from a few days to a few months. A degenerating disk may cause low-grade, persistent discomfort that is exacerbated during acute flare-ups. Patients with osteoarthritis, inflammatory conditions, or cancer usually develop chronic persistent symptoms.

C. **Time of day.** Inflammatory conditions produce greater back pain and stiffness in the morning; mechanical disorders typically cause pain that increases with the day's activities. Most individuals with spinal cancer complain of back pain that is worse during the night.

D. **Location of pain.** Most mechanical and medical disorders result in pain localized to the LS spine and surrounding areas. Nerve root irritation (eg, from a herniated disk, spinal stenosis, or spondylolisthesis) is signaled by pain that radiates from the back to the lower leg or is felt exclusively in the lower leg. Poorly localized pain along nonanatomic routes suggests the presence of social or psychological distress.

    E. Aggravating and alleviating factors. Pain caused by mechanical disorders typically improves with recumbency and worsens with activity, whereas patients with back pain caused by inflammatory diseases or tumor often feel worse with bed rest. Relief of pain only with absolute immobility is often a sign of acute infection or a compression fracture.

IV. Signs. The purpose of the physical examination of a patient with LBP is to supplement information obtained in the medical history in searching for serious underlying spinal pathology (eg, cancer) or possible neurologic compromise. The basic elements of the examination are:

    A. Vital signs. The presence of fever or weight loss may indicate infection or cancer.

    B. Inspection. An **antalgic** gait, resulting from avoidance of weight bearing on the involved leg, may be a sign of nerve root irritation.

    C. Spinal range of motion. Very limited range of motion suggests the possibility of a spinal infection, but this finding is also common in patients without infection.

    D. Palpation. Most patients with back strain will exhibit **local tenderness** or **muscle spasm.** These signs, however, are neither highly sensitive nor specific. **Point tenderness** over bony landmarks is a sensitive but nonspecific sign of infection. It is also commonly seen in patients with arthritis or cancer. Pain from percussion of the sacroiliac joints is suggestive but not diagnostic of ankylosing spondylitis.

    E. Neurologic evaluation. This examination emphasizes ankle and knee reflexes, ankle and great toe dorsiflexion strength, and distribution of sensory complaints.

        1. Diminished or absent ankle reflex, calf weakness or atrophy, and **sensory loss along the lateral aspect of the foot** are caused by compression of the first sacral nerve root (S-1).

        2. Weakness of dorsiflexors of the ankle or great toe and **sensory loss along the medial foot** are caused by compression of the fifth lumbar root (L-5).

        3. Diminished knee jerk is caused by compression of the fourth lumbar nerve root (L-4). This is a relatively uncommon finding.

        4. Pain during a **straight leg raising test** indicates nerve root irritation or compression. The examiner raises the affected leg of the supine patient by the heel while keeping the knee fully extended. In a positive test, pain below the knee occurs when the leg is raised 30–60 degrees.

    F. Abdominal, rectal, and pelvic examination. A mass detected on abdominal examination may indicate cancer or aortic aneurysm. A rectal and pelvic examination is especially important if cancer or infection is suspected, or if the patient is new to the practice or has not been examined in the recent past.

    G. Anatomically "inappropriate" signs. These signs elicited on examination often identify psychological distress as a result, or as an amplifier, of LBP. Such signs include back pain from downward pressure applied to the skull, patient overreaction during the examination, or marked discrepancy between the examination and the patient's ability to dress or move about.

V. Laboratory Tests. For most patients with acute LBP, x-rays, imaging studies, and laboratory tests are unnecessary. Table 44–1 lists the signs/symptoms on the initial history and physical examination that suggest a need for immediate testing. Testing is also indicated if significant improvement of LBP is not seen after 2–4 weeks of conservative treatment.

TABLE 44–1. SIGNS/SYMPTOMS THAT SUGGEST A NEED FOR EARLY IMAGING IN ADULT PATIENTS WITH ACUTE LOW BACK PAIN

Finding	Rationale for Early Imaging
Major trauma (eg, fall, MVA)	Possible fracture
Age >50 years	Greater risk of cancer, compression fracture
History of cancer	Greater risk of underlying malignancy
Unexplained weight loss	Greater risk of cancer or infection
Fever, immunosuppression, human immunodeficiency virus, IV or injection drug use	Risk for spinal infection
Saddle anesthesia, bladder or bowel incontinence	Possible cauda equina syndrome
Severe or progressive neurologic deficit	Possible cauda equina syndrome or severe nerve root compression

IV, intravenous; MVA, motor vehicle accident.

A. Radiologic evaluation should be used selectively and the results interpreted with care. **Plain films** of the back do not rule out significant LS spine disease and may give false-negative results in as many as 40% of patients with known vertebral cancer. Moreover, conditions such as degenerative arthritis, narrowed disk space, mild scoliosis, facet subluxation, and minor congenital abnormalities (eg, spina bifida occulta) detected radiographically may be unrelated to back pain, since these conditions are noted with the same frequency in symptomatic and asymptomatic individuals.

Bone scan should be considered for patients with signs or symptoms suggestive of cancer, infection, or occult fractures of the vertebrae, conditions for which bone scans are more sensitive detecting than plain films. However, positive scan results almost always need to be confirmed using other tests.

For patients at risk (Table 44–1), whose symptoms persist despite normal plain films, and those who fail to improve within 6 weeks of conservative treatment, **magnetic resonance imaging (MRI)** is a logical next imaging step. **Computerized tomography (CT),** however, is less expensive and almost as accurate in identifying most serious conditions, making it a reasonable alternative. The clinician should be aware, however, that many abnormalities found on MRI or CT of the back, including herniated or "bulging" disks, are also found in normal, asymptomatic persons. Fear may become more disabling for some patients with LBP than any organic condition, and irrelevant radiographic findings probably contribute to this fear.

B. Simple **clinical screening tests** such as the **erythrocyte sedimentation rate** and **serum alkaline phosphatase** can be used to evaluate patients with LBP at risk of having malignancy or an acute infectious or inflammatory process (Table 44–1). Abnormalities of the **urinalysis** may help identify those patients suspected of having referred back pain of urinary origin. However, **serologic tests** (eg, antinuclear antibodies, rheumatoid factor, and HLA-B27) should not be used for routine screening of patients with LBP since the common spondyloarthropathies affecting the back are seronegative conditions.

C. Electromyography is occasionally useful in assessing a patient with leg symptoms that are possibly back-related and of more than 3–4 weeks' duration. Test results are not reliable before this time.

VI. Treatment

A. Acute LBP. When back pain is found to result from medical conditions such as cancer or infection, specific treatment should be directed at the underlying disease. Treatment for almost all other causes of acute LBP (including early treatment of minor neural compression) should be conservative, aimed at relieving pain, maintaining or restoring function, and reassuring the patient that the acute symptoms are self-limited.

   1. Activity. Staying active within the limits permitted by the acute pain leads to a more rapid recovery than either bed rest or specific back-mobilizing exercises. Prolonged periods of sitting and activities stressful to the back (eg, lifting) may need to be limited temporarily. The goal, however, is for the patient to be back to normal activities as soon as possible. Neither prolonged bed rest (ie, more than a few days) nor spinal traction has any proven efficacy in the treatment of acute LBP.

   2. Medication. Nonsteroidal anti-inflammatory drugs (NSAIDs), such as ibuprofen (1600 mg/day), are effective for short-term symptomatic relief in patients with acute symptoms. There is no evidence that any particular NSAID has superior efficacy. **Acetaminophen** (2600 mg/day, every 4–6 hours) is a reasonably safe and effective alternative for patients who are intolerant of NSAIDs. **Muscle relaxants,** such as cyclobenzaprine (10–20 mg every 8 hours for 7 days), appear to be as effective as NSAIDs in relieving back symptoms, although drowsiness (which occurs in up to 30% of patients) may limit the patient's ability to ambulate or participate in other activities. There is no added benefit when muscle relaxants are used in combination with NSAIDs. Sedation is also a major problem with **opioids,** such as codeine (30–60 mg every 4–6 hours), although these drugs may be required for a fixed period of time by patients with severe or radicular pain not relieved by NSAIDs. **Epidural corticosteroid injections** (in consultation with a pain management specialist) may be useful in the treatment of leg pain and sensory deficits early in the course of sciatica secondary to a herniated lumbar disk. Their use should be based on clinical findings rather than imaging results. There is no evidence that injections into facet joints or trigger points improve pain relief or function.

3. **Physical modalities.** **Spinal manipulation** has been shown in some studies to be effective in reducing LBP (and perhaps in speeding recovery) within the first month of symptoms. Other modalities such as diathermy, ultrasonography, or massage treatments have no proven effect on longer-term outcomes.
4. **Exercise.** The patient should be encouraged to begin low-impact aerobic exercise (eg, short walks, swimming, or cycling) as soon as possible. More rigorous exercise programs to improve abdominal and paraspinal muscle tone should be delayed for at least 2 weeks following the onset of symptoms.
5. **Patient education.** In addition to assuring the patient that in over 80% of cases the acute LBP will resolve or improve significantly within 4–6 weeks, the clinician should focus on the patient's general physical condition. A program of weight loss, exercise, and cessation of smoking can help prevent recurrence of symptoms, which occurs in as many as 75% of patients with occupationally related acute episodes of LBP. Patients should also be instructed in body mechanics, such as appropriate work stance and the best ways to lift and carry objects. Job design/redesign to avoid pain-inducing movements may also help prevent recurrences. It is often useful for the clinician to assist the patient in identifying and addressing significant psychosocial stresses or family dysfunction that may contribute to slow recovery or recurrence of back pain.
6. **Surgery.** The only absolute indication for early lumbar disk surgery is an acute disk herniation associated with either a cauda equina compression or progressive neurologic deficits. Patients with significant pain and unequivocal, disk-related neurologic signs and symptoms may be treated either medically or surgically, depending on individual patient preferences. Surgical diskectomy may substantially improve the short-term symptoms and quality of life for carefully selected patients with painful herniated lumbar disks, although long-term outcomes do not appear to be superior to medical treatment. Surgical consultation is not needed, however, for patients with acute LBP alone who have neither sciatica nor evidence of cancer, infection, or fracture. Surgical treatment of spinal stenosis or spondylolisthesis should be considered only after an adequate trial of conservative therapy (see sections VI,A,1–5) has failed.
B. **Chronic LBP.** For the approximately 20% of patients whose acute symptoms persist longer than 3 months, other treatment options should be considered. The most important objectives in treating chronic LBP are to prevent or reduce disability, both physically and mentally, and to limit sick leave for employed patients. Although evidence on long-term effects is lacking, there is strong evidence of the short-term effects of several interventions:
   1. **Individualized exercise programs** (through physical therapy or a qualified exercise trainer) aimed at increasing endurance and strength of the back to perform specific tasks required on a daily basis at home or work.
   2. **Behavioral therapy** geared toward improving symptoms and disability.
   3. **Multidisciplinary pain treatment programs.**
   4. **Back schools** in occupational settings. There is no evidence that other interventions (such as antidepressants, steroid injections, traction, and acupuncture) are effective.
   Management of chronic LBP should focus not only on the problems that patients have with activities of daily living, but also on any emotional problems, depression, or other psychosocial factors that may be playing a role in the symptoms of the individual patient.

REFERENCES

Deyo RA, Weinstein JN: Low back pain. N Engl J Med 2001;**344:**363.
Jarvik JG, Deyo RA: Diagnostic evaluation of low back pain with emphasis on imaging. Ann Intern Med (October 1) 2002;**137**(7):586.
Saal JS: General principles of diagnostic testing as related to painful lumbar spine disorders: A critical appraisal of current diagnostic techniques. Spine (November 15) 2002;**27**(22):2538.
van Tulder M, Koes B: Low back pain and sciatica: Acute. Clin Evid (June) 2002;**7:**1018.
van Tulder M, Koes B: Low back pain and sciatica: Chronic. Clin Evid (June) 2002;**7:**1032.
Watson KD, Papageorgious AC, Jones GT, et al: Low back pain in school children: The role of mechanical and psychosocial factors. Arch Dis Child (January) 2003;**88**(1):12.

45   Lymphadenopathy

Mari Egan, MD, MHPE

KEY POINTS

- Most patients who present to primary care physicians with lymphadenopathy have benign, easily identifiable causes. The prevalence of malignancy in these patients has been found to be as low as 1.1%.
- Lymphadenopathy is classified as either localized or generalized. Generalized lymphadenopathy occurs if nodes are involved in two or more noncontiguous anatomic areas; localized lymphadenopathy involves a single anatomic area. Three fourths of patients will present with localized lymphadenopathy.
- Localized lymphadenopathy in a patient with benign signs and symptoms can be observed for a month. Generalized adenopathy should always prompt investigation.
- Lymph nodes >1 cm in diameter are considered to be abnormal. Location of the lymphadenopathy and age of the patient are two of the most important determinants of the cause of the problem and the likelihood that it is malignant.

I. **Definition.** Lymph nodes are found throughout the body and serve as a site for the filtering of lymphatic fluid for microorganisms and abnormal proteins. The normal immune response to acute or chronic infectious or noninfectious stimuli may lead to lymph node enlargement. In children with constant exposure to new antigens, palpable cervical, axillary, and inguinal lymph nodes are normal. **Lymphadenopathy** is defined as an abnormality in the size, character, or number of lymph nodes.

II. **Common Diagnoses** (Table 45–1). Lymphadenopathy is a common finding in primary care caused by a vast array of conditions. In the primary care setting, unexplained lymphadenopathy is rare, occurring in only 0.6% of the general population in one study. Of these patients, 3.2% required a lymph node biopsy and only 1.1% were found to have a malignancy. Additional studies have supported this low prevalence of malignancy.

III. **Symptoms.** The patient's history often guides clinical evaluation.
   A. **Age** is an important predictor of diagnosis. The most common causes of enlarged lymph nodes in children are infectious or benign. Malignant or granulomatous causes of lymphadenopathy are more likely in older patients.

TABLE 45–1. COMMON CAUSES OF LYMPHADENOPATHY IN PRIMARY CARE

Diagnosis	Etiologies
1. Infectious	Viral infections: infectious mononucleosis, cytomegalovirus (CMV), rubella, herpes simplex, infectious hepatitis, adenovirus, rubeola, and human immunodeficiency virus (HIV). Nonviral infectious causes: scarlet fever, cat scratch disease, brucellosis, tuberculosis, atypical mycobacterial syphilis, histoplasmosis, leptospirosis, tularemia, malaria, toxoplasmosis, typhoid fever, and pyogenic bacterial infections
2. Immunologic	• Connective tissue disorders (eg, systemic lupus erythematosus and rheumatoid arthritis, Sjögren syndrome) • Immunologic reactions (eg, serum sickness and drug reactions [eg, to phenytoin or propylthiouracil]) • Benign reactive hyperplasia
3. Metabolic	Gaucher's disease, Niemann-Pick disease, hyperthyroidism
4. Malignant	Leukemia, lymphomas (Hodgkin's and non-Hodgkin's), skin neoplasms, Kaposi's sarcoma, metastatic cancers, malignant histiocytosis
5. Miscellaneous disorders	Kawasaki disease, sarcoidosis, and chronic pseudolymphomatous lymphadenopathy

B. Duration. Lymphadenopathy that lasts <2 weeks is usually infectious. Malignant causes are usually present for >2 weeks and increase in size over time.

C. Constitutional systemic symptoms such as fatigue, fever, weight loss, unusual rashes, or arthralgias may suggest cancer, systemic infection, or connective tissue disease.

D. Localized symptoms may suggest the cause of lymphadenopathy (ie, sore throat and cervical lymphadenopathy).

E. Personal/social or family history such as travel, exposure to animals, occupation, dietary habits, hobbies, sexual history and orientation, drug use, infectious contacts, and environmental and family history may help in the diagnosis. For example, travelers to a tropical area have an increased risk of tuberculosis, scrub typhus, and leishmaniasis; hunters may have an increased risk of tularemia; and patients with a family history of dysplastic nevus syndrome may have a neoplastic cause of lymphadenopathy from melanoma.

IV. Signs. If lymph nodes are detected, several characteristics should be noted.

A. Size. Lymph nodes >1 cm in diameter are considered abnormal. Exceptions are epitrochlear nodes, which are abnormal if larger than 0.5 cm, and inguinal nodes, which need to be >1.5 cm to be abnormal. There is little information supporting diagnosis based on size alone. However, in one study, only 8% of patients with nodes from 1 cm^2 to 2.25 cm^2 had cancer, but this number increased to 38% in patients with lymph nodes larger than 2.25 cm^2. In another study of patients aged 9–25 years, lymph node diameter >2 cm distinguished malignant or granulomatous diagnoses from other causes.

B. A hard **texture** to the lymph node is consistent with cancer. Softer (fluctuant) nodes are more often infectious or inflammatory.

C. Pain. Although nonspecific, tenderness on node palpation is characteristic of an inflammatory cause, and absence of pain makes tuberculosis or malignancy more likely.

D. Location of the lymphadenopathy can be helpful in diagnosis (Table 45–2). Three fourths of patients in primary care will present with localized lymphadenopathy: 55% in the head and neck region, 14% in the inguinal region, 5% in the axillary region, and 1% in the supraclavicular region.

E. In patients with **lymphadenopathy and splenomegaly,** the diagnosis of infectious mononucleosis, lymphoma, leukemia, or sarcoidosis is more likely than others. Since most localized lymphadenopathy is cervical, physical examination should include ears, nose, and throat examination.

V. Laboratory Tests (Figure 45–1). The critical task is to determine which patients with lymphadenopathy have benign, self-limited conditions and which ones have malignancy or another serious condition requiring specific treatment. A careful history and physical examination should allow the physician to determine if careful observation, treatment, or additional testing is needed.

A. Lymph node biopsy should be considered when simple measures have failed to provide a diagnosis or if there is a clinical suspicion of a therapeutically important cause such as tuberculosis, sarcoidosis, or neoplasm.

1. Certain clinical features suggest **the need for an early biopsy.** These features include a diameter >2 cm, hard texture of the node, lack of pain or tenderness over the node, patient age older than 40 years, an abnormal chest x-ray result (adenopathy or infiltrate), associated signs and symptoms (such as weight loss or hepatosplenomegaly) that suggest a serious disorder, an absence of upper respiratory tract symptoms, an enlargement of a supraclavicular node, or a cervical node in a smoker.

2. Small lymph nodes, an upper respiratory tract infection, positive viral serology, or a normal chest x-ray result argue against the need for a biopsy.

3. During follow-up for undiagnosed lymphadenopathy, nodes that remain constant in size in 4–8 weeks or fail to resolve in 8–12 weeks should have a biopsy specimen taken.

4. If a biopsy result is nondiagnostic, careful observation of the patient is still important. As many as 25% of patients with persistent lymphadenopathy who undergo a second biopsy have cancer.

B. Imaging studies such as ultrasonography or computerized tomography (CT) of the involved area may differentiate lymphadenopathy from nonlymphatic causes. CT is also

TABLE 45–2. DIFFERENTIAL DIAGNOSIS OF LYMPHADENOPATHY BY LOCATION

Location	Diagnosis
Cervical • The most common area of lymphadenopathy. Most cases are caused by infections.	*Infections:* Viral upper respiratory infections, bacterial pharyngitis, infectious mononucleosis, cytomegalovirus, toxoplasmosis, mycobacterial diseases, rubella *Malignancy:* Non-Hodgkin's lymphoma, Hodgkin's disease, head and neck malignancy *Others:* Kawasaki syndrome, sarcoidosis, Kikuchi's disease, oral injuries, dental lesions
Supraclavicular • This location has the highest risk of malignancy; 90% of patients older than 40 years will have a malignancy when lymphadenopathy is localized here	• Left supraclavicular node (Virchow's node) pathology in the abdomen or thorax. Common causes: breast cancer, lymphoma, and other malignancies • Right supraclavicular node drains the mediastinum, lungs, and esophagus and is associated with pathology in these areas • Chronic fungal (histoplasmosis) and mycobacterial infections
Axillary • Usually secondary to infection or malignancy	*Infections:* Staphylococcus and strep infections of the arm, tularemia, cat scratch disease, toxoplasmosis *Malignancy:* Breast cancer, lymphoma, melanoma
Epitrochlear • Rare in healthy patients	*Infections:* Infectious mononucleosis, HIV, secondary syphilis, leprosy, rubella, tularemia, and leishmaniasis *Malignancy:* Lymphoma and leukemia
Inguinal • Most adults will normally have some degree of inguinal enlargement, and there is a low suspicion of malignancy	*Infections:* Sexually transmitted diseases, bubonic plague *Malignancies:* Squamous cell carcinoma of the penis/vulva, lymphoma, or melanoma
Generalized • Lymphadenopathy found in two or more distinct anatomic regions • Usually needs prompt specific testing	It is more likely to result from serious infections (ie, HIV), autoimmune disease (ie, systemic lupus erythematosus), hematologic malignancies (ie, leukemia), and metastatic cancers

useful to demonstrate the presence of mediastinal, mesenteric, or retroperitoneal lymph nodes.

   C. A **bone marrow examination** is indicated for patients with severe anemia, neutropenia, thrombocytopenia, or a peripheral smear with malignant blast cells.

VI. Treatment

   A. **Viral infections.** Treatment of viral infections is primarily limited to symptomatic treatment such as warm compresses, analgesics, and the avoidance of trauma to the swollen node (see Chapters 55 and 57).

   B. **Cat scratch disease.** This disease is usually self-limited, requiring only symptomatic treatment. Aspiration of suppurative glands may reduce swelling and discomfort. Incision and drainage should be avoided to prevent sinus tract formation. For typical cat scratch disease, there is no proven response to antibiotics.

   C. **Neoplasm.** Neoplastic disease should be referred to an oncologist for treatment.

   D. **Mycobacterial disease.** Nodes affected with atypical mycobacteria are treated by surgical excision. A positive culture result or the demonstration of acid-fast bacilli is the most direct method of diagnosis, although treatment of *Mycobacterium tuberculosis* can be initiated on the basis of the clinical presentation and a positive skin test. (See Chapter 13.)

   E. **Acute lymphadenitis.** Initial therapy should be directed toward staphylococcal and streptococcal infections. Oral cephalexin (25–50 mg/kg in divided doses up to 500 mg four times a day), erythromycin (30–50 mg/kg up to 500 mg four times a day), or a semisynthetic penicillinase-resistant penicillin such as dicloxacillin (25–50 mg/kg up to 500 mg four times a day for 7–10 days) is useful.

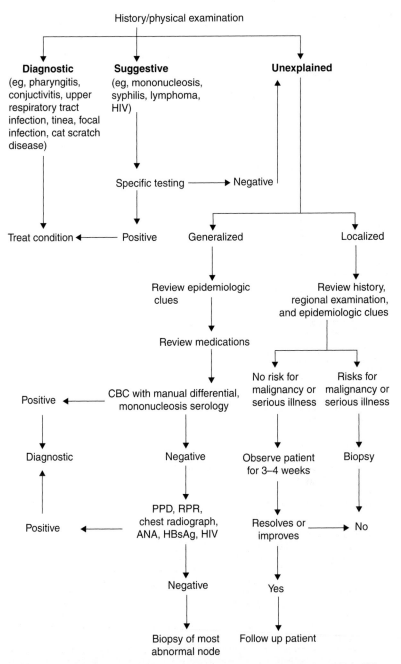

FIGURE 45–1. Algorithm for the evaluation of a patient with lymphadenopathy. ANA, antinuclear antibody; CBC, complete blood count; HBsAg, hepatitis B surface antigen; HIV, human immunodeficiency virus; PPD, purified protein derivative; RPR, rapid plasma reagin.

REFERENCES

Allhiser JN, McKnight TA, Shank CJ: Lymphadenopathy in a family practice. J Fam Pract 1981;**12**:27.
Bazemore AW, Smucker DR: Lymphadenopathy and malignancy. Am Fam Physician 2002;**66**:2103.
Ferrer R: Lymphadenopathy: Differential diagnosis and evaluation. Am Fam Physician 1998;**58**:1313.
Habermann TM, Steensma DP: Lymphadenopathy. Mayo Clin Proc 2000;**75**:723.
Lipsky MS: A systematic approach to evaluating pediatric lymphadenopathy. Fam Pract Recertification 1987;**9**:23.
Pangalis GA, et al: Clinical approach to lymphadenopathy. Semin Oncol 1993;**20**:570.
Twist CJ, Link MP: Assessment of lymphadenopathy in children. Pediatr Clin North Am 2002;**49**:1009.

---

46   Myalgia

Tomás P. Owens, Jr., MD

KEY POINTS

- Most common causes of myalgia can be diagnosed through careful history and examination, without laboratory testing.
- Ischemia should be considered in localized myalgia, especially with suggestive risk factors and normal muscle examination.
- Drug-induced rhabdomyolysis should be considered as a potential cause of myalgia.

I. **Definition.** Myalgia is defined as generalized or localized pain perceived as originating in skeletal muscle tissue, usually characterized as a deep, aching sensation but sometimes as a burning or electric sensation. Myalgia can be classified as acute (lasting less than 1 month) or chronic (lasting more than 3–6 months); localized (one or a few muscle groups), or generalized (involving more than 4 areas), or symmetric or asymmetric.

II. **Common Diagnoses.** As many as one third of patients presenting in an ambulatory primary care setting complain of muscle pain in an extremity or the back. In the general population, as many as 60% of adults have musculoskeletal pain lasting more than 1 month or caused by identified trauma. In one study, 9% of primary care visits were for myofascial pain syndrome.

   A. **Viral syndromes** (and other infectious causes). Most **viral syndromes** have seasonal variations, with a winter peak in temperate climates. Arbovirus myalgic syndromes such as West Nile virus predominate between June and October, paralleling the mosquito vectors. Children are particularly at risk for viral syndromes, but myalgia in children is less common than in adults. A rare form of localized myalgia is staphylococcal myositis, which can accompany cellulitis.

   B. **Major or minor trauma.** Accumulated metabolic waste products cause myalgia with strenuous exercise in a deconditioned patient. Direct blunt or minor repetitive trauma occurs with occupational hazards (faulty ergonomics, repetitive acts of a monotonous nature), recreational pursuits ("weekend warrior syndrome," with poor conditioning or inappropriate training), or substance abuse (repetitive accidental or self-inflicted trauma), and results in hemorrhage within the muscle tissue and muscle fiber or fascial tears. Trauma also causes muscle spasm or cramping.

   C. **Fibromyalgia and myofascial pain** (8–10% of all visits to a primary care outpatient practice).

   1. **Fibromyalgia syndrome (FMS**—former name: fibrositis) affects 5–10% of the US population at some point in their lives. It is more common in women than in men (10:1), particularly in women aged 20–50 years (with a peak incidence at age 35). **FMS** is the second most common disorder in American rheumatology practices. It has been associated with a history of sexual abuse during childhood, drug use, and eating disorders, but no causal relationship has been established. Depression, personality disorders, and anxiety are also strongly associated. In FMS there is

clear evidence of regional blood flow abnormalities in the thalamus and caudate nucleus associated with low pain-threshold levels (hyperalgesia) and allodynia, occurring spontaneously or as a neuroimmune response to viral, physical, or psychological trauma. Biochemical abnormalities are inconsistent and muscle biopsies are unrevealing.

2. Less generalized **myofascial pain syndromes** (not fulfilling **FMS** diagnostic criteria) are seen in up to 50% of the population, are equally common in men and women, and have a much better prognosis with appropriate therapy.

D. **Collagen vascular diseases** (about 15% in the general population and over 1 million newly afflicted patients each year). **Inflammatory articular diseases** such as rheumatoid arthritis and lupus occur primarily in women between ages 20 and 50 years. **Inflammatory nonarticular diseases** such as **polymyositis** and **dermatomyositis** are more common in children and occur equally in men and women, but a particular form occurs in men older than 40 years in association with malignancy of other organ systems. **Polymyositis** may be postviral; it is especially common following enteroviral infections (particularly Coxsackie) or parasitic infection such as trichinosis. Polymyalgia rheumatica **(PMR)** occurs equally in men and women, usually older than age 65 years. Myalgia from these conditions is due to immune-mediated inflammation of periarticular structures or muscle.

E. **Vascular insufficiency** (<1% of patients with myalgia) has a strong association with older age, smoking, hypertension, hyperlipidemia, and diabetes mellitus and is due to insufficient arterial perfusion.

F. **Primary muscle malignancy** is an extremely rare cause of myalgia in primary care, has no specific risk factors, and causes pain from rapid tumor growth with compression of surrounding structures.

G. **Substance-induced** (an emerging cause of myalgia).

1. The **"statins"** class of lipid-lowering agents has rarely been associated with generalized myalgia by direct toxicity to the muscle (rhabdomyolysis), the so-called **statin-induced myalgia (SIM)**. The synchronous use of gemfibrozil or cyclosporine potentiates the effect significantly, as does pre-existing renal insufficiency. It is believed that lipid-soluble statins are more likely to produce the syndrome and one has been withdrawn from the market for that reason (cerivastatin).

2. Excipients in some batches of Λ-tryptophan (eg, "peak X") produce a complex immunologic response called **eosinophilia-myalgia syndrome (EMS)**.

3. Other drugs causing myopathy or myalgia but not discussed further here include amphotericin B, chloroquine, cimetidine, clofibrate, glucocorticoids, oral contraceptives, and zidovudine.

III. **Symptoms and Signs**

A. Myalgia from **viral syndromes** is relatively mild; the time course parallels the course of the illness and is often accompanied by other systemic viral infection symptoms (malaise, weakness, and any combination of the following: headache, nausea, vomiting, diarrhea, and upper respiratory symptoms, including fever). Viral myalgia is usually generalized, but many patients complain of pain in larger, proximal muscle groups and in the back (particularly the upper back, trapezius, neck, and shoulders). Many experts believe that acute viral infection can precipitate progression to chronic fibromyalgia, in which case patients report a deep, aching discomfort, an inability to be comfortable in any position, and localized, palpable pain. **Well-localized inflammation in relation to cellulitis** is the hallmark of staphylococcal myositis.

B. Myalgia due to **trauma** is localized and specific to the trauma history.

1. Patients sometimes report the **relatively acute onset of localized pain** without associated illness or obvious trauma, but further probing usually reveals some new activity or minor repetitive act (eg, lifting furniture, gardening, painting, or new work responsibility).

2. The **pain of major trauma** (eg, a motor vehicle accident) or overuse usually starts several hours after the event and reaches a peak at 48 hours. The pain may persist for days or weeks, particularly if the offending activity is not identified and stopped. The patient may report some loss of function or pain with a specific movement or position, which sometimes reminds the patient of the precipitating event.

3. **Tenderness on palpation of the specific muscle,** sometimes with crepitus, decreased active range of motion, and erythema, is a common finding. Blunt trauma

may cause ecchymosis, hematoma, superficial abrasions, pain on palpation, or decreased active and passive range of motion of the involved muscle.

C. **FMS and myofascial pain syndrome**

1. With **FMS,** pain is worse after even minimal activity and may include generalized symptoms such as diffuse myalgia, fatigue, a low-grade fever, muscle tension, headache, and skin sensitivity. Sleep disturbance is a particularly prominent and nearly universal complaint. The American College of Rheumatology (1990) diagnostic criteria require the patient to have at least 11 of 18 possible tender points on digital examination and a history of widespread pain (Figure 46–1).

2. **Myofascial pain syndrome** includes localized muscle pain in such common areas as the paraspinous regions of the upper and middle back, trapezius, levator scapulae, neck, shoulders, arms, glutei, and legs, often manifesting as **trigger points** (excruciatingly painful foci of muscle from which diffuse pain and spasm emanate).

D. The myalgia associated with a **collagen vascular disease** parallels the course of the primary disease and is increased with muscle palpation.

1. Signs of the primary rheumatic disease dominate, including joint erythema and swelling or effusion, Raynaud's phenomenon, vasculitis, conjunctivitis, urethritis, or uveitis.

2. The onset of **polymyositis** may be acute, particularly in children, and may include fever. In polymyositis of any cause, the patient reports loss of muscle function either from pain or loss of functioning neuromuscular units. Primary idiopathic **dermatomyositis** can present with multiple abdominal complaints (eg, pain or dysphagia) and a classic lilac-colored (heliotrope) rash.

3. The pain and stiffness of inflammatory articular disorders such as **rheumatoid arthritis** or lupus are more severe in the morning upon arising.

4. Patients with **PMR** complain of stiffness, weakness, and pain, particularly in the hip and shoulder girdle, along with systemic symptoms such as malaise, fatigue, and headache due to temporal (giant cell) arteritis.

E. **Vascular insufficiency** causes the most severe myalgia, is intermittent, and physical examination of the muscle is often normal.

1. The pain associated with **arterial insufficiency** (intermittent claudication) occurs with exercise of a predictable type and intensity, is almost always in the lower extremity, and can be described precisely by the patient. It resolves shortly after cessation of the activity. With severe ischemia, rest pain may be present. Peripheral pulses are delayed, decreased, or absent, and extremity blood pressures are asymmetric, with a decreased leg:arm ratio (see Chapter 42). Marked hair loss, dry skin, decreased capillary refill, and pronounced pachyonychia are commonly present.

2. In **thoracic outlet syndrome,** pain, weakness, paresthesias, and claudication occur in one of the upper extremities. Abducting the affected arm and externally rotating the shoulder may precipitate pain with or without cyanosis and pulselessness.

3. The pain of **venous insufficiency** is more vague in onset, nature, and cessation, but is often related to a dependent position of the affected extremity (almost always the leg). Signs may include increased circumference, edema, erythema, brawny hyperpigmentation, and ulceration of dependent areas, particularly the lower legs and ankles ("venous stasis"). Rarely, a **superior vena cava syndrome** will produce symptoms in the upper extremities. These findings are accompanied by facial swelling, cyanosis, and neck vein distention.

F. The pain of **primary muscle malignancy** is gradual in onset and vague in nature, but patients usually report associated weakness and an enlarging, localized mass in the body of the muscle.

G. Generalized, slowly progressive pain, asthenia, and weakness/tenderness of major muscle groups are characteristic of **SIM.** The onset of **EMS** can be abrupt or insidious. Early manifestations include low-grade fever, fatigue, cough, dyspnea, arthralgias, muscle cramping, and myalgia. Arthritis and evanescent erythematous rashes ensue thereafter. Months later, scleroderma-like skin changes, an ascending polyneuropathy with cognitive impairment and, rarely, pulmonary hypertension can develop.

IV. **Laboratory Tests** (Figure 46–1). Laboratory evaluation is not usually indicated in cases of viral syndrome, trauma, or clear-cut myofascial pain or **FMS,** but tests may be indicated in patients with rheumatic symptoms or who have impressive systemic symptoms; whose

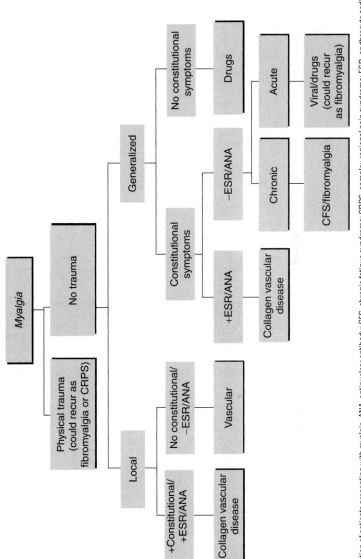

FIGURE 46–1. Evaluation of patients presenting with myalgia. ANA, antinuclear antibody; CFS, chronic fatigue syndrome; CRPS, complex regional pain syndrome; ESR, erythrocyte sedimentation rate. (From Klippel JH (editor): *Primer on the Rheumatic Diseases*, 12th ed. Arthritis Foundation; 2001.)

symptoms have persisted despite conservative, nonspecific therapy for several weeks; who
have joint effusions; or whose disease has caused significant disability.

A. **Complete blood cell count.** The white blood cell count may show a neutropenic or inflammatory (leukocytosis) reaction with a viral syndrome, although the **erythrocyte
sedimentation rate (ESR)** is usually normal. The ESR helps differentiate fibromyalgia
(normal) from collagen vascular diseases (ESR >50 mm/hr). A high ESR may prompt
further testing (eg, antinuclear antibody, rheumatoid factor, and more comprehensive
rheumatologic panels) (Chapter 39.) Parasitic infection may cause eosinophilia. Mild
anemia and thrombocytosis are common in rheumatic diseases.

B. **Culture of specific infectious lesions** (eg, primary herpes simplex) should be performed only in appropriate clinical situations. Routine throat swabs and blood cultures
are usually unrevealing with viral syndromes.

C. **X-rays** may be required to rule out bony pathology as a result of known or unknown
trauma (particularly relating to the hip or pelvis in older persons), or they may be helpful in patients with localized muscle or tendon pain that is difficult to differentiate from
bone pain (eg, lateral epicondylitis).

D. **An empiric trial of a low daily dose (10–20 mg orally) of prednisone** usually has a
dramatic positive effect on almost all collagen vascular diseases and thus has some
diagnostic value pending more definitive studies. Unfortunately, corticosteroid use can
produce a sense of well-being in patients with almost any pathology. Therefore, empiric
corticosteroid use must be adapted to each clinical situation.

E. **Impedance Doppler studies** are required in patients with evidence of vascular insufficiency (see Chapter 42). These may be followed or, in some instances, supplanted
by **arteriography** or **venography.**

F. **Muscle biopsy** should be arranged for any enlarging painful muscle mass not explain-
able by specific trauma. Abnormal histology on muscle biopsy is the only specific laboratory abnormality in patients with primary muscle tumors.

G. In **SIM,** marked elevations of creatine phosphokinase (CPK) are noted. In **EMS,** the
eosinophil count is higher than 1000/mm^3 and biopsy results show eosinophilic fasciitis.

V. **Treatment**

A. Myalgia due to **viral syndromes** is relieved by treatment with nonsteroidal anti-
inflammatory drugs (NSAIDs). **Aspirin,** 650–1000 mg orally every 4 hours, is as effective as a prescription NSAID. **Ibuprofen,** 600 mg orally every 6 hours, or **naproxen,**
375–500 mg orally every 8–12 hours, is an excellent substitute for the anti-inflammatory
effects of aspirin, but each is less effective as an antipyretic agent. **Acetaminophen,**
650–1000 mg orally every 4 hours, can be used in addition to the NSAID and, for
severe myalgia (particularly associated with severe headache), can be combined
with **codeine,** 15–30 mg (eg, Tylenol No. 2 or No. 3), one to two tablets orally every
4 hours.

B. Myalgia due to **blunt trauma** or repetitive minor trauma is best treated with rest of the
affected muscle, ice and cold therapy (particularly after use of the muscle injured by
overactivity or inappropriate athletic training), heat therapy (particularly for generalized
myalgia or for localized myalgia with muscle weakness or dysfunction), and immobilization (for localized myalgia due to trauma with significant dysfunction). Immobilization can be accomplished with either soft (eg, felt) or rigid (eg, commercial plastic or
metal) splints for only a few days to prevent atrophy and weakness. A more specific diagnosis of the cause of repetitive overuse injuries (recreational or occupational) may
lead to specific exercises, strengthening, or avoidance/modification of certain activities
in the workplace (ergonomics evaluation) or during leisure time.

C. For myalgia due to **fibromyalgia,** prescribed reading may give the patient hope by
naming the problem and informing the patient that the problem is manageable, and it
may help in controlling health care–seeking behavior for the multitude of associated
symptoms. Support groups may have similar benefit.

1. An **exercise and stretching program** should be similar to that for rehabilitation of
a postmyocardial infarction patient, with specific submaximal heart rate targets
(70–80% of maximum heart rate), frequency (three to five times weekly), and duration (30–40 minutes with appropriate warm-up and cool-down).

2. **Antidepressant therapy** (eg, **imipramine** or **amitriptyline,** 75–100 mg orally
1–2 hours before bedtime, selective serotonin reuptake inhibitors, heterocyclics,
or bupropion) is used in a moderate dosage, primarily for regulation of sleep rather
than in the full dosage used for major depressive disorder (see Chapter 92).

3. **Trigger point injection** can be performed as often as necessary with local anesthetic, but preferably no more than four or five injections per year should be given if corticosteroids are used. The trigger point should be carefully palpated to determine the point of most exquisite pain. This point is injected intramuscularly using a long 25- or 27-gauge needle that contains 0.5–1.0 mL of a long-acting local anesthetic such as bupivacaine 0.25%. There is some evidence of benefit from moving the needle around and pulling back into different parts of the trigger point ("needling"). A corticosteroid, such as 0.5 mL of **triamcinolone,** 40 mg/mL, can be added to the injection, but no evidence exists that the injection will be more effective than any of the local anesthetics or even normal saline.
4. **Cognitive behavioral therapy** is very useful in many patients. Minimal intervention (paradoxical approach) has also been effective, particularly in the outpatient setting. Disability claims, with legal and financial repercussions and tremendous secondary gain, make the management of this syndrome complicated in some patients.
5. **Alternative, integrative, complementary,** or **balanced medicine** approaches, including biofeedback, yoga, meditation, tai chi, qi gong, spray-and-stretch techniques, acupuncture, and acupressure, may be helpful, but strong research supporting their efficacy is scarce.

D. Myalgia due to **collagen vascular diseases** is managed according to the underlying disease, usually with rheumatologic consultation (see Chapter 39).
1. **PMR,** though self-limited, is treated with low-dose (10–20 mg) oral prednisone daily for symptomatic relief. If the patient is not nearly asymptomatic in a few days, the diagnosis should be reconsidered. Treatment should continue for 1 year and the disease can be followed clinically, without regard to ESR, tapering off the prednisone over a few weeks and restarting if the pain recurs. Most people are asymptomatic in 24 months, rarely 36 months. Some patients have recurrences early or in a few years, and they respond well to retreatment.
2. If the patient has symptoms of **giant cell arteritis,** treatment with 60 mg of prednisone daily should start immediately to prevent ischemic events, which occur in 20% of all nontreated patients. If the diagnosis is uncertain, a biopsy of the affected arterial segment should be done within a few days. Response to prednisone is rapid and complete in about 3–4 days. In 4–6 weeks the ESR should be normal. Prednisone dose is decreased by 10% per month while continuing a monthly check of the ESR, until a dose of 10 mg per day is reached. That dose is continued for at least 2 years. About 10% of patients may require 3 or more years of therapy. Some patients have recurrences or may require very long or permanent low-dose therapy. Side effects of prednisone include weight gain, worsening of glucose intolerance, and Cushingoid features.

E. Myalgia due to **vascular insufficiency** (see Chapters 23 and, 42).
F. Myalgia resulting from **primary muscle malignancy** is relieved by excision of the malignant tumor, in consultation with a surgeon and oncologist.
G. In **SIM,** full resolution of symptoms and normalization of laboratories can be expected within days of drug withdrawal. Intense hydration and loop diuretics are recommended with CPKs higher than 2000. Chronic renal insufficiency can occur secondary to the myoglobinuria. **EMS** has been successfully treated during the acute phase with oral prednisone, 1–2 mg/kg/day, for days to weeks. In the late phase of the illness, no treatment has been helpful. Most symptoms and signs of the illness are resolved in 2–3 years, except for cognitive impairment and peripheral neuropathy.

REFERENCES

Buskila D: Fibromyalgia, chronic fatigue syndrome, and myofascial pain syndrome. Curr Opin Rheumatol (March) 2001;**13**(2):117.

Klippel JH (editor): *Primer on the Rheumatic Diseases,* 12th ed. Arthritis Foundation; 2001.

Sim J, Adams N: Systematic review of randomized controlled trials of nonpharmacological interventions for fibromyalgia. Clin J Pain (September/October) 2002;**18**(5):324.

Sprott H: What can rehabilitation interventions achieve in patients with primary fibromyalgia? Curr Opin Rheumatol (March) 2003;**15**(2):145.

Taylor RR, Friedberg F, Jason LA: *A Clinician's Guide to Controversial Illnesses: Chronic Fatigue Syndrome, Fibromyalgia, and Multiple Chemical Sensitivities.* Professional Resource Press (Sarasota, FL); 2001.

47   Nausea & Vomiting

Frances Emily Biagioli, MD, & Jay A. Swedberg, MD

KEY POINTS

- Nausea and vomiting are common complaints that are usually self-limited.
- Serious etiologies can be ruled out with a thorough history and a directed examination.
- Once any necessary tests show negative results, treatment can be directed toward symptom control and dehydration precautions.

I. **Definition. Nausea** is an unpleasant sensation of impending vomiting. **Retching** is a strong, involuntary effort to vomit without bringing up emesis. **Vomiting** is the forceful expulsion of stomach contents in a series of involuntary, spastic movements. **Regurgitation** is often confused with vomiting especially in infants; it is the nonforceful retrograde flow of esophageal contents. Vomiting occurs when the neuroreceptors in the emetic center are stimulated. The emetic center is located in the reticular formation of the medulla oblongata and is rich in histamine (H_1) receptors, muscarinic (M) cholinergic receptors, and serotonin ($5HT_3$) receptors. The emetic center can be stimulated through:

   A. **Stomach** or **biliary duct distention** via vagal afferents.

   B. **Vestibular dysfunction** via H_1 and M receptors.

   C. **Metabolic derangements, toxins, and some medications** (cardiac glycosides, chemotherapy, and opiates) via the chemoreceptor trigger zone (CTZ), which is rich in $5HT_3$ and dopamine (D_2) receptors.

   D. **Inflammation or ischemia** of the heart, pericardium, liver, pancreas, gallbladder, or peritoneum.

II. **Common Diagnoses.** Nausea and vomiting are common presenting symptoms in a variety of ailments. Because of lost function, nausea and vomiting inflict significant costs on the patient, their employers, and society.

   A. **Vomiting in infants** may be associated with acute gastroenteritis or any acute illness (eg, urinary tract infections, otitis media, or asthma), feeding disorders, hypertrophic pyloric stenosis, or intussusception. Pyloric stenosis is the most common surgical condition in the first 2–4 weeks of life; risk factors include male sex (1 : 150 males, 1 : 750 females) and a positive family history. Intussusception occurs between 6 and 18 months of life, but a small percentage occurs after age 3 years. Regurgitation (spitting up) often is a normal variant and should be distinguished from vomiting.

   B. **Vomiting in children,** in addition to the above diagnoses, may be from abdominal migraines (cyclic vomiting syndrome). They occur in as much as 1% of all children, at the mean age of 5 years; male incidence is higher in younger children, but male:female incidence equalizes as children grow older. Cyclic vomiting has a familial component and may be associated with migraine headaches.

   C. **Vomiting in women** is common during the first trimester of normal pregnancy. It may occur with hyperemesis gravidarum, hydatidiform molar pregnancy, and extrauterine pregnancy.

   D. **Vomiting in adolescents and adults** occurs most commonly in association with the disorders below (listed in the approximate order of frequency).

      1. **Acute gastroenteritis,** usually viral (rotavirus, reovirus, adenovirus, Norwalk) and is self-limited. It is most common between ages 20–29 years and occurs most often in autumn and winter. Bacterial etiologies include include *Staphylococcus aureus, Salmonella, Bacillus cereus,* and *Clostridium perfringens.*

      2. **Reaction to drugs** (Table 47–1), **toxins** (environmental exposures, alcohol, illicit drugs), or **tumor-produced peptides.**

      3. **Gastrointestinal tract inflammation or infection.** Gastroesophageal reflux disease **(GERD)** and **peptic ulcer disease** are more common with excessive caffeine, alcohol, or nicotine use. **Pancreatitis** occurs with alcohol, hypertriglyceridemia, or cholelithiasis. Risk factors for **cholecystitis** and **cholelithiasis** include obesity,

TABLE 47–1. MEDICATIONS ASSOCIATED WITH NAUSEA AND VOMITING

Pain medications
Aspirin
Nonsteroidal anti-inflammatory drugs
Opiate analgesics (codeine, morphine, etc)
Anti-gout drugs

Infectious disease treatments
Erythromycin or tetracycline
Nitrofurantoin
Sulfa drugs
Acyclovir
Tuberculosis medications

Cardiac medications
Digoxin
Antiarrhythmics
Antihypertensive medications (diuretics, beta blockers, calcium channel blockers)

Gastrointestinal medications
Sulfasalazine
Azathioprine

Other medications
Theophylline
Anticonvulsants
Nicotine
Chemotherapy agents
Lithium
Quinidine
Oral contraceptives
Oral diabetes medications

rapid weight loss, pregnancy, being female, and being older than age 40. Other diagnoses include **hepatitis, appendicitis, pyelonephritis, Reye's syndrome** (a complication of aspirin use in children with viral illnesses, especially with influenza or varicella), and **postgastrectomy states** (often associated with bile reflux or the inability to digest and clear foods normally).

4. **Motility disorders,** diabetic gastroparesis and postvagotomy states, as well as intestinal pseudo-obstruction (gastroduodenal motor dysfunction occurring in patients with neuromuscular disorders).

5. **Gastrointestinal obstruction,** such as gastric outlet obstruction, small-bowel obstruction, incarcerated hernia (femoral or inguinal), volvulus, and achalasia. Risk factors and related diagnoses include having prior abdominal surgeries, being elderly, or having hernias or cancer.

6. **Vestibular disorders,** such as motion sickness, Meniere's disease, or labyrinthitis.

7. **Increased intracranial pressure** associated with meningitis or space-occupying lesions (eg, tumors or subdural hematomas).

8. **Metabolic disorders,** including severe electrolyte derangements, uremia, diabetic ketoacidosis, hypercalcemia, adrenal insufficiency, and thyrotoxicosis.

9. **Psychogenic vomiting** associated with syndromes of physical or sexual abuse, post-traumatic stress, and eating disorders.

III. **Symptoms** (Table 47–2). Because there are many diagnoses associated with nausea and vomiting, an accurate history is essential to determining the underlying cause. Details about the **timing** of symptoms (time of day and any association with eating), **characteristics of the vomitus** (digested chyme, bilious, etc), any **associated symptoms** (abdominal pain or other symptoms), **associated past history,** and **duration of symptoms** are important.

A. **Duration of symptoms.** Chronic nausea and vomiting is defined as the persistence of symptoms for longer than 1 month. Acute nausea and vomiting usually lasts for days, but later can be found to be the presentation of chronic symptoms. Acute symptoms are most often due to toxins, infections (gastroenteritis, systemic, etc), inflammation (cardiac, gastrointestinal, etc), or obstruction. Chronic nausea and vomiting poses a more challenging diagnostic dilemma.

TABLE 47–2. DIAGNOSIS USING SYMPTOMS OF NAUSEA AND VOMITING IN ADULTS

Timing	Characteristics of Vomitus	± Associated Symptoms	± Associated Past Medical History	Possible Diagnoses
Before breakfast		Breast tenderness, fatigue		Pregnancy
	Projectile	Headache, dizziness		Increased intracranial pressure
		Headache, shakiness		Alcohol
			Kidney disease	Uremia
Delayed (>1 hour after meal)	Digested food	Early satiety, nonpainful	Diabetes	Gastroparesis
	Nonbilious, undigested	Painless or colicky pain		Achalasia, Zenker's diverticula, or gastric outlet obstruction
	Bilious, feculent	Colicky pain		Small-bowel obstruction
After meals		Abdominal pain		Ulcerative disease
		Abdominal or back pain		Pancreatitis
		RUQ abdominal pain		Cholecystitis
Immediately after meals (but can make it to the toilet)		No dysphagia	Psychiatric disorders	Bulimia, anorexia nervosa, or psychoneurotic vomiting
Intermittent attacks			Migraine headache	Cyclic vomiting syndrome (usually initially diagnosed in childhood)

    B. Timing and relationship to eating. Intermittent discrete attacks (typically eight attacks per year) of chronic cyclic nausea and vomiting lasting usually 20 hours with intervening asymptomatic periods occurs with **cyclic vomiting syndrome.**

        1. In infants or children, a **feeding disorder** (overfeeding or too-rapid feeding) should be considered when there is no weight loss or abdominal distention or when bilious emesis is absent.

        2. Delayed vomiting (more than 1 hour after eating) occurs with **gastric outlet obstruction, gastroparesis,** or **esophageal disorders.**

        3. Vomiting in the early morning hours before eating is associated with **pregnancy, uremia, alcohol withdrawal,** and **increased intracranial pressure** (eg, meningitis or space-occupying lesions).

        4. Nausea and vomiting without any clear relationship to meals can be from any cause but are most likely related to **metabolic disorders, vestibular disorders,** or **drugs and toxins.**

IV. Signs. The physical examination is unremarkable in many cases of nausea and vomiting, especially when associated with motility disorders, metabolic disorders, or drugs and toxins.

    A. Vomiting in infants

        1. If there is no fever, no weight loss, and no abdominal distention and the child does not appear ill, the cause may be a **feeding disorder** or **normal regurgitation.**

        2. Hypertrophic pyloric stenosis presents with weight loss, dehydration, and occasionally a palpable "olive" mass in the epigastric area in male infants younger than 7 weeks old.

        3. Children with **intussusception** usually have significant abdominal pain, possibly a palpable sausage-shaped mass, and loose stools that are heme-positive and described as "currant jelly."

    B. Gastrointestinal tract obstruction

        1. Small-bowel obstruction gives high-pitched bowel sounds with occasional visible peristalsis.

2. **Incarcerated hernia** is a painful inguinal hernia, occasionally with bowel sounds in the hernia sac.
3. **Volvulus** is associated with acute abdominal distention and periumbilical tenderness.
4. **Gastric outlet obstruction** may have distention and an epigastric succussion splash present more than 4 hours after eating.

C. **Increased intracranial pressure**
1. Focal neurologic signs are usually present with **space-occupying central nervous system lesions.**
2. A change in mental status, fever, and stiffness of the neck occur frequently with **meningitis.**

D. For a discussion of signs associated with the following causes of nausea and vomiting, see the chapters indicated below.
1. Vestibular disorders (Chapter 17).
2. Pregnancy (Chapter 97).
3. Gastroenteritis (Chapter 16).
4. Gastritis (Chapter 19).
5. Appendicitis (Chapter 1).
6. Hepatitis (Chapter 43).
7. GERD (Chapter 19).

V. **Laboratory Tests.** Diagnostic tests should be directed by the history and the physical examination. Figure 47–1 is a flow diagram aiding in the choice of diagnostic testing. The history will guide the examiner toward one or more broad classes of diagnoses. Specific testing can then be directed toward likely etiologies. Pregnancy should be considered and ruled out for all patients of childbearing age. Once this is done, if the symptoms are severe, diagnostic tests should be done to determine the patient's electrolyte status, hydration status/kidney function (blood urea nitrogen and creatinine), and if infection is likely, a complete blood count with differential. Further urgent diagnostics may be needed if symptoms, risk profiling and examination suggest severe etiologies such as increased intracranial pressure, obstruction, meningitis, or drug overdosing.

If the symptoms become chronic (4 weeks), the history and examination should be reviewed for elusive diagnoses. If the cause remains cryptic or symptoms persist or worsen, more complex diagnostic testing or gastroenterology referral may be necessary. Additional points to remember:

A. If a patient presents with significant pain, obstruction must be considered. **Supine and upright abdominal x-ray series** should be done to look for obstruction, perforation, or ileus.

B. **Upper gastrointestinal series, barium enemas, small-bowel follow-through,** and **small-bowel enema** will detect obstruction, masses, and large ulcers, but low-grade obstruction and smaller mucosal lesions may not be seen. Because smaller lesions may be missed, a **computerized tomographic scan of the abdomen** may be necessary to fully evaluate obstruction.

C. **Endoscopy** (ie, sigmoidoscopy, colonoscopy, or esophagogastroduodenoscopy) is useful for evaluating anatomic lesions, especially if biopsy is required. Endoscopy is not reliable in diagnosing physiologic gastrointestinal motility disorders.

D. Nasogastric tube aspiration showing significant **gastric residual** after an overnight fast suggests gastric outlet obstruction.

E. **Formal psychiatric assessment** should be considered in unexplained chronic nausea and vomiting and when psychogenic vomiting is suspected.

F. **Specialized testing. Radionuclide testing** measures gastric emptying rate. **Antroduodenal manometry** and **electrogastrography** measure gastric motility and rhythmic functions.

VI. **Treatment.** An underlying disorder should be identified and treated if possible. During diagnostic testing, management is usually symptomatic, including electrolyte and fluid replacement. If gastrointestinal obstruction is evident, hospitalization for skilled nursing, close monitoring, and surgical consultation are needed. If appropriate testing has been done and diagnosis is still uncertain, symptoms may be controlled with a combination of nonpharmacologic measures and antiemetics.

A. **Nonpharmacologic treatment** consists of clear liquids sipped slowly, foods served cool or at room temperature, bland foods (ie, avoidance of very sweet, fatty, salty, and spicy foods), and minimization of visual, auditory, and olfactory stimulation.

B. **Pharmacologic treatment** (Table 47–3).
1. **Phenothiazines, butyrophenones,** and **metoclopramide** are effective for vomiting secondary to drugs (eg, chemotherapy, cardiac glycosides, or opiates), as

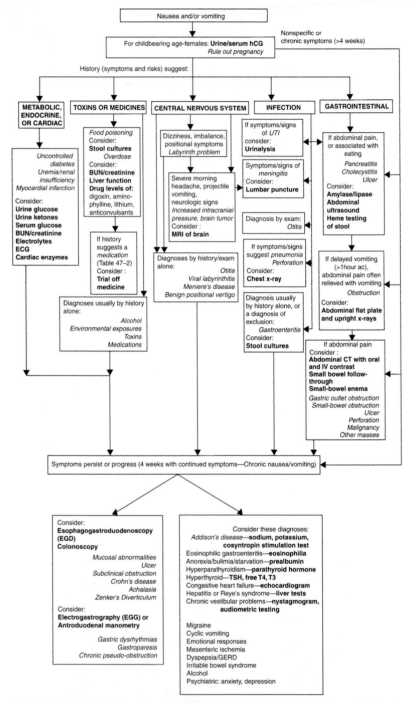

FIGURE 47–1. Evaluation of nausea and vomiting. BUN, blood urea nitrogen; ECG, electrocardiogram; GERD, gastroesophageal reflux disease; hCG, human chorionic gonadotropin; IV, intravenous; MRI, magnetic resonance imaging; TSH, thyroid-stimulating hormone; UTI, urinary tract infection.

TABLE 47–3. PHARMACOLOGIC TREATMENT FOR NAUSEA AND VOMITING

Agents—Receptor Antagonist[1]—Usual Dose Range	Main Use Situations for This Class	Common Side Effects of This Class
Phenothiazines—D_2		
Prochlorperazine (Compazine) 5–10 mg PO/IM q4–6, 25 mg PR q6	Chemotherapy, cardiac glycoside, or opiate reactions	Drowsiness
Promethazine (Phenergan) 12.5–25 mg PO/IM q4–6, 12.5–25 mg PR q6	Radiation therapy effects	Dry mouth
Chlorpromazine (Thorazine) 10–50 mg PO q4–6, 25–50 IM q3–4, 100 mg PR q 6–8	Postoperative effects	Dizziness, hypotension
Thiethylperazine (Torecan) 10 mg PO/IM q4–6, 10 mg PR q6	Compazine also is used in migraines	Extrapyramidal reactions (more in children)
Perphenazine (Trilafon) 4–8 mg PO q6, 5 mg IM q6		
Butyrophenones—D_2		
Haloperidol (Haldol) 0.5–2 mg q6–12, 2–3 mg IM q4–6	Chemotherapy reactions	Less commonly, hypotension
		Extrapyramidal reactions at higher doses
Serotonin receptor antagonists—$5\text{-}HT_3$		
Dolasetron (Anzemet)—100 mg PO once, 100 mg IV once	Chemotherapy reactions	Dizziness, headache
Ondansetron (Zofran)—8 mg PO twice, 32 mg IV once	Postoperative effects	Less commonly: prolonged ECG intervals
Granisetron (Kytril)—2 mg PO once or 1 mg PO bid, 10 μg/kg IV	Radiation therapy effects	
	Adjunctively used with steroids	
Prokinetic agents—D_2		
Metoclopramide (Reglan)—5–10 mg before meals and qhs, 10 mg IV over 2 min q6	Gastroparesis	Diarrhea
	Gastroesophageal reflux disease	Extrapyramidal reactions
Cisapride (Propulsid)[2]—No longer on the market		
Ethanolamine-antiemetics—H_1, Anticholinergic		
(trimethobenzamide—unknown receptor)	Chronic nausea patients	Drowsiness, dizziness, hypotension
Trimethobenzamide[3] (Tigan)—250 mg PO qid, 200 IV/PR qid	Gastroenteritis	May potentiate opiates or other sedatives

(continued)

TABLE 47-3. (*Continued*)

Agents—Receptor Antagonist[1]—Usual Dose Range	Main Use Situations for This Class	Common Side Effects of This Class
Promethazine (Phenergan)—12.5–25 mg PO/PR q4–6	Less effective, but, fewer side effects than phenothiazines	
Antihistamines—H₁		
Dimenhydrinate (Dramamine)—50–100 mg q6–8, 50–100 mg q12 Meclizine (Antivert, Bonine) 12.5–25 mg q8	Best with vestibular disturbances Motion sickness (best when used in prevention) Meniere's disease	Drowsiness *Elders:* Confusion *Children:* Paradoxical CNS stimulation
Anticholinergics—M		
Scopalamine[4] (Transderm Scop)—1 patch 4 hours before travel, replace q3 days; for postoperative nausea apply patch the night prior to surgery Hyoscine—150–300 µg q8	Prevention of motion sickness Less effective: postoperative and chemotherapy effects	Dry mouth Fewer side effects when used transdermally
Others		
Diphenidol hydrochloride[5] (Vontrol)—not on market—Inhibits conduction in vestibular pathways Dronabinol (Marinol)—Cannabinoid—5 mg/m² q1–3 Aprepitant (Emend)—Substance P/neurokinin 1—80–125 mg qam	Diphenidol—Use in closely monitored patients, for post-operative, chemotherapy or radiation therapy effects, or labyrinth disturbances Dronabinol—When other treatments fail Aprepitant—Use with other antiemetics	Diphenidol—Auditory and visual hallucinations, disorientation, hypotension Dronabinol—Euphoria, dizziness, paranoia Aprepitant—Asthenia/fatigue, dizziness

[1] Serotonin receptor, 5-HT₃; dopamine receptor, D₂; histamine receptor, H₁; muscarinic cholinergic receptor, M.
[2] Cisapride was removed from the market because of serious cardiac arrhythmias and death. It is available by protocol for patients not responsive to other medications.
[3] Trimethobenzamide's receptor is unknown. It is believed to inhibit the chemoreceptor trigger zone.
[4] Transdermal patch behind the ear every 72 hours (removed and reapplied, if necessary).
[5] Diphenidol hydrochloride is only available by calling the manufacturer.
CNS, central nervous system; ECG, electrocardiogram.

well as nausea and vomiting associated with radiation therapy, gastrointestinal causes, and postoperative effects. **Ondansetron hydrochloride** (Zofran) and **dolasetron** (Anzemet) are antiemetics used primarily for prevention of nausea and vomiting associated with chemotherapy.

When one is treating nausea and vomiting associated with chemotherapy, ondansetron is often used in combination with steroids (eg, dexamethasone, 4–8 mg orally or 10 mg IV with chemotherapy, or methylprednisolone, 4 mg orally three times daily for 3 days).

2. **Prokinetic agents. Metoclopramide** (Reglan) is helpful in treating motility disorders, such as diabetic gastroparesis and postvagotomy states. **Metoclopramide,** in addition to D_2 antagonism, directly stimulates gastrointestinal smooth muscle, increasing motility.

3. **Agents to prevent motion sickness and vertigo** (eg, **meclizine, dimenhydrinate,** and **scopolamine**) affect the vestibular system, and probably the emetic center, through antagonism of H_1 and M (muscarinic cholinergic) receptors. These agents are most effective if administered prior to the onset of nausea and vomiting.

REFERENCES

American Gastroenterological Association: American Gastroenterological Association medical position statement: Nausea and vomiting. Gastroenterology 2001;**120**(1):261.

Axelrod RS: Antiemetic therapy. Compreh Ther 1997;**23**(8):539.

Longstreth GF: Approach to the patient with nausea and vomiting. UpToDate online 11.1, 2003. www.uptodate.com

Longstreth GF, Hesketh PJ: Characteristics of antiemetic drugs. UpToDate online 11.1, 2003. www.uptodate.com

Quigley EM, Hasler WL, Parkman HP: AGA Technical review on nausea and vomiting. Gastroenterology 2001;**120**(1):263.

48   Neck Pain

Michael P. Rowane, DO, MS, FAAFP, FAAO

KEY POINTS

- Over 50% of adults experience neck pain at some time.
- A careful history and physical examination are usually sufficient to establish a diagnosis, yet in most cases no definable pathology is found.
- Laboratory investigations play a minor role in most cases of neck pain, but they may help confirm a diagnosis.
- Treatment of problems arising primarily from neck joints and associated ligaments and muscles successfully alleviates symptoms, whereas treatment of problems involving the cervical nerve roots or spinal cord often does not achieve complete pain relief.

I. **Definition.** Neck pain is associated with the vertebral column, surrounding muscle, and connective tissue. Neck pain may be classified as:
- **Mechanical,** including nontraumatic (neck strain/torticollis, spondylosis, and myelopathy) and traumatic (whiplash, disk herniation, cervical fracture, neck sprain, and stinger).
- **Nonmechanical** (rheumatologic/inflammatory, neoplastic, infectious, neurologic, and referred).
- **Miscellaneous** (eg, sarcoidosis and Paget's disease).

II. **Common Diagnoses.** (Table 48–1). The lifetime prevalence of at least one episode of significant neck pain is estimated at 40–70%, whereas nonspecific neck pain over the last 6 months is reported by 40% of adults. Neck pain is most commonly mechanical or due to age-related changes in the cervical spine.

TABLE 48–1. DIFFERENTIAL DIAGNOSIS OF COMMON CAUSES OF NECK PAIN

Condition	Risk Factors	Symptoms	Signs	Testing
Acute nonspecific neck pain	Young adults under some stress	Typically, unilateral neck pain that radiates to the top of the shoulder and periscapular area	Limited ROM; widespread tender/trigger points suggest fibromyalgia	C-spine radiographs show decrease or reversal of cervical lordosis (nonspecific)
Chronic mechanical neck pain	Older individuals	Intermittent acute attacks super-imposed on chronic pain; pain often radiates to scapular region and top of arms	Limited ROM, tenderness to palpation	Typical **C-spine radiographic findings** (loss of posterior disk height, irregular disk margins, subchondral sclerosis, osteophytes) correlate poorly with incidence/severity of neck pain;
Spondylosis/osteoarthritis	Individuals >50 years, history of OA (osteophytes)	Neck stiffness after rest, possible paresthesias/numbness	Limited ROM, neurologic changes with progression	**CT** can assess for spinal stenosis (older individual with axial stiffness and paresthesias over several dematones);
Cervical nerve root irritation	History of spondylosis, osteophytes	Discomfort worsening when turning head toward the side of neck pain; paresthesias, weakness	Abnormal Spurling maneuver	**MRI** provides the best anatomic assessment of disk herniation and soft tissue/spinal cord abnormalities; **EMG** is helpful in localizing radiculopathy/ myelopathy.
Acceleration injury/whiplash	Rear-end or side-impact motor vehicle accidents	Acute pain and stiffness within hours, headache	Limited ROM	**C-spine radiographs** may be indicated (Table 48–4)
Torticollis	History of congenital or acquired fixed head or C-spine rotation	Usually painless if congenital; usually painful if acquired	Limited ROM; neck is laterally flexed and rotated	

CT, computerized tomography; EMG, electromyogram; MRI, magnetic resonance imagery; OA, osteoarthritis; ROM, range of motion.

TABLE 48-2. "RED FLAGS" IN NECK PAIN (CLUES TO POTENTIAL SERIOUS UNDERLYING DISEASE)

1. **Fracture** (significant trauma; osteoporosis history)
2. **Infection** (fever, alcohol, or drug abuse)
3. **Tumor** (history of cancer; unexplained weight loss; age >50 years, failure to improve with treatment)
4. **Radiculopathy** (lower extremity spasticity, bowel/bladder incontinence)

III. **Symptoms** (Table 48–1).
   A. **Pain.** **Acute torticollis** is a recent sudden onset of unilateral muscular pain, whereas **cervical sprain/whiplash** is a severe generalized discomfort in the neck and upper back after acute trauma. When pain is aggravated by movement, worse after activities, and there is a dull ache in the base of the neck or interscapular region, **osteoarthritis (cervical spondylosis)** should be considered.
   B. **Loss of motion.** Mechanical pain is typically worse on movement and relieved by rest.
   C. **Headache.** Patients with **whiplash** (cervical flexion-extension injuries) frequently have headaches, along with associated nausea, blurred vision, or vertigo.
   D. **Radiating symptoms.** Mechanical pain frequently radiates to the shoulder blades or the top of the arm without any nerve root or spinal cord involvement. **Cervical root irritation** should be considered with radiation of symptoms down the arms, or weakness, numbness, or paresthesias in the arms. With bilateral radicular symptoms, a **cervical cord compression syndrome** should be considered.
   E. **Precipitating factors.** Tension and stress, along with frequent bouts of pain and depression, may suggest an underlying behavioral or psychiatric diagnosis.
   F. **Difficulty walking,** which could be the presenting symptom of **cervical myelopathy.**
   G. **Other.** A **whiplash injury** especially may be accompanied by anxiety, loss of sleep, dizziness, paresthesias, or nerve root pain. Table 48–2 lists findings suggesting significant underlying disease.
IV. **Signs** (Table 48–1). A focused examination of the patient presenting with neck pain should include **inspection** (for posture, asymmetry, and deformity); **palpation** (for localized tenderness); passive/active/resisted **range of motion (ROM)** (for restrictions and severity of disease); and **provocative maneuvers/neurologic testing** (for radiculopathy).
   A. **Tenderness to palpation. Tender points** are common in nonspecific acute neck pain. Associated widespread tender points, which are sometimes referred to as trigger points, may be indicative of fibromyalgia (see Chapters 39 and 46). Muscle spasm occurs in acute nonspecific neck pain, whiplash injury, and torticollis.
   B. **ROM.** Normal neck ROM includes rotation 60–90 degrees, flexion 60–90 degrees, extension 60–90 degrees, and lateral flexion (side-bending) 30–60 degrees. ROM normally decreases with age. Loss of motion is common in acute nonspecific and chronic mechanical neck pain.
   C. **Neurologic testing/provocative maneuvers** (Table 48–3). Evaluation for possible levels of sensory and motor involvement, including weakness of the upper extremities, may suggest lesions of the nerve roots, brachial plexus, or muscles. A **Spurling test,** or the neck compression test, requires side-bending and rotating the patient's head

TABLE 48-3. EVALUATION FOR CERVICAL NERVE ROOT LESIONS

Nerve Root	Disk Level	Muscle Weakness/ Movement Affected	Reflex	Paresthesia	Site of Pain
C-5	C-4/5	Shoulder abduction, elbow flexion	Biceps	Shoulder	Shoulder, lateral arm
C-6	C-5/6	Wrist extension/pronation	Brachioradialis and biceps	Thumb	Deltoid, rhomboid muscle areas
C-7	C-6/7	Elbow/finger extension	Triceps	Middle finger	Dorsolateral upper arm, superomedial angle of scapula
C-8	C-7/T-1	Wrist/finger extension	Triceps and finger	Ring and little finger	Scapula, ulnar side of upper arm

toward the side of radicular pain and exerting downward pressure. This maneuver reproduces symptoms in the affected upper extremity. The Spurling test has a high specificity but low sensitivity for cervical radiculopathy. Nonspecific mechanical pain should be considered when a Spurling test or contralateral neck motion result only in neck discomfort.

V. **Laboratory Tests** are usually not necessary. Testing should be considered if a careful history and physical examination do not clearly suggest a diagnosis, or to guide management (eg, surgical consultation).

  A. **Plain C-spine radiographs** (Table 48–1). A cervical spine injury is unlikely in the absence of neck pain/tenderness, neurologic signs/symptoms, loss of consciousness, and distracting injury, and with a normal mental status examination. The Canadian Cervical Spine Rules (Table 48–4) are a validated tool to determine which patients with neck pain require radiographic evaluation.

  B. In the presence of neurologic abnormalities, **other imaging techniques** should be used to resolve lesion anatomy (Table 48–1).

    1. A **bone scan** can appraise osseous pathology, including osteomyelitis and neoplastic lesions in bone.

    2. **Bone densitometry** diagnoses suspected osteoporosis.

  C. **Blood tests** are rarely indicated. Erythrocyte sedimentation rate and complete blood count with differential may help evaluate for suspected serious disorders, including tumor, infection, or inflammatory arthritis, especially with "red flag" history or physical examination (Table 48–2).

VI. **Treatment.** The management of neck pain is aimed at relieving symptoms and maintaining good function. Neck pain usually resolves within days or weeks. Approximately 10% of acute neck pain becomes chronic and 5% of patients experience severe disability.

  A. **Uncomplicated neck pain without severe neurologic deficit, including acute nonspecific neck pain and chronic mechanical neck pain**

    1. Manual manipulation/mobilization, active physiotherapy, pulsed electromagnetic field treatment, and exercise are likely to be beneficial. Therapeutic exercises, initiated either in the office or in consultation with a physical therapist, include ROM, isometrics, dynamic exercises, postural training, and general fitness programs.

    2. Pharmacologic treatment (Table 48–5), behavioral interventions/biofeedback, patient education, application of heat/cold, home or office cervical traction, acupuncture, spray and stretch, laser treatment, and soft collars/special pillows have unknown effectiveness, yet are common conservative treatments.

  B. **Spondylosis/osteoarthritis.** Treatment must involve reducing pain and stiffness, while minimizing risk (see Chapter 80). Fashionable complementary techniques include transcutaneous electrical nerve stimulation (TENS) units, acupuncture, and a variety of heat, light, magnetic, or filing therapies, but there are little data to support their efficacy.

  C. **Cervical nerve root irritation/radiculopathy.** In patients followed up for over a year, there currently are no data supporting surgery compared to conservative treatment. Conservative modalities include local heat, analgesics, cervical collar in the acute phase, and consideration of cervical traction. Pharmacologic treatment, including oral medications (Table 48–5) and referral for epidural steroid injections, have unknown effectiveness.

TABLE 48–4. CANADIAN CERVICAL SPINE RULES

1. Is there one high-risk factor that mandates immobilization:
   - Age ≥ 65 years old, or dangerous mechanism (fall from 1 meter or greater, axial load to head, motorized recreational vehicles, bicycle collision, or motor vehicle collision (MVC) with high speed, rollover, or ejection); or
   - Numbness/tingling in extremities
2. Is there one low-risk factor to allow safe assessment of range of motion:
   - Simple rear-end MVC; or
   - Ambulatory at any time at scene, or
   - No neck pain at scene, or
   - Absence of midline C-spine tenderness
3. Is patient able to voluntarily actively rotate neck 45 degrees to the left and right when requested, regardless of pain?

An answer "yes" to the first question or "no" to the second or third question requires radiography.

TABLE 48-5. ORAL MEDICATIONS COMMONLY USED FOR NECK PAIN

Medication	Dosage (mg)	Frequency	Comment
Acetaminophen	325–500	Every 4–6 hours	
NSAIDs			• Caution with this class, especially in elderly, as renal and GI side effects can be dangerous
• Ibuprofen	400–800	Every 6–8 hours	• Consider taking with food
• Naproxen	375–500	Every 12 hours	
COX-2 inhibitors			• An expensive alternative to NSAIDs for patients intolerant or at high risk for side effects
• Celecoxib	100–200	Daily–twice daily	• Acute pain = 400 mg × 1, then 200–400 mg daily
• Rofecoxib	12.5, 25, and 50	Daily	• Acute pain = 50 mg
• Valdecoxib	10–20	Daily	• OA/RA 10 mg daily
Muscle relaxants			
• Cyclobenzaprine	10	Three times daily	• Appropriate for torticollis (Cyclobenzaprine should be avoided in the elderly)
• Metaxalone	400	2 pills three to four times daily	• Abuse potential
• Carisoprodol	350	Three to four times daily	
Nutritional supplements			
• Glucosamine	500–750	Two to three times daily	• Limited studies demonstrate effective treatment of OA and RA with almost no side effects
			• All studies at 1500 mg/day dose

GI, gastrointestinal; NSAIDs, nonsteroidal anti-inflammatory drugs; OA, osteoarthritis; RA, rheumatoid arthritis.

D. Acute whiplash injury. Likely beneficial interventions include early mobilization and return to normal activity, electrotherapy (diathermy and TENS units), and multimodal treatment. Multimodal or combined therapy typically refers to intensive programs incorporating exercise as well as pharmacologic, behavioral, and psychosocial interventions.

E. Chronic whiplash injury. Outcomes are no different comparing physiotherapy alone and multimodal treatment. One study showed significant numbers of pain-free patients 6 months after undergoing percutaneous radiofrequency neurotomy. Another demonstrated significant pain reduction in those undergoing percutaneous radiofrequency neurotomy combined with other modalities, compared to those treated with single modalities.

F. Torticollis in adults is managed with physical therapy, stretching techniques, gentle manual manipulation, judicious use of a soft cervical collar, and ice/heat. Muscle relaxants are primary medications, along with analgesics and nonsteroidal anti-inflammatory drugs (Table 48–5).

REFERENCES

Binder A: Neck pain. In: Godlee F (editor): *Clinical Evidence Concise* (June) 2003;**9**:243.

Devereaux MW: Neck and low back pain. Med Clin North Am (May) 2003;873.

Klippel JH, Dieppe PA, Ferri FF: *Neck Pain in Primary Care Rheumatology.* Mosby International Limited (London); 1999:201–214.

Swezey RL (editor): Neck Pain (issue theme). Phys Med Rehabil Clin N Am (August) 2003;**14**(3).

Tsang I: Rheumatology: 12. Pain in the neck. Canadian Medical Association Journal (Journal de l'Association médicale canadienne) 2001;**164**(8):1182.

---

49   Palpitations

D. Mike Hardin, Jr., MD

KEY POINTS

- Most causes of palpitations are benign and do not require extensive work-up or treatment.
- Palpitations that are sustained or associated with syncope or presyncope require further work-up, electrophysiologic evaluation, or both.
- In general, palpitations are insensitive indicators of arrhythmias.

I. Definition. Palpitations are an awareness of the heartbeat, are usually benign, and may be due either to intrinsic cardiac conditions or to noncardiac conditions impacting cardiac rate, rhythm, or force (Table 49–1).

II. Common Diagnoses. Palpitations are a common chief complaint, accounting for up to 16% of outpatient visits. Relative incidence and risk factors for common causes of palpitations follow:

A. Cardiac (43% of cases). Factors increasing the likelihood for a cardiac etiology of palpitations include (1) male sex; (2) description of an irregular heartbeat; (3) history of heart disease; or (4) event duration >5 minutes. Patients with three predictors have a 71% chance of a cardiac etiology, those with two predictors, a 48% chance; those with one predictor, a 26% chance; and those with zero predictors, a zero percent chance of cardiac etiology. The most common cardiac cause is benign supraventricular or ventricular ectopy.

B. Psychiatric (31% of cases). Palpitations may be a feature of panic attacks, generalized anxiety disorder, somatization, and depression. Because these disorders are common, they may coexist with other causes of palpitations.

C. Ten percent of palpitations are due to a **variety of defined causes** such as endocrinologic disorders (eg, hyperthyroidism), cardiac stimulants (eg, caffeine, over-the-counter sympathomimetics, illicit drugs), and anemia.

D. In 16% of cases, the cause of palpitations is **unknown.**

TABLE 49-1. ETIOLOGIES OF PALPITATIONS

Cardiac	**Habits**
Arrhythmia	Cocaine
Sinus tachycardia	Amphetamines
Ventricular premature contractions	Caffeine
Atrial premature contractions	Nicotine
Re-entrant atrial tachycardias	
Atrial fibrillation or flutter	**Metabolic disorders**
Sinus bradycardia	Thyrotoxicosis
Sick sinus syndrome	Hypoglycemia
Atrioventricular nodal block	Pheochromocytoma
Conduction defects	Mastocytosis
Ventricular tachycardia	Scombroid food poisoning (eg, tuna fish)
Ventricular fibrillation	**High-output states**
Cardiac and extracardiac shunts	Anemia
Valvular heart disease	Pregnancy
Pacemaker	Paget's disease
Atrial myxoma	Fever
Cardiomyopathy	
	Catecholamine excess
Psychiatric disease	Stress
Panic attack and disorder	Exercise
Generalized anxiety disorder	
Somatization	
Depression	
Medications	
Sympathomimetic agents	
Vasodilators	
Anticholinergic drugs	
Beta blocker withdrawal	

Adapted with permission from Zimetbaum P: Overview of Palpitations (from www.UpToDate.com, online version 11.1).

III. **Symptoms.** Because palpitations can be difficult to characterize, it may be helpful for the patient to tap out the rhythm or for the physician to tap out examples of different rhythms. Important historical features of the palpitations include the following.

A. **Description**

1. **Rate and rhythm.** A **rapid and regular** rhythm suggests paroxysmal supraventricular tachycardia (PSVT) or ventricular tachycardia (VT); **rapid and irregular** suggests atrial fibrillation or atrial flutter with a variable block.

2. A **"flip-flopping"** sensation suggests **ventricular or atrial premature contractions** (VPCs, APCs) with a pause followed by a forceful contraction (postextrasystolic potentiation of ventricular inotropy).

3. A description of **"rapid fluttering in the chest"** may represent a **sustained ventricular or supraventricular rhythm,** including sinus tachycardia.

4. A **"pounding in the neck"** sensation is due to cannon A waves resulting from atrial contractions against a closed tricuspid or mitral valve in **atrioventricular dissociation.** Irregular neck palpitations are seen in VPCs, complete heart block, or VT. **Rapid and regular neck pulsations** are typical of atrioventricular reentrant tachycardia (AVNRT).

B. **Onset and offset**

1. **Random, episodic,** and last an instant: Premature beats.

2. **Gradual onset and offset:** Sinus tachycardia.

3. **Abrupt onset/termination:** PSVT or VT.

4. Patient able to **terminate with vagal maneuver:** PSVT (especially AVNRT).

C. **Positional**

1. Initiated by **standing up straight after bending over,** aborted by lying down: AVNRT.

2. **Augmented by supine or left lateral decubitus position:** VPC or APC, secondary to greater awareness of heart activity while relaxed or due to the proximity of the heart to the chest wall.

D. Syncope or presyncope
  1. VT.
  2. PSVT, secondary to vasodilation at the onset of the arrhythmia.
E. Reliability of reported palpitations. Although the classic descriptions noted above can be helpful, a recent review of the accuracy of patient awareness of cardiac activity found that:
  1. The vast majority of arrhythmias are unrecognized by patients as symptoms.
  2. Of those reporting palpitations, patients with psychiatric disease (eg, somatization, hypochondriasis) were less accurate historians.
  3. Palpitations are insensitive indicators of arrhythmias.
IV. Signs. The physical examination should search for:
  A. Cardiovascular abnormalities that could serve as a substrate for arrhythmias:
    1. Mitral valve prolapse: Midsystolic click (associated with many arrhythmias).
    2. Hypertrophic obstructive cardiomyopathy: Harsh, holosystolic murmur along the left sternal border that increases with Valsalva's maneuver (associated with atrial fibrillation, VT).
    3. Dilated cardiomyopathy and heart failure: Diffuse and laterally displaced apical impulse, ventricular (S_3) and atrial (S_4) gallops (associated with VT, atrial fibrillation).
  B. Signs of other medical disorders such as hyperthyroidism or pheochromocytoma.
V. Laboratory Tests (Figure 49–1). Most palpitations have a benign etiology and extensive evaluation is usually not necessary. The history, physical examination, electrocardiogram (ECG), and limited laboratory tests will yield a diagnosis in over one third of patients; only a small portion of the remaining cases will require further testing (see sections V,C and V,D).
  A. Laboratory. Limited laboratory tests to rule out hyperthyroidism (thyroid-stimulating hormone), anemia (hemoglobin/hematocrit), and electrolyte disturbances (potassium, magnesium) are sufficient.
  B. ECG. An episode of palpitations is rarely captured on a routine ECG. Certain ECG findings, however, may suggest the etiology of the palpitations (Table 49–2).
  C. Ambulatory ECG monitoring (AECG). Further AECG testing is used to rule out a serious condition, identify treatable causes of arrhythmias, or reassure a patient.
    1. A **Holter (24-hour) monitor** is useful only if a patient has daily palpitations.
    2. The **continuous loop event recorder,** activated by the patient at time of symptoms, is currently the preferred study for investigating palpitations. Two weeks of monitoring is usually adequate and more cost-effective than the traditional 4 weeks.
    3. An **exercise stress test** is useful only for exertional arrhythmias.
  D. Electrophysiologic testing is reserved for patients with a high pretest likelihood of serious arrhythmia (eg, structural heart disease or sustained or poorly tolerated arrhythmia).
VI. Treatment
  A. Patients with **sustained supraventricular tachycardia (SVT) or VT.** These patients should be referred to an electrophysiologist (a cardiologist specializing in the pharmacologic and invasive management of arrhythmias) for consideration of radiofrequency ablation (SVT), medical therapy, or implantable defibrillator.
  B. Nonsustained ventricular tachycardia (NSVT). NSVT is defined as three or more consecutive beats at a rate of >120 beats per minute with a duration of less than 30 seconds. In patients without underlying heart disease, it is a benign finding and no treatment is necessary. Patients with heart disease should be referred to electrophysiology for treatment recommendations.
  C. Benign supraventricular or ventricular ectopy. Reassure the patient and remove precipitating causes (eg, caffeine, drugs). If symptoms are incapacitating, consider treatment with a beta blocker to relieve symptoms. (Treatment, however, may not necessarily suppress the arrhythmia, just its symptoms.)
  D. Atrial fibrillation (AF). There are four principal issues regarding the treatment of AF:
    1. Reversion to normal sinus rhythm (NSR)
      a. Urgent electrical cardioversion is indicated in **unstable patients** (those with active ischemia, hypotension, or a pre-excitation syndrome with an extremely rapid ventricular rate).
      b. In the **stable patient,** rate control is first attained with a calcium channel blocker, beta blocker, or digoxin (Table 49–3).
      c. Factors that guide drug selection include the patient's medical condition, the presence of concomitant heart failure, the characteristics of the medicine, and

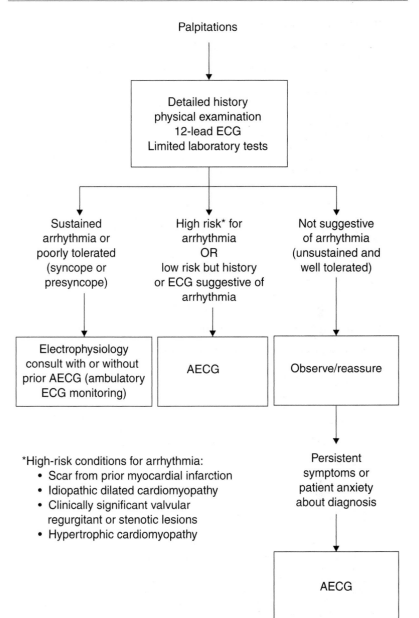

FIGURE 49–1. Decision tree for evaluation of palpitations. AECG, ambulatory electrocardiogram; ECG, electrocardiogram.

the physician's experience with specific drugs. Digoxin is currently recommended as a second-line treatment for rate control, except in heart failure.

d. Recent trials have shown that either rhythm or rate control is acceptable in managing AF. Thus, the decision to perform **elective pharmacologic or electrical cardioversion** should be made in consultation with cardiology

TABLE 49–2. ELECTROCARDIOGRAPHIC CLUES TO THE CAUSE OF PALPITATIONS

ECG Findings	Condition	Suggested Etiology
Short PR interval, delta waves	Wolff-Parkinson-White syndrome	Atrioventricular re-entrant tachycardia
P mitrale, left ventricular hypertrophy (LVH), atrial premature depolarizations	Left atrial abnormality	Atrial fibrillation
Marked LVH, deep septal Q waves in I, aVL, and V4–6	Hypertrophic obstructive cardiomyopathy	Atrial fibrillation
Ventricular premature depolarizations, left bundle-branch block with positive axis (in patients without structural heart disease)		Idiopathic VT, right ventricular outflow tract type
Ventricular premature depolarizations, right bundle-branch block with positive axis (in patients without structural heart disease)		Idiopathic VT, left ventricular type
Q waves	Prior myocardial infarction	VPCs, nonsustained or sustained VT
Complete heart block	Complete heart block	VPCs, polymorphic VT (torsade de pointes)
Long QT interval	Long QT syndrome	Polymorphic VT
Inverted T wave in V_2, with or without epsilon wave	Arrhythmogenic right ventricular dysplasia	VT

VT, ventricular tachycardia; VPC, ventricular premature contractions.
Adapted with permission from Zimetbaum P: Overview of Palpitations (from www.UpToDate.com, online version 11.1).

TABLE 49–3. DRUGS USED FOR RATE CONTROL IN PATIENTS WITH ATRIAL FIBRILLATION

Drug	Loading Dose	Usual Maintenance Dose
Digoxin (Lanoxin)	**IV:** 0.25 mg IV every 2 h, up to 1.5 mg **PO:** 0.25 mg every 2 h, up to 1.5 mg	**IV:** 0.125–0.25 mg daily **PO:** 0.125–0.375 mg daily
Calcium channel blockers		
Diltiazem (Cardizem, Dilacor, Tiazac)	**IV:** 0.25 mg/kg IV over 2 min **PO:** NA	**IV:** 5–15 mg/h infusion for <24 hours **PO:** 120–360 mg/24 hours (divided doses or slow-release forms available)
Verapamil (Calan, Isoptin, and others)	**IV:** 0.075–0.15 mg/kg over 2 min **PO:** NA	**IV:** NA **PO:** 120–480 mg/24 hours (divided doses or SR forms available)
Beta blockers (only two representative members of the class are listed here— others may be used as well)		
Metoprolol (Lopressor, Toprol)	**IV:** 2.5–5 mg IV bolus over 2 min; up to 3 doses **PO:** NA	**IV:** NA **PO:** 25–100 mg/24 hours (divided doses or SR forms available)
Propranolol (Inderal)	**IV:** 0.15 mg/kg (typically 1–3 mg) **PO:** NA	**IV:** NA **PO:** 80–240 mg/24 hours (divided doses or SR forms available)

IV, intravenous; NA, not applicable; PO, oral; SR, sustained release.
Adapted from Fuster V, et al: ACC/AHA/ESC guidelines for the management of patients with atrial fibrillation: Executive summary. A report of the American College of Cardiology/American Heart Association Task Force on Practice Guidelines and the European Society of Cardiology Committee for Practice Guidelines and Policy Conferences (Committee to develop guidelines for the management of patients with atrial fibrillation). Developed in collaboration with the North American Society of Pacing and Electrophysiology. J Am Coll Cardiol 2001;**38**:1231.

after consideration of the risks and benefits. Successful reversion to and maintenance of NSR is more likely if:

   (1) The AF has been present less than 1 year.
   (2) The left atrium is not enlarged (diameter ≤4.0 cm).
   (3) A reversible etiologic factor of the AF is present.

2. **Maintenance of NSR**
   a. After successful cardioversion, only 20–30% of patients maintain NSR without therapy.
   b. Class IA (quinidine, procainamide, disopyramide), IC (flecainide, propafenone) and III (amiodarone, sotalol, ibutilide, dofetilide) drugs are used to maintain NSR. Although cardiology may initiate this therapy, family physicians are often involved in its maintenance and should be familiar with the numerous drug interactions of antiarrhythmics.

3. **Rate control in chronic AF** is achieved using calcium channel blockers, beta blockers, or digoxin (Table 49–3).

4. **Anticoagulation** for prevention of systemic embolization:
   a. While restoring NSR. If AF is present for more than 48 hours, patients should receive 3–4 weeks of warfarin (eg, Coumadin) therapy (target international normalized ratio 2.5, range 2.0–3.0) prior to cardioversion and continued for 4 weeks after cardioversion. Recent trials have suggested that long-term anticoagulation may be recommended even after cardioversion due to a 50% risk of recurrent AF. Contraindications to warfarin therapy include systemic or intracranial bleeding, noncompliance, or a significant risk of falls.
   b. Chronic AF. Determination of a patient's risk for an embolic event guides the selection of anticoagulant therapy (Table 49–4). Risk factors include age, left ventricular dysfunction, hypertension, thyrotoxicosis, and diabetes.

TABLE 49–4. RISK-BASED APPROACH TO ANTITHROMBOTIC THERAPY IN ATRIAL FIBRILLATION (AF)

Patient Features	Antithrombotic Therapy
Age <60 years No heart disease (lone AF)	ASA 325 mg daily or no therapy
Age <60 years Heart disease but no risk factors[1]	ASA 325 mg daily
Age ≥60 years No risk factors[1]	ASA 325 mg daily
Age ≥60 years With diabetes or CAD	Warfarin (INR 2.0–3.0) Addition of ASA 81–162 mg/day optional
Age ≥75 years, especially women	Warfarin (INR ~2.0) Warfarin (INR 2.0–3.0)
Any age patient with: Heart failure LVEF ≤35% Thyrotoxicosis Hypertension Rheumatic heart disease (mitral stenosis) Prosthetic heart valves Prior thromboembolism Persistent atrial thrombus on TEE	Warfarin (INR 2.5–3.5 or higher may be appropriate)

[1]Risk factors for thromboembolism include heart failure, LVEF less than 35%, thyrotoxicosis, or history of hypertension.
AF, atrial fibrillation; ASA, aspirin; CAD, coronary artery disease; INR, international normalized ratio; LVEF, left ventricular ejection fraction; TEE, transesophageal echocardiography.
Adapted from Fuster V, et al: ACC/AHA/ESC guidelines for the management of patients with atrial fibrillation: Executive summary. A report of the American College of Cardiology/American Heart Association Task Force on Practice Guidelines and the European Society of Cardiology Committee for Practice Guidelines and Policy Conferences (Committee to develop guidelines for the management of patients with atrial fibrillation). Developed in collaboration with the North American Society of Pacing and Electrophysiology. J Am Coll Cardiol 2001;**38**:1231.

REFERENCES

Arnsdorf MF: Nonsustained VT in the absence of apparent structural heart disease. www.UpToDate.com, online version 11.1.

Arnsdorf MF, Podrid PJ: Overview of the presentation and management of atrial fibrillation. www.UpToDate.com, online version 11.1.

Barsky AJ: Investigating selected symptoms: Palpitations, arrhythmias, and awareness of cardiac activity. Ann Intern Med 2001;**134**:832.

King DE, Dickerson LM, Sack JL: Acute management of atrial fibrillation: Part I. Rate and rhythm control. Am Fam Physician 2002;**66**:249.

Zimetbaum P: Overview of palpitations. www.UpToDate.com, online version 11.1.

---

50   Pediatric Fever

Sanford R. Kimmel, MD

KEY POINTS

- Evaluation of the young child with fever is a common but often challenging task for the family physician.
- Most febrile illnesses are viral and self-limited. However, the physician must detect those children with a potentially serious bacterial illness.
- Careful observation and examination along with judicious laboratory testing and close follow-up enable family physicians to evaluate and manage most febrile children.

I. **Definition.** Fever is an elevation of body temperature above the normal range. The normal range for temperature of the body varies according to the age of the child, method of measurement, and time of day. A rectal temperature >37.8 °C (100 °F) in newborns or 38 °C (100.4 °F) in older infants denotes fever, as does an oral temperature of 37.8 °C in older children. Rectal temperature most consistently reflects the body's core temperature and is used in this chapter.

Fever occurs when exogenous pyrogens such as viruses, bacteria, fungi, toxins, drugs, malignancies, metabolic disorders, and antigen-antibody complexes induce release of endogenous pyrogens, such as interleukin (IL) 1β and IL-6. These stimulate the production of hypothalamic prostaglandin E_2 (PGE_2) that raises the "set point" of the body's thermostat. Heat is generated or conserved through shivering or peripheral vasoconstriction. The resulting fever may increase leukocyte migration and antibacterial activity as well as T-cell and interferon production. However, the risk of dehydration also increases, since the body's basal metabolic rate increases 10% for each degree Celsius above normal.

II. **Common Diagnoses.** During the first 2–3 years of life, children have an average of four to six acute infections per year. Viral infections cause most febrile episodes, but serious bacterial infections are present in 10–15% of febrile infants younger than 3 months old with a temperature 38 °C or higher and in 13% of children ages 3 months to 3 years old presenting with a fever >39 °C (102.2°F) and a white blood count >15,000 cells/μL.

   A. **Upper respiratory infections (URIs)** (eg, viral infections, otitis media, pharyngitis, and sinusitis) account for about one third of all visits children younger than 15 years make to family physicians, while **lower respiratory infections (LRIs)** (eg, bacterial and viral pneumonias, bronchitis, and bronchiolitis) are less common but significant causes of pediatric fever. Exposure to ill siblings, day-care attendance, and parental smoking are some risk factors for respiratory infections.

   B. **Gastroenteritis** causes over 20 million episodes of diarrhea annually in children in the United States younger then 5 years old. Rotavirus infects almost all children by 3 years of age, especially during the winter months in temperate climates in the United States. The ingestion of contaminated food or water are risk factors for bacterial gastroenteri-

tis caused by *Salmonella* species, *Campylobacter* species, enterotoxigenic *Escherichia coli,* and *Shigella* species.
C. **Bacteremia** occurs in about 2–3% of febrile children aged 2–36 months seen in the emergency room. In addition to young age, risk factors for bacteremia include immunodeficiency or immunosuppression, anatomic or functional asplenia, and household or day-care contact with invasive bacterial disease. *Streptococcus pneumoniae* now causes most cases of occult bacteremia, whereas invasive disease due to *Haemophilus influenzae* type b (Hib) has become rare in areas with high immunization rates.
D. **Urinary tract infections (UTIs)** occur in 5–7% of girls younger than age 2 presenting with fever and no localizing signs. Uncircumcised male infants have a 10 times greater incidence of UTIs (1%) during the first year of life than do circumcised infants (0.1%). The prevalence of bacteremia is higher in young infants with UTIs.
E. **Bacterial meningitis** can occur throughout the year, but *S pneumoniae* and *Neisseria meningitidis* usually occur during the winter months. If one child has meningococcal meningitis, the rate of a simultaneous case occurring in that family is 1% without chemoprophylaxis. Gram-negative enteric bacteria, group B streptococci, and *Listeria monocytogenes* are important causes of bacterial meningitis in infants younger than 3 months of age. Invasive Hib disease has significantly decreased due to the Hib vaccine. **Viral meningitis** occurs during the summer and fall in temperate climates. Enterovirus is the most common cause and is spread from person to person by fecal-oral and respiratory routes and by fomites.
F. About 50% of cases of childhood **osteomyelitis** occur in children younger than 5 years. *Staphylococcus aureus* is the most common cause, but gram-negative bacteria such as *Salmonella* may cause recurrent osteomyelitis in children with hemoglobinopathies such as sickle cell disease, whereas *Pseudomonas aeruginosa* usually causes disease due to puncture wounds of the foot. About 75% of childhood cases of **septic arthritis** occur in children younger than 5 years. Most cases are caused by *S aureus*, but *Neisseria gonorrhoeae* often causes disease in sexually active or abused adolescents. Group B streptococci and enteric gram-negative bacilli are important causes of septic arthritis and osteomyelitis in neonates; Hib may cause bone and joint infections in inadequately immunized children.
G. **Febrile exanthems. Roseola** is caused by human herpesvirus type 6 and usually affects children between ages 6 and 24 months, seldom occurring after 3 years of age. **Measles** is transmitted by direct contact with infectious airborne droplets, predominantly during the winter and spring in temperate climates. Measles cases in the United States have declined as a result of a second measles immunization given prior to school entry. **Scarlet fever** is usually associated with erythrogenic exotoxin-producing group A streptococcal pharyngitis and follows close contact with respiratory secretions of infected individuals. **Varicella** usually occurs by direct contact with persons who have varicella or zoster, and occasionally by airborne spread from respiratory secretions. It is highly contagious among susceptible contacts and is most common during late winter and early spring.
III. **Symptoms.** The febrile child often demonstrates some degree of lethargy, loss of appetite, or irritability.
A. **Respiratory symptoms** include sore throat, nasal congestion, otalgia, cough, and wheezing.
B. **Diarrhea** and **vomiting** usually indicate a gastrointestinal infection, although these symptoms occasionally occur in acute otitis media or UTI.
C. **Fever** may be the only symptom of a UTI in young infants, but older infants and children may **cry with urination or refuse to urinate.**
D. Persistence or worsening of **lethargy** and **irritability** may indicate meningitis.
E. **Refusal to bear weight** or use an extremity may be seen with septic arthritis or osteomyelitis.
F. A transient red maculopapular rash appearing after defervescence of several days of high fever is characteristic of **roseola.** Cough, coryza, and conjunctivitis accompany the confluent red rash of **measles.** A strawberry tongue may be seen with the characteristic sandpaper-like rash of **scarlet fever.** The croplike spread of different stages of macules, papules, and vesicles from the face and trunk to the extremities (but sparing the palms and soles) denotes varicella. **Smallpox** begins on the oral mucosa, face, and upper extremities, then spreads to the trunk and lower extremities, often involving the palms and soles. The initial papules evolve simultaneously into vesicles and then umbilicated pustules.

IV. Signs

    A. The **degree of temperature reduction in response to acetaminophen** is generally not helpful in differentiating viral from bacterial infection.

    B. **Observation** of the child's appearance and interaction with the parent or caregiver often determine whether the physician needs to have a high or low index of suspicion of serious underlying disease.

        1. McCarthy and associates (1982) developed six key criteria for serious illness based on observation and interaction with the febrile child seated on the caregiver's lap, prior to antipyretic therapy (Table 50–1).

        2. A serious underlying disease was found in 92% of children with an acute illness observation scale (AIOS) score of 16 or more and in 26% of those with a score of 11–15. Only 2.7% of children with a score of 10 or less had a serious illness.

        3. No child who smiled normally had a serious illness. In another study, the presence of a social smile did not always exclude the possibility of a serious bacterial illness.

        4. The AIOS is most useful in children 2 months of age or older. In infants 4–8 weeks old, the AIOS detected <50% of those with a serious illness in one study. The sensitivity and positive predictive value of the AIOS also decrease as the prevalence of bacteremia in the population decreases.

    C. **Physical findings** associated with specific diseases are presented in Table 50–2.

V. Laboratory Tests

    A. **Screening laboratory tests** help determine if further diagnostic studies are needed for moderately ill-appearing children (eg, an AIOS score of 11–15) who do not have an obvious focus of infection or for well-appearing children with high or persistent fever.

        1. In infants older than 28 days, the following conditions suggest an underlying or occult bacterial illness.

            a. White blood cell count (WBC) of ≥15,000 cells/μL.

            b. Absolute band count >1500 cells/μL.

            c. Absolute neutrophil count >10,500 cells/μL.

        2. The positive predictive value of the above tests for serious bacterial illness (SBI), such as pneumonia or meningitis, is about 10–30%. Thus, many children with a positive screening test result will not have an underlying SBI.

        3. No test will detect bacteremia or other serious illnesses in all children. Some children with meningitis may have a WBC of <15,000/μL, and some children with overwhelming sepsis may have a WBC of <5000/μL.

TABLE 50–1. ACUTE ILLNESS OBSERVATION SCALES

Observation Item	Normal—1	Moderate Impairment—3	Severe Impairment—5
Quality of cry	Strong cry with normal tone, or contented and not crying	Whimpering or sobbing	Weak cry, moaning, or high-pitched cry
Reaction to parental stimulation	Cries briefly and then stops, or is contented and not crying	Cries off and on	Cries continually or hardly responds
State variation	If awake, stays awake, or if asleep and then stimulated, awakens quickly	Closes eyes briefly when awake, or awakens with prolonged stimulation	Falls asleep or will not arouse
Color	Pink	Pale extremities or acrocyanosis	Pale, cyanotic, mottled, or ashen
Hydration	Normal skin and eyes, moist mucous membranes	Normal skin and eyes, slightly dry mouth	Doughy or tented skin, dry mucous membranes or sunken eyes
Response (talk, smile) to social overture	Smiles, or "alert" (≤2 months)[1]	Smiles briefly, or "alert" briefly (≤2 months)[1]	No smile, anxious face, dull expression, or does not "alert" (≤2 months)[1]

[1] "Alert" applies to children younger than 2 months of age, since these young infants do not have a social smile.

Adapted with permission from McCarthy PL, et al: Observation scales to identify serious illness in febrile children. Pediatrics 1982;**70**:806, as used in Kimmel SR, Gemmill DW: The young child with fever. Am Fam Physician 1988;**37**:196.

TABLE 50–2. PHYSICAL FINDINGS AND CLINICAL CLUES TO ILLNESSES IN FEBRILE CHILDREN

Body Region or System	Physical Findings	Potential Disease(s)
Skin	Petechial rash	Meningococcemia
	Maculopapular rash, followed by petechial rash	Rocky Mountain spotted fever
Head	Bulging fontanelle, nuchal rigidity	Meningitis (later manifestation in child younger than 2 years of age)
Eyes	Conjunctivitis	Associated otitis media, Kawasaki disease, or measles with cough, coryza
	Redness or swelling around eye	Periorbital cellulitis
Ears	Red, dull, nonmobile tympanic membrane	Otitis media
	Swelling and tenderness behind ear	Mastoiditis
Nose	Purulent rhinorrhea	Sinusitis
	Nasal flaring	Pneumonia or any condition producing respiratory distress
Throat	Stridor	Laryngotracheobronchitis (croup)
	Stridor with drooling, dysphagia, or aphonia	Epiglottitis
	Petechiae on soft palate and uvula	Streptococcal pharyngitis
	Vesicles or ulcers on soft palate and tonsillar pillars	Herpangina
	Vesicles or ulcers on tongue, lips, and buccal mucosa	Herpes stomatitis
	Strawberry tongue	Streptococcal pharyngitis or Kawasaki disease
Chest	Tachypnea, retractions, decreased breath sounds, rales (may not be present)	Pneumonia
	Rhonchi	Bronchitis
	Wheezing	Bronchiolitis, asthma (inhaled foreign body or other causes)
Heart	Murmur	Subacute bacterial endocarditis, rheumatic fever (or normal due to increased cardiac output)
Abdomen	Local tenderness worsening with movement	Appendicitis or condition producing peritoneal irritation
Rectal	Fluctuant mass	Ruptured appendix or perirectal abscess
Musculoskeletal	Refuses to bear weight or use extremity	Septic arthritis or osteomyelitis, especially in the hip

Reprinted with permission from Kimmel SR, Gemmill DW: The young child with fever. Am Fam Physician 1988;**37**:202.

4. Careful clinical assessment of the child is necessary in interpreting screening tests. A positive test result is more likely to be significant in an ill-appearing child or one who has underlying risk factors than in one who looks well.

B. Further diagnostic tests (Table 50–3) should be considered in febrile children who appear moderately or severely ill (AIOS score >10) or who have an abnormal screening test result.

VI. Treatment (Figure 50–1).

A. Hospitalization is indicated in the following circumstances.

1. Infants 0–28 days old with a fever of >38 °C (100.4 °F) require a sepsis work-up and parenteral antibiotics pending culture results.

2. Febrile children 29–90 days of age not fulfilling the Rochester low-risk criteria (Table 50–4) are at risk for bacteremia or SBI based on their clinical appearance, physical findings, and laboratory studies. These children should be hospitalized for further evaluation and treatment.

3. Hospitalization is also required for any immunosuppressed or severely ill febrile child (eg, AIOS score ≥16), or one having an underlying condition placing him or her at high risk of overwhelming infection.

TABLE 50–3. DIAGNOSTIC STUDIES IN FEBRILE CHILDREN WITHOUT AN OBVIOUS FOCUS OF INFECTION

Test	Indications	Comments
Chest x-ray	Fever of sudden onset, tachypnea, decreased breath sounds, or WBC >20,000/μL	Pneumonia may lack usual auscultatory findings
Urinalysis (UA) with culture and sensitivity (C&S)	Boys ≤6 months or uncircumcised boys <12 months of age. Girls ≤2 years old	Bladder tap newborn; catheterize older children; negative UA does not rule out infection
Lumbar puncture	Child ≤3 months of age or very irritable or lethargic, feeds poorly, has seizures, bulging fontanelle, or nuchal rigidity	Use needle with stylet; consider hospital admission
Blood culture	Age ≤3 years at high risk of bacteremia, acute illness observation score (AIOS) ≥11 ± WBC ≥15,000/μL	Draw 0.5–2 mL of blood; one test sufficient for outpatient use
Stool for polymorphonuclear cells (PMNs) with C&S	Abrupt onset or bloody diarrhea, greater than four stools per day, and no vomiting before diarrhea	Positive if ≥5 PMNs/hpf

AIOS, acute illness observation scale; hpf, high-power field.

B. Ambulatory management

1. Specific therapy should be initiated for conditions diagnosed and amenable to outpatient treatment (see Chapter 13, for LRIs; Chapter 16, for gastroenteritis; Chapter 22, for otitis media; Chapter 55, for sinusitis; and Chapter 57, for pharyngitis).

2. Infants aged 29–90 days old who fulfill **all** the Rochester low-risk criteria may be managed as outpatients, provided they have reliable caregivers who are able to contact their physician by telephone and obtain medical care within 30 minutes. Parents must be instructed to call or seek immediate medical attention if the child demonstrates worrisome signs such as poor feeding, vomiting, excessive fussiness or sleepiness, skin rash, or color changes. The child must be re-evaluated within 24 hours after blood and catheterized urine cultures are obtained (Figure 50–1). A lumbar puncture should be considered prior to empiric antibiotic treatment (see section VI,B,4).

3. Febrile children without localizing signs who are 3 months of age or older may be followed up as outpatients if their caretakers are reliable and the children can be re-evaluated within 24–48 hours.

4. Intramuscular ceftriaxone (Rocephin) at a dose of 50 mg/kg intramuscularly once daily up to 1 g maximum is preferred if the child is given empiric treatment. Amoxicillin–potassium clavulanate (Augmentin) may also decrease the risk of focal infection in bacteremic children, but there is less experience using this antibiotic for this purpose.

   a. Presumptive antibiotic therapy may be begun after obtaining a blood culture and other appropriate diagnostic studies if the child is between 3 months and 3 years of age, the fever is 39 °C (102.2 °F) or more, the AIOS score is 11–15, or the WBC is ≥15,000/μL. Antibiotic therapy might be withheld if the child appears nontoxic and has completed a primary series of conjugate pneumococcal vaccine or if prompt reporting of positive blood cultures and callback of the child is feasible.

   b. Therapy should be directed against *S pneumoniae*, which is the most common cause of occult bacteremia, as well as *H influenzae* and meningococcus.

5. Follow-up of the older child who has fever and no obvious focus must occur by re-examination or telephone in 24–48 hours.

   a. If the child is better or cultures are negative after 48 hours, antibiotic therapy should be discontinued.

   b. If the child's condition is improved and blood culture grows *S pneumoniae*, outpatient antibiotic therapy should be continued for 10 days under close observation. A follow-up blood culture should be obtained to confirm clinical cure.

   c. If the child is improved and afebrile but the urine culture is positive, outpatient antibiotic therapy based on culture results should be continued for 7–14 days. Clinical pyelonephritis should be treated for 14 days. A urine culture should be obtained after 48 hours of treatment if the child is not improving, sensitivity test-

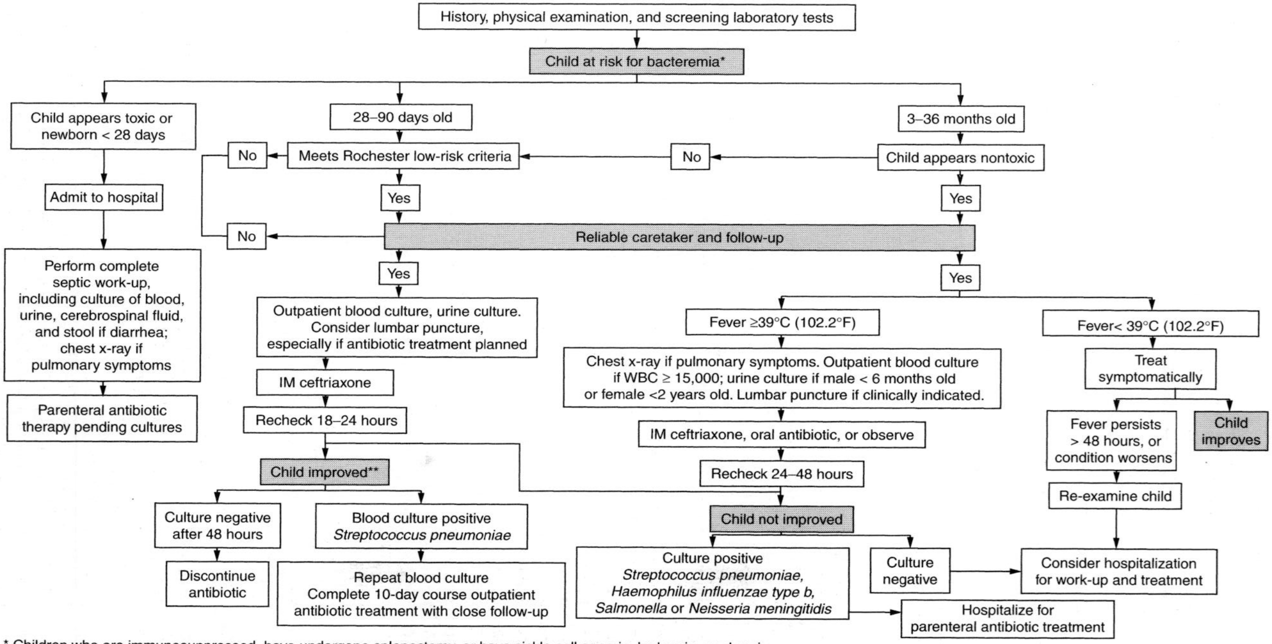

FIGURE 50–1. Guidelines for the management of children with fever without localizing signs. IM, intramuscular; WBC, white blood cell count.

History, physical examination, and screening laboratory tests

Child at risk for bacteremia*

28–90 days old

Child appears toxic or newborn < 28 days

- No → Meets Rochester low-risk criteria
  - No → Admit to hospital
    - Perform complete septic work-up, including culture of blood, urine, cerebrospinal fluid, and stool if diarrhea; chest x-ray if pulmonary symptoms
    - Parenteral antibiotic therapy pending cultures
  - Yes → Reliable caretaker and follow-up
    - Yes → Outpatient blood culture, urine culture. Consider lumbar puncture, especially if antibiotic treatment planned
      - IM ceftriaxone
      - Recheck 18–24 hours
      - **Child improved****
        - Culture negative after 48 hours → Discontinue antibiotic
        - Blood culture positive *Streptococcus pneumoniae* → Repeat blood culture. Complete 10-day course outpatient antibiotic treatment with close follow-up

3–36 months old

Child appears nontoxic

- Yes → Reliable caretaker and follow-up
  - Yes
    - Fever ≥39°C (102.2°F)
      - Chest x-ray if pulmonary symptoms. Outpatient blood culture if WBC ≥ 15,000; urine culture if male < 6 months old or female <2 years old. Lumbar puncture if clinically indicated.
      - IM ceftriaxone, oral antibiotic, or observe
      - Recheck 24–48 hours
      - **Child not improved**
        - Culture positive *Streptococcus pneumoniae, Haemophilus influenzae type b, Salmonella* or *Neisseria meningitidis* → Hospitalize for parenteral antibiotic treatment
        - Culture negative → Consider hospitalization for work-up and treatment
    - Fever < 39°C (102.2°F)
      - Treat symptomatically
        - **Child improves**
        - Fever persists > 48 hours, or condition worsens → Re-examine child → Consider hospitalization for work-up and treatment

* Children who are immunosuppressed, have undergone splenectomy, or have sickle cell anemia, leukemia, nephrosis, and other conditions placing them at high risk for overwhelming bacterial infection should be managed like toxic children.
**Nontoxic, nonbacteremic, afebrile children with otitis media or urinary tract infection may be treated with outpatient antibiotics.

311

TABLE 50–4. ROCHESTER CRITERIA FOR LOW-RISK INFANTS

1. Infant appears generally well
2. Infant has been previously healthy
   Born at term (≥37 weeks' gestation)
   Did not receive perinatal antimicrobial therapy
   Was not treated for unexplained hyperbilirubinemia
   Had not received and was not receiving antimicrobial agents
   Had not been previously hospitalized
   Had no chronic or underlying illness
   Was not hospitalized longer than mother
3. No evidence of skin, soft tissue, bone, joint, or ear infection
4. Laboratory values
   Peripheral blood WBC count 5.0–15.0 × 10^9 cells/L (5000–15,000/mm³)
   Absolute band form count ≤1.5 × 10^9 cells/L (≤1500/mm³)
   ≤10 WBCs per high-power field (×40) on microscopic examination of a spun urine sediment
   ≤5 WBC per high-power field (×40) on microscopic examination of a stool smear (only for infants with diarrhea)

WBC, white blood cell.
Jaskiewicz JA, McCarthy CA, Richardson AC, et al, and the Febrile Infant Collaborative Study Group: Febrile infants at low risk for serious bacterial infection—an appraisal of the Rochester criteria and implications for management. Reproduced with permission from *Pediatrics*, Vol. **94**, page 391, 1994.

ing is not performed, or bacteria are intermediate or resistant to the chosen antibiotic. A structural evaluation of the urinary tract by renal ultrasound followed by voiding cystourethrography (VCUG) should be done in all children 2 months to 2 years old. The child should continue to receive therapeutic or prophylactic antimicrobial therapy pending the VCUG.

   d. If the blood culture grows Hib, *N meningitidis, Salmonella,* or other pathogenic organisms, the child should be hospitalized for parenteral antibiotic therapy and evaluated for focal sites of infection.
   e. If the child is worse or not improved at follow-up, repeat history, physical examination, and laboratory studies should be performed. Hospital admission is often indicated at this time.

6. The primary reason to treat fever symptomatically is to make the child more comfortable. Parents should be instructed as follows.
   a. Fever of 38.9 °C (102 °F) or greater should be treated with **acetaminophen,** 10–15 mg/kg every 4 hours up to a maximum of five doses per day. **Ibuprofen,** 5–10 mg/kg every 6–8 hours, may also be used for fever reduction in children aged 6 months or older.
   b. Children with a temperature ≥40 °C (104 °F) and no response to acetaminophen or ibuprofen should be sponged with lukewarm water. Alcohol or cold water should not be used.
   c. Children should be covered with light blankets and encouraged to drink liquids.
   d. Fever itself is seldom dangerous. It is a symptom of an underlying illness. Observation of children's behavior is even more important than a record of their temperature.

REFERENCES

Alpern ER, et al: Occult bacteremia from a pediatric emergency department: Current prevalence, time to detection, and outcome. Pediatrics 2000;**106**:505.
American Academy of Pediatrics. In: Pickering LK (editor): *2003 Red Book: 2003 Report of the Committee on Infectious Diseases,* 26th ed. American Academy of Pediatrics; 2003.
American Academy of Pediatrics Committee on Quality Improvement, Subcommittee on Urinary Tract Infection. Practice parameter: The diagnosis, treatment, and evaluation of the initial urinary tract infection in febrile infants and young children. Pediatrics 1999;**103**:843.
Baraff LJ: Management of fever without source in infants and children. Ann Emerg Med 2000;**36**:602.
Nelson JD: Osteomyelitis and suppurative arthritis. In: Behrman RE, Kliegman RM, Jenson HB (editors): *Nelson Textbook of Pediatrics,* 16th ed. Saunders; 2000:776–780.
Powell KR: Fever without a focus. In: Behrman RE, Kliegman RM, Jenson HB (editors): *Nelson Textbook of Pediatrics,* 16th ed. Saunders; 2000:742–747.

51   Pelvic Pain

Maria V. Gibson, MD, PhD

KEY POINTS

- Pelvic pain originates below the umbilicus of the female and may be acute (<6 months' duration) or chronic (>6 months' duration).
- Pelvic inflammatory disease, ectopic pregnancy, appendicitis, urinary tract infection, and adnexal mass rupture/torsion/hemorrhage are the most common causes of acute pelvic pain.
- Treatment of chronic pelvic pain is empiric, unless the causative agent is found.

I. **Definition.** Pelvic pain (PP) occurs below the female umbilicus. **Acute pelvic pain (APP)** refers to pain for <6 months. **Chronic pelvic pain (CPP)** lasts >6 months. PP may originate in the lower abdominal organ systems in women. **Gynecologic** pain includes ectopic pregnancy, acute and chronic pelvic inflammatory disease (PID), adnexal mass, endometriosis, dysmenorrhea, uterine leiomyoma, and chronic pelvic congestion. **Gastrointestinal** pain includes gastroenteritis, irritable bowel syndrome, appendicitis, intestinal obstruction, hernia, diverticulitis, perirectal abscess, mesenteric ischemia, mesenteric adenitis, and inflammatory bowel disease. **Urologic pain** includes interstitial cystitis, urolithiasis, and pyelonephritis. Pain from **musculoskeletal disorders** includes hematoma of the abdominal wall, spontaneous rectus sheath hematoma, ilioinguinal and iliohypogastric nerve entrapment, and incarcerated hernia. Pain also could be referred from other organs or be psychogenic. This chapter will focus on gynecologic causes of pelvic pain; for other causes see Chapters 1 (Abdominal Pain), 21 (Dysuria in Women), and 46 (Myalgia).

II. **Common Diagnoses.** PP is a major health problem. It is the reason for 10% for all outpatient visits, 10% of gynecologic referrals, 12% of hysterectomies, and over 40% of laparoscopies. The annual prevalence of PP in the primary care setting (38 of 1000 patients) was found to be comparable to that of asthma and back pain. Women with PP have a high incidence of concomitant depression, somatization, and substance abuse potentiating PP symptoms. The relative frequency of the causes of PP is influenced by patient population risk factors. For example, in young women with a high prevalence of sexually transmitted diseases, acute and chronic PID are most common causes of PP. Reproductive-age patients have a higher prevalence of endometriosis, urinary tract infections, and ovarian cysts. Postmenopausal women have a higher frequency of gastrointestinal and genitourinary disorders, and adnexal masses in this age group are most likely malignant.

A. **Acute pelvic pain (APP).** Five percent of ambulatory primary care visits are for APP. Ten percent of these patients require urgent surgery.

1. **Pelvic inflammatory disease (PID).** The incidence of PID is 7.2/1000, and nearly 400,000 patients a year present to primary care offices with PID. Risk factors for PID include multiple sex partners, a symptomatic partner, age 15–25 years, African American ethnicity, history of previous PID, and intrauterine medical device (IUD) contraception.

2. **Adnexal mass torsion.** Risk factors for adnexal torsion (16% of APP) include reproductive age, prior pelvic surgery, history of ovarian cyst or PID, pedunculated uterine leiomyoma, and prior tubal ligation.

3. **Ectopic pregnancy** (1–2% of APP) occurs in 30.2 to 94.8 of 100,000 women aged 15–44 years. Predisposing factors include a history of tubal surgery, tubal pathology, PID, in-utero diethylstilbestrol exposure, infertility, multiple sexual partners, and vaginal douching. Contraceptive types influence the risk of ectopic pregnancy, ranging from 0.005/1000 with oral contraceptive pills (OCP) to 0.020/1000 for IUDs and 0.318/1000 for tubal ligation.

4. **Uterine leiomyoma.** Thirty to 40% of women older than 30 years have uterine leiomyomas, making this the most common gynecologic tumor in reproductive-age

women; leiomyoma occurs in one in four white women and one in two African American women. Other risk factors include family history, history of hypertension, infectious complications of PID and IUD use, heavy consumption of red meat, nulliparity, and sedentary lifestyle. Acute degeneration or torsion of pedunculated leiomyoma may cause APP.

B. Chronic pelvic pain (CPP) is present in 15% of women seeking medical care. The incidence of CPP is 38.3/1000 women aged 12–70 years. In 61% of cases the cause of CPP is not identified.

1. **Endometriosis** is found in 45–50% of women with CPP. Prevalence ranges from 2% to 18% and is higher in infertile women (5–50%). Risk factors for endometriosis include genetic abnormalities, immune disorders, Asian ancestry, cigarette smoking, alcohol consumption, lack of exercise, vaginal or cervical stenosis, and uterine anomalies (noncommunicating uterine horn, coelomic metaplasia). The incidence of endometriosis is inversely related to body mass index.

2. **Mittelschmerz** is experienced by 25% of ovulating females, and the major risk factor for mittelschmerz is the presence of a follicular cyst, which usually ruptures during the midcycle.

3. **Dysmenorrhea** (15% of CPP). Approximately 50% of all women experience dysmenorrhea, and 15% are incapacitated for 1–3 days of each month because of severe symptoms. See Chapter 18.

4. The prevalence of **dyspareunia** (35% of CPP) ranges from 8% to 30.6% and increases in postpartum and postmenopausal women. Risk factors for dyspareunia include a history of vulvar and perineal surgeries, sexual abuse, vaginal dryness, and vaginismus.

5. **Adhesions** are diagnosed in 25% of women with CPP, but their causative role remains controversial. CPP due to adhesions is experienced by 2.9 women per 100 operations, with risk influenced by surgical site—the colon and rectum have the highest incidence, followed by the ovaries. The postoperative adhesion rate does not appear to be different between laparotomy and laparoscopy.

6. **Psychogenic pain.** Women with a history of somatization disorder, sexual abuse, post-traumatic stress disorder, and depression frequently experience CPP. The prevalence of sexual abuse history in CPP is 50%. Depression coexists with CPP in 50% and anxiety in 31% of women.

III. Symptoms (Tables 51–1 to 51–3).

A. Location and quality

1. **APP**
   a. Unilateral sharp moderate/severe pain occurs with ureteral colic and diverticulitis.
   b. Bilateral diffuse sharp pain occurs with intra-abdominal hemorrhage and intestinal obstruction.
   c. Dull, pressure pain commonly occurs with mesenteric lymphadenitis, mesenteric ischemia, and diverticulitis.

2. **CPP**
   a. Dull and deep pain characterizes interstitial cystitis and irritable bowel syndrome.
   b. Reproducible trigger points confined to one anatomical region on the abdomen and back are found in patients with myofascial syndrome.

B. Onset/chronology

1. **APP**
   a. Sudden onset of pain suggests acute perforation of hollow viscus or intraperitoneal hemorrhage; gradual onset characterizes inflammation or obstruction.
   b. Most patients with appendicitis present within 48 hours of pain onset.

2. **CPP**
   a. Pain associated with abdominal wall contraction suggests abdominal wall hematoma, tear, or nerve entrapment.
   b. Pain associated with food intake and relieved after defecation is characteristic of irritable bowel syndrome.

C. Associated symptoms

1. Nausea/vomiting/anorexia is common for intestinal obstruction, gastroenteritis, and irritable bowel syndrome.
2. Sexual dysfunction is a prominent feature in 28% of women with endometriosis, dyspareunia, and irritable bowel syndrome.

TABLE 51–1. FINDINGS WITH COMMON CAUSES OF ACUTE PELVIC PAIN

Diagnosis	Location/Quality/Chronology of Pain	Other Symptoms	Signs
Ovarian cyst	Unilateral dull, pressure-like; severe/diffuse low abdominal (rupture) Within 7 days of menses, worse with strenuous physical activity	Delayed/scanty menses if lutein cyst	Smooth mobile adnexal mass/fullness; peritoneal signs if ruptured
Pelvic inflammatory disease	Lower abdominal with gradual unset, usually bilateral, worse perimenstrually	Fever, vaginal discharge, dysuria, abnormal vaginal bleeding	See Table 51–3
Adnexal torsion	Unilateral moderate/severe pain; sudden onset, within 24–48 hours of presentation	Nausea/vomiting	Adnexal mass and tenderness on the affected side, rebound, guarding may be present
Appendicitis	Initial vague epigastric progressed to RLQ/flank/suprapubic; develops over 24–48 hours	Anorexia/nausea/mild diarrhea	Low-grade fever, McBurney's point tenderness, peritoneal and obturator signs
Ectopic pregnancy	Diffuse or localized, colicky or dull lower abdominal, radiating to the shoulder if hemoperitoneum	Amenorrhea or abnormal vaginal bleeding (metrorrhagia/menorrhagia) nausea/breast tenderness	Adnexal tenderness/mass, uterus slightly enlarged, peritoneal signs, abdominal distention and shock if significant hemorrhage
Urinary tract infection	Variable, midline, suprapubic	Urinary frequency, urgency, dysuria	Suprapubic tenderness occasionally, often none
Uterine leiomyoma	Low midline pressure, back pain; moderate to severe pain with torsion/degeneration	Menorrhagia; metrorrhagia, nausea/vomiting with torsion, dysuria (if large), infertility	Enlarged, nodular uterus, tender if degeneration/torsion

RLQ, right lower quadrant.

315

TABLE 51–2. CLINICAL FINDINGS WITH COMMON CAUSES OF CHRONIC PELVIC PAIN

Diagnosis	Location/Quality/ Chronology of Pain	Other Symptoms	Signs
Endometriosis	Variable midline suprapubic, premenstrual/menstrual	Dyspareunia, painful defecation, infertility, hematuria	Often none; palpable cysts and nodules on uterosacral ligament
Mittelschmerz	Suprapubic, dull to sharp Midcycle; lasts hours to 3 days	None	None
Psychogenic	Variable	Depression, anxiety, back pain, fatigue, nausea	Signs of depression or anxiety, normal pelvic examination, occasional pelvic tenderness
Dysmenorrhea	Low abdominal starting prior/with menses, dyspareunia, radiates to the rectum	Painful defecation, nausea/vomiting, anorexia, headache, occasional diarrhea	None
Dyspareunia	Dull pain on vaginal entry or deep pelvic pain during sexual intercourse	Anxiety, depression, sexual dysfunction, vaginal dryness	Anxiety, depression, PTSD
Adhesions	Colicky diffuse or localized	Bloating, nausea	Diffuse abdominal tenderness without masses

PTSD, post-traumatic stress disorder.

TABLE 51–3. DIAGNOSTIC CRITERIA FOR PELVIC INFLAMMATORY DISEASE

Minimum diagnostic criteria: Uterine, adnexal, or cervical motion tenderness.

Additional diagnostic criteria: Oral temperature >38.3 °C, cervical sampling positive for *Chlamydia trachomatis* or *Neisseria gonorrhoeae*, white blood cells saline microscopy, elevated erythrocyte sedimentation rate, elevated C-reactive protein (CRP), and cervical discharge.

Definitive diagnostic criteria: Endometrial biopsy with histopathologic evidence of endometritis, transvaginal ultrasonography or magnetic resonance imaging scan showing thick fluid-filled fallopian tubes, laparoscopic abnormalities consistent with pelvic inflammatory disease.

From the Centers for Disease Control and Prevention recommendations, 2002.

3. Substance abuse, somatization, depression, and post-traumatic stress disorder are present in 60–70% of women with CPP. Up to 25% of these patients have a history of physical or sexual abuse. Thirty-one percent of women with CPP have anxiety disorder.

IV. **Signs** (Tables 51–1 to 51–3). Also see the sidebars on chronic endometritis, adnexal mass, pelvic congestion syndrome, and ovarian remnant syndrome.

CHRONIC ENDOMETRITIS

Chronic endometritis in nonpregnant women is usually due to infections (PID, tuberculosis), IUD, submucosal leiomyoma, or radiation therapy. CPP, menorrhagia or metrorrhagia, mucopurulent vaginal discharge, and tender enlarged uterus are characteristic findings. Recommended treatment includes removal of an IUD and use of doxycycline (100 mg orally twice a day for 10 days) for *Chlamydia trachomatis* or unknown etiology; *Mycobacterium tuberculosis* should be treated with combination drug therapy for 9–12 months (See Chapter 13).

ADNEXAL MASS

A family history of reproductive malignancy (uterine, breast, ovarian), presence of the BRCA gene, nulliparity, early menarche, and late menopause are risk factors for ovarian tumors. Eighty percent of ovarian masses in girls younger than 15 years are malignant. Thirty to 60% of adnexal masses in postmenopausal women are malignant as well. Adnexal masses can cause APP through adnexal mass torsion or ovarian cyst rupture or hemorrhage, and rupture of small (<4 cm) cysts is usually asymptomatic. The approach to a discovered adnexal mass depends on the patient's age and cyst size. Because of high oncogenic potential (germ cell tumors) in premenarchial patients, all adnexal masses in these individuals should be evaluated by transvaginal ultrasound (TVU) and referred for surgical removal. In reproductive-age women, adnexal masses are commonly follicular or lutein cysts or complications of PID (hydrosalpinx and tubo-ovarian abscess). If pain is not acute or recurrent, palpable cysts <6 cm in women of childbearing age may be monitored with repeat pelvic examination in 6 weeks. Any persistent or increasing mass on serial observation or a mass initially >6 cm should be evaluated by TVU. Adnexal masses in postmenopausal women have a high risk of malignancy (surface epithelial or stromal tumors) and should be evaluated with TVU, tumor markers (CA-125) and possibly computerized tomography scanning.

Management of adnexal masses is referral to gynecology for further evaluation and removal, unless a mass in a reproductive-age woman is cystic, small (<6 cm), and does not persist or increase in size.

PELVIC CONGESTION SYNDROME

Pelvic congestion syndrome is caused by overdistention of pelvic vasculature and is commonly associated with pelvic, vulvar, and thigh varicosities and psychogenic disorders (depression, anxiety, and post-traumatic stress disorder). Patients present with dull, aching CPP after prolonged standing or nonorgasmic intercourse. Nutcracker syndrome (mesoaortic compression of the left renal vein) should be suspected in women with pelvic congestion symptoms and hematuria. Evaluation for suspected pelvic congestion includes transvaginal ultrasound (TVU) with Doppler flow study and pelvic venography (the gold standard for evaluation of pelvic congestion). First-line treatment includes continuous progestins (eg, medroxyprogesterone acetate, 30 mg orally daily for 6 months); antidepressants (eg, paroxetine [Paxil], 20 mg orally daily), and elastic compression stockings. Second-choice agents include gonadotropin-releasing hormone (GnRH) analogues such as goserelin (Zoladex), 3.6 mg a month subcutaneously for 6 months. Surgical stripping and ligation of the ovarian vein or transcatheter embolization is recommended when pelvic varicosities are found on venogram. Internal or external stenting as well as gonadocaval bypass are effective treatments for nutcracker syndrome.

OVARIAN REMNANT SYNDROME

Ovarian remnant syndrome is a rare condition, which develops when functional ovarian tissue is left after intended bilateral oophorectomy. Clinical presentation includes cyclic or constant CPP and dyspareunia, with or without adnexal mass. Patients deny menopausal symptoms. Follicle-stimulating hormone and luteinizing hormone typically are in premenopausal range. Transvaginal ultrasound or computerized tomographic scanning helps to identify an adnexal mass. Gonadotropin-releasing hormone analogues such as goserelin (Zoladex), 3.6 mg subcutaneously, may be used once to identify functioning ovarian tissue prior to surgery, which is the treatment of choice.

V. **Laboratory Tests** (Tables 51–4 and 51–5).
    A. **Pregnancy test** (urine or serum) must be performed in all patients with APP or CPP who are of reproductive age with an intact uterus.
        1. Most currently available **urine pregnancy tests** can detect human chorionic gonadotropin (hCG) levels of 15–100 U/mL 3–4 days after conception. Dilute urine may

TABLE 51–4. TESTS HELPFUL IN DIAGNOSING COMMON CAUSES OF ACUTE PELVIC PAIN

Suspected Diagnosis	Tests
PID	β-hCG, CBC, cervical sampling for *Neisseria gonorrhoeae* and *Chlamydia trachomatis*, ESR, vaginal wet preparation, endometrial biopsy, TVU, laparoscopy, LFT if perihepatitis
Ectopic pregnancy	Serum β-hCG, CBC, TVU, laparoscopy
Adnexal mass torsion	TVU with Doppler flow study, CT
Appendicitis	CBC, CT
UTI	UA, urine culture

CBC, complete blood count; CT, computerized tomography; ESR, erythrocyte sedimentation rate; hCG, human chorionic gonadotropin; LFT, liver function tests; PID, pelvic inflammatory disease; TVU, transvaginal ultrasound; UA, urinalysis.

decrease sensitivity. Most current urine pregnancy tests are 84–94% sensitive by the first day of the expected period. By 1 week after the first day of the missed period, sensitivity for urinary hCG is 97%.

2. **Quantitative serum β-hCG** is detected at the level of 2–25 mLU at 7 days after conception and doubles every 2 days during the first 4 weeks after implantation. With ectopic pregnancy, quantitative serum β-hCG levels off (plateau) or decreases.

B. **Complete blood cell count.** Fifty-six percent of patients with PID and 36% of patients with acute appendicitis have a normal white blood cell count.

C. **The cervical DNA probe** has a specificity of 99% and a sensitivity of 86% for *Neisseria gonorrhoeae* and a specificity of 98% and a sensitivity of 93% for *C trachomatis*.

D. The sensitivity for adnexal mass detection by **transvaginal pelvic ultrasonography (TVU)** is 60–84%, and specificity is 90–98%. TVU with Doppler flow study adds diagnostic efficiency for endometrioma, pelvic congestion syndrome, and ovarian neoplasm.

E. **Magnetic resonance imaging (MRI)** improves visualization of small cystic lesions, which are undetectable on TVU (eg, endometriomas). The sensitivity and specificity of MRI are 71% and 82%, respectively. The fat suppression technique increases sensitivity and specificity to 90% and 98%, respectively. In women desiring future pregnancy, MRI can differentiate between a single leiomyoma (candidate for uterus-preserving interventions) and adenomyosis (necessitating hysterectomy).

F. The sensitivity of **computerized tomography (CT)** is 92% for diagnosis of peritoneal lesions (eg, endometriosis or ovarian metastasis). MRI and CT are equally accurate, but more sensitive than TVU for staging of ovarian cancer and localization of endometriosis.

TABLE 51–5. USEFUL TESTS FOR EVALUATING COMMON CAUSES OF CHRONIC PELVIC PAIN

Suspected Diagnosis	Tests
Adenomyosis	TVU, MRI
Endometriosis	TVU, MRI, laparoscopy, CA-125
Abdominal wall nerve entrapment	Nerve conduction study
Diverticular disease	Barium enema radiography, CT
Dyspareunia	*Neisseria gonorrhoeae* and *Chlamydia trachomatis* study, vaginal wet preparation, vaginal pH, UA, urine culture
Hernias	Abdominal wall ultrasonography, CT
Urethral syndrome	Urine culture, *Neisseria gonorrhoeae* and *Chlamydia trachomatis* probes, urodynamic study

CT, computerized tomography; MRI, magnetic resonance imaging; TVU, transvaginal ultrasound; UA, urinalysis.

G. **Laparoscopy** is the gold standard for evaluation of CPP. It is reserved for patients with equivocal diagnosis (eg, surgical emergency, tubal pregnancy), those unresponsive to treatment (eg, with PID), or when tissue diagnosis is necessary (eg, in endometriosis). Patients with endometriosis may require therapeutic laparoscopy for electrocoagulation or laser ablation of lesions.

H. **Erythrocyte sedimentation rate** is elevated in 75% of patients with PID.

VI. Treatment

A. APP

1. **Treatment of PID** should provide coverage for likely etiologic agents (*N gonorrhoeae, C trachomatis,* anaerobes, enteric gram-negative rods, *Mycoplasma hominis,* and *Ureaplasma urealyticum*), treatment of underlying disease (acute endometritis, salpingitis, or peritonitis), as well as prevention of complications: tubo-ovarian abscess (15% of cases) Fitz-Hugh-Curtis syndrome/perihepatitis (30% of cases), and septicemia.

   a. **Inpatient treatment** of PID with parenteral antibiotics is recommended for pregnant women, patients with severe illness with fever and vomiting, cases where surgical emergencies (appendicitis, tubo-ovarian abscess) cannot be excluded, or when there is intolerance or poor response to outpatient antimicrobial regimens. Parenteral therapy such as cefotetan (Cefotan), 2 g intravenously every 12 hours, OR cefoxitin (Mefoxin), 2 g intravenously every 6 hours plus doxycycline (Vibramycin), 100 mg orally or intravenously every 12 hours, may be discontinued 24 hours after clinical improvement; oral therapy should continue for 14 days.

   b. **Outpatient treatment** (Table 51–6) may start presumptively while awaiting culture results.

2. **Ectopic pregnancy**

   a. Gynecologic consultation and surgery (laparotomy or laparoscopy) is indicated for ruptured ectopic pregnancy, especially in hemodynamically unstable patients; women unable to comply with monitoring after medical treatment; failure of medical treatment; tubal size >3 cm; serum β-hCG greater than 5000 mIU, or fetal cardiac activity on TVU.

   b. Otherwise, women with ectopic pregnancy are managed either with **methotrexate (Mexate)** or expectantly. Methotrexate is less expensive and effective in 86–94% of patients without indications for surgery.

      (1) The oral outpatient protocol includes methotrexate (1 mg/kg/day) with folic acid (Folvite) (0.1 mg/kg/day) for one to four doses, depending on response to treatment.

      (2) Alternatively, a single intramuscular (IM) dose of methotrexate (50 mg/m^2 body surface area) can be given. Weekly monitoring of serum hCG, complete blood cell count with differential, aspartate aminotransferase, creatinine, blood type, and Rhesus (Rh) is required. A second IM dose of

---

TABLE 51–6. OUTPATIENT THERAPY FOR PELVIC INFLAMMATORY DISEASE

Regimen A
Ofloxacin (Floxin), orally 400 mg twice daily for 14 days,
or
Levofloxacin (Levaquin), 500 mg daily for 14 days **with or without** metronidazole (Flagyl), orally 500 mg twice daily for 14 days

Regimen B
Ceftriaxone (Rocephin), 250 mg IM once
or
Cefoxitin (Mefoxin), 2 g once, plus oral **probenecid** (Benemid), 1 g,
plus
Doxycycline (Vibramycin), 100 mg orally twice daily for 14 days **with or without** oral **metronidazole** (Flagyl), 500 mg twice daily for 14 days

From the Centers for Disease Control and Prevention recommendations, 2002.

methotrexate (50 mg/m^2) is recommended if the hCG titer decreases less than 15% by 4 days after the first injection.

(3) Methotrexate side effects include stomatitis, diarrhea, leukopenia, thrombocytopenia, anemia, nephrotoxicity, hepatic dysfunction, alopecia, and dermatitis; these are mild and reported in 34% of patients.

3. Urgent gynecologic referral is indicated for **adnexal torsion** and **necrosis of pedunculated leiomyoma.** Torsed ovary may be salvaged by detorsion if pedunculated. Myomectomy and hysterectomy are optional treatments for pedunculated leiomyoma.

B. Specific causes of **CPP** should be identified and treated; otherwise, empiric therapy is indicated.

1. Dysmenorrhea (See Chapter 18).

2. **Uterine leiomyoma** should be treated only if symptomatic. Stable leiomyoma can be managed medically with nonsteroidal anti-inflammatory drugs (NSAIDs) such as oral ibuprofen (Motrin), 400 mg every 6 hours. Women unresponsive to medical therapy may require gynecologic referral for surgery (myomectomy or hysterectomy). Preoperative GnRH agonists such as leuprolide (Lupron), 3.75 mg IM monthly, are often given to increase hemoglobin, reduce uterine size, and decrease intraoperative blood loss. Long-term (>6-month) treatment with GnRH agonists is not recommended, because of significant bone loss. Another option for leiomyoma treatment is interventional radiology referral for uterine artery embolization.

3. **Mittelschmerz** usually requires only patient education and reassurance. Oral NSAIDs such as mefenamic acid (Ponstel) may be prescribed for symptoms. OCPs also may be helpful (Chapter 95).

4. Gynecologic referral for surgery may be required for treatment of **adhesions.** Hysterectomy is effective in some cases; however, 40% of women continue to experience CPP after hysterectomy. The success rate for adhesiolysis ranges from 0% to 65%.

5. **Symptomatic therapy**

   a. Pharmacologic methods include:

      (1) Oral NSAIDs (eg, ibuprofen or mefenamic acid).

      (2) Oral opioids and acetaminophen such as hydrocodone with acetaminophen (eg, Vicodin, 7.5/500 mg) every 4–6 hours as needed.

      (3) Antidepressants such as oral paroxetine (eg, Paxil), 20 mg once daily; amitriptyline (Elavil), 25–50 mg at bedtime; or both.

      (4) Continuous oral progestins, such as medroxyprogesterone acetate (eg, Provera), 5 mg daily, have been reported to improve symptoms in 73% of patients (Chapter 95).

      (5) Oral contraceptive pills (OCPs) or Depo-Provera.

      (6) Failure to improve symptoms within 3 months mandates laparoscopic confirmation of clinical diagnosis and trial of GnRH agonists: leuprolide (eg, Lupron), 3.75 mg IM every month, or nafarelin (Synarel), 200 µg intranasally twice daily.

   b. **Nonpharmacologic approaches** include counseling, acupuncture, behavioral and relaxation feedback therapies, and social interventions, as well as neuroablative treatments. Neuroablative therapies employed in consultation with a pain management specialist or surgeon include presacral neurectomy, uterosacral neurotomy, paracervical denervation, uterovaginal ganglion excision, injection of neurotoxic chemicals, laser treatment, cryotherapy, or thermocoagulation.

REFERENCES

Gambone JC, et al: Consensus statement for the management of chronic pelvic pain and endometriosis: Proceedings of an expert-panel consensus process. Fertil Steril 2002;**78**:961.

Howard FM: Chronic pain. Obstet Gynecol 2003;**101**:594.

Lifford KL: Diagnosis and management of chronic pelvic pain. Urol Clin North Am 2002;**29**(3):637.

Ryan KJ: *Kistner's Gynecology & Women's Health,* 7th ed. Mosby; 1999.

Sexually Transmitted Diseases Treatment Guidelines 2002. MMWR Morbid Mortal Wkly Rep 2002; **51**:RR-6.

52   Perianal Complaints

Kalyanakrishnan Ramakrishnan, MD

KEY POINTS

- Although benign anorectal diseases such as hemorrhoids, fissures, pruritus ani, and perianal infections are common, a high index of suspicion for colorectal cancer should be maintained in the presence of perianal complaints, especially in elderly people.
- In young individuals with bleeding-associated defecation and no family history, anoscopy and flexible sigmoidoscopy are sufficient testing. In people older than 50 years, and especially in the presence of fatigue, weight loss, or anemia, double-contrast barium enema or colonoscopy is required.
- Most treatment measures for perianal pathology (banding of hemorrhoids, sphincterotomy for fissures, drainage of perianal and pilonidal infections) can be performed as office procedures under local or no anesthesia.

I. **Definition** (Figure 52–1). The **musculature of the anal canal** consists of the **internal sphincter,** the downward continuation of the involuntary circular smooth muscle of the rectum, and the **external sphincter,** an elliptical cylinder of voluntary skeletal muscle that surrounds the anal canal and runs continuously upward with the **levator ani,** which forms the greater part of the pelvic floor. Sympathetic and parasympathetic nerves, both of which are inhibitory, supply the internal sphincter.

    The anal mucosa is lined by columnar epithelium above the undulating **dentate line** and supplied by sympathetic nerves (L-1–L-3); the squamous epithelium below the dentate line

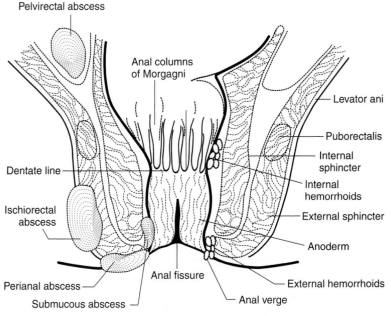

FIGURE 52–1. Anatomy and pathology of the anal canal.

is supplied by somatic nerves. Above the dentate line are longitudinal folds, 6 to 14 in number, the **columns of Morgagni.** The anal glands, 3–10 in number, open directly into an anal crypt at the dentate line.

Perianal complaints include irritation, soreness, or discomfort in the region surrounding the anal canal. Hemorrhoids, fissures, anorectal and pilonidal infections, and pruritus ani are all common causes.

Hemorrhoids are fibrovascular cushions with arteriovenous connections that bulge into the lumen of the anal canal. Their anchoring and supporting connective tissue system deteriorates with aging. Chronic straining secondary to constipation leads to prolapse, thinning, and friability of the overlying mucosa, and results in bright-red rectal bleeding. **Perianal hematoma** is a painful swelling, secondary to thrombosis within a saccule of the hemorrhoidal venous plexus.

Anal fissure is a laceration in the vertical axis of the anal canal due to repeated trauma by hard stool. Internal sphincter spasm impairs healing.

Anorectal abscesses arise from blockage of the anal glands followed by superimposed polymicrobial aerobic and anaerobic infection.

Fistula-in-ano is a tract lined with granulation tissue connecting a primary opening inside the anal canal to a secondary opening in the perianal skin and is most often caused by rupture or drainage of an anorectal abscess.

Pilonidal cysts develop through in-growth of hair or through trauma to the sacrococcygeal region.

The pain of **proctalgia fugax** results from puborectalis muscle spasm. Suggested causes include laxity of the anal sphincter, levator muscle tension resulting in spasm, and increased contractile activity of the sigmoid colon.

Proctitis, which arises from rectal inflammation (within 15 cm of the dentate line), is due to inflammatory bowel disease (IBD), sexually transmitted diseases (STDs)—ie, *Neisseria gonorrhoeae,* syphilis, *Chlamydia trachomatis, Herpes simplex* virus or cytomegalovirus, or from bacterial infections. It may also be due to prior antibiotic use (*Clostridium difficile* proctitis), radiotherapy, or diversion colostomy or ileostomy in patients with an intact rectum. **Pruritus ani** can be caused by benign anorectal diseases causing a discharge, premalignant lesions (Paget's and Bowen's disease), and nonprimary anal diseases (contact dermatitis, fungal infections, diabetes, pinworm infestations, psoriasis, and seborrhea).

II. **Common Diagnoses**

   A. **The incidence of hemorrhoids** is high (about 40%), with equal sexual prevalence, and peak incidence between 45 and 65 years. Symptomatic hemorrhoids are associated with aging, pregnancy, pelvic tumors, prolonged sitting and straining, and chronic diarrhea or constipation.

   B. **Anal fissures** affect both genders equally; risk factors include the passage of hard stool, chronic diarrhea, habitual use of laxatives, anal trauma during intercourse or examination.

   C. **Anorectal infections**

      1. **Anorectal abscess.** The peak incidence is the third to fourth decades. Male-to-female predominance is 2:1 to 3:1. One third of patients report a similar past history. Risk factors include immunosuppression, diabetes mellitus, IBD (predisposes to recurrent/multiple abscesses) and pregnancy.

      2. The incidence of **fistula-in-ano** is 8.6 cases per 100,000, and the mean age of occurrence is 38.3 years. Risk factors include trauma, Crohn's disease, fissures, carcinoma, radiation, actinomycoses, tuberculosis, and chlamydial infections.

      3. Incidence of **pilonidal disease** is approximately 0.7% and the incidence in men is twice that in women. Precipitants include hyperhidrosis associated with sitting and buttock friction, poor personal hygiene, obesity, and local trauma, and buttock hair characteristics such as kinking, coarseness, and rapid growth rate.

   D. **Levator ani syndrome** occurs in 6–7% of the general population, slightly more often in women than in men.

   E. **Proctalgia fugax** occurs in about 13% of adults and is two to three times more common among women. Stress and anxiety are precipitants. Many patients have other functional bowel symptoms.

   F. **Proctitis** occurs predominantly in adults, more in men. Risk factors include high-risk sexual behavior (anal sex, homosexuality, multiple partners), autoimmune disorders, radiation therapy, immunocompromised state, and fecal diversion. Following radiation, 5–20% of patients develop proctitis, within 3–24 months.

G. Idiopathic **pruritus ani** (most common type) is seen more often in men and is typically worse at night. Less common causes include benign anorectal diseases, premalignant lesions, and nonprimary anal diseases.

III. Symptoms. The common symptoms of perianal pathology include pain, bleeding, perianal mass, prolapse, pruritus, and discharge.

A. The most common lesions causing **anorectal pain** are **fissure, abscess, and thrombosed external hemorrhoid.** Anal pain of any etiology may be aggravated by bowel movements.

1. In **anal fissure,** pain occurs during and after defecation and is most acute over the first 2–3 days, resolving over a 7- to 10-day period.
2. A dull ache, or throbbing pain in the perianal area worsened by coughing, sneezing, sitting, and relieved by defecation, suggests an **anorectal abscess.** Pain intensifies as the abscess increases in size and becomes superficial.
3. **Perianal hematoma** (external hemorrhoid) appears as a painful swelling soon after straining. **Strangulation** of internal hemorrhoids also causes severe pain, bleeding, and occasionally signs of systemic illness.
4. **Proctalgia fugax** is characterized by the sudden onset of severe pain in the anus lasting several seconds or minutes, which then disappears completely. About one third of patients suffer attacks following defecation, and some following sexual activity.
5. Tenesmus, an uncomfortable desire to defecate, is associated with inflammatory conditions. Tenesmus with urgency of evacuation suggests **proctitis.**
6. The **levator ani syndrome** is associated with chronic or recurrent episodes of rectal pain or aching lasting 20 minutes or longer occurring for at least 3 months, precipitated by prolonged sitting, or by defecation. Some patients have dyschezia or a sense of incomplete evacuation.

B. Bleeding

1. **Hemorrhoids** and **fissures** cause bright red blood on stool, toilet paper, or the toilet bowl with, or following, bowel movements. Dark or clotted blood mixed with the stool suggests sources proximal to the anus. Hemorrhoids cause painless bleeding; bleeding with painful defecation suggests a fissure.
2. Drainage of blood or pus with associated pruritus and pain suggests a **fistula.**
3. Bleeding with a painful lump not exclusively related to defecation suggests a thrombosed external hemorrhoid; bleeding with tenesmus suggests **proctitis.**

C. Prolapse. Prolapse occurs in second- and third-degree hemorrhoids, usually with a bowel movement, or during walking or heavy lifting, and is associated with an uncomfortable fullness, which resolves on spontaneous or manual reduction.

D. Perianal mass. A painful perianal lump is an abscess, a thrombosed external hemorrhoid, or a strangulated prolapsed internal hemorrhoid. **Pilonodal abscess** presents with a painful swelling overlying the coccyx, purulent drainage, fever, and constitutional symptoms.

E. Discharge. Blood-stained discharge mixed with mucus, pus, or both is a feature of proctitis, thrombosed or prolapsed hemorrhoids, perianal or pilonidal abscess, fistula, or neoplasm.

F. Miscellaneous. Fever and other constitutional symptoms (anorexia, nausea, vomiting, or diarrhea) may accompany strangulated hemorrhoids, perirectal and pilonidal abscesses, inflammatory bowel disease, and proctitis.

IV. Signs

A. Inspection. Skin changes suggestive of psoriasis, seborrhea, ulcerations, or lichenification may indicate the existence of **pruritus ani.** In **pilonodal infections,** a sinus, swelling, and redness overlying the coccyx or purulent drainage may be seen. **Perianal hematoma** presents as a bluish mass at the anal verge and **anorectal abscess,** with localized erythema, purulent drainage, or perianal edema. In **anal fistulas,** external (secondary) openings are seen. Findings in **proctitis** can range from a mild mucoid exudate to marked infection with spontaneous bleeding, purulent discharge, and erosions (in human immunodeficiency virus patients). Papules, vesicles, shallow ulcerations, and crusts around the anal and genital areas may be seen in **herpetic infections.**

B. Palpation (including digital rectal examination)

1. A tender fluctuant mass may be palpated at the anal verge (perianal abscess), sacrum (pilonidal abscess), or through the rectal wall (ischiorectal abscess) (Figure 52–1).

2. Most **fissures** are posterior (Figure 52–1), and can be observed with gentle lateral retraction around the anus or on anoscopy. Anterior fissures have an incidence of 1% in men and 10% in women. **Acute fissures** appear as a fresh laceration, whereas **chronic fissures** have raised edges, exposing the white horizontally oriented fibers of the internal sphincter. The sphincter tone is markedly increased and digital examination or anoscopy reproduces the extreme pain associated with defecation. When fissures are lateral, infections such as syphilis, tuberculosis, occult abscesses, herpes, acquired immunodeficiency syndrome, carcinoma, and IBD should be considered. Secondary changes such as a sentinel pile, induration of the fissure edge, and anal stenosis, due to spasm or a fibrotic internal sphincter, may be seen.

3. Palpable tenderness of overly contracted levator ani muscles may be noticed in the **levator ani syndrome,** as the examining finger moves from the coccyx posteriorly to the pubis anteriorly.

4. Uncomplicated internal hemorrhoids are not palpable.

C. **Anoscopy.** This procedure is performed with the patient in the left lateral position. The instrument is well lubricated to ease insertion. A side-viewing anoscope is inserted with the open portion in the right anterior, then right posterior, and finally the left lateral position to look for hemorrhoidal masses, which will bulge into the anoscope.

1. **Hemorrhoids** are classified as internal, external, or combined intero-external. **External hemorrhoids** originate below the dentate line; **internal hemorrhoids** originate above it (Figure 52–1). Internal hemorrhoids are found in the right anterior, right posterior, and left lateral positions within the anal canal, and graded as first degree—bleeding without prolapse; second degree—prolapse on straining, reducing spontaneously; third degree—prolapse requiring manual reduction; and fourth degree—strangulated, irreducible prolapse.

2. **Fissures** may also be seen, with the characteristics as stated above.

3. Internal openings may be identified in **fistulas.** The **Goodsall rule** states that fistulas with an external opening anterior to a plane passing transversely through the center of the anus will follow a straight radial course to the dentate line. Fistulas with their openings posterior to this line will follow a curved course to the posterior midline.

4. Proctitis due to *C trachomatis* and *N gonorrhoeae* cause erythema, discharge, and swelling in the anal canal.

V. **Laboratory Tests**

A. **Tests for pruritus ani and proctitis**

1. In pruritus ani, skin scrapings (potassium hydroxide preparation) are useful to detect tinea cruris and yeast infections.

2. In proctitis, diagnosis is confirmed in 92% of patients by anoscopic smears and culture for bacterial, fungal, and viral pathogens, Tzanck testing for multinucleate giant cells, and stool testing for *C difficile* toxin. Syphilis can be confirmed by finding spirochetes on dark-field examination of rectal discharge, and *N gonorrhoeae* through appearance of gram-negative diplococci on Gram staining. If warranted, cultures for *C difficile, N gonorrhoeae, C trachomatis,* and *H simplex,* and serologic testing for syphilis (RPR), should be obtained.

B. **Skin biopsy.** Visible abnormalities in the perianal skin may necessitate a skin biopsy (excision or punch biopsy) to rule out Paget's or Bowen's disease.

C. **Endoscopy**

1. Rectal bleeding in people older than 50 years warrants a **colonoscopy** to rule out colorectal neoplasm.

2. Younger individuals with bleeding-associated defecation, and no family history of colon cancer, require only **flexible sigmoidoscopy.**

3. **Flexible sigmoidoscopy or colonoscopy** may be performed to exclude more proximally located inflammatory disorders with which **anal fistulas** or **perianal pruritus** may be associated. Endoscopic biopsy may show crypt abscesses or other features of inflammatory bowel disease.

D. **Miscellaneous**

1. **Endoanal ultrasound** or **magnetic resonance imaging (MRI)** is useful before surgery to determine the existence, extent, and location of **anorectal abscesses.**

2. **Ultrasound, fistulography, computerized tomography (CT), and MRI** may be helpful in identifying an occult cause of **recurrent fistula.**

3. **Electromyography** studies may be used to differentiate the **levator ani syndrome** from pelvic floor dyssynergia, a relaxation abnormality associated with dyschezia and straining.

VI. Treatment

A. **Hemorrhoids** causing minor bleeding can be managed with dietary and lifestyle modifications to minimize constipation and straining (see Chapter 12). More symptomatic hemorrhoids (eg, third- or fourth-degree) are likely to require operative intervention.

1. **Office procedures**

   a. **Rubber band ligation** is indicated in first-, second-, and third-degree hemorrhoids. After rectal examination, the anoscope is inserted and the hemorrhoid to be banded is identified (the largest hemorrhoid is banded first) and grasped with a modified Allis forceps placed through the ligator. In the absence of discomfort, the band is applied by depressing the trigger on the hemorrhoid ligator. Multiple hemorrhoids can be banded at one sitting, or sequentially. A dull persistent ache is common following banding. Significant anal pain due to band placement below or close to the dentate line requires removal and reapplication. An **anoscope/ligator,** attached to wall suction, is an alternative to traditional banding methods. Complications with both methods are rare (5%) and include urinary retention, bleeding, band slippage, pain, ulceration, thrombosis, and perineal sepsis. Bleeds are self-limited and occur immediately after banding, or 7–10 days later. Up to 25% of patients require repeat banding over 5 years.

   b. **Infrared coagulation** is most beneficial in first- and second-degree hemorrhoids. The coagulator is applied through the anoscope for 1.5 seconds, thrice to the apex of each hemorrhoid.

   c. **Sclerotherapy** involves the injection of a sclerosant (sodium morrhuate, 5% phenol, and hypertonic saline) through the anoscope into the submucosa at the apex of the hemorrhoid. This causes ischemia, induces fibrosis, and fixes the hemorrhoid to the rectal wall, decreasing bleeding and prolapse. It is performed as an office procedure and requires no special training or equipment. Misplacement may result in perianal infection, anal ulceration, and fibrosis.

   d. Most patients with **perianal hematoma** respond to conservative measures (sitz baths twice a day, stool softeners, and analgesics). Surgical excision under local anesthesia is an office procedure. It is considered for patients presenting during the first 2–3 days, if ulceration or rupture has occurred, or if medical treatment has failed and symptoms persist. The anoderm overlying the swelling is infiltrated with plain lidocaine and incised with a #15 blade, evacuating the clot. Bleeding is controlled with sutures or packing, and conservative measures are continued.

2. **Hemorrhoidectomy** is reserved for large third- and fourth-degree hemorrhoids. This is usually performed by a surgeon as a day-case under local anesthesia; patients are generally able to return to work within 2 weeks.

B. **Anal fissures**

1. Acute (superficial) fissures can be managed with fiber supplementation, bulk laxatives, sitz baths, and topical corticosteroid or local anesthetic creams (eg, Anusol H, Proctosedyl, or 5% lidocaine ointment applied twice daily).

2. Other successful topical therapies are nifedipine 0.3% with lidocaine ointment 1.5%, every 12 hours for 6 weeks, and diltiazem gel 2%, three times a day for 8 weeks.

3. Botulinum toxin A, a potent inhibitor of acetylcholine release from nerve endings, injected into the anal sphincter as an outpatient procedure, improves healing in chronic fissures.

4. If medical measures fail, a lateral sphincterotomy can be offered as an office procedure performed by a surgeon or a family physician with requisite training.

C. **Anorectal abscess**

1. Outpatient incision and drainage (I&D) under local anesthesia is reasonable in a healthy patient with a localized abscess. The skin over the abscess is cleaned with Betadine and infiltrated with anesthetic, and a #11 blade is used to enter the cavity. The skin edges are debrided and the cavity is syringed with saline or hydrogen peroxide, then packed with iodoform gauze. Conscious sedation is useful in excessive pain or anxiety. Analgesics, sitz baths, and stool softeners are continued. Frequent dressing changes may be necessary, until granulation is well advanced.

Complications of drainage include perianal fistula (most common), sepsis, Fournier's gangrene, and rarely death due to sepsis.

2. Drainage in the operating room is advisable in poorly localized infection, septic patients, and in immunocompromised states such as diabetes.

3. The need for routine use of antibiotics has not been established; intravenous antibiotics may be needed in patients who are immunocompromised, septic, or have heart valve abnormalities or valve replacements or prostheses.

D. Initial management of **perianal fistulas** should be directed at resolving acute infection (including proctitis in IBD). Both outpatient fistulotomy for simple fistulas and more extensive excision in complicated fistulas (postradiation, complicated anatomy) may require a surgical referral.

E. **Pilonidal sinus disease**

1. **Conservative, nonexcisional therapy** (shaving the gluteal cleft, improving perineal hygiene, I&D of localized abscesses) effectively controls pilonidal sinus disease in most patients. This requires minimal equipment and leads to early recovery. Abscesses are drained under lidocaine infiltration anesthesia after skin preparation with Betadine, with a #15 blade. The wound is then syringed and packed as described earlier.

2. **Excisional therapy** should be considered for more extensive or recurrent disease and requires a surgical referral.

F. Treatment options for the **levator ani syndrome** include digital massage of the levator ani muscles three to four times a week, sitz baths at 40 °C, and biofeedback. Recalcitrant cases may benefit from a referral to a gastroenterologist for electrogalvanic stimulation through a rectal probe. Surgical division of the puborectalis muscle is associated with a high rate of fecal incontinence and hence is not recommended.

G. Reassurance of the benign nature of **proctalgia fugax,** warm baths, and massage are often all that is necessary. In severe cases, inhaled albuterol, one or two puffs every 3 hours, or oral diltiazem, 2.5–5 mg every 6 hours as necessary, may help.

H. **Proctitis**

1. In suspected STD, oral doxycycline (100 mg twice daily) or trimethoprim-sulfamethoxazole double strength (160/800 mg twice daily, or ciprofloxacin (500 mg twice daily) for 7 days, is therapeutic.

2. *Clostridium difficile* proctitis is treated with oral metronidazole (250 mg orally four times a day) or vancomycin (250 mg four times a day) for 7–10 days.

3. In radiation proctitis, rectal corticosteroids as foam (hydrocortisone 90 mg) or enema (hydrocortisone 100 mg or methylprednisolone 40 mg) twice daily for 3 weeks, or mesalamine 4 g enema at bedtime or as suppositories 500 mg once or twice a day for 3–6 weeks, are useful. Oral mesalamine (800 mg three times a day) and sulfasalazine (500–1000 mg four times a day) for ~3 weeks alone or in combination with topical therapy may also be effective. Systemic steroids are reserved for patients unresponsive to these forms of therapy.

I. Treatment of **pruritus ani** depends on recognizing the cause, ruling out other potential diagnoses, addressing precipitating or exacerbating conditions, and relieving the itch/scratch cycle.

1. Excessive cleaning, and particularly the use of brushes and caustic soaps, should be avoided.

2. The perianal region should be washed liberally with water to remove any soap after bathing. Following defecation, water-moistened cloths or toilet paper should be used. In between defecation, cotton balls placed next to the anal orifice may help to absorb sweat. Moisture barriers, such as zinc oxide, may ameliorate symptoms.

3. Dietary modifications (restriction of caffeinated or carbonated beverages, dairy products, alcohol, tomato-based food products, cheese, and chocolate) may be useful.

4. A short course of topical steroids (hydrocortisone 1%) may also provide symptom relief, though long-term use should be avoided because of skin atrophy. Anesthetic ointments should also be avoided.

5. *Tinea* and *Candida* respond well to 1% clotrimazole cream applied twice daily for up to 4 weeks.

6. **Pinworms** are treated with one 100-mg dose of mebendazole or a 1-g dose of pyrantel pamoate.

7. **Condyloma acuminata** can be treated effectively with liquid nitrogen or 10% podophyllin. Podofilox applied by the patient every 12 hours for 3 consecutive days is an alternative. Application may be repeated after 4 days.
8. Improvement in symptoms has been noted with the subcutaneous injection of 30 cc of 0.5% of methylene blue.

REFERENCES

Kaiser AM, Ortega AE: Anorectal anatomy. Surg Clin North Am 2002;**82:**1125.
Pfenninger JL, Zainea GG: Common anorectal conditions: Part I. Symptoms and complaints. Am Fam Physician 2001;**63:**2391.
Pfenninger JL, Zainea GG: Common anorectal conditions: Part II. Lesions. Am Fam Physician 2001;**64:**77.
Vincent C: Office management of common anorectal problems. Primary Care Clinics in Office Practice 1999;**26:**52.

---

53 Proteinuria

Aamir Siddiqi, MD

KEY POINTS

- Asymptomatic persistent proteinuria on dipstick test needs further evaluation and possible referral to nephrology.
- Urine dipsticks are usually sensitive only to albuminuria and give false-negative results with other urinary proteins.
- Transient proteinuria is a nonpathologic condition.
- Taking a good medication history is an important step in the work-up of proteinuria.

I. **Definition.** Proteinuria is the presence of urinary protein in concentrations >0.150 g/day in adults and >0.1 mg/m^2/24 hours in children. Protein excretion of >3.5 g/day is defined as a **nephrotic** level of proteinuria. **Microalbuminuria** is defined as excretion of 30–150 mg of protein per day.

II. **Common Diagnoses**
   A. **Transient proteinuria** defined as isolated, self-limited proteinuria is by far the most common, occurring in 4% of males and 7% of females on a single examination. Stressors such as fever and exercise have been considered as potential causes.
   B. **Orthostatic proteinuria** appears when a person is upright and accounts for up to 60% of all proteinuria seen in children and adolescents.
   C. **Persistent proteinuria** occurs in 5–10% of patients with isolated proteinuria. This is commonly associated with underlying extrarenal causes, such as diabetes or hypertension. After the development of proteinuria, as many as 50% of these patients may develop hypertension during the next 5 years, and as many as 20% may develop renal insufficiency during the next 10 years.
   D. **Primary renal diseases,** including acute glomerulonephritis, acute renal failure, acute tubular necrosis, and anomalies such as polycystic kidneys, may cause proteinuria.
   E. **Drugs** and **toxins,** including antibiotics, analgesics, anticonvulsants, antihypertensives, and heavy metals, may lead to proteinuria (Table 53–1).
   F. **Systemic illnesses** (Table 53–2). About one third of type I diabetics and one quarter of type II diabetics develop persistent proteinuria. **Overload proteinuria** occurs in systemic diseases, which cause production of abnormal and excessive low molecular weight proteins, as in multiple myeloma.
   G. **Nephrotic syndrome** is primarily caused by minimal change disease, focal segmental glomerulosclerosis, membranous glomerulonephritis, membranoproliferative glomerulonephritis, and mesangial proliferative glomerulonephritis. The most common cause in children is minimal change disease; membranous glomerulonephritis is the most common

TABLE 53–1. DRUGS AND TOXINS CAUSING PROTEINURIA

Acute interstitial nephritis	**Cyclosporine toxicity**
Cephalosporins	**Heavy metals**
Penicillins	Gold
Sulfonamides	Lead
Aminoglycoside toxicity	Mercury
Analgesic nephropathy	**Heroin**
Nonsteroidal anti-inflammatory drugs	**Lithium**
Anticonvulsants	**Penicillamine**
Phenytoin	
Trimethadione	**Probenecid**
Antihypertensive agents	**Sulfonylureas**
Angiotensin-converting enzyme inhibitors	Tolbutamide

cause in adults. In children, it is most common from age 2 to 6. Males are slightly more likely to be affected than females.

III. **Symptoms.** It is rare to find any symptoms of proteinuria except in patients with the nephrotic syndrome, in whom swelling may be prominent. Characteristic symptoms of primary renal disease or systemic illness may appear in a patient with proteinuria that is caused by the pathologic process of an underlying disease.

A. **Red or cola-colored urine** can be a presenting symptom of acute glomerulonephritis.

B. **Polydipsia or polyuria** can indicate uncontrolled diabetes.

C. **Joint stiffness or pain** may be the presenting complaint of lupus erythematosus.

D. **Fatigue, weakness, anorexia, and malaise** may be associated with chronic renal insufficiency.

E. **Bone pain especially in the back or chest** may be associated with multiple myeloma.

IV. **Signs.** If the patient excretes <2 g of protein daily, signs will usually be absent.

A. **Periorbital edema, peripheral edema, ascites,** or **pleural effusions** may result from a decrease in serum albumin level and plasma oncotic pressure from nephrotic levels of proteinuria.

B. **Elevated blood pressure** may aggravate proteinuria in patients with primary renal disease.

C. A **toxic neuropathy** may indicate heavy metal poisoning.

TABLE 53–2. SYSTEMIC ILLNESSES CAUSING PROTEINURIA

Infections	**Multisystem diseases**
Acute poststreptococcal glomerulonephritis	Amyloidosis
Bacterial	Cryoglobulinemia
Endocarditis	Diabetes mellitus
Syphilis	Goodpasture's syndrome
Tuberculosis	Henoch-Schönlein syndrome
Parasitic	Polyarteritis
Malaria	Pre-eclampsia
Toxoplasmosis	Sarcoidosis
Viral	Systemic lupus erythematosus
Cytomegalovirus	Transplant rejection
Epstein-Barr virus	
Hepatitis B	
Human immunodeficiency virus	
Cancers	
Carcinoma	
Leukemia	
Lymphoma—Hodgkin's disease	
Multiple myeloma	

D. Fever may be present with infection.

E. A **heart murmur** may accompany bacterial endocarditis.

F. Characteristic signs of systemic illness may appear in patients whose proteinuria is caused by such illness.

    1. Adenopathy, organomegaly, and **masses** can occur with cancer.

    2. Malar rash and **joint inflammation** are usually present with lupus erythematosus.

    3. Diabetic retinopathy is strongly associated with proteinuria in diabetics.

V. Laboratory Tests (Figure 53–1).

  A. The **initial screen** for proteinuria is a **dipstick** performed on a random clean-catch urine sample. This is a colorimetric test (quantitative chemical analysis using color) detecting urine protein concentration of >10–30 mg/dL, giving positive results if used in relatively concentrated samples.

    1. False-positive dipstick test results can occur with highly concentrated urine, gross hematuria, contamination with antiseptics, or highly alkaline urine (pH >8.0). Radiographic contrast media, analogues of cephalosporin or penicillin, or metabolites of tolbutamide or sulfonamide can give false-positive tests.

    2. False-negative qualitative test results may occur with dilute urine. Dipstick qualitative urine tests are relatively insensitive to proteins other than albumin and may give a false-negative result for nonalbumin proteins such as Bence Jones proteins.

    3. Sulfosalicylic acid test is a turbidometric test in which one part of supernatant urine is mixed with sulfosalicylic acid. The turbidity is then graded according to a scale. The advantage of this test is detection of proteins besides albumin. This is especially helpful if myeloma kidney is suspected.

    4. A negative qualitative test result on a first-morning specimen (recumbent) followed 2 hours later by a positive test on second sample (upright) indicates orthostatic proteinuria. This can be confirmed by a split urine test in which a 16-hour upright collection is obtained between 7 AM and 11 PM, with the patient performing normal activities and finishing the collection by voiding just before 11 PM. A separate overnight 8-hour collection is obtained between 11 PM and 7 AM. The diagnosis of orthostatic proteinuria is made if urinary protein excretion is normal in the supine collection (<50 mg/8 hours).

  B. A **24-hour urine test** for protein and creatinine levels will verify a repeated positive qualitative test result.

    1. Urinary creatinine validates an adequate urinary collection; normal creatinine range is 16–26 mg/kg body weight per day for males and 12–24 mg/kg body weight per day for females. A 24-hour urine creatinine allows calculation of creatinine clearance, which is a good measure of renal function. An alternative to measuring 24-hour urine protein is to measure spot urinary protein to creatinine ratio. In a healthy person the ratio seldom exceeds 0.1 (100 mg protein per gram creatinine).

    2. A normal 24-hour **urinary protein** level indicates a false-positive qualitative test result or transient proteinuria.

  C. Urinalysis of a clean-catch midstream specimen is needed to diagnose primary renal disease.

    1. Positive urine culture indicates infection.

    2. Red blood cell casts indicate glomerulonephritis.

    3. White blood cell casts indicate an inflammatory process such as pyelonephritis or interstitial nephritis.

  D. Blood tests should be performed when systemic disease is suspected.

    1. Serum creatinine and **blood urea nitrogen (BUN)** levels should be determined in order to evaluate renal function. Creatinine clearance is more accurate, especially in elderly patients with decreased muscle mass.

    2. Blood glucose or a **glycolysated hemoglobin test** is helpful in the detection of diabetes mellitus. Risk factors for these patients include symptoms of polydipsia, polyuria, and a strong family history of diabetes.

    3. Protein electrophoresis or **immunoelectrophoresis** of urine and serum may assist in the diagnosis of multiple myeloma or other monoclonal gammopathies. These patients are usually elderly and may complain of bone pain and fatigue.

    4. Complement studies may be helpful in the diagnosis of immune complex diseases. These include autoimmune diseases such as rheumatoid arthritis, systemic lupus erythematosus, and dermatomyositis.

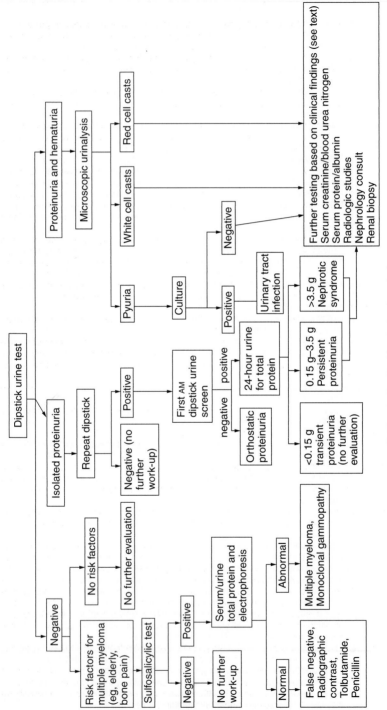

FIGURE 53–1. Algorithm for evaluation of proteinuria.

5. **Antistreptococcal enzyme titers** can help the physician diagnose poststreptococcal glomerulonephritis. This is most common in children younger than age 7
   and may be preceded by a skin infection or pharyngitis.
6. **Fluorescent antinuclear antibody tests** may indicate the presence of systemic
   lupus erythematosus. Patients usually have arthritis and fatigue and may present
   with the classic malar rash.
7. **Serum albumin levels** will be decreased in patients with nephrotic syndrome.
   These patients usually have significant facial and pedal edema and may have
   hypertension.
8. **Complete blood cell count** will help in determining infection or the anemia of renal
   insufficiency. Systemic infections will cause an elevation of the white cell count.
   Anemia, if present, is usually characterized by normocytic and normochromic red
   blood cells.

E. **Radiographic evaluation** may detect congenital, obstructive, or malignant disease.
   This should be considered in patients complaining of abdominal pain and hematuria.
   1. **Intravenous pyelography** or **computerized tomographic scans** of the kidney
      can show structural or obstructive pathology. Caution should be observed using
      contrast media in patients with diabetes, renal insufficiency, or multiple myeloma
      because of the risk of renal failure.
   2. **Renal ultrasonography** can be of value in determining renal size, obstruction, and
      congenital cysts. This should be considered if abdominal examination reveals a mass.
   3. **Voiding cystourethrogram** is useful in documenting reflux. This is usually per-
      formed in children who may present with recurrent urinary tract infections.

F. **Renal biopsy** is reserved for diagnosing and differentiating the glomerulonephropathies
   and is also performed on most patients with nephrotic-range proteinuria.

VI. **Treatment** of proteinuria is directed at the underlying cause.

   A. **Transient proteinuria** requires no further evaluation or follow-up, as no harmful seque-
      lae have been documented.
   B. **Orthostatic proteinuria** is mostly a benign condition. Patients with this problem have
      a 50% chance of remission over 10 years. Follow-up of this problem should occur every
      1–2 years, if proteinuria persists, and should involve a blood pressure check as well as
      urinalysis.
   C. **Removal of toxins or medications** (Table 53–1) can reverse or at least prevent pro-
      gression of proteinuria.
   D. **Appropriate antibiotics** can resolve proteinuria associated with urinary tract infections
      (see Chapter 21).
   E. **Primary renal disease**
      1. **Supportive therapy,** including **sodium** and **fluid restriction** (2 g/day, 1 L/day, re-
         spectively) may help relieve fluid retention.
      2. **Loop diuretics** such as **furosemide,** 20–400 mg/day, can be used to treat circu-
         latory congestion, edema, and hypertension. These agents have not been shown
         to alter the course of acute renal failure or to improve the patient's chance of sur-
         vival, however.
      3. **Dietary protein restriction** may prevent progression of renal disease and usually
         comprises 20–40 g (0.5 g/kg) of protein per day, with 100 g of carbohydrate per
         day if azotemia is present.
      4. **Corticosteroids** such as **prednisone,** 1–1.5 mg/kg/day, and cytotoxic drugs such
         as **cyclophosphamide,** 1–2 mg/kg/day, may be of benefit to patients with certain
         types of nephrotic syndrome and primary glomerulonephritis. These should be pre-
         scribed in consultation with nephrology.
      5. **Renal dialysis** is indicated for patients with progressive renal failure and should be
         initiated when any of the following conditions exist: volume overload refractory to di-
         uretics, pericarditis, or uremia (BUN >80–100 mg/dL or creatinine >8–10 mg/dL).
      6. **Renal transplantation** should be considered when a poor quality of life or health
         exists despite dialysis with end-stage renal disease.
   F. **Specific treatment of underlying systemic illness** (Table 53–2, Chapters 74, 76, and
      84) may resolve or improve proteinuria.
      1. **Persistent proteinuria** is associated with a high mortality and risk of death from
         renal disease. Patients with persistent proteinuria from any cause should be re-
         ferred to nephrology. This should be followed up every 6 months to 1 year with uri-
         nalysis, blood pressure, and renal function studies.

2. **Antihypertensive therapy** in a patient with nephropathy characterized by proteinuria can delay progression of renal failure.
3. **Corticosteroids** and cytotoxic drugs may improve proteinuria from lupus nephritis.

REFERENCES

Burton C, Harris KP: The role of proteinuria in the progression of chronic renal failure. Am J Kidney Dis 1996;**27**:765.

Hogg RJ, et al: National Kidney Foundation's Kidney Disease Outcomes Quality Initiative clinical practice guidelines for chronic kidney disease in children and adolescents: Evaluation, classification, and stratification. Pediatrics 2003;**111**:1416.

House AA, Cattran DC: Nephrology: 2. Evaluation of asymptomatic hematuria and proteinuria in adult primary care. CMAJ Canadian Medical Association Journal 2002;**166**:348.

Mahan JD, Truman MA, Mentser MI: Evaluation of hematuria, proteinuria, and hypertension in adolescents. Pediatr Clin North Am 1997;**44**:1573.

Roth KS, Amaker BH, Chan JC: Nephrotic syndrome: Pathogenesis and management. Pediatr Rev 2002;**23**:237.

Wingo CS, Clapp WL: Proteinuria: Potential causes and approach to evaluation. Am J Med Sci 2000; **320**:188.

---

54   The Red Eye

Victor Alejandro Diaz, Jr., MD, & Deborah K. Witt, MD

KEY POINTS

- Red eye is the most common ocular problem encountered in ambulatory primary care settings.
- Symptoms suggestive of a medical emergency include eye pain, persistent blurred vision, photophobia, symptoms >1 week in duration, and proptosis.
- Topical corticosteroids or corticosteroid-antibiotic combinations are contraindicated when treating the red eye.

I. **Definition.** An appreciation of normal eye anatomy is the foundation for understanding the differential diagnosis of red eye (Figure 54–1). The arterial blood supply of orbital structures originates from the ophthalmic artery, which supplies the glands, upper eyelids, ciliary structures, and musculature. The eyelids contain eyelashes and meibomian glands, which secrete a sebaceous substance that prevents the upper and lower lids from adhering to one another.

"Red eye" describes a group of distinct inflammatory or infectious diseases involving one or more ocular structures, that is, **conjunctiva** (viral/bacterial/chlamydial/allergic conjunctivitis, pterygium, pingueculum), **cornea** (abrasion, keratitis), **sclera/episclera** (scleritis, episcleritis), **lids** (blepharitis), **uveal tract** (iritis, uveitis), and **anterior chamber** (acute angle-closure glaucoma).

II. **Common Diagnoses.** The most likely source of red eye is the anterior segment, which consists of conjunctiva, cornea, anterior chamber, and iris (Figure 54–1). Conjunctivitis is the most common eye disease worldwide.

   A. **Conjunctivitis** can be due to the following causes:
      1. **Infectious**
         a. **Viral**
            (1) **Adenovirus.** Approximately 85% of viral conjunctivitis is caused by *Adenovirus,* which is highly contagious.
            (2) **Herpes** is the least common cause of viral conjunctivitis and can be due to *Herpes simplex* virus type 1 or type 2. It is usually a disease of young children in the setting of primary infection or during recurrent episodes.
         b. **Bacterial.** Only 15% of conjunctivitis is bacterial.

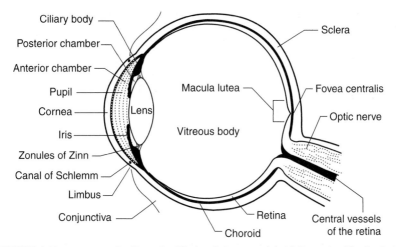

FIGURE 54–1. The eye—cross section. The zonules of Zinn keep the lens suspended, while the muscles of the ciliary body focus the lens. The ciliary body also secretes aqueous humor, which fills the posterior chamber, passes through the pupil into the anterior chamber, and drains primarily via the canal of Schlemm. The iris regulates the light entering the eye by adjusting the size of its central opening, the pupil. The visual image is focused on the retina, the fovea centralis being the area of sharpest visual acuity. The conjunctiva ends abruptly at the limbus. The cornea is covered with an epithelium that differs in many respects from the conjunctival epithelium. (From Beers MH, Berkow R (editors): *The Merck Manual of Diagnosis and Therapy*, 17th ed. Merck & Co.; 1999:701. Copyright 1999 by Merck & Co., Inc., Whitehouse Station, NJ.)

    c. *Chlamydia trachomatis* is the leading cause of preventable blindness worldwide and is a major public health concern in rural and developing countries. Inclusion conjunctivitis is usually bilateral and spread by direct contact with family members. Spread is often associated with epidemics of bacterial conjunctivitis. **Inclusion conjunctivitis of the newborn,** due to exposure during vaginal delivery from an infected mother, is the most common cause of conjunctivitis in neonates.
    2. Noninfectious or **allergic** conjunctivitis occurs in individuals with seasonal, environmental (eg, dust pollen, animal dander) or chemical (eg, drugs, chemicals, or cosmetics) sensitivities.
  B. Corneal abrasion, loss of a portion of superficial epithelium, occurs most commonly in individuals who frequently participate in outdoor activities or certain occupations (eg, tree trimmers, metal shop workers).
  C. Blepharitis is a common inflammatory lesion affecting eyelid margins.
  D. Subconjunctival hemorrhage, spontaneous rupture of small conjunctival vessels, usually results from sudden increase in intrathoracic pressure (eg, sneezing, coughing, defecating) especially in the elderly, but is also seen with minor trauma, hypertension, and blood dyscrasias and is common in neonates following vaginal delivery.
  E. Acute angle-closure glaucoma, a rare ophthalmic emergency associated with suddenly elevated intraocular pressure (IOP), comprises 10–15% of glaucoma cases in whites and about 5–10 % of all glaucoma cases.
III. Symptoms and Signs (Table 54–1). In ambulatory primary care, patients commonly present with the complaint of "pink eye" or "red eye."
  A. Viral conjunctivitis has an incubation period of 7–10 days and can remain contagious for up to 4–6 weeks on fomites. Viral conjunctivitis is usually mildly symptomatic, resolves in 10–14 days, and is distinguished from bacterial infection by presence of a palpable preauricular lymph node.
  B. Epidemic keratoconjunctivitis (EKC) is inflammation of the cornea, which produces significant pain, photophobia, and blurred vision. EKC may be difficult to differentiate from other viral forms because it also is associated with preauricular lymphadenopathy, subconjunctival hemorrhage, and purulent discharge.

TABLE 54–1. DIFFERENTIAL DIAGNOSIS OF COMMON CAUSES OF RED EYE

Condition	Risk Factors	Symptoms	Signs	Testing
Viral conjunctivitis	Highly contagious, epidemic, person-to-person (eg, day care, school, swimming pool, medical instruments). HSV—neonates with primary or recurrent herpes infection.	Mildly symptomatic: URI/sore throat/ itching or FB sensation HSV—photophobia, pain	Unilateral or bilateral, injected sclera, watery discharge, fever; **palpable preauricular lymph node.** HSV—grouped pinpoint vesicles on eyelids.	None usually indicated. Conjunctival scrapings: predominant **lymphocytes and monocytes.** HSV—corneal dendrites with fluorescein staining.
Bacterial conjunctivitis	*Neisseria gonorrhoeae*—neonates via infected birth canal and sexually active patients *Staphylococcus aureus*—Adults *Streptococcus pneumoniae/ Haemophilus influenzae*—children	Pain and photophobia Gritty sensation	Beefy red conjunctivae; matted lids; constant, copious purulent discharge	None usually indicated. Conjunctival scrapings: predominant **poly-morphonuclear (PMN) leukocytes.** Gram stain/culture if severe and persistent, but not always reliable.
Chlamydial conjunctivitis	Spread by direct contact from other family members. Newborn—via infected birth canal.	Tearing/photophobia/pain/burning Neonate—onset first 10 days of life	Mucopurulent discharge, redness. Herbert's pits Neonate—also with tearing and swollen eyelids	DNA amplification testing if needed. Conjunctival scrapings: predominant mixed PMN, lymphocytes; **intracyto-plasmic inclusion bodies** in epithelial cells.
Noninfectious conjunctivitis	Seasonal allergies. Exposure to chemicals, cosmetics, dust, animal dander, etc.	Itchy/burning/watery discharge; associ-ated allergic rhinitis symptoms	Conjunctival injection with swelling; may have a cobblestone appearance.	None usually needed. Conjunctival scrapings: predominant **eosinophils.**
Corneal abrasion	Frequent outdoor activities. Occupational risks (eg, wood and metal workers)	Acute discomfort/tearing/blurred vision/ FB sensation	Lacrimation	Ulcerations with fluorescein staining. Topical anesthetic (tetracaine 0.5%) may facilitate examination.

Blepharitis	Patients with seborrheic dermatitis	Bilateral lids Chronic itching/scaling/burning Foreign body sensation	Ulcerative eyelash folliculitis; scaling/crusting lids. Associated scalp eyebrow/ ear seborrhea Meibomian glands involved	Culture if ulcerative lesion (commonly *S aureus*).
Subconjunctival hemorrhage	Elderly; trauma, HTN, blood dyscrasia. Neonate—vaginal delivery.	Painless/unilateral	Localized, sharply circumscribed hemorrhage.	Coagulation profile, CBC and platelets, protein C and S levels if recurrent or other abnormal bleeding
Inflamed pingueculum	Sun/wind exposure (farmers, lifeguards, fishermen, welders)	Mild ocular discomfort	Hyperemic, yellowish, conjunctival nodules at 3 and 9 o'clock on bulbar conjunctiva.	No testing indicated
Pterygium	Heat/dust/wind exposure (farmers, fishermen, equatorial environment).	Usually painless, normal or blurred vision	Triangular, yellowish, fleshy, injected bulbar conjunctival lesion; extension from canthus with possible corneal encroachment	No testing indicated
Acute angle closure glaucoma	Middle age/older, especially Asians, Eskimos; hyperopia; + FHx; small anterior chambers or altered iris structure; mydriatic use or eye surgery.	Acute photophobia, periocular pain, unilateral; "haloes" around light, N/V, headache; often spontaneous onset in dark environment (eg, theater); rapidly progressive loss of vision	Decreased VA Ciliary flush, hazy cornea Dilated pupil, poor light reaction	Preferably and more accurately tested with applanation tonometry, slit-lamp and gonioscopy elevated IOP: 50–100 mm Hg. (normal IOP: 10–20 mm Hg)

CBC, complete blood count; DNA, deoxyribonucleic acid; FB, foreign body; FHx, family history; HSV, herpes simples virus; HTN, hypertension; IOP, intraocular pressure; N/V, nausea/vomiting; URI, upper respiratory infection; VA, visual activity.

SCLERITIS AND EPISCLERITIS

Scleritis and **episcleritis** are uncommon conditions, which may occur in association with autoimmune or inflammatory conditions (eg, rheumatoid arthritis, Wegener's granulomatosis, lupus, polyarteritis nodosa, or herpes zoster). In episcleritis and scleritis, the palpebral conjunctiva is spared, thus distinguishing it from conjunctivitis. Episcleritis more commonly affects young adults, whereas scleritis tends to affect women in the fourth to sixth decades. Both **scleritis** and **episcleritis** present with eye pain; the pain is more severe in scleritis. In addition, patients with **simple episcleritis** have photophobia and focal bright red conjunctival injection, whereas **nodular episcleritis** presents as a hyperemic papule. **Scleritis** pain is deep and boring and often interrupts sleep; erythema and decreased visual acuity may be sudden or gradual, unilateral or bilateral. A bluish hue indicates scleral thinning.

Application of phenylephrine 2.5% eye drops causes vascular blanching in episcleritis, but not in scleritis. Testing for suspected underlying diseases may include complete blood cell count, erythrocyte sedimentation rate, uric acid, rapid plasma reagent, fluorescent treponemal antibody-absorption, rheumatoid factor, antinuclear antibody, fasting blood glucose, angiotensin converting-enzyme, anti-neutrophil cytoplasmic antibodies (ANCA), and CH 50 and C3 and C4 complement levels. Other tests to consider, if suspicious, include purified protein derivative of tuberculin (PPD) with anergy panel and x-rays of the chest and sacroiliac joints. Mild and nonrecurrent episcleritis may be treated symptomatically with artificial tears, with resolution expected over 1–2 weeks; moderate cases can be managed with a trial of oral nonsteroidal drugs (eg, naproxen, 250–500 mg twice daily) or ophthalmic steroids (eg, prednisolone acetate, 0.12% susp., 2 gtt every hour for 24–48 hours, then 1–2 gtt twice to four times daily until resolved). Recurrent and more severe episcleritis and all scleritis should be managed by an ophthalmologist.

KERATITIS

Keratitis is superficial or interstitial (deeper layers) corneal inflammation due to infection, trauma, decreased tearing, topical medications, ultraviolet exposure, contact lens use, eyelid disorders, or immunosuppression. Interstitial keratitis may also be associated with congenital syphilis or Cogan syndrome (interstitial keratitis, tinnitus, vertigo, and deafness). Keratitis presents with blurred vision, photophobia, periocular pain, gritty foreign body sensation, and ciliary flush (circumcorneal conjunctival injection), sometimes associated with corneal opacification or fragmented corneal light reflection.

Fluorescein staining often reveals multiple punctate corneal lesions; definitive diagnosis requires ophthalmologic referral for slit-lamp examination and appropriate corneal testing (culture, scraping, or biopsy). Other testing (eg, serologic testing for syphilis, PPD, ESR, rheumatoid factor, antinuclear antibodies, chest radiographs) may also be indicated.

ACUTE ANTERIOR UVEITIS

Acute anterior uveitis (iritis, iridocyclitis is an uncommon condition affecting young or middle-aged persons either idiopathically or via autoimmune reaction in conjunction with ankylosing spondylitis (up to 50% of patients), juvenile rheumatoid arthritis (up to 20% of patients), Reiter's syndrome, or sarcoid, herpes simplex or zoster, or Behçet's disease. **Anterior uveitis** presents with periocular achy pain, photophobia, normal or blurred vision, tearing, violaceous ciliary flush, and possibly a constricted, irregular pupil that reacts more slowly to light than the unaffected eye. Occasionally a white or yellow-white purulent anterior chamber layer (a **hypopion**) may be noted.

Ophthalmologic referral for further evaluation and management of suspected acute anterior uveitis is indicated; if serologic testing indicates underlying autoimmune disease, rheumatology consultation is also indicated.

CILIARY FLUSH

Ciliary flush is a term used to describe the concentrated injection of the circumcorneal (limbal) conjunctiva that is characteristic of several red eye conditions such as keratitis, acute angle-closure glaucoma, and acute anterior uveitis.

IV. **Laboratory Tests** (Table 54–1). **Conjunctivitis** is generally a self-limited condition that does not require special testing.

APPLANATION TONOMETRY

Applanation tonometry is preferred over Schiøtz tonometry in the diagnosis of glaucoma, but requires more training. A Schiøtz is portable and easy to learn and use, but requires thorough cleaning between uses. A shallow anterior chamber in a red eye suggests acute angle-closure glaucoma.

V. **Treatment**
   A. **Conjunctivitis**
      1. **Viral conjunctivitis** is treated with supportive measures including cold compresses and lubricating drops (eg, artificial tears 1–2 gtts as needed). Preventive measures include frequent handwashing, especially in environments (medical offices, daycare centers) where transmission risk is high. Due to serious ocular side effects (increased duration of viral shedding, risk of corneal ulcerations and perforation), topical corticosteroids are contraindicated in conjunctivitis (see the sidebar).
      2. **Herpes conjunctivitis** can be indistinguishable from adenovirus, which is an important reason to avoid topical steroid use. Herpes conjunctivitis can be treated with trifluridine, 1% ophthalmic solution (1 gtt every 2 hours while awake until re-epithelialization takes place in 7–14 days, then reduce frequency for 7 more days) or vidarabine, 3% ophthalmic ointment ($\frac{1}{2}$ inch in the lower conjunctival sac five times daily every 3 hours until re-epithelialization occurs in 7–21 days, then reduce to twice daily for 7 more days).

TOPICAL CORTICOSTEROIDS AND CONJUNCTIVITIS

Due to serious ocular side effects, topical corticosteroids are contraindicated in treatment of conjunctivitis. Studies document increased duration of viral shedding, prolongation of infectious period, possible corneal ulcerations, and perforations.

      3. **Bacterial conjunctivitis** is usually self-limited, resolving within 7–10 days.
         a. **Broad-spectrum topical antibiotics** can be used for severe, profusely exudative infections. Eye drops are preferred for all patients except infants and young children, for whom ointment is preferable. Examples include bacitracin-polymyxin B (Polysporin oph oint, $\frac{1}{2}$ inch every 3–4 hours for 7–10 days), trimethoprim (Polytrim oph soln, 1 gt every 3 hours for 7–10 days), aminoglycosides (gentamicin or tobramycin, 0.3%, 2 gtt or $\frac{1}{2}$ inch ointment every 1 hour for 24–72 hours around the clock, then a slow reduction to three to four times daily as condition improves), or quinolones (ciprofloxacin or ofloxacin, 0.3%, 1–2 gtt every 2–4 hours for 2 days, then four times daily for 5 more days).
         b. **Ophthalmologic referral** is indicated for persistent symptoms beyond 10 days.
         c. *N gonorrhoeal infection* is a medical emergency requiring ophthalmologic referral. If untreated it can lead to corneal ulceration or perforation within 24 hours.
      4. **Chlamydial conjunctivitis is treated with** oral erythromycin, 250 mg four times daily, or doxycycline, 100 mg twice daily for 14–21 days. Sexual partners must also be treated.

5. **Allergic conjunctivitis.** Avoidance of offending allergens, application of artificial tears (1–2 gtt as needed), or administration of a topical vasoconstrictor (naphazoline, 0.025%, 1–2 gtt four times daily), topical antihistamines (olopatadine HCl, 0.1%, 1 gtt twice daily at 6- to 8-hour intervals), or topical mast cell stabilizer (cromolyn sodium, 4%, 1–2 gtt four to six times daily) can provide symptomatic relief.

B. **Corneal abrasion.** Primary treatment goals are to restore patient comfort, assist in rapid healing, and prevent secondary infections. The corneal epithelium regenerates rapidly, and healing is usually complete within 24–48 hours. Although soft pressure patches are often used, they are usually not necessary. Contact lens wearers should not receive eye patches at all as this can promote serious corneal/conjunctival infections (eg, *Pseudomonas*).

   1. **Topical cycloplegic drops** (atropine ophthalmic soln. 1%, 1–2 gtt each eye once) relieve the pain caused by reflex ciliary body muscle spasm. A cycloplegic (eg, atropine) is a mydriatic medication that is used in both the diagnosis and treatment of certain ocular conditions by dilating the pupil and paralyzing the muscles of accommodation.

   2. **Oral analgesics with codeine** (Tylenol #3, 1–2 tablets every 3–4 hours as needed for pain) may occasionally be prescribed.

   3. A **topical ophthalmic antibiotic** (see section V,A,3,a) can also be applied. Under no condition should topical anesthetic solutions be prescribed to the patient for pain relief because of their toxic effects on the corneal epithelium.

C. **Blepharitis.** Washing with baby shampoo once daily is an effective way of treating the seborrheic form. An antistaphylococcal antibiotic or topical sulfacetamide, 10% (Bleph-10 ointment, ½ inch every 3–4 hours and at bedtime for 7–10 days) can be used in the ulcerative form. Most cases are chronic and require long-term therapy. Posterior (meibomian gland) blepharitis may require long-term, low-dose, systemic antibiotics (tetracycline, 250 mg twice daily, or erythromycin, 250 three times daily) and short-term, low-potency, topical steroids (prednisolone, 0.125% twice daily).

D. **Subconjunctival hemorrhage.** No treatment is usually required, as hemorrhage spontaneously clears in 2–3 weeks. If episodes are recurrent, underlying high blood pressure or bleeding disorder should be treated and elective aspirin or nonsteroidal anti-inflammatory drug use discontinued. Artificial teardrops (1–2 gtt as needed) may help for mild irritation. If diagnosis is in doubt or some other abnormality becomes evident on examination, referral to an ophthalmologist is appropriate.

E. **Inflamed pingueculum.** Topical vasoconstrictors (naphazoline, 0.025%, 1–2 gtt four times daily) work well. Nonurgent referrals to ophthalmology are appropriate for lesions unresponsive in 1 week. Surgical removal is not necessary. Topical vasoconstrictors are to be used with caution, especially if redness is not relieved promptly or if other significant problems occur.

F. **Pterygia** require nonurgent referral to an ophthalmologist for possible surgical excision if the cornea is involved. No medical treatment is necessary for a long-standing, unchanging, asymptomatic growth. Protective sunglasses are recommended for at-risk individuals to prevent recurrences.

G. **Acute angle-closure glaucoma** is an ophthalmic emergency requiring referral for urgent lowering of IOP to preserve vision.

   1. Since intraocular beta blockers, osmotic agents, cholinergics, and carbonic anhydrase inhibitors can impact fluid/electrolyte status, it is important to inform consultants of underlying cardiovascular disease or medications potentially adversely interacting with ophthalmologic drugs.

   2. Since glaucoma is inherited, patients with the disease should alert first-degree relatives, who may require screening.

REFERENCES

Kanski JJ: *Clinical Ophthalmology,* 4th ed. Butterworth-Heinemann; 1999:151–268.
Leibowitz HM: Primary care: The red eye. N Engl J Med 2000;**343**(5):345–351.
Patel SJ, Lundy DC: Ocular manifestations of autoimmune disease. Am Fam Physician 2002;**66**:991.
Rhee DJ, Pyfer MF: *The Wills Eye Manual: Office and Emergency Room Diagnosis and Treatment of Eye Disease,* 3rd ed. Lippincott Williams & Wilkins; 1999.
Trobe JD: *Physician's Guide to Eye Care,* 2nd ed. American Academy of Ophthalmology; 2000.
Vaughan DG, Asbury T, Riordan-Eva P: *General Ophthalmology,* 15th ed. Appleton & Lange; 1999.

55   Rhinitis & Sinus Pain

Vanessa A. Diaz, MD, MS, Arch G. Mainous III, PhD, & Pieter J. de Wet, MD

KEY POINTS

- Allergic rhinitis is a common condition that can be managed in the primary care setting with medications and lifestyle interventions.
- Acute sinusitis should be diagnosed using specific criteria in order to decrease overdiagnosis and inappropriate use of antibiotics.
- Most patients with acute sinusitis or rhinitis do not benefit from laboratory tests or imaging studies.

I. **Definition. Rhinitis** is an inflammation of the nasal mucous membrane frequently resulting in edema of the mucous membranes, vasodilatation, and rhinorrhea. Common causes include **viruses** and other **infectious agents; type I hypersensitivity reactions** to antigens such as pollens, molds, and animal danders; **autonomic hyperresponsiveness; rebound congestion** from intranasal or certain systemic medications; or **atrophy** of the nasal mucosa.

Five main groups of paranasal sinuses drain into the nasal cavity: the maxillary, frontal, anterior ethmoid, posterior ethmoid, and sphenoid. The maxillary and ethmoid sinuses are present at birth, whereas the sphenoid sinuses develop by age 3 and the frontal sinuses appear by age 5. Maxillary sinuses are noted radiographically by age 4, sphenoid sinuses by age 6, and frontal sinuses by age 7. However, the sinuses are often asymmetrical and may not be fully developed in as many as 5% of adults.

Sinusitis is an inflammatory process in one or more of the paranasal sinuses, associated with obstruction of the sinus ostea. It is usually due to **infection.** Viral infections are the most common cause, bacterial infections are usually due to *Staphylococcus pneumoniae* or *Haemophilus influenzae,* and fungal infections are rarely seen except in poorly controlled diabetic patients or the immunocompromised. Infection of the sphenoid sinus can lead to serious complications due to its proximity to the apex of the orbital cavity, optic nerve, hypophysis, and cavernous sinus. Other factors predisposing to sinusitis include **allergies; anatomic abnormalities** (eg, nasal polyps, septal deviation, foreign bodies, or adenoidal hypertrophy); **irritants** (eg, tobacco, smog, chemicals); **low humidity;** and **systemic diseases** such as cystic fibrosis (abnormally thick mucus), Kartagener's syndrome (immobile cilia within the respiratory tract), and congenital or acquired immunodeficiency syndrome.

II. **Common Diagnoses**
   A. **Common cold or viral upper respiratory infection.** There are nearly 62 million cases annually, resulting in 22 million school days lost. Common colds peak in the winter and occur more commonly in families with children aged 2–7 years. The average preschool child has six to 10 colds per year; the average adult, two to four. Hand-to-hand contact as well as contact with wet fomites are risk factors for spread of the virus.
   B. **Allergic rhinitis** is the most common cause of chronic rhinitis. Twenty to 40 million Americans are affected and 9 million visits to office-based physicians each year are attributed to allergic rhinitis. The peak incidence occurs in the late teenage years, with another peak between the ages of 30 and 40. It is more common in those with a family history of allergies and is often associated with atopy. It may be seasonal or perennial, depending on the types of allergens involved. The seasonal allergens are mostly encountered outdoors and include pollens and, less commonly, mold spores. The perennial allergens are more likely to be encountered indoors and include dust mites, many mold spores, cockroach feces, and animal dander.
   C. **Vasomotor rhinitis** occurs most commonly in the third to fifth decades but is occasionally seen in childhood and adolescence. Vasomotor rhinitis of pregnancy occurs most frequently from the second trimester on and resolves spontaneously by the fifth postpartum day.

D. **Atrophic rhinitis** occurs mainly in elderly adults. Risk factors for its development include chronic granulomatous nasal infections, chronic sinusitis, irradiation, trauma, or radical nasal surgery.

E. **Rhinitis medicamentosum** usually affects young to middle-aged adults, although cases have been reported in children as young as 4 years. Abusers of topical nasal decongestants are at risk, and rebound congestion may occur after decongestant use more frequently than every 3 hours or for longer than 3 weeks. In some individuals, a form of rhinitis medicamentosum occurs with the use of certain antihypertensive agents (eg, beta blockers, guanethidine, methyldopa, or reserpine); aspirin; and oral contraceptives.

F. **Sinusitis** is commonly overdiagnosed and is often confused with other conditions, such as the common cold and allergic rhinitis, so its overall incidence is unclear. Approximately 32 million adults are told by a physician that they have sinusitis annually. Chronic sinusitis leads to 11.6 million office-based doctor visits annually. The incidence peaks in winter, when viral upper respiratory infections are common.

G. **Conditions that can mimic sinus pain** include migraine headaches and temporal arteritis (see Chapter 34), periapical dental abscesses of the maxillary teeth, and nasal polyps. **Other causes** of rhinitis not discussed in this chapter include pregnancy (see Chapter 97), endocrine disorders including hypothyroidism (see Chapter 87), nonallergic rhinitis with eosinophilia (NARES), nasal foreign bodies, cocaine snorting, nasal neoplasms, and menstruation-induced rhinitis.

III. **Symptoms** (Table 55–1).

A. Intense, unrelenting **nasal congestion** occurs in patients with rhinitis medicamentosum, usually without significant rhinorrhea.

B. **Postnasal drip/drainage** is often present in patients with allergic rhinitis, the common cold, and sinusitis and can exacerbate cough and asthma, especially at night.

C. **Associated symptoms** of the common cold and sinusitis are **general malaise, fatigue, sore throat, hoarseness, cough,** and **headache.** Additionally, **acute sinusitis** is associated with **anosmia** or **hyposmia, maxillary toothache** (painful mastication), intrafacial **pressure sensation,** and **halitosis** that lasts more than 3 days but <4 weeks. Other symptoms include facial pain above or below both eyes when leaning forward and "**double sickening,**" which refers to patients who start out with a cold and begin to improve, only to have symptoms return. **Subacute sinusitis** is characterized by the similar symptoms but lasts 4–12 weeks. **Recurrent acute sinusitis** is more than four episodes of acute sinusitis per year lasting at least 7 days with apparent complete resolution of symptoms between bouts. Patients with **chronic sinusitis** present with the same symptoms that persist for 3 months or more. **Headache** in chronic sinusitis is often worse in the morning and with head movement. The symptoms of sinusitis may mimic and overlap those of other diseases, ranging from the common cold to allergic rhinitis. Sinusitis should be suspected when symptoms of these common conditions are prolonged and interfere with daily living or when these symptoms are severe rather than mild or moderate.

D. The most common cause of **sinus pain** is sinusitis, with numerous other conditions that can mimic this symptom (see section II,G). Patients may complain of vague tension-type headaches with sinusitis, or they may complain of pain or pressure over the affected sinuses, specifically facial pain with **maxillary sinusitis,** pain between the eyes with **ethmoid sinusitis,** frontal headaches with **frontal sinusitis,** and vertex headache with **sphenoid sinusitis.**

E. **Epiphoria,** or watery discharge from the eyes, is common with allergic rhinitis. The sensation of **nasal congestion** and a complaint of a constant bad smell (**ozena**) in the nose are common symptoms in patients with atrophic rhinitis.

F. Nasal congestion and complete nasal obstruction are common symptoms of **nasal polyps.** Other symptoms of nasal polyps (in decreasing order of frequency) include hyposmia, rhinorrhea, sneezing, postnasal drip, facial pain, and ocular itching.

IV. **Signs** (Table 55–1). Examination of the nose begins with inspection of the anterior and inferior surfaces, which is aided by a **nasal speculum** and a strong light source. Abnormalities of the nasal mucosa and septum and presence of exudates can help diagnose common causes of rhinitis. A **nasopharyngeal mirror** is required for detection of posterior abnormalities.

Examination of the paranasal sinuses begins with **inspection** of the overlying skin for erythema, which can be associated with infection, **followed by palpation for tenderness** of the maxillary and frontal sinuses. **Transillumination** of the sinuses should be performed in a darkened room. A strong, narrow light source is placed snugly under each brow, close

TABLE 55–1. SIGNS AND SYMPTOMS OF VIRAL URI, SINUSITIS, ALLERGIC RHINITIS AND VASOMOTOR RHINITIS

Sign/Symptom	Viral URI	Sinusitis	Allergic Rhinitis	Vasomotor Rhinitis
Sneezing	Common	Sometimes	Common	Uncommon
Cough	Common	Common[2]	Common	Uncommon
Rhinorrhea and nasal congestion	Common, usually mucoid but may become mucopurulent after 1–3 days. Usually resolve in 7–10 days.	Common, often purulent and yellow to green, continues for >7 days, responds poorly to decongestants. Most often bilateral but may be unilateral. May not have drainage in chronic sinusitis due to occlusion.	Common, usually watery or mucoid	Commonly have unrelenting congestion, rhinorrhea usually very watery
Nasal obstruction/ blockage	Uncommon	Common[1]	Uncommon	Uncommon
Nasal and conjunctival itching	Uncommon	Uncommon	Common	Uncommon
Nasal mucosa	Erythematous and swollen	Marked erythema and swelling if acute, varies with chronic. May have nasal or post-nasal discharge/ purulence.[2]	Pale and boggy or bluish, may have nasal polyp	Bright and red to bluish
Fever	Unusual in adults, more common in children	Usually <101°F, but may be higher with aggressive sinusitis[1]	None	None
Pain or pressure over sinuses	Uncommon	Common[1]	None	None
Hyposmia/anosmia	Uncommon	Common[1]	Uncommon	Uncommon
Headache	Sometimes	Sometimes[2]	Sometimes	None
Halitosis	Uncommon	Sometimes[2]	Uncommon	None
Fatigue	Sometimes	Common[2]	Uncommon	None
Dental pain	None	Common[2]	None	None
Ear pain/pressure	Sometimes	Common[2]	Uncommon	None

[1]Major criteria (pain/pressure and fever are not major criteria in the absence of another major criterion).
[2]Minor criteria.
The presence of two or more major criteria, one major and two or more minor criteria, or nasal purulence on examination constitutes a diagnosis of sinusitis.

to the nose. A dim red glow should be seen as the light is transmitted through the air-filled frontal sinus to the forehead. The maxillary sinuses are transilluminated by shining light downward from just below the inner aspect of each eye while asking the patient to tilt his head back with the mouth wide open. A reddish glow seen at the hard palate indicates a normal air-filled sinus. Asymmetrical or poor transillumination is consistent with sinusitis, although it may also be due to nonpathologic hypoplastic or aplastic sinuses.

Physical examination of children should include evaluation of several key components. The child's **general appearance** should be assessed for lethargy and respiratory distress, which are worrisome signs. The **skin** should be examined for atopic dermatitis, often associated with allergic rhinitis. The **nasal cavity** and **oropharynx** should also be examined for mucosa and anatomy, specifically for nasal obstruction and discharge.

A. Marked erythema or even a hemorrhagic appearance and swelling of the nasal mucosa are typical in patients with rhinitis medicamentosum. In chronic sinusitis, the appearance of the mucous membranes depends on the underlying cause—pale or bluish and edematous in allergic rhinitis or even relatively normal with anatomic causes, such as choanal atresia or septal deviation.

B. **Nose wrinkling, nose rubbing** (also known as the allergic salute), and **allergic "shiners"** (dark rings under the eyes) are especially common in children with allergic rhinitis.

C. In patients with allergic rhinitis, the **conjunctiva** may appear inflamed, the palpebral conjunctiva may have an edematous and cobblestone appearance, and nasal polyps may be present.

D. **Nasal crusting,** a shrunken-appearing nasal mucosa, and enlarged nasal cavities suggest atrophic rhinitis. Patients may also present with **epistaxis.** Despite the sensation of nasal congestion, there is no increase in airflow resistance in most of these cases.

E. **External signs** of sinusitis include erythema overlying the sinuses. The bony structures overlying the maxillary, frontal, or ethmoid sinuses may be tender to palpation, and eyelid puffiness (chemosis) may be present, especially with maxillary and ethmoid sinusitis.

F. **Sinus transillumination** has very low sensitivity and specificity because of the great variability in sinus anatomy, including asymmetry and underdevelopment. Only normal findings are useful in ruling out maxillary or frontal sinusitis.

G. **Signs of complications** of sinusitis include periorbital erythema, proptosis, and edema. Cranial nerve deficits, especially an abducens nerve palsy, can indicate invasive infection. Meningitis should be considered in patients with signs of severe acute sinusitis.

V. **Laboratory Tests** may be indicated if medical therapy fails, if there are symptoms and signs of complications, or if there is a serious underlying condition.

A. **Study of nasal secretions** is not necessary for diagnosis but may help identify the etiology of rhinitis. Nasal secretions are obtained and placed on a glass slide, stained with Hansel, Wright's, or Giemsa stain and examined microscopically. Eosinophils are seen in allergic rhinitis, NARES, and nasal polyposis; large numbers of neutrophils are seen with infection.

B. **Cultures of nasal secretions** from nasal swabs are of limited value because they do not correlate well with bacteria aspirated directly from the sinuses. Endoscopically guided microswab cultures from the middle meatus correlate 80–85% with central puncture cultures. Cultures are indicated when acute sinusitis is resistant to one or two courses of antibiotic therapy and in immunocompromised individuals. Cultures are also obtained during most surgical procedures on the sinuses if persistent sinus infection is suspected. Aerobic and anaerobic cultures should be obtained, and fungal cultures should be added if a fungal origin is suspected.

C. **Fiberoptic rhinoscopy** can reveal the presence of nasal polyps, septal deviation, or mucopurulent secretions, and can be used to obtain microswab cultures.

D. **Allergy tests**

1. **Allergen skin testing** is helpful in diagnosing allergic rhinitis and identifying specific allergens for which avoidance measures, allergen immunotherapy, or both are warranted. It should be considered in patients who fail medical therapy or have perennial rhinitis that is moderate to severe. These tests are relatively inexpensive and fairly reliable. They are not useful in children younger than 3 years because the very young produce inadequate amounts of histamine.

a. Groups of allergens or single allergens are selected for testing based on the most likely causes of the patient's allergy.

b. Allergens are introduced into the skin by intradermal injection (which is most accurate but carries a greater risk of anaphylaxis), skin prick test (the easiest, most widely used, and reasonably accurate), or scratch test. *Note:* Methylxanthines and antihistamines should be discontinued before skin testing.

2. **Radioallergosorbent (RAST) testing** is the determination of serum allergen-specific IgE levels by immunoassay. This test is useful in young children, who might not tolerate multiple skin pricks; those with skin conditions such as dermatographia and severe eczema; and those receiving medications that might affect the reliability of skin testing (eg, antihistamines). However, it is relatively more expensive, is less sensitive, and can test for fewer antigens than skin testing.

E. **Imaging studies**

1. **Sinus films** may be helpful in uncertain or recurrent cases, but not for initial evaluation, since up to 40% of sinus films may be abnormal in viral rhinosinusitis if obtained within 7 days of symptom onset. Four views constitute the sinus series: Water's view (maxillary sinuses), the Caldwell view (ethmoid and frontal sinuses), the submental vertex view (sphenoid sinuses), and the lateral view. A single Water's view has a high level of agreement with the complete sinus series. A normal series has a negative predictive value of 90–100%, particularly for the maxillary and frontal sinuses. A sinus film is read as abnormal if there is mucosal thickening >6 mm, air-fluid levels, > 33% loss of air space volume, or opacification of one or more sinuses on one or more views. The positive predictive value is 80–100%, but sensitivity is only 60%.

2. The computerized tomography (**CT scan**) has superior sensitivity (95–98%) and specificity compared to sinus films. The CT scan is particularly valuable in assessing obstruction of the sinus ostia. CT scanning is indicated when medical therapy has failed, to establish the diagnosis of chronic sinusitis in equivocal cases before starting long-term antibiotic therapy or when complications are suspected. A complete series sinus CT scan is required prior to sinus surgery. More than 80% of scan results may be abnormal in viral rhinosinusitis if obtained within 7 days of illness onset.

3. **Magnetic resonance imaging** is used when fungal sinusitis and tumors are suspected. It is not used for routine evaluation of sinusitis.

VI. Treatment
A. Treatment of **common colds** is largely palliative and may include the following strategies.

1. For **fever and headache, acetaminophen** (eg, Tylenol), 325 mg, one or two tablets orally every 4–6 hours for adults (maximum 4 g/24 hours) or 10–15 mg/kg every 4–6 hours for children younger than 12 years, or **ibuprofen** (eg, Advil), 200 mg, one or two tablets every 4–6 hours for adults (maximum 1200 mg/24 hours) or 5–10 mg/kg every 6–8 hours for children (maximum 50mg/kg/day) may be used.

2. For **nasal congestion and rhinorrhea,** oral decongestants such as **pseudoephedrine** (eg, Sudafed), 30 mg, one or two tablets every 4–6 hours for adults and children older than age 12, or 0.5–1 tsp every 4–6 hours of the liquid for children younger than 12 years, may be used. Short-term use (up to a maximum of 3–4 days) of topical decongestants such as **phenylephrine hydrochloride** (eg, Neo-Synephrine), 0.125% or 0.25%, two or three sprays in each nostril up to every 4 hours for children and the same dosing schedule of the 0.5% spray for adults, may be helpful. These medications can cause insomnia, nervousness, loss of appetite, and urinary retention in males. They should be used with caution in patients with certain conditions, such as arrhythmias, hypertension, and hyperthyroidism.

3. For **cough,** syrups containing **dextromethorphan** (eg, Robitussin DM) or **codeine** (eg, Robitussin AC), 0.5–2 tsp every 4 hours (the exact dose depends on the patient's age), can be prescribed, with **benzonatate** (eg, Tessalon Perles), 100 mg three times daily for adults, a potentially helpful alternative.

4. **Watery rhinorrhea** may be treated with the anticholinergic nasal spray **ipratropium bromide** (eg, Atrovent 0.06%).

5. **Antihistamines** have not been shown to be beneficial, nor are antibiotics indicated or helpful in these patients.

6. **Alternative therapies**
   a. **General supportive measures** in the treatment of **common colds** and **allergies** include adequate sleep, increased fluids, cool vapor steam, and rest. Certainly, adequate fluids (especially water and soups) improve mucous membrane and ciliary function and may also enhance immune function.
   b. The use of other alternative therapies, such as **homeopathic medicines, vitamins, acupuncture,** and **herbs,** is controversial. Although **vitamin C** in high doses (up to 1 g daily) does not seem to prevent illness, it does reduce the duration of symptoms. **Zinc** may also be effective in shortening the duration of symptoms when taken within 24 hours of their onset. Studies indicating **Echinacea** preparations stimulate the immune system, thereby reducing the severity and duration of infection, are debated, although effects appear generally positive.

B. Allergic rhinitis
1. **Environmental control.** Avoidance of inciting factors is fundamental.
   a. For **pollen allergy,** patients should keep doors and windows closed, limit the amount of time spent outdoors, and use air conditioners and a high-efficiency particle air (HEPA) filter.
   b. For **dust mite allergy,** patients should cover bedding (including pillows) with plastic covers, eliminate wall-to-wall carpets (especially in bedrooms), use

acaricides such as tannic acid solutions regularly to kill dust mites, avoid or regularly wash stuffed animals in hot water, keep home humidity below 40%, and use HEPA filters.

c. Patients with **mold allergies** should decrease mold exposure by wiping vulnerable surfaces (eg, those in the bathroom) with household bleach, keeping indoor humidity below 40%, using air filters, avoiding piles of leaves in the fall, and cutting grass to reduce exposure outside.

d. **Cat dander** (saliva) is by far the most frequent cause of allergies to animals. If sensitivity develops, contact with the animal should be minimized. The cat should be washed at least once every 2 weeks to remove the antigen-containing cat saliva from its coat.

e. Elimination of **food allergens** may be beneficial. However, ingested allergens rarely cause isolated rhinitis without involvement of other organ systems. Relatively common food allergens include dairy products, chocolate, wheat, citrus fruits, and food additives such as artificial dyes and preservatives.

2. **Pharmacologic therapy** includes the following.

a. **Steroid nasal sprays** are more effective than antihistamines in the treatment of allergic rhinitis. Available preparations include **beclomethasone** (eg, Beconase or Vancenase), one spray per nostril two or three times daily; **flunisolide** (eg, Nasalide), two sprays per nostril twice daily; **triamcinolone acetonide** (eg, Nasacort), two to four sprays per nostril daily; **budesonide** (eg, Rhinocort), two to four sprays per nostril daily; and **fluticasone** (eg, Flonase), one or two sprays daily. Other steroid nasal sprays have good long-term safety records. Local side effects are minimal with proper use, although nasal irritation, bleeding, mucosal erosions, and perforation may occur. Since some nasal corticosteroid preparations have been reported to reduce linear growth (at least temporarily), growth should be monitored when used in children. **Oral steroids** should be avoided, except in severe cases of refractory allergic rhinitis, in rhinitis medicamentosum while topical decongestants are discontinued, and in obstructive nasal polyposis. If used in these situations, short-acting steroids should be used (eg, in adults, prednisone, 30 mg orally for 3–7 days).

b. **Antihistamines** (Table 55–2) reduce sneezing, rhinorrhea, and nasal and ocular pruritus associated with allergic rhinitis, but are less effective for nasal congestion. They are effective when used occasionally for episodic symptoms, but work best when administered on a regular basis. If economic factors are less important, the newer-generation antihistamines are usually preferred, because they have fewer anticholinergic side effects and especially cause less sedation. These agents include **desloratadine** (Clarinex), **fexofenadine** (Allegra), **cetirizine** (Zyrtec), and **loratadine** (Claritin), which is currently the only one available over the counter. **First-generation antihistamines** are effective and less expensive than newer agents, but tend to cause more side effects, such as sedation, dry mouth, and fatigue. Even more serious side effects can occur, such as urinary obstruction and slowed reaction times, which can potentially lead to accidents. **Levocabastine** (Livostin 0.05%), one drop into each affected eye four times daily, or **Patanol (olopatadine 0.1%), 1–2 drops in each affected eye twice a day,** can be very helpful in the treatment of allergic conjunctivitis. **Intranasal antihistamines** (eg, azelastine) offer no therapeutic benefit over conventional treatment.

c. **Antihistamine-decongestant combinations** such as **Claritin-D 12 Hour, Claritin-D 24 Hour, Tavist-D,** and **Allegra-D** are also useful, especially if nasal congestion is a prominent symptom. The dose is one tablet twice daily for all except Claritin-D 24 hour, which is taken once daily.

d. **Mast cell–stabilizing agents** such as **cromolyn sodium** (eg, Nasalcrom), one spray per nostril three or four times per day, can be useful. Ideally, these agents should be started before major symptoms develop because they may take several weeks to be effective.

e. **Anticholinergic agents** such as **ipratropium bromide** (eg, Atrovent 0.03% nasal spray), one or two sprays in each nostril every 6 hours, may reduce rhinorrhea. Ipratropium bromide can also alleviate symptoms of vasomotor rhinitis and cold air–induced rhinorrhea.

TABLE 55–2. ANTIHISTAMINES USEFUL IN THE TREATMENT OF ALLERGIC RHINITIS

Class	Generic Name	Sample Trade Name	Dose[1]	Sedative Effects	Anticholinergic Effects
First generation					
Ethanolamines	Diphenhydramine	Benadryl[2]		Marked	Mild
		Allergy tablets	A: 25–50 mg qid		
		Syrup	C: 12.5 mg/5 mL		
			5–10 mL q 4–6 hours		
	Clemastine	Tavist			
		Tablets	A: 1.32–2.68 mg bid		
		Syrup	C: 0.5 mg/5 mL		
			5–10 mL bid		
Alkylamines	Chorpheniramine	Chlor-Trimeton		Mild	Mild
		tablets	A: 4 mg qid		
		Triaminic[2] syrup	C: 1 mg/5 mL		
			1.5–10 mL q 4 hours		
Phenothiazines	Promethazine	Phenergan		Marked	Mild
		Tablets	A: 25–50 mg qid		
		Syrup	C: 6.25 mg/5 mL		
			5–10 mL tid–qid		
Piperidines	Cyproheptadine	Periactin tablets	A: 4 mg qid	Moderate	Mild
			C: 2 mg/5 mL		
			5–15 mL bid–tid		
	Azatadine	Trinalin tablets	A: 1 bid		
Piperazine	Hydroxyzine	Atarax		Moderate	Mild
		Tablets	A: 10–50 mg qid		
		Syrup	C: 10 mg/5 mL		
			5–15 mL tid–qid		
Second generation					
	Cetirizine	Zyrtec		Mild	None
		Tablets	A: 10 mg qd		
		Syrup	C: 5–10 mL qd		
			(1 mg/mL)		
	Fexofenadine	Allegra tablets	A: 60 mg bid	None	None
	Loratadine	Claritin (OTC)			
		Tablets	A: 10 mg qd	None	None
		Syrup	C: 10 mL qd		
			(1 mg/mL)	None	None
	Desloratadine				
	Clarinex	Tablets	A: 5 mg qd	None	None

Children's dosages are listed for those medications with available pediatric suspensions. Be aware that a range of dosages are listed. Look up the exact dosages by age before prescribing these medications for children.
[1]A, adults' dose (mg); C, children's dose (mL).
[2]A decongestant is added to this formulation.

3. **Immunotherapy** is useful especially in severe or refractory cases and in those patients with year-round symptoms (perennial allergic rhinitis). It is the only method demonstrated to favorably modify the long-term course of allergic rhinitis. Criteria for treatment include a history of at least moderate symptoms of allergic rhinitis for ≥2 years or severe symptoms for at least 6 months responding poorly to symptomatic treatment. Other considerations in choosing immunotherapy include comorbidities and failure or unacceptability of alternative treatments. Selection of antigen injection is based on the presence of specific IgE antibodies (see section V,D) and the patient's history. The patient receives weekly injections of antigen(s), with increasing doses at weekly intervals until a maintenance dose is achieved; injections are then given every 3–6 weeks for 3–5 years. If therapy does not significantly relieve symptoms within 12 months, immunotherapy should be terminated.
4. **Patient education** should include information about environmental controls to minimize antigen exposure, management options, and complications.

5. Alternative therapies
   a. For more information on **common supportive measures,** see section VI,A,6,a.
   b. **Other alternative therapies, such as vitamin C, quercetin, homeopathy, acupuncture, and hypnosis, require further study.**
C. Treatment of **vasomotor rhinitis** consists mainly of symptomatic therapy with oral decongestants such as **pseudoephedrine** (eg, Sudafed), 60 mg three or four times a day. Anticholinergic agents such as **ipratropium bromide** (eg, Atrovent nasal spray) (see section VI,B,2,e) can be very helpful in alleviating profuse watery rhinorrhea. **Intranasal steroids** (see section VI,B,2,a) may be helpful in treating troublesome exacerbations unresponsive to the therapies listed above. **Intranasal antihistamines** (eg, azelastine, two sprays per nostril twice daily) are also effective. Severe nonresponsive cases may require surgical resection of the inferior turbinate. Patients should be educated to avoid irritants that may exacerbate this condition; these include tobacco and fireplace smoke, strong perfumes, chemical and gasoline fumes, and wood dust. Sudden changes in temperature or humidity should also be avoided when possible.
D. In **rhinitis medicamentosum,** topical decongestants should be discontinued. Oral decongestants or a short course of a topical nasal steroid may be helpful (see section VI,B,2,a). A short course of systemic steroids (eg, **prednisone,** 40 mg orally initially, tapered over 7–10 days) may be required if other methods are ineffective. The problem usually resolves in 2–3 weeks without long-term sequelae. Patients should be educated about the causes of the condition and discouraged from further abuse of topical decongestants.
E. Treatment of **atrophic rhinitis** is directed toward moistening the nasal mucosa. A mucolytic such as **guaifenesin,** 600–1200 mg twice daily, can be used in conjunction with nasal preparations such as **Alkalol liquid,** an OT Coral or intranasal mucolytic, **or intranasal saline** (eg, Afrin saline), two to six sprays in each nostril every 2 hours. **Pulsed irrigators** can also be helpful in helping to cleanse and moisten areas deeper within the nasal cavity. Systemic estrogens in menopausal women may alleviate rhinitis symptoms. Surgical reductions of nasal cavity patency are used only as a last resort. It is important to educate patients that treatment is directed at relieving symptoms and is sometimes only partially successful.
F. **Sinusitis** can usually be managed in the outpatient setting. Acute sinusitis resolves without antibiotic treatment in most cases. Antibiotic therapy should be reserved for patients with moderately severe symptoms who meet the criteria for the clinical diagnosis of acute bacterial sinusitis and for those with severe sinusitis symptoms, regardless of duration of illness, or for those who do not improve or worsen with supportive measures (see section VI,A). Hospital admission is necessary for complicated sinusitis (sinusitis associated with serious complications such as otitis media, asthma, bronchiectasis, fungal infection, multiple antibiotic allergies, or sinusitis that compromises quality of life) or when there is a high risk of complications from a serious underlying disease and close outpatient monitoring is not feasible.
   1. Antibiotics (Table 55–3).
      a. The standard has been to treat adults and children with uncomplicated acute sinusitis for a minimum of 7–10 days. Recent data show as little as 3 days of antibiotic treatment (ie, with **trimethoprim-sulfamethoxazole [TMP-SMX]**) may be as effective as treatment for 10 days. Thus, the duration of treatment is currently a controversial topic. Antibiotics should be changed if there is no improvement after 3 days of therapy.
      b. For initial treatment, the most narrow-spectrum agent active against the likely pathogens, *S pneumoniae* and *H influenzae,* should be used. Appropriate first-line therapy in otherwise healthy patients with uncomplicated acute sinusitis who have not received antibiotics in the previous month and are in an area with <30% prevalence of drug-resistant pneumococcus includes high-dose **amoxicillin, TMP-SMX, cefuroxime axetil, cefdinir,** and **cefpodoxime.** For patients with penicillin/cephalosporin allergies, other treatment options include **clarithromycin, azithromycin, doxycycline,** or **quinolones.**
      c. If the response to first-line therapy is poor, if there is at least a 30% prevalence of drug-resistant pneumococcus, or if the patient is immunocompromised, reasonable alternative antimicrobials include **amoxicillin-clavulanate** and **quinolones.** Quinolones should only be used in individuals 18 years or older. The American Academy of Pediatrics recommends that for moderate to more severe

TABLE 55-3. AMBULATORY ANTIBIOTIC REGIMENS IN THE TREATMENT OF UNCOMPLICATED SINUSITIS

Antibiotic	Dose	Relative Cost
Amoxicillin (Amoxil)[1]	Adult: 500 mg tid Child: (high-dose) 90 mg/kg/day divided bid or tid	$
Trimethoprim-sulfamethoxazole (TMP-SMX)[1] (Bactrim, 160 mg of TMP and 800 mg of SMX per DS tablet; Septra, 8 mg of TMP and 40 mg of SMX per tsp)	Adult: one DS tablet bid Child: 8–12 mg/kg/day TMP and 40–60 mg/kg/day SMX divided bid	$
Clarithromycin (Biaxin)[2]	Adult: 500 mg bid or 1 gm qd if extended release Child: 15 mg/kg/day bid	$$$
Amoxicillin-clavulanate (Augmentin)[2]	Adult: 875/125 mg bid Child: (high-dose) 90 mg/kg/day amoxicillin com- ponent divided bid	$$$
Cefuroxime axetil (Ceftin)[1]	Adult: 250 mg bid Child: 30 mg/kg/day bid	$$$
Cefpodoxime proxetil (Vantin)[1]	Adult: 200 mg bid Child: 10 mg/kg/day bid	$$$
Azithromycin (Zithromax)[2]	Adult: 500 mg day 1, 250 mg days 2–5 Child: 10 mg/kg/day 1, 5 mg/kg days 2–5	$$
Levofloxacin (Levaquin)[2]	Adult: 500 mg qd	$$$

[1]First-line treatment.
[2]Second-line treatment.

sinusitis, if a child has recently received antibiotics or attends day care, therapy should be initiated with high-dose amoxicillin-clavulanate (80–90 mg/kg/day of amoxicillin component in two divided doses).

   d. For chronic sinusitis, antibiotic therapy should continue for at least 3 weeks and until the patient is well for 7 days. Antibiotics with good staphylococcal coverage are often preferred; these include **cloxacillin, dicloxacillin, cephalexin, cefadroxil monohydrate, erythromycin, clarithromycin, amoxicillin-clavulanate,** and **cefuroxime axetil.** With complicated sinusitis, hospital admission for parenteral antibiotics is indicated. If mucormycosis is suspected, parenteral **amphotericin B** should be used.

2. **Humidification** with cool steam and increased oral intake of water helps thin nasal secretions.

3. **Oral decongestants** or short-term use (3–5 days) of **topical nasal decongestants** (see section VI,A,2) decrease nasal congestion and mucosal edema that can block the sinus ostea.

4. **Oral decongestant–antihistamine combinations** (section VI,B,2,c) may be helpful in patients with underlying allergic rhinitis.

5. **Guaifenesin** in high doses (1200 mg twice daily) may thin tenacious secretions and therefore promote sinus drainage.

6. **Nasal irrigation** with a normal saline solution is recommended to liquefy secretions. It is especially helpful in infants and young children.

7. **Other therapies**
   a. **Topical corticosteroids** may be effective adjuncts to antibiotic therapy, but objective data are lacking. The short-term use of **oral corticosteroids** is reasonable in patients with nasal polyps or severe mucosal edema.
   b. **Surgery** should be considered for patients who have frequent recurrences of sinusitis (ie, three or more attacks in 1 year) despite adequate medical treatment, who have chronic sinusitis responding inadequately to medical therapy alone, or who have an anatomic obstruction amenable to surgery. Functional endoscopic sinus surgery (FESS) has supplanted older surgical techniques. FESS leads to a significant improvement of symptoms in 80–90% of patients. It is typically

directed at the removal of locally diseased ethmoid tissue to improve ventilation and drainage. When polyps are present and cause marked mechanical obstruction, polypectomy may be indicated. Adenoidectomy may be indicated primarily in younger children with moderate to severe nasal obstruction secondary to adenoidal hyperplasia and may decrease recurrence of sinusitis.

8. **Dental referral** is indicated in patients in whom a tooth abscess is suspected as the underlying cause of maxillary sinusitis.

9. **Patient follow-up**
   a. There are no clear recommendations for follow-up of acute sinusitis; however, it is reasonable to see a patient 10–14 days after therapy is initiated to establish whether symptoms and signs of sinusitis have completely resolved.
   b. **Complications** of sinusitis are uncommon. They occur more frequently in children and in patients with immunodeficiency disorders. Patients should be instructed to return to the physician immediately if symptoms worsen or if new symptoms such as visual disturbance, neck stiffness, or lethargy develop. Complications of sinusitis can be **local, orbital,** or **intracranial.**
      (1) **Local complications** include mucoceles or mucopyoceles. Mucoceles occur most frequently in the frontal sinus, and patients often present complaining of diplopia because the affected eye is displaced.
      (2) **Orbital complications** are the most common, and children with acute ethmoid sinusitis are the most prone to this complication. Preseptal or orbital cellulitis can occur; the latter is more severe because it involves orbital structures. Signs of orbital cellulitis include swelling and inflammation of the eyelids and proptosis of the affected eye. Complete ophthalmoplegia, impairment of vision, and chemosis indicate likely orbital abscess.
      (3) **Intracranial complications** include cavernous sinus thrombosis (signs include bilateral orbital involvement, ophthalmoplegia, progressive and severe chemosis, retinal engorgement, fever, and prostration); meningitis; subdural empyema; and brain abscess.

REFERENCES

American Academy of Pediatrics. Subcommittee on Management of Sinusitis and Committee on Quality Improvement. Clinical practice guideline: Management of sinusitis. Pediatrics 2001;**108**:798.

Dykewicz MS: Rhinitis and sinusitis. J Allergy Clin Immunol 2003;**111**:S520.

Gilbert DN, Moellering RC, Sande MA (editors): *The Sanford Guide to Antimicrobial Therapy 2003.* Antimicrobial Therapy, Inc. (Hyde Park, Vermont); 2003.

Hickner JM, et al: Principles of appropriate antibiotic use for acute rhinosinusitis in adults: Background. Ann Intern Med 2001;**134**:498.

Jaber R: Respiratory and allergic diseases: from upper respiratory tract infections to asthma. Prim Care; Clin in Office Pract 2002;**29**:231.

Schoem SR, et al: Why won't this child's nose stop running? Cont Ped. 2002;**19**(12):48.

Snow V, Mottur-Pilson C, Hickner JM: Principles of appropriate antibiotic use for acute sinusitis in adults. Ann Intern Med 2001;**134**:495.

Spector SL, et al: Parameters for the diagnosis and management of sinusitis. J Allergy Clin Immunol 1998;**102**:S107.

---

56   Scrotal Complaints

John A. Heydt, MD, & Ted D. Epperly, MD

KEY POINTS

- A firm grounding in scrotal anatomy is helpful in approaching the patient with scrotal complaints.
- Scrotal complaints affect 0.1–0.3% of the male population each year; most causes can be determined by history and limited testing.
- Scrotal pain can have an insidious (>48 hours) or acute (<48 hours) onset; a limited history and physical examination, with or without selective testing, will pinpoint the diagnosis.

I. Definition. Scrotal pain refers to discomfort, pain, or an unpleasant sensation originating or referred to the scrotum.

Knowledge of scrotal anatomy (Figure 56–1) is fundamental to diagnosing scrotal complaints.

II. Common Diagnoses
  A. Testicular causes
  1. **Epididymitis** most commonly occurs in sexually active males from retrograde spread of prostatitis or urethral secretions through the vas deferens, but may also occur in prepubertal boys with urologic abnormalities such as ectopic ureters, or congenital/acquired urethral strictures.
      a. In **sexually active men younger than 35 years,** epididymitis is usually associated with urethritis and caused by *Neisseria gonorrhoeae* or *Chlamydia trachomatis* but may be due to *Ureaplasma* or mycoplasma infections.
      b. In **sexually monogamous men older than 35 years,** epididymitis is usually caused by enteric gram-negative rods (*Enterobacter*) and may occur in association with prostatitis or prostatitis with cystitis.
  2. **Orchitis** is most commonly viral. Approximately 20–35% of males who contract mumps develop orchitis, and 35% of those affected have involvement of both

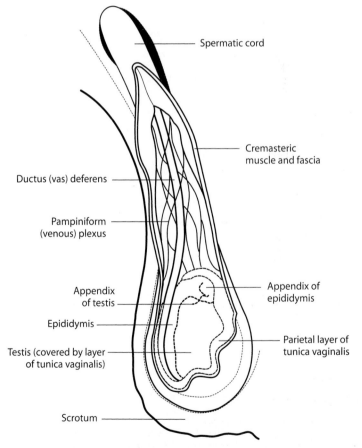

FIGURE 56–1. Testicular anatomy.

testes. Other viral infections known to cause orchitis include influenza, Epstein-Barr, varicella, echo, and Coxsackie. Orchitis can also be associated with a bacterial epididymitis or epididymo-orchitis.

3. **Torsion**
    a. **Testicular torsion** occurs most frequently in neonates and pubertal boys. It is rare over age 30. The overall risk of a male having either testicular torsion or torsion of the testicular appendage by age 25 is 1 in 160. Predisposing conditions include the "bell clapper deformity," small testicles, excessive exercise, straining, cremasteric spasm, sexual activity, a sudden scare, immersion in cold water, attempted reduction of an inguinal hernia, or trauma.
    b. **Incidence of torsion of the testicular appendage** peaks at age 10, almost always occurs prior to puberty, and shares risk factors with testicular torsion.
4. With **traumatic injuries,** severe scrotal trauma is uncommon and results from either the testicle being compressed against the pubic bone or from straddle injury.
5. **Testicular neoplasms** are the third most common tumors in men between ages 20 and 34 years (incidence of 2–3 per 100,000 men per year). A history of undescended testicle(s), even with correction, increases the risk 2.5–20 times over those without such a history.

CRYPTORCHIDISM

Undescended testicle(s) (cryptorchidism) occur in 3–5% of term newborns and up to 30% of premature males. Most descend spontaneously, so the prevalence is 1% of boys by age 1 year. Because of the associated risk of testicular neoplasms and decreased fertility, urologic consultation for orchiopexy is indicated between ages 6 months and 1 year.

B. **Extratesticular causes** can produce scrotal pain and swelling.
    1. **Hernias** can be direct or indirect and are common in all ages. Congenital defects, straining, or both are predisposing factors.
    2. **Prostatitis** (see section II,A,1,b) can refer pain to the scrotum via the same sensory nerve fibers innervating the testicles.
    3. **Renal colic** from urinary tract lithiases also causes referred scrotal pain. Risk factors include a positive family history, decreased fluid intake, and residency in the southeastern United States.
    4. **Hydrocele,** a fluid-filled mass in the scrotal sac, is usually an idiopathic congenital condition; new-onset hydroceles in young men may be associated with testicular tumor.
    5. **Varicocele,** dilatation and tortuosity of the pampiniform plexus, rarely occurs before age 10 years and is found in up to 15% of adult males.
    6. **Spermatocele** is a small cystic mass just above the testis.
III. **Symptoms** (Table 56–1).
    A. **Testicular causes.** Thirty-three to 50% of males with torsion will have experienced similar transient pain in the past. Torsion rarely occurs after trauma, but a history of trauma does not exclude the possibility of torsion.
    B. **Extratesticular causes**
        1. **Renal colic** can produce severe intermittent flank pain, but the pain can radiate to the abdomen, pubic area, or scrotum. Nausea, vomiting, fevers, chills, and urinary frequency may be present.
        2. **Prostatitis** presents with fever; chills; dysuria; urinary frequency; myalgias; or scrotal, perineal, or back pain. Patients may also experience pain with ejaculation and defecation.
IV. **Signs** (Table 56–1).
    A. **Testicular causes**
        1. **Acute epididymitis** can be difficult to distinguish from testicular torsion.
            a. The **cremasteric reflex** (elicited by stroking or pinching the inner thigh, causing the ipsilateral testicle to retract toward the inguinal canal) is present in epididymitis, but not testicular torsion.

TABLE 56–1. DIFFERENTIAL DIAGNOSIS OF COMMON SCROTAL COMPLAINTS

Diagnosis	History	Examination	Tests
Epididymitis	Fevers, chills, rigors, unilateral scrotal swelling and pain	Swollen/tender upper posterior testicle, presence of cremasteric reflex, Prehn's sign	UA, urethral smear, color Doppler if diagnosis unclear; VCU and renal/bladder US in prepubertal boys
Orchitis	Unilateral/bilateral testicular pain/swelling; if mumps, occurs 4–10 days after parotitis	Unilateral or bilateral testicular swelling/tenderness	None; color Doppler US if diagnosis unclear
Torsion	Acute onset, unilateral swelling and pain, nausea and vomiting, ± previous symptoms, no constitutional symptoms	Unilateral testicular swelling and retraction transversely— "bell clapper" deformity; no testicular cremasteric reflex or Prehn's sign	Radionuclide scan/testicular scintigraphy or color Doppler if diagnosis unclear or symptoms >12 hr
Torsion of the testicular appendage	Moderate pain, acute onset, swelling; no constitutional symptoms	Firm tender nodule upper pole of epididymis; "blue dot sign"	No tests necessary; color Doppler if diagnosis unclear
Traumatic epididymitis	Trauma a few days prior, pain and swelling	Possible ecchymosis, unilateral or bilateral edema; cremasteric reflex and Prehn's sign present	No tests necessary; color Doppler if diagnosis unclear
Testicular hematomas/ hematocele	Trauma, pain, swelling, nausea or vomiting	Ecchymosis and enlargement of affected testicle	Color Doppler US
Testicular rupture	Trauma history, pain, swelling, nausea or vomiting	Ecchymosis and enlargement of affected testicle	Color Doppler US
Testicular neoplasms	Enlarging scrotal mass/testicular nodule; occasional pain if hemorrhage	Palpable nodule or enlarged testicle; gynecomastia or left supraclavicular node	Scrotal US/tumor markers, biopsy
Inguinal hernia	Variable pain, enlargement in scrotum, or bulge of abdominal wall	Palpable hernia on abdominal wall or through inguinal ring; increases with Valsalva's maneuver	None or CT of abdomen and pelvis
Hydrocele	Painless testicular swelling	Minimally tender transilluminating swelling around testicle	Scrotal US
Varicocele	Swelling, dull scrotal heaviness, worse with exercise	"Bag of worms" supratesticular, collapsing with supine position	No tests necessary; color Doppler US if uncertain
Spermatocele	Asymptomatic	Painless nodule above testicle (spermatic cord)	No tests necessary; US if diagnosis unclear

CT, computerized tomogram; UA, urinalysis; US, ultrasound; VCU, voiding cystourethrogram.

    b. Prehn's sign is relief of pain on elevation of the testicle when the patient is supine. This may occur with epididymitis but not with testicular torsion. This maneuver is not specific to epididymitis.
  2. Torsion
    a. The "bell clapper" deformity, in which the testicle lacks attachment to the tunica vaginalis and hangs freely, may be noted in older children at risk for testicular torsion. With torsion, the testicle rapidly becomes firm and tender and enlarges with the epididymis into a solitary mass. The scrotum can become erythematous and edematous similar to epididymitis.
    b. A small bluish discoloration (the "**blue dot sign**") may be seen through scrotal skin near the upper testicular pole. Coupled with pain, this finding is pathognomonic for appendiceal torsion.
 B. Extrascrotal causes
  1. Renal colic may present with hematuria, there may be tenderness of the flank and hyperparesthesias of the skin of the abdomen, but examination of the scrotum is unremarkable.

2. In **prostatitis,** a warm, tender, spongy, enlarged prostate can be palpated on rectal examination.
V. **Laboratory Tests** (Table 56–1). Scrotal complaints can often be diagnosed with a careful history and physical examination, maintaining a high index of suspicion for serious conditions, such as testicular torsion, acute infectious epididymitis, or acute incarcerated inguinal hernia.
　A. **Urinalysis** detects pyuria or bacteriuria with epididymitis or prostatitis and microscopic or gross hematuria in urinary lithiasis. Urinalysis is normal in testicular torsion or torsion of the testicular appendix.
　B. **Urethral smear** produced by inserting a small sterile cotton-tipped probe into the urethra for one turn, then layering the secretions on a microscope slide for Gram stain and microscopic examination, is helpful in evaluation of epididymitis in sexually active males younger than age 35 or with suspected sexually transmitted epididymitis. The smear may demonstrate white blood cells (WBCs) and bacteria.
　C. An elevated **WBC count** and **erythrocyte sedimentation rate** may occur in febrile patients; an elevated WBC count can occur in torsion, most likely as a stress reaction.
　D. **Doppler studies** measure testicular blood flow.
　　1. For most clinicians, **color Doppler ultrasonography** is the preferred diagnostic test, with sensitivity of approximately 90% and specificity of 100% in testicular torsion. It is indicated when testicular pain has been present >12 hours or the diagnosis of torsion is uncertain. Color ultrasonography can also diagnose incarcerated hernia, varicocele, hematoma, or testicular rupture and can differentiate testicular appendiceal torsion (increased blood flow) from testicular torsion (decreased/absent blood flow) if the diagnosis is uncertain.
　　2. **Doppler stethoscope** and **conventional gray-scale ultrasonography** are not as accurate as color ultrasonography and should not be used.
　E. **Radionuclide testicular scan** or **testicular scintigraphy** demonstrates decreased blood flow to the affected testicle within a few hours in torsion (sensitivity/specificity >90% for acute torsion when performed by an experienced physician) and increased blood flow with epididymitis. Scintigraphy's main limitation is the delay in results compared to color ultrasonography.
　F. **Scrotal ultrasound** is extremely accurate in distinguishing between solid and fluid-filled masses.
　G. In prepubertal boys with epididymitis/urinary tract infection, **renal/bladder ultrasound and voiding cystourethrogram** are indicated to evaluate for urinary tract anomalies.
VI. **Treatment**
　A. **Testicular conditions**
　　1. In **acute epididymitis,** treatment goals include pain relief and addressing underlying infection. In most cases, this is feasible in the outpatient setting.
　　　a. **Pain relief** is best accomplished by ice packs for 24–48 hours, bed rest, scrotal support, and oral medications, such as ibuprofen, 600–800 mg three to four times daily (mild/moderate pain); acetaminophen with codeine, 325/30 mg; or hydrocodone, 5 mg four times daily (severe pain). A cord block with 5–8 mL of a 50/50 mixture or 1% lidocaine and 0.5% bupivacaine can be helpful if administered by an experienced physician.
　　　b. **Antibiotic** selection is based on age and sexual history. Generally speaking, in sexually active males older than 35 years the treatment of choice is either a single intramuscular dose of ceftriaxone (Rocephin), 250 mg, plus doxycycline, 100 mg orally twice daily for 10 days; OR ofloxacin, 300 mg orally for 10 days. In males older than 35 and at low risk for sexually transmitted diseases, treatment options include ciprofloxacin (eg, Cipro), 500 mg orally twice daily, or ofloxacin, 300 mg orally daily for 10–14 days.
　　　c. Hospitalization may be required for males with high fevers, intractable pain, toxic appearance, or suspicion of scrotal abscess.
　　　d. **Surgical drainage, orchiectomy, or both** is warranted when severe epididymo-orchitis results in abscess formation.
　　　e. **Urologic consultation** and **surgical exploration** are indicated when the diagnosis is unclear or if testicular torsion is suspected (see section VI,A,3).
　　2. The pain of **orchitis** can be managed similarly to that of epididymitis (see section VI,A,1,a).

3. Torsion

a. If **testicular torsion** is confirmed or high clinical suspicion is present, immediate surgical referral should be made. If detorsion is accomplished by 10 hours, 70–100% of testicles remain viable, after 10–12 hours viability drops to 20%, and at 24–48 hours 0% of testicles are viable. No testicle is viable after 48 hours. In patients with torsion, bilateral orchiopexy is necessary, because the "bell clapper" deformity usually exists in both testicles.

b. **Testicular appendage torsion** is managed conservatively with analgesics, ice, and scrotal elevation. Activity may worsen symptoms, so it should be restricted. If pain and swelling are severe and the diagnosis is clear, urologic consultation for local nerve block may control pain. If the diagnosis is unclear, prompt diagnostic testing (see section V,D,1), referral for exploration, or both should be made.

4. Trauma

a. For **testes rupture** emergent referral should be made for repair; **testicular hematoma** and hematocele also require surgical consultation.

b. **Traumatic epididymitis,** which occurs a few days after trauma, is managed conservatively with anti-inflammatory medications, elevation, and ice.

5. **Testicular neoplasms** should be managed in consultation with a urologic oncologist.

B. Extratesticular causes

1. **Inguinal hernias** require urgent surgical consultation if incarcerated or strangulated and elective repair if reducible.

2. **Renal colic** (see Chapter 36).

3. **Prostatitis** is generally managed with antibiotics (see Chapter 61).

4. **Hydroceles** in infants usually spontaneously resolve during the first 1–2 years of life. Hydroceles persisting beyond age 1–2 years, accompanied by hernia, or occurring in males beyond infancy require surgical consultation for repair.

5. Because **varicoceles** can affect testicular growth and fertility, consultation with a urologist for elective spermatic vein ligation is prudent. A noncollapsible varicocele raises suspicion for retroperitoneal tumor and requires appropriate imaging study (eg, abdominal magnetic resonance imaging scan or computerized tomography) and specialist consultation based on findings.

6. Only large **spermatoceles** require urologic consultation for excision.

REFERENCES

Docimo SG, Silver RI, Cromie W: The undescended testicle: Diagnosis and management. Am Fam Physician 2000;**62:**2037.

Galejs LE, Kass EJ: Diagnosis and treatment of the acute scrotum. Am Fam Physician (February 15) 1999;**59:**817.

Gilbert DN, Moellering RC Jr, Sande MA: *The Sanford Guide to Antimicrobial Therapy.* Jeb C. Sanford; 2003:17, 18.

Jimenez C: Advantages of diagnostic nuclear medicine, Part 2. Physician Sports Med 1999;27(13):51.

Nusbaum MR: Sexually transmitted infections. In: Sloane PD, et al: *Essentials of Family Medicine,* 4th ed. Lippincott Williams & Wilkins; 2002:674–5.

---

57 Sore Throat

L. Peter Schwiebert, MD

KEY POINTS

- Most sore throats encountered in ambulatory family medicine are due to viruses or irritants.
- Clues to a diagnosis of strep throat include a temperature >38°C, absence of cough, tender anterior cervical adenopathy, or tonsillar exudate/swelling.
- Antibiotics are not indicated in most patients with sore throat.

I. **Definition.** Sore throat is a pharyngeal sensation of scratchiness or pain due to a wide spectrum of causes, including endogenous/exogenous irritants (eg, gastroesophageal reflux, allergens, tobacco smoke, low humidity) and infections (viral or bacterial).

II. **Common Diagnoses.** In ambulatory primary care, up to 8% of patient visits per year are for a sore throat. Common causes include:

A. **Irritants.** Thirty to 65% of individuals with sore throat have no specific causative pathogen. Irritants are causative in an undetermined number of these cases. Those at risk include smokers (tobacco is the most common environmental irritant), those whose clinical picture is compatible with allergies or gastroesophageal reflux disease (GERD) (see below), or who are exposed to irritants (eg, dust, low humidity, animals, textiles, solvents) in their environment.

B. **Viral infections** (30–60% of cases), including common cold viruses (rhinovirus, coronavirus, respiratory syncytial virus, parainfluenza virus); herpesvirus; adenovirus; coxsackievirus; and infectious mononucleosis (IM) viruses (cytomegalovirus and Epstein-Barr virus). Sore throat is more likely due to common cold viruses during community outbreaks in colder months of the year; adenoviral infections are frequent (up to 19%) causes of exudative pharyngitis in children younger than 6 years, and coxsackievirus infections are also most common in young children during the summer and fall. IM is most common in upper-socioeconomic-class adolescents (industrialized societies) living in close contact with one another (eg, students living in college dormitories).

C. **Group A β-hemolytic streptococcal infection (GABHS)** (5–10% of cases in adults and up to 30% of children). GABHS is most common in 5- to 15-year-olds during the winter/spring months and may, like other infections, occur as epidemics.

III. **Symptoms**

A. **Sore throat**

1. Scratchy, dry throat is most common with irritants or common cold viruses.

2. Painful sore throat with dysphagia is typical of streptococcal infection, IM, coxsackievirus, herpesvirus, or adenovirus.

B. **Other symptoms**

1. Patients with **allergies** classically present with paroxysms of sneezing, watery, itchy eyes, and rhinorrhea associated with exposure to the allergen, although these symptoms may be absent (see Chapters 54 and 55).

2. Individuals with sore throat due to **GERD** often give a history of heartburn/sour eructations, worsening symptoms after a large meal or with recumbency, associated nonproductive cough, and relief with over-the-counter histamine-2 blockers or antacids.

3. The presence of cough, rhinorrhea, conjunctivitis, or diarrhea decreases the likelihood of streptococcal infection and increases the likelihood of irritants, allergies, or viral infection.

4. Individuals with **streptococcal infection** may complain of associated symptoms of chills, malaise, headache, mild neck stiffness, and some gastrointestinal symptoms, though these symptoms are not specific for this diagnosis.

IV. **Signs.** Since GABHS pharyngitis is the only common cause of sore throat for which antibiotics are indicated and since sore throat and patient requests for antibiotic treatment are common, researchers have investigated clinical scoring systems to predict the likelihood of streptococcal infection. The best-known system is the Centor Strep Score, and McIsaac et al validated this scoring system in a family medicine population of children and adults (Table 57–1). (Also see the sidebars on epiglottitis, retropharyngeal abscess, peritonsillar abscess, and carotidynia.)

A. The ability of an individual symptom or sign to predict a diagnosis of strep throat is limited. For example:

1. **Exudative pharyngitis** also occurs with viral infections (53% of children younger than 6 years with this sign had adenoviral infection, as do 50% of patients with IM).

2. Fifty-six percent of pediatric patients with adenoviral infection present with fever and temperature >40 °C (104 °F); moderate to high fever is also associated with coxsackievirus and initial outbreaks of herpesvirus infections.

3. More than 90% of patients with IM have **cervical lymphadenopathy** (posterior chain).

B. **Other signs characteristic of common causes of sore throat. Coxsackievirus** infections are associated with erythematous-based small vesicles or ulcers in the pharynx and may be associated with similar papulovesicles on the palms and soles. The shallow, erythematous-based vesicles and ulcers of **herpesvirus** can occur anywhere on the pharynx, gingiva, or vermilion border.

TABLE 57–1. MCISAAC MODIFICATION OF THE CENTOR STREP SCORE

1. Add points for patient

Symptom or sign	Points
History of fever or measured temperature >38°C (100.4°F)	1
Absence of cough	1
Tender anterior cervical adenopathy	1
Tonsillar swelling or exudates	1
Age <15 years	1
Age ≥45 years	−1

2. Find risk of strep

Points	LR	% with Strep (patients with strep/total)
−1 or 0	0.05	1 (2/179)
1	0.52	10 (13/134)
2	0.95	17 (18/109)
3	2.5	35 (28/81)
4 or 5	4.9	51 (39/77)

EPIGLOTTITIS

Epiglottitis should be considered when there is a rapidly worsening sore throat, fever, muffled voice, and dysphagia. Epiglottitis is usually due to *Haemophilus influenzae* (but pediatric incidence of this organism has decreased due to Hib immunization, such that the incidence now peaks between ages 20 and 45 years); *Streptococcus pyogenes, Staphylococcus aureus,* or viruses may also be causative. Lateral neck radiographs are 90% sensitive and show an enlarged epiglottis ("thumb sign") with hypopharyngeal distention. Due to the danger of critical airway obstruction, suspected epiglottitis requires parental antibiotics in an intensive care setting where immediate intubation is available.

RETROPHARYNGEAL ABSCESS

Retropharyngeal abscess is a complication of infected retropharyngeal lymph nodes (usually due to GABHS) and is more common in pediatric than adult populations. Presenting symptoms of dysphagia and a lateral neck radiograph showing an increased prevertebral space are characteristic.

PERITONSILLAR ABSCESS

Peritonsillar abscess (quinsy), a suppurative complication of superficial tonsillitis, is most common in 20- to 40-year-olds and presents with worsening sore throat, fever, and dysphagia/odynophagia. Likely agents include *S pyogenes, S aureus, H influenzae,* or anaerobes. Examination reveals a muffled "hot potato" voice, trismus (difficulty opening the mouth), and an erythematous, swollen tonsil pushing the uvula to the opposite side. The gold standard for diagnosis is needle aspiration of pus from the abscess (should only be performed with proper training), and the currently recommended treatment is twice-daily clindamycin or a second- or third-generation cephalosporin.

CAROTIDYNIA

Carotidynia is an idiopathic inflammation of the carotid sheath and is a not-uncommon cause of "sore throat," which, on examination, is actually tenderness over the common carotid sheath. Carotidynia responds rapidly to nonsteroidal drugs (eg, indomethacin, 25–50 mg three times a day with food, continued 5–7 days or until symptoms resolve, whichever occurs first).

V. Laboratory Tests. Based on clinical findings alone, one can arrive at a presumptive diagnosis in many patients presenting with sore throat. In those with irritant exposure or a common cold viral infection, no further laboratory work-up of sore throat is indicated, and one can proceed with treatment.

   A. Streptococcal testing. A decision on which patients with pharyngitis should have a streptococcal screen depends on the physician's goals—minimizing total cost, minimizing risks associated with a missed diagnosis, or minimizing the cost of a missed diagnosis and unnecessary use of antibiotics. The following strategy, which is more cost-effective than mass screening but minimizes chances of missing a case of streptococcal pharyngitis, is recommended. A rapid streptococcal screen should be performed on patients with a sore throat and an intermediate pretest likelihood of streptococcal pharyngitis (Table 57–2).

   1. **Rapid streptococcal screen** is a 10-minute test for streptococcal antigens that has a sensitivity of 80–90% and a specificity of >90% for detection of streptococcal pharyngitis. Proper collection requires that the swab contact both tonsils or tonsillar fossae and the posterior pharyngeal wall. Because of its test characteristics and rapid turnaround time, it is the test of choice in confirming suspected streptococcal pharyngitis and should be used in patients with an intermediate pretest likelihood of this diagnosis (Table 57–2). With appropriate test selection, therapeutic decisions can confidently be based on a positive result. However, a negative screen result in the context of clinical suspicion of streptococcal pharyngitis should be followed up with blood agar plate (BAP) culture.

   2. **Throat culture.** The BAP culture is 95% sensitive and has a low false-positive rate in diagnosing streptococcal pharyngitis, but it requires 24 hours' incubation. BAP culture should be performed if rapid streptococcal screen result is negative with high suspicion of streptococcal infection or in high-risk, low-prevalence situations (Table 57–2).

   3. A **follow-up screen** to test for cure is not recommended or indicated in patients who respond clinically to antibiotic therapy within 5 days. However, in patients with a history of rheumatic fever, post-treatment cultures should be done to ensure eradication of GABHS.

   4. The **carrier state** (positive strep screen or BAP with low pretest likelihood or without GABHS antigenemia) usually represents low infectivity. In certain situations, the carrier state warrants treatment; these include a history of rheumatic fever, community outbreak of rheumatic fever or nephritogenic streptococcal infection, or "Ping-Pong" spread of GABHS in a family or other closed community, such as military barracks, prisons, or college dormitories.

   B. Heterophile antibody test. The Monospot test, which rapidly detects heterophile antibodies, compares favorably with the sensitivity and specificity of older heterophile antibody tests in diagnosing IM. A complete blood cell count (CBC) with differential smear

---

TABLE 57–2. TESTING PATIENTS WITH SORE THROAT BASED ON PRETEST LIKELIHOOD OF STREPTOCOCCAL PHARYNGITIS

Signs	Season	
	Winter/Spring	Summer/Fall
Temperature >38°C (101°F), enlarged erythematous tonsils with exudates, enlarged tender anterior cervical nodes	No testing necessary; begin treatment[1]	Rapid streptococcal screen[2]
Patient with two of the above signs, or all three signs with cough, rhinorrhea, or hoarseness	Rapid streptococcal screen[2]	Blood agar plate culture (BAP)
Patient with one of the three signs or with no signs but in a high-risk group[3]	BAP[4]	No testing necessary unless in a high-risk group[3]

[1]High pretest likelihood (>50%).
[2]Intermediate pretest likelihood (20–50%).
[3]Such patients include those who have diabetes mellitus, have a history of rheumatic fever, or present during a community outbreak of nephritogenic streptococcal infection.
[4]Low pretest likelihood (<20%).

showing at least 50% lymphocytes and at least 10% atypical lymphocytes also confirms this diagnosis.

C. **Other tests**

1. Though not common, *Neisseria gonorrhoeae* should be suspected in patients with pharyngitis and a history of oral-genital sexual relations; in such cases, pharyngeal, endocervical, and urethral cultures for gonorrhea and chlamydia should be done.

2. **Liver function tests,** including serum aspartate aminotransferase (AST) and serum alanine aminotransferase (ALT) as well as serum bilirubin, CBC, platelet count, and Coombs' test, should be performed in patients with IM. These patients are at risk for developing hepatitis, hemolytic anemia, granulocytopenia, and thrombocytopenia (see Chapter 45). Severe hepatitis is indicated by an ALT or AST of >1000 U/L or a serum bilirubin of >10 mg/dL.

VI. Treatment. Because 80–90% of cases of pharyngitis are caused by viruses or irritants, antibiotics are not indicated for most patients with this complaint. Despite this finding, studies have shown that antibiotics are prescribed for 75% of adults with acute pharyngitis. Dangers of this practice include unnecessary cost, possible allergic reaction, and development of resistant bacterial strains. To avoid these drawbacks, it is important to base antibiotic use on strict criteria and use nonantibiotic treatment in cases not meeting these criteria.

A. **Environmental irritants** should be avoided if possible. In particular, patients should be encouraged to stop smoking, avoid allergens or dusty environments, and humidify low-humidity environments. Treatment of allergies is discussed in Chapter 55, and management of GERD is discussed in Chapter 19.

B. **Viral infections** (eg, common cold, adenovirus, coxsackievirus, and herpesvirus) are self-limited, lasting from a few days to 2 weeks. Patients may obtain symptomatic relief with the following regimens.

1. **Topical pain relief** may be provided by as-needed lozenges (eg, Cepastat or Chloraseptic) or saline nasal spray or gargles, made by mixing $\frac{1}{4}$ tsp of salt in 4 oz of warm water. Oropharyngeal lesions of coxsackievirus or herpes simplex virus may benefit from viscous Xylocaine 2% or benzocaine 15%, applied to lesions every 3–4 hours with a cotton-tipped applicator; soothing rinses ($\frac{1}{4}$ tsp of baking soda in 4 oz of warm water or saline, swished orally, then expectorated three or four times daily); or a variety of coating agents (eg, diphenhydramine elixir, 12.5 mg/5 mL, mixed with an equal volume of either kaolin and pectin [Kaopectate] or aluminum-magnesium hydroxide antacid [Maalox], 1 tsp swished intraorally for 2 minutes every 2 hours).

2. **Fluid intake** should be increased to up to 2–3 quarts of water or juice per day.

3. **Analgesic drugs** include either aspirin, 650 mg every 4–6 hours orally in teenagers or adults, or acetaminophen, 5–10 mg/kg/day every 4–6 hours orally in children. Codeine relieves more severe discomfort; the dosage is 30–60 mg orally every 4–6 hours in adults or 3 mg/kg/day orally every 4–6 hours in children.

4. **Decongestants** (see Chapter 55).

C. **Streptococcal infections.** Antibiotic therapy instituted within 2–3 days of onset of symptoms hastens symptomatic improvement in patients with positive culture results or a high likelihood of streptococcal infection, as well as decreasing contagion (especially if the patient lives in close contact with others). The incidence of suppurative complications (eg, peritonsillar abscess) and immune complications (eg, glomerulonephritis) is low, regardless of whether antibiotics are used or not.

1. **Indications**

a. Patients with a positive result on rapid streptococcal screen, throat culture, or both.

b. Patients with a high probability of having streptococcal infection (Table 57–1).

c. Some clinicians initiate antibiotic therapy in high-risk patients pending throat culture results (see section V,A,2), although studies have demonstrated that delaying therapy for 48 hours does not interfere with the antibiotic's reduction in risk of rheumatic fever.

2. **Regimens**

a. **Penicillin** is the drug of choice (in non–penicillin-allergic patients); there is no evidence of resistance (eg, resurgence of rheumatic fever due to lower rates of GABHS elimination by penicillin).

(1) **Oral penicillin V potassium,** 500 mg two to three times daily for 10 days, is the treatment for adults; children should receive 30–50 mg/kg/day in two or three divided doses, also for 10 days.

    (2) Penicillin G benzathine may be preferred for patients in whom compliance with the oral regimen or follow-up is questionable. Adults and children weighing >27 kg (60 lb) should receive 1.2 million U intramuscularly, and those weighing <27 kg should receive 600,000 U. A mixture of 900,000 U of benzathine and 300,000 U of procaine penicillin (eg, **Bicillin C-R**) is also effective and causes less local reaction than penicillin G benzathine alone.

  b. Erythromycin (eg, Ery-Tab, Eryc, or E-Mycin) is the drug of choice for penicillin-allergic patients. Adults should receive 500 mg orally twice daily for 10 days. The pediatric dosage is 30–50 mg/kg/day, given in two or four divided doses. Another macrolide, **azithromycin** (eg, Zithromax), 500 mg orally on day 1 and 250 mg on days 2–5, is also effective for adults; the dosage for pediatric patients older than 2 years is 12 mg/kg/day for 5 days.

  c. The following oral **5-day regimens** have proved clinically and bacteriologically comparable to 10 days' penicillin V in a large pediatric study: **amoxicillin/clavulanate** (eg, Augmentin) three times daily at 37.5 mg/kg/day (maximum, 1875 mg/day); ceftibuten (eg, Cedax) daily at 9 mg/kg/day (maximum 400 mg/day); **cefarixone axetil** (eg, Ceftin) twice daily at 20 mg/kg/day (maximum 500 mg/day); **loracarbef** (eg, Lorabid) twice daily at 15 mg/kg/day (maximum 400 mg/day); or **clarithromycin** (eg, Biaxin) twice daily at 15 mg/kg/day (maximum, 500 mg/day). Shorter regimens may improve compliance; disadvantages include higher cost and broader spectrum, which may foster bacterial resistance.

3. Follow-up

  a. Failure to improve. Antibiotic therapy should improve symptoms within 12–24 hours; persistence of symptoms for a week after initiation of antibiotics may be due to noncompliance with the drug regimen, penicillin tolerance, destruction of penicillin by β-lactamase–producing organisms, missed diagnosis, or an undiagnosed second cause of pharyngitis, particularly IM. In addition to evaluating for noncompliance, the following may help:

    (1) Appropriate tests for IM should be performed (see sections V,B and C).

    (2) Antibiotic regimens for penicillin tolerance should be instituted. **Amoxicillin-clavulanate potassium** (eg, Augmentin), 500–875 mg orally twice daily (adults) or 40 mg/kg/day orally in three divided doses (children); or a cephalosporin (eg, **cefadroxil,** 1 g orally in one dose for adults or 30 mg/kg/day orally in two doses for children) have been shown to be effective in eradicating streptococci in those patients who do not respond to repeated courses of oral penicillin.

  b. Recurrent episodes of acute pharyngitis raise the issue of whether **acute streptococcal pharyngitis** or **acute viral pharyngitis with streptococcal carrier state** is occurring. **Viral pharyngitis** is suggested by clinical or epidemiologic findings consistent with viral infection, failure to improve on antistreptococcal antibiotics, no rise in antistreptolysin-O (ASO) titers, or positive throat cultures between episodes of pharyngitis. **Acute recurrent streptococcal infection** is suggested by appropriate clinical or epidemiologic findings, dramatic response to antibiotic therapy, a rise in ASO titers, or negative throat cultures between episodes of acute pharyngitis.

  c. When eradication of the carrier state is appropriate (see section V,A,4), the following regimens are effective: clindamycin (eg, Cleocin), 20 mg/kg/day orally in three doses for 10 days, OR rifampin (Rifadin), 20 mg/kg/day orally in two doses for 4 days, *plus* the standard regimen of phenoxymethyl *or* penicillin G benzathine.

4. IM

  a. Ninety-five percent of patients with **IM** recover uneventfully, and supportive treatment will suffice. Such therapy includes avoidance of contact sports or heavy lifting in the first 2–3 weeks of illness (especially if the patient has splenomegaly), adequate rest, and analgesics (see section VI,B,3).

  b. Corticosteroids may be necessary in the following circumstances: impending airway obstruction, severe hepatitis, thrombocytopenia, hemolytic anemia, or granulocytopenia. Treatment should be initiated with prednisone (or any equivalent), 60–80 mg/day orally in divided doses, tapered over 1–2 weeks.

REFERENCES

Adam D, Scholz H, Helmerkung M: Short-course antibiotic treatment of 4782 culture-proven cases of group A streptococcal tonsillopharyngitis and incidence of poststreptococcal sequelae. J Infect Dis 2000;**182**:509.

Bisno AL: Acute pharyngitis. N Engl J Med 2001;**344**:205.

Ebell MH, et al: Does this patient have strep throat? JAMA 2000;**284**:2912.

Hayes CS, Williams H Jr: Management of group A beta-hemolytic streptococcal pharyngitis. Am Fam Physician 2001;**63**:1557.

McIsaac WJ, et al: The validity of a sore throat score in family practice. CMAJ 2000;**163**:811.

Ressel G: Principles of appropriate antibiotic use: Part IV. Acute pharyngitis. Am Fam Physician 2001;**64**(5):870.

---

58   Syncope

Dennis P. Lewis, MD, Brian H. Halstater, MD, & Felix Horng, MD, MBA

KEY POINTS

- Most syncope is from neurally mediated reflex mechanisms (eg, vasovagal or situational).
- Cardiac syncope is associated with a much higher 1-year mortality than all other types and its detection is the primary focus of laboratory evaluation.
- Most patients with syncope (ie, those without identified cerebrovascular or cardiac causes) can be effectively managed by the primary care physician.

I. **Definition.** Syncope is a simultaneous loss of consciousness and postural tone due to cerebral hypoperfusion, which can occur with interruption of cerebral blood flow for as few as 6–8 seconds. This can be due to decreased cardiac output, cerebrovascular disease, or neurally mediated reflexes. **Decreased cardiac output** can be from hypovolemia, structural heart disease, or arrhythmias. **Neurally indicated syncope** results from reflex decrease in heart rate, blood pressure, or both.

Syncope is a symptom, not a disease, and must be differentiated from conditions that may at first appear to be syncope. Nonsyncopal disorders that may present with real or apparent loss of consciousness include seizure disorders, psychogenic "syncope," and metabolic disorders such as hypoglycemia or hyponatremia.

II. **Common Diagnoses** (Table 58–1). At least 3% of the population will have a syncopal event within a 26-year period, and of those patients, 30% will have a recurrence. The prevalence of syncope increases with age, and the annual incidence in the elderly approaches 6%. In the United States, syncope accounts for approximately 3% of emergency room visits and 6% of hospital admissions annually. Approximately 1 million patients are evaluated for syncope each year, at a cost of $750 million. Syncope can be classified as **neurally mediated, cardiac, cerebrovascular, miscellaneous differentiated causes,** and **idiopathic** (unknown cause). Roughly half of syncope is either cardiac or neurally mediated, although multiple causes may coexist. A Mayo Clinic study of 987 syncopal patients referred to an electrophysiologic studies service revealed multiple causes in 18.4%, with an increased likelihood of multiple causes in the elderly, those with atrial fibrillation, those taking cardiac medications, or those in New York Heart Association classes II–IV.

  A. **Neurally mediated** reflex syncope accounts for 20–58% of syncope.
   1. **Vasovagal syncope** accounts for most reflex syncope.
   2. **Situational syncope** is similar, but beta or calcium channel blockers, angiotensin-converting enzyme inhibitors, sedatives, alcohol, or other central nervous system depressants may contribute to **situational syncope.**

  B. **Cardiac syncope** (9–23% of cases) has a higher mortality rate than all other etiologies (20–30% at 1 year, compared to 6% for all other etiologies).

TABLE 58–1. DIFFERENTIAL DIAGNOSIS OF SYNCOPE

Category	Risk Factors	Symptoms	Signs	Testing
Neurally mediated vasovagal	Young women; exposure to stress, pain, enclosed space	Unpleasant stimulus Prodrome (nausea/lightheadedness/ palpitations/tunnel vision/warmth) Syncope	Examination is noncontributory	ECG, tilt-table testing
Neurally mediated situational	Elderly, autonomic dysfunction, dehydration, prolonged recumbency, certain medications	Preceded by micturition/cough/ swallow/defecation	Orthostatic hypotension	ECG
Neurally mediated carotid sinus	Elderly, atherosclerotic disease	Syncope after head rotation/neck extension	Hypotension or ventr. Asystole with carotid sinus massage	ECG
Cardiac—arrhythmia	Sick sinus, A–V block medications, pacemaker malfunction; recent MI, supra- or ventricular tachycardia, WPW	No prodrome, occurrence while supine	Often normal; may note irregular heart rhythm	ECG, Holter monitor, ambulatory loop ECG
Cardiac—structural	VHD, FHx sudden unexplained cardiac death	Occurrence with exertion, change in position, acute shortness of breath	Heart murmur, signs of CHF	ECG, echocardiogram, Holter monitor, EP testing
Cerebrovascular	HTN, dyslipidemia, diabetes mellitus, old age, cigarette use	Vertigo, dysarthria, diplopia; excessive arm exercise	Carotid bruit, focal neurologic deficit, asymmetric upper extremity BPs	ECG, Consider carotid Doppler; EEG if seizure-like activity; brain CT or MRI for focal deficits
Miscellaneous differentiated	20–40 yr old with frequent "fainting," alcohol abuse	Anxiety or depression; multiple somatic complaints	Normal examination or signs of anxiety/depression	ECG
Idiopathic		Absence of classic symptoms of other types of syncope	No specific findings	ECG, Holter monitor

A–V, atrioventricular; BP, blood pressure; CHF, congestive heart failure; CT, computerized tomographic scan; ECG, electrocardiogram; EEG, electroencephalogram; EP, electrophysiologic; FHx, family history; HTN, hypertension; MI, myocardial infarction; MRI, magnetic resonance imaging; VHD, valvular heart disease; WPW, Wolff-Parkinson-White syndrome.

1. **Arrhythmia** underlies most cardiac syncope.
   a. Risk factors for **bradyarrhythmia** include use of certain medications that delay atrioventricular (A-V) conduction (commonly beta and calcium channel blockers).
   b. Risk factors for **tachyarrhythmia** include use of certain medications that increase A-V conduction (pseudophedrine and other stimulants, both legal and illicit).
2. In patients with no known **structural heart disease,** a family history of unexplained sudden cardiac death increases the likelihood of hypertrophic obstructive cardiomyopathy.

C. **Cerebrovascular syncope** (2–3% of syncope) most commonly results from vertebrobasilar artery insufficiency, transient ischemic attack (TIA), stroke (cerebrovascular accident, or CVA), or subclavian steal syndrome. Risk factors for **subclavian steal syndrome** are the same as for CVA and TIA, but also include vigorous use of an upper extremity, and, when it occurs in younger populations, a congenital anatomic variant.
D. **Miscellaneous differentiated causes** most commonly include psychiatric disorders (roughly 2% of all syncope).
E. Eighteen to 60% of cases of syncope are considered **idiopathic.**

III. **Symptoms** (Table 58–1). A careful history is essential to accurate assessment of syncope. This should include patient age, details of the syncopal event (timing and onset of the syncope, association with activity, presence of associated symptoms such as palpitations or chest pain), and previous occurrences and circumstances surrounding these episodes. Risk factor assessment should include chronic diseases, family history, and medication use/substance abuse (see section II).
A. **Neurally mediated reflex syncope**
   1. **Vasovagal syncope** typically occurs after a sudden unexpected, usually unpleasant sight, smell, or sound, or with pain or fear. Vasovagal syncope also occurs with prolonged standing.
   2. **Situational syncope** may have the same premonitory symptoms as vasovagal syncope.
B. **Cardiac syncope.** In **structural heart disease,** the history commonly reveals an association with acute shortness of breath or chest pain (pulmonary embolism, myocardial infarction). This type of syncope may also occur with **exertion** (aortic stenosis, pulmonary hypertension, mitral stenosis, hypertrophic obstructive cardiomyopathy, coronary artery disease) or with a **change of position** such as lying down/bending over/turning over in bed (atrial myxoma or thrombus).

IV. **Signs** (Table 58–1). Physical examination should focus on the **cardiovascular** and **neurologic** systems. Vital signs should be recorded, including bilateral supine and standing blood pressures and pulses. Cyanosis or pallor should be noted. Cardiopulmonary auscultation should be performed and carotid/peripheral pulses palpated. Neurologic examination should include orientation and cranial nerves, motor, sensory, and cerebellar testing (gait and Romberg testing). A digital rectal examination should be performed for occult blood.
A. **Neurally mediated syncope**
   1. **Situational.** In patients with **orthostatic hypotension,** standing in place for 2–5 minutes decreases systolic blood pressure ≥20 mm Hg, diastolic blood pressure ≥10 mm Hg, or both. Volume-depleted patients may also manifest a postural increase in heart rate of ≥30 beats per minute.
   2. In **carotid sinus hypersensitivity,** 5–10 seconds of carotid sinus massage produces ventricular asystole for ≥3 seconds or fall in systolic pressure of ≥50 mm Hg. This maneuver should not be done if carotid bruits are present, if the patient has a history of ventricular tachycardia, or with recent stroke or myocardial infarction. A false-positive test may occur in the absence of historical risk factors for carotid sinus hypersensitivity.
B. **Cardiac syncope.** With **structural heart disease,** cardiac examination is less likely to be normal than with arrhythmia-induced syncope. Auscultation may reveal murmurs of mitral regurgitation/aortic stenosis/hypertrophic obstructive cardiomyopathy, or murmurs with change in position such as lying down/bending over/turning over in bed (suggestive of atrial myxoma/thrombus), or findings of pulmonary hypertension (right ventricular lift, loud P2, prominent A-wave in jugular venous pulse).
C. In **cerebrovascular syncope,** carotid bruit may be noted (indicating significant generalized atherosclerosis), **focal neurologic deficit** may be uncovered (after a CVA, but possibly absent after a TIA), or an **asymmetric blood pressure or pulse** between upper extremities may be noted (suggesting subclavian steal syndrome or aortic dissection). In

patients at risk, upper extremity activity could reveal pulse discrepancy between extremities (subclavian steal syndrome).

V. Laboratory Tests (Table 58–1). A systematic history and examination alone can elucidate the cause of syncope in up to 75% of cases. Since **cardiac syncope** has a 20–30% 1-year mortality compared with 6% for all other causes, testing is directed at differentiating cardiac from noncardiac causes.

In one prospective study, a limited evaluation (hematocrit, serum creatinine kinase, glucose, electrocardiogram [ECG], carotid massage, orthostatic blood pressure, and evaluation of pulses) yielded a diagnosis in 76% of patients with syncope. Pregnancy testing should also routinely be performed in women of childbearing age at risk for pregnancy. Further testing (Holter monitor, echocardiography, ambulatory loop ECG, and tilt-table testing) produced a diagnosis in only an additional 5% of patients.

A. All patients with syncope should have an **ECG** even though the diagnostic yield is low (5%), since the test is essentially risk-free and relatively inexpensive. In addition to revealing certain structural heart diseases (eg, previous myocardial infarction (MI) or left ventricular hypertrophy), ECG is primarily helpful in uncovering arrhythmogenic causes of syncope, including **long QT interval, conduction delay/block, bundle branch block, fascicle block** (possible bradycardia); atrial and ventricular **ectopy** (nonspecific indicator of arrhythmogenic substrate); **bradycardia** (nonspecific indicator of conduction system disease); and **ventricular pre-excitation/delta wave** (Wolff-Parkinson-White syndrome).

B. An **echocardiogram** is recommended in all patients whose evaluation is suggestive (eg, for valvular heart disease with auscultated murmur or for hypertrophic cardiomyopathy with history of exertional syncope).

C. Stress testing (eg, exercise treadmill testing or stress echocardiography) is indicated in syncopal patients whose history and risk factors suggest ischemic heart disease.

D. 24-hour Holter monitoring is recommended in suspected arrhythmogenic syncope (eg, syncope without prodrome or syncope preceded by palpitations) and with suspected structural heart disease, abnormal ECG, or syncope of unknown cause.

E. Long-term ambulatory loop ECG is a noninvasive method of cardiac monitoring indicated in syncopal patients with a structurally normal heart but abnormal ECG or 24-hour Holter monitor.

F. Referral to a cardiac electrophysiologist for **intracardiac electrophysiologic studies** is indicated in syncope with structural heart disease (eg, history of MI, congestive heart failure, cardiomyopathy, coronary artery anomaly), identified arrhythmogenic syncope (eg, Wolff-Parkinson-White or long Q-T syndrome, ventricular tachycardia, refractory sinus bradycardia/A-V block or supraventricular tachycardia); and also for exertional syncope, syncope with family history of sudden death, and syncope whose cause remains unclear despite less invasive testing.

G. Tilt-table testing is recommended in patients with unexplained recurrent syncope in whom cardiac causes of syncope, including arrhythmias, have been excluded. An abnormal result suggests vasovagal syncope, but reproducibility and yield are highly variable. Some centers recommend pregnancy testing in women of childbearing age, and stress testing in men older than 45 years and women older than 55 years, with positive/abnormal tests precluding tilt-table testing.

H. Neurologic testing should be reserved for patients with neurologic signs or symptoms or carotid bruits.

    1. Carotid or transcranial Doppler ultrasonography is indicated for bruits or with suggested vertebrobasilar insufficiency (prolonged loss of consciousness, diplopia, nausea, or hemiparesis).

    2. Focal neurologic signs mandate brain imaging, usually with **computerized tomography (CT)** or **magnetic resonance imaging (MRI).**

    3. With evidence of seizure activity, **electroencephalography (EEG)** may be useful. Cardiac syncope evaluation (see section V,A–F) should be done in patients with seizure activity, normal EEG, and no postictal symptoms, as well as patients with seizures unresponsive to anticonvulsants.

VI. Treatment of syncope is directed at the underlying cause. The prognosis is very good (6% 1-year mortality) even without intervention in those with noncardiac syncope; in cardiac syncope, identification and treatment of underlying causes can reduce the 20–30% 1-year mortality.

A. Hospitalization is indicated for patients with syncope who have known or suspected cardiac ischemia or arrhythmia, structural heart disease, cardiopulmonary circulatory disease (pulmonary embolus, pulmonary hypertension, atrial myxoma), or stroke. Hospitalization should be considered for diagnostic evaluation of syncope with known or suspected significant heart disease, ECG abnormalities suggesting arrhythmogenic syncope, syncope occurring while supine or with exertion, associated severe injury, family history of sudden death, frequent recurrences, or age older than 60 years.

B. **Cardiology consultation** is indicated for syncope with underlying structural or valvular heart disease, or underlying coronary artery disease. The multicenter automatic defibrillator implantation trial II (MADIT-II) study suggests that patients with a history of MI and ejection fraction <30% have reduced mortality with automatic defibrillator implantation, regardless of electrophysiologic study results. Cardiology consultation for consideration of pacemaker implantation may benefit patients with carotid sinus hypersensitivity and a systole or carotid sinus massage.

C. **Neurologic consultation** is indicated for those suspected of a seizure disorder or TIA.

D. **Vascular surgery** consultation for carotid endarterectomy is clearly beneficial in symptomatic patients with ≥70% carotid artery stenosis and may also benefit those symptomatic with 50–65% stenosis. Benefits of endarterectomy vs. aspirin therapy are unclear in asymptomatic individuals with significant (>60%) stenosis; such patients have a 10–15% CVA risk over the ensuing 3–5 years.

E. **Psychiatric evaluation** should be considered in young, otherwise healthy patients who faint frequently without any associated injury and in patients presenting with many unassociated nonspecific symptoms such as nausea, lightheadedness, numbness, fear, and dread.

F. **Neurally mediated reflex syncope (situational, vasovagal, or carotid sinus hypersensitivity)**
  1. Patients should be counseled to:
     a. Avoid situations that may trigger fainting, such as hot, crowded rooms or prolonged standing.
     b. Avoid stressful events that predispose to fainting, such as venipuncture in the upright position, or exposure to blood, pain, fear, or highly emotional settings.
     c. Avoid dehydration, ensure adequate fluid and salt intake with proper attire (possibly compression hose), and provide ventilation, especially during exercise.
     d. Minimize situations that trigger syncope, such as coughing excessively or wearing tight collars.
     e. Be aware of warning signs, such as feeling nauseated, sweaty, dizzy, or lightheaded, and sit or lie down to prevent loss of consciousness.
  2. Additional helpful measures include:
     a. Discontinuing, if possible, medications (eg, vasodilating antihypertensives) that increase susceptibility to fainting spells.
     b. Considering pharmacotherapy for syncope resistant to the foregoing; such therapy may include salt tablets; fludrocortisone, 0.1–0.2 mg orally daily; vasoconstrictors (ephedrine, 15–30 mg, or midodrine, 2.5–10 mg orally three times daily), beta blockers (eg, metoprolol starting at 50 mg orally twice daily); anticholinergic agents (eg, transdermal scopolamine, 1.5 mg changed every 3 days); and selective serotonin reuptake inhibitors (eg, fluoxetine, starting at 20 mg orally daily).
  3. In **orthostatic hypotension,** treatment is directed at the underlying disorder (eg, dehydration, medications, endocrine disorders, or neuropathies). In many cases, rising slowly and crossing the legs while standing, combined with use of compression stockings, is helpful. Potentially, beneficial pharmacotherapy in refractory cases includes fludrocortisone, ephedrine, midodrine (see section VI,F,2,b), theophylline (starting at 300 mg/day orally in two to three doses), or caffeine.

G. If a thorough history, physical examination, ECG, and other appropriate tests fail to suggest a cause, the patient should be counseled to return for further evaluation if syncope recurs.

REFERENCES

Farwell D, Sulke N: How do we diagnose syncope: J Cardiovasc Electrophysiol 2002;**13**(suppl):S9.

Goldschlager N: Approach to the patient with syncope: History and physical are key. Adv Stud Med 2003;**3**(5):265.

Goldschlager N, et al: Etiologic considerations in the patient with syncope and an apparently normal heart. Arch Intern Med 2003;**163:**151.

Kapoor WN: Current evaluation and management of syncope. Circulation 2002;**106**:1606.
Kenny RA, et al: Carotid sinus syndrome: A modifiable risk factor for nonaccidental falls in older adults (SAFE PACE). J Am Coll Cardiol 2001;**38**:1491.
Soteriades ES, et al: Incidence and prognosis of syncope. N Engl J Med 2002;**347**:878.
Task Force on Syncope, European Society of Cardiology. Guidelines on management (diagnosis and treatment) of syncope. Eur Heart J 2001;**22**:1256.

---

59   Tremors & Other Movement Disorders

Goutham Rao, MD

KEY POINTS

- The systematic evaluation of tremor should include a thorough history to identify age at onset, rate of progression, family history of tremor, symptoms of complex disease syndromes of which tremor is a part (Wilson's disease), and identification of precipitants (eg, certain medications). The physical examination should identify key features of the tremor (eg, rest or action) and other signs of complex disease syndromes (eg, bradykinesia in patients with Parkinson's disease).
- Levodopa alone or in combination with a COMT inhibitor, and dopamine agonists alone or in combination with levodopa, are acceptable forms of pharmacotherapy for patients with Parkinson's disease who are functionally impaired.
- Propanolol and primidone are both effective treatments for essential tremor.

I. **Definition.** A **movement disorder** is any condition that disrupts normal voluntary movements of the body or one that consists of one or more abnormal movements. Movement disorders characterized by overall slowness of movement are classified as **hypokinesias;** those characterized by extra or exaggerated movements are classified as **hyperkinesias.** Tremors are the most common hyperkinesias.

    Tremor can be defined as a rhythmical, involuntary oscillatory movement of one or more body parts. A practical classification system divides tremors into rest tremors and action tremors. **Rest tremors** occur in a body part that is not voluntarily activated and is fully supported by gravity. **Action tremors** appear when muscles are voluntarily contracted. Action tremors can be further divided into **postural tremors** (tremor that occurs while maintaining a position against gravity) and **kinetic tremors** (tremor occurring during voluntary movement). There are four principal types of kinetic tremors. This typological classification is outlined in Table 59–1.

TABLE 59–1. TYPOLOGICAL CLASSIFICATION OF TREMORS

Rest Tremor	Tremor occurring in a body part that is not voluntarily activated and is supported completely against gravity.		
Action Tremors	Postural tremor		Tremor that occurs while voluntarily maintaining a position against gravity.
	Kinetic tremors (Tremor occurring during any voluntary movement)	(1) Simple kinetic tremor	Tremor occurring during voluntary movements that are not target-directed.
		(2) Intention tremor	Tremor whose amplitude increases during visually guided movements (eg, finger-to-nose test).
		(3) Task-specific kinetic tremor	Tremor that appears or is exacerbated by specific tasks (eg, writing).
		(4) Isometric tremor	Tremor that occurs during voluntary muscle contraction against a rigid stationary object (eg, squeezing examiner's hand).

II. Common Diagnoses. The prevalence of tremor varies by disease and by population. The list of causes of tremor is very long. A useful starting point is to be able to distinguish among the three most common causes of tremor (Table 59–2). (Also see the sidebars on tic disorders, chorea, myoclonus, dystonia, Wilson's disease, and ataxia.)

    A. Essential tremor is the most common of all movement disorders. It affects 1.3–5% of people older than 60 years. A family history of tremor is common among affected patients. Alcohol may temporarily attenuate essential tremor.

    B. Parkinson's disease has several characteristic features and affects 1% of those older than age 65 and 2% of those older than 85. Most patients have tremor.

    C. Physiologic tremor is present in all subjects to differing degrees. It can be enhanced by stimulants such as caffeine, nicotine, and some illicit drugs as well as medications such as bronchodilators, lithium, neuroleptics, valproate sodium, and tricyclic antidepressants.

III. Symptoms. The evaluation of a patient with first presentation of tremor begins with a thorough history that includes age at onset, rate of progression, and family history of tremor, medication history, and history of neurologic symptoms other than tremor.

    A. Both essential tremor and the tremor of Parkinson's disease usually begin after age 50 and are progressive in severity.

    B. Enhanced physiologic tremor may appear at any age and does not progress in severity.

    C. Associated symptoms

        1. In addition to tremor, patients with Parkinson's disease may present with bradykinesia (slowness of movement) and rigidity. Such patients may complain of loss of balance and difficulty with tasks such as turning in bed, rising from a chair, and opening jars.

        2. Hyperthyroidism may "enhance" physiologic tremor among patients with other features of the disease such as heat intolerance and weight loss.

IV. Signs. The focused history should be followed by a physical examination with the goal of (1) identifying the key features of the tremor and (2) identifying features other than tremor that can help establish the diagnosis. A useful first step is to determine if the tremor occurs at rest or during action. A **rest tremor** can be observed by having the patient position his hands on his lap. Postural tremor can be elicited by holding up an arm against gravity. A **kinetic tremor** may be apparent during purposeful movements such as using a spoon, writing, performing a finger-to-nose test, or squeezing an examiner's hand.

    A. Parkinson's disease. Obvious tremor at rest should raise suspicion of Parkinson's disease. Other common signs of this disease should be elicited.

        1. Rigidity can be detected by passively flexing and extending the patient's elbow several times. Resistance to movement can be smooth or interrupted (cog wheeling).

        2. Bradykinesia can be detected by asking the patient to perform any one of a number of repetitive movements such as tapping the fingers or pinching the index finger and thumb repetitively. Obvious slowness in performing such maneuvers increases the likelihood of Parkinson's disease.

        3. The **glabella tap reflex** is tested by percussing the patient's forehead. The orbicularis oculi muscle reflexively contracts, causing both eyes to blink. The blinking normally stops after 5–10 repeated taps. Persistence of blinking is a positive test (Myerson's sign) and is more common among patients with Parkinson's disease.

        4. A sample of writing in a patient with Parkinson's disease may reveal **micrographia** (writing that becomes smaller across a page).

        5. Late in the course of disease, many patients develop **postural instability.** It becomes difficult for patients to maintain a particular posture. Asking a patient to

TABLE 59–2. THREE COMMON TREMOR SYNDROMES

Tremor of Parkinson's Disease	Slow frequency (4–6 per second) tremor at rest. Tremor inhibited during movement and sleep. Aggravated by emotional and physical stress. "Pill rolling quality."
Classic Essential Tremor	Bilateral, usually symmetric postural or kinetic tremor. Family history of tremor is common. Attenuated by alcohol.
Physiologic Tremor	Present to differing degrees in all normal subjects. Enhanced form is easily visible, mainly postural, and has a high frequency (8–12 per second). No evidence of underlying neurologic disease. Cause is usually reversible (eg, caffeine).

History:

Inquire about age at onset, rate of progression, family history of tremor. If age of onset > 21 years, consider primary dystonia or Wilson's disease. Lack of progression suggests enhanced physiologic tremor. Family history of tremor suggests essential tremor.

↓

Inquire about use of medications, stimulants, illicit drugs, and alcohol—all secondary causes of tremor.

↓

Inquire about other symptoms of tremor syndromes and medical illnesses (eg, bradykinesia in patients with Parkinson's disease, symptoms of hyperthyroidism.)

Physical Examination:

Determine key characteristics of tremor: amplitude, frequency, when it occurs (rest, postural kinetic).

↓

If rest tremor, assess for other signs of Parkinson's disease: bradykinesia detected by slowness of repetitive movements, rigidity of extremities, positive glabella tap test, and festination.

FIGURE 59–1. Systematic approach to the evaluation of tremor.

walk may reveal a tendency to fall or involuntary acceleration forward or backward (festination.)

B. Figure 59–1 outlines a rational approach to systematic evaluation of tremor.

V. Treatment. Therapy for most forms of tremor should target the underlying cause. Specific treatment for Parkinson's disease and essential tremor is discussed below.

A. **Parkinson's disease** (Table 59–3). Pharmacological therapy has been shown to reduce morbidity and mortality but requires careful monitoring to determine the optimal dosage.

1. *Neuroprotective* protective therapy is designed to slow or stop disease progression. The monoamine oxidase B inhibitor (MAO-B) **selegiline** has been shown to delay functional impairment and disease progression. It is unclear whether this is secondary to its neuroprotective effect or its effect on symptoms, which may mask disease progression. **Rasaligine,** another MAO-B inhibitor, is now being studied as a neuroprotective agent.

2. Most patients with Parkinson's disease are treated with *symptomatic* therapy when they begin to experience functional impairment. Factors to consider before instituting symptomatic therapy include whether the patient's symptoms affect the patient's dominant hand, whether symptoms interfere with work or other activities, and which features of Parkinson's disease are present. Bradykinesia, for example, is usually more disabling than tremor.

    There are currently three commonly used types of symptomatic therapy.

    a. The dopamine precursor **levodopa** is the most widely used and effective drug. To prevent its conversion to dopamine outside the blood-brain barrier, it is combined with the decarboxylase inhibitor, **carbidopa.** Levodopa is associated with serious adverse effects that increase in severity with prolonged use. These include nausea, vomiting, anorexia, orthostatic hypotension, cardiac arrythmias, and psychosis.

    b. Even when combined with carbidopa, only 10% of levodopa reaches the brain. Much of it is converted to an inert metabolite by the enzyme catechol-*O*-methyl transferase (COMT). The COMT inhibitors **tolcapone** and **entacapone** can be administered with levodopa to increase its effectiveness.

TABLE 59–3. AVAILABLE PHARMACOTHERAPY FOR PARKINSON'S DISEASE

Type of Therapy	Class	Agent	Trade Name(s)	Starting Dose	Titration/Maximum Dose/ Special Instructions
Neuroprotective	Monoamine oxidase B inhibitor	Selegiline	Eldepril, Deprenyl	5 mg orally twice daily	5 mg orally twice daily
Symptomatic	Dopamine precursor	Carbidopa-levodopa	Sinemet, Sinemet CR	Carbidopa 25 mg/ levodopa 100 mg two to four times daily	Carbidopa 200 mg/ levodopa 2000 mg per day
	COMT inhibitors	Tolcapone	Tasmar	100 mg–200 mg three times daily	Consider ↓ levodopa dose upon initiation of tolcapone
		Entacapone	Comtan	200 mg orally with each dose of carbidopa-levodopa	1600 mg/day
	Dopamine agonists	Bromocriptine	Parlodel	1.25 mg orally twice daily	Increase by 2.5 mg/day every 2–4 weeks to maximum of 90 mg per day.
		Pergolide	Permax	0.05 mg orally once daily	Increase by 0.1 or 0.15 mg/day every 3 days for first 12 days and by 0.25 mg/day every 3 days until optimal therapeutic response attained. Maximum dosage is 5 mg/day
		Pramipexole	Mirapex	0.125 mg orally three times daily	Increase by 0.375 mg/ day every 5–7 days until optimal therapeutic response attained. Maximum dosage is 4.5 mg/day

COMT, catechol-*o*-methyltransferase.

    c. The third class of available pharmacotherapy is the dopamine agonists such as **bromocriptine, pergolide,** and **pramipexole.** They stimulate dopamine receptors and have a very favorable side effect profile. Dopamine agonists can be used for initial symptomatic therapy or as adjuncts to therapy with levodopa.
    3. Surgical treatment of Parkinson's disease is emerging as an effective option for patients in whom pharmacotherapy fails.
        a. **Ablation** of tissue in specific areas of the brain including the ventral intermediate nucleus of the thalamus (Vim nucleus) and globus pallidus pars interna (Gpi) with radio waves, heat, or chemicals is associated with significant improvement.
        b. **Deep brain stimulation** of the Vim nucleus, Gpi, or subthalamic nucleus with an electrode connected to a pulse generator placed subcutaneously over the chest wall is also effective.
        c. **Transplantation of fetal dopaminergic neurons** into the substantia nigra has shown some promise but remains a controversial and experimental procedure.
    4. **Supportive care** is an important component of management. The clinical manifestations of the disease itself are frequently accompanied by a profound psychological and social impact. Depression and insomnia are common among patients

with Parkinson's disease. Stress among caregivers is a significant concern. Health care providers should be sensitive to these problems. Patients with Parkinson's disease and their families should also receive counseling about the clinical features, prognosis, and impact of the disease. A number of support groups are helpful in this regard.

B. Essential tremor

1. Mild essential tremor need not be treated if it causes no functional impairment. Functional impairment as assessed by the severity of symptoms and ability to perform daily tasks (eg, writing, buttoning) should always be used as a guide to initiate or adjust therapy. Careful monitoring for side effects of medications is essential.

2. **Pharmacological therapy**

   a. The beta blocker **propanolol (Inderal)** and the anticonvulsant **primidone (Mysoline)** are used as first-line treatments for more severe tremor. Both are roughly equally effective. Propanolol is initiated at a dose of 20–40 mg orally twice daily. Maintenance doses are usually 120–320 mg per day. Patients on propanolol should be carefully monitored for side effects of fatigue, headaches, bradycardia, impotence, and depression. Primidone should be started at a dose of 25 mg orally once daily and slowly increased as needed to a maximum of 750 mg per day given in three divided doses. Long-term treatment with primidone is well tolerated, but some patients will have an acute reaction consisting of nausea, vomiting, or ataxia.

   b. The anticonvulsant **gabapentin (Neurontin)** is also effective, but experience with it as a treatment for essential tremor is limited. It can be initiated at a dose of 100 mg orally once daily and increased until tremor is under good control to a maximum of 2400 mg a day (divided into three doses).

   c. Other classes of medications including benzodiazepines, calcium channel blockers, and theophylline should not be routinely used.

TIC DISORDERS

A tic is a brief, intermittent, repetitive, nonrhythmic, unpredictable, purposeless movement or sound. Tics are preceded by a conscious urge to execute them. Stress results when a tic is suppressed. Stress is relieved upon executing the tic. Tics have a number of causes. Tourette syndrome is the most common tic disorder, affecting roughly 5–10 of every 10,000 children. Boys are disproportionately affected. Tourette syndrome is frequently accompanied by attention deficit hyperactivity disorder. Dopamine receptor blockers, such as pimozide and haloperidol, and alpha-receptor agonists such as clonidine provide effective treatment for the tics. Behavioral approaches have also shown some success.

CHOREA

Chorea is an unpredictable, irregular, nonrhythmic, brief, jerky flowing or writhing movement. Chorea can be consciously incorporated into voluntary movements, such that patients exhibit "semipurposeful" movements known as parakinesias. Chorea has several causes, including Wilson's disease, stroke, and as part of an immunologic reaction after streptococcal infection (Sydenham's chorea). Huntington disease is a hereditary form inherited in an autosomal dominant pattern. Symptoms typically appear between ages 35 and 50.

Haloperidol (Haldol) and fluphenazine (Prolixin) are effective in treating chorea but can impair voluntary movements. Both are initiated at a dose of 0.5 or 1.0 mg orally once daily and can gradually be increased to a maximum daily dose of 6–8 mg/day. The dopamine-depleting drugs reserpine (Serpalan) and tetrabenazine (Nitoman) and the benzodiazepine clonazepam (Klonopin) are also effective. Reserpine is initiated at a dose of 0.1 mg orally once daily (maximum dose, 3 mg/day). Tetrabenazine is started at 25 mg orally once daily (maximum dose, 100 mg/day). Klonopin is started at a dose of 0.5 mg orally once daily (maximum dose, 4 mg/day). Wrist weights can improve function by decreasing the amplitude of chorea.

MYOCLONUS

Myoclonus is a brief, sudden movement caused by involuntary muscle contractions or lapse of muscle contraction (*asterixis*). **Generalized myoclonus** refers to synchronous "jerks" in many body parts; **focal myoclonus** affects a single body part. Physiologic myoclonus is benign and includes "sleep jerks" that occur while falling asleep. Essential myoclonus is disabling and can be treated with clonazepam (starting dose of 0.25 mg orally twice daily, increasing over 3 days to 1 mg/day). Most causes of myoclonus are secondary and include drugs such as lithium, toxins, advanced liver disease, infections including human immunodeficiency virus, dementia, and brain lesions. Treatment should target the underlying disorder.

DYSTONIA

Dystonia is a syndrome that includes sustained muscle contractions that cause twisting, repetitive movements and abnormal postures. Progressively severe tremor is also common. Primary dystonia is an inherited form that appears before age 21. Dystonic movements are involuntary but can be diminished by specific maneuvers. In spasmodic torticollis that affects the neck, for example, placing a hand on the chin or side of the face reduces the severity of dystonia. Primary dystonia is generally hereditary and can be treated successfully with high doses of trihexyphenidyl (Artane) alone (starting dose of 1 mg orally per day, increasing gradually to 6–80 mg/day until symptoms are well-controlled), or in combination with baclofen (Lioresal) (starting dose of 10 mg orally once daily; maximum dose of 30–120 mg/day). The list of secondary causes includes Wilson's disease, metachromatic leukodystrophy, Lesch-Nyhan syndrome, stroke, and encephalitis.

WILSON'S DISEASE

Wilson's disease is a rare inherited disorder of copper metabolism that, in addition to hepatic manifestations, often also presents with neuropsychiatric features including progressive tremor and dystonia. Symptoms and signs of Wilson's disease may appear at a young age. Tremor in a young patient, therefore, should raise suspicion of primary dystonia or Wilson's disease.

ATAXIA

Ataxia is a wide-based, unsteady gait associated with cerebellar dysfunction, proprioceptive defects, or both. Inherited forms include Friedreich's ataxia and spirocerebellar ataxia. Ataxia can occur secondary to stroke, trauma, alcoholic degeneration, multiple sclerosis, vitamin B_{12} deficiency, and hydrocephalus. Treatment, when possible, should target the underlying cause.

REFERENCES

Bagheri MM, Kerbeshian J, Burd L: Recognition and management of Tourette's syndrome and tic disorders. Am Fam Physician 1999;**59**(8):2263.
Louis ED: Essential tremor. N Engl J Med 2001;**345**(12):887.
Olanow CW, Watts RL, Koller WC: An algorithm (decision tree) for the management of Parkinson's disease (2001): Treatment guidelines. Neurology 2001;**56**(11 suppl 5):S1.
O'Brien CF: Movement disorders for the primary care physician. Fam Practice Issues in Neurology 1999;**10**(2). URL: http://www.thecni.org/reviews/10-2-p04-obrien.htm
Rao G, et al: Does this patient have Parkinson disease? JAMA 2003;**289**:347.

60   Urinary Incontinence

Karen D. Novielli, MD, & Barry D. Weiss, MD

KEY POINTS

- Urinary incontinence is extremely common in older patients, particularly older women.
- Middle-aged and older patients should be asked routinely about urinary incontinence, because they are unlikely to spontaneously mention the condition.
- Treatment is based on the cause of urinary incontinence, and behavioral management is often the most effective treatment.

   I. **Definition.** Urinary incontinence is the involuntary leakage of urine at undesired or inappropriate times. Since micturition is controlled through both the central and peripheral nervous systems as well as local anatomic support, incontinence can be caused by numerous conditions affecting the brain, spine, and pelvis.
  II. **Common Diagnoses.** Urinary incontinence becomes more frequent with advancing age and is often associated with poor general health and functional status. Among ambulatory, community-dwelling persons older than age 65, urinary incontinence occurs in 17–55% of females and 11–34% of males. About 14% of older women and 4% of older men are incontinent on a daily basis.
      A. **Transient (reversible) incontinence** may be present in as many as 20% of incontinent patients and is more likely when incontinence is of recent onset. See Table 60–1 for common causes of reversible incontinence.
      B. **Urge incontinence** accounts for approximately 50–75% of irreversible incontinence in older individuals. Urge incontinence results from uncontrolled contractions of the detrusor muscle. Although most cases are idiopathic, patients with neurologic disorders (including dementia) are at particularly high risk.
      C. **Stress incontinence** occurs because of an incompetent urethral sphincter and most commonly is found in parous women, but a similar syndrome can occur in nulliparous women, in patients with neuropathic disorders that denervate the urethral sphincter, or in post-prostatectomy patients whose sphincter mechanisms have been surgically damaged.
      D. **Overflow incontinence** accounts for <5% of incontinence in women but, because of the prevalence of prostate disorders, accounts for 30–50% of incontinence in older men. Overflow incontinence is caused either by obstruction of urinary outflow or impaired detrusor contractility.
      E. **Mixed incontinence** occurs when two or more of the above causes are present simultaneously, most often urge incontinence in combination with another cause. Mixed incontinence is very common and may occur in as many as 50% of incontinent patients.
      F. **Functional incontinence** is the inability or unwillingness to toilet because of physical, cognitive, psychological, or environmental factors (eg, such as a patient with severe depression or who is physically restrained). Functional incontinence is common in the hospital and nursing home settings.
 III. **Symptoms.** Basic elements of the history include duration, frequency, and severity of urine loss; precipitating factors (such as coughing, change in position); and associated symptoms.
      A. **Urgency** is the primary symptom of uncontrolled bladder contractions (ie, urge incontinence). The sensitivity of the symptom of urgency in identifying patients with true urge incontinence, in comparison to formal urodynamic testing, is approximately 80%.
      B. **Loss of urine with coughing,** descending stairs, sneezing, and so on is a classic symptom of stress incontinence. The positive predictive value of these symptoms exceeds 85% for identifying patients with true stress incontinence and exceeds 95% when accompanied by physical examination findings typical of stress incontinence. However, symptoms similar to those of stress incontinence can occur in patients with urge in-

TABLE 60–1. CONDITIONS COMMONLY ASSOCIATED WITH TRANSIENT (REVERSIBLE) URINARY INCONTINENCE

Obstructions of bladder outflow
Fecal impaction
Prostate enlargement
Medications that increase sphincter tone
    α-Adrenergic agonists
    β-Adrenergic antagonists

Decreased contractility of the bladder detrusor muscle
Medications that decrease detrusor tone
    Anticholinergics
    Prostaglandin inhibitors
    Calcium channel-blocking agents
    Narcotic analgesics

Irritability of the bladder detrusor muscle
Acute urinary tract infection
Atrophic vaginitis or urethritis
Bladder neoplasms and stones
Excessive urine production
    Diuretic medications
    Glycosuria or hypercalciuria
    Excessive fluid intake

Impairment of urethral contraction
Medications (α-adrenergic blockers)

Central nervous system depression
Medical or psychiatric illness (eg, hypoxia, delirium, or depression)
Medications (eg, sedative-hypnotics or narcotics)

Temporary impairments of mobility
Injury, medical illness

    continence (pseudo-stress incontinence), because in urge incontinence the bladder is "irritable" and may contract when stimulated by repetitive increases in intra-abdominal pressure, such as from repetitive coughing.

  C. Dribbling is a symptom of overflow incontinence, and it may occur with sphincter weakness, especially when it is caused by sphincter denervation. It usually increases with postural change or with Valsalva's maneuver.

  D. Abdominal discomfort may be present in patients with overflow incontinence because of bladder distention, particularly if urinary retention and overflow are of recent onset.

IV. Signs. Physical examination should include an evaluation of the functional and cognitive status of the patient in addition to a thorough neurologic, abdominal, and pelvic evaluation.

  A. Abnormal mental status (eg, dementia) indicates decreased function of cerebral inhibitory centers associated with urge incontinence.

  B. Abnormal reflex, motor, or sensory function suggests the presence of a neurologic disorder leading to neuropathic sphincter, detrusor denervation, or cerebral dysfunction and associated urge incontinence.

  C. Abdominal distention or **palpable bladder** is suggestive of urinary retention and associated overflow incontinence.

  D. Atrophic vaginitis indicates the possibility of urge incontinence due to estrogen-responsive irritable bladder.

  E. Prolapse of pelvic organs is frequently associated with stress incontinence.

  F. Prostate enlargement or masses suggest the possibility of overflow incontinence secondary to bladder outflow obstruction.

  G. Impacted rectal stool suggests overflow incontinence from obstruction of urethral outflow by the fecal impaction.

V. Laboratory Tests. Some patients may have pre-existing conditions warranting specialized evaluations not discussed in this chapter (Figure 60–1).

  A. Basic evaluation (for all incontinent patients)

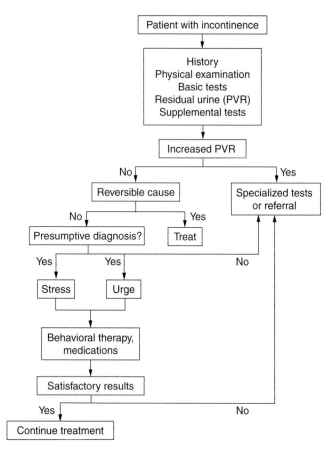

FIGURE 60–1. Urinary incontinence—diagnostic and management strategy for primary care physicians. Note that patients with certain conditions may need specialized evaluation and should not be diagnosed and managed exclusively according to this algorithm. Such patients are those with (1) hematuria or pyuria in the absence of infection, (2) recent (within 2 months) onset of irritative voiding symptoms, (3) previous anti-incontinence surgery or radical pelvic surgery, (4) severe pelvic prolapse, (5) suspicion of prostate cancer, or (6) neurologic abnormalities. PVR, postvoid residual urine.

1. **Urinalysis.** *Pyuria* or *bacteriuria* suggests infection, and a culture can confirm the diagnosis. *Hematuria* may indicate neoplasm or calculi, necessitating further evaluation with cystoscopy, renal ultrasound, or radiography.
2. **Postvoid residual urine (PVR)** volume should be measured to exclude overflow incontinence. Normal PVR is <50 mL; PVR of 200 mL or more is abnormal and indicates outflow obstruction or diminished detrusor contractility. PVRs between 50 and 200 mL are equivocal, and the test should be repeated on another occasion.
   a. **Postvoid catheterization** is the most common method for determining PVR. A sterile catheter is inserted into the patient's bladder immediately after the patient voids, and the volume of collected urine is recorded. Inability to pass the catheter suggests obstruction from urethral stricture, prostate enlargement, etc.
   b. **Ultrasound** measurement of bladder volume is a noninvasive method for determining the presence of residual urine. Where it is available, ultrasonography may be preferable to catheterization, especially in men with suspected

prostate enlargement, because ultrasound involves no risk of infection or urethral trauma, both of which can occur with catheterization.

3. A **cough stress test** should be performed on all females. With the patient in the lithotomy position and with a full bladder, the patient coughs while gauze or a menstrual pad is held over the perineum. Instantaneous leakage onto the pad during coughing suggests stress incontinence. Delayed leakage suggests urge incontinence. If there is no leakage, the test should be repeated with the patient in the standing position.

B. **Supplemental tests** can be performed if a presumptive diagnosis cannot be reached with a history, physical examination, and the aforementioned tests.

1. **Office cystometrography** (Table 60–2) is a simple office procedure that is useful for detecting the presence of uncontrolled bladder contractions associated with urge incontinence. Cystometrography is safe; urinary infection develops in <5% of patients who undergo this test. Compared to formal urodynamic testing, several studies have shown that the sensitivity of simple office cystometrography for diagnosing detrusor instability is between 75% and 100%, the specificity is 69–89%, and the positive predictive value is 74–91% in patients for whom reversible causes of incontinence have been excluded.

2. **Urinary flow determination** can be useful in male patients suspected of having prostate enlargement causing outflow obstruction. Decreased flow is indicated by either straining or an interrupted stream, or abnormally low flow measurement with a commercially available urine flowmeter. Flow rates in older men are usually >20 mL/s; rates <10–15 mL/s are abnormal.

C. **Specialized tests** can be performed in selected patients with specific indications or in those for whom a presumptive diagnosis cannot be reached after history, physical examination, and basic and supplemental tests.

1. **Complete urodynamic testing** (including full cystometrography, perineal electromyography, urethral pressure profilometry, and other measurements) is commonly performed when a presumptive diagnosis cannot be made, when patients do not respond to treatments for the presumptive diagnosis, when the PVR is increased, and when surgical interventions are being considered.

2. **Endoscopic and imaging studies** of the urinary tract may be indicated in patients with hematuria, sterile pyuria, or recent onset of irritative voiding symptoms (ie, symptoms of urge incontinence that developed within the previous 2 months). In such patients, these tests may detect neoplasms, stones, diverticuli, etc.

VI. **Treatment.** After the basic and supplemental evaluations described above, in most cases a presumptive diagnosis can be made as to the cause and type of incontinence. Treatment, as outlined below, can be administered based on the presumptive diagnosis. If treatment is unsuccessful, the diagnosis should be re-evaluated, and more specialized tests may be indicated to better define the cause of incontinence. The patient can keep a **voiding diary,** in which symptoms and information on the frequency and circumstances of incontinent episodes are recorded. The diary is useful for defining the patient's symptoms and determining the baseline frequency of incontinence to judge efficacy of therapy.

TABLE 60–2. PERFORMANCE OF OFFICE CYSTOMETROGRAPHY

1. Have the patient empty his or her bladder by voiding in the toilet, and then have him or her assume the dorsal lithotomy position.
2. Insert a sterile nonballooned No. 12–14 French catheter, and empty the patient's bladder. Measurement of postvoid residual and collection of urinalysis may be performed at this time.
3. Insert the syringe (50 mL, with the plunger removed) into the end of the catheter, and position it 15 cm above the urethra.
4. Fill the bladder by pouring sterile water through the open end of the syringe in 25- to 50-mL aliquots.
5. Record the cumulative total fluid instilled into the bladder, and note the volume at which the patient first reports having the urge to void. Severe urge to void at <300–350 mL is suggestive of detrusor overactivity (urge incontinence).
6. Continue adding fluid slowly until the fluid level (meniscus) in the syringe rises, indicating contraction of the detrusor muscle with transmission of intrabladder pressure to the syringe.
   a. The rise in fluid level may be either gradual or explosive.
   b. Detrusor contractions at <300–350 mL of bladder volume are generally indicative of urge incontinence.

A. Transient causes of urinary incontinence are managed by treating the identified cause. If incontinence does not resolve, other causes of transient incontinence should again be considered. If none are found, the patient is then treated for the type of irreversible incontinence (eg, urge or stress) presumptively diagnosed based on the testing described above.

B. Urge incontinence

1. **Behavioral therapies** are the first-line treatment because they are safer and generally more effective than drug therapy. Two principles underlie behavioral treatments for urge incontinence: (1) keep the bladder volume low by frequent voiding; (2) inhibit detrusor contractions by retraining cerebral and pelvic continence mechanisms.

   a. **Bladder training** is the treatment of choice for urge incontinence. It involves progressively lengthening the interval between voiding and encouraging the patient to postpone voiding for increasing lengths of time. Several randomized controlled studies have demonstrated bladder training to be effective. At least one study found it superior to drug therapy in cognitively intact women. Most patients experience improvement in their incontinence symptoms, and most studies indicate cure rates exceeding 50%.

   b. **Pelvic muscle exercises (Kegel exercises)** can also improve symptoms of urge incontinence (see section VI,C,1,a), especially when supplemented with biofeedback.

2. **Medications** are a second-line treatment for urge incontinence.

   a. **Oral medications** for urge incontinence act by diminishing bladder contractions. **Oxybutynin** is an antimuscarinic agent that has a direct antispasmodic effect on the bladder. It is used at doses ranging from 2.5 mg at bedtime to 5 mg four times per day. An extended-release preparation is also available that permits once daily dosing and fewer side effects. **Tolterodine** is an anticholinergic drug that has similar efficacy to oxybutynin and may have a lower incidence of dry mouth. The dose of tolterodine ranges from 0.5 mg at bedtime to 2 mg twice a day. Both oxybutynin and tolterodine have significant anticholinergic side effects that may limit their use, particularly in older individuals with comorbid illnesses. Urinary retention, in particular, should be considered in patients with worsening incontinence. There are insufficient data to support the use of other agents including propantheline, tri-cyclic antidepressants, and calcium channel blockers.

3. **Other treatments**

   a. **Electrical stimulation** with both implantable and nonimplantable electrodes may improve urge incontinence in some patients. This therapy is used in many centers but is considered investigational.

   b. **Surgical treatment** of urge incontinence with procedures such as augmentation cystoplasty is effective, but is used only in selected patients. Bladder denervation, which reduces detrusor contractility, can be accomplished with subtrigonal phenol injections and a variety of other methods. Cure rates with bladder denervation are low.

C. Stress incontinence

1. **Behavioral therapies** are effective in some patients with stress incontinence.

   a. **Pelvic muscle (Kegel) exercises** may lessen the severity of sphincter weakness in stress incontinence. Patients are instructed to contract the pelvic muscles for 10 seconds at a time, 30–80 times per day, and continue the exercises indefinitely. On average, incontinence is improved in about 75–85% of patients and eliminated in about 10–15%. Instruction in proper technique for pelvic muscle exercises is important to improved patient outcomes.

   b. **Adjuncts to pelvic muscle exercises** include **biofeedback** and **vaginal cones.** Each may further improve the effectiveness of treatment, although further research is necessary to quantitate the additional benefit.

   c. **Bladder training** (as described in section VI,B,1,a for urge incontinence) can result in additional improvement in symptoms of stress incontinence.

2. **Medications**

   a. **α-Adrenergic agonists,** which cause urethral sphincter contraction, may be tried if no contraindication (eg, hypertension) exists. **Pseudoephedrine** (30 mg orally up to four times a day) is the alpha agonist of choice. Up to 50% of patients are improved, and about 10% are cured.

    b. Estrogen, oral, vaginal, or transdermal, can be administered in conjunction with alpha agonists and may result in more improvement than alpha agonists alone. Estrogen alone may improve symptoms of urge or stress incontinence in women with atrophic vaginitis; however, studies to date have not shown a beneficial effect.

  3. Surgery is the most effective treatment for women with stress incontinence. The appropriate surgical treatment is dictated by whether the patient's symptoms are caused by hypermobility (ie, descent) of the urethra or by intrinsic weakness of the sphincter muscle (intrinsic sphincter deficiency). Surgery can eliminate incontinence in 70–85% of patients with stress incontinence. For men with stress incontinence, such as occurs after prostatectomy, injections of periurethral bulking agents (eg, collagen) or surgical implantation of an artificial urethral sphincter can improve or eliminate incontinence. When men are treated with periurethral bulking injections or artificial sphincters, cure (ie, complete elimination of incontinence) occurs in 20% and 50%, respectively.

  4. Devices are also available for treating stress incontinence. For women, these include pessaries, suction devices that occlude urethral outflow, and ballooned inserts that lie within the urethral orifice. For men, penile clamps are sometimes used on a temporary basis; clamps sometimes result in injury to the urethra or penile skin.

D. Overflow incontinence must be treated by draining the bladder. Failure to drain retained urine may result in hydronephrosis and subsequent renal damage.

  1. Intermittent catheterization, performed by patients or their caretakers, is the treatment of choice. The catheter must be clean, but not necessarily sterile, although sterile catheters are recommended for immunocompromised patients. The interval between catheterization varies, depending on how often the individual patient's bladder becomes distended.

  2. Chronic indwelling catheterization (ie, Foley catheter) is generally used if intermittent catheterization is not possible.

    a. Urinary tract infection. Bacterial colonization is universal among chronically catheterized patients. Antibiotic treatment results in selection of antibiotic-resistant organisms; therefore, only symptomatic urinary tract infections should be treated.

    b. Leakage around the catheter is generally caused by encrustation of the catheter lumen and orifice with calculo-proteinaceous debris, with subsequent drainage of urine around the sides of the catheter. A larger catheter should not be used in an attempt to prevent leakage. Instead, the catheter should be replaced at a frequency dictated by the development of encrustation and leakage. **Acidification of urine** decreases build-up of encrusted material and lengthens the interval between catheter changes. Several medications can acidify urine, for example, **methenamine hippurate** (1 g orally twice a day), **ascorbic acid** (500 mg orally every day), and **acetic acid** (0.25% or less) lavage of catheter and bladder, performed anywhere from once per week to every other day, as needed to prevent encrustation.

    c. Mortality from septic complications is increased among patients who require chronic bladder catheterization.

  3. Suprapubic catheterization is useful in selected patients for whom neither intermittent nor chronic urethral catheterization is appropriate.

E. Intractable incontinence exists when incontinence from any cause cannot be adequately controlled by the above measures. As noted above, irreversible overflow incontinence always requires catheter drainage. When other forms of incontinence are intractable, the following treatment options are available.

  1. Behavioral techniques may be sufficient to decrease incontinence episodes and improve hygiene in some chronically incontinent patients.

    a. Habit training involves identification of the patient's natural voiding schedule and ensuring that toilet facilities are available at that time. This technique is used at nursing homes and is superior to placebo and as effective as drug therapy in reducing episodes of incontinence.

    b. Prompted voiding involves asking patients whether they need to void and providing them with toilet facilities if they answer affirmatively. It also is used for institutionalized patients and is effective at reducing the frequency of incontinence.

    c. **Routine or scheduled toileting** involves bringing the patient to the toilet on a fixed schedule. It also reduces the frequency of incontinent episodes.
2. **Incontinence underpants** and absorbent pads are useful for collecting and absorbing incontinent urine. The absorbent garment or pad is changed at intervals dictated by the frequency of incontinence.
3. **Condom catheters** may sometimes be useful in male patients, especially on a short-term basis. Condom catheters increase the risk of skin problems and urinary tract infections.
4. **Intermittent catheterization,** if logistically feasible, can be used to control intractable incontinence from any cause.
5. **Chronic bladder catheterization** may be used in patients whose incontinence cannot be managed by other means.
6. **Diverting ureteroileostomy** may be appropriate for controlling incontinence in carefully selected patients.

REFERENCES

Burgio KL, et al: Behavioral vs drug treatment for urge urinary incontinence in older women: A randomized controlled trial. JAMA 1998;**280:**1995.

Culligan PJ, Heit M: Urinary incontinence in women: Evaluation and management. Am Fam Physician 2000;**62:**2433.

Fantl JA, et al: *Urinary Incontinence in Adults: Acute and Chronic Management.* Clinical Practice Guideline No. 2, 1996 Update; AHCPR Publ. No. 96-0682. US Department of Health and Human Services, Public Health Service, Agency for Health Care Policy and Research; 1996.

Parazzini F, et al: Prevalence of overactive bladder and urinary incontinence. J Fam Pract 2002; **51:**1072.

Thom D: Variations in estimates of urinary incontinence prevalence in the community: Effects of differences in definition, population characteristics, and study type. J Am Geriatr Soc 1998;**46:**473.

Weiss BD: The diagnostic evaluation of urinary incontinence in geriatric patients. Am Fam Physician 1998;**57:**1675.

---

61   Urinary Symptoms in Men

Linda L. Walker, MD & Steven E. Reissman, DO

KEY POINTS

- Younger men are more likely to present with infectious processes such as urethritis and acute prostatitis.
- Older men are prone to more insidious conditions such as benign prostatic hypertrophy, chronic prostatitis, and cancers of the prostate and bladder.
- Simple cystitis is not the norm in men; underlying causes of urinary tract infection symptoms should be sought.

I. **Definition.** Common urinary symptoms in men include voiding pain or discomfort, abnormal urine flow, hematuria, and urethral discharge. Pain is generally due to infection or inflammation (eg, urethritis, or acute or chronic prostatitis.) Flow is influenced by abnormal tone and physical obstruction (eg, benign prostatic hypertrophy [BPH], prostate cancer, or urethral strictures). Hematuria is pathologic if from bladder or other cancers, but may be due to BPH or infection. Urethral discharge is nearly always infectious.

II. **Common Diagnoses**

    A. **Urethritis** is pervasive, affecting over 4 million males each year, primarily sexually active younger men with multiple partners. There is a resurgence in the number of **gonococcal** cases due to male-to-male transmission. However, **nongonococcal urethritis (NGU)** (commonly due to *Chlamydia trachomatis, Mycoplasma* and *Ureaplasma, Trichomonas* and, infrequently, *Herpes simplex* virus-2) predominates as the **most com-**

mon sexually transmitted disease in men. It can be transmitted from asymptomatic partners, and recurrence is widespread. Anal intercourse increases risk for urethritis from enteric pathogens.

B. Prostatitis/chronic pelvic pain syndromes (CPPS). Twenty-five percent of adult males presenting with genitourinary symptoms have some form of **prostatitis,** and up to 50% of all men experience symptoms in their lifetime. This disease spectrum results in more than 100,000 hospitalizations per year. Risk factors for prostatitis include reflux of urine due to bladder, prostate, or urethral abnormalities; anal intercourse; epididymitis; urinary catheters; and urinary tract surgery.

Recently the National Institutes of Health (NIH) classified and redefined prostatitis as follows:

1: **Acute bacterial prostatitis**—a fairly uncommon condition primarily affecting men aged 30–50 years, consisting of <5% of all prostatitis cases overall.

2: **Chronic bacterial prostatitis**—also uncommon, making up 5–10% of cases, affecting men older than age 50.

3: **Chronic pelvic pain syndrome (CPPS)**—subdivided into two categories, both conditions of men aged 30–50 years.

3A: **Inflammatory CPPS**—known also as **nonbacterial prostatitis,** is the largest category of prostatitis syndromes, comprising 40–65% of cases overall. The NIH postulates that it is the most prevalent prostate condition, even outnumbering BPH. The cause is unknown.

3B: **Noninflammatory CPPS**—known previously as **prostatodynia,** is also very frequently seen, occurring in 20–40% of cases. It also has uncertain etiology, but may be related to internal sphincter failure and pelvic floor relaxation.

4. **Asymptomatic inflammatory prostatitis**—an incidental laboratory finding.

C. BPH is the most common neoplastic and urologic disorder of older men. Twenty-five percent eventually seek care for symptoms, leading to nearly 2 million patient visits each year. The prevalence is 8% in the fourth decade, 40–50% in the fifth decade, and > 80% in the ninth decade of life, reflecting a probable cumulative androgen trophic effect on the prostate. Medications exacerbating BPH obstructive symptoms include antihistamines, anticholinergics, decongestants, and tranquilizers.

D. The most common (nondermal) malignancy in males is **prostate cancer,** affecting 10% of all men. Over 180,000 new cases are diagnosed each year and approximately 30,000 people die annually in the United States of this cancer, which is 3% of adult male mortality. However, most men with prostate cancer die of other causes. Aging is the strongest risk factor and long-term androgens may stimulate neoplastic development, as prostate cancer is unknown in eunuchs. Having one, two, or three first-degree relatives with prostate cancer confers a 2-fold, 5-fold, or 11-fold increased risk, respectively. African Americans may have the highest lifetime risk of developing prostate cancer worldwide. At an incidence rate of 200 cases per 100,000, their risk is 1.5 times greater than Caucasians for acquiring the disease and 2 times greater for dying from it. Asian Americans have a lower risk than Caucasians. A diet high in fat or red meat may increase risk. Nutritional practices that may prove protective include intake of antioxidants, lycopenes, soy, garlic, and selenium.

E. Bladder cancer is also age-dependent; 80% of cases occur in individuals older than age 50. It is the fourth most commonly diagnosed cancer in men and the second most prevalent. More than 50,000 people are diagnosed with bladder cancer yearly, and about 12,000 die of it. The greatest risk factor is tobacco use; other risk factors include exposure to dyes and chemicals in metal- and leather-working occupations, long-term urinary catheter use, chronic urinary tract infection, bladder calculi, and pelvic irradiation.

III. Symptoms

A. Urethral discharge is copious, purulent, and yellow-green in **gonococcal urethritis,** developing 1–14 days after exposure. In **NGU,** the incubation period is 1–3 weeks, and the discharge is scantier and more mucoid. The marked **dysuria** associated with urethritis is perceived most strongly at the meatus.

B. Symptoms of **urinary flow abnormalities** in an older man without other complaints most commonly suggest **BPH.** Urinary flow symptoms are divided into two types, and most BPH patients have both.

1. **Obstructive symptoms** include **hesitant or interrupted stream, decreased stream force/caliber, straining, terminal dribbling, incomplete emptying,** or **frank urinary retention** with possible **overflow incontinence** of small volumes of

urine. (*Note:* obstructive symptoms are so described because of subjective characteristics and cannot be directly correlated with objective findings on urodynamic testing.)

2. **Irritative symptoms** comprise **frequency, urgency, urge incontinence,** and **nocturia.** These occur in BPH, prostatitis, urinary tract infections (UTIs), and malignancies and with polyuria in systemic diseases (eg, diabetes mellitus, congestive heart failure, or nephritic syndrome).

The American Urological Association (AUA) recommends using a symptom index score (Table 61–1) if patients are to be considered for medication for BPH. These symptoms are not unique to BPH, and the index is a monitoring and not a diagnostic tool.

3. When **pain** is a component of flow abnormalities, then **infectious, inflammatory, and malignant conditions** are higher in the differential diagnosis.

C. **Pain and discomfort** characterize inflammatory and infectious conditions of the prostate.

1. **Acute prostatitis** usually has an unambiguous appearance presenting in a younger man who is **febrile, toxic, and acutely ill,** with **moderate to severe pelvic, perineal, and low back pain.**

2. **Chronic prostatitis and CPPS** present with gradual onset of **vague pelvic fullness** or pain, **ejaculatory or penile pain** (or both), and perhaps **testicular or scrotal aching,** along with irritative voiding and occasionally obstructive symptoms. A key component in the history of patients with chronic prostatitis is **recurrent prior UTIs** or previous bouts of prostatitis. These individuals often have **anxious or depressive symptoms when CPPS impairs their quality of life.**

D. **Painless hematuria** can be due to **BPH** or **bladder cancer.** Urolithiasis and renal cell carcinoma are less common causes. When present in BPH, the blood tends to be seen at the beginning and end of the urine stream. In bladder cancer, the urine is typically uniformly bloody. Patients presenting with more advanced bladder cancer may have irritative voiding symptoms, **flank pain,** or **leg edema.**

IV. **Signs**

A. **Acute urinary retention** is typically due to severe **BPH** exacerbated by medications precipitating sudden obstruction, or from **acute prostatitis.** The **abdominal examination** will reveal **suprapubic tenderness** and a **distended bladder** that may hold >1 L of urine, percussable or palpable nearly to the umbilicus.

B. **Digital rectal examination of the prostate** should be done in all men with urinary symptoms to evaluate for prostate size, consistency, symmetry, and masses.

1. In **acute prostatitis** the gland will be **swollen, boggy, and exquisitely tender.** To decrease the risk of bacteremia and sepsis, the examination should be gently performed in the toxic, ill-appearing patient.

TABLE 61–1. AMERICAN UROLOGICAL ASSOCIATION SYMPTOM INDEX

Questions—Over the past month, how often have you:	Score
1. . . . had a sensation of not emptying your bladder completely after you finished urinating?	Not at all—0 <1 time in 5—1
2. . . . had to urinate again in less than 2 hours after you had finished urinating?	< half the time—2 About half the time—3
3. . . . found you stopped and started again several times when you urinated?	> half the time—4
4. . . . found it difficult to postpone urination?	Almost always—5
5. . . . had a weak urinary stream?	
6. . . . had to push or strain to begin urination?	
7. . . . Over the past month, how many times did you most typically get up to urinate from the time you went to bed at night until the time you got up in the morning?	0–5 points maximum scored here per time reported

Score 7 or less = Mild.
Score 8–19 = Moderate.
Score 19 or more = Severe.

    2. **Mild tenderness, sponginess,** or **induration** may be noted in **chronic prostatitis/ CPPS.** The gland is massaged firmly, in a rolling motion of the examiner's finger-pad, from the lateral margins of the prostate to the midline, to collect expressed secretions at the meatus for analysis and culture.

    3. The gland can be normal or smooth, rubbery, and enlarged in **BPH.**

    4. **Carcinoma** may be palpable as **lobular asymmetry, induration,** or **mass.**

  C. The anus, penis, testes, scrotum, and inguinal region should be evaluated for tenderness, masses, adenopathy, or lesions that could be the source of the patient's genital, urinary, or pelvic complaints (eg, anal fissure, genital ulcer, inguinal hernia, phimosis.)

  D. **Neurologic examination** should focus on anal sphincter tone (may correlate with bladder sphincter tone) and on any neurologic deficits (eg, sudden onset of urinary or fecal incontinence, urinary retention, back pain, extremity weakness, or symmetric extremity or trunk sensory deficits) indicative of spinal cord compression if metastatic prostate cancer is suspected.

V. Laboratory Tests. Most common nonmalignant urologic conditions in men can be diagnosed using symptoms, physical findings, and laboratory testing available in the primary care setting. Typical patient presentations with clinical strategies for evaluation follow.

  A. In **a sexually active young man with a urethral discharge, a urethral swab should be sent for culture,** or for the less expensive **DNA probe assay.** The latter is 99% sensitive for gonorrhea and *Chlamydia.*

    1. According to the Centers for Disease Control and Prevention (CDC) guidelines, urethritis in the above setting can also be diagnosed by:

      a. Observed **urethral discharge.**

      b. **Gram staining a urethral swab.** If gram-negative intracellular diplococci are seen, gonococcal infection is present. This is the most rapid and sensitive method for diagnosing **gonorrhea.** At least 5 WBCs per oil immersion field indicates the presence of pus, supporting the diagnosis of **NGU.**

      c. A positive **leukocyte esterase dipstick test** of the first voided urine specimen of the day. This test is equivalent to detecting pus in the urethra.

      d. At least **10 WBCs per high-power field** and absence of significant bacteriuria on the first voided urine specimen of the day.

    2. In the absence of the above CDC criteria, urethritis cannot be diagnosed, pending culture or DNA probe assay.

  B. A **toxic-appearing man** in his thirties with the **acute onset of fever and chills, dysuria, severe perineal pain, obstructive symptoms and a swollen, boggy, very tender prostate** has **acute prostatitis;** prostatic massage is contraindicated, and testing should include a **urinalysis (UA) and culture.** Marked pyuria will be present, and the culture will typically be positive for urethritis organisms in younger men and coliforms in older men.

    1. **Blood cultures** should be done in hospitalized, septic-appearing patients.

    2. Possible acute urinary retention is evaluated with **abdominal ultrasound;** catheterization for residual urine is very painful and could cause bacteremia, so it should only be done with urologic consultation.

  C. A **middle-aged to older aged man** with the **insidious complaints of mixed irritative and obstructive voiding symptoms** along with **numerous genitourinary pain complaints and mildly tender or spongy prostate gland** is presumed to have **chronic prostatitis** or one of the two types of **CPPS.** All such patients should have a **UA and culture** performed. **Expressed prostatic secretions (EPS)** are examined microscopically for white blood cell counts (WBCs) and sent for **culture.**

    1. In chronic bacterial prostatitis, urinary and EPS cultures are often recurrently positive, with at least 10 WBCs per high-power field in the EPS. Pyuria may also be present.

    2. In **inflammatory CPPS,** only WBCs are seen.

    3. Culture and WBCs are absent in secretions in **noninflammatory CPP.**

  D. An **older man with typical lower urinary tract symptoms (LUTS)** as reported on the American Urological Association symptom index (Table 61–1) and a digital rectal examination consistent with **BPH** is diagnosed on clinical grounds alone. All such patients should have a UA, as a simple screen for other contributing urinary abnormalities (eg, hematuria, which, if found, demands evaluation—see section VI,E).

    1. **Prostate-specific antigen (PSA)** testing should be performed only in men expected to live at least 10 years longer and if the test results would impact clinical management (see section VI,F).

2. No evidence supports evaluating blood urea nitrogen and creatinine in the absence of clinical suspicion. Elderly men have a high incidence of elevated serum creatinine, not necessarily attributable to their uncomplicated LUTS.

3. **Urinary ultrasound (US)** detects asymptomatic obstructive hydronephrosis in <2% of otherwise healthy men with BPH and **is not recommended as a screening test** in these individuals.

4. **Postvoid residual (PVR)** urine volume can be measured by "in-and-out" or Foley catheterization; >350 mL is a typical threshold for diagnosis of urinary retention. However, no correlation exists between PVR volume and symptom severity, urodynamics, or outcomes. (With *acute* urinary retention, a Foley catheter should be left in place because retention recurs in hours to days without a catheter, even if precipitants, such as medications, are corrected.)

5. Referral to urology is necessary for patients with atypical or complex symptoms, when surgical therapy is contemplated, or whenever cancer of the urinary tract is suspected. The urologist decides whether to perform **urodynamic tests (uroflowmetry, cystometrography,** and **pressure flow studies).** The urologist may also perform **cystoscopy** to visualize the urothelium and obtain tissue biopsy.

E. **An elderly man with a significant smoking history and hematuria** should be evaluated for **bladder cancer.**

1. Evaluation of an otherwise asymptomatic, low-risk patient with hematuria includes UA and culture, urine cytology, and bladder/renal ultrasound.

2. Patients with hematuria and risk factors for bladder cancer, persistent refractory irritative voiding symptoms, or both require further investigation, including cytology on a spontaneously voided urine specimen, an **intravenous pyelogram** for upper tract cancers, stones, or obstruction (or **retrograde pyelography** if there is a contrast dye allergy), and referral for cystoscopy. **Cystoscopic biopsy** definitively diagnoses bladder cancer. High-risk patients with a negative initial evaluation need ongoing surveillance for malignancy in consultation with a urologist.

F. When a **patient with BPH requests PSA testing,** he needs thorough counseling on the pros and cons of testing. The AUA and the American Cancer Society (ACS) recommend annual screening for men aged 50 years and older with a life expectancy of at least 10 years. The ACS recommends African American men and those with two affected first-degree relatives begin annual screening at age 35, and the AUA recommends African Americans and those with one affected relative begin annual screening at 40. The American Academy of Family Physicians (AAFP) recommends counseling about the potential benefits and harms of PSA screening and making individualized patient decisions. The United States Preventive Services Task Force (USPSTF) recommends against PSA screening.

1. **Normal PSA levels (<4 ng/mL)** are found in 25% of prostate cancer cases.

2. **Mild elevations (4–10 ng/mL)** are frequently found and in 75% of cases are due to benign conditions, usually BPH. Urologic evaluation of these patients with **transrectal ultrasound (TRUS) and biopsy** risks detecting latent microscopic disease, with an unknown natural history and significant treatment-related morbidity (namely, urinary incontinence and erectile dysfunction—see section VI,G). It is possible that screening in these patients results in detection and treatment of cancer that may never have caused any health problems during the patient's lifetime, but causes considerable anxiety and lifestyle changes from knowledge of test results and decision-making relating to treatment.

G. **Advanced prostate cancer.** A minority of men with prostate cancer present with symptoms of advanced disease, including **advanced urinary symptoms, a markedly abnormal prostate examination, gross hematuria, bone pain, elevated alkaline phosphatase (highly suggestive of bony metastases), and generally markedly elevated PSA.** Prostate cancers in these men are felt to be so rapidly growing that early laboratory diagnosis is impossible, and patients are only diagnosed clinically relatively late in the course of their illness. With PSA >10, there is at least a 75% chance of prostate cancer, and the risk rises exponentially with PSA values (in advanced cancer the PSA is >100). PSA is monitored for a decrease indicating response to treatment or rise in refractory cases. All such patients are referred to a urologist for evaluation and management.

H. **If a prostate nodule is detected** in an otherwise asymptomatic or LUTS patient, he is neither in the screening nor the advanced prostate cancer category. A PSA should be ordered and regardless of results, urologic referral is indicated for further evaluation.

Statistically, there is at least a 50% chance that the mass is prostate cancer, which often has spread beyond the gland and is incurable.

VI. Treatment

   A. Urethritis. Unless results of rapid assays are available, patients with urethritis (and their sexual partners) should be treated for both NGU and gonococcal urethritis.

1. For **NGU,** the most common regimen is oral **doxycycline,** 100 mg twice daily for 7 days. **Azithromycin,** 1 g once orally, is more expensive but has the advantage of improved compliance. Alternative oral regimens (for allergy or refractory cases presumed due to resistant mycoplasma or *Ureaplasma*) are metronidazole, 2 g once orally with **erythromycin,** 500 mg four times daily for 7 days; or various fluoroquinolones such as **ofloxacin,** 300 mg orally every 12 hours for 7 days.

2. **Gonorrhea** is effectively treated with **ceftriaxone,** 125 mg intramuscularly (IM) once; or **cefixime,** 400 mg orally; or single oral doses of fluoroquinolones such as **ofloxacin,** 400 mg.

   B. Acute prostatitis

1. Men younger than 35 years are treated with oral **ofloxacin,** 400 mg initially, then 300 mg twice daily for 10 days; or **ceftriaxone,** 250 mg IM, then oral **doxycycline** 100 mg twice daily for 10 days.

2. In older men, coliforms are presumed present and longer regimens are used. Currently recommended are oral **ciprofloxacin,** 500 mg twice daily for 10–14 days, or **trimethoprim-sulfamethoxazole (TMP-SMX DS),** twice daily for 10–28 days.

3. Oral **nonsteroidal anti-inflammatory drugs (NSAIDs),** such as **ibuprofen,** 400–800 mg three times daily, are helpful for analgesia. **Opiates,** such as hydrocodone-APAP 5 mg/500 mg (eg, Vicodin), 1–2 tablets orally every 4–6 hours as needed, may be used for severe pain. Acute urinary retention may be precipitated by opiate use if the prostate is severely swollen. Opiate side effects of constipation and straining to stool can markedly increase pelvic symptomatology.

4. **Hospitalization** for **intravenous antibiotics** may be necessary for severely ill patients.

   C. Optimal treatment for **chronic bacterial prostatitis and CPPS** is being investigated in numerous ongoing clinical trials.

1. **Chronic bacterial prostatitis** is treated with the antibiotics listed for acute bacterial prostatitis, in prolonged courses lasting 4–6 weeks for quinolones, and up to 12 weeks for TMP-SMX, repeated as necessary.

   a. If recurrences are frequent, data support symptomatic use of oral α-**adrenergic blockers.** These include **doxazosin (eg, Cardura),** titrated up to 8 mg over several weeks; **tamsulosin (eg, Flomax),** 0.4 mg once daily, titrated to 0.8 mg after 2–4 weeks, can also be used.

   b. Recent clinical data support the benefit of repetitive **prostatic massage** and **frequent ejaculation.**

   c. For severe symptoms (Table 61–1) persisting despite medical therapy, urologic consultation for possible surgery (laser or transurethral needle ablation, balloon dilation, or heat therapy) may be beneficial.

2. **CPPS.** Because WBCs are seen in prostatic secretions in **inflammatory CPPS, antibiotics** as above are tried for 4 weeks.

   a. For the obstructive symptoms of either type of CPPS, at least a 12-week trial of α-**adrenergic blockers** is recommended.

   b. Pain symptoms are treated with oral **NSAIDs**—either over-the counter products such as **ibuprofen (eg, Motrin IB),** 200 mg four times daily; or a **COX-2 inhibitor** such as **rofecoxib (Vioxx),** 25 mg once daily for at least a 6-week trial. If symptoms persist, patients are re-evaluated for further therapy.

   c. Standard **phytotherapy** consists of **quercetin**—a bioflavenoid (eg, **Prosta-Q),** sold as a dietary supplement, taken orally as a 540-mg capsule three times daily for at least 6 weeks.

   d. Men older than 40 years with inflammatory CPPS can be offered a long-term trial of oral **finasteride (Proscar),** 5 mg daily, or **dutasteride (Avodurt),** 0.5 mg daily. These drugs are **5α-reductase** inhibitors, blocking testosterone conversion in the prostate, used primarily in BPH to shrink enlarged tissue, and can be continued long-term if the patient gets symptomatic relief.

   e. **Supportive counseling and psychological treatment** may be necessary for patients severely impacted by lifestyle limitations of their condition. It is especially important that any fears patients have about contagion or cancer be addressed and allayed.

    f. Current recommendations for CPPS patients with refractory voiding symptoms include a trial of **Pentosan (Elmiron)**, 100 mg orally three times a day for a limited course of 3–6 months, usually under urologic supervision.

    g. As in chronic prostatitis, urologists can offer various surgical interventions as a last resort.

    h. Biofeedback, acupuncture, and **neurostimulation** of the pelvic floor muscles are therapeutic adjuncts without proven benefit.

D. BPH

    1. Watchful waiting is recommended for patients with mild symptom scores; symptom scores should be monitored annually (Table 61–1). **Lifestyle changes** should include **restriction of caffeine and bedtime fluids, and limitation of any sympathomimeter (eg, decongestants) and anticholinergic medications. Frequent, regular voiding** may improve quality of life.

    2. Drug therapy. In patients with moderate or severe symptoms, medications should also be considered.

        a. Patients with mild to moderate symptom scores wishing to begin medication should initially be offered α**-blockers.** These drugs block the reversible component of obstructive symptoms (prostatic smooth muscle contraction), providing fairly prompt relief. Traditionally, α_1**-blockers** (eg, **terazosin** or **doxazosin**) have been used. The α_{1A}**-blockers**, (eg, **tamsulosin [Flomax]**), are a newer class. This drug has effects within days instead of weeks and causes less hypotension than the α_1-blockers, but is more expensive.

        b. Oral 5α**-reductase** inhibitors such as **finasteride (Proscar)** or **dutasteride (Avodurt)** gradually reduce gland mass up to 50%. (PSA values while taking these medications may be doubled.) Androgen deprivation slowly relieves symptoms over months to years; thus it is often used with or after α-blockade trials for larger glands, and for patients with moderate to severe symptom scores. 5α-reductase inhibitors cost more than α-blockers but considerably less than surgery and can delay the need for surgery up to several years. Side effects include erectile dysfunction, decreased libido, decreased ejaculatory volume, and testicular pain.

        c. Saw palmetto helps voiding symptoms in 50% of users, without affecting prostate size, PSA levels, or voiding measurements. A typical dose is 160 mg twice daily.

    3. Urologic referral is indicated for BPH patients with marked urinary retention, recurrent UTIs, refractory gross hematuria, bladder calculi, or renal insufficiency caused by obstruction. Surgical interventions include **transurethral resection of the prostate (TURP); transurethral incision of the prostate (TUIP);** or **ablation by microwave, laser, or electrode.** The latter procedures are less invasive, with lower complication rates, but provide no surgical specimens to evaluate for occult malignancy. TURP is very effective in relieving symptoms long-term, but retrograde ejaculation ensues in most men. Less frequently seen are impotence, UTIs, and incontinence.

E. Prostate cancer management is based on the symptoms; histologic grading of the tumor (glandular disorganization based on the Gleason system); and clinical staging based on tumor size, local extension, spread to pelvic lymphatics, and metastases to bone, lungs, or liver. The patient's overall expected longevity should be considered based on his his other medical conditions. The course of prostate cancer is quite variable, from a slow, indolent disease lasting years or decades (most common) to a rapid, invasive illness causing mortality in a few years or less. The 10-year survival rate for localized disease is 85%, and survival for several years is not uncommon in metastatic disease.

    1. In **localized lesions, radical prostatectomy** or **radiation** is offered, in consultation with urology and a radiation oncologist. Risks to be weighed include postoperative urinary incontinence, radiation bowel injury, and erectile dysfunction.

    2. In more **advanced disease, surgery** can relieve obstruction, and radiation can ameliorate urinary and metastatic symptoms, such as bone pain.

    3. Widespread disease is often treated **palliatively,** as no cytotoxic chemotherapy prolongs survival. Various methods are used in succession to cause tumor regression by inducing androgen deprivation. **Orchiectomy** is frequently performed;

leuprolide injections inhibit pituitary gonadotropins and are often given with oral **flutamide** (an androgen receptor competitor). **Finasteride** may be used, and rarely, **DES (diethylstilbestrol),** at risk of thromboembolism. Once the cancer becomes hormone refractory, the median survival is only 1 year.

F. As with prostate cancer, **bladder cancer** management should be coordinated by a urologist knowledgeable in oncology.

1. **Superficial bladder cancer** can be treated by **local resection.** Bacille Calmette-Guérin **(BCG) infusions** into the bladder are given for patients at high risk for recurrence, and **intravesical chemotherapy** infusions are used to prevent and treat recurrence.
2. For **locally invasive disease, radical cystectomy** offers up to a 5-year survival rate. **Radiation** is an acceptable alternative.
3. **Chemotherapy** is the treatment for metastatic bladder cancer; median survival is at least 12 months.

REFERENCES

Bremnor JD, Sadorsky R: Evaluation of dysuria in adults. Am Fam Physician 2002;**65:**1589.
Dull P, Reagan RW Jr, Bahnson RR: Managing benign prostatic hyperplasia. Am Fam Physician 2002;**66:**77.
Nickel C: Managing chronic prostatitis: A modern approach. Ur Times; April 1, 2003.
Rubenstein E, Federman D (editors): Infections of the urinary tract. Sci Am Medicine 2002;**7:**XXIII.
Rubenstein E, Federman D (editors): Bladder, renal and testicular cancer. Sci Am Medicine 2003;**12:**XIV.
Walsh PC, et al (editors): *Campbell's Urology,* 8th ed.; 2002.

---

62   Urticaria

Charles F. Margolis, MD

KEY POINTS

- The etiology of urticaria is most commonly not apparent after a careful history, physical examination, and full laboratory investigation.
- One phenomenon aggravating urticaria in many cases is dermographism; in some cases, dermographism is the primary cause of urticaria, occurring, for example, where clothing binds the skin.
- Unless history or physical examination suggests laboratory evaluation because of concern over additional conditions, laboratory evaluation is usually unnecessary.

I. **Definition.** Urticaria are **transient,** circumscribed, raised skin lesions, which are usually intensely pruritic and characterized by areas of erythema and edema of varying size and duration. **Angioedema** ("giant hives") is more commonly nonpruritic than urticaria, is characterized by nonpitting edema, and often involves oral and respiratory mucosae. The lesions of **urticarial vasculitis** appear similar to urticaria but last longer than 24 hours, are more intensely symptomatic, and may leave residual bruising and be associated with immune complex–mediated disease elsewhere.

Urticaria and angioedema are caused by localized vasodilation and transudation of fluid from capillaries and small blood vessels. The locus of vascular permeability is deeper in angioedema than in urticaria. Urticaria and angioedema often occur at the same time in patients and differ little in demographic features or apparent cause. Chemical mediators released by mast cells and basophils cause increased vascular permeability. Histamine is the most prominent mediator, but substances such as leukotrienes, prostaglandins, kinins, and others also play a role. The variety of mediators may account for different patterns of urticaria and varying individual responses to medications. Triggers of mediator release include physical and

immunologic factors and certain substances causing direct release of histamine by degranulation of mast cells. Immunologic mechanisms are probably involved more often in **acute** than
in **chronic** urticaria (recurrent urticaria lasting longer than 6 weeks).

The characteristic appearance of urticaria is usually readily apparent, making the diagnosis obvious. Edema is sometimes transient, leading the clinician to suspect other erythematous rashes.

II. **Common Diagnoses.** Urticaria is among the most common skin conditions encountered
by family physicians. The annual incidence of urticaria in an urban US family practice center was found to be 0.27%, and the lifetime incidence is 15–20% of the population. Acute
urticaria is more than twice as common as chronic urticaria. Females are three times as
likely as males to present with urticaria. Urticaria and angioedema may occur at any age,
but the incidence is highest in young adults.

Uncovering the cause of urticaria is more difficult than diagnosing it. In 60–70% of cases
of urticaria, careful evaluation fails to reveal a cause. A specific cause is more likely to be
identified in patients with acute urticaria than in those with chronic urticaria.

Specific causes of urticaria include:

A. **Physical factors** (5–10% of cases) (Table 62–1).

  1. **Dermographism** ("skin writing") is the occurrence of whealing and erythema within
     minutes of exposure to pressure or mechanical irritation such as stroking or scratch-
     ing. It occurs in about 5% of the general population, although wheals may occur in
     anyone if the pressure stimulus is great enough. Patients with **symptomatic der-
     mographism** develop urticaria in sites where minor pressures associated with ac-
     tivities of daily living have been applied. Common sites are the waist and the neck,
     where tight-fitting garments are the pressure source. Scratching wheals already
     present may lead to the formation of additional wheals. Symptomatic dermographism
     accounts for two of every three cases of urticaria caused by physical factors.

  2. Other physical causes are more unusual. **Cold urticaria,** which may be recognized
     in the patient who urticates on the face and the extremities in cold weather, can be
     demonstrated by the application of an ice cube to the skin. **Cholinergic urticaria,**
     induced by heat, emotional stress, or exercise, results in 2- to 3-mm scattered
     wheals surrounded by large erythematous flares.

B. **Infections** (10–15% of cases). Streptococcal infection has been considered a common
   cause in children in the past, but some now consider the relationship to be less causal
   and more likely due to the co-occurrence of two common conditions, streptococcal infection and urticaria. Nonspecific viral infections, hepatitis B, and infectious mononucleosis are all thought to cause many cases of urticaria, whereas sinusitis and parasitic
   and dermatophytic infections are considered unusual causes of urticaria.

C. **Medications** (5–10% of cases). Medications may cause urticaria. The most common
   causes include penicillins, cephalosporins, and sulfa drugs. **Aspirin** and nonsteroidal
   anti-inflammatory drugs, which may facilitate urticaria caused by other factors, and
   codeine, which may cause direct degranulation of mast cells, deserve special mention.
   Angiotensin-converting enzyme inhibitors may cause urticaria and angioedema,
   which may occur months or years after initiation of treatment, or with long symptom-
   free intervals between multiple episodes.

D. **Foods** and **food additives** used for color, preservation, and taste may also cause urticaria. Nuts, seafood, eggs, and strawberries are among the foods implicated. Penicillin is commonly fed to livestock and may appear in small quantities in milk and meat.

E. Urticaria can uncommonly be a sign of **collagen vascular disease, cancer, hyperthyroidism,** and **familial, hereditary conditions.** Inhalant allergens and insect bites
   or stings may also cause urticaria. Contact with substances such as foods, fibers, radiocontrast media, chemicals, and cosmetics may induce urticaria by direct degranulation
   of mast cells in the skin. **Papular urticaria** is a hypersensitivity reaction to the bites of

TABLE 62–1. TYPES OF PHYSICAL URTICARIA

Symptomatic dermographism	Solar urticaria
Cold urticaria	Vibratory urticaria
Cholinergic urticaria	Aquagenic urticaria
Heat urticaria	Decompression urticaria

fleas, mosquitoes, chiggers, and mites. The appearance of the lesions is papular, and they are more persistent than typical urticaria.

  F. Physicians and patients have felt that many cases of urticaria are strongly influenced by **emotional and psychogenic factors.** Although case studies support the significance of psychogenic factors, it has been difficult to prove that these factors are the sole cause of urticaria in individual patients.

III. Symptoms. Pruritus is usually present with urticaria in varying degrees of severity. The intensity of the pruritus, like urticaria itself, is affected by external factors such as temperature, alcohol, and emotional distress.

IV. Signs. The characteristic skin lesions of urticaria are evanescent, well demarcated, and raised. Erythema surrounds edematous central areas. Where the skin has been scratched, lesions are more prominent. While examining the patient, the physician should test for dermographism by stroking the patient's skin and should test for other causes of physical urticaria when the patient's history indicates that further testing would be appropriate.

V. Laboratory Tests. Extensive laboratory evaluation usually provides little information beyond that suggested by the patient's history and physical examination, and tests are not routinely required.

  A. When patients are seen initially with urticaria, laboratory evaluation might include testing children for streptococcal infection and evaluating all patients for causes suggested by the history or the physical examination.

  B. If urticaria persists, the tests shown in Table 62–2 may be helpful.

VI. Treatment (Figure 62–1). Removal of the offending agent or management of the underlying cause is the treatment of choice when possible. Even after treatment has begun, continuing efforts should be made to establish a cause for urticaria if the cause was not apparent at the first visit.

  A. Patient education. If the cause of urticaria cannot be established during the office visit, the patient should be educated about possible offending agents, ideally with the help of a printed handout. The patient should be asked to think about possible associations after the office visit. The patient's observations and additional insights are one of the physician's best sources of information in determining the cause of this condition.

  B. General measures

  1. The patient should avoid vasodilating influences such as heat, emotional stress, exertion, or alcohol.
  2. Cool compresses, Aveeno baths, and antipruritic lotions may provide some relief.
  3. Aspirin use probably should be discontinued.
  4. Urticaria and angioedema, like other skin conditions, are highly visible to the patient. The visibility of the condition contributes to the patient's anxiety, which can aggravate the condition. The physician should **reassure the patient** that the condition usually resolves in a few days or weeks and that it is usually associated with a benign outcome.

TABLE 62–2. LABORATORY EVALUATION OF URTICARIA

Initial tests
Complete blood cell count and sedimentation rate
Urinalysis
Multichemistry screening panel
Thyroid function tests
Throat and urine cultures[1]

Further tests to be considered if urticaria persists
Stool for ova and parasites
Vaginal smear for *Candida* and *Trichomonas* spp
Sinus or chest radiographs
Serum complement, antinuclear antibody, and immunoglobulin analysis
Hepatitis B tests
Elimination diets and skin tests
Skin biopsy

[1]Testing for streptococcal infection, either culture or rapid antigen testing, should be performed on children upon initial presentation with urticaria.

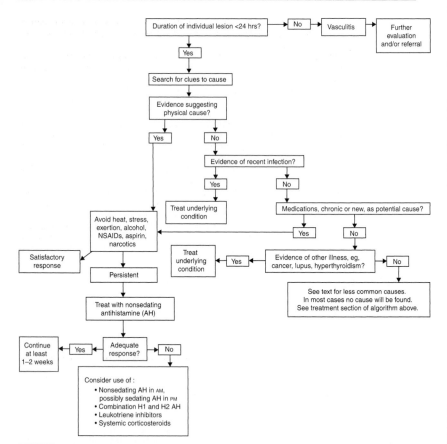

FIGURE 62–1. Approach to the patient with new-onset urticaria. H_1, H_2, histamine-1, histamine-2 blocking medication; NSAIDs, nonsteroidal anti-inflammatory drugs.

5. Follow-up care is required when the condition is prolonged, when the condition intensifies rather than improves, or when new symptoms supervene.

C. **Medications**

1. Oral **antihistamines,** including ones likely to cause sedation such as **hydroxyzine, diphenhydramine, chlorpheniramine, and loratadine** and relatively nonsedating ones such as fexofenadine and **cetirizine,** have been commonly used. There is some individual variation in response.

a. **Hydroxyzine** and **cetirizine** are sometimes more effective than other antihistamines. Cetirizine is less likely to cause sedation than hydroxyzine but may occasionally lead to some sedation. The usual dose of hydroxyzine is 25 mg every 4–6 hours, and cetirizine's usual dose is 10 mg once daily, but higher doses may be used to control symptoms if the patient can tolerate them. In children, the starting dose of diphenhydramine is 2 mg/kg/day, dosed every 4–6 hours, and cetirizine may be prescribed at doses of 2.5–5 mg once daily for ages 6 months to 2 years, 5 mg once daily for ages 2–5 years, and 10 mg daily for children 6 years and older.

b. **Loratadine** (10 mg once daily for adults and children 6 years of age and older, 5 mg for children ages 2–5 years) and **fexofenadine** (180 mg once daily for ages 12 and older and 30 mg twice daily for ages 6–11 years) are especially useful because they are generally nonsedating. In some patients the combination of a nonsedating antihistamine in the morning and a sedating one in the evening will be beneficial.

c. **Diphenhydramine** (25 mg four times a day), **chlorpheniramine** (4–12 mg twice a day), and loratadine are available without a prescription, which may represent an advantage for some patients.

2. **Other medications** that are occasionally used include the following.

a. **Systemic corticosteroids** are useful in severe and poorly responsive cases of urticaria. **Prednisone** may be given for 10 days, starting at 40–60 mg and tapering orally to 5–10 mg on the last day, and should be added to antihistamine therapy. Benefit and risk must be weighed in considering the use of systemic corticosteroids. Topical corticosteroids have very little value in the treatment of urticaria.

b. **Leukotriene inhibitors** may be useful in some cases of urticaria. They have been shown to provide benefit in placebo-controlled trials.

c. The subcutaneous injection of **epinephrine** (0.3 mL) may be used to confirm the transient nature of the lesions, to provide temporary relief to the acutely symptomatic patient, and in cases of anaphylaxis.

d. Cimetidine and other H_2 antihistamines sometimes provide benefit when added to H_1 antihistamine treatment but are of little value when used alone. The use of **ephedrine, terbutaline, doxepin, nifedipine, colchicine,** and **dapsone** has been reported to benefit some patients.

REFERENCES

Kaplan AP: Chronic urticaria and angioedema. N Engl J Med 2002;**346:**175.
Mahmood T: Physical urticarias. Am Fam Physician 1994;**49:**1411.

---

63 Vaginal Bleeding

Judith Anne Kerber, MD, & Clark B. Smith, MD

KEY POINTS

- Patients of childbearing age with abnormal vaginal bleeding must have a negative pregnancy test result before further work-up is pursued.
- Perimenopausal patients with vaginal bleeding need an endometrial biopsy to rule out a tumor before starting treatment.
- A normal Pap smear (for **cervical** cancer) can never ensure that the patient's uterus (**endometrium**) is normal.

I. **Definition.** A **normal menstrual cycle** involves the sequential stimulation and withdrawal of ovarian hormones that affect the uterine endometrium. Immediately after menses, the endometrial layer is thinned and new growth is ready to occur. During the **proliferative phase,** ovarian estradiol 17-β secretion causes spiral arterial elongation and endometrial thickening. Endometrial hyperplasia develops as the epithelium becomes taller. With ovulation, progesterone is secreted by the ovarian corpus luteum (**early secretory phase**). Estradiol levels decrease as progesterone increases, causing coiled arteries to become progressively more tortuous, culminating (**late secretory phase**) in arterial vasoconstriction and ischemia, which in combination with progesterone withdrawal causes the endometrium to slough (**menses**). Normal menstrual cycles are established approximately 2 years after menarche at average age 12–13 (range: 10–16 years); cycle length averages 28 days (normal range: 21–35 days), with menses lasting 2–8 days (average, 4–6 days) and blood loss between 25 and 60 cc/cycle. This translates into about 25 pads or 30 tampons (1 box); however, since some women change pads before saturation, pad counts may not provide an accurate assessment of menstrual blood loss.

Abnormal bleeding is cycle length <21 days or >35 days, irregular/noncyclic, or heavy (>80 mL per cycle) bleeding. Commonly, this is due to deviations from sequential estrogen/progesterone stimulation and withdrawal just described. Such deviations have many causes as described in the next section.

II. **Common Diagnoses.** The literature suggests that 10–20% of women have abnormal uterine bleeding at some time in their lives.

   A. **Dysfunctional uterine bleeding (DUB)** is abnormal uterine bleeding not caused by other pathology or systemic disease.

   1. **Anovulatory bleeding,** continuous unopposed endometrial estrogen stimulation, accounts for 95% of DUB in women younger than 20 years of age. This incidence falls to less than 20% in women between 20 and 40 years and then rises again to about 90% beginning 2–3 years prior to menopause.

   2. **Ovulatory bleeding,** due to fluctuations in estrogen or progesterone levels, occurs in about 10% of patients with DUB. More than 50% of women have microscopic midcycle spotting due to midcycle decreases in circulating estrogen.

   B. **Pregnancy and its complications** occur most frequently between ages 18–35. Abnormal vaginal bleeding (VB) may complicate up to 1 in 5 pregnancies. Common causes included placenta previa, placenta pathology, and spontaneous abortions.

   C. **Medications** cause abnormal VB. Oral contraceptives cause VB in 10% of users. Depot medroxyprogesterone acetate (Depo-Provera), an injectable progestin, frequently causes irregular vaginal bleeding or the first three injections. Other medication culprits include antidepressant, antihypertensive, anticoagulant, and anticholinergic drugs and digitalis, phenothiazines, steroids, tamoxifen, vitamins, and illegal drugs.

   D. **Sexually transmitted diseases (STDs)** produce VB through cervicitis or endometritis (*Neisseria gonorrhoeae, Chlamydia trachomatis*) or necrosis when blood supply is outstripped (condyloma acuminata). Risk factors include prior history of STDs, multiple sexual partners, and lack of condom use.

   E. **Tumors**

   1. Uterine leiomyomas (fibroids), endometrial polyps, and adenomyomas (adenomyosis) are the most common **benign** tumors of the uterus, are usually seen in the 25- to 45-year age group and cause bleeding by distorting the endometrial cavity or when the tumor outstrips its blood supply.

   2. **Malignant growth,** hyperplasia, or endometrial carcinoma accounts for 10–15% of postmenopausal bleeding. Chronically anovulatory women have 3 times the average risk, and women taking tamoxifen have a sevenfold increased risk of endometrial hyperplasia/carcinoma. Other high-risk groups include those who are obese, diabetic, or hypertensive. Vaginal adenosis and adenocarcinoma are uncommon but are often seen in patients who had intrauterine exposure to diethylstilbestrol (DES).

   F. **Trauma and foreign bodies** are not uncommon in children. Sexual abuse of children and young teens frequently presents as abnormal bleeding. Foreign bodies may include objects that can cause abrasions or lacerations.

   G. Blood dyscrasias are very uncommon. Ten percent of women with blood dyscrasia have abnormal uterine bleeding. Twenty-five percent of women with a hereditary coagulation disorder (thrombocytopenic purpura or von Willebrand's disease) have a negative family history. In adolescents, coagulation disorders cause up to 19% of acute menorrhagia, 25% of severe menorrhagia (hemoglobin <10 g/dL), 33% of menorrhagia requiring transfusion, and 50% of menorrhagia presenting at menarche.

   H. **Chronic or acute conditions** that can affect VB include weight changes, emotional problems, chronic illness, and endocrine disorders. Less frequent causes include adrenal disorders, central nervous system (CNS) tumors, and organ failure.

III. **Symptoms.** The history should include the **age of menarche, menstrual pattern**/timing (including last menstrual period and previous menstrual period), **duration** (ie, number of bleeding days), and estimated **amount of menstrual bleeding.**

   A. **Menstrual pattern**

   1. **Amenorrhea** preceding the abnormal bleeding, without signs or symptoms of pregnancy or recent oral contraceptive use, suggests anovulatory bleeding, particularly in the adolescent or perimenopausal patient. In the perimenopausal or

postmenopausal patient, a period of amenorrhea preceding abnormal bleeding suggests endometrial carcinoma.
2. **Unpredictable bleeding** suggests anovulatory bleeding.
3. **Midcycle predictable spotting** suggests midcycle estrogen deficiency.
4. Predictable **late cycle** spotting or bleeding suggest persistent corpus luteum or luteal phase defect.
5. Irregular bleeding is not uncommon in the **first 3 months of oral contraceptive pill use.**

B. **Premenstrual symptoms** (eg, breast tenderness, mood swings, and bloating) tend to be associated with ovulatory cycles.
C. **Fever,** particularly if associated with pelvic or abdominal pain or dyspareunia may suggest an STD, pelvic inflammatory disease (PID), or sepsis associated with abortion.
D. A history of **easy bruising** may indicate coagulation defects, drug or medication use, or dietary extremes. **Multiple injuries** may indicated trauma, which can include spouse or child abuse.
E. History of **maternal drug use during pregnancy** (eg, DES), particularly in adolescents with abnormal bleeding, suggests congenital anomalies of the genitourinary tract, including carcinoma of the upper vagina.
F. **Headaches** and **visual changes** may suggest a CNS cause, such as a pituitary neoplasm.

IV. Signs. The physical examination should include a pelvic examination, which may require anesthesia in very young girls or those who have not used tampons. Rectal bimanual examination is not a substitute for pelvic examination, since the rectal examination fails to reveal most vaginal or cervical causes or to allow for adequate evaluation of the uterus or adenexal structures.
A. **Pallor** not associated with tachycardia or signs of hypovolemia suggests **chronic** excessive blood loss such as that found in anovulatory bleeding, adenomyosis, uterine myomas, or blood dyscrasia.
B. If **signs of shock** or impending shock are present, the blood loss is likely related to pregnancy (including ectopic pregnancy).
C. **Pelvic masses** may represent pregnancy, uterine or ovarian neoplasia, pelvic abscess, or hematoma.
D. **Fever, leukocytosis,** and **pelvic tenderness** strongly suggest PID.
E. Fine, **thinning hair** and **hypoactive or slow-reactive reflexes** suggest hypothyroidism.
F. **Ecchymoses** or **multiple bruises** may indicate trauma (including sexual abuse or incest), coagulation defects, drug use, medication effects, or dietary extremes.

V. Laboratory Tests (Figure 63–1) should be directed by history and physical findings. For detailed evaluation of the following causes of vaginal bleeding, see the chapters indicated: PID, Chapter 51; child abuse, Chapter 91; contraceptives, Chapter 95; and pregnancy and complications, Chapter 97.
A. **Endometrial biopsy (EB)** is an easy office procedure to sample tissue for pathological evaluation.
1. **Indications**
a. Frequent or exceptionally heavy or prolonged **bleeding refractory to a course of cyclic hormonal therapy.**
b. **Risk factors for endometrial cancer** (ie, unopposed estrogen or patients who are diabetic, hypertensive, or obese).
c. **Women older than 30** years with irregular bleeding or any postmenopausal patient with VB.
d. **Unexplained vaginal bleeding.**
2. **Contraindications to EB** include pregnancy, acute infection, PID, or known bleeding disorder (including coumadin use).
3. **Timing and patient preparation.** With irregular sporadic menses, EB should be performed on the presumed first or second day of menses; EB can be performed at any time in women with continuous bleeding. Premedication with a nonsteroidal anti-inflammatory drug (NSAID) such as ibuprofen, 1600 mg, taken orally about 2 hours before the procedure, is adequate to control postprocedure cramping. Antibiotic prophylaxis is unnecessary for endometrial sampling. A signed consent must be obtained and potential complications (ie, pain, bleeding, infection, uterine perforation, bowel or bladder injury) explained prior to the procedure. Since this is a blind procedure, a poor sample may be obtained, necessitating repeat of

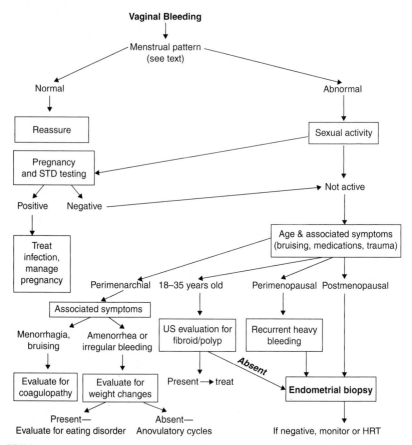

FIGURE 63–1. Primary care evaluation of vaginal bleeding. HRT, Hormone replacement therapy; STD, sexually transmitted disease; US, ultrasound.

the procedure. There must be documentation in the chart that the risks were explained to the patient.

4. **The procedure** begins with the patient in lithotomy (Pap smear) position. A manual examination will tell the size and orientation of the uterus. A sterile speculum is then placed and the cervix cleaned with povidone iodine. This is easier if ring forceps are used with cotton balls or 4×4s. A topical anesthetic (eg, Hurricane or benzocaine) can be applied to the cervix for patient comfort. A tenaculum is placed on the upper portion of the cervix for counter traction. A sterile sound is gently inserted into the endocervical canal to measure the depth of the uterus; normal is 6–8 cm. Pulling the cervix up and outward by placing gentle traction on the tenaculum can facilitate this. If the sound cannot be inserted, a dilator may be necessary to enlarge the cervical canal. The sterile pipette is then inserted through the os and advanced to the depth measured by the sound. At this point the piston on the pipette is pulled back to aspirate a sample. This process is repeated as the pipette is moved to sample multiple areas of the endometrium, in a clockwise fashion. The sample is then evacuated into a specimen cup with formalin preservative. Large volumes of aspirate may necessitate reinserting the pipette and repeating the above procedure, being cautious not to touch the pipette tip to the specimen cup. Blood clots may be

seen in the sample; endometrial tissue will be denser. After adequate sample is obtained, the tenaculum and the speculum are removed. Patients should be cautioned to expect slight bleeding and cramping (like a menstrual period).

5. **Cytologic evaluation** provides information about endometrial cycle stages.

   a. **Endometrial hyperplasia with cytologic atypia** progresses to endometrial carcinoma in about 25% of cases; without atypia, fewer than 2% progress to carcinoma.

   b. **Adenomatous endometrial hyperplasia** means a superficial carcinoma is present.

   c. **Other cytologic findings** include infection, proliferative vs. secretory endometrium, endometrial hyperplasia, or atrophic endometrium and neoplasia.

B. **Hysteroscopy** is a visualization of the endometrium. It is an office procedure but requires special training and equipment. If performed prior to endometrial sampling, hysteroscopy reveals abnormalities missed by endometrial sampling or dilation and curettage (D&C) alone in up to 30% of patients. Hysteroscopy is easier to perform when the patient is not bleeding, but it can be done at any time.

C. **Transabdominal and transvaginal ultrasound** may help delineate **pelvic masses** and can provide information regarding endometrial thickness, uterine size, and the presence of small ovarian cysts such as a persistent corpus luteum cyst that may be significant.

D. Patients with palpable or ultrasound-proven **pelvic masses** require **computerized tomography** or **magnetic resonance imaging scans**.

VI. **Treatment.** Treatment of abnormal vaginal bleeding should be directed at the underlying cause. Symptomatic treatment depends on the amount of bleeding. A hemoglobin (Hgb) <7 g/dL requires hospitalization for stabilization, parenteral hormone therapy, and blood transfusion. If Hgb is between 7 and 10 g and the patient is symptomatic (tachycardia, hypoxia, or positive tilt test), hospitalization should also be considered. If Hgb is >10 g and vital signs are stable, treatment may be with one of the following regimens.

A. **Outpatient therapy** for acute bleeding.

   1. **Progestins** such as medroxyprogesterone acetate (Provera), 20 mg orally initially followed by 10 mg twice daily for 7 days, or aqueous medroxyprogesterone acetate (Depo-Provera), 200 mg intramuscularly.

   2. **Oral contraceptives** such as Lo-Ovral, four times daily for 4 days, tapered over 7–10 days.

B. Once acute bleeding is controlled, **subsequent hormonal therapy** can include:

   1. Provera, 10 mg orally each day for the first 10 days of each calendar month (or from days 16–25 of the menstrual cycle) for 3–6 months. Alternatively, **oral contraceptives** can be used for a period of 3–6 months. However, if bleeding is due to anovulation, oral contraceptives may prolong the problem.

   2. **Estrogen replacement therapy** can be considered in the menopausal patient symptomatic from estrogen deficiency once endometrial or other pelvic malignancy has been excluded. See Chapter 78.

   3. **Gonadotropin-releasing hormone (GnRH) therapy and uterine fibroid embolization** may be used for fibroids. See Chapter 51.

   4. **Hysterectomy** or other surgical treatment may be appropriate in patients with neoplasms, endometriosis, adenomyosis, or chronic PID.

   5. With infrequent, asymptomatic bleeding and normal complete blood cell count, reassurance and an accurate explanation of the physiology of the cause are sufficient. Additional oral iron supplementation should be used in anemic patients until iron stores are replenished (see Chapter 4). Forty percent of chronic menorrhagia patients may also respond to a D&C. Oral NSAIDs, such as ibuprofen, 600–800 mg three times daily for 5 days, effectively reduce blood loss in chronic menorrhagia but are ineffective for acute bleeding episodes or in regulating noncyclic bleeding.

REFERENCES

The endometrium and decidua menstruation and pregnancy. In: Cunningham FG, Gant NF, Leveno KJ (editors): *Williams Obstetrics,* 21st ed. McGraw-Hill; 2001:66–83.

Oriel KA, Schrager S: Abnormal uterine bleeding. Am Fam Physician 1999;**60:**1371.

Schranger S: Abnormal uterine bleeding associated with hormonal contraception. Am Fam Physician 2002;**65:**2073.

Smith SJ: Uterine fibroid embolization. Am Fam Physician 2000;**61:**3601.

Zuber T: Endometrial biopsy. Am Fam Physician 2001;**63:**1131, 1137, 1139.

64   Vaginal Discharge

L. Peter Schwiebert, MD

KEY POINTS

- A careful history, physical examination, and office laboratory studies allow arrival at an appropriate diagnosis for common causes of vaginal discharge.
- Sexually transmitted diseases often coexist; the presence of risk factors for one should prompt screening for others.
- It is important to base treatment of vaginal discharge on solid clinical documentation to avoid inappropriate treatment and resulting drug resistance, excessive cost, and iatrogenic vaginitis.

I. **Definition.** From menarche to menopause, estrogen stimulates proliferation and glycogen production by vaginal squamous epithelial cells on which lactobacilli depend; these lactobacilli produce hydrogen peroxide (toxic to most vaginal pathogens) and lactic acid, resulting in a vaginal pH of 3.5–4.5. Normal (physiologic) discharge varies among women and with the stage of a woman's menstrual cycle; normal cervical discharge is clear to slightly opaque.

This chapter focuses on vaginal discharge that is unusual in amount or odor, or causes symptoms, such as itching or burning, and these are often due to alterations in the physiologic vaginal environment. Such unusual or symptomatic discharge may be related to:

- **Hypoestrogenic states** (in prepubertal or postmenopausal women), which thin the vaginal epithelium, decrease glycogen levels, raise pH to >5.0, and create a mixed vaginal flora.
- **Sexually transmitted pathogens** (eg, *Neisseria gonorrhoeae, Chlamydia trachomatis, Trichomonas vaginalis*), which stimulate inflammatory response, raise vaginal pH, or both.
- **Irritants** (eg, douching, some spermicides), which can alter physiologic vaginal pH and create a favorable environment for pathogens.
- **Immunocompromise or suppression of normal flora by antibiotics,** which permits overgrowth of opportunistic organisms (eg, *Candida* species). (*Candida* also grows well in the glycogen-rich vaginas of reproductive-age women, but has no such substrate in premenarchial or postmenopausal females and is therefore rare in these groups.)

II. **Common Diagnoses.** In the ambulatory primary care setting, vaginal discharge is the 10th to 15th most common presenting complaint, resulting in over 10 million physician office visits annually. These figures underestimate the true prevalence of the problem, however, since many women with discharge or odor do not seek medical attention. Up to 90% of all cases of vaginitis are due to bacterial vaginosis (BV), vulvovaginal candidiasis (VVC), or *Trichomonas.*

A. **BV** accounts for up to 40–50% of cases of vaginitis, with prevalence varying, depending on the population studied (ie, 15–19% of ambulatory gynecology patients and 24–40% of patients attending sexually transmitted disease (STD) clinics). Risk factors for BV include >1 sexual partner over the previous 3 months, use of intrauterine device (IUD), douching, and pregnancy.

B. **VVC** (approximately 20% of cases) is the second most common cause of vaginitis in the United States and the most common cause in Europe. Up to 75% of women have an episode of VVC at some point and up to 5% have recurrent episodes. Risk factors for VVC include recent antibiotic use (especially penicillins, tetracycline, or cephalosporins); oral contraceptive pill (OCPs) or systemic glucocorticoid use; pregnancy; poorly controlled diabetes mellitus; obesity; immunocompromised state; or diaphragm or spermicide use. *Candida albicans* is the pathogen in 80–90% of VVC, with increased likelihood of non-*albicans* infection (eg, *C glabrata* or *Candida tropicalis*) with immunocompromise, long-term anticandidal treatment, or >4 documented episodes of VVC over a year.

C. *Trichomonas* **vaginitis** (10–25% of cases), a true STD, is the third most common cause of vaginitis; risk factors include IUD or tobacco use or multiple sex partners. Twenty to 50% of women with *T vaginalis* are asymptomatic, and 23% of patients with this infection are also infected with *N gonorrhoeae.*

TABLE 64-1. SYMPTOMS AND SIGNS OF VAGINAL DISCHARGE

Condition	Complaint	Appearance of Discharge and Mucosa
Bacterial vaginosis	Odor or vaginal discharge	Thin, watery, grayish discharge; minimal mucosal erythema
Candida vaginitis	Vulvar itching or burning (50% specificity), external dysuria	Curdy white discharge; sometimes erythematous vaginal epithelium
Cervicitis	Mucoid discharge, intermenstrual spotting, dyspareunia	Yellow, mucoid endocervical discharge; inflamed cervix with focal hemorrhage
Trichomonas vaginitis	Discharge, vulvar itching	Typically copious, frothy; green or yellow discharge; punctate cervical hemorrhage sometimes present; vulvar and vaginal erythema
Physiologic discharge	Discharge without itching or odor	Clear to slightly opaque cervical discharge
Atrophic vaginitis	Discharge, burning, or dyspareunia, or all three	Thin and inflamed with loss of rugal folds; discharge, if present, is watery and may be foul-smelling

    D. Cervicitis, due to *C trachomatis,* herpes simplex virus (HSV), or *N gonorrhoeae,* accounts for up to 20–25% of cases of vaginal discharge. Risk factors include recent new sex partners, lack of contraceptive use (including barrier contraceptives), and age younger than 24 years.

    E. Physiologic discharge (10% of cases) is due to normal variations in cervical or vaginal mucus production.

    F. Atrophic vaginitis (10–40% of postmenopausal women) is due to natural or induced (eg, radiation/chemotherapy, oophorectomy, antiestrogenic medications) hypoestrogenic states.

    G. Allergic vaginitis (frequency unknown) is due to topical sensitizers or irritants, such as synthetic tampons, spermicides, hygienic sprays, soaps, perfumes, povidone-iodine solution, latex condoms, or douches.

III. Symptoms and Signs (Table 64–1).

IV. Laboratory Tests (Table 64–2) A careful history and examination, coupled with office laboratory studies, allows confident assessment of common causes of vaginal discharge.

    A. A wet preparation is made by adding a drop of normal saline to a drop of vaginal discharge on a glass slide and then examining the slide with a microscope.

    B. A potassium hydroxide (KOH) preparation is made similarly using a drop of 10% KOH solution instead of saline.

    C. Nitrazine paper changes color in response to changes in the pH of vaginal discharge. A 1- to 2-inch strip of Nitrazine paper is applied to secretions on the vaginal walls or pooled in the posterior fornix.

TABLE 64-2. OFFICE LABORATORY FINDINGS IN VAGINAL DISCHARGE

Condition	pH (from Vaginal Walls, Not Cervix)/Color of Nitrazine Paper	Wet and Potassium Hydroxide (KOH) Preparations
Bacterial vaginosis	>4.5/green to purple	Clue cells (bacteria obscuring epithelial cell border in 90% of cases), few WBCs on wet preparation amine "fishy" odor on addition of KOH (>90% sensitive)
Candida vaginitis	3.5–4.5/yellow to green	Spores and hyphae on KOH preparation (21% sensitive)
Cervicitis	>4.0/yellow to purple	Mature squames, >10 WBCs (50–70% sensitive) on wet preparation
Trichomonas vaginitis	>4.5/green to purple	Mature squames with many WBCs on wet preparation, motile protozoa can be seen in 60% of cases
Physiologic discharge	<4.0/yellow	Normal superficial epithelial cells, lactobacilli, no WBCs or spores on wet preparation
Atrophic vaginitis	>5.0/green to purple	Wet preparation shows many WBCs, small round epithelial cells (parabasal cells) which are immature squames unexposed to sufficient estrogen

WBCs, white blood cells.

D. The Hansel stain is a modified Wright-Giemsa stain that enhances eosinophils. This test should be considered in women with persistent discharge in whom the usual tests are normal and no other diagnosis is obvious. In one unpublished study of 50 patients with vaginal discharge, 12% had no evidence of infection and also had more than 25% eosinophils in their discharge using the Hansel stain.

E. Cultures. Because of the fairly low sensitivity of wet and KOH preparations in diagnosing *Candida* vaginitis, *Trichomonas* vaginitis, and cervicitis, cultures for *Candida, Trichomonas, N gonorrhoeae,* and *C trachomatis* should be performed in high-risk patients (see sections II,A–D) if KOH and wet preparations show negative results. In addition, all pregnant women should be screened for *C trachomatis* and *N gonorrhoeae.*

    1. Culture results for *C trachomatis* are unavailable for 4–7 days. Recently, direct immunofluorescence and enzyme immunoassays have become available. The positive predictive value (PPV) depends on the prevalence of *C trachomatis* studied in the population. So far, studies indicate that direct immunofluorescence has a better PPV than the enzyme immunoassay in populations at intermediate risk. The PPV of neither test has been adequately studied in populations with a low prevalence of *C trachomatis* infection.

    2. Culture for cure following treatment of cervicitis with a recommended regimen (see section V,E,1) is not necessary. However, cultures should be repeated 1–2 months after finishing treatment to detect reinfection.

F. Serologic **syphilis test (eg, VDRL), human immunodeficiency virus (HIV) testing (eg, enzyme-linked immunosorbent assay [ELISA]),** and counseling should be offered to patients with documented *N gonorrhoeae* infection.

V. Treatment

A. General measures. The patient should be instructed to do the following.

    1. Discontinue irritating agents (eg, sprays or bubble baths).

    2. Wear nonocclusive, absorbent clothing (cotton rather than nylon underclothing).

    3. Use barrier contraceptives (eg, condom or diaphragm) to prevent recurrence. (Oil-based intravaginal creams and suppositories may weaken latex condoms and diaphragms and risk unintended pregnancy.)

    4. Restore a normal vaginal environment (ie, pH and flora). Some clinicians recommend use of lactobacillus suppositories or oral yogurt.

    5. Practice good perineal hygiene (ie, wiping from front to back).

B. BV is diagnosed (90% sensitivity) if three of the following four criteria are met: (1) homogeneous gray discharge adherent to vaginal walls, (2) vaginal pH of >4.5, (3) positive "whiff test" (fishy odor on addition of KOH to wet prep), or (4) clue cells are present (Amsel's criteria). Other scoring systems (Nugent, Spiegel) focus on the mix of bacterial morphotypes, with the likelihood of BV increasing with decreasing prevalence of lactobacilli (long gram-positive rods).

    1. Metronidazole (eg, Flagyl or Protostat), 500 mg orally twice a day for 7 days, has been the standard therapy. Single-dose therapy (2 g) is the least expensive treatment and an effective option when compliance is a problem. Other effective regimens are metronidazole vaginal gel 0.75% (eg, MetroGel), 5 g vaginally twice daily for 5 days, or clindamycin (eg, Cleocin), 300 mg twice a day orally or applied vaginally as a 2% cream for 7 days.

    2. Although BV is associated with sexual activity, there is currently no evidence that treatment of sex partners prevents recurrences.

    3. BV is associated with adverse pregnancy outcomes (preterm labor, premature ruptured membranes, chorioamnionitis, preterm birth, postpartum endometritis, postcesarean section wound infection). However, the US Preventive Services Task Force (USPSTF) currently cites insufficient evidence to recommend for or against routine intrapartum screening for BV, especially in average-risk, asymptomatic patients. Although to date there is no evidence of teratogenic or mutagenic effects of metronidazole on newborns, its use is still recommended only after the first trimester. Dosing with it or clindamycin is as in nonpregnant women. The USPSTF recommends against using intravaginal agents, especially clindamycin, during pregnancy.

C. VVC (Table 64–3). A growing issue in management of VVC is the availability and heavy use of over-the-counter (OTC) medications (VVC preparations are the 10th best-selling OTC products in the United States). In one study, only 28% of women who thought they had VVC actually did and only 11% of women responding to another survey recognized the classic symptoms of VVC. This results in inappropriate treatment, increasing inci-

TABLE 64–3. TREATMENT OF VULVOVAGINAL CANDIDIASIS

Medication	Proprietary Name	Formulation	Dosage[1]
Clotrimazole	Gyne-Lotrimin, Mycelex Mycelex-7[2] Mycelex-G	100-mg vaginal suppository 1% vaginal cream 500-mg tablet	1 daily for 7 days or twice daily for 3 days 1 applicatorful daily for 7–14 days 1 tablet for 1 day
Miconazole	Monistat 7[2] Monistat 7[2] Monistat 3[2] Monistat 3 Combination[2]	2% vaginal cream 100-mg vaginal suppository 200-mg vaginal suppository 200-mg suppository, 2% cream	1 applicatorful daily for 7 days 1 tablet for 7 days 1 daily for 3 days 1 suppository daily for 3 days; cream prn
Butoconazole	Femstat 3[2] Mycelex-3[2]	2% cream	1 applicatorful daily for 3 days
Tioconazole	Vagistat-1[2]	6.5% ointment	1 applicatorful for 1 day
Terconazole	Terazol 3 Terazol 7 Terazol 3 suppository	0.8% cream 0.4% cream 80-mg vaginal suppository	1 applicatorful daily for 3 days 1 applicatorful daily for 7 days 1 daily for 3 days
Nystatin	Mycostatin	100,000-U vaginal tablet	1 daily for 14 days
Fluconazole	Diflucan	150-mg tablet	1 orally for 1 day
Ketoconazole	Nizoral	400-mg tablet	1 orally twice a day for 5 days
Itraconazole	Sporanox	200-mg tablet	1 orally either twice a day for 1 day or daily for 3 days

[1]Unless otherwise indicated, the route of administration is intravaginal; for daily doses, the preferred administration time is at bedtime.
[2]Available over the counter.

dence of resistant *Candida* strains and, in some situations, induction of irritant vaginitis. In light of this evidence, it is desirable to rely on documentation by a knowledgeable health care provider to diagnose acute or recurrent VVC.

1. **Uncomplicated infection** (healthy host, infrequent occurrences, mild to moderate symptoms).
   a. Imidazole creams, ointments, or suppositories share similar efficacy (>80%) in curing uncomplicated VVC.
   b. Tioconazole and terconazole are effective against a broader spectrum of *Candida* species than butoconazole, clotrimazole, or miconazole.
   c. Single-dose fluconazole (eg, Diflucan) is less expensive, better tolerated, and at least as effective as standard 3- to 7-day intravaginal regimens. Treatment with oral azoles is contraindicated during pregnancy; topical agents should be used.
2. For **complicated VVC** (moderate or severe symptoms or risk factors—see section II,B), extending standard therapy to 10–14 days for acute symptoms may be effective.
3. For **recurrent VVC** (>4 microscopically or culture-documented episodes in a year), the following may be effective.
   a. Because of the increased likelihood of non-*albicans* infection in recurrent VVC, culture is advisable.
   b. Medication should be prescribed for 10–14 days, with efficacy confirmed by negative post-treatment fungal culture.
   c. This should be followed by a 6-month maintenance regimen; options include ketoconazole, 100 mg daily; itraconazole, 100 mg/day; fluconazole, 100–200 mg/week; or clotrimazole, 500 mg vaginally per week. *Note:* Chronic daily use of the foregoing oral medications can interact with other medications (eg, theophylline, anticonvulsants, anticoagulants, OCPs), can be hepatotoxic, and may be teratogenic.
   d. Repopulating vaginal lactobacillus using yogurt douches may be effective.
   e. If non-*albicans* infection is documented, intravaginal terconazole or oral itraconazole may be more effective than standard regimens; other beneficial

medications in these patients include boric acid vaginal suppositories (600 mg/day for 14 days) or topical flucytosine (Ancoban) cream.

D. ***Trichomonas* vaginitis**
   1. **Standard regimen.** Metronidazole, 500 mg orally twice daily for 7 days, or a single 2-g dose for both the patient and her sex partner(s).
   2. **Treatment of pregnant patients.** Approximately 30% of symptomatic patients in the first trimester obtain relief with clotrimazole vaginal suppositories (100 mg at bedtime for 7 days). After the first trimester, metronidazole may be given in standard dosing.
   3. **Recurrent *Trichomonas* vaginitis.** Metronidazole-resistant *T vaginalis* has been documented. As of yet, there is no proven effective treatment for it; however, metronidazole, 500 mg orally twice daily for 14 days or 2 g orally for 3 days, may be effective.

E. Cervicitis. Empiric therapy for *C trachomatis* or *N gonorrhoeae* can be instituted in high-risk individuals while awaiting culture results.
   1. Because of the coprevalence of *N gonorrhoeae* and *C trachomatis* infection, patients should be treated with ceftriaxone (eg, Rocephin), 250 mg intramuscularly (one dose) and doxycycline, 100 mg orally twice daily for 7 days. Alternatives to ceftriaxone for *N gonorrhoeae* include cefixime (eg, Suprax), 400 mg, or ciprofloxacin (eg, Cipro), 250 mg, or ofloxacin (eg, Floxin), 400 mg orally for one dose. Alternatives to doxycycline for *C trachomatis* include azithromycin, 1.0 g orally for one dose, or erythromycin base 500 mg, or erythromycin ethylsuccinate, 800 mg orally four times daily for 7 days. **Pregnant or breast-feeding women should receive ceftriaxone plus erythromycin.**
   2. **Acyclovir,** or a similar nucleoside analogue, should be given in standard doses for HSV (see Chapter 31, genital lesions).

F. No treatment other than reassurance is necessary for **physiologic discharge.**

G. Seventy-five to 90% of patients with **atrophic vaginitis** obtain relief with standard oral estrogen replacement, with added benefits of relief of vasomotor symptoms and osteoporosis prevention. (However, such benefits must be weighed against potential risks of combined estrogen/progestogen therapy found in the Women's Health Initiative study released in July 2002). Other therapeutic options include transvaginal estrogen creams, pessaries, or a hormone-releasing ring (eg, Estring). The latter offers advantages of only needing replacement every 3 months, not being messy, and allowing consistent estrogen release at levels low enough to avoid endometrial stimulation. Topical vaginal lubricants (eg, Vagisil, Replens) can also provide some relief for symptoms of atrophic vaginitis.

H. Treatment for **allergic vaginitis** is elimination of likely sensitizers.

REFERENCES

Bachmann GA, Nevadunsky NS: Diagnosis and treatment of atrophic vaginitis. Am Fam Physician 2000;**61:**3090.
Egan ME, Lipsky MS: Diagnosis of vaginitis. Am Fam Physician 2000;**62:**1095.
Nyirjesy P: Chronic vulvovaginal candidiasis. Am Fam Physician 2001;**63:**697.
US Preventive Services Task Force. Screening for bacterial vaginosis in pregnancy: Recommendations and rationale. Am Fam Physician 2002;**65:**1147.

---

65   Wheezing

Judith Anne Kerber, MD

KEY CONCEPTS

- The *cause* of wheezing should be identified based on the patient's age, and diseases other than asthma should be considered.
- **Respiratory distress** (cyanosis, retractions, apnea, or stridor) should be assessed immediately.
- **Chest x-ray** should be done in patients who present with new-onset wheezing.

I. **Definition.** Wheezing is a high-pitched musical sound produced by the lungs when airways become narrowed. Wheezing produces a sound similar to deep breathing with a child's party kazoo in the mouth.

II. **Common Diagnoses**
   A. **Infants younger than 2 years**
      1. **Acute viral respiratory tract infection (RTIs)** cause up to 50% of wheezing. Risk factors for RTIs include fall or winter season, child younger than 2 years, history of atopy (allergies or allergic skin conditions), hospitalization, school-aged siblings, day care attendance, passive smoke from parents or caregivers, and bottle-feeding.
      2. **Acute bronchitis and pneumonia** causes 33–50% of wheezing in infants. Most cases are caused by viral infection. Risk factors include passive smoke exposure from caregivers, viral upper respiratory infection (URI), and impaired gag reflex.
      3. **Bronchiolitis** is due to viral infections, especially respiratory syncytial virus (RSV), and accounts for <5% of wheezing. RSV is the most important cause of bronchiolitis and pneumonia in children younger than 2 years. It is epidemic in winter and spring in temperate climates. RSV is seen in all age groups, but preterm infants are at greater risk.
      4. **Aspiration** is seen in 1 in 300 infants. Gastroesophageal reflux (GER) is physiologic. It peaks at 1–4 months of age and usually resolves by 12 months. True gastroesophageal reflux disease (GERD) is pathologic. It presents with persistent respiratory symptoms, poor weight gain, and esophagitis. Other risk factors include anatomic abnormalities (pyloric stenosis, hiatal hernia, webs, malrotation, etc.).
      5. **Cystic fibrosis (CF)** has an incidence of 1/3500 births in whites. It is an inherited autosomal recessive trait that predisposes the patient to respiratory infections. Risk factors include white race and family history.
      6. **Anaphylaxis or hypersensitivity** requires that the patient must have had a prior exposure to the offending agent, often a drug (aspirin), food, bee sting, or exercise.
   B. **Children (age 2 years–teenager)**
      1. **RTIs**
      2. **Acute bronchitis and pneumonia**
      3. **Anaphylaxis or hypersensitivity**
      4. **Asthma** causes 10–15% of wheezing in children (see Chapter 68.) Risk factors for asthma include viral URI, family history, environmental exposures, passive smoke, age older than 2 years, and allergic rhinitis. Asthma in patients younger than age 2 may be called hyperreactive airway disease.
   C. **Young adult–middle age**
      1. **RTIs**
      2. **Acute bronchitis and pneumonia**
      3. **Asthma**
      4. **Anaphylaxis or hypersensitivity**
   D. **Elderly (age older than 50 years)**
      1. **RTIs**
      2. **Acute bronchitis and pneumonia**
      3. **Chronic obstructive pulmonary disease (COPD)** (see Chapter 70) affects more than 14 million Americans. Risk factors include current or prior smoking history of >20 pack-years, air pollution, environmental exposures, α_1-antitrypsin deficiency, and family history.
      4. **Congestive heart failure (CHF)** (see Chapter 72) affects over 5 million people in the United States. Risk factors include hypertension, glucose intolerance, smoking, cardiomegaly, atrial fibrillation, electrocardiogram abnormalities, coronary artery disease, and valvular heart disease.
      5. **Aspiration**
      6. **Anaphylaxis or hypersensitivity**
      7. **Pulmonary embolus** is rare and causes wheezing due to clot obstruction of pulmonary vessels. Risk factors include hypercoagulable state, prolonged bed rest, and CHF.

III. **Symptoms** (Table 65–1).
   A. Every symptom may not be present in each case.
   B. Additional symptoms may also be present.

IV. **Signs.** Systematic chest examination is essential and may provide clues to the cause of wheezing.

TABLE 65-1. SYMPTOMS WITH COMMON CAUSES OF WHEEZING

	Wheeze	Fever	Cough	Sore Throat	Rhinorrhea	Lethargy	Onset	Other
Acute viral infection	x	x	x	x	x		Rapid	Coryza
Pneumonia/ bronchitis	x	x	x				Rapid	
Bronchiolitis	x	x	x	x	x	x	Rapid	
GER/GERD	x		x				Gradual	Hoarseness
CF	x					x	Gradual	Irritability Poor feeding Meconium ileus Pancreatic insufficiency
Anaphylaxis	x		x				Rapid	Urticaria Stridor Chest discomfort Lump in throat Flushing N/V/D
Asthma	x		x		x		Gradual	Evening wheezing or coughing
COPD	x		Chronic				Gradual	Recurrent bronchitis Barrel chest
CHF	x		x				Gradual	Lower extremity swelling JVD
PE	x		x				Rapid	Acute shortness of breath Increased respiratory rate

CF, cystic fibrosis; CHF, congestive heart failure; COPD, chronic obstructive pulmonary disease; GER, gastroesophageal reflux; GERD, gastroesophageal reflux disease; JVD, jugular venous distention; N/V/D, nausea/vomiting/diarrhea; PE, pulmonary embolism.

A. **Inspection**
  1. **Respiratory rate** should be determined. (Normal is approximately 12–20 breaths per minute in adults; the normal rate in children varies with age.)
  2. **Intercostal retractions,** irregular abdominal breathing motions, are clues to respiratory distress.
  3. A so-called **barrel chest** is often associated with COPD, asthma, and CF.
B. **Percussion.** Symmetrical resonance is normal, whereas either dullness or hyperresonance may indicate asthma.
C. **Auscultation**
  1. A **prolonged expiratory phase** suggests constricted airways. It is noted by a continued exhale beyond normal duration.
  2. **Localized rhonchi** may signify pneumonia.
D. **Associated nonpulmonary findings** in wheezing patients.
  1. **Dennie's pleats** (a crease under the under the eyes from repeated rubbing) and **allergic shiners** (dark circles under the eyes) are often seen in patients with allergic rhinitis or asthma.
  2. **Jugular venous distention** and bilateral dependent edema are associated with CHF. (See Chapter 72.)
V. **Laboratory Tests**
  A. Posteroanterior and lateral views (PA and lat) **chest radiographs (CXR).**
    1. **Patients with a first episode of wheezing** require a CXR.

    a. Consolidations suggest pneumonia. A CXR may not show an infiltrate until 3 days into the disease.

    b. Cardiomegaly (an enlarged heart) may indicate CHF.

    c. Hyperexpansion, noted by >10 ribs showing and flat diaphragms, may indicate either asthma or COPD.

    d. A **diffuse hazy pattern** is seen in most viral illnesses.

  2. Known asthmatic patients do not require a CXR with every episode. If the patient has a fever, rhonchi, or sputum, a CXR is indicated to look for pneumonia.

B. Lung function tests

  1. Peak flow. This reading can be done in the office or at home. It involves the patient standing upright, placing a peak flowmeter in the mouth, inhaling, then exhaling rapidly and forcefully into the flowmeter. The meter is graduated and will record the FEV_1 (forced expired lung volume in 1 second). It measures how much air patients can rapidly move out of their lungs in 1 second.

    a. Results vary by height, sex, and age.

    b. Peak flow testing **does not** confirm a diagnosis, but is used to monitor the status of lung disease.

    c. Peak flow decreases with obstruction (airway narrowing seen in COPD or asthma) and is a good early indicator of worsening or improving obstruction.

  2. Pulmonary function tests (PFTs) can be performed in some clinic settings but are usually done in a pulmonary laboratory. These tests differentiate obstructive from restrictive lung disease, are useful in patients with recurrent lung problems (asthma, COPD), and provide more information than peak flow alone.

C. Complete blood count (CBC)

  1. Elevated white blood cell count (WBC) can indicate infection.

    a. Elevated lymphocytes indicate viral infection.

    b. A CBC with differential will include a band count, but it must be ordered specifically. **Elevated band count** or total polymorphonuclear cells (PMNs) [segs + bands] indicates a bacterial infection (a "left shift").

    c. WBC count can be **falsely elevated** in patients taking intravenous or oral steroids. (Watch for this in asthmatic patients or COPD patients on steroid tapers.)

  2. Low hemoglobin or hematocrit is often seen in patients with chronic diseases (anemia of chronic disease) and decreases oxygen-carrying capacity.

D. Nasopharyngeal wash (NP wash) is also called FA-5 (depending on the institution) and identifies five viruses causing bronchiolitis in infants/children—RSV, adenovirus, influenza A, influenza B, and parainfluenza. The test is performed by placing 2–3 cc of normal saline in a syringe; attaching 2–3 inches of plastic tubing, such as used for a butterfly venipuncture kit with the needle removed; making sure the patient is upright; and injecting all the saline into one of the patient's nostrils, then quickly pulling back on the plunger so the fluids re-enter the syringe. The syringe contents are then emptied into a media test tube, which must be kept on ice and sent to the virology laboratory for evaluation.

    Regular RSV NP wash takes approximately 24 hours to process; a rapid RSV test has recently become available, is used in emergency departments, and takes approximately 1–1.5 hours for results.

E. Other tests

  1. CF testing

    a. Sweat sodium and chloride testing is usually performed in a hospital setting. It is elevated in 90% of CF patients.

    b. Genetic testing is also indicated to identify CF carriers.

  2. GER/GERD testing

    a. The gold standard in a pediatric patient is a **24-hour pH probe.** (The patient is taken to the endoscopy laboratory for placement, then the device is left in the patient for 24 hours to assess for decreases in pH indicative of reflux.)

    b. Upper gastrointestinal barium swallow study reveals structural defects.

    c. Endoscopy is very invasive, requires sedation to perform, and usually is reserved for patients unresponsive to medical management.

VI. Treatment

A. Acute viral respiratory infection (see Chapters 55 and 57).

B. Acute bronchitis/pneumonia (see Chapter 13 for cough).

C. **Bronchiolitis**
1. **Prevention is best.** Premature infants may benefit from using either palivizumab (Synagis) or RSV immune globulin, which should be administered just prior to RSV season.
2. **Acute infection** necessitates supportive treatment.
    a. **Some patients may need to be hospitalized** if they cannot maintain acceptable oxygen saturation.
    b. **If they are stable enough to be at home,** they may benefit from nebulizer albuterol treatments, 2.5–5 mg every 8 hours, to relieve bronchial constriction. Outpatient treatment is preferred for otherwise healthy children.
    c. There is no evidence that ribavirin or antibiotics help.
D. **Aspiration**
1. **Reflux precautions** include thickening feeds (1 tbsp rice to 1 oz formula); sitting the infant upright and prone; giving small feeds (feed 1 oz, then burp the baby and repeat after every ounce consumed).
2. **GERD**
    a. Patients may need oral medications such as H_2 **blockers** (eg, ranitidine, 75–150 mg twice daily for adults); children aged 1 month to 16 years use 1–2 mg/kg twice daily. A **prokinetic agent** (eg, metoclopramide, 10–15 mg every 6 hours) may also help control GERD.
    b. In adolescents and adults, caffeine, alcohol, and smoking should be avoided.
E. Patients with **CF** should be referred to a CF clinic for a team approach to management.
F. **Anaphylaxis.** Immediate treatment includes epinephrine injections and H_1 antagonists (loratadine or fexofenadine). Prevention of recurrences includes behavior modification before another episode occurs.
G. **Asthma** (see Chapter 68).
H. **COPD** (see Chapter 70).
I. **CHF** (See Chapter 72).
J. **Pulmonary embolus** requires emergent hospitalization for anticoagulation and supportive care.

REFERENCES

American Academy of Pediatrics. Respiratory syncytial virus. In: Pickering LK (editor): *Red Book: 2003 Report of the Committee on Infectious Diseases,* 26th ed. American Academy of Pediatrics; 2003: 523–528.
Hosey R, Carek P, Goo A: Exercise-induced anaphylaxis and urticaria. Am Fam Physician 2001; **64:**1367.
Jung A: Gastroesophageal reflux in infants and children. Am Fam Physician 2001;**64:**1853.
Knutson D, Braun C: Diagnosis and management of acute bronchitis. Am Fam Physician 2002; **65:**2039.
Seidel H, et al (editors): *Mosby's Guide to Physical Examination,* 5th ed. Mosby; 2003:365–413.

SECTION II. Chronic Illnesses

66   Acne Vulgaris

Martin Quan, MD

KEY POINTS

- Classification of acne is the prime determinant of management and is based primarily on the number of lesions, the predominant type of lesion present, and the presence of scarring.
- Patients need to understand that cosmetic improvement is not likely to be apparent until 3–6 weeks after the initiation of therapy.
- Topical retinoids are the most effective agents for treating obstructive acne.
- Mild to moderate inflammatory acne can be treated with benzoyl peroxide plus a topical antibiotic or a topical retinoid.
- Oral contraceptives are indicated for the treatment of mild to moderate inflammatory acne.
- Moderate to severe inflammatory acne can be treated with a topical retinoid plus an oral antibiotic.
- Isotretinoin is a powerful acne agent whose indications include severe recalcitrant nodulocystic acne and patients with moderate to severe inflammatory acne unresponsive to conventional therapy.
- Isotretinoin is associated with numerous side effects and, because of its teratogenicity, must be prescribed with extreme caution in women of reproductive age.

I. **Introduction**
A. **Definition.** Acne vulgaris is a chronic, polymorphic skin disease of pilosebaceous units located on the face, chest, and back. It is generally a self-limited condition that begins during adolescence; however, acne can persist into adulthood.
B. **Epidemiology**
1. An estimated 17 million Americans are affected by acne vulgaris. The National Health Survey has found the prevalence of significant acne vulgaris to be as follows: in the 12- to 17-year age group, 250 per 1000; in the 18- to 24-year age group, 191 per 1000; in the 25- to 34-year age group, 84 per 1000; in the 35- to 45-year age group, 25 per 1000; and in the 45- to 54-year age group, 9 per 1000.
2. The incidence and severity of acne vulgaris are lower in Asians than in whites, and severe acne is less common in blacks than in whites.
3. Acne vulgaris tends to be familial, although its exact genetic pattern remains undetermined.
C. **Pathophysiology**
1. Although the cause of acne remains unknown, its manifestations arise from the interaction of the following four pathogenic events.
a. **Increased sebum production** caused by androgenic stimulation of sebaceous glands.
b. **Outlet obstruction** of the pilosebaceous follicle caused by follicular hyperkeratinization, an abnormal keratinization process characterized by increased cohesiveness and turnover of follicular epithelial cells.
c. **Proliferation of *Propionibacterium acnes,*** an anaerobic diphtheroid residing in the pilosebaceous follicle.
d. **Inflammation** mediated by the irritant action of sebum leaking into the dermis, as well as the production of chemotactic factors and enzymes produced by *P acnes.*
2. **Impaction of the pilosebaceous follicle** is the primary pathologic event in acne vulgaris, giving rise to the microcomedo. When this obstruction occurs, the continued production of sebum and keratin gives rise to visible lesions, which include closed and open comedones. Leakage or rupture of the contents of closed comedones into the dermis causes inflammatory acne lesions, including papules, pustules, nodules, and cysts.

II. Diagnosis. Clinical manifestations of acne vulgaris follow the pathophysiologic progression described above and include obstructive, inflammatory, and severe acne.

   A. Obstructive acne

      1. The **closed comedo,** or "**whitehead,**" is a flesh-colored or whitish, slightly palpable lesion that is approximately 1–3 mm in diameter.

      2. The **open comedo,** or "**blackhead,**" is a flat or slightly raised, brownish or black lesion that measures up to 5 mm in diameter.

   B. Inflammatory acne

      1. **Acne papules** are red, tender, elevated lesions that are as large as 5 mm in diameter. **Pustules** are superficial papules containing visible pus.

      2. **Acne nodules** are solid, inflammatory lesions that exceed 5 mm in diameter and are situated deeper than papules in the dermis.

      3. The **acne "cyst"** is actually a large nodule that has suppurated and become fluctuant.

      4. **Acne scars** are sequelae of inflammatory acne and may appear as small, deep, punched-out pits ("ice pick" scars), atrophic macules, hypertrophic scars, or broad, sloping depressions.

   C. Severe acne variants

      1. **Acne conglobata** is a disfiguring, highly inflammatory form of acne found predominantly in males. It is characterized by the presence of multiporous comedones, nodules, cysts, abscesses, and draining sinus tracts on the face, upper trunk, and posterior neck.

      2. **Acne fulminans** is an uncommon systemic disease characterized by sudden eruptions of large, highly inflammatory, encrusted, ulcerative acne lesions on the trunk, accompanied by other systemic features, including fever, polyarthritis, leukocytosis, anemia, and weight loss.

III. Treatment. Scarring is an important physical and psychosocial sequela of acne that occurs in a small percentage of patients with severe inflammatory acne. The treatment of acne is directed toward minimizing scarring and providing the patient with the best appearance possible by reducing the frequency and severity of exacerbations. Attempts at scar revision should be limited to patients with significant scarring whose acne is quiescent or well controlled. Scars should be permitted to evolve to their final appearance for at least 1 year before revision is considered.

   A. Obstructive acne. The treatment of patients with predominantly obstructive acne includes applying topical comedolytic agents, extracting comedones, and avoiding comedogenic products.

      1. Comedolytic agents and exfoliating agents

         a. Benzoyl peroxide is an antibacterial, oxidizing agent that possesses mild comedolytic properties and is available in a variety of concentrations (2.5%, 5%, or 10%) and formulations, including lotions, creams, and gels. A thin film of a low-strength (2.5% or 5%) preparation is applied once or twice daily. Preparation strength is increased as needed every 1–2 months. Mild redness and scaling frequently develop during the first few weeks of therapy but usually diminish with continued use. The liquid and cream preparations are less irritating, but the gel formulation is more effective. Contact allergy occurs in 1–2% of patients.

         b. Tretinoin (topical retinoic acid) is commercially available as Retin-A gel (0.01% or 0.025%), Retin-A cream (0.025%, 0.05%, or 0.1%), Retin-A liquid (0.05%), Retin-A gel microsphere (0.1%), and Avita polymer cream (0.025%). It is applied lightly once a day at bedtime; patients must take care to avoid the eyes, nose, and mouth.

           A highly effective topical comedolytic agent, tretinoin accelerates follicular epithelial cell turnover and reduces the cohesiveness of epidermal cells. Beneficial effects may not be seen for up to 12 weeks. Skin irritation is the major side effect of tretinoin, and an apparent exacerbation of inflammatory lesions may occur during the early weeks of therapy. Treatment for patients with fair or sensitive skin should be initiated with the cream preparation (0.025%) on an every other day or twice-weekly basis, since this preparation is the least irritating. Retina-A Micro and Avita cream are two new formulations of tretinoin with novel delivery systems designed to minimize irritative effects. The liquid preparation is the most irritating and therefore should be reserved for patients with recalcitrant lesions. The skin should be completely dry before tretinoin is applied, and the patient should minimize sun exposure and use a protective sunscreen (sun protection factor >15).

c. **Combined benzoyl peroxide and tretinoin.** Combination therapy may be tried in patients who continue to form comedones despite monotherapy with either benzoyl peroxide or tretinoin. Benzoyl peroxide is generally applied in the morning and tretinoin in the evening. It is best to initiate therapy by using each medication on alternating days and advancing to day and night applications in accordance with the patient's tolerance.

d. **Adapalene** is a synthetic retinoid analogue that is commercially available as Differin gel (0.1%). In addition to providing comedolytic activity, adapalene possesses anti-inflammatory activity and appears to be less irritating. It is applied once a day (at bedtime) as a thin film, to affected areas, avoiding the eyes, lips, and mucous membranes. Its therapeutic effect is typically seen 8–12 weeks after the initiation of treatment, and patients should be advised that their acne may actually worsen during the first few weeks of therapy. Skin irritation is seen in 10–40% of patients, and the use of sunscreen and the avoidance of excessive sun exposure should be recommended.

e. **Tazarotene** is a synthetic acetylenic retinoid that is commercially available as Tazorac gel (0.1% and 0.05%). It is a potent anticomedonal agent that is more irritating than tretinoin and adapalene. It is applied as a thin film once a day in the evening to affected areas. In addition to having US Food and Drug Administration (FDA) approval for the treatment of mild to moderate acne, it is also indicated for the treatment of stable plaque psoriasis.

f. **Azelaic acid** is a naturally occurring dicarboxylic acid that possesses a combination of antimicrobial and comedolytic properties. Although a less potent comedolytic than the retinoids, it may be useful in patients with obstructive acne who are unable to tolerate these agents. It is commercially available as Azelex cream (20%) and is approved by the FDA for the topical treatment of mild to moderate inflammatory acne. It is applied as a thin film that is massaged into the affected areas twice daily, after the skin is thoroughly washed and patted dry. Azelaic acid is not associated with photosensitivity and causes minimal skin irritation in 1–5% of patients. Clinical improvement in inflammatory lesions is typically seen by the fourth week of therapy.

g. **Exfoliating agents,** such as salicylic acid, elemental sulfur, and resorcinol, are less effective than benzoyl peroxide or tretinoin and are best used only in cases in which patients are unable to tolerate the latter preparations.

2. **Comedo extraction.** Both open and closed comedones can be extracted manually by applying gentle pressure with a comedo extractor or with the opening of an eyedropper. Prior to extraction, the pore may be enlarged with a 25-gauge needle.

B. **Inflammatory acne.** Antibiotics are the mainstay of treatment of inflammatory acne. Topical antibiotics are generally favored as first-line therapy for patients who have mild to moderate acne or as maintenance therapy during the tapering and withdrawal of systemic antibiotics. Systemic antibiotics are indicated for patients who have moderate to severe inflammatory acne as well as for those who fail topical therapy. Tretinoin and benzoyl peroxide, either singly or in combination, and intralesional steroid injections are important ancillary measures.

1. **Topical antibiotics.** These antibiotics work by inhibiting the growth and activity of *P acnes* within the follicle.

a. Commonly used preparations include **clindamycin** (Cleocin T 1%, available as a solution, lotion, or gel formulation); **erythromycin** (eg, A/T/S 2% gel and solution, Akne-mycin 2% ointment, Emgel 2% gel, Erycette 2% solution, and T-stat 2% solution); **tetracycline** (Topicycline 2.2% solution); and sodium sulfacetamide (eg, Klaron 10% solution, Sulfacet-R 5% and 10% solution). Combining benzoyl peroxide with a topical antibiotic offers several potential advantages including a synergistic antimicrobial action as well as reduced risk for the development of antibiotic resistance. Combination products include gel formulations containing 3% erythromycin and 5% benzoyl peroxide (eg, Benzamycin) as well as gel formulations containing 1% clindamycin and 5% benzoyl peroxide (eg, Duac, BenzaClin, Clindoxyl).

b. The usual dosage is applied twice daily to affected areas.

     c. The most common side effects of topical antibiotics are skin dryness and irritation. Antimicrobial-associated colitis is a rare complication resulting from topical clindamycin use. Topical tetracycline can produce fluorescence under ultraviolet light. Sodium sulfacetamide products may rarely cause hypersensitivity.

  2. Systemic antibiotics. Clinical experience of nearly four decades has shown such therapy to be effective in the treatment of acne.

     a. The antibiotics most commonly prescribed for acne are **tetracycline** and **erythromycin.**

     b. The initial daily dosage is 1–2 g in two to four divided doses, continued until beneficial effects occur (generally 1–2 months). This dose is then gradually reduced over 2–4 months to the lowest maintenance dose sufficient to maintain control. Patients should increase their dose to 1–2 g at the first sign of a flare-up.

     c. Side effects are infrequent, consisting primarily of gastrointestinal upset and vaginal candidiasis. Gram-negative folliculitis is a superinfection seen in 1–4% of patients on long-term antibiotic therapy.

     d. Tetracycline is contraindicated in pregnant patients and in children younger than 9 years of age because it may stain developing teeth.

     e. Antibiotics less frequently prescribed in acne include doxycycline, minocycline, and trimethoprim-sulfamethoxazole. Doxycycline, which is prescribed at a dose of 75–200 mg/day, is a second-generation tetracycline agent with a similar side effect profile as tetracycline except for a higher risk of phototoxicity. Minocycline (Minocin), in a daily dosage of 100–200 mg, is another tetracycline derivative that is usually reserved for inflammatory acne unresponsive to conventional oral antibiotic therapy. Side effects limiting its use include dizziness and, rarely, pigmentary changes in the skin. Trimethoprim-sulfamethoxazole (eg, Bactrim or Septra), administered as a double-strength tablet once or twice a day, is usually prescribed for severe cases refractory to other antibiotics and for gram-negative folliculitis.

  3. Intralesional corticosteroid injection is an important adjunct in the management of nodulocystic acne lesions. It often produces a rapid reduction in inflammation and reduces the likelihood of scarring.

     a. A 30-gauge needle is used to inject a solution containing **triamcinolone acetonide** (0.63–2.5 mg/mL), formed by diluting the preparation with either normal saline or lidocaine. Approximately 0.05–0.3 mL is injected into the cavity of the acne lesion so as to slightly distend it. Injections can be repeated after 3 weeks.

     b. The risk of steroid-induced skin changes (eg, atrophy, telangiectasia, and pigmentary changes) can be reduced by using the dilute solution and injecting the minimum amount required. Adrenal suppression can be avoided by administering no more than 20 mg at a time.

  4. Combined oral contraceptives. Birth control pills that combine ethinyl estradiol with a progestin agent with low androgenicity (ie, norgestimate, desogestrel) can improve acne by raising sex hormone–binding globulin and lowering serum free testosterone levels in females.

     a. Birth control pills represent a particularly valuable option in female patients with acne who need an effective contraceptive method and have no medical contraindications to their use.

     b. Ortho Tri-Cyclen was the first birth control pill to have FDA approval for use in the treatment of acne. FDA approval has subsequently been granted to Estrostep.

C. Severe inflammatory acne. Patients with severe nodulocystic acne refractory to standard therapy as well as patients with severe acne variants are generally best managed by a dermatologist. Treatment options include oral isotretinoin, spironolactone, and systemic corticosteroids.

  1. Oral isotretinoin. Isotretinoin (Accutane), a highly effective treatment for acne that often produces prolonged remissions following a successful course of therapy, is the only acne treatment that can alter the natural history of the disease. It is indicated for patients with acne that is unresponsive to conventional therapy who have either severe nodulocystic acne or moderate to severe noncystic, inflammatory acne that has the potential for scarring. Isotretinoin causes an involution of sebaceous glands, lowers intrafollicular bacterial counts, reverses retention hyperkeratosis, and directly decreases inflammation.

    a. The recommended daily dosage of isotretinoin is 0.5–1.0 mg/kg. A dose of 2 mg/kg should be used in resistant cases. During treatment, the dose can be modified according to the clinical response, the appearance of side effects, or both; most of these are dose related. The drug should be taken once or twice daily for 15–20 weeks.

    b. Adverse reactions to isotretinoin are frequent. Mucocutaneous side effects, which include cheilitis, conjunctivitis, dry mucous membranes of the nose and mouth, xerosis, and photosensitivity, are the most common and can generally be managed by the use of topical emollients, artificial tears, or dose reduction. Other side effects include arthralgias and myalgias as well as central nervous system side effects such as headache, nyctalopia, and pseudotumor cerebri. Laboratory changes associated with isotretinoin include hypertriglyceridemia, elevated total cholesterol, and reduced high-density lipoprotein levels, as well as abnormalities in liver function tests and hematologic parameters.

    c. Isotretinoin is a teratogen, resulting in a 25-fold increase in major fetal malformations (eg, hydrocephalus, microcephalus, external ear abnormalities, facial dysmorphia, and cardiovascular abnormalities). It is imperative that female patients of reproductive age understand the risk of these severe birth defects and observe **strict contraceptive precautions** during therapy and for at least 1 month following completion of therapy. A pregnancy test should be performed prior to starting therapy as well as monthly during therapy.

    d. To improve pregnancy avoidance in women taking this teratogen, physicians prescribing isotretinoin are required to participate in the S.M.A.R.T. (System to Manage Accutane-Related Teratogenicity) program. This program, which was implemented by Roche Pharmaceuticals in April 2002, calls for documentation of a negative pregnancy test to the pharmacy before the prescription is filled, monthly pregnancy testing as well as the commitment of sexually active women to simultaneously use two reliable forms of contraception for at least 1 month before, during, and 1 month after isotretinoin therapy.

2. Spironolactone

    a. Spironolactone is an antiandrogen agent whose role in acne is generally limited to selected females with difficult-to-treat acne.

    b. It is administered at a dose of 50–100 mg a day in two or three divided doses.

    c. Menstrual irregularities are the most common side effects associated with its use. Less common adverse effects include breast tenderness, breast enlargement, reduced libido, and hyperkalemia.

3. Other agents. Although **dapsone** (diacetyl diaminodiphenylsulfone) and systemic **corticosteroids** have been used in patients with severe inflammatory acne because of their powerful anti-inflammatory properties, these agents are rarely prescribed because of significant side effects associated with long-term use.

IV. Management Strategies. Successful acne management has its roots in patient education and compliance. Sufficient time should be allotted at the initial visit to explain the pathogenesis of acne and the rationale behind its treatment. It is important that the patient be involved as an active participant in his or her own care and that the physician be viewed as a caring and interested ally. Follow-up visits should be routinely scheduled at regular intervals and used to monitor therapy and to respond to questions or concerns that may arise. Important points of information that warrant discussion include the following items.

A. Acne vulgaris is a **chronic skin disorder** likely to run a waxing and waning course. Although treatment generally controls acne, it does not cure it.

B. Long-term therapy is required to control acne. Therefore, therapy must be continued even after the patient's skin clears. **Topical therapy** should be applied to all affected areas, not just individual lesions. **Oral antibiotics** (particularly tetracycline) should generally be taken on an empty stomach, either 1 hour before or 2 hours after meals.

C. Significant improvement of the patient's appearance may not be apparent for 3–6 weeks after the initiation of therapy, and maximum benefit may not be seen for several months.

D. Acne is not caused by poor **hygiene.** Obsessive scrubbing can actually exacerbate the condition. Picking and popping pimples serve only to increase inflammation and the likelihood of scarring.

E. There is no relationship between acne and **masturbation, sexual activity,** or **venereal disease.**

F. Oil-based cosmetics and moisturizers can be comedogenic and should be avoided.

G. Research studies have failed to substantiate the need for rigid **dietary restrictions** in acne management. Patients are advised to eat a healthy diet, avoiding only those foods that have consistently resulted in aggravation of acne.

REFERENCES

Cunliffe WJ, Gollnick HPM: *Acne: Diagnosis and Management.* Martin Dunitz; 2001.
Liou DC: Management of acne. J Fam Pract 2003;**52:**43.
Oberemok SS, Shalita AR: Acne vulgaris. II: Treatment. Cutis 2002;**70:**111.
Russell JJ: Topical therapy for acne. Am Fam Physician 2000;**61**(2):357.
Thiboutot D: New treatments and therapeutic strategies for acne. Arch Fam Med 2000;**9:**179.

---

67   Acquired Immunodeficiency Syndrome (AIDS)

Jennifer Cocohoba, PharmD, & Ronald H. Goldschmidt, MD

KEY POINTS

- Assess risk for human immunodeficiency virus (HIV) and sexually transmitted diseases in all patients.
- Consider the diagnosis of acute HIV infection in patients presenting with fever, rash, and myalgias. Assess risk factors for HIV.
- Consider HIV infection for patients presenting with thrush, pneumonia, and herpes infections.
- Do not initiate antiretroviral therapy in acutely hospitalized patients.
- Antiretroviral therapy should be initiated only for patients who are prepared for lifelong multidrug treatment. Consultation with experts in HIV treatment is helpful.
- Do not discontinue antiretroviral therapy in acutely hospitalized patients unless severe toxicity is apparent.
- Antiretroviral drug failure can be the result of nonadherence with treatment regimens or virologic resistance. Resistance testing can be helpful in guiding treatment choices.

I. Introduction

A. Definition. Human immunodeficiency virus (HIV) disease is a chronic progressive disease caused by a retrovirus, the **human immunodeficiency virus. Acquired immunodeficiency syndrome (AIDS),** as defined by characteristic opportunistic infections (eg, *Pneumocystis carinii* pneumonia [PCP]), cancers (eg, Kaposi's sarcoma), neurologic conditions (eg, HIV-related encephalopathy), a CD4+ lymphocyte count below 200 cells per microliter, or all of these, is the advanced stage of HIV disease.

1. **Acute syndrome.** This syndrome, which usually occurs about 2–4 weeks following HIV infection, is difficult to identify because of its nonspecific nature. The symptoms and signs are similar to those of many viral syndromes and can include fever, maculopapular rash, sore throat, lymphadenopathy, oral and genital ulcers, headache, malaise, arthralgias, and myalgias. Oral ulcers in the setting of acute viral symptoms and compatible risk factors for HIV infection are considered pathognomonic pending laboratory confirmation. Sometimes abdominal cramps and diarrhea are present. (Aseptic meningitis, encephalopathy, and neuropathies rarely occur.) The acute HIV syndrome usually resolves spontaneously within 1–2 weeks.

2. **Asymptomatic HIV infection.** After infection, an asymptomatic phase lasting 5–10 years occurs. Although infection persists and the virus continues to proliferate, the immunologic system remains relatively intact.

3. **Symptomatic HIV infection.** Conditions such as oral candidiasis (thrush), oral hairy leukoplakia, generalized lymphadenopathy, thrombocytopenia, and weight loss generally precede the development of clinical AIDS. These conditions can also occur in persons who are not infected with HIV, however, so their presence alone does not define HIV infection.

4. AIDS. Clinical AIDS is characterized by advanced immunodeficiency with specific opportunistic infections, wasting, cancers, and encephalopathy. AIDS is also defined by the finding of a CD4$^+$ (T helper) lymphocyte count of <200 cells per microliter.

5. AIDS in children

  a. Infants and children with AIDS present with recurrent bacterial infections, lymphadenopathy, pneumonia, failure to thrive, loss of developmental milestones, or behavioral problems. Consultation with pediatric AIDS specialists is generally necessary to guide therapy and arrange for clinical trials.

  b. Immunization schedules for children with HIV differ from the standard schedules found in Chapter 101. Oral polio vaccine should not be used in children with AIDS or in families with children who are either infected or suspected of being infected with HIV.

B. Epidemiology

  1. Prevalence. An estimated 750,000 Americans are infected with HIV; more than 650,000 of these persons have developed clinical AIDS. As of December 2001, more than 8000 children were infected through vertical transmission in the United States. Because of extensive testing and treatment, fewer than 200 new vertical transmissions have occurred annually since 2000.

  2. Transmission of HIV requires the exchange of body fluids. HIV, which is not spread by casual contact, can be transmitted in the following ways.

   a. Intimate sexual contact.

   b. Intravenous drug use involving sharing of needles.

   c. Transfusion of HIV-infected blood products. Since the introduction of HIV antibody screening in 1985, blood products have become extremely safe (approximately 1 in 40,000 units is infected). Organ transplantation, once a means of HIV transmission, is also very safe.

   d. Perinatal transmission from mother to child.

   e. Occupational exposures from needlesticks.

  3. The **average period between initial infection and development of clinical AIDS** has been estimated to be about 8–11 years among homosexual males. AIDS takes less time to develop in children and among intravenous (IV) drug users.

  4. Prior to the use of highly active antiretroviral therapy (HAART), the **average length of survival** was <15 years. In the era of HAART, opportunistic infections and other complications of AIDS have declined and the average length of survival has increased dramatically.

C. Pathophysiology

  1. HIV, a retrovirus, invades CD4$^+$ lymphocytes, macrophages, monocytes, and certain other tissue cells, causing their destruction and dysfunction. Immunodeficiency results from the destruction of the CD4$^+$ lymphocytes and associated abnormalities of the immune system.

  2. Opportunistic infections and cancers can occur in virtually any organ system during this state of impaired immune function.

II. Diagnosis. Most patients are diagnosed by screening tests rather than by history of opportunistic infections or other manifestations. Early stages of AIDS can be similar to diseases of specific organ systems or nonspecific illnesses such as influenza. Advanced AIDS, with the combination of wasting, infections, and cancers, is rarely confused with other diseases. AIDS complications can be confused with other disorders, so risk assessment, counseling, and HIV testing must be considered.

A. Symptoms and signs

  1. Nonspecific symptoms such as weakness, anorexia, fever, and weight loss are most commonly caused by HIV or opportunistic infections and cancers. Such symptoms can also be caused by bacterial or fungal sepsis or *Mycobacterium avium–intracellulare* complex (MAC) disease or tuberculosis. Cultures can help determine the cause of significant fevers. Treatment of infections caused by MAC can relieve associated fever and other symptoms, although treatment can be more toxic than helpful in some cases.

  2. Common opportunistic infections and cancers

   a. Skin conditions

    (1) Kaposi's sarcoma (KS) of the skin or oral mucosa appears as red to purple lesions, usually >0.5 cm in diameter.

     (2) **Maculopapular rashes** are exceedingly common and are often associated with drug treatment (either prescription or over-the-counter drugs).
- b. **Eye diseases.** Yellow-white or hemorrhagic patches on the retina can indicate sight-threatening **cytomegalovirus (CMV) retinitis.**
- c. **Oral cavity**
  - (1) White plaques or erosive (erythematous) areas suggest **oral candidiasis.** Thrush is common in advanced symptomatic HIV infection and is seen almost universally in clinical AIDS.
  - (2) Painless, white, somewhat hairlike lesions on the lateral borders of the tongue indicate **hairy leukoplakia.** This condition, which is caused by the **Epstein-Barr virus,** will disappear and may recur. It requires no treatment.
- d. **Lymph nodes.** Lymph nodes are frequently enlarged, usually reflecting a generalized response to HIV infection. Hard, asymmetrical, or extremely prominent nodes may require biopsy to exclude fungal infection or cancer.
- e. **Pulmonary** involvement is the most common condition in patients with AIDS. *P carinii* is the most common pathogen, and **PCP** is the most common pulmonary disease. Bacterial pneumonias, fungal and mycobacterial infections, and KS are also important causes of pulmonary diseases.
  - (1) Patients with pulmonary disease may present with symptoms that range from mild shortness of breath or nonproductive cough to severe respiratory distress. Acute PCP is most commonly characterized by shortness of breath, dry cough, and fever. Chest x-rays usually show patchy infiltrates or diffuse interstitial disease, although 5% of chest x-rays of patients with pulmonary disease may be normal. Sputum production is uncommon unless bacterial pneumonia is present.
  - (2) Evaluation of pulmonary disease generally requires examination of induced sputum, bronchial washings, or biopsies. Careful microscopic examination and cultures for *P carinii, Mycobacterium tuberculosis,* bacteria, and fungi are essential.
- f. **Gastrointestinal conditions**
  - (1) **Esophagitis.** Dysphagia, odynophagia, and substernal burning pain are symptomatic of **esophagitis.** Esophagitis can be caused by *Candida albicans,* CMV, or herpes simplex virus. When an empiric trial of antifungal-medications for patients with concurrent oral candidiasis fails, endoscopy with biopsies and cultures is essential to establish a diagnosis and direct treatment.
  - (2) **Diarrhea,** often copious and frequently associated with malabsorption, can be caused by *Isospora belli, Cryptosporidium, Entamoeba histolytica, Campylobacter,* and other enteric pathogens. Diarrhea from HIV infection alone can occur and requires symptomatic treatment. Diarrhea can also be a complication of HIV medications.
  - (3) **Liver disease.** Increased alkaline phosphatase levels commonly indicate liver infection by *M avium–intracellulare* or *M tuberculosis* or liver involvement by KS or lymphoma. Acute and chronic **viral hepatitis** and **drug-induced hepatitis** can also occur. Biopsy, although rarely helpful, can be considered in some cases in which *M tuberculosis* infections or other treatable conditions may be present.
- g. **Neurologic problems**
  - (1) **Peripheral neuropathies** can result in painful dysesthesias of the feet and the legs. Cranial neuropathies can also occur. Presumably, HIV involvement of neural tissue causes this condition.
  - (2) **AIDS dementia complex** is characterized by behavioral changes, deficits in cognitive function, and lack of coordination. Although HIV appears to be the principal cause, other pathogenic conditions (eg, cryptococcal meningoencephalitis or cerebral toxoplasmosis) can also be involved.
  - (3) **Meningoencephalitis,** most often caused by *Cryptococcus neoformans* infection, is characterized by headache (usually slight, although at times severe), fever, and decreased mental functioning. Neck pain and nuchal

rigidity can be present. Cryptococcal antigen determination from serum and cerebrospinal fluid is positive in most cases.

(4) **Mass lesions in the central nervous system** may result in encephalopathic symptoms, seizures, or focal neurologic deficits. These lesions can be caused by *Toxoplasma gondii* infection, lymphomas, and, rarely, other opportunistic infections.

B. **Laboratory tests**

1. **Screening for HIV.** A reactive screening test (eg, enzyme-linked immunoabsorbent essay [ELISA]) plus a positive specific test (eg, Western blot or immunofluorescent antibody) confirm HIV infection. Generally, these tests become positive within 1 month of infection; almost all infected persons display positive HIV tests within 3–6 months of infection. In most cases, these tests will remain positive indefinitely.

2. **Indicators of progression of HIV disease**

   a. A person with advanced HIV disease usually has a **CD4+ count** of <200 cells per microliter. Normal levels of CD4+ cells usually exceed 800 cells per microliter.

   b. Quantitative plasma **HIV RNA (viral load)** testing is used for staging and monitoring response to therapy. Current tests can now detect viral particles down to 20–50 copies/mL. After a baseline test is obtained (two tests 2 weeks apart), viral load testing should be checked every 3–4 months. A significant change in viral burden is measured as a threefold increase and can be caused by disease progression, failure of antiretroviral therapy, active infection, or immunizations. Conversely, a threefold decrease from baseline after therapy has been instituted is considered a significant drop in viral burden.

3. **Laboratory evaluation of specific organ systems** includes hematologic tests, examination of body fluids, invasive diagnostic tests to obtain cultures and tissues, and imaging studies.

4. **Drug resistance testing** may be useful for individual patient management.

III. **Treatment.** *Drug therapy for HIV disease is rapidly changing and is complex. US Public Health Service guidelines are updated regularly (www.aidsinfo.nih.gov) and serve as the most important single source of comprehensive guidance for HIV care. Starting or changing regimens may have far-reaching implications that may affect the availability and efficacy of future therapy. Before one prescribes any medications, consultation with an HIV expert is recommended.*

A. **HIV antiretroviral (ARV) treatment strategies.** All patients with AIDS and patients symptomatic with any level of viremia should be offered therapy.

1. **Initiating ARV therapy.** The best time to initiate ARV therapy for asymptomatic patients is not clearly established. Current standards recommend that ARV therapy be initiated when CD4+ cell counts fall below 200–cells/mm^3. When the viral load is >55,000 copies per milliliter, ARV therapy should be considered. Patients whose CD4+ count is >350 cells/mm^3 have the option to delay therapy. Note that initiating ARV therapy can induce an **immune reconstitution syndrome** within days or weeks. The manifestations of this syndrome are generally the activation of a quiescent opportunistic infection (such as CMV retinitis, *M tuberculosis* infection, PCP, and many other opportunistic infections).

2. **Constructing an ARV regimen**

   a. First-line therapy consists of a backbone of two nucleoside reverse transcriptase inhibitors (nRTIs) combined with single or dual ("boosted") protease inhibitors (PI), a non-nucleoside reverse transcriptase inhibitor (nNRTI), or a third nucleoside nRTI.

   b. Potent regimens should not be a random selection of agents from different antiretroviral classes. Clinically proven combinations should be considered in conjunction with potential for toxicity, drug-drug interactions, and cross-resistance patterns.

   c. Certain combinations should be avoided because of poor virologic outcomes or overlapping toxicities. These include all monotherapies and the following nRTI combinations: stavudine + zidovudine, didanosine + stavudine, zalcitabine + didanosine, and zalcitabine + lamivudine.

3. **Classes of antiretroviral agents.** There are currently five classes of antiretroviral agents that can be used in combination (Table 67–1).

TABLE 67-1. HIV ANTIRETROVIRAL AGENTS

Class	Drug	Dosing	Adverse Effects	Administration/Other Notes
Nucleoside/nucleotide RT inhibitors (nRTIs)	Abacavir *(ABC, Ziagen)*	300 mg po bid	Nausea, vomiting, diarrhea, headache, rash, rare hypersensitivity syndrome (2–5%)	Hypersensitivity usually occurs during the first 6 weeks of therapy. Symptoms include fever, rash, nausea/vomiting, and flu-like symptoms. If a patient experiences a hypersensitivity reaction, abacavir should be discontinued. Fatalities have occurred upon rechallenge.
	Didanosine *(ddI, Videx Videx EC)*	200 mg po bid (>60 kg, buffered) 125 mg po bid (<60 kg, buffered) 400 mg po qd (>60 kg, *Videx EC*) 250 mg po qd (<60 kg, *Videx EC*)	Peripheral neuropathy, pancreatitis, diarrhea, GI upset	2 tablets per dose of buffered didanosine must be given to ensure proper absorption. Interactions may occur with drugs impaired by buffered agents.
	Emtricitabine *(FTC, Emtriva)*	200 mg po qd	Headache, nausea, skin discoloration, diarrhea, rash	Very similar to lamivudine, even in resistance patterns
	Lamivudine *(3TC, Epivir)*	150 mg po bid or 300 mg po qd	Headache, fatigue, insomnia	No known drug interactions. Also used to treat hepatitis B.
	Stavudine *(d4T, Zerit)*	40 mg po bid if >60 kg 20 mg po bid if <60 kg	Peripheral neuropathy, pancreatitis	Stavudine should not be combined with zidovudine due to antagonism.
	Tenofovir *(TDF, Viread)*	300 mg po qd	Nausea, vomiting, diarrhea, flatulence, headaches	Lower dose of didanosine if given in combination with tenofovir
	Zalcitabine *(ddC, Hivid)*	0.75 mg po tid if >60 kg 0.375 mg po tid if <60 kg	Peripheral neuropathy, pancreatitis, stomatitis, GI upset, aphthous ulcers	This medication is less potent than other NRTIs
	Zidovudine *(AZT, Retrovir)*	300 mg po bid	Bone marrow suppression, myositis, GI upset, headache	Beware of drug interactions with probenecid and ribavirin
Fusion inhibitors	Enfuvirtide *(T-20, Fuzeon)*	90 mg sq bid	Injection-site reactions, fever, asthenia	Reconstituted doses are stable for 24 hours. Patients must be taught to self-inject. Availability may be limited.

	Drug	Dosing	Adverse effects	Comments
Non-nucleoside RT inhibitors (nNRTIs)	Efavirenz (EFV, Sustiva)	600 mg po qd	Dizziness, difficulty concentrating, vivid dreams, dysphoria, rash, LFT elevations, hepatitis	Avoid high-fat meals. Monitor for drug interactions.
	Nevirapine (NVP, Viramune)	200 mg po qd × 2 weeks, then ↑ to 200 mg po bid	Rash, LFT elevations, nausea, vomiting, diarrhea, fulminant hepatotoxicity, Stevens-Johnson syndrome	Fulminant hepatotoxicity (black box warning) may occur during the first 8 weeks of therapy. Dose escalation may reduce incidence of rash. Monitor for drug interactions.
	Delavirdine (DLV, Rescriptor)	400 mg po tid	Rash, nausea, headache, LFT elevations	Monitor for drug interactions. Separate delavirdine and antacids by 1–2 hours.
Protease inhibitors (PIs)	Ritonavir (RIT, Norvir)	600 mg po bid or 100–200 mg qd–bid as a "boosting" agent	Nausea, vomiting, diarrhea, anorexia, fatigue, hepatitis, lipid disturbances	Used in small doses to boost the serum levels of other PIs. Monitor for drug interactions.
	Saquinavir (SQV, Invirase Fortovase)	1600 mg po tid or 1600 mg (+200 mg ritonavir) qd or 1000 mg (+100 mg ritonavir) bid	Headache, confusion, nausea, GI upset	Fortovase has improved absorption if used alone. If boosted, Invirase and Fortovase have equal absorption. Monitor for interactions.
	Indinavir (IND, Crixivan)	800 mg po tid or 800 mg (+100 mg ritonavir) bid	Diarrhea, GI upset, nephrolithiasis, asymptomatic increases in bilirubin	Best on empty stomach unless boosted. Patients should consume at least 6 glasses of water per day to avoid nephrolithiasis. Separate from buffered didanosine and antacids by 1–2 hours. Monitor for drug interactions.
	Nelfinavir (NFV, Viracept)	1250 mg po bid or 750 mg po tid	Diarrhea, nausea, vomiting, GI upset	Monitor for drug interactions. Diarrhea may require symptomatic treatment with loperamide or Lomotil.
	Amprenavir (AMP, Agenerase)	1200 mg po bid or 600 mg (+100 mg ritonavir) bid or 1200 mg (+200 mg ritonavir) qd	Rash, nausea/vomiting, diarrhea, perioral paresthesias	Avoid high-fat meals and vitamin E. Sulfa drug. Monitor for drug interactions.
	Lopinavir/ritonavir (LOP/r, Kaletra)	3 capsules (400/100) po bid	Diarrhea, headache, rash, asthenia	Fixed dose combination capsules. Monitor for drug interactions
	Atazanavir (ATV, Reyataz)	400 mg po qd with food	Nausea, vomiting, diarrhea, rash, increased bilirubin	Monitor for drug interactions

GI, gastrointestinal; LFT, liver function tests.

411

    a. **Nucleoside and nucleotide reverse transcriptase inhibitors (nRTIs)** work by inhibiting HIV viral DNA synthesis. Two nRTIs in combination form the "backbone" of most HIV regimens. All nucleoside/nucleotide agents can cause nausea, vomiting, liver function test (LFT) elevations, lipoatrophy, and lactic acidosis with hepatic steatosis.

    b. **Non-nucleoside reverse transcriptase inhibitors (nNRTIs)** inhibit HIV viral DNA synthesis. A single nNRTI can be combined with a nucleoside backbone to form a complete regimen. As a class, nNRTIs commonly cause LFT elevations, hepatitis, rash, and drug interactions.

    c. **Protease inhibitors (PIs)** inhibit formation of HIV viral proteins. PI serum levels are often "boosted" by the addition of a small amount of ritonavir. A single or boosted protease inhibitor is combined with a nucleoside backbone to form a complete regimen. Protease inhibitors as a class may cause nausea, vomiting, hepatitis, and various metabolic disturbances including lipid, glucose, fat accumulation, and bone disturbances. Medications should be screened for drug interactions with protease inhibitors.

    d. **Fusion/entry inhibitors** are typically reserved for patients who have failed multiple antiretroviral regimens.

4. Preferred initial regimens

    a. Therapy should be initiated in consultation with a clinician experienced in managing antiretroviral regimens. Regimen selection should be based on several factors including potency, durability, tolerability, and the patient's ability to adhere. The US Department of Health and Human Services recently published guidelines containing two preferred initial regimens a clinician may consider starting in an ARV-naïve patient. For information regarding the dose of each ARV agent, please refer to Table 67–1.

        (1) Option #1: Efavirenz (Sustiva) *PLUS* lamivudine (Epivir) *PLUS EITHER* zidovudine (Retrovir) *OR* tenofovir (Viread) *OR* stavudine (Zerit). Potential acute side effects include rash, nausea, vomiting, flatulence, anemia, and drug-induced hepatitis. This combination is contraindicated in pregnant patients.

        (2) Option #2: Lopinavir/ritonavir (Kaletra) *PLUS* lamivudine (Epivir) *PLUS EITHER* zidovudine (Retrovir) *OR* stavudine (Zerit). Potential acute side effects from this regimen include but are not limited to nausea, vomiting, anemia, drug-induced hepatitis, and metabolic disturbances in lipids and glucose.

5. Adherence. Optimal adherence to antiretroviral therapy is key in achieving and maintaining durable viral suppression. Patients should be counseled on the risks of developing resistance if adherence is less than excellent. Tools such as pill boxes or watch alarms can be used to help enhance adherence.

B. Opportunistic infections and other manifestations

  1. Prophylaxis to prevent opportunistic infections is indicated when CD4+ levels decrease to specific threshold values, as described in Table 67–2.

  2. Kaposi's sarcoma (KS) of the skin and oral mucosa does not require treatment unless the lesions are uncomfortable or cosmetically disturbing. Widespread disease can be treated with chemotherapeutic agents. Radiation therapy and direct injection with chemotherapeutic agents are effective for some localized disease. Treatment does not appear to prolong life. Antiretroviral treatment may improve KS.

  3. CMV retinitis. Ganciclovir, foscarnet, cidofovir, or oral **valganciclovir** administered for an induction period of 14–21 days followed by lifelong maintenance therapy, is effective in retarding the progression of CMV retinitis. Selection of drug therapy depends on clinical toxicity variables and availability of supportive care. Valganciclovir is dosed at 900 mg orally twice daily during the induction period, followed by 900 mg orally once daily for maintenance therapy. Ganciclovir is dosed at 5 mg/kg IV every 12 hours during the induction period and 5 mg/kg IV once daily for maintenance therapy. Alternative medications include foscarnet, 90 mg/kg IV every 12 hours (induction), followed by 90 mg/kg IV once daily (maintenance); and cidofovir, 5 mg/kg IV once weekly (induction), followed by 5 mg/kg IV once every 2 weeks. All four medications must be dose-adjusted for renal impairment.

TABLE 67-2. PRIMARY PROPHYLAXIS FOR OPPORTUNISTIC INFECTIONS[1]

CD4+ Count	Provide Prophylaxis for
<200	*Pneumocystis carinii* pneumonia
<100	Toxoplasmosis
<50	*Mycobacterium avium–intracellulare* complex (MAC)

[1] If antiretroviral therapy results in a CD4+ count increase above prophylaxis thresholds for 6 months, primary prophylaxis can be discontinued.

4. **Oral candidiasis** is readily treated with **fluconazole,** 50–100 mg by mouth daily. Standard antifungal troches or solutions such as **clotrimazole** troches, 10 mg five times daily, or vaginal suppositories, 100 mg once or twice daily, or **nystatin,** 5 mL swish-and-swallow every 6 hours or 500,000-U vaginal tablets dissolved in the mouth every 6 hours, are–suitable alternative therapies.

5. *Pneumocystis carinii* **pneumonia (PCP)**
   a. **Acute PCP.** Three weeks of uninterrupted treatment is successful in most episodes of acute PCP. Clinical and radiologic evidence of response to therapy usually takes 3–7 days. Acute PCP can be treated on an inpatient or outpatient basis. Outpatient therapy is preferred when the disease appears mild and adequate home support is available.
      (1) **Trimethoprim-sulfamethoxazole (TMP-SMZ),** administered intravenously or orally, is the drug of choice in treating acute PCP. TMP-SMZ has the advantage of providing additional treatment against most bacterial pulmonary pathogens. The dosage is 15 mg of TMP and 75 mg of SMZ per kilogram daily, divided into four equal doses or two double-strength TMP-SMZ tablets orally every 8 hours. Two- to 3-week therapy is recommended. Skin rashes are common; when the rash is mild and does not involve the mucous membranes, TMP-SMZ treatment can usually be continued with the addition of antihistamine therapy. Nephrotoxicity and hepatotoxicity can also occur.
      (2) **Other agents can be effective against PCP. Clindamycin,** 300–450 mg orally every 6 hours, plus 15 mg of **primaquine** base orally every 6 hours; **dapsone,** 100 mg orally once daily plus **trimethoprim,** 5 mg/kg orally three times daily; or **atovaquone,** 750 mg orally twice daily, can be used for mild to moderate PCP. **Pentamidine** at 4 mg/kg IV daily is an alternative for severe PCP.
   b. **PCP prophylaxis.** Patients with a CD4+ lymphocyte count <200 cells per microliter should receive **primary PCP prophylaxis.**
      (1) **TMP-SMZ** is the drug of choice. The dosage is one double-strength tablet twice daily, or three times per week.
      (2) **Dapsone,** 50–100 mg orally daily, is a suitable alternative.

6. **Esophagitis** caused by *C albicans* can be treated with oral **fluconazole,** 100–200 mg daily, or **ketoconazole,** 400 mg daily. Failure to respond necessitates endoscopic evaluation for herpes esophagitis or CMV esophagitis. Intravenous **acyclovir,** 5 mg/kg every 8 hours, followed by oral acyclovir suppression, is effective against herpes simplex esophagitis. **Ganciclovir,** 5 mg/kg IV twice daily for 2 weeks, followed by 5 mg/kg IV daily maintenance; **foscarnet,** 60 mg/kg IV every 8 hours for 2 weeks, followed by 60 mg/kg IV daily maintenance; or **valganciclovir,** 900 mg orally twice daily for 2 weeks followed by 900 mg orally once daily maintenance, may be used to control CMV esophagitis.

7. **Diarrhea** caused by specific bacterial or parasitic organisms may respond to standard therapy. Symptomatic treatment should be offered when antimicrobial therapy is not effective or when no causative organisms can be identified.

8. **Peripheral neuropathies** may respond to **gabapentin** (300–3600 mg/day in three divided doses), or **tricyclic antidepressant drugs** (eg, amitriptyline, 25–150 mg orally daily), or may require **narcotic analgesics.**

9. **Cryptococcal meningitis** and other cryptococcal infections should be treated acutely with **amphotericin B,** 0.7–1 mg/kg daily, in combination with **flucytosine (5-FC)** at 75–100 mg/kg/day. If the patient is clinically well after receiving 7.5 mg/kg

of amphotericin B, **fluconazole** at 400 mg by mouth daily can be given to complete a 10- to 12-week course. Long-term suppressive therapy with fluconazole should be given.

10. **Toxoplasmosis of the central nervous system** can be treated with **pyrimethamine,** 25 mg by mouth daily, plus **sulfadiazine,** 1 g by mouth four times daily. **Clindamycin,** 600–900 mg by mouth four times daily, can be substituted for sulfadiazine in patients who are allergic to sulfa drugs.

11. **Mycobacterium avium complex (MAC)** can cause a wide range of localized or systemic problems, including hepatic or other gastrointestinal disease, fevers, weight loss, and anemia. Treatment with ethambutol, 15 mg/kg by mouth daily, plus either clarithromycin, 500 mg by mouth twice daily, or azithromycin, 500 mg by mouth daily, can be effective. Prophylaxis against MAC disease should be offered to all patients with CD4+ counts <50 cells/mL; azithromycin (1200 mg by mouth once weekly) or clarithromycin (500 mg orally twice daily) are the preferred agents.

IV. **Management Strategies.** Patients with HIV infection require comprehensive primary care. A team of physicians, public health or visiting nurses, social workers, hospice workers, and family members that is organized around the care of the patient is essential to the treatment of patients with HIV disease.

A. **Prevention.** Comprehensive sexual and drug histories are key tools for both diagnosis and prevention of HIV and other transmitted diseases. In addition, education with HIV-positive individuals regarding ways of preventing transmission is an essential component of HIV care.

B. **Psychosocial problems.** Special attention to the psychosocial impact of HIV disease is essential to the development of therapeutic strategies. Especially important interventions include discussions about transmission of HIV, treatment strategies, and consideration of the quality of life. Aftercare for the family of a patient who has died of AIDS is also very helpful.

C. **Primary care for persons living with HIV.** Ideally, one primary physician who is responsible for health care maintenance, early intervention, and treatment of common opportunistic infections should be identified. Consultation with specialists for specific problems can augment primary care.

V. **Prognosis.** Because of the effectiveness of combination ARV therapy, the prognosis for persons living with HIV infection continues to improve dramatically.

A. **The mean survival** of HIV-infected persons in the United States before the advent of effective ARV therapy was approximately 11 years from time of infection. The CD4+ count and viral load at the time of diagnosis were closely correlated with the prognosis, with persons with high viral loads and CD4+ counts <200 cells/μL having an 80% likelihood of developing AIDS within 3 years, whereas persons with high viral loads but CD4+ cell counts >350 cells/μL having a 40% chance of developing AIDS within 3 years. In contrast, the patient with a CD4+ cell count >500 cells/μL and viral load <20,000 has less than a 20% chance of developing AIDS within 3 years. These data continue to apply to persons with HIV disease who are not receiving effective combination ARV therapy, including the nearly 300,000 persons in the United States infected with HIV disease but unaware of their HIV diagnosis.

B. **The life expectancy** of most HIV-infected persons who receive effective combination ARV therapy has increased by many years, but the average number of years remains to be determined. Deaths from AIDS have decreased dramatically, and clinical manifestations of HIV infection and AIDS have partially or completely resolved in many patients. The quality of life for persons receiving effective combination ARV therapy can improve dramatically. However, the pill burden and side effects from ARV drugs can be considerable, so quality of life is not invariably improved. The clinician, therefore, needs to help each patient make the best possible decisions about their use of ARV therapy.

REFERENCES

Because advances in HIV/AIDS occur frequently, the principal Federal Guidelines that represent current standards in treatment are continually updated. The essential Guidelines in HIV are:

Centers for Disease Control and Prevention. Guidelines for using antiretroviral agents among HIV-infected adults and adolescents: Recommendations of the Panel on Clinical Practices for Treatment of HIV. MMWR 2002;**51**(No. RR-7).

Centers for Disease Control and Prevention. Guidelines for preventing opportunistic infections among HIV-infected persons—2002 recommendations of the U.S. Public Health Service and the Infectious Diseases Society of America. MMWR 2002;**51**(No. RR-8).

Centers for Disease Control and Prevention. Updated U.S. Public Health Service guidelines for the management of occupational exposures to HBV, HCV, and HIV and recommendations for postexposure prophylaxis. MMWR 2001;**50**(No. RR-11).
These and other Guidelines can be downloaded from many sites, including:
www.aidsinfo.nih.gov
www.cdc.gov
Additional resources can be found at www.hivinsite.com and www.hopkins-aids.edu

68   Asthma

Jonathan MacClements, MD, FAAFP, & Paul W. Wright, MD

KEY POINTS

- Effective control of asthma is necessary to prevent fibrosis of the basement membrane and remodeling of the airways, which can lead to irreversible obstructive lung disease. This control is accomplished by use of anti-inflammatory agents, most commonly inhaled corticosteroids.
- Successful control of asthma requires high-quality ongoing patient education in which the patient understands his or her medications and how to avoid factors that aggravate asthma.
- Common precipitating factors include house dust mites, tobacco smoke, mold, and animal allergens (cat and dog dander and cockroach and rodent products).
- HEPA (high-efficiency particulate air) filtration has become less expensive, more available, and more effective in providing protection from airborne allergens.
- Patients with asthma are at significant risk of high morbidity and death and should be monitored in a systematic and careful manner by their primary care provider. Spirometry and patient-monitored peak flowmeters play an important role in this management.

I. Introduction

A. Definition. Asthma is a disease of the airways, manifested by recurrent or persistent inflammatory and obstructive processes, or both, secondary to multifactorial stimuli, and not infrequently eventuates in irreversible loss of lung function and major disability. The terms describing the severity of asthma are mild intermittent, mild persistent, moderate persistent, and severe persistent, defined by frequency and severity of symptoms (Table 68–1).

B. Epidemiology

1. **Onset** is before age 5 in 75–90% of cases, with peak prevalence between 10 and 12 years of age.
2. **Risk factors** include a family history of asthma or atopy, parental smoking, ambient air pollution, and viral respiratory infections, especially bronchiolitis from respiratory syncytial virus. Males and blacks are at greater risk.

TABLE 68–1. DESCRIPTION OF ASTHMA SEVERITY

Degree of Severity	Daytime Symptoms	Nighttime Symptoms	Pulmonary Function
Mild intermittent	Symptoms ≤2/week	≤2/month	Within 20% of normal; asymptomatic between episodes
Mild persistent	≤3 episodes/week <1/day	≤3 episodes/month	PEFR within 20% of normal
Moderate persistent	≥2/week to daily episodes	>1 episode/week	FEV_1/PEFR 60–80%
Severe persistent	Continual symptoms with limited physical activity	Frequent	FEV/PEFR ≤60%

FEV_1, forced expiratory volume in 1 second; PEFR, peak expiratory flow rate.

3. The **prevalence** of asthma in the United States has increased during the last two decades, and the condition currently affects 14–15 million persons including 4.8 million children. Five percent to 10% of all children experience the disease during childhood. Asthma is second only to acute respiratory infection as a cause of pediatric hospital admissions and illness-related school absenteeism.

C. Pathophysiology

1. **Expiratory airflow obstruction** is initiated by bronchial wall inflammation, resulting in bronchospasm, bronchial gland mucus exudation, airway edema, and airway remodeling.

2. **Resultant pathophysiologic changes** include increased airway resistance and hyperinflation.

3. The **etiology** is not completely understood but encompasses a wide variety of genetic, immunologic, infectious, and environmental factors.

II. Diagnosis. The patient's history is most important. Although patients with asthma typically present with recurrent episodes of wheezing, not all asthma is characterized by wheezing—and not all wheezing indicates asthma. Undiagnosed asthma is a common reason for referral to pediatric and adult pulmonary outpatient departments.

A. Symptoms and signs

1. **Symptoms** usually include wheezing, coughing, dyspnea, chest tightness, and sometimes sputum production. Most patients report symptom-free intervals, but a rapidly changing and variable clinical picture is common.

    a. **Coughing** may be the initial symptom of asthma and is essentially the only symptom in cough-variant asthma. This form of asthma presents with nonproductive cough occurring both day and night. Pulmonary function studies tend to be normal. Therapy is similar to standard asthma treatment.

    b. **Atelectasis,** often misdiagnosed on chest x-ray as pneumonia, is a common clue to undiagnosed asthma.

    c. A **patient history of atopy** or a family history of atopy or asthma supports the diagnosis.

2. **Signs** may be absent in the asthmatic patient, especially early in the disease and during asymptomatic intervals. Forceful expiration occasionally uncovers otherwise unnoticed end-expiratory wheezing.

    a. **Severe asthma** may be characterized by both expiratory and inspiratory wheezing, prolongation of the expiratory phase, thoracic cage retractions, tachypnea, cyanosis, accessory muscle recruitment, and apprehension.

    b. **Pulsus paradoxus** (a pulse pressure that markedly decreases in size during inspiration), a silent chest, or chest wall crepitus caused by subcutaneous emphysema may signify severe airway obstruction requiring emergent care.

    c. **Chronic changes** may include such chest wall deformities as pectus carinatum or an increased anterior-posterior diameter. Clubbing is rarely associated with asthma and should suggest a diagnosis of cystic fibrosis or cancer.

B. Diagnostic tests

1. A **peripheral blood smear** and a **sputum examination** showing eosinophilia may suggest allergic asthma.

2. **Allergy skin tests, allergen-specific IgE,** and the **radioallergosorbent test (RAST)** can be used to test specific allergens. These tests may identify specific allergens that can be avoided or treated with immunotherapy desensitization. Skin tests are the least costly of the three tests. RAST and IgE blood tests are usually reserved for patients who cannot undergo skin testing because of a history of severe reaction or other intolerance. Positive tests should be correlated with the patient's history of allergies. Total IgE levels are usually elevated in atopic asthma.

3. The **chest x-ray** is useful for selected patients in ruling out other diseases. It may show hyperinflation, atelectasis, pneumonia, or, rarely, pneumomediastinum. Criteria for ordering chest films include tachypnea (>60 breaths per minute), tachycardia (>160 beats per minute), localized rales, localized decreased breath sounds, or cyanosis. Lateral chest films are helpful in acute pediatric pulmonary disease and should be ordered when the posterior-anterior view requires clarification, such as when the physician suspects that a posterior-inferior lung infiltrate is concealed behind the cardiac silhouette.

4. **Pulmonary function tests (PFTs)**
   a. **Indications** for PFTs include confirmation of the diagnosis of asthma, objective measurements of the response to therapy, and measurement of pulmonary dysfunction.
   b. **Forced expiratory volume in 1 second (FEV$_1$)** is very useful in assessing acute asthma, but the **peak expiratory flow rate (PEFR)** parallels the FEV$_1$ and is usually easier to obtain. Devices that measure PEFR are inexpensive and can be prescribed to allow patients with asthma to monitor their progress at home. Patients with a PEFR below 70% of their baseline value should be carefully evaluated. An FEV$_1$ or PEFR below 40% after aggressive therapy indicates severe obstruction, and the patient should be hospitalized. The accuracy of peak flowmeters varies, however, and can deteriorate over time.
   c. The **peak flow-zone system** allows patients to monitor the PEFR and make clinical decisions about their asthma—under the physician's supervision.
      (1) The **green zone** (PEFR = 80–100% of the patient's best score) indicates that the patient can continue the usual course of medicine.
      (2) The **yellow zone** (PEFR = 50–80%) is a warning to the patient to take additional medicine or call the physician.
      (3) The **red zone** (PEFR <50%) indicates that the patient should both use the inhaler and call the physician immediately.
5. **Provocative testing** with either methacholine or histamine is indicated for the rare patient for whom a definitive diagnosis is sought when the clinical picture is unclear. These tests carry a minimal risk of producing life-threatening bronchospasm. They must be performed under experienced supervision with resuscitative support immediately available.
6. **Arterial blood gases** are indicated for patients who have poor respiratory status or a poor response to therapy. Impending respiratory failure should be suspected—even when the Pco$_2$ is normal or slightly elevated (>40 mm Hg) in the presence of hypoxia (Po$_2$ <70 mm Hg). Pulse oximetry monitoring is noninvasive and very useful in monitoring the oxygenation of asthmatic patients.
7. **Nitric Oxide Test System (NIOX)** monitors exhaled nitric oxide levels, which seem to correlate well with lung inflammation. This test may prove beneficial in monitoring the response of lung inflammation with asthma treatment, but is still experimental.

C. **Differential diagnosis**
   1. **Common diseases** to be excluded are bronchiolitis, cystic fibrosis, foreign bodies, chronic bronchitis, and congestive heart failure.
   2. **Less common diseases** to be considered are vocal cord dysfunction, bronchopulmonary dysplasia, allergic bronchopulmonary mycoses, and bronchiolitis obliterans.

III. **Treatment.** Goals include maintenance of normal activities (including exercise) and optimal pulmonary function values while minimizing symptoms, exacerbations, and adverse drug effects. Long-term therapy directed at suppressing inflammation early in the course of illness is now felt to be necessary to modify the disease process and prevent irreversible lung dysfunction.

A. **Environmental control** can provide significant relief by avoiding the triggers identified in the clinical history and known to produce deleterious effects.
   1. **Inhaled allergens** can be totally avoided only rarely, but much of the exposure can be eliminated.
      a. **Tobacco smoke** should be banned from the home and automobile. The use of nonsmoking hotel rooms, rental cars, and restaurants is very beneficial.
      b. **House dust mites** are difficult to eradicate. Frequent household cleanings can help reduce their numbers.
         (1) **Rooms,** when practical, should be free of carpets, stuffed toys, and other dust-collecting items.
         (2) **Central air-conditioning systems** should have frequently cleaned mechanical or electrostatic air filters. Portable electrostatic air filters can be used in patients' bedrooms.
         (3) **Nonallergenic mattress covers** should be used.
      c. **Other irritants** to be avoided include pets, flowering plants, molds, perfumes, hair sprays, paints, and aerosolized chemicals.

2. **Emotional factors** may play a significant role in triggering asthma in some patients and must be minimized.
   a. **Parents** should avoid overcompensating behavior that can create opportunities for manipulation by the asthmatic child. They should also avoid the other extreme of ignoring the child's plight.
   b. The **home** should offer the child support, consistency, and loving parental guidance.
3. **Exercise** and exposure to cold air frequently aggravate asthma. Acute exacerbations resulting from exercise may be lessened by appropriate premedication and by restricting activities to participation in such sports as water sports, which typically cause less bronchial irritation than do other athletic activities.

B. **Drug therapy** involves two groups of drugs: long-term-control and quick-relief medications.
   1. **Long-term-control medications** are usually given daily over the long term to control persistent asthma. They include corticosteroids, cromolyn and nedocromil, long-acting bronchodilators, leukotriene modifiers, and theophylline.
      a. **Corticosteroids** are very effective anti-inflammatory drugs for treating acute and chronic asthma, but can cause many serious adverse effects. In children, suppression of linear growth and adverse effects on the hypothalamic-pituitary-adrenal axis are of major concern. In adults, bone demineralization, cataract formation, gastrointestinal hemorrhage, and psychiatric problems sometimes occur with systemic usage. Corticosteroids should be initiated early in the course of treatment and in adequate doses for patients with severe asthma. The mode of action of corticosteroids is unclear, but the current consensus suggests that they improve airflow by decreasing inflammatory activity in the arachidonic acid, leukotriene, prostaglandin, and inflammatory cell systems and by increasing smooth muscle responsiveness to β-agonists.
         (1) **Inhaled corticosteroids** are first-line drugs and are often prescribed with inhaled β-agonists. Inhaled corticosteroids available in metered-dose inhalers (MDIs) include budesonide (Pulmocort), fluticasone (Flovent), beclomethasone (Vanceril or Beclovent), triamcinolone (Azmacort), and flunisolide (AeroBid).
            (a) **Administration** is by MDI and dosages are listed in Table 68–2. These preparations are not available in nebulized solutions.
            (b) **Significant adverse effects** of inhaled corticosteroids are much less than those of systemic corticosteroids. The safety of long-term treatment with inhaled budesonide with respect to children's growth has been well documented in a recently published study in 2000. The newer drugs, budesonide and fluticasone, are considered to be more potent and have less gastric absorption and less-active metabolites than the older drugs. Minor adverse effects include oropharyngeal candidiasis, cough, and, rarely, dysphonia, but they are seldom severe enough to warrant discontinuation. The use of spacer devices and oral rinses after inhalation can lessen these side effects. Budesonide and fluticasone are available also in powder MDI preparations. Budesonide is also available in solution for updraft inhalation.
         (2) **Systemic steroids** are indicated when other modes of therapy fail to control severe asthma.
            (a) **Oral steroids**—prednisone, methylprednisolone, and prednisolone—are given in doses of 1–2 mg/kg/day (usually 20–80 mg/day) and gradually reduced over 1–3 weeks, depending on disease severity.
            (b) **Liquid preparations** of prednisolone include Prelone (15 mg/5 mL) and Pediapred (5 mg/5 mL). Liquid preparations of prednisone include Liquid Pred Syrup (5 mg/5 mL) and Prednisone Intensol (5 mg/1 mL).
      b. **Cromolyn sodium and nedocromil**
         (1) **Cromolyn sodium,** an anti-inflammatory medication used prophylactically to control chronic asthma and exercise-induced asthma, inhibits both early- and late-response allergic reactions. Although cromolyn's mechanism of action is not fully understood, it probably stabilizes mast cells, preventing their degranulation and release of inflammatory mediators.

TABLE 68–2. COMMONLY PRESCRIBED ASTHMA DRUGS

Drug	Mode of Administration	Adult Dosage	Relative Cost per Month[1]
β₂-agonists			
Albuterol	MDI	90 µg/puff 1–2 puffs q4–6 h prn	+
	Rotocaps	200 µg/cap 1 cap q4–6 h prn	++
Levalbuterol	Nebulizer solution	0.63–1.25 mg q 6–8 hours prn	++++++
Salmeterol	MDI	21 µg/puff 1–2 puffs bid	+++++
	Dry powder	50 µg/puff 1 puff bid	+++++
Formoterol	Dry powder	12 µg/cap 1 puff q 12 hours	+++++
Mast cell stabilizers			
Cromolyn sodium	MDI or nebulizer solution	800 µg/puff 3–4 puffs tid–qid	++++++
Nedocromil sodium	MDI	1.75 mg/puff 2 puffs qid	++++
Inhaled corticosteroids			
Beclomethasone	MDI	42/84 µg/puff 6/12–10/20 puffs per day	+++
Budesonide	MDI	200 µg/puff; 1 puff bid to tid	++++++
	Nebulized solution	0.25–0.5 mg/2 mL bid	++++++
Flunisolide	MDI	250 µg/puff 4–8 puffs per day	++++
Fluticasone	MDI	44/110/220 µg/puff 2–6 puffs per day	+++/++++/+++++
	Dry-powder inhaler	50/100/250 µg/puff 2–6 puffs per day	+++/++++/+++++
Triamcinolone	MDI	100 µg/puff 4–20 puffs per day	++++
Methylxanthines			
Theophylline	Extended-release tablets or capsules	300–600 mg/day	+
Leukotriene modifiers			
Montelukast	Tablets	5 mg–10 mg daily	+++++
Zafirlukast	Tablets	20 mg bid	+++++
Zileuton	Tablets	600 mg qid	++++++

[1] Cost per month per average dose: + less than or equal to $25; ++ less than or equal to $40; +++ less than or equal to $60; ++++ less than or equal to $80; +++++ less than or equal to $80; ++++++ more than $100.
MDI, metered-dose inhaler.

    (a) **Adverse effects** are few, but cromolyn requires dedicated patient compliance, since an adequate therapeutic response may not occur until after 4–6 weeks of therapy. Children appear to respond to cromolyn better than adults do.

    (b) **Preparations** of cromolyn (Intal) include an MDI, an aerosolized solution that can be combined in an aerosol with a β₂ drug, and an inhaled powder capsule. The recommended dosage is two inhaled metered sprays (800 μg per spray) four times a day at regular intervals. It seems more effective in children with asthma.

    (2) **Nedocromil** (Tilade) is an anti-inflammatory drug available as an MDI. Its action is similar to cromolyn in that it stabilizes mast and other inflammatory cells, but it provides significant clinical improvement within 2–4 days. Similar to cromolyn, its adverse side effect profile is very low. It is considered first-line therapy along with β_2-agonist agents in mild and moderate asthma in children 6 years of age and older. Up to 20% of patients experience an unpleasant taste with nedocromil.

c. Long-acting β_2-agonists

    (1) **Salmeterol** (Seravent), available as an MDI and inhaled powder, is a longer-acting (every 12 hours) β-agonist indicated for maintenance therapy and contraindicated for acute treatment. It is approved for children 6 years and older. Salmeterol acts as a bronchodilator, relaxing smooth muscle by adenylate cyclase activation and increase in cyclic AMP production. Its onset of action is 15–30 minutes and the duration of action is greater than 12 hours. It is especially useful for controlling nocturnal symptoms.

    (2) **Formoterol** (Foradil Aerolizer) is a dry powder inhaler (DPI), which is similar to salmeterol and is dosed at 12 μg every 12 hours.

    (3) **Albuterol, sustained-release** (Proventil Repetabs), is an oral sustained-release form of albuterol that tends to have more side effects than the inhaled long-acting β_2-agonists.

d. The combination of inhaled fluticasone and salmeterol (Advair Diskus, DPI) offers the advantage of improved compliance and may also enhance efficacy through drug synergy. It is dosed one puff every 12 hours with 100, 250, or 500 μg of fluticasone combined with 50 μg of salmeterol.

e. Theophylline is a methylxanthine bronchodilator that is usually well absorbed from the gastrointestinal tract. Theophyllines are considered second-line agents and are used as adjuncts with anti-inflammatory and other bronchodilator drugs.

    (1) **Dosage requirements** of theophylline vary considerably with age and the individual patient. Blood levels should be monitored and maintained between 5 and 15 μg/mL. When possible, therapy should be initiated slowly to minimize side effects. Children tend to clear the drug significantly more rapidly than adults do.

    (2) **Adverse effects** are similar to those of caffeine and include nervousness, anorexia, irritability, nausea, vomiting, enuresis, insomnia, poor school performance, and behavioral problems. Factors that may increase serum levels of theophylline and give rise to toxicity include impaired liver function, age older than 55 years, chronic heart and lung disease, sustained high fever, viral illnesses, and drug interactions, including those with cimetidine, allopurinol, ciprofloxacin, erythromycin, rifampin, propranolol, oral contraceptives, phenytoin, clarithromycin, and lithium carbonate.

    (3) **Overdosage** usually manifests as nausea and vomiting but also can cause arrhythmias, seizures, and, very rarely, death. Patients and their family members should be taught to recognize signs of theophylline toxicity.

    (4) **Oral preparations** of theophylline include liquid, tablets, and capsules. Capsules (Theo-Dur Sprinkle, Slo-bid, Slo-Phyllin, and others) can be given to young children by sprinkling the medication on food to facilitate administration and accurate dosing.

f. Leukotriene modifiers are indicated for the treatment of mild to moderate nonacute asthma by modifying the inflammatory effects of leukotrienes.

    (1) **Preparations** include orally administered zileuton (Zyflo), a 5-lipooxgenase inhibitor, zafirlukast (Accolate), and montelukast (Singulair), leukotriene receptor antagonists. These drugs offer better compliance because of their oral administration, especially with montelukast's once-a-day dosing. However, they are less effective than inhaled corticosteroids, being indicated for mild intermittent and mild persistent asthma, and are less well supported in their ability to block lung inflammation and sequelae.

    (2) **Adverse effects** include drug-drug interactions, hepatic toxicity with zileuton, and rare Churg-Strauss vasculitis with zafirlukast and montelukast.

g. Other drugs used to treat asthma

(1) **Antihistamines,** which formerly were believed to have adverse effects on asthma, are now considered safe. These agents act as weak bronchodilators.

(2) **Antiviral agents,** such as ribavirin for respiratory syncytial virus, may be helpful.

(3) **Antibacterial drugs** are useful for the treatment of patients with pneumonia, bacterial sinusitis, and other specific bacterial infections. Antibiotics are frequently misused in the treatment of patients with asthma, especially when atelectasis is confused with pneumonia.

(4) **Expectorants** and **mucolytics** (eg, guaifenesin and iodides) have not been proven effective. Aerosolized acetylcysteine (Mucomyst) is contraindicated in asthma, since it may cause severe bronchospasm. Sedatives and anxiolytic agents are also contraindicated.

(5) **Immunosuppressive** drugs such as methotrexate, cyclosporine, and hydroxychloroquine have been considered as therapy, but are not well accepted due to their potential toxicity, low efficacy, or both. Omalizumab (Xolair), a humanized monoclonal antibody that blocks IgE, was recently approved by the US Food and Drug Administration (FDA). It has shown promise in reducing corticosteroid dosage in patients with persistent and severe allergic asthma who are 12 years of age and older. It is administrated subcutaneously every 2–4 weeks, but may cost $5,000–$10,000 per year.

h. **Immunotherapy,** also called desensitization, allergy injection therapy, or allergen immunotherapy, remains controversial, inconvenient, and expensive but may benefit a few selected patients with allergic asthma. Immunotherapy also involves a small but significant risk of anaphylaxis and even death.

i. **Complementary alternative medicine** includes relaxation techniques, herbal medicines, vitamin supplements, dietary changes, acupuncture, homeopathy, and chiropractic spinal manipulation. Although these alternative healing processes are not recommended as substitutes for conventional pharmacologic therapy, they are used in up to 40% in asthma patients in the United States and continue to grow in popularity.

(1) **Herbal remedies** used to treat asthma have a worldwide origin involving hundreds of plants as well as minerals, animals, and mixtures of all three.

(a) The **herb ma huang (ephedra)** contains ephedrine (a bronchodilator) and is perhaps the most commonly used agent in alternative medicine. This drug was formerly included in several asthma prescriptions and over-the-counter preparations. However, ephedrine is no longer recommended to treat asthma due to its adverse effects including sudden death, high blood pressure, nephrolithiasis, and hyperglycemia.

(b) **Traditional Chinese medicine** is widely used in the United States and involves the use of many unfamiliar herbs, some having been used for hundreds of years. The typical Chinese remedy may contain 10 or more herbs, including ma huang, gingko extracts, Cordyceps, licorice, magnolia, and others. While some of these have some efficacy, their clinical value remains unproved.

(2) **Hydrotherapy (cold baths)** are commonly used in Japan to open constricted airways.

(3) **Acupuncture** is very popular, especially in Europe, and has been investigated in a number of controlled studies. It has not been shown to be as effective as conventional therapy, but may be helpful, especially for quick relief of asthma. However, avoidable deaths have been reported in patients with asthma who relied only on acupuncture and refused conventional therapy. Furthermore, acupuncture carries some risk, including organ puncture or infection from contaminated needles.

(4) **Relaxation techniques** are designed to relieve stress, which is believed to aggravate asthma. These include yoga and biofeedback training, especially emphasizing breathing techniques.

2. **Quick-relief medications**

a. **Short-acting inhaled β_2-agonists** are most frequently delivered as aerosols through MDIs and, less commonly, as solutions via compressed-air nebulizers

(Pulmo-Aide, among others). The MDI delivery system should be enhanced by the use of reservoir spacer devices (eg, AeroChamber, Inhal-Aid, InspirEase, or Brethancer). Some spacers have masks that allow for infant and toddler use. Inhaled β_2-agonists are most commonly prescribed as needed, rather than with firm dosage times, because of concerns about tachyphylaxis and adverse side effects.

    (1) Preparations include albuterol (Ventolin, Proventil), levalbuterol (Xopenex), metaproterenol (Alupent, Metaprel, Pro-Meta), bitolterol (Tornalate), pirbuterol (Maxair), and terbutaline (Brethine, Bricanyl).

        (a) Albuterol (Ventolin or Proventil) is available in syrup, tablets, MDI, nebulizer solutions, and powdered capsules for inhalation.

        (b) Terbutaline (Brethaire, Brethine, or Bricanyl) is available in tablets, MDI, nebulizer solution, and an aqueous solution for subcutaneous injection. It is classified as an FDA category B drug in pregnancy.

        (c) Levalbuterol (Xopenex), the *R*-enantiomer of racemic albuterol, is available for nebulization (0.63 mg and 1.25 mg per three mL unit-dose vials). Availability as an MDI is anticipated in the near future. Levalbuterol may offer fewer adrenergic effects than albuterol while providing excellent bronchodilatation.

    (2) Indications include the rapid relief of acute bronchospasm and prevention of exercise-induced bronchospasm. These drugs are generally recommended to be administered on a need basis rather than on a regularly scheduled daily basis. The inhaled route is preferred because of faster onset of action, fewer adverse effects, and greater effectiveness.

    (3) Adverse effects include tachycardia, nervousness, irritability, tremor, headache, hypokalemia, and hyperglycemia. The less selective β_2-agonists (epinephrine, metaproterenol, isoproterenol, isoetharine) are no longer recommended for therapy. Patients should be warned against overuse of these drugs (eg, >200 puffs of albuterol per month) and encouraged to use more of their anti-inflammatory medications.

  b. Ipratropium bromide (Atrovent), an anticholinergic quaternary derivative of atropine, is indicated for the relief of acute cholinergically mediated bronchospasm. This drug is frequently used with a β_2-agonist but has a slightly slower onset of action. It is the treatment of choice for bronchospasm due to the effects of beta-blocker therapy.

  c. Systemic corticosteroids (methylprednisolone, prednisolone, prednisone) are indicated in doses of 1–2 mg/kg for patients with acute exacerbations of moderate or severe asthma. They are usually given for 3–10 days and are continued until the patient's PEFR is 80% of his personal best value. Prolonged therapy, >1–2 weeks, requires tapering of the dosage to prevent pituitary-adrenal-cortical dysfunction, but tapering per se does not prevent relapse of symptoms of asthma.

IV. Management Strategies

  A. Education is a critical tool in the care of the patient with asthma. Family members, teachers, and athletic coaches must understand the disease process. Asthma support groups and camps for asthmatic children can be very helpful also.

    1. Patient compliance is much better when patients are given the opportunity to acquire an adequate understanding of both the disease process and the prescribed medications.

    2. Office counseling should be provided to patients and their families, especially to those patients with special educational or behavioral problems.

    3. Referral to an outside counselor may occasionally be necessary to provide parents with additional help in the management of the troubled asthmatic child.

  B. Treatment guidelines. The 2002 (National Asthma Education and Prevention Program) expert committee recently applied evidence-based methods to review the scientific literature and update the 1997 consensus panel's asthma management guidelines. New recommendations now encourage the earlier use of inhaled steroids as one of the preferred methods of management for mild persistent and more severe asthma.

    1. Patients with **mild intermittent asthma** have acute episodes of illness separated by symptom-free intervals occurring no more than twice weekly. These patients have normal PEFR and no symptoms between exacerbations. They can usually be managed with inhaled β_2-agonists given on an as-needed basis.

2. Patients with **mild persistent asthma** have symptoms more than twice weekly but less than daily. Their exacerbations may affect their daily activities, but their PEFR is at least 80% of predicted. They are usually managed with one inhaled anti-inflammatory drug or oral leukotriene modifier and augmented with an inhaled β_2-agonist for quick relief. Low-dose inhaled corticosteroids are now preferred.

3. Patients with **moderate persistent asthma** have daily symptoms requiring daily use of inhaled short-acting β_2-agonists. They have exacerbations at least twice weekly, which affect their activities and may last for days. Their PEFR values are 60 to 80% of predicted. They are preferably managed with medium-dosed inhaled corticosteroids and long-acting inhaled β_2-agonists (eg, salmeterol plus low- to medium-dose inhaled corticosteroid) in addition to quick-acting relief, as-needed short-acting β_2-agonists. Alternative treatment may include medium-dose inhaled corticosteroids with either a leukotriene modifier or theophylline.

4. Patients with **severe persistent asthma** have continual symptoms, limited physical activity, frequent exacerbations, and PEFR less than 60% of predicted. They usually require high-dose inhaled corticosteroids, long-acting bronchodilators, and sometimes augmentation with oral corticosteroids in addition to quick relief with as-needed short-acting β_2-agonists.

5. **Nocturnal asthma** is now easier to manage with the use of longer-acting agents such as inhaled salmeterol, sustained-release preparations of theophylline or albuterol tablets, or the leukotriene modifiers. Nocturnal asthma may be associated with gastrointestinal reflux disease, even with minimal symptoms of the latter. In patients with nocturnal asthma who respond poorly to therapy, diagnosis and therapy for gastrointestinal reflux should be considered.

V. **Prognosis**
   A. **Total remission** of symptoms occurs in as few as 16% of patients with asthma by late adolescence or early adulthood. Most patients retain airway hyperreactivity (as demonstrated by provocative testing).
   B. **Onset** of disease is not a reliable factor in predicting either the length or the severity of symptoms.
   C. **Initial severity** of the illness, especially the length of the episode and the need for hospitalization, is a more reliable factor than the time of onset in predicting whether the child's asthma will persist into adulthood.
   D. **Persistence of reduced pulmonary function** and the presence of atopy (eczema, allergic rhinitis, and skin test reactivity to antigens) are associated with continued and more severe disease.
   E. **Control** of the disease process through good pharmacotherapy is not a known predictor of future disease. The relationship of childhood asthma and adult emphysema is unclear.
   F. **Mortality** of patients with asthma in the United States continues to decline, with less than 5000 deaths reported in 2000. Mortality rates are higher in blacks, females, the elderly, and patients with coexistent chronic obstructive pulmonary disease. Historical events of concern for potential fatal outcome include previous history of respiratory acidosis with or without intubation, history of episodes of cyanosis, frequent hospitalizations, multiple emergency room visits during a short period, episodes of loss of consciousness, minimal response to a major therapeutic regimen, and presence of severe anxiety and depression.

REFERENCES

Agertoft L, Pedersen S: Effect of long-term treatment with inhaled budesonide on adult height in children with asthma. N Engl J Med 2000;**343:**1064.

American Lung Association, Epidemiology and Statistic Unit, Research and Scientific Affairs, March 2003: Trends in asthma morbidity and mortality. http://www.lungusa.org/dat/asthma/asthma1.pdf.

Beasley R, et al: Epidemiology and genetics of asthma. J Allergy Clin Immunol 2000;**l05:**S466.

Bousquet J, et al: Asthma from bronchoconstriction to airways inflammation and remodeling. Am J Respir Crit Care Med 2000;**161:**1720.

Bush RK: Asthma. Med Clin North America 2002;**86:**925.

Huntley A, Ernst E: Herbal medicines for asthma: A systematic review. Thorax 2000;**55:**925.

Jadad AR, et al: Systematic reviews and meta-analyses on treatment of asthma: Critical evaluation. BMJ 2000;**320:**537.

Lenfant C: Guidelines for the diagnosis and management of asthma. J Allergy Clin Immunol 2002; **110:**S141.

Weinberger M: Clinical patterns and natural history of asthma. J Pediatr 2003;**142:**S15.

Wenzel SE: The pathobiology of asthma implications for treatment. Clin Chest Med 2000;**21:**213.

69   Chronic Pain

Michael P. Temporal, MD

KEY POINTS

- The biopsychosocial context is important in the assessment and management of chronic pain conditions to understand both the perception of severity and the effect of treatment.
- Pain scales and pain medication contracts help to decrease the risk of inappropriate pain medication prescription.
- A multidisciplinary approach using multiple modalities is usually needed to manage chronic pain.
- Routine, rather than as-needed, dosing of medications results in better pain control.
- Nonsteroidal anti-inflammatory (NSAID) agents have equivalent efficacy and are used as first-line medications. COX-2 inhibitors may have a role as an alternative in older patients or when first-line NSAIDs fail.
- Narcotic pain medications should be used when patients have failed NSAID therapy alone. They should not be used as a sole agent and should be titrated to the most effective dose and then changed to long-acting preparations when available.
- Adjuvant medications can be particularly helpful for chronic, relapsing pain. Antidepressants are also useful for both the emotional component of pain and analgesia.

I. Introduction

A. Pain is the most common reason people seek medical care. **Pain** is an unpleasant sensory and emotional experience associated with actual or potential tissue damage. **Chronic pain** is defined as recurrent or persistent pain lasting more than 3 months. Chronic pain complaints affect 15% of the population. Annual US monetary loss due to lost productivity from chronic pain is over $60 billion.

B. Chronic pain may be classified as nociceptive or neuropathic. While acute pain can be protective, a reflexive response to limit further tissue destruction, chronic pain does not have a similar useful purpose.

   1. **Nociceptive pain** stems from ongoing tissue damage such as arthritis or tumor. Pain signals are transmitted through nonmyelinated c-fiber nerves mediated by calcium and sodium. Chronic nociceptive pain is related to *N*-methyl-D-aspartate (NMDA) receptors that are both more easily stimulated and require higher antinociceptive activity to quiet. Released endorphin and enkephalin binding to mu and gamma opioid receptors reduce nociceptive pain.

   2. **Neuropathic pain** results from the sustained transmission of pain signals in the absence of ongoing tissue damage. Injury or damage to the sensory nerves or central ganglia has occurred. Common descriptions of this chronic pain include numbness (hypoesthesia), pins-and-needles sensation (paresthesia), or severe pain from usually innocuous stimuli (allodynia). It is more difficult to treat and usually does not respond to treatment with NSAIDs or acetaminophen alone.

II. Diagnoses

A. The **assessment of pain** must include the type, severity, onset, location, duration, and previous history. Chronic pain may have variable duration (less than once per week, multiple times per week, daily, or constant). Within a psychosocial context, more intense pain may be associated with certain activities, emotions, or events (work, mood, menstrual cycle).

B. An important **measure of chronic pain** is the associated impairment or loss of function. Associated symptoms such as nausea, dizziness, diaphoresis, and weakness should be sought as well as comorbid conditions such as diabetes mellitus, connective tissue disease, and psychiatric illness (which may affect treatment response) as well as hepatic disease, renal disease, history of gastrointestinal (GI) bleeding, and medication sensitivity (which may limit treatment choices). Previous treatment strategies (including complementary and alternative therapies) and response to those strategies provide important historical information and can guide the current management.

C. **Pain rating scales** allow quantification of baseline and relative response to pain therapies. The simplest range from 0 (no pain) to 10 (worst pain possible). Mild pain ranges from 1 to 3, moderate pain ranges from 4 to 6, severe pain from 7 to 9. While developed for palliative care, the Edmonton Symptom Assessment System scale has the patient rate on a 0 to 10 scale additional domains, including tiredness, nausea, depression, anxiety, drowsiness, appetite, well-being, shortness of breath, and other problems to give a multidimensional perspective.

D. Physical assessment can give more objective data to the necessarily subjective sensation of pain. However, instability of vital signs or alterations of consciousness seen in acute pain situations may be blunted in chronic pain. Important functional information of endurance, range of motion, and palpable inflammation, point tenderness, or spasm should be identified.

III. Treatment

A. **Physical.** Physical therapy has been used in the management of acute pain to help with stretching, strengthening, and improving endurance. The primary impairments—due directly to the injury—may or may not be responsive to physical therapy. The secondary impairments—lack of exercise, poor body alignment, shortening and weakening of the joint structures, and over-guarding of the injured area—which can exacerbate daily functioning and the perception of pain and suffering, often are responsive in the motivated patient. Physical reconditioning in a gradual, directed program will help the patient who has been immobile. With the goal of increasing function, decreasing disability, and establishing effective pain coping and management skills, exercise programs can include the following: aerobic exercise to 65–80% of predicted maximal heart rate; stretching exercises for shortened muscles; endurance exercise for major postural muscles; and coordination and stabilization exercises.

1. **Transcutaneous electrical nerve stimulation (TENS)** has been helpful in mild to moderate pain. It works through counterstimulation of the pain-transmitting nerves.
2. Scheduled use of **ice or heat** may provide a similar benefit.
3. **Occupational therapy** can be used to help moderate total activity and develop compensatory techniques for activities of daily living. The provision of adaptive equipment can enhance the effectiveness of other treatment modalities.
4. **Biofeedback, self-hypnosis,** and **relaxation** can also be taught to help manage the sensation of pain.

B. **Cognitive.** Understanding the pain cycle and how the individual is affected can be a step toward moving the focus away from the pain and more toward adaptive behaviors. Cognitive therapies seek to bring an awareness of the triggers and responses the body has to pain in the context of daily life activities. Educating the patient and the family regarding pain, tension, and the physiologic response is a therapeutic intervention. Reframing the language and associations of pain may bring control for a person who has not had control of pain for a long time. Relaxation techniques, stress management, and pain diary records help to respond productively to pain.

C. **Medical**
1. **Conventional agents**
   a. Acetaminophen is an excellent analgesic for mild to moderate nociceptive pain. In the treatment of osteoarthritis, doses to 4 g/day (500 mg, 2 tablets orally four times daily) have been associated with long-term efficacy comparable to nonsteroidal agents. Although it has no anti-inflammatory properties, acetaminophen is thought to work through NMDA receptors and substance P.
   b. **Nonsteroidal anti-inflammatory agents (NSAIDs)** are effective agents for mild to moderate pain with an inflammatory component. They work at the peripheral site of action and are effective in the chronic management of arthritides and myalgias. They also can be effectively combined with centrally acting opioid medications for other chronic pain. No one NSAID is superior to others for chronic pain, but periodic substitution between classes may afford an improved response. The risks of NSAIDS are related to prostaglandin inhibition and include gastric irritation, bleeding, and renal dysfunction. Allergic reactions including angioneurotic edema, asthma, and hypotension have been reported. Due to sodium retention, caution is advised in the setting of congestive heart failure. Choices include:
      (1) Ibuprofen, 200–800 mg orally three times daily.
      (2) Naproxen, 250–500 mg orally twice daily.
      (3) Piroxicam, 20 mg orally every day.

   c. **COX-2 inhibitors** are newer medications that inhibit cyclooxygenase-2 and have comparable efficacy to that of NSAIDs. They are reported to have less GI toxicity and bleeding, but ulcers and bleeding have occurred. Another potential risk is cardiovascular complications (ie, thrombosis). These medications are often used as first-line agents in the elderly or when first-line NSAIDs fail. Choices include:

      (1) Celecoxib, 100–200 mg orally every day to twice daily.

      (2) Rofecoxib, 12.5–25 mg orally every day.

      (3) Valdecoxib, 10–20 mg orally every day to twice daily.

   d. Tramadol (Ultram) is a centrally acting, synthetic opioid agonist oral analgesic useful in moderate to severe pain. It is discussed here because it is a non-scheduled medication. It binds to mu-opioid receptors and inhibits serotonin and norepinephrine reuptake. Starting doses are 50 mg every 4–6 hours and ranges to 300–400 mg/day. Like codeine, it can cause nausea, constipation, or drowsiness, but reportedly has less of these effects and it is not associated with the GI and renal effects of NSAIDS. Serious reactions include seizures, angioedema, and Stevens-Johnson syndrome.

2. **Psychopharmacologic agents.** The majority of patients with chronic pain will be prescribed an antidepressant. In chronic pain, antidepressants have a dual role of treating mood disorders and independently addressing pain symptoms. Tricyclic antidepressants work through various degrees of inhibition of norepinephrine and serotonin reuptake. Selective serotonin reuptake inhibitors are effective and have a more favorable side effect profile than older agents. Atypical antidepressants include norepinephrine and dopamine reuptake inhibitors, serotonin-norepinephrine reuptake inhibitors, and serotonin-2 antagonist reuptake inhibitors. These agents have analgesic qualities and are used for chronic pain but have not been proven in randomized control trials.

   a. **Tricyclic antidepressants** have analgesic properties in low doses, but maximal analgesic affect is achieved at increased doses. Dosing then should be titrated over weeks and increased to maximum efficacy as dose-related side effects will allow. Typical agents include tertiary amines imipramine (Tofranil), amitriptyline (Elavil), clomipramine (Anafranil), and doxepin (Sinequan). Each has various degrees of anticholinergic activity, and hypotension and sedation are common side effects. Amitriptyline (0.1 mg/kg/day titrated over a few weeks to maximum 150 mg/day) and imipramine (0.2–3 mg/kg/day up to 100 mg/day maximum in elderly or 300 mg/day) have chronic pain indications. The quaternary amines may be better tolerated in older patients and tend to have less central activity and hypotension. These include desipramine (Norpramin), nortriptyline (Pamelor), protriptyline (Vivactil), and amoxapine (Asendin). Blood counts should be monitored for agranulocytosis or thrombocytopenia.

   b. Selective serotonin reuptake inhibitors were introduced in the late 1980s as a novel antidepressant. They were soon found to be useful in a variety of conditions including panic disorder, generalized anxiety, chronic fatigue, premenstrual syndrome, and chronic pain. Common side effects include headache; stimulation or sedation; cardiac effects (bradycardia or tachycardia); GI effects (increased or decreased appetite, nausea, vomiting, bloating, diarrhea); sedation; fine tremor; and tinnitus. They variably affect libido. Agents include fluoxetine (Prozac), fluvoxamine (Luvox), paroxetine (Paxil), sertraline (Zoloft), citalopram (Celexa), and escitalopram (Lexapro). See Chapter 92 on depression for further dosing information.

   c. Currently, the only serotonin-norepinephrine reuptake inhibitor available is venlafaxine (Effexor). Duloxetine is expected to be available late 2004 with an indication for chronic pain.

3. **Opioid agents** (Table 69–1). Whereas opioid medications are readily accepted in the management of cancer pain, their use in chronic, nonmalignant pain is characterized by provider fear of regulatory scrutiny, fostering addiction and overuse. However, the use of opioids is appropriate when usual modalities have failed to provide adequate analgesia. In cancer pain, opioid dose is titrated to patient response and limited by side effects such as respiratory depression. In chronic nonmalignant pain, there is evidence that continued escalating doses results in wors-

TABLE 69-1. OPIOID THERAPY

Drug	Equianalgesic Dose (mg)	Starting Oral Dose (mg)/frequency	Duration of Action (hours)
Morphine	10 IM, 30 po	15–30/q 2–4 h	3–4
Codeine	75 IM, 130 po	60/q 4–6 h	3–4
Oxycodone	15 IM, 30 po	15–30/q 4–6 h	2–4
Hydromorphone	1.5 IM, 7.5 po	2–4/q 4–6 h	2–4
Levorphanol	2 IM, 4 po	4–8/q 6–8 h	4–8
Methadone	10 IM, 20 po	5–10/q 8–12 h	4–8
Fentanyl patch	25 µg/h = 1 mg/hr	25 µg/q 72 h	72

ened analgesic response. This is because NMDA receptors are upregulated and lead to tolerance, while pain receptors become more sensitive to similar stimuli. Low to moderate total dosage of opioid agents may have the best response in chronic pain. Short-acting agents can be used initially to titrate quickly to effect, then converted to long-acting agents for chronic use. In situations of tolerance to medication with a desire to change receptor response, it is appropriate to switch from one opioid agent to another, usually starting at half the equivalent dose of the alternate medication.

4. **Adjuvant therapies.** Randomized, controlled trials have shown the efficacy of tricyclic antidepressants and other agents for management of the pain of diabetic neuropathy, postherpetic neuralgia, trigeminal neuralgia, and peripheral neuropathy. These same agents have been tried for other chronic pain conditions.

   a. **Anticonvulsants.** Stabilizing neuronal membranes; alteration of sodium, calcium, and potassium ion channels; and effects on other neurotransmitters (norepinephrine, gamma-aminobutyric acid, serotonin, etc) have been proposed mechanisms for anticonvulsants.

      (1) **Gabapentin** has been used for a variety of neuropathic pain conditions. It has relatively few side effects and its absorption is not affected by food. The starting dose is 300 mg at bedtime, gradually increased to 300 mg three times daily, then titrated based on response, to a maximum of 900 mg three times daily, although up to 900 mg four times daily has been used. Leukopenia is a serious reaction to monitor. Common side effects include somnolence, dizziness, and fatigue. The dose should be adjusted in renal insufficiency.

      (2) **Phenytoin** can be started at 100 mg three times daily and titrated to patient response. Serum levels can be monitored; >20 µg/mL are considered toxic. It should be taken after meals to decrease GI irritation. Folate (1 mg/day) supplementation should be given to decrease risk of drug-induced peripheral neuropathy and megaloblastic anemia.

      (3) **Carbamazepine** may be started at 200 mg/day and increased by 200 mg every 1–3 days to a maximum of 1500 mg/day, with therapeutic response typically at 800–1200 mg/day. It should be taken with food. Sedation, nausea, diplopia, and vertigo are common side effects; slower titration may minimize them. Monitoring of the complete blood count and liver function studies are important to monitor for aplastic anemia, agranulocytosis, thrombocytosis, and jaundice.

      (4) **Valproic acid** can be started at 15 mg/kg/day in divided doses and increased weekly by 5–10 mg/kg/day to clinical response or a maximum dose of 60 mg/kg. Baseline and periodic liver function tests should be monitored. GI side effects will often improve over time.

      (5) **Clonazepam** is a benzodiazepine with anticonvulsant activity. It may be started at 0.5 mg three times daily and increased by 0.5 mg every 3–4 days until adequate response (typically 1–4 mg/day) or a maximum dosage of 6 mg/day is reached. Typical effects of benzodiazepines can be expected. Abrupt cessation of this medication can result in a withdrawal syndrome.

   b. **Local anesthetics.** Local anesthetics have been used as blocking agents subcutaneously, along nerve roots, and at the spinal cord for acute conditions and procedures. In chronic pain, they may be helpful for continuous and lancinating pain, neuropathic pain of herpes zoster, phantom limb pain, and diabetic neuropathy. The mechanism of action is direct stabilization of nerve membranes and decreased ion flux in sodium channels. A trial with intravenous lidocaine (under appropriate cardiac monitoring) can be infused at 1–2 mg/kg over 10–15 minutes. During the infusion, the patient may experience tinnitus, perioral numbness, a metallic taste in the mouth, or dizziness. A reported 50% or greater reduction in pain based on pre and post infusion questionnaires warrants a trial of mexiletine. Oral mexiletine may be given as 150 mg at bedtime, increased weekly to 150 mg three times daily, then up to a maximum dose of 10 mg/kg/day or 1200 mg/day. Side effects may include dizziness, tremor, hypotension, ataxia, dyspepsia, or rash.

   c. **Antispasmodics** are often used to treat spasticity associated with chronic conditions, but they are also believed to have analgesic properties that may augment opioid-induced analgesia.

   (1) **Baclofen** has been useful for painful spasticity, trigeminal neuralgia, and lancinating neuropathic pain. Oral dosing begins at 5 mg three times daily and increased by 5-mg increments every few days to a maximum 80 mg/day. Side effects include central nervous system depression, fatigue, dizziness, orthostatic hypotension, headaches, insomnia, and headache.

   (2) **Cyclobenzaprine** (Flexeril) relieves muscle spasm without interfering with muscle function. It should not be used for more than 2–3 weeks, so it may not be a good choice for chronic conditions. Typical doses range from 20 to 40 mg/day. It should not be given with monoamine oxidase inhibitors, and side effects include arrhythmia, hyperthyroidism, and urinary obstruction.

   (3) **Tizanidine** (Zanaflex) is an α_2-agonist that decreases sympathetic transmission at the level of the dorsal horn and is indicated for sympathetic maintained pain as well as pain described as lancinating, electrical, or burning. Dosing begins with 1–2 mg orally at bedtime and then is switched to three-times-daily dosing with the usual range 4–12 mg/day; it should not exceed 36 mg/day. Side effects include dry mouth, sedation, dizziness, and weakness.

   d. **Clonidine.** Through α-adrenergic receptor stimulation in the brain stem, decreased sympathetic outflow results in decreased peripheral resistance, heart rate, and blood pressure. Thus, this drug has been used for sympathetically maintained pain. The transdermal patch is associated with more consistent blood levels and easier administration. Dizziness is a common side effect, as well as dry mouth, drowsiness, fatigue, and headache. Clonidine should be used with caution in the patient with already low blood pressure. The 0.1-mg patch (TTS-1) worn daily for a week is the typical starting dose and can be titrated to a maximum of two TTS-3 patches per week.

D. **Complementary and alternative therapies.** Patients in chronic pain are usually willing to try anything to help relieve their pain. Complementary approaches including homeopathy, naturopathy, and spiritual healing may have a therapeutic effect on the patient, although randomized, controlled trials have not been conducted. The provider must find the balance between maintaining hope while limiting potential harm to the patient.

E. **Surgical therapies** include implanted nerve stimulators, injected anesthetics, and nerve ablation. Specialized anesthesiologists can assist in these techniques.

IV. **Management Strategies**

   A. Effective care of chronic pain is best delivered using multidisciplines and modalities. The biochemical pain may respond better to usual or adjuvant pharmacotherapies. The physical pain may respond to massage, cold/heat, and medication. The emotional pain response may depend on the effective communication of the provider as much as any other treatment. Caregivers must be included in discussions and may be a critical component to implementing care plans.

   B. The patient and care provider must negotiate and agree on the goals of treatment: the reduction rather than elimination of pain; the improvement or restoration of function; the ability to resume social activities; or the improvement of mood. They must also discuss possible limitations including medication side effects (sedation, confusion) or tolerance and risk of addiction. Both patient and provider must be willing to acknowledge when a

TABLE 69-2. COMPONENTS OF A NARCOTIC MEDICATION PAIN CONTRACT

- The risks, side effects, and benefits have been discussed in detail.
- Only one physician will be responsible for prescribing narcotic pain medications.
- Other providers caring for the patient must be aware of the pain medication plan.
- Patient must make regular scheduled visits at least every 2 months to receive prescriptions.
- Narcotic prescriptions will not be mailed.
- Patient agrees to random urine or blood tests to assess compliance.
- Lost, misplaced, destroyed, or stolen medications will not be replaced. Refills will not be given early for any reason.
- If there is no observed improvement in quality of life or function for the patient, narcotic pain medication will be tapered.

particular treatment is not working and should be abandoned. With the use of chronic opioid pain medications, a pain contract should be initiated (Table 69–2).

REFERENCES

American Geriatrics Society. The management of persistent pain in older persons. J Am Geriatr Soc 2002;**50**(6 suppl):S205.

American Pain Society: *Principles of Analgesic Use in the Treatment of Acute Pain and Cancer Pain,* 5th ed. American Pain Society; 2003.

Ballantyne J (editor): *The Massachusetts General Hospital Handbook of Pain Management.* Lippincott, Williams & Wilkins; 2002.

Ballantyne J, Mao J: Opioid therapy for chronic pain. N Engl J Med 2003;**349**(20):1943.

Guidelines for using the Edmonton Symptom Assessment System (ESAS). http://www.palliative.org/PC/clinicalinfo/assessmenttools?easa.pdf

McCarberg BH, Dachs R: *Managing Pain: Dispelling the Myths.* American Academy of Family Physicians; 2003.

70 Chronic Obstructive Pulmonary Disease

H. Bruce Vogt, MD

KEY POINTS

- Chronic obstructive pulmonary disease (COPD) is the fourth leading cause of death in the United States, and the mortality rate continues to rise.
- COPD is divided into two types—emphysema and chronic bronchitis. Although additional risk factors have been identified, cigarette smoking accounts for 80–90% of cases.
- The primary differential diagnoses for COPD are asthma bronchiectasis and congestive heart failure. In acute exacerbations, the physician must consider comorbid disorders causing or contributing to the respiratory deterioration such as infection (pneumonia, purulent bronchitis); congestive heart failure; cardiac dysrhythmias; pneumothorax; pulmonary embolism; and myocardial infarction.
- Spirometry is required to make the diagnosis of COPD, assess disease severity, and monitor response to treatment.
- Bronchodilators via metered-dose inhalers—either anticholinergic (ipratropium [Atrovent]) or β_2-adrenergic agents (eg, albuterol [Ventolin, Proventil]; salmeterol [Serevent, Serevent Diskus]; formoterol [Foradil])—are the initial drugs used in the management of COPD. Ipratropium (Atrovent) is considered by many as the drug of first choice for maintenance therapy. The starting dose is two puffs four times daily. Albuterol (Proventil, Ventolin) is also typically started as two puffs four times daily and, given its quicker onset of action, is preferred as a "rescue" drug for acute bronchospasm. Salmeterol (Serevent, Serevent Diskus) and formoterol (Foradil) are long-acting agents. They must only be given twice daily and are not appropriate for acute bronchospasm. Combivent is a combined preparation of ipratropium and albuterol commonly used for patients requiring both drugs.

I. Introduction

A. Definition. Chronic obstructive pulmonary disease (COPD) is a disease state characterized by airflow obstruction that is generally progressive, although it may be partially reversible. It is associated with an inflammatory response of the lung to noxious particles or gases and may be accompanied by airflow hyperreactivity. COPD is manifested clinically as emphysema, chronic bronchitis, or both.

Chronic bronchitis is defined clinically as the presence of a chronic productive cough for 3 consecutive months in 2 successive years. **Emphysema** is defined morphologically as permanent enlargement of airspaces distal to the terminal bronchioles due to destruction of alveolar walls.

B. Epidemiology. COPD affects 16 million persons in the United States. It is the fourth leading cause of death and mortality rates continue to rise. The usual age of diagnosis is between 55 and 65 years. The predominant form is chronic bronchitis. Although more common in men, the prevalence of COPD has increased in women as smoking rates in women have increased.

C. Pathophysiology

1. Cigarette smoking, usually at least a 20 pack-year history, is the major cause of COPD, accounting for 80–90% of cases, although only about 15–20% of smokers develop clinically significant COPD. The age of onset of smoking, total pack-years, and current smoking status are predictive of mortality from COPD. The role of passive smoking (secondhand smoke) is unclear.

2. Urban air pollution is harmful to persons with lung disease, but its role in the etiology of COPD is uncertain. Occupational exposure to hazardous airborne substances, when intense or prolonged, is an independent risk factor for COPD and, when associated with smoking, increases the risk of disease.

3. α_1-Antitrypsin deficiency is a rare genetic abnormality that accounts for less than 1% of COPD. More than 95% of severely deficient individuals are monozygous for the Z allele (PiZZ). Screening for this problem should be considered in patients who present with COPD prior to age 50; a predominance of basilar emphysema in a smoker with dyspnea; unremitting asthma; unexplained hepatic cirrhosis; or a family history of the disorder.

II. Diagnosis

A. Differential diagnosis

1. The primary differential diagnoses for COPD are asthma, bronchiectasis, and congestive heart failure. Asthma and congestive heart failure are discussed in Chapters 68 and 72, respectively. Bronchiectasis is a disease in which destruction of the structural components of the bronchial walls leads to permanent dilation of bronchi. Infection is the primary cause. Clinical features include persistent cough productive of purulent sputum and episodic exacerbations of increased sputum production and fever.

B. Symptoms and signs

1. Dyspnea is the cardinal symptom of patients presenting with emphysema, whereas chronic productive cough is the key symptom of patients with chronic bronchitis. In the latter, cough with sputum production initially occurs only in the morning ("smoker's cough"). Sputum is usually mucoid except during exacerbations, when it may become purulent.

2. Other symptoms of COPD include wheezing, chest tightness, and recurrent respiratory infections. Weight loss is common in emphysema.

3. COPD is characterized by acute exacerbations, with the intervals between episodes decreasing over time as the disease progresses.

4. The physical examination may be entirely normal or reveal only prolonged expiration or wheezing on forced expiration with early or mild disease.

5. With later-stage disease, hyperinflation is manifested by a barrel-shaped chest, hyperresonance to percussion, decreased breath sounds, and distant heart sounds. Crackles may be heard, particularly in chronic bronchitis, and wheezing is common. In advanced disease, there is dyspnea at rest and there may be cyanosis. The patient often uses pursed lip breathing during expiration and the accessory muscles of respiration are employed. While sitting, the patient may lean forward and rest on his or her elbows to increase use of the accessory muscles (*tripoding*).

6. Physical findings unrelated to heart failure may include a palpable but normal-sized liver due to chest hyperexpansion and neck vein distention due to increased intrathoracic pressure. When right heart failure is present, increased jugular venous distention, tender hepatomegaly, and peripheral edema are typical.

C. **Diagnostic tests**

1. **Office spirometry** is necessary to make the diagnosis, assess disease severity, and monitor response to treatment. In addition, it is indicated in COPD patients who will be undergoing an operation. Measurements of airflow include forced vital capacity (FVC), forced expiratory volume in 1 second (FEV_1), forced expiratory flow rate over the interval from 25% to 75% of the total FVC ($FEF_{25-75\%}$), and the calculated FEV_1/FVC ratio. Lung volume measurements (total lung capacity [TLC]), functional residual capacity [FRC], and residual volume [RV]) are not routinely used in the office management of COPD. They are important, however, for the accurate diagnosis of restrictive lung disease. It is logical that an active lung infection, active hemoptysis, unstable angina, and a recent myocardial infarction are among the contraindications to spirometry.

   a. **Spirometry** results are interpreted as percentages of predicted values based on gender, age, and height. An FVC, FEV_1, and $FEF_{25-75\%}$ 80% or more of predicted and a FEV_1/FVC ratio (a more sensitive measure) 70% or more of predicted are considered normal. If initial testing indicates airflow obstruction, a short-acting inhaled bronchodilator should be administered and the testing repeated in 10 minutes. A 15% or greater increase in the FEV_1 or a 30% or greater increase in the $FEF_{25-75\%}$ indicates a significant component of reversibility. For daily monitoring by the patient and during office follow-up visits, the peak expiratory flow rate (PEFR)—which correlates well with FEV_1 in an individual patient—can be easily measured with use of an inexpensive peak flowmeter. The American Thoracic Society classifies the severity of COPD based on the percent of predicted FEV_1 (Stage I = ≥50%; Stage II = 35–49%; Stage III = <35%). Another classification system adopted by the World Health Organization and the National Heart, Lung and Blood Institute is depicted in Table 70–1.

2. **Arterial blood gas measurements** are usually normal in early or mild COPD. They should be obtained in patients with an FEV_1 <40% of predicted, findings suggestive of respiratory or right heart failure, polycythemia, dysrhythmias, or an altered mental state. A Pao_2 <60 mm Hg (hypoxia) with or without a $Paco_2$ of >45 mm Hg (hypoventilation, respiratory acidosis) on room air indicates respiratory failure. An O_2

TABLE 70–1. CLASSIFICATION OF COPD BY SEVERITY

Stage	Characteristics
0: At Risk	• Normal spirometry • Chronic symptoms (cough, sputum production)
I: Mild COPD	• FEV_1/FVC <70% • FEV_1 ≥80% predicted • With or without chronic symptoms (cough, sputum production)
II. Moderate COPD	• FEV_1/FVC <70% • 30% ≤ FEV_1 <80% predicted 　　(IIA: 50% ≤ FEV_1 < 80% predicted) 　　(IIB: 30% ≤ FEV_1 < 50% predicted) • With or without chronic symptoms (cough, sputum production, dyspnea)
III. Severe COPD	• FEV_1/FVC <70% • FEV_1 <30% predicted or FEV_1 <50% predicted plus respiratory failure or clinical signs of right heart failure

FEV_1, forced expiratory volume in one second; FVC: forced vital capacity; respiratory failure: Pao_2 less than 60 mm Hg with or without $Paco_2$ greater than 50 mm Hg while breathing room air at sea level.

Adapted with permission from Pauwels RA, et al: Global strategy for the diagnosis, management and prevention of chronic obstructive pulmonary disease. NHLBI/WHO Global Initiative for Chronic Obstructive Lung Disease (GOLD) workshop summary. Am J Respir Crit Care Med 2001;**163**(5):1256.

saturation of <90% also indicates hypoxia. Arterial blood gases should also be obtained at the time of initiation of oxygen and periodically thereafter. Finger or ear pulse oximetry, which measure oxygen saturation, may be used to follow up on patients both in the hospital and in the outpatient setting, but is less reliable.

3. **Complete blood counts** are indicated to screen for polycythemia and when the patient is febrile or a superimposed infection is suspected. Eosinophilia suggests allergies and possibly an element of reversible bronchospasm (ie, allergic asthma).

4. **Chest x-rays** are unremarkable in early disease, but abnormalities are apparent with advanced disease. Findings include hyperexpansion characterized by a low and flat diaphragm, increased anteroposterior diameter of the thorax, hyperlucency, increased retrosternal airspace, and a vertically positioned, narrow heart shadow. Bullae may or not be seen and, if present, may only indicate focal severe disease, not necessarily diffuse disease. High-resolution computerized tomographic scans of the chest have a much greater sensitivity and specificity, but are not part of routine care unless the diagnosis is in doubt or if a surgical procedure (eg, bullectomy) is considered.

5. In patients with long-standing COPD, an electrocardiogram may show low voltage, right axis deviation, poor R wave progression, and—when cor pulmonale is present—may demonstrate right atrial enlargement (P pulmonale) and right ventricular hypertrophy with strain.

III. **Treatment. Treatment goals** include prevention of progression; correction of any reversible component; increasing respiratory muscle function; controlling symptoms (optimum therapy); and minimizing respiratory infections and exacerbations. The various components of treatment are discussed below. A typical drug regimen for treating COPD is outlined in Figure 70–1.

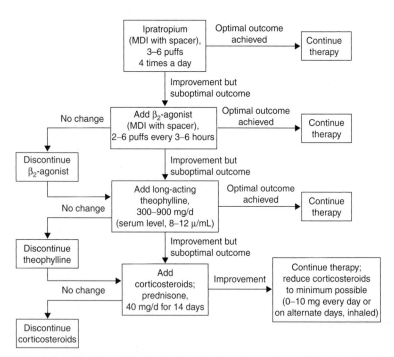

FIGURE 70–1. A typical regimen for treating chronic obstructive pulmonary disease. MDI, metered-dose inhaler. (Adapted with permission from Ferguson GT, Cherniak RM: Management of chronic obstructive pulmonary disease. N Engl J Med 1993;**328**:1017. Copyright © 1993 Massachusetts Medical Society.)

A. Nutrition

1. Patients with COPD, particularly emphysematous patients, are prone to nutritional deficiencies. They have below-normal muscle mass, including respiratory muscles. Although weight loss is more frequent in emphysematous patients, the difference in body weight between the two types of patients relates to a difference in fat mass. That is, there is a depletion of fat-free mass in both conditions. Weight loss may be due to reduced caloric intake and hypermetabolism. Nutritional depletion affects both muscle strength and endurance.

2. Inhaled bronchodilators, as well as chest physiotherapy if part of a patient's treatment plan, should be scheduled 1 hour before or after meals to prevent or reduce nausea.

3. For the patient with advanced disease, having frequent small meals avoids loss of appetite and adverse metabolic and ventilatory effects of a high caloric load.

4. An adequate protein intake (approximately 20% of calories or 1.2–1.5 g of protein per kilogram) is important to maintaining muscle mass. Liquid high-calorie protein supplements can enhance caloric intake. Vitamin supplementation, particularly A, B complex, C, and E, should be considered.

5. Sodium restriction is appropriate in patients with cor pulmonale or congestive heart failure.

6. Fluid intake should be adequate to maintain good hydration and help thin secretions, thereby promoting expectoration. Limiting fluids with meals decreases early satiety.

7. Consultation with a nutritionist may be helpful in developing a plan tailored to the patient and in identifying psychosocial impediments to adequate intake.

B. Exercise

1. Exercise has both physiologic and psychological benefits.

2. A combination of muscle strength and endurance training is beneficial. Programs should relate to daily activities such as walking and use of the arms. Recommendations for frequency vary from two to five times per week with the intensity and duration based on baseline functional status, needs, and goals. Relative contraindications to exercise include resting tachycardia greater than 110 beats per minute, $Paco_2$ >55 mm Hg, FEV_1 <0.5 L, frequent or symptomatic premature ventricular contractions, and right heart failure.

3. Regular lower extremity exercise improves exercise tolerance, particularly endurance, enhances performance of daily activities, and reduces dyspnea. Walking, jogging, bicycling, stair climbing, and swimming are examples of aerobic (endurance) exercise. Treadmills, Exercycles, and stair steppers are also effective devices, as well as cross country ski and rowing machines, which provide the added benefit of upper extremity exercise.

4. Upper extremity exercise is associated with a higher ventilatory and metabolic demand than lower extremity exercise. Upper extremity training—endurance and strength—improves arm muscle endurance and sense of well-being.

5. Resistance training (eg, weightlifting) is the mainstay of strengthening.

6. Breathing retraining and respiratory muscle training are discussed below.

C. Bronchodilators.
Although most patients with COPD do not have a large reversible component to their disease, an increase of 10–20% in FVC or FEV_1 after administration of a bronchodilator is not unusual. β-Adrenergic agents produce sympathetic-mediated bronchodilation, whereas anticholinergic agents reduce parasympathetic-mediated bronchoconstriction. The methylxanthines (eg, theophylline) also have a bronchodilatory effect but primarily decrease dyspnea by enhancing diaphragmatic function. These medications are either given on a routine basis to prevent or decrease symptoms or as needed for relief of acute or persistent symptoms. Inhaled bronchodilators are preferred due to potential theophylline toxicity. Long-acting agents are more convenient but more expensive. Combining drugs with different mechanisms of action (eg, β-adrenergic with an anticholinergic with/without theophylline) may improve bronchodilation and exercise tolerance with equivalent or even less prominent side effects. Increasing the number of drugs, however, usually increases cost. Therefore, increasing the dose of one agent is an appropriate strategy as this may offer a similar benefit, assuming side effects are not a problem.

1. **Anticholinergic agents** have an effectiveness at least as good as that of β-adrenergic agents in improving the pulmonary function of patients with COPD.

Side effects (dry mouth and a metallic taste have been reported) also are less troublesome. They have fewer cardiac side effects and tremor. They are supplied as either metered-dose inhalers (MDIs) or aerosols for use with nebulizers. Ipratropium (Atrovent) is the only agent currently available. Given a number of studies demonstrating that anticholinergic agents produce significantly greater bronchodilation than β-adrenergics, and the fact they reduce mucous hypersecretion, have fewer side effects even at high doses, and do not cause tachyphylaxis, many consider ipratropium (Atrovent) as the initial agent of choice for maintenance therapy. The drug has a slower onset of action than short-acting β_2-agonists and, therefore, is not suited for "rescue" when a rapid response is required. There is some benefit, however, for patients with acute dyspnea when delivered as an aerosol via nebulizer. The standard dosage of an ipratropium (Atrovent) MDI is two to four puffs four times daily, but higher doses (six to eight puffs) may be required and tolerated in selected patients with severe exacerbations. A combined preparation of ipratropium and albuterol available as an MDI (Combivent) or as a solution for nebulization (Duo Neb) has been found to produce greater and more sustained improvements in FEV_1 than either agent alone.

2. **β-Adrenergic agents** are available in inhaled (via MDI or nebulizer), oral, and subcutaneous preparations. Selective β_2 agents are preferred to minimize the likelihood of β_1 (cardiac) side effects. Inhalation via MDI or nebulizer-delivered aerosol is preferential to oral preparations due to their ability to present a high concentration of drug to target receptors with minimal systemic effects. Short-acting (albuterol [Ventolin, Proventil]; levalbuterol [Xopenex]) and long-acting (salmeterol [Serevent, Serevent Diskus]; formoterol [Foradil]) agents are available. The usual regimen for short-acting agents given via an MDI is two puffs four times daily. Salmeterol inhalation aerosol (Serevent) is given as two puffs twice daily, whereas, salmeterol inhalation powder (Serevent Diskus) and formoterol (Foradil) are given as one puff twice daily. They must not be given more often due to their duration of action. Salmeterol (Serevent, Serevent Diskus) and formoterol (Foradil) are excellent choices for the patient with nocturnal symptoms. The short-acting agents are required for "rescue" in the scenario of acute bronchospasm with dyspnea. In severe exacerbations, nebulized aerosol can deliver a high concentration of medication; however, the repeated use of an MDI has equivalent effects, particularly when a spacer is employed. Routine use of a spacer is always preferable, but particularly in the setting of an acute exacerbation or for patients who are not facile with use of an MDI. The potential for cardiac dysrhythmias necessitates careful monitoring in patients with known cardiac disease, although complications are rare with usual doses. Levalbuterol (Xopenex) is the R-isomer of racemic albuterol and is available only in a solution for nebulized delivery. Although promoted as safer than albuterol, and with less affect on heart rate, there appears to be no significant clinical advantage and it is considerably more expensive. See Table 70–2 for inhaled bronchodilator preparations and dosages. Oral β_2 drugs should only be prescribed for patients unable to use inhaled agents, and when employed, should be administered in small doses that are gradually increased. If inhaled dosage is adequate, little additional bronchodilation is gained from an added oral agent. See Table 70–3 for oral bronchodilator preparations and dosages. A subcutaneous preparation of terbutaline (Brethine, Bricanyl) is available with a recommended dose of 0.25–0.5 mg every 4–8 hours.

3. **Theophylline** is effective in COPD through more than one mechanism. Although a bronchodilator, it also improves diaphragmatic function and stimulates the respiratory center. The fact that theophylline can improve cardiac output, decrease pulmonary vascular resistance, and improve the perfusion of ischemic cardiac muscle offers advantages to COPD patients with associated cor pulmonale or cardiac disease. It, however, is not a first-line drug and carries the risk of significant toxicity. Added to a regimen of a β_2-agonist and ipratropium, theophylline produces enhanced bronchodilation, improved pulmonary function, and improved health status. It is indicated in patients who remain symptomatic despite optimum inhalation therapy and in patients who have difficulty with or are noncompliant with MDIs. Potential toxicities include gastrointestinal intolerance (eg, anorexia, nausea, vomiting, abdominal cramping, diarrhea); headache; tremors; cardiac side effects (eg, sinus

TABLE 70–2. COMMON INHALANT BRONCHODILATORS

Class	Drug	Formulation/Adult Dosage	Cost[4]
Anticholinergic	Ipratropium Bromide[1] (Atrovent)	MDI/2–4 puffs qid	$$
		Nebulized/0.5 mg tid–qid	$$
β₂-agonists[2]	Albuterol (Proventil, Ventolin)	MDI/2–4 puffs q 4–6 h	$
		Nebulized/2.5 mg tid–qid	$
	Levalbuterol (Xopenex)	Nebulized/0.63–1.25 mg q 6–8 h	$$$$
	Metaproterenol (Metaprel, Alupent)	MDI/2–4 puffs q 3–6 h	$$
		Nebulized/0.3 mL q 3–6 h	$$
	Pirbuterol (Maxair)	MDI/2 puffs q 4–6 h	$$
	Salmeterol (Serevent)[3]	MDI/2 puffs bid	$$$
	Salmeterol (Servent Diskus)[3]	MDI/1 puff bid	$$$
	Formoterol (Foradil)[3]	MDI/1 puff bid	$$$
	Terbutaline (Brethine)	MDI/2 puffs q 4–6 h	$$
Combination anticholinergic-β₂-agonist	Ipratropium-Albuterol (Combivent)	MDI/2–3 puffs qid	$$
	(DuoNeb)	Nebulized/3 mL qid	$$$$

[1] Considered drug of first choice in COPD; Slower onset of action than β₂-agonists, making the latter preferable for acute bronchospasm.
[2] Given there are some β₁ receptors in cardiac muscle, a significant cardiovascular effect can occur in some patients, particularly at high dosages.
[3] Long-acting, therefore, only given bid; not used for acute bronchospasm.
[4] Range of average monthly cost from $ (low) to $$$$ (high).

tachycardia, premature ventricular contractions, ventricular tachycardia); and seizures. Ventricular tachycardia and seizures tend to occur at high serum concentrations (>35 mg/L). Toxicities are more likely in patients who do not metabolize the drug well (eg, liver disease) and when drug interactions increase the level of theophylline.

a. **Dosage.** The usual starting dose, based on lean body weight, for a nonsmoking patient is 10–12 mg/kg/day of a long-acting preparation given twice a day. How-

TABLE 70–3. COMMON ORAL BRONCHODILATORS

Class	Drug	Supplied As	Adult Dosage	Cost[2]
Methylxanthines	Theophylline (generic)	100,125,200,300, 450 mg SR	10–12 mg/kg/day[1]	$
	Theophylline (Theo 24)	100,200,300, 400 mg SR	10–12 mg/kg/day[1]	$–$$
	Theophylline (Theo-Dur)	100,200,300, 450 mg SR	10–12 mg/kg/day[1]	$
	Theophylline (Uniphyl)	400,600 mg SR	10–12 mg/kg/day[1]	$$–$$$
β₂-agonists	Albuterol (Proventil, generic)	2,4 mg tablets 2 mg/5 mL syrup	2–4 mg tid–qid (maximum 32 mg/day)	$
	Albuterol (Proventil Repetabs)	4 mg SR tablets	4–8 mg q 12 h (maximum 32 mg/day)	$$$
	Albuterol (Volmax Extended Release)	4,8 mg SR tablets	4–8 mg q 12 h (maximum 32 mg/day)	$$$–$$$$
	Metaproterenol (Alupent, Metaprel, generic)	10,20 mg tablets 10 mg/5 mL	10–20 mg q 6–8 h	$$$
	Terbutaline (Brethine, Bricanyl)	2.5,5 mg tablets	2.5–5 mg q 6–8 h (maximum 15 mg)	$$$

[1] Based on lean body weight for a nonsmoking adult. Higher dosage required in smokers (12–18 mg/kg/day); lower dosage needed in patients with hepatic insufficiency (<5 mg/kg/day), cor pulmonale (4–7 mg/kg/day), and heart failure (4–7 mg/kg/day).
[2] Range of average monthly cost from $ (low) to $$$$ (high).
SR, sustained-release.

ever, the most appropriate dose depends on many factors including age, lean body weight, smoking status (speeds rate of metabolism), liver function, associated congestive heart failure, and concomitant drug use. A conservative approach is to start with 400 mg/day given as 200 mg twice a day and to increase the dose every 3–5 days. Use of a long-acting preparation in the evening reduces overnight declines in FEV_1 and morning dyspnea. The therapeutic window is narrow and serum levels must be checked on a regular basis. Clinical judgment, along with subjective and objective improvement (spirometry), is very important as some patients require drug levels below or above the therapeutic range to achieve maximum improvement with minimal side effects. Patients with daily fluctuations in symptoms may benefit from peak and trough theophylline levels. Rapid metabolizers, such as smokers, who require 900 mg/day or more, may benefit from doses given three times a day in order to achieve steady levels. Patients with a history of gastrointestinal intolerance to medications may benefit from starting at a lower dose and gradually increasing the dose.

D. **Corticosteroids** are most useful in patients who do not respond adequately to bronchodilators or during acute exacerbations. They are most beneficial in patients whose COPD has an asthmatic component or who have a 15% improvement in FEV_1 with a bronchodilating agent. Steroids enhance responsiveness to bronchodilators, inhibit the release of proteases from leukocytes, and reduce mucosal edema. A 6-week to 3-month trial of inhaled corticosteroids is recommended to identify COPD patients who may benefit from long-term use. For acute exacerbations, oral corticosteroids are effective, but it is important to either discontinue high doses within a few days or taper the dose to discontinuance over a period of approximately 2 weeks. Long-term use of oral corticosteroids is not routinely recommended as there is no evidence that they are beneficial. If there is objective evidence of a response (20–25% improvement in FEV_1), however, maintenance therapy can be tested with the corticosteroid tapered to the lowest dose that maintains the improvement. Alternate-day administration may be sufficient. If FEV_1 does not improve or is not maintained, steroids should be tapered and discontinued. Parenteral steroids are commonly used during acute exacerbations treated in the hospital setting. A study employing parenteral methylprednisolone (Solu Medrol) reported more rapid improvement of FEV_1 over the first 72 hours in patients treated with steroids compared with those who were not. The Systemic Corticosteroids in COPD Exacerbations clinical trial demonstrated that patients treated with systemic steroids had fewer treatment failures, better spirometry, and shorter hospital stays.

1. **Dosage/route**
   a. **Oral administration.** For acute exacerbations, **prednisone** can be started in doses as high as 40–60 mg/day for 5 days and discontinued or tapered by 10 mg every 1–2 days over a 1- to 2-week period and then discontinued. The risk of significant side effects is low if the equivalent of 10 mg/day or less of prednisone is used or if higher-dose treatment is limited to 2 weeks.
   b. **Parenteral administration.** An appropriate intravenous dose of methylprednisolone (Solu Medrol) is 125 mg given every 6 hours for 3 days as used in the Systemic Corticosteroids in COPD Exacerbations trial referred to above. In this trial, parenteral therapy was followed by oral prednisone tapered over 2 weeks.
   c. **MDI administration.** This route allows the use of smaller dosages, since the medication is delivered directly to its site of action. The usual dosage range is two to four puffs administered two to four times a day. Four to 8 weeks of use may be needed before subjective or objective benefits are noted. Available preparations include beclomethasone (Beclovent, Vanceril, QVAR), flunisolide (AeroBid, AeroBid-M), fluticasone (Flovent, Flovent Rotadisk), triamcinolone (Azmacort), and budesonide (Pulmicort Turbuhaler). A combination of fluticasone and salmeterol (Advair Diskus, 100/50, 250/50, or 500/50) is available for patients who respond well to long-acting β_2-adrenergics and who demonstrate long-term improvement with inhaled steroids. The usual dosage is one puff twice daily.

2. **Side effects.** Side effects from long-term oral administration include steroid myopathy (which contributes to muscle weakness and respiratory failure in patients with advanced disease), as well as cataract formation, diabetes mellitus, osteoporosis, avascular necrosis, and immune suppression. Oral candidiasis is the most common

side effect reported with use of a steroid MDI and can be prevented by use of a spacer and by rinsing the mouth with water after use.

E. Antibiotics are indicated for acute exacerbations of COPD because infections—purulent bronchitis and pneumonia—are the most common causes of exacerbations. The smaller airways of patients with COPD are often colonized with bacteria (up to 50%) and, therefore, their presence does not necessarily indicate infection. Symptoms suggestive of infection include increased sputum volume, increased sputum purulence, and increased dyspnea. These symptoms, however, may occur whether the causative organism is bacterial or viral. The proportion of exacerbations associated with viral infection has been estimated to be from 7% to 63%, the large discrepancy due to differences in study design. Influenza, parainfluenza, coronavirus, and rhinovirus are common isolates. Bacteria may either be the cause of an infection or represent a secondary infection of what originated as a viral syndrome. Because many sputum cultures fail to reveal a predominant organism and because of the issues of bacterial colonization and the difficulty in distinguishing a viral from a bacterial infection, the choice of whether to use an antibiotic and which antibiotic to use can be difficult. The emergence of drug resistance also demands thoughtful consideration in selection. Pending culture results, initial therapy is directed against the most likely bacterial pathogens: *Haemophilus influenzae, Streptococcus pneumoniae,* and *Moraxella (Branhamella) catarrhalis. Mycoplasma pneumoniae* and *Chlamydia pneumoniae* have also been reported. It should be noted, however, that in patients with a baseline FEV_1 of 35% or less of predicted, gram-negative bacteria (eg, *Enterobacteriaceae, Pseudomonas*) play a more significant role in the etiology of exacerbations. First-line, less expensive antibiotics include amoxicillin, sulfa-trimethoprim, tetracycline, doxycycline, and erythromycin. Second-line agents offer broader coverage but are more expensive. Table 70–4 lists first- and second-line oral antibiotics commonly used during exacerbations of COPD. The effectiveness of long-term antibiotics for prophylaxis is controversial and their routine use is not recommended. With recurrent infections, however, a prolonged course—either continuous or intermittent—may be useful.

TABLE 70–4. COMMON ORAL ANTIBIOTICS FOR CHRONIC OBSTRUCTIVE PULMONARY DISEASE EXACERBATIONS

	Drug	Dosage (10-day course)	Cost[1]
First-line agents			
	Amoxicillin (generic, Amoxil, Polymox, Trimox)	500 mg tid	$
	Sulfamethoxazole/Trimethoprim[2] (generic, Bactrim, Septra, Sulfatrim)	160 mg/800 mg bid	$
	Tetracycline (generic, Sumycin)	500 mg qid	$
	Doxycycline (generic, Vibramycin, Doryx, Monodox)	100 mg bid	$
	Erythromycin (generic, Eryc, E-mycin, EES)	1000–2000 mg/day divided dose (bid–tid) depending on agent	$
Second-line agents	Amoxicillin/Clavulanate Potassium (Augmentin)	875 mg/125 mg bid or 500 mg/125 mg tid	$$$
	Cerfuroxime (Ceftin)	250–500 mg bid	$$$
	Ceprozil (Cefzil)	500 mg bid	$$$
	Cefixime (Suprax)	400 mg/day (single dose or divided dose)	$$$
	Cefpodoxime (Vantin)	200 mg bid	$$$
	Azithromycin (Zithromax)[3,4]	500 mg day 1, then 250 mg days 1–4	$$
	Clarithromycin (Biaxin)[4]	500 mg bid	$$$
	Levofloxacin (Levaquin)[4]	500 mg daily	$$$

[1] Range of daily cost from $ (low) to $$$$ (high).
[2] Available in single-strength (80 mg/400 mg) or double-strength (160 mg/800 mg) tablets.
[3] Five-day course.
[4] Caution must be taken when using macrolides or levofloxacin (Levaquin) in a patient on theophylline because of drug level increases of the latter.

F. Mucokinetic agents are commonly given to thin and improve the mobilization of secretions, although objective evidence of their benefit is lacking. Their widespread use cannot be recommended. Hydration (oral, intravenous) and moisture administered by nebulization may be useful.

G. Chest physiotherapy is of no benefit during acute exacerbations unless there is sputum production of >25 mL/day or mucus plugging with resultant lobar atelectasis.

H. Antitussives must be used judiciously as cough has a significant protective role. If prescribed, a nonnarcotic agent such as dextromethorphan should be tried. Codeine and other narcotics should be avoided because they cause respiratory depression and may worsen hypercapnia.

I. Other treatments

1. **Respiratory stimulants** such as doxapram and almitrine bismesylate are not currently recommended in stable COPD patients.

2. **Antioxidants** such as *N*-acetylcysteine have been shown to reduce the frequency of exacerbations, but ongoing trials must be completed prior to recommending their routine use.

3. **Antiproteases** for aerosol or MDI administration may eventually be available to restore the protease-antiprotease balance, which may retard the progression of COPD. Human α_1-proteinase inhibitor is available for patients with emphysema from a congenital deficiency of this enzyme. The efficacy of human α_1-proteinase inhibitor administered intravenously on a weekly basis is being studied; treatment is very expensive.

4. **Nitric oxide** can worsen gas exchange and is thus contraindicated.

5. **Psychoactive agents** to treat depression, insomnia, or anxiety can be helpful to improve the quality of life for patients with COPD. Benzodiazepines are generally safe to use in patients with mild or moderate COPD. Their use must be closely monitored in patients with severe COPD to prevent respiratory depression, especially during sleep. Sedating antihistamines and chloral hydrate are safer hypnotics for use in insomnia. In addition to their primary use, antidepressants can help improve sleep and relieve chronic pain.

6. **Surgery** can be considered in carefully selected patients. Bullectomy, which allows greater lung expansion, is effective in reducing dyspnea and improving pulmonary function. **Lung volume reduction surgery (LVRS)** is a promising technique requiring further study. LVRS involves volume reduction in one or both lungs by stapler resection, laser, or both. The National Emphysema Treatment Trial was conducted to determine whether the addition of LVRS to medical therapy improves survival and exercise capacity. In a recently published article of the study's results, investigators reported that at 24 months, 15% of surgical patients had improved exercise capacity and 33% improved health-related quality of life compared to 3% and 9%, respectively, in medically treated patients. There was a statistically significant difference in the mortality rates (mean follow-up of 29.2 months) in the surgical and medical groups depending on the primary distribution of the lung disease. Patients with predominantly upper lobe emphysema and low baseline exercise capacity had significantly lower mortality with surgery (19%) compared with medical treatment (34%). This contrasted with high mortality in the surgical group (25%) vs. the medical group (13%) in patients with predominantly non–upper lobe disease and high exercise capacity. Additional trials have been advocated. Lung transplantation (single or double) has been shown to improve quality of life and functional capacity in COPD patients with very advanced disease. Appropriate patient selection is important. Perioperative mortality is 7–10%, with 1- and 5-year survival rates of approximately 75% and 45%, respectively. The average waiting period for single lung transplant is 1–2 years.

V. Management Strategies. The primary care physician should develop an individualized plan for the patient and coordinate the care given by others.

A. Smoking cessation. This is often the most difficult challenge faced by the patient with COPD but also the most important, as overcoming dependency on tobacco is the best way to change the course of COPD. Smoking cessation decreases cough and sputum production, slows the decline of FEV_1, and reduces the risk of respiratory failure. It also can lower the patient's risk of contracting other smoking-related illnesses. The physician needs to be persistent in educating patients about the benefits of and methods for discontinuing smoking. Since there are various factors that foster smoking, success in cessation often involves combined approaches. Practical counseling, behavior modification, self-help materials, group cessation programs, social support, and pharmacotherapies all have a place in assisting the patient (see Chapter 100).

B. Hospitalization. The physician should consider hospitalization for the patient with COPD under the following circumstances:

1. Acute exacerbations failing to improve symptomatically or objectively despite aggressive treatment in the office or hospital's emergency department.

2. New-onset or worsening cor pulmonale unresponsive to outpatient treatment.

3. New-onset (uncompensated) respiratory acidosis or marked deterioration of blood gases from the patient's baseline levels.

4. Significant comorbidities, both pulmonary (eg, pneumothorax, pleural effusion, pneumonia, pulmonary contusion) and nonpulmonary (eg, rib or vertebral body fracture, severe steroid myopathy).

5. New-onset cardiac dysrhythmias.

6. Gradual decline in pulmonary function unresponsive to outpatient management or rapid decline that results in a loss of independence.

7. Lack of sufficient home support either by family or supplementary home care services.

8. Planned surgical or diagnostic procedure requiring analgesics or sedatives that may adversely affect pulmonary function.

9. **Discharge criteria** for patients who require hospitalization include clinical stability (including arterial blood gases) for 12–24 hours; inhaled bronchodilators required no more often than every 4 hours; the ability to walk across the room (if previously ambulatory); home care addressed; and follow-up appointment with the physician arranged.

C. Environmental control

1. Patients with COPD should avoid exposure to secondhand tobacco smoke and should remain indoors during air pollution or smog alerts.

2. Patients who are sensitive to extremes of humidity and temperature may find that use of a humidifier in the winter and a dehumidifier or air conditioner in the summer improves symptoms.

3. Air cleaners, whether directed against indoor or outdoor generated air contaminants, are ineffective.

4. Patients with chronic hypoxemia generally should not travel to altitudes above 4000 feet. Studies have shown decreased survival rates among patients who live at altitudes above 3500 feet. Commercial aircraft are usually pressurized to between 5000 and 7000 feet. Patients with COPD may require supplemental oxygen during flights. It is recommended that PaO_2 be maintained above 50 mm Hg. In patients with O_2 saturations of 88–92% at sea level, 1–2 L per nasal cannula may be sufficient to achieve this. The flow rate for patients ordinarily on oxygen should also be increased by 1–2 L. The Federal Aviation Administration requires a physician statement for patients to receive continuous oxygen during flights. Patients should contact their travel airline to learn of the specifics necessary to make such arrangements. Patients should avoid flying in unpressurized aircraft.

D. Home oxygen therapy. Reversing hypoxemia improves the patient's survival, decreases hospitalization, increases exercise capacity and endurance, enhances neuropsychological function, increases cardiac output, reverses secondary polycythemia, and decreases pulmonary vascular resistance. Oxygen is the most potent treatment for cor pulmonale and mitigates right heart failure secondary to it. The prevention of tissue hypoxia is the ultimate concern and involves all aspects of oxygen transport and delivery. The concern that oxygen therapy may lead to respiratory acidosis due to respiratory center depression has been overemphasized. Most evidence does not show a decrease in minute ventilation or respiratory drive. Although CO_2 retention may occur, it is often caused by ventilation-perfusion mismatch rather than suppression of respiratory drive. Correcting hypoxemia is critical as it is the only intervention that has been demonstrated to improve survival in patients with severe COPD.

1. **Guidelines**

   a. PaO_2 ≤55 mm Hg or SaO_2 ≤88% (waking values), with or without hypercapnia; OR PaO_2 between 55 mm Hg and 60 mm Hg or SaO_2 of 89% with pulmonary hypertension, cor pulmonale, peripheral edema suggesting congestive heart failure, impaired mental status, or polycythemia (hematocrit >55%). At least two arterial blood gas measurements should be obtained while the patient is breathing room air for a minimum of 20 minutes.

    b. The goal is to increase baseline PaO_2 to 60–65 mm Hg or SaO_2 to 90–94% using the lowest liter flow rate possible. Start with 1 L per minute by nasal cannula. The flow rate should be adjusted upward by 1 liter over baseline for exercise and sleep.

  2. Delivery systems are outlined in Table 70–5.

  3. Monitoring. A patient should initially be assessed via arterial blood gases. Pulse oximetry is insufficient and, of course, does not determine acid-base status. Monitoring may then be accomplished by either arterial blood gases or by pulse oximetry done periodically. This is particularly important in the patient with worsening symptoms and after changes in oxygen dose. A patient who continues to have symptoms at night should be monitored by pulse oximetry or formal sleep laboratory evaluation.

  4. Regular education on the proper use of equipment and supervision during the first 3 months of use increases patient acceptance of home oxygen therapy.

E. Pulmonary rehabilitation is a multidisciplinary approach to the care of patients with chronic respiratory illnesses with goals of reducing symptoms, preventing complications, improving quality of life, and achieving the individual's maximum level of independence and functioning in the community. Major components of rehabilitation include education, nutrition counseling, exercise training, breathing re-training, and inspiratory muscle training. Documented benefits include symptomatic improvement, increased exercise tolerance, less depression, and a reduction in sick days, including hospitalization. Baseline and outcome assessments (eg, exercise tolerance, health status, inspiratory/expiratory muscle strength, limb strength) document gains and identify areas for continued improvement.

  1. Participation. COPD patients most likely to benefit from rehabilitation are those under optimal medical management, who have no cardiac disease and are symptomatic at rest or with mild exertion. Family support increases the likelihood of success.

  2. Breathing retraining should be part of a rehabilitation program with the aim of helping the patient relieve and control dyspnea and of counteracting physiologic abnormalities such as hyperinflation. Pursed-lip and diaphragmatic breathing assist in slowing the respiratory rate and increasing tidal volume, while inhibiting airspace collapse and enhancing gas exchange. Both help alleviate dyspnea. Leaning forward and resting the arms on one's thighs or on a table (*tripoding*) may also help relieve dyspnea. **Inspiratory muscle training** has been shown to decrease dyspnea for some patients; however, no benefit has been demonstrated when

---

TABLE 70–5. ADVANTAGES AND DISADVANTAGES OF HOME OXYGEN SYSTEMS

System	Liquid Portable	Concentrators	Compressed Gas
Advantages	Lightweight Long-range portable canister Most practical ambulatory system Valuable for pulmonary rehabilitation	Lower cost Convenient for home use Attractive equipment Widely available	Lower cost in general (cost may equal liquid in continuous situation) Widely available
Disadvantages	Expensive; more costly than O_2 concentrators used alone Limited availability in small or rural communities	Requires electricity (car/truck adapters available) May need backup tank system Not portable; not useful for ambulation or pulmonary rehabilitation Noisy	Multiple tanks needed unless transfilling from a large tank can be done at home Frequent deliveries needed Heavy, unsightly tanks

Adapted with permission from Celli BR, Petty TL: Pulmonary rehabilitation. In: Murray JF, et al: (editors): *Textbook of Respiratory Medicine*, 3rd ed. WB Saunders; 2000:2512. Copyright 2000, with permission from Elsevier.

compared with aerobic lower extremity conditioning. Thus, additional research is required to determine its role.

F. Personalized patient education should address the disease process and provide information about medications (eg, rationale, side effects, inhaler technique). Patient education and patient-physician agreement on short- and long-term goals improves adherence to the therapeutic regimen. This should include helping identify a way for the patient to monitor progress toward goals. Sensitive issues such as sexual activity should be addressed. Education of family members, particularly those involved in the patient's care, is also important and, given the considerable adaptation they must make in their own lives, caregivers may need supportive therapy themselves.

G. Immunization for influenza is recommended on an annual basis for all COPD patients. The value of pneumococcal immunization has also been demonstrated. The vaccine covers more than 80% of pneumococcal strains. Revaccination is not currently recommended except for patients who receive the vaccine before age 65. In such cases, a booster should be given after age 65 and at least 5 years after the initial vaccination.

VI. Prognosis

A. Death rate. There was a dramatic increase in the age-adjusted COPD death rates (52%) between 1979 and 1998. Although death rates have always been higher in men, between 1979 and 1998 death rates in women increased 159% compared to 9% in men. This reflects an increased smoking rate in women. The difference in the age-adjusted death rates of whites and African Americans has also narrowed.

B. COPD is characterized by a progressive decline in pulmonary function. Although variable, FEV_1 decreases by an average of 45 mL/year in smokers and by 50–75 mL/year in patients with COPD, compared to 25–30 mL/year (beginning at about age 35) in nonsmokers without pulmonary disease. Age, lifetime smoking, and the number of cigarettes currently smoked are all risk factors for more rapid decline in pulmonary function. Dyspnea with moderate exertion is usually noticeable when FEV_1 falls to about 1.5 L. Dyspnea with any exertion is usually present at a FEV_1 of 1 L. Patients with a FEV_1 of 0.5 L or less are usually invalids. Besides age, FEV_1 is the best predictor of mortality. Other indicators of poor prognosis include resting tachycardia, severe hypoxemia, severe atrial hypoxia, severe hypercapnia, hypoalbuminemia, and cor pulmonale. In severe COPD, death is related to recurrent episodes of hypoxia, leading to the development of pulmonary vascular hypertension and cor pulmonale. Acute respiratory failure, severe pneumonia, pneumothorax, pulmonary embolism, and cardiac dysrhythmias are medical complications often responsible for death. The mortality rate 10 years after diagnosis is >50%.

C. Regular follow-up is important to the successful management of the patient with COPD. The purpose of such visits includes supporting the patient in smoking cessation, monitoring and modifying as necessary the therapeutic regimen, monitoring changes in pulmonary function, early identification of complications, ongoing education, and emotional support. Attention to the pulmonary illness must not entirely supplant addressing other health promotion/disease prevention issues. Advance directives should also be reviewed periodically.

REFERENCES

American Thoracic Society: Standards for the diagnosis and care of patients with chronic obstructive pulmonary disease. Am J Respir Crit Care Med 1995;**152**:S77.

Beeh K-M, Welte T, Buhl R: Anticholinergics in the treatment of chronic obstructive pulmonary disease. Respiration 2002;**69**:372.

Kirby M, Thomson BD, Vogt HB: *COPD Reference Guide,* 7th ed. American Board of Family Practice; 2001.

MacIntyre NR: Chronic obstructive pulmonary disease management: The evidence base. Respir Care 2001;**46**(11):1294.

Madison JM, Irwin RS: Chronic obstructive pulmonary disease. Lancet 1998;**352**:467.

Pauwels RA, et al: Global strategy for the diagnosis, management, and prevention of chronic obstructive pulmonary disease. NHLBI/WHO Global Initiative for Chronic Obstructive Lung Disease (GOLD) workshop summary. Am J Respir Crit Care Med 2001;**163**(5):1256; Respir Care 2001;**46**(8):798.

National Emphysema Treatment Trial Research Group: A randomized trial comparing lung-volume-reduction surgery with medical therapy for severe emphysema. N Engl J Med 2003;**348**:2059.

Rochester CL (guest editor): Chronic obstructive pulmonary disease. Clinics in Chest Medicine 2000;**21**(4).

71   Cirrhosis

Mari Egan, MD, MHPE, & Mark C. Potter, MD

KEY POINTS

• Cirrhosis is the 10th leading cause of death in the United States. Alcohol abuse is the most common cause of cirrhosis, followed by hepatitis C.

• Treatment for hepatitis C is indicated for patients with biopsy-proven active hepatitis and detectable serum levels of hepatitis C RNA. The current regimen of first choice is pegylated interferon alfa 2b (PEG-Intron), 1.5 µg/kg subcutaneously weekly, or pegylated interferon alfa 2a (Pegasys), 180 µg subcutaneously weekly with ribavirin (Rebetol), 600 mg orally twice daily for up to 48 weeks' treatment duration.

• Other treatments for underlying causes of cirrhosis include Hepatitis B treatment, consisting of interferon alfa-2b, 5 million IU subcutaneously or intramuscularly (IM) daily; OR 10 million IU subcutaneously or IM three times per week; OR lamivudine, 100 mg orally daily; OR Adefovir dipivoxil, 10 mg orally daily. Treatment for primary biliary cirrhosis is ursodeoxycholic acid, 13–15 mg/kg orally daily. Treatment for Wilson's disease is D-penicillamine, 250–500 mg orally three times daily, OR trientine, 250–500 mg orally four times daily. Treatment for hemochromatosis is phlebotomy (removing 500 mL of blood) weekly.

• In patients with cirrhosis, the primary care physician should monitor for signs of encephalopathy, fluid retention, infection, and gastrointestinal bleeding. The physician should also use prophylaxis against rebleeding in patients with a history of variceal bleeding with beta blockers. The usual starting dose is propranolol, 10 mg three times daily. In addition, vaccinations should be administered (influenza and pneumococcus) and education given on avoiding medical toxicity (eg, acetaminophen), eating a low-salt, 1 g protein per kg/day diet, and being aware of increased risks for infection.

• Patients with cirrhosis are at an increased risk for hepatocellular carcinoma. Patients should be screened for cancer with a serum α-fetoprotein test and liver ultrasound every 6–12 months.

I. Introduction

A. Cirrhosis is characterized by diffuse liver injury, which progresses with nodular regeneration to eventual irreversible fibrosis. Due to loss of normal hepatocytes and distorted hepatic architecture, the liver is unable to perform its synthetic or metabolic functions normally. Also blood flow is diverted around the liver rather than through it (portosystemic shunting). This process has major effects on all other organ systems, which manifests as the important complications of cirrhosis.

B. Cirrhosis is a frequent cause of death in the United States and is most prevalent in the 36- to 54-year-old age group. This age range is affected because chronic liver disease progresses from hepatitis to cirrhosis over 20–40 years. With progressive liver decompensation, liver transplantation is the only treatment that extends life. There are four times the number of patients who need liver transplants in the United States than will eventually get one.

C. When a physician first evaluates a patient with liver disease, it is important to assess risk factors. History should be elicited of prior blood transfusions, hemodialysis, hemophilia, organ transplants, sexual practices, multiple sexual partners, problem drinking, hepatotoxic drugs (prescription and over-the-counter drugs and vitamins and herbal remedies), occupational exposures, family history, and other systemic disease.

D. In patients with cirrhosis, the physician is also managing complications of the liver damage. However, not all patients with cirrhosis will develop life-threatening complications. In 40% of patients with cirrhosis, the diagnosis will be made at autopsy.

E. Among patients infected with hepatitis C virus (HCV), 20–30% will develop cirrhosis in 20–40 years.

II. Diagnosis

A. Symptoms and signs. The clinical presentation of patients with cirrhosis varies widely. It ranges from asymptomatic patients found incidentally to have liver disease to patients presenting with multiple end-stage findings.

The symptoms and signs of cirrhosis can be separated into the three major groups below.

1. **Symptoms and signs of hepatocellular dysfunction.** These include fatigue, weakness, weight loss, jaundice, nausea and vomiting, coagulopathy, palmar erythema, gynecomastia, testicular atrophy, menstrual dysfunction, loss of pubic hair, muscle waisting, spider angiomas, and parotid and lacrimal gland hypertrophy.

2. **Signs and symptoms of portal hypertension.** These are due to increased intrahepatic vascular resistance, which causes ascites, edema, splenomegaly, esophageal and gastric varices, and dilated abdominal wall veins (caput medusa).

3. **Signs and symptoms caused by the disease underlying the cirrhosis.** These include withdrawal symptoms and signs in chronic alcoholics and cardiomyopathy or arthropathy in patients with hemochromatosis.

B. Diagnosis of diseases that cause cirrhosis. A complete diagnostic work-up should be undertaken in all patients with cirrhosis to identify all contributing underlying causes. In some types of cirrhosis, treatment can slow the progression of further injury.

1. **Viral hepatitis. Chronic hepatitis C, chronic hepatitis B, and coinfection with hepatitis D** are major causes of cirrhosis. Most patients with chronic viral hepatitis are asymptomatic or have nonspecific symptoms. Some patients will present with complications of cirrhosis as the earliest signs of infection. Patients presenting with cirrhosis should be tested for hepatitis B surface antigen, surface antibody core antibody, and hepatitis C antibody. Patients with chronic hepatitis C infection will have a positive test for anti-HCV antibody. Patients with a positive anti-HCV antibody test and low or intermediate risk for hepatitis C infection based on risk history should have the presence of HCV RNA confirmed with either a quantitative (preferred if treatment likely) or a qualitative polymerase chain reaction test. Patients with positive anti-HCV antibody with a high risk history for hepatitis C infection (eg, injection drug users) can be assumed on the basis of the anti-HCV antibody test to have true hepatitis C infection and proceed to liver biopsy if they are a candidate for treatment. Persistently elevated alanine aminotransferase (ALT) may be seen, though ALT levels often fluctuate, may have periods in the normal range even with persistent viral infection, and are not a reliable guide as to the severity of liver injury. A positive test for hepatitis D virus indicates coinfection by hepatitis D.

2. **Alcoholic cirrhosis** usually occurs 10 or more years after a period of excessive alcohol ingestion. Between 8 and 20% of chronic alcoholics develop cirrhosis. Laboratory evidence in patients who are currently drinking can show a ratio of aspartate aminotransferase (AST) to ALT greater than 1 and usually greater than 2. Hypoalbuminemia is commonly seen in malnourished alcoholics as well as hyponatremia, hypomagnesemia, hypophosphatemia, low blood urea nitrogen levels, and elevated mean corpuscular volume. Other toxins (eg, industrial cleaning solvents) and drugs (eg, methotrexate, isoniazid, acetaminophen, and estrogen) can cause cirrhosis.

3. **Primary biliary cirrhosis** is a chronic, progressive autoimmune disease of the liver characterized by destruction of the intrahepatic bile ducts. The disease chiefly affects women, with an onset from age 30–50 years. More than half of patients are asymptomatic when diagnosed, although pruritus with fatigue is a common presenting symptom. Hepatomegaly is seen in 50% of patients, and 10–50% will have splenomegaly. Laboratory tests may show an isolated elevation of serum alkaline phosphatase often more than twice the upper limit of normal with no other abnormal liver function test findings. Patients will also be positive for antimitochondrial antibodies with high titers. Other autoimmune diseases known to cause cirrhosis are autoimmune hepatitis (associated with anti–smooth muscle antibodies and elevated antinuclear antibody tests) and primary sclerosing cholangitis.

4. **Hereditary diseases** can be the cause of cirrhosis. **Wilson's disease** is a rare autosomal recessive disorder of copper metabolism. Cirrhosis occurs if it is untreated in children and adolescents. Central nervous system damage also occurs. Kayser-Fleischer rings, a deposition of copper in the cornea, are detected by slit-lamp examination when making the diagnosis. Patients are found to have reduced serum levels of ceruloplasmin, increased urine copper excretion, and increased hepatic

copper concentrations. **Hemochromatosis** is a more common autosomal recessive disorder that is associated with increased absorption of iron and deposition of the iron in the liver and other organs. Clinical symptoms of the disease are not seen until after age 40, when the body iron stores reached 4–10 times the normal amount. The disease affects men more often than women and at an earlier age. Most patients are asymptomatic when diagnosed, but symptoms of diabetes mellitus, cutaneous hyperpigmentation, fatigue, arthralgias, and impotence are seen. Laboratory tests reveal elevated serum transferrin saturation and an elevated ferritin concentration. Another hereditary disease that can cause cirrhosis is α_1-antitrypsin deficiency.

5. **Other causes of cirrhosis** include chronic biliary obstruction, cardiac cirrhosis, postnecrotic cirrhosis, and nonalcoholic steatohepatitis. In 10% of patients, there is no identifiable cause of the liver damage, and this is called **cryptogenic cirrhosis.**

C. **Laboratory tests.** Common laboratory findings in cirrhotic patients include mild anemia, normal or slightly decreased white blood cell count, elevated serum globulins, reduced albumin, and moderate thrombocytopenia.

1. **Liver enzymes** (ALT and AST) assess liver injury. They are usually moderately increased in cirrhosis, although they may be minimally elevated or normal in as many as 10% of patients. Paradoxically, the enzymes may be virtually normal in severe liver disease, since many of the normal liver cells have been replaced by fibrous tissue. ALT is found predominantly in the liver and is a more sensitive indicator of liver damage.

2. **Lactate dehydrogenase** is a marker of hepatocyte injury, although less specific than AST or ALT. It is elevated disproportionally after ischemic injury to the liver.

3. **Alkaline phosphatase** originates mostly from liver and bones. Elevated levels are seen when there is a blockage of the bile ducts or impaired bile formation. It also is elevated when there is injury to the bile ducts. It is elevated disproportionately to AST or ALT in primary and secondary biliary cirrhosis as well as primary sclerosing cholangitis.

4. **Serum bilirubin levels, albumin levels, and prothrombin time** represent hepatic function rather than acute hepatocellular injury. Liver disease inhibits the secretion and conjugation of bilirubin. The conjugated **bilirubin** level will not become elevated until the liver has lost more than 50% of its excretory capacity. **The serum albumin** is often depressed in cirrhosis and can serve as a gauge of the liver's synthetic function. Because the liver manufactures the blood-clotting factors, the **prothrombin time** can be prolonged in cirrhosis. A prolonged prothrombin time that does not correct after parenteral vitamin K (10 mg subcutaneously every day for 3 days) suggests severe liver damage.

5. **Serum ammonia** is often measured in patients with hepatic encephalopathy. Although elevated serum ammonia levels do suggest a hepatic cause for encephalopathy, the ammonium concentration does not correlate tightly with the level of stupor or coma.

6. A **radionucleotide scan of the liver and spleen** in cirrhotic patients will show decreased patchy uptake in the liver and increased uptake in the spleen and bone marrow. This noninvasive test is useful in clinically equivocal cases of cirrhosis and is also useful for assessing liver function.

7. An **ultrasound examination or computerized tomography** of the abdomen is helpful in detecting the presence and cause of secondary biliary cirrhosis. Ultrasonography is very sensitive for detecting ascites and can detect as little as 100 mL of peritoneal fluid.

8. **Liver biopsy.** A liver biopsy provides information on the grade (inflammatory severity) and stage (degree of fibrosis) of liver disease. A liver biopsy is indicated if a treatable cause of cirrhosis, such as Wilson's disease, is suspected. This procedure may also be used to help establish a prognosis or to determine whether a patient with antibody evidence of hepatitis B or C infection would benefit from interferon therapy.

III. **Treatment.** The treatment of cirrhosis consists of managing the potential complications of cirrhosis, preventing further liver damage, and, if possible, treating the underlying cause.

A. **Diet.** Diet is an important component of managing patients with cirrhosis. A nutritious low-salt diet is desirable because cirrhotic patients have increased sodium retention. A negative salt balance can be achieved by restricting sodium intake to 2 g/day. In early cirrhosis with muscle-wasting malnutrition, a diet containing 1–1.5 g of protein per kilogram per day is optimal. With worsening cirrhosis and increased risk of encephalopathy, protein should be restricted to no more than 1 g/kg/day. A patient with cirrhosis should also eat a low-fat diet to prevent or reverse the development of fatty liver disease. In some patients, weight loss with exercise will be beneficial in preventing the progression of liver disease.

B. **Avoidance of alcohol and drug toxicity.** Safe levels of alcohol consumption in cirrhosis have not been established, so complete abstinence is the most prudent recommendation. Alcohol also acts synergistically with hepatitis C, so abstinence from alcohol should also be recommended to those with chronic hepatitis C even without established cirrhosis. The liver is also vulnerable to injury from medications, vitamins, and herbs. Common hepatotoxic medications include tricyclic antidepressants, muscle relaxants, lipid-lowering drugs, antidiabetic agents, isoniazid, nitrofurantoin, antifungal agents, and anticonvulsant agents. Nonsteroidal anti-inflammatory drugs are especially important to avoid in cirrhosis. Because they inhibit platelet function, they may exacerbate coagulopathy. In addition, as a prostaglandin inhibitor, they may decrease renal blood flow and precipitate renal failure. Acetaminophen should be used with caution if at all, and should be restricted to a dose of 500 mg four times a day in well-nourished patients who are not actively consuming alcohol. Patients and physicians should attempt to assess all vitamins and herbal therapies for hepatotoxicity.

C. **Folic acid supplementation** (1 mg/day) may be desirable, particularly in alcoholics. Niacin, iron, and high doses of vitamin A should be avoided due to being potentially hepatotoxic.

D. **Vaccinations against hepatitis A and B viruses** should be performed in patients with cirrhosis if they are not already immune. Superinfection with these viruses can worsen liver disease. In addition, the pneumococcal and influenza vaccines should be given.

E. **Ascites** in patients with cirrhosis is an indication that liver disease is progressing. Evaluation for liver transplant should be undertaken when ascites develops. Restriction of sodium intake is the cornerstone of therapy. Sodium intake should be limited to less than 2 g/day. Diuresis can be initiated with **spironolactone,** 100 mg as a single daily dose, if salt restriction alone is ineffective. If there is no effect after 1 week, the daily dose of spironolactone may be increased by 100 mg every 3–5 days until a total dose of 400–600 mg/day is reached.

   If diuresis remains inadequate, **furosemide** can be added in gradually increasing doses, starting with 20 mg/day. Care must be taken to avoid intravascular depletion. Weight loss should be limited to no greater than 0.5 kg/day for patients with ascites and 1 kg/day for patients with both ascites and edema.

   Repeated large-volume therapeutic paracentesis is safe and useful for patients with diuretic-resistant ascites. If more than 5 L of fluid is withdrawn, giving 25–50 g of albumin intravenously is helpful to avoid intravascular depletion.

   Restriction of fluid intake to 1500 mL/day may be necessary for treating ascites in patients with sodium levels less than 125 mEq/L.

F. **Spontaneous bacterial peritonitis (SBP)** is one of the major potential complications of cirrhosis. Patients with ascites that is new in onset should have a diagnostic paracentesis performed. Symptoms may include fever, hypotension, abdominal pain, decreased bowel sounds, and an abrupt onset of hepatic encephalopathy. Ascitic fluid with a total white blood cell count of >500/mL or a neutrophil count >250 cells per mm^3 or a positive culture is diagnostic for bacterial peritonitis. Hospitalization and treatment with broad-spectrum antibiotics are required. Several sources have recommended prophylaxis antibiotics to prevent secondary recurrences of SBP.

G. **Hepatic encephalopathy** should be considered when the cirrhotic patient exhibits a change in mental status. Common symptoms are forgetfulness, impaired arousability, and asterixis (flapping tremor). Infection, gastrointestinal bleeding, medications, and increased protein intake are common precipitants of encephalopathy. Dietary protein should be restricted. **Lactulose,** 30 mL orally every 4–6 hours, with subsequent adjustment to allow for two or three soft stools a day, is indicated for encephalopathy that is incompletely controlled by diet alone. Antibiotics are added if symptoms worsen. **Amoxicillin, 4 g/day, or neomycin,** 1–4 g orally in four divided doses, are used. However, chronic usage of neomycin may result in ototoxicity and nephrotoxicity.

H. **Coagulopathy** may be improved by vitamin K, 10 mg subcutaneously every day for 3 days.

I. Varices occur secondary to chronic high pressure in the portal veins. Bleeding from varices is the most common cause of death in the cirrhotic patient. Sixty percent of patients with cirrhosis will have varices on endoscopic examination. Patients with cirrhosis should be endoscopically screened for varices. Nonselective beta blockers are used for primary prophylaxis against bleeding. The usual dose is propranolol, 10 mg three times a day, or nadolol, 20 mg once daily. Isosorbide mononitrate is a second-line therapy and is given in a dosage of 20 mg twice daily. Endoscopic sclerotherapy or esophageal banding is effective for variceal bleeding.

J. Specific treatment may be helpful for underlying diseases that have caused cirrhosis.

   1. Treatment for primary biliary cirrhosis is ursodeoxycholic acid (UDCA), 13–15 mg/kg/every day. The **pruritus of primary biliary cirrhosis** may be improved by cholestyramine, 4 g mixed with food or juice with each meal.
   2. **Hemochromatosis** is treated when there is evidence of iron overload with an elevated serum ferritin concentration. Removing 500 mL of blood weekly by phlebotomy until the hemoglobin is found to be lower than 12 g/dL and the ferritin level is no higher than 50 ng per mL is effective.
   3. Treatment for **Wilson's disease** is D-penicillamine, 250–500 mg orally three times daily; OR trientine, 250–500 mg orally four times daily.
   4. **Alcoholic liver disease** patients may have disease progression slowed and longevity increased by using colchicine, 0.6 mg orally twice daily.
   5. **Treatment for chronic hepatitis B** is indicated when the ALT level is two times normal, HBV DNA is positive, and HBe antigen is positive. Hepatitis B treatment consists of interferon alfa 2b, 5 million IU subcutaneously or IM daily OR 10 million IU subcutaneously/IM three times per week for 16 weeks; OR lamivudine, 100 mg daily for up to 1 year; or Adefovir dipivoxil, 10 mg daily for up to 48 weeks.
   6. **Treatment for chronic hepatitis C** therapy is indicated when the ALT level > two times normal, or when HCV RNA is positive or there is evidence of inflammation, fibrosis, or cirrhosis on liver biopsy (or both). Medications consist of pegylated interferon alfa 2b (PEG-Intron), 1.5 µg/kg subcutaneously weekly, or pegylated interferon alfa-2a (Pegasys), 180 µg subcutaneously weekly with or without ribavirin (Rebetol), 600 mg twice daily for up to 48 weeks' treatment duration. The HCV viral load should be assessed after 24 weeks of therapy. Detection of viremia at 24 weeks predicts viral persistence, and therapy should be discontinued.

IV. Management Strategies. Management of cirrhosis not only consists of treatment but also of monitoring for complications, deciding when hospitalization is required, providing education for the patient, and, if needed, referring the patient for liver transplantation.

A. Monitoring

   1. **Laboratory parameters** to be followed include liver function tests, prothrombin times, serum albumin, and bilirubin. The patient should be checked clinically for ascites, signs of volume depletion, bleeding, and encephalopathy.
   2. **Hospitalization** is indicated for gastrointestinal bleeding, worsening encephalopathy, increasing azotemia, or intractable ascites.
   3. **Diagnostic paracentesis** should be considered for new-onset or worsening ascites.
   4. A **hepatoma** should be considered in patients with an unexplained clinical deterioration of chronic cirrhosis.
   5. Patients with cirrhosis from **hepatitis B** and **C infection** require regular screening every 6 months with ultrasonography and tests of α-fetoprotein levels because of the high incidence of hepatoma in this group.

B. Patient support for adherence to diet is essential. Abstinence from alcohol is also essential; most patients will require considerable skill and support from the primary care physician in order to abstain (see Chapter 88).

C. Liver transplantation

   1. A physician should consider referring a patient for a liver transplant when death from cirrhosis is expected in 3–6 months, no alternative therapy is available, and the patient is otherwise in reasonably good health. Hepatitis C is the most common reason for liver transplantation today.

   Absolute contraindications to liver transplantation include portal vein thrombosis, severe medical illness, malignancy, hepatobiliary sepsis, or lack of patient understanding. Among the **relative contraindications** are active alcoholism, human immunodeficiency virus (HIV) positivity, hepatitis B surface antigen positivity, extensive previous abdominal surgery, and lack of a family or personal support system.

V. Prognosis. Cirrhosis is the eighth leading cause of death among males and the 10th leading cause of death among females. The prognosis for cirrhosis is determined by the cause and the presence of complications. Complications of cirrhosis include portal hypertension, variceal bleeding, splenomegaly, ascites, edema, and hepatic encephalopathy.

  A. Prognosis related to complications of cirrhosis
    1. **Portal hypertension.** Portal hypertension contributes to the development of splenomegaly, varices, and ascites and caries a significant negative prognosis.
    2. **Hepatic encephalopathy** is a complex neuropsychiatric disorder most likely caused by one or more substances of intestinal origin that are not metabolized because of hepatocellular dysfunction and portal systemic shunting. As a late-stage finding in cirrhosis, unless an acute reversible liver insult is identified and removed, hepatic encephalopathy tends to recur.
  B. Patients without gastrointestinal bleeding, encephalopathy, low albumin, and ascites have a better prognosis than those with such complications.
  C. The prognosis of alcoholic cirrhosis is dependent on abstinence. The 5-year survival rate is 60% or greater for patients who abstain, compared to 40% for patients who continue to drink alcohol.
  D. In a 20-year prospective study of cirrhotic individuals, liver failure, hepatoma, and gastrointestinal hemorrhage accounted for three quarters of the deaths. The 5-year survival rates were 14% for cryptogenic cirrhosis and 60% for chronic active hepatitis.

REFERENCES

Gross JB: Clinician's guide to Hepatitis C. Mayo Clin Proc 1998;**73:**355.

Lai CL, et al: A one year trial of lamivudine for chronic hepatitis B: Asia Hepatitis Lamivudine Study Group. N Engl J Med 1998;**339:**61.

Management of Hepatitis C. NIH Consensus Statement. 1997;Mar 24–26;**15**(3):1.

Moseley RH: Evaluation of abnormal liver function tests. Med Clin North Am 1996;**80:**887.

---

72 Congestive Heart Failure

Philip M. Diller, MD, PhD

KEY POINTS

- Heart failure (HF) is a common progressive terminal condition with a poor prognosis; the prevalence of HF is increasing with the aging of the population.
- Optimal management of the HF patient identifies the stage of HF (A–D) and the type of HF (systolic vs. diastolic) and uses therapies that slow the progression of cardiac remodeling (angiotensin-converting enzymes and beta blockers), achieve euvolemia (diet and diuretics), and maintain or improve quality of life (exercise, digitalis).
- Angiotensin-converting enzymes, beta blockers, aldosterone, and angiotensin II receptor blockers have been shown to reduce mortality rates in clinical trials of HF patients with left ventricular systolic dysfunction.
- Diastolic HF therapies are directed to the underlying cause—typically ischemia, hypertension, and rate control if a tachycardia is present.

I. Introduction
  A. Definition. Heart failure (HF) is a clinical syndrome of symptoms and signs that may include fatigue, exercise intolerance, dyspnea, peripheral edema, and pulmonary congestion. Heart failure signs and symptoms result when the heart is unable to fill with or eject blood sufficient to perfuse body tissues and meet metabolic demands. "Heart failure" is preferred over the older term "congestive heart failure" (CHF) because up to one third of ambulatory patients with HF do not manifest pulmonary or systemic congestion.

B. **Classification.** In clinical practice HF is commonly classified according to left ventricular ejection fraction (LVEF): **systolic** if **LVEF <40%** or **diastolic** if LVEF >45–50% and documented diastolic dysfunction. In addition to this differentiation, a new classification scheme for HF was recently introduced that emphasizes the early, often asymptomatic, onset of HF and its progression to more advanced stages.
  - **Stage A:** The patient who is at risk of developing HF but has no structural disorders of the heart.
  - **Stage B:** The patient with a structural disorder of the heart but who has never developed symptoms of HF.
  - **Stage C:** The patient who is experiencing or has experienced the HF syndrome and has underlying structural heart disease.
  - **Stage D:** The patient with end-stage disease who requires specialized treatment approaches.
    This staging system underscores the important role of preventing HF for the primary care physician.
C. **Epidemiology**
  1. **Prevalence.** Close to 5 million people in the United States have HF, with nearly 500,000 new cases diagnosed annually. HF is the primary reason for over 1 million hospital admissions each year and is the most common reason for hospital admission among persons older than 65 years. Approximately 300,000 HF-related deaths occur each year in the United States, and the number increases despite advances in treatment. Approximately 6–10% of people older than 65 years of age have HF.
    In primary care practice approximately 40% of patients present with signs and symptoms of HF and have normal systolic dysfunction; the other 60% have left ventricular systolic dysfunction. HF causes with a normal LVEF are shown in Table 72–1.
  2. **Etiology.** Underlying the signs and symptoms of HF are diverse causes that lead to an inability of the heart to perfuse tissues and meet the metabolic demands of the body. Some of the most important predisposing factors include the following:
    a. **Hypertension.** From the Framingham study, 5143 adults without HF at baseline were followed up for an average of 14 years. Of 392 persons who developed HF, 357 (91%) had hypertension that antedated initial HF diagnosis. Hypertension accounted for 39% of new HF cases in men and 59% of new cases in women. Chronic hypertension that leads to left ventricular hypertrophy (LVH) is a common pathway in the development of HF.
    b. **Coronary artery disease (CAD).** CAD is the cause of HF in two thirds of patients with left ventricular (LV) systolic dysfunction. Measurable decreases in systolic function may be present for months or years before overt HF symp-

TABLE 72–1. COMMON CAUSES OF HEART FAILURE WITH NORMAL LVEF

Inaccurate diagnosis of HF (eg, COPD)
Inaccurate measurement of LVEF
LV systolic function overestimated by LVEF (eg, mitral regurgitation)
Episodic LV systolic dysfunction, normal at the time of evaluation (severe hypertension, ischemia, tachycardia, infection, volume overload, spontaneous variability of EF)
Obstruction of LV inflow (mitral stenosis)
Diastolic dysfunction due to:
  Abnormal LV relaxation
  Ischemia
  Hypertrophy
  Cardiomyopathies
  High-output states
  Volume overload
  Aging
  Diabetes mellitus
  Amyloidosis
  Pericardial disease

COPD, chronic obstructive pulmonary disease; EF, ejection fraction; HF, heart failure; LV, left ventricular; LVEF, left ventricular ejection fraction.
Adapted from Dauterman KW, Massie BM, Gheorghiade M: Heart failure associated with preserved systolic function: A common and costly clinical entity. Am Heart J 1998;**135**:S310.

toms develop. Acute myocardial ischemia and myocardial infarction can result in sudden changes in systolic and diastolic ventricular function and acute HF with systemic congestion.

c. **Other causes of cardiomyopathy.** Viral infections, diabetes mellitus, and excessive alcohol intake have direct effects on the myocardium and can lead to cardiomyopathy and ventricular dysfunction.

d. **Valvular disease.** Significant valvular stenosis, regurgitation, or both, particularly in the mitral or aortic valves, are well-documented factors that contribute to ventricular dysfunction.

e. **Cardiovascular changes that occur with normal aging** help explain why HF incidence and prevalence increase with age. Arterial stiffening with increased afterload and peripheral resistance occurs with advancing age even in normotensive individuals. An increase in left ventricular mass that often occurs with aging may lead to impaired ventricular diastolic filling.

3. **Prevention of HF.** The common etiologic factors leading to HF suggest potentially useful strategies to prevent HF. Preventive measures include adequate blood pressure control using medications known to limit or reverse LVH, smoking cessation, aggressive lipid lowering, achieving target blood sugar control in patients with diabetes, alcohol abstention, surgical valve replacement when indicated, improvement of coronary blood flow with appropriate revascularization strategies, and use of angiotensin-converting enzyme inhibitors (ACEIs) for patients with asymptomatic LV systolic dysfunction.

D. **Pathophysiology**

1. **The HF syndrome is a heterogeneous, progressive condition** caused by various combinations of central and peripheral pathophysiologic mechanisms. These mechanisms are often dynamic, leading to wide fluctuations in measured ventricular function and physical impairment that may be observed over time in individual patients.

2. **Central/cardiac factors.** HF begins with some injury to or stress on the myocardium that leads to impaired ventricular function during systole, diastole, or both. Initially, the effects of inadequate cardiac output may only be experienced with physical exertion, but eventually in advanced HF dyspnea at rest occurs. This progression of symptoms correlates with changes in the geometry of the left ventricle: dilatation, hypertrophy, and assumption of a more spherical shape. Such cardiac remodeling leads to inefficient hemodynamic performance that is sustained and progressive.

3. **Peripheral factors.** Peripheral compensatory responses to diastolic or systolic LV dysfunction or both may initially help maintain cardiac function and organ perfusion, but eventually they lead to worsening HF signs and symptoms.

a. **Renin-angiotensin-aldosterone system (RAAS).** In response to LV dysfunction, the RAAS is activated, resulting in increased levels of angiotensin II, aldosterone, increased preload and afterload, and sodium and water retention. Initially, RAAS activation may help maintain or even improve LV function, but continued increases in intravascular volume and peripheral resistance become detrimental to LV function and lead to volume overload.

b. **The sympathetic nervous system.** This system is also activated in response to LV dysfunction in order to maintain blood pressure and organ perfusion. Prolonged sympathetic activation causes chronic elevations in afterload and eventual worsening of LV function. Elevated resting plasma norepinephrine levels are independent predictors of clinical outcomes and mortality among patients with severe HF.

c. **Natriuretic peptides and other parahormones.** Atrial natriuretic peptide (ANP) and brain natriuretic peptide (BNP) are produced from myocytes in response to increased pressures in the cardiac chambers. These peptides initially promote natriuresis and diuresis, but resistance occurs to these effects over time in chronic HF. Endothelins are endogenous peptides with strong vasoconstrictor and vasopressor activities and are found at high levels in patients with HF. Elevated levels of the natriuretic and endothelin peptides correlate with worsening HF and higher mortality rates among HF patients. Measurement of BNP is helpful when the diagnosis of HF is unclear (see section II,C,1).

II. **Diagnosis.** HF diagnosis requires first, the recognition of the clinical syndrome based on the characteristic constellation of clinical signs and symptoms, and second, the determination of the underlying structural abnormality of the heart that produced those symptoms. Clinical criteria used to aid in the diagnosis of HF include the Framingham Criteria and the Boston Criteria (Table 72–2). These criteria may not identify individuals with LV dysfunction who have mild or intermittent symptoms. More recently, determination of plasma BNP levels can assist in the differentiation between cardiac and noncardiac causes of dyspnea.

A. **Clinical symptoms and signs**
   1. **Symptoms**
      a. **Shortness of breath** can range from mild to severe. **Exertional dyspnea** may occur with any level of activity, depending on the severity of the HF syndrome. With **orthopnea,** patients will report feeling short of breath while lying flat, may be using pillows to prop themselves up at night, or may need to sleep sitting up if HF is severe. With **paroxysmal nocturnal dyspnea (PND) or nighttime cough,** waking from sleep because of dyspnea or experiencing dry cough only while lying down are suggestive of HF. **Dyspnea at rest** occurs in advanced HF or during acute exacerbations and volume overload.
      b. **Fatigue and weakness.** These symptoms are nonspecific and are in part due to abnormal autoregulation of blood flow to the extremities and muscle deconditioning.
   2. **Clinical signs**
      a. **Tachycardia** is present in many patients with HF and reflects increased adrenergic activity. Other symptoms related to increased adrenergic activity are pallor and coldness of the extremities and cyanosis of the digits (peripheral vasoconstriction).

TABLE 72–2. CRITERIA USED FOR DIAGNOSIS OF CONGESTIVE HEART FAILURE (CHF) IN CLINICAL STUDIES

The Framingham Heart Study Criteria	The Boston Scale Criteria
Major criteria	**Category I: History**
• Paroxysmal nocturnal dyspnea	• Rest dyspnea (4 points)
• Neck vein distension	• Orthopnea (4 points)
• Rales	• Paroxysmal nocturnal dyspnea (3 points)
• Cardiomegaly	• Dyspnea climbing (1 point)
• S₃ gallop	
• Increased venous pressure (> 16 cm)	**Category II: Physical examination**
• Circulation time ≥ 25 s	• Heart rate: 91–110 (1 point): > 110 (2 points)
• Hepatojugular reflux positive	• Jugular venous pressure elevation: > 6 cm H₂0 plus hepatomegaly or leg edema (3 points)
Minor criteria	• Lung rales: Basilar (1 point); more than basilar
• Ankle edema	(2 points)
• Night cough	• Wheezing (3 points)
• Hepatomegaly	• Third heart sound (3 points)
• Pleural effusion	
• Vital capacity reduced by one third from predicted	**Category III: Chest radiography**
• Tachycardia (≥ 120)	• Alveolar pulmonary edema (4 points)
	• Interstitial pulmonary edema (3 points)
Major or minor criterion	• Bilateral pleural effusion (3 points)
• Weight loss of more than 4.5 kg over 5 days in response to treatment	• Cardiothoracic ratio ≥ 0.50 (3 points)
	• Upper zone flow redistribution (2 points)
Definite CHF	**Determine score**
• Two major criteria or one major and two minor criteria	• Point value within parentheses and no more than 4 points from each category allowed. The maximum possible is 12 points.
	Definite CHF
	• 8–12 points
	Possible CHF
	• 5–7 points

Adapted from McKee PA, Castelli WP, McNamarra PM, et al: The natural history of congestive heart failure: The Framingham study. N Engl J Med 1971;**285**:1441; and Remes J, Miettenen H, Rennanen A, et al: Validity of clinical diagnosis of heart failure in primary health care. Eur Heart J 1991;**12**:315; and Young JB: The heart failure syndrome. In: Mills RM, Young JB (editors): *Practical Approaches to the Treatment of Heart Failure.* Williams & Wilkins; 1998.

  b. Moist crackles, usually heard in both lung bases, are a consequence of transudation of fluid into the alveoli. Pleural effusion collecting in the bases may lead to dullness on percussion. If the bronchial mucosa are congested, then bronchospasm and associated high-pitched wheezes may also be present.

  c. Systemic venous hypertension is suggested by a jugular venous pressure level higher than 4 cm above the sternal angle when the patient is examined sitting at a 45-degree angle. In advanced cases, venous pressure is so high that peripheral veins on the dorsum of the hand are dilated and fail to collapse when elevated above the shoulder.

  d. Hepatojugular reflux is helpful in differentiating hepatomegaly resulting from HF from other conditions. The neck veins are observed, and then the right upper quadrant of the abdomen is compressed continuously for 1 minute. The patient is instructed to breathe normally. This maneuver increases venous return to the heart. In HF patients, the jugular veins expand during and immediately after compression, because of the inability of the heart to respond to the increased venous supply.

  e. Hepatomegaly is due to congestion of the liver. If this occurs acutely, the liver may be tender to palpation. With advanced HF, the liver is still enlarged, but typically nontender.

  f. Peripheral edema is a nonspecific yet very common sign in HF. A corresponding symptom of weight gain may often be elicited from patients. The edema is typically bilateral and symmetrical in the dependent portions of the body. For ambulatory patients, the edema worsens as the day progresses and resolves after a night's rest.

  g. Cardiomegaly is also a nonspecific yet very common sign in HF patients. A normal apical impulse is located in the 4th or 5th intercostal space and is a brief tap. It is only palpable in about 50% of HF patients. If the apical impulse involves more than one intercostal space, cardiomegaly is present. Precordial percussion is more sensitive than the apical impulse for detecting abnormal LV size. A percussion dullness distance greater than 10.5 cm in the 5th intercostal space has a sensitivity of 91% and a specificity of 30% for increased LV size.

  h. The presence of an S_3 gallop occurs from ventricular vibration with rapid diastolic filling. It is a low-pitched sound that is best heard with the bell of the stethoscope over the apical impulse. Having the patient in the 45-degree left lateral decubitus position doubles the yield.

B. Chest roentgenogram. Findings in HF patients may include the following:

  1. Cardiomegaly. A cardiothoracic ratio ≥0.5 on an anteroposterior chest x-ray.

  2. Pulmonary edema marked by equalization of the caliber of blood vessels in the apex and the lung bases, interstitial edema (development of Kerley's B lines, sharp linear densities of interlobular interstitial edema), and alveolar edema (central butterfly or cloudlike appearance of fluid around the hili).

C. Laboratory testing in a patient with a new HF diagnosis should include an electrocardiogram (ECG); a complete blood count; a urinalysis; tests of levels of serum creatinine, potassium, and albumin; and thyroid studies (T4, thyroid-stimulating hormone). Screening evaluation for arrhythmias using Holter monitoring is not routinely warranted.

  1. Measuring BNP in HF patients. BNP is elevated in both systolic and diastolic HF. BNP can be helpful when the physician is unclear if the patient has dyspnea due to HF or to other noncardiac causes. Using a cutoff level of 100 pg/mL, BNP has a sensitivity of 90%, a specificity of 76%, and a positive predictive value of 83% in identifying patients with LV dysfunction compared to the Framingham clinical criteria, which have a sensitivity of 83%, a specificity of 67%, and a positive predictive value of 73%. Elevated pulmonary hypertension and pulmonary embolus can also cause elevations of BNP, so if these conditions are suspected based on clinical presentation, then appropriate tests should be obtained to diagnose these disorders.

D. Diagnosing the heart's structural abnormality (the type of HF) helps outline the physiologic goals of treatment and individualize pharmaceutical therapy.

  1. Two-dimensional echocardiography coupled with Doppler flow studies allows the physician to determine whether the structural abnormality is myocardial, valvular, or pericardial, and if myocardial, whether the dysfunction is systolic or diastolic. Measurement of LVEF is determined with this study; patients with LVEF <40% have systolic dysfunction. Physiologic goals and the evidence base for specific therapeutic decisions differ for patients with LV systolic dysfunction and those who have normal LVEF and isolated diastolic dysfunction. Doppler flow measures of diastolic filling need to be interpreted in the context of the individual patient, since they are often abnormal in healthy elderly patients without Hf and may be deceivingly normal in patients with progressively restrictive filling patterns or difficult to assess in obese patients.

   E. **Assessing the level of HF severity. The level of physical impairment** from HF is a strong prognostic marker, allows the physician to monitor the effects of treatment, and determines whether patients will benefit from certain therapies (see section V). **The New York Heart Association (NYHA) Functional Classification** is the simplest and most widely used tool for assessing physical functioning (Table 72–3).

III. **Treatment.** The heterogeneous nature of HF mandates an individualized approach to treatment with attention to etiology, type of HF, noncardiac comorbid conditions, and if systolic HF, the stage. Most of the large clinical trials that have influenced the treatment of HF have only included patients with systolic dysfunction. The treatment of diastolic HF continues to be based on the underlying pathophysiologic mechanism(s).

   A. **Treatment of specific underlying cardiac factors** may significantly improve ventricular function and HF symptoms. Special attention should be given to surgical correction of significant valvular disease when appropriate and reversal of myocardial ischemia with transluminal angioplasty, stent placement, or surgical bypass when indicated. Ventricular rate control and conversion to sinus rhythm may improve ventricular function for patients with atrial fibrillation and HF.

   B. A number of **noncardiac comorbid conditions** may affect the proper diagnosis and clinical course of HF and should be carefully assessed and treated:
      1. **Chronic obstructive pulmonary disease (COPD).** Dyspnea, exercise intolerance, nighttime cough, and other symptoms of chronic pulmonary disease may be misinterpreted as HF symptoms. Treatment of COPD should be optimized.
      2. **Diabetes mellitus** may predispose patients to silent myocardial ischemia that worsens LV function, "stiff" ventricles, and diastolic dysfunction. For both types of HF, diabetes control is an important goal.
      3. **Renal insufficiency** will influence fluid and electrolyte problems in HF and may limit usefulness or lead to changes in dosing for HF medications, particularly ACEIs and diuretics.
      4. **Significant arthritis** may further limit physical activity and worsen the skeletal muscle changes that occur in HF patients. nonsteroidal anti-inflammatory drugs and COX-II inhibitors can cause sodium retention and peripheral vasoconstriction, leading to reduced efficacy, and can potentially enhance the toxicity of diuretics and ACEIs. Such anti-inflammatory drugs are used cautiously in HF patients.
      5. **Depression and poor social support** have been shown to be important predictors of clinical outcomes, hospitalizations, and deaths among patients with ischemic heart disease. Depression is common is HF patients.
      6. **Substance abuse.** Smoking cessation should be encouraged. Patients with a component of LV dysfunction resulting from alcohol abuse may show significant functional improvement with abstention from alcohol.
      7. **Hypothyroidism or hyperthyroidism** may aggravate HF symptoms.

TABLE 72–3. NEW YORK HEART ASSOCIATION FUNCTIONAL CLASSIFICATION

Class I	No limitation of activity.
	Ordinary activity does not cause undue fatigue, palpitation, dyspnea or anginal pain.
Class II	Slight limitations of physical activity.
	Patient is comfortable at rest. Ordinary activity results in fatigue, palpitation, dyspnea, or anginal pain.
Class III	Marked limitation of physical activity.
	Patient is comfortable at rest, but less than ordinary activity causes fatigue, palpitation, dyspnea, or anginal pain.
Class IV	Inability to carry out physical activity without symptoms.
	Symptoms of heart failure often present at rest. Increased symptoms or discomfort with even minor physical activity.

Adapted from Criteria Committee, New York Heart Association: *Nomenclature and Criteria for Diagnosis of Diseases of the Heart and Great Vessels*, 9th ed. Boston: Little, Brown; 1994:253–256.

    8. Nephrotic syndrome, hypoalbuminemia, or both may worsen volume overload in HF.

C. Treatment of systolic dysfunction HF. The treatment of systolic HF is guided by stage. For stage A (asymptomatic, high risk for developing HF), stage B (structural dysfunction without HF symptoms), stage C (LV dysfunction with symptomatic HF), and stage D (refractory HF requiring specialized interventions), the treatment recommendations are shown in Table 72–4.

The centerpiece of these recommendations for the stage C HF patient is the use of ACEIs and beta blockers to reduce mortality in all patients with systolic HF. Additional mortality reductions are possible with the addition of aldosterone antagonists in patients with severe HF. These physiologic goals of treatment for stage C patients and how they can be achieved include the following:

    1. Achieving and maintaining optimal volume status. Although ACEIs should be considered first-line therapy for chronic HF resulting from systolic dysfunction, the initial presentation of the HF patient with pulmonary and systemic congestion dictates acute treatment with diuretics to lessen fluid overload and rapidly improve symptoms.

        a. The loop diuretic furosemide is the most frequently prescribed diuretic for treatment of volume overload in HF. Initial oral doses of 10–40 mg once a day should be administered to patients with dyspnea on exertion and signs of volume overload who do not have indications for acute hospitalization. Severe overload and pulmonary edema are indications for hospitalization and intravenous furosemide. Other considerations for prescribing diuretics in HF include the following:

            (1) Some patients with mild HF can be treated effectively with thiazide diuretics. Those who have persistent volume overload on 50 mg of hydrochlorothiazide per day should be switched to an oral loop diuretic.

TABLE 72–4. TREATMENT RECOMMENDATIONS ACCORDING TO HEART FAILURE STAGE

Stage A. At risk for heart failure but without structural heart disease or symptoms of HF
–Treat hypertension
–Encourage smoking cessation
–Treat lipid disorders
–Encourage regular exercise
–Discourage alcohol intake, illicit drug use
–ACE inhibition in appropriate patients

Stage B. Structural heart disease but without symptoms of HF
–All measures under Stage A
–ACE inhibitors in appropriate patients
–Beta blockers in appropriate patients

Stage C. Structural heart disease without prior or current symptoms of HF
–All measures under Stage A
–Drugs for routine use:
    Diuretics
    ACE inhibitors
    Beta blockers
    Digitalis
–Dietary salt restriction

Stage D. Refractory HF requiring specialized interventions
–All measures under Stages A, B, and C
–Mechanical assist devices
–Heart transplantation
–Continuous (not intermittent) intravenous inotropic infusions for palliation
–Hospice care

ACE, angiotensin-converting enzyme.
Adapted from Hunt SA, et al: ACC/AHA guidelines for the evaluation and management of chronic heart failure in the adult: A report of the American College of Cardiology/American Heart Association Task Force on Practice Guidelines; 2001. http://www.acc.org/clinical/guidelines/failure/hf_index.htm

    (2) Oral absorption of furosemide is diminished by physiologic changes in HF, particularly if the oral dose is taken on a full stomach. Torsemide is an alternative loop diuretic that is extremely well absorbed from the gastrointestinal tract in HF patients.

    (3) HF patients with poor oral absorption, renal insufficiency, or both may require much higher doses of a loop diuretic to reach a threshold level for diuresis, up to a maximum of 240 mg twice a day of furosemide.

    (4) Important adverse effects of diuretics that require periodic monitoring include orthostatic hypotension, prerenal azotemia, hyponatremia, hypomagnesemia, and hypokalemia. Most patients taking 40 mg or more of furosemide daily should supplement their oral potassium intake through dietary changes, prescribed potassium supplements, or both.

    (5) Once volume overload is corrected and an ACEI is initiated, the diuretic dose can often be carefully decreased or even eliminated. Some patients may only need intermittent diuretic therapy when symptoms and increases in daily weights signal a return of excess fluid volume.

b. Adding a second diuretic is sometimes necessary to maintain optimal fluid balance. Adding **metolazone,** 2.5–10 mg per day, to a daily furosemide dose can significantly increase diuresis for outpatient treatment of moderate volume overload. Prolonged combined therapy with metolazone should be avoided because of the increased risk of electrolyte depletion.

c. Spironolactone can also be added to standard regimens (diuretics, ACEI, digoxin, and a beta blocker) to increase diuresis, but this medication is reserved for NYHA class III or IV patients and those who have a serum potassium level <5.0 mmol/L. This medication and a more specific aldosterone antagonist, eplerenone (starting dose, 25 mg orally) may improve survival for patients with moderate to severe systolic dysfunction HF.

d. Sodium restriction. Patients should limit sodium intake to 2–3 g per day or less by avoiding salty-tasting foods, not adding salt at the table, and reading nutritional labels to choose lower-sodium food options. A sudden increase in dietary sodium intake is a frequent cause of acute fluid overload, pulmonary congestion, and hospitalization.

e. Patients should **weigh themselves daily,** record their weight, and report any gain or loss of more than 3 lbs from their baseline weight. Baseline weight is determined when the patient is at optimal fluid balance on a stable medical regimen. Reliable patients may be instructed to increase daily diuretic dose for 2–4 days when they see an increase in daily weights.

2. Decreasing preload and afterload by blunting the exaggerated peripheral compensatory response has, as its foundation, treatment with ACEIs, which should be considered first-line therapy for HF resulting from systolic dysfunction.

a. Angiotensin-converting enzyme inhibitors (ACEIs). Many clinical trials have provided consistent evidence that ACEIs result in decreased symptoms, improved quality of life, fewer hospitalizations, and reductions in mortality for patients with NYHA class II–IV HF. In addition, ACEIs slow the progression to HF among patients with asymptomatic LV systolic dysfunction. All HF patients with LV systolic dysfunction should be prescribed ACEIs unless they have a contraindication to these drugs.

    (1) Contraindications to ACEI use include pregnancy, bilateral renal artery stenosis, angioedema or other allergic responses, or documented persistent intolerance to ACEI (symptomatic hypotension, severe renal dysfunction, hyperkalemia, or cough).

    (2) The positive effects of ACEI probably apply to all available drugs in this class, but preference should be given to drugs with the most evidence for improved clinical outcomes. Enalapril, captopril, lisinopril, and ramipril have the strongest evidence for mortality reductions.

    (3) To minimize the risk of symptomatic hypotension, one half the normal starting dose should be given to patients with hyponatremia (<135 mEq/L), recent increase in diuretic dose, serum creatinine levels >1.7 mg/dL, and patients older than 75 years. Patients at high risk for symptomatic hypotension should be given a test dose of a short-acting ACEI (captopril, 6.25 mg) and be observed in the physician's office for 2 hours before starting daily ACEI therapy.

(4) Blood urea nitrogen (BUN), serum creatinine and potassium concentrations, and blood pressure should be determined before starting ACEI therapy, 1–2 weeks after initiating therapy, after changes in dose, and every 3–4 months thereafter. The average increase in creatinine is 0.4 mg/dL, with most of the change observed in the first 6 weeks. The reversible renal function caused by ACEIs may resolve with a careful decrease in diuretic dose. As long as creatinine stabilizes at approximately 3.5 or less, and hyperkalemia or symptomatic hypotension is not persistent, ACEIs should be continued and titrated up to target doses (Table 72–5). If target doses are not tolerated, lower doses should be used because they also appear to confer some benefit. Systolic blood pressure of 90–100 should not deter the physician from titrating to target doses unless hypotension becomes symptomatic.

(5) Nonproductive cough is a common adverse effect of ACEIs, secondary to increased bradykinin levels. Cough may not be attributable to ACEIs in a given HF patient, since it is a common HF symptom. Only 1–2.5% of patients in clinical trials discontinued ACEI because of cough. For patients with cough on an initial ACEI trial, switching to an alternative ACEI may diminish cough symptoms.

(6) Concomitant use of aspirin may attenuate the hemodynamic actions of ACEIs and their effects on survival, whereas clopidogrel does not. However, there is not enough evidence to justify not using aspirin and ACEIs together in appropriate patients.

b. For patients unable to use ACEIs, a trial of **hydralazine and isosorbide dinitrate (HYD-ISDN)** should be initiated to decrease preload and afterload (Table 72–5). Patients at high risk for symptomatic hypotension should receive lower initial doses and be monitored for adverse effects. The HYD-ISDN combination has shown decreased mortality in HF clinical trials, but compliance with this combination is poor due to the high number of tablets needed and the high incidence of adverse effects (headache and gastrointestinal complaints).

c. **Angiotensin II receptor blockers (ARBs)** are an alternative therapy for patients who cannot use ACEIs. ARBs do not affect bradykinin levels and thus do not induce angioedema and cough to the same extent as ACEIs. Evidence is mounting that these medications alone confer mortality reductions equivalent to ACEIs, and that addition of ARBs to standard regimens of ACEIs and beta blockers reduces hospitalizations for HF. A recent study suggests that addition of ARBs to patients taking ACEIs and a beta blocker may also lead to further mortality reductions. It is not clear yet if ARBs should be included in all patients with systolic dysfunction HF.

TABLE 72–5. TARGET DOSES FOR ACEIS AND HYD-ISDN COMBINATION

	Initial Dose (mg)	Target Dose (mg)	Recommended Maximum Dose (mg)
Preferred ACEIs (see text)			
Captopril[1]	6.25–12.5 tid	50 tid	100 qid
Enalapril	2.5 bid	10 bid	20 bid
Lisinopril	5 qd	20 qd	40 qd
Ramipril	1 bid	5 bid	10 bid
Other ACEIs indicated for heart failure			
Fosinopril	5 qd	20 qd	40 qd
Quinapril	5 bid	20 bid	20 bid
Hydralazine-ISDN combination			
Hydralazine (HYD)	25 tid	75 qid	150 qid
Isosorbide dinitrate (ISDN)	10 tid	40 tid	80 tid

[1] Give a single dose of captopril 6.25 mg with observation of the patient for 2 hours for patients at high risk for symptomatic hypotension.
ACEIs, angiotensin-converting enzyme inhibitors.

    d. The first- and second-generation **calcium channel blockers** such as nifedipine, diltiazem, and nicardipine may worsen systolic dysfunction symptoms because of their negative inotropic effects. Amlodipine is better tolerated, with evidence of a neutral if not beneficial effect on HF survival. Amlodipine can be considered for patients with continued hypertension who take ACEI and diuretics, or those with symptomatic ischemia not controlled by nitrates, beta blockers, or both.

    e. Exercise training is an effective intervention that reverses some of the exaggerated peripheral compensatory changes in patients with stable mild to moderate (class I–III) systolic dysfunction HF. A series of randomized trials have shown improvements in a number of peripheral hemodynamic parameters, with diminished symptoms and improved physical functioning. Most trials have used supervised aerobic exercise on treadmills or stationary cycles. A single study evaluating the long-term effect of exercise training showed a reduction in hospitalization and deaths. Exercise training should be considered for all stable HF patients.

  3. Delaying the clinical progression of systolic dysfunction HF and further improving symptoms may be accomplished with two other pharmaceutical interventions. One has been a part of HF treatment for some 200 years (cardiac glycosides/digoxin), while the other has gained acceptance only in recent years (beta blockers).

    a. Beta blockers inhibit the adverse effects of sympathetic nervous system activation (eg, cardiac hypertrophy and apoptosis, provoked arrhythmias, increased ventricular volumes) in HF patients. Three drugs have been studied in clinical trials involving >10,000 patients: β_1-adrenergic receptor selective blockers (bisoprolol and metoprolol) and α_1, β_1, and β_2-adrenergic receptor blocker (carvedilol). The collective experience indicates that treatment with beta blockers in systolic dysfunction HF patients reduces HF symptoms, improves quality of life, reduces the risk of death by 35%, and prevents hospitalizations. The patients in these trials were also taking ACEIs, diuretics, and digoxin; thus, the benefits of beta blockers were in addition to those already seen with the ACEIs. Beta blockers should be prescribed in all patients with stable HF due to left ventricular systolic dysfunction unless they have a contraindication (symptomatic bradycardia, allergy) or are unable to tolerate them (asthmatic patients).

    (1) Starting beta blockers should be delayed in patients who are not euvolemic. Volume overload should be treated before starting a beta blocker.

    (2) The starting dose of the medication should be at very low doses, followed by a gradual up-titration once the lower dose is well tolerated (~ every 2–4 weeks). If fluid retention occurs, then the diuretic can be increased until the weight returns to its pretreatment levels. The goal is to get the patient to the target doses achieved in the clinical trials. Table 72–6 shows the starting and target doses for beta blockers in HF patients.

    (3) Patients should be monitored for the most common complications of beta blockade: hypotension/poor perfusion, bradycardia or atrioventricular block, and bronchospasm.

    (4) Patients should be informed that achieving benefit and desired clinical response might take 2–3 months. Fatigue is a common side effect and usually resolves spontaneously after several weeks except in a small percentage of patients.

TABLE 72-6. STARTING AND TARGET DOSES FOR BETA BLOCKERS

Drug	Initial Dose (mg)	Target Dose (mg)	Recommended Maximum Dose (mg)
Bisoprolol	1.25 mg qd	10 mg qd	20 mg
Carvedilol	3.125 mg bid	25 mg bid	50 mg bid
Metoprolol			
Immediate release	6.25 mg bid	75 mg bid	225 mg bid
Extended release	12.5–25 mg qd	200 qd	400 mg qd

    b. Digoxin is considered the preferred agent among a number of available cardiac glycoside preparations. Digoxin neither improves nor worsens HF survival but does decrease symptoms, increase exercise capacity, and decrease the need for hospitalization in systolic dysfunction HF. Digoxin is particularly appropriate for patients who remain symptomatic on ACEI, beta blockers, and diuretics, and for patients with atrial fibrillation and rapid ventricular response.

      (1) Loading doses are generally unnecessary. A daily oral dose of 0.125–0.25 mg will lead to steady-state serum levels in 1–2 weeks.

      (2) Once a steady state is reached, a serum digoxin level, an ECG, BUN/creatinine levels, and serum electrolytes should be obtained.

      (3) Results of the Digitalis Investigation Group (DIG) trial suggest that a serum concentration in the lower therapeutic range (0.7–1.2 ng/mL) retains the clinical benefit of digoxin while avoiding toxicity. Levels should be checked yearly and at the time of significant changes in HF symptoms or renal function.

D. Isolated diastolic dysfunction. In comparison to the large evidence base for treating systolic dysfunction, there are minimal data available to guide the treatment of HF resulting from diastolic dysfunction. Treatment is largely empiric and directed toward reversing presumed underlying pathophysiology. There are a number of ongoing trials of ACE, beta blockers, and ARBs in HF patients with preserved systolic function.

    1. The methods for achieving and maintaining optimal fluid balance are similar to those described for systolic dysfunction. Rapid or over-diuresis should be avoided since small changes in intravascular volume may cause significant decreases in diastolic filling and cardiac output.

    2. Treatment of cardiac ischemia may improve diastolic function. Nitrates, beta blockers, and calcium channel blockers may all be useful, but there is little direct evidence for their effectiveness in treating diastolic dysfunction.

    3. Effective treatment of hypertension is indicated with drugs that may limit or even reverse LVH and thus improve the compliance of the ventricle. Beta blockers are attractive in this regard in addition to their anti-ischemic and rate-limiting properties, all of which may improve diastolic filling. ACEIs are often appropriate, but compared with systolic dysfunction there is no evidence for specific indications for diastolic dysfunction HF.

    4. Conversion of atrial fibrillation to sinus rhythm will restore the atrial component of diastolic filling and may improve cardiac output. If conversion to sinus rhythm is not feasible, then ventricular rate control with a rate-limiting calcium channel blocker or digoxin may allow more complete ventricular filling in diastole.

    5. Attention to controlling the heart rate is important in managing HF patients with diastolic dysfunction. Slowing the heart rate will improve cardiac output in HF patients with diastolic dysfunction who have tachycardia. Over-diuresis often leads to tachycardia in these patients, compounding the problem of dyspnea in the acute setting.

    6. Theoretically digoxin would not be indicated for patients with diastolic dysfunction; however, a subgroup analysis of the recent DIG clinical trial showed surprising improvement in clinical outcomes for the small number of patients in the study who had normal LVEF. Until more evidence is available, however, digoxin should be reserved for diastolic dysfunction patients who have a separate indication such as atrial fibrillation.

IV. Management Strategies

A. Patient education and self-care are important components of maintaining clinical stability. Topics include explanation of symptoms, causes, and prognosis; activity recommendations including exercise prescription when appropriate; proper use of medications; sodium restriction; daily weights; and instructions for monitoring symptoms and when to contact the patient's physician (Table 72–7).

B. Case management strategies such as the MULTIFIT program have been shown to improve quality of life and decrease the need for hospitalization. Nurse case managers work with patients to improve patient education, promote adherence to medication and dietary regimens, improve home-based self-monitoring, and coordinate, medical, community, and social support resources.

C. Consultation or referral to a cardiologist or HF specialty clinic should be considered for patients who remain symptomatic on standard HF therapy, have underlying valvular or pericardial infiltrative disease, or have potentially reversible ischemic heart disease. Patients may also benefit from co-management with a cardiologist to ensure reaching

TABLE 72–7. SPECIFIC INSTRUCTIONS FOR PATIENTS ABOUT WHEN TO CONTACT A PHYSICIAN'S OFFICE

Weight gain ≥ 3 lbs, not responding to predesignated diuretic change
Uncertainty about how to increase diuretics
New swelling of the feet or abdomen
Worsening shortness of breath with mild exercise
Onset of inability to sleep flat in bed or awakening from sleep because of shortness of breath
Worsening cough
Persistent nausea/vomiting or inability to eat
Worsening dizziness or new spells of sudden dizziness not related to sudden changes in body position
Prolonged palpitations
If you, the patient, experience any sudden severe symptoms, you may need to call 911 or the equivalent emergency
phone number to arrange a trip to the emergency room. (These sudden severe symptoms may include **but are not
limited to** chest pain, severe shortness of breath, loss of consciousness not due to sudden standing, new cold or
painful arm or foot, sudden new visual changes, or impairment of speech or strength in an extremity.)

Note: This is only a sample list and is not intended to include all potential problems for which a patient with heart failure should
seek urgent medical advice.
Reprinted with permission from Goldman L, Braunwald E: *Primary Cardiology.* Philadelphia: Saunders; 1998:326.

target doses of an ACEI or to initiate beta blocker therapy. Those with symptomatic atrial
or ventricular tachyarrhythmias should also be assessed by a cardiologist. Evaluation
for possible cardiac transplantation includes exercise evaluation with measurement of
maximal oxygen uptake (VO_2max). Patients with VO_2max <14 mL/kg/min and no severe
comorbid conditions may be candidates for transplantation.

V. Prognosis
  A. Exacerbations and hospitalization frequently occur in HF. More than 40% of hospi-
    talized HF patients require readmission to the hospital within 6 months of discharge. Pa-
    tients often experience a fluctuating clinical course marked by periods of fluid overload
    and diminished exercise tolerance. Common preventable reasons leading to hospital-
    ization include poor adherence to sodium restriction or medication regimens, inadequate
    social support systems, or failure to seek medical attention when symptoms worsen or
    daily weights increase. Hospital rates are similar for patients with systolic and diastolic
    dysfunction HF.
  B. Mortality risk for HF patients is substantial, with annual rates as high as 50% mortality
    for patients with advanced disease (NYHA class IV). LVEF is one of the most consistent
    predictors of mortality, with a marked increase in mortality risk for patients with LVEF
    less than 20%. Hyponatremia, elevated plasma norepinephrine levels, BNP levels, and
    significant ventricular arrhythmias are also independent markers for increased mortality
    risk. Mortality rates are lowest for HF patients with normal LVEF.

REFERENCES

Abraham WT, Scarpinato L: Higher expectations for management of heart failure: Current recommen-
  dations. J Am Board Fam Pract 2002;**15**:39.
Dauterman KW, Massie BM, Gheorghiade M: Heart failure associated with preserved systolic function:
  A common and costly clinical entity. Am Heart J 1998;**135**:S310.
DiBianco R: Update on therapy for heart failure. Am J Med 2003;**115**:480.
D.I.G. (The Digitalis Investigation Group): The effect of digoxin on mortality and morbidity in patients
  with heart failure. N Engl J Med 1997;**336**:525.
Diller PM, Smucker DR: Management of heart failure due to diastolic dysfunction. Clin Fam Med 2001;
  3(4):857.
Hunt SA, et al: ACC/AHA guidelines for the evaluation and management of chronic heart failure in the
  adult: A report of the American College of Cardiology/American Heart Association Task Force on
  Practice Guidelines. 2001. http://www.acc.org/clinical/guidelines/failure/hf_index.htm
Jong P, et al: Angiotensin receptor blockers in heart failure: Meta-analysis of randomized controlled
  trials. J Am Coll Cardiol 2002;**39**:463.
Krum H: Beta-blockers in chronic heart failure: What have we learned? What do we still need to know?
  Curr Opin Pharmacol 2003;**3**:168.
Nohria A, Lewis E, Stevenson LW: Medical management of advanced heart failure. JAMA 2002;
  287:628.
West JA, et al: A comprehensive management system for heart failure improves clinical outcomes and
  reduces medical resource utilization (MULTIFIT). Am J Cardiol 1997;**79**:58.

73   Dementia

Richard J. Ham, MD

KEY POINTS

- "Dementia" is a syndrome in which memory loss and at least one other cognitive deficit is persistent and severe enough to interfere with daily function; it is *not* a final diagnosis (Table 73–1).
- Most *progressive* dementias are caused by Alzheimer's disease (AD). AD is extremely slow in its onset, so its early symptoms are frequently subtle or only present at times of stress. Memory loss, typically one of the early symptoms, is often misattributed to "normal aging."
- **Age** is the single most potent risk factor for AD; over 45% of individuals age 85 and older have clinical AD.
- Earlier diagnosis of AD is crucial to management for ensuring safety, relieving family stress, providing early education of caregivers, clarifying advance directives (and a will) while the patient can still participate, and initiating potentially stabilizing treatment while the symptoms are still mild.
- Early treatment, as soon as the diagnosis is a strong probability, with an acetylcholinesterase inhibitor (AChEI) is strongly recommended (Table 73–2). Vitamin E (2000 IU daily), early education of family caregivers, and early involvement with the Alzheimer's Association are recommended (Contact the Alzheimer's Association at 1-(800)-272-3900 or www.alz.org or find a local chapter).

I. Introduction

A. **Dementia** is an extremely common syndrome, particularly in the elderly. Two careful US studies, sampling whole populations, confirm the prevalence of clinical AD to be approximately 45% at age 85+ years. It is estimated that 4.5 million Americans currently have AD and that the prevalence will increase by 27% by 2020, 70% by 2030, and near 300% by 2050, when it is estimated that approximately 13.2 million Americans will be afflicted. Even allowing for the longevity of women, more women have AD than men (the ratio is 3:2).

B. The pathophysiology of the main cause of progressive dementias (AD) is increasingly well-defined. The basic histopathology (and still the definitive pathologic diagnostic technique, usually at autopsy) is as described by Alzheimer in 1907: plaques, with beta-amyloid, and neurofibrillary tangles. However, these classical changes do not in themselves explain the extensive neuronal degeneration that ultimately takes place in the illness. Inflammatory changes around the lesions may play a role. Estrogen interferes in the processes preceding the formation of both plaques and tangles. Considerable research continues to be carried out on the formation of the beta-amyloid in the plaques. An experimental vaccine to prevent the formation of the amyloid had to be discontinued because of the occurrence of encephalopathy in some subjects. However, stopping beta-amyloid formation may not stop the disease process. Research also focuses on the dephosphorylation of tau protein, which is an initial step leading to the neurofibrillary tangles.

TABLE 73–1. WHAT IS DEMENTIA?

- Multiple cognitive deficits, ie, memory impairment and one or more of aphasia, apraxia, agnosia or disturbed executive functioning (ie, planning, organizing, sequencing, abstracting)
- The deficits impair occupational or social function **and** represent a decline from prior status **and** do not only occur during a delirium

Modified from DSM-IV, American Psychiatric Association, 1997.

TABLE 73–2. ALZHEIMER'S MANAGEMENT PRINCIPLES

Diagnose it earlier Name it, name the proxy	**Care for the caregivers** Training, support, respite
Treat it persistently Cholinesterase inhibitors, vitamin E, memantine	**Develop community resources** Use them, promote them
Manage it comprehensively Cognition, function, behavior	

C. Deficits in a number of neurotransmitters, most especially acetylcholine and recently glutamate and others, are well documented. The "cholinergic hypothesis" (that reducing the known decline in cholinergic neuronal activity might be therapeutic) has an extensive literature stretching back over 20 years. Medications (the AChEIs) that inhibit acetylcholinesterase, thus preventing the breakdown of naturally occurring acetylcholine, have been available for nearly 10 years and offer symptomatic treatment, allowing optimal functioning of the deteriorating nerve cells. As well as having a quite persistent effect on cognition, function, and behavioral symptoms, they postpone nursing home care. They do not effect the disease process itself.

D. Genetic "risk factors" appear crucial. Familial clusters due to specific genes have been defined, but apolipoprotein epsilon 2, 3, and 4 alleles were shown in 1994 to be "risk" (apo-E 4) and "protective" (apo-E 2) factors in typical "late-onset" AD. The National Institute on Aging is currently conducting a study to find the predicted three or more other genetic "risk factors." However, being genetically "at risk," or even having the presence of plaques and tangles pathologically, does not correlate fully with symptoms. All Down syndrome patients apparently develop the plaques and tangles of AD, but only about half have evidence of progressive dementia in late life. A reasonable theory is that there is genetic risk, which is precipitated into clinical symptomatology by other factors or events.

E. Cerebrovascular disease (and possibly vascular disease elsewhere, such as systolic hypertension), and head injury (especially serious head injury earlier in life) are strongly associated with increasing the risk of clinical AD. Hypercholesterolemia and diabetes mellitus have more recently been described as potential "risk factors" (Table 73–3.)

F. No environmental factor has yet been shown to influence the emergence of AD, but chemicals that adversely affect mitochondria (eg, insecticides, pesticides, and some horticultural and agricultural agents) could be factors.

II. Diagnosis
    A. Symptoms and signs
        1. It is vital for all primary care physicians to realize that early dementia is frequently unreported, not presented for care, denied, or unrecognized. This last characteristic—being unrecognized not only by the family and the patient, both of whom will often attribute early changes to "aging," but also by ourselves, the physicians, and other clinicians who are in contact with the patient—occurs because it is characteristic of AD (the main cause of dementia) that the symptoms (initially memory loss, often manifested as functional decline, or by recurrent or persistent behavioral changes) are extremely *insidious* in their onset. And many early AD patients retain good social function and speech and look fine in the familiar setting of their own doctor's office.

TABLE 73–3. RISK FACTORS (AND PROTECTIVE FACTORS) FOR AD

Risk Promoting	Possibly Protective
Age	Estrogen use
Family history	Higher education
Apolipoprotein E4	Apolipoprotein E2
Head trauma	Anti-inflammatory drugs
Female gender	Statins
Cerebrovascular disease	Antioxidants
Chromosome abnormalities (eg, 14 and 21)	
Down syndrome	
Diabetes mellitus	

TABLE 73–4. EARLY WARNINGS OF AD: SYMPTOMS

- Memory loss that is getting worse
- Losing things
- Repetitive questions
- "Slowing down"
- Driving problems
- Financial mistakes
- Aggressive or inappropriate behavior (eg, shoplifting, sexuality, explosive outbursts)
- "Depressed"
- Weight loss
- Poor hygiene
- Irritability
- Suspiciousness

For the primary care physician, then, the information contained in Tables 73–4 through 73–6 is crucial. There are "hints" that early dementia may be present (Tables 73–4 and 73–5). There are also specific medical events (Table 73–6) which, if they occur in a person who does not have a history suggestive of progressive decline, imply that screening for dementia should be carried out up to 6 months after the incident or event, and possibly at intervals thereafter. The same questionnaires and "work-up" recommended to confirm that a dementia is present in the more typical clinical picture, of slowly progressive decline, should be used.

2. There are many reasons for making an accurate early diagnosis of an apparent dementia (Table 73–7). Exposing the patient (and others, if driving is the issue) to avoidable dangers, as well as the marital and familial disharmony of blaming someone for annoying symptoms that are apparently under the person's own control, are examples of the ways in which early dementia patients can suffer as a result of nonrecognition of their illness. Table 73–8 summarizes the process, from early recognition to a working diagnosis.

3. "Screening" people who, due to age or predisposing factors, are at increased risk, in order to detect dementia at an earlier stage than merely waiting for it to present itself, appears reasonable in clinical practice. Exactly who to ask and what to ask is not proven, however. Mass screening of asymptomatic people has recently been *not* recommended by the US Preventive Services Task Force, focusing on lack of data and the creation of unnecessary anxiety. However, asking a simple review-of-symptoms (ROS)-type question, such as "how is your memory?" or (of a relative, ideally with the patient's expressed permission) "how is his/her memory?" when the patient is at increased risk (or there have been some potential AD symptoms) is reasonable in practice.

4. The **past medical history** may be helpful in the differential diagnosis, and the cardiovascular history must be carefully established. Head injury should be specifically inquired after, for its connection to the development of AD is certainly not yet well recognized by the public (or many professionals).

5. The **family history** is significant, given the genetic risk factors for AD described above. Having a first-degree relative (especially a sibling) with clinical AD (even if not autopsy-proven) would increase the likelihood of AD as the diagnosis. A fam-

TABLE 73–5. EARLY WARNINGS OF AD: OBSERVATIONS

- Cannot remember recent information
- Defers to caregiver
- Dresses inappropriately
- Has poor hygiene or grooming
- Has trouble expressing thoughts
- Is persistently a "no show" or comes at wrong day/time
- Is noncompliant
- Procrastinates excessively
- Has failure to thrive

TABLE 73–6. EARLY WARNINGS OF AD: CONDITIONS TO FOLLOW UP AND SCREEN FOR AD

- Delirium
- Depression
- Head injury
- Stroke
- Catastrophic reaction

ily history of one or two isolated clinical cases, more distantly related (rarely is there autopsy evidence to support the diagnosis in such cases) does not increase an individual's risk much and should not be allowed to cause family anxiety. A family history of Down syndrome has some weight as a risk factor and should be specifically sought. All Down syndrome patients do apparently develop Alzheimer's-type pathology late in life (late 50s/early 60s). However, only about half appear to develop symptoms suggesting a dementia developing in their final years. This may be simply because the pathology precedes the dementia by a fairly long interval.

6. A thorough **medication history** is also required. Patients with early dementia may mix up their medications and worsen an already bad situation. Seldom, medications alone will be the cause of apparent dementia. AD patients are of course sensitive to the anticholinergic side effects of many over-the-counter allergy medications (eg, diphenhydramine [Benadryl]), and occasionally a patient will present following abrupt confusion with the use of them, often as a result of their inclusion in an over-the-counter respiratory remedy.

7. A general **physical examination** should be done if (as is likely) the patient has not been seen lately, and indeed throughout the illness, **health maintenance** will have been neglected. Thus the examination must include a look for signs of common problems at the patient's age, including abuse or neglect or unreported falls, as well as hearing loss and issues of poor balance or gait (Table 73–9). The **review of systems (ROS)** can be done at the same time as the physical examination, in order to improve the chance of the patient recalling unreported problems. (A family member should be interviewed for the ROS as well.)

B. **Confirming dementia and differential diagnosis.** Progressive dementias like AD can present for "first-time" diagnosis at any stage. Sometimes the changes have been so insidious, or the patient's verbal ability and social skills have been so well preserved, that the patient's decline has truly been unnoticed, or it has been slow enough that the family has been able to "deny" that there is decline. Sometimes a patient declining because of one or more chronic and progressive illnesses, in becoming more and more dependent, is able to cope, despite the cognitive decline, or it is overlooked, in part from the pressure to manage the other medical problems, or the decline is attributed to the illness itself. For example, the patient with progressive chronic obstructive pulmonary disease may well get anxious and confused at times, disguising a quietly evolving, progressive dementia. Hypoxia could contribute to this cognitive decline, but if the patient is elderly, it is often simply because another chronic illness has set in: a progressive dementia. (Remember that in the elderly, multiple conditions are characteristic; so our traditional training to tie in all the symptoms to one or two diagnoses does not apply!!)

It is clinically useful to describe the manifestations of all dementias in three domains: cognitive, functional, and behavioral.

At whatever stage the dementia presents, but especially in the earliest stages, it is useful both for diagnosis and management to confirm examples of characteristic symp-

TABLE 73–7. WHY DIAGNOSE ALZHEIMER'S EARLY?

- Safety (eg, driving, compliance, cooking)
- Family stress and misunderstanding (eg, blame, denial)
- Caregiver education re early coping skills (eg, choices, getting started)
- Advance planning while patient is competent (will, proxy, power of attorney, advance directives)
- Patient's and family's right to know
- Stabilizing treatments now available

TABLE 73–8. ESTABLISHING THE AD DIAGNOSIS EARLIER: THE PROCESS

- Be alert to hints, clues, and early warning signs
- Question patient and family about memory
- When suspicious:
  - Confirm history: How long? How abrupt? Getting worse? How fast?
  - Are there other typical early AD symptoms?
  - Test cognitive status (MMSE, clock drawing test)
  - Record functional status (FAQ)
  - In most cases, diagnosis now established
  - Investigate for contributors, causes, and concurrent conditions

FAQ, Functional Activities Questionnaire; MMSE, Mini-Mental State Examination.

toms from these three domains, asking direct questions if necessary, while recognizing that all the early symptoms may be in only one or two domains. In distinguishing slowly progressive dementias like AD, dementia of Lewy body type, and true vascular dementia from other dementias, such as those that can follow anoxic/hypoxic brain injury (eg, following cardiopulmonary resuscitation in the community), and in differentiating illnesses that mimic dementia such as a delirium or a major depressive episode (MDE, popularly called "clinical depression"), there are "three plus" questions to ask about the history of the memory or other cognitive or functional changes observed by the patient or family (Table 73–10).

1. **Mild cognitive impairment (MCI)** is a term being increasingly used, although it is not truly a diagnostic entity and is not in ICD-9 or DSM-IV. It is a syndrome defined in order to research those patients who we used to reassure as having "benign forgetfulness," who have mild symptoms, generally memory loss, not convincingly progressive, and insufficient to cause significant functional impairment. (If they did have impairment, provided there were any other cognitive deficits, however mild, then the patient would be described as having a "mild" dementia.) Research on such patients indicates a wide range of "conversion" rates to "clinical AD" (ranging from 10% to 15% or more per year in differing clinical series). On this basis, it is wrong to reassure patients, particularly if they are somewhat elderly, that memory loss is to be accepted as "normal." Such a patient should be scheduled for follow-up visits, and called if he or she is a "no show," in order that formal cognitive testing, as later described, could be done at intervals of 6 months or more. This would be done in hopes that any developing cognitive decline would be found as early as possible, and the diagnosis changed, and treatment begun, for what would be reasonably described as early probable AD.

2. **Confirmation that a dementia is present** should be carried out objectively. The most widely recommended instrument (questionnaire) for the objective recording of **cognitive symptoms** is the Mini-Mental State Examination (MMSE), a straightforward, easy-to-administer test, which briefly assesses orientation to time and place, registration and short-term recall, visuospatial skills, reading and obeying a written command, naming of objects, and sequencing skills and language skills (writing a sentence and repeating a well-known phrase) (Figure 73–1). The MMSE is not a very sensitive instrument, nor was it designed for the uses to which it has

TABLE 73–9. PHYSICAL EXAMINATION IN DEMENTIA

- Nutritional status?
- Hearing loss?
- Visual loss?
- Neglect of mouth, feet, perineum?
- Physical abuse or neglect?
- Appears safe when standing up or walking?
- Localizing or lateralizing motor signs?
- Signs of parkinsonism?
- Review of systems while examining patient

TABLE 73–10. THREE PLUS QUESTIONS IN ALL MEMORY DISORDERS

- How long has this been going on?
- How abruptly did it start?
- Are the symptoms progressing, and if so, how fast?

i. Orientation (Maximum score: 10)
"What is today's date" Then ask specifically for parts omitted, such as
and "you also tell me what season it is"

Date (e.g. January 21) ..... 1 ___
Year................................. 2 ___
Month.............................. 3 ___
Day (e.g. Monday) .... 4 ___
Season .... 5 ___

"Can you tell me the name of this hospital"
"What floor are we on?"
"What town (or city) are we in?"
"What country are we in?"
"What state are we in?"

Hospital........................... 6 ___
Floor................................ 7 ___
Town/City........................ 8 ___
Country............................ 9 ___
State...............................10 ___

ii. Registration (Maximum score: 3)
Ask the patient if you may test his memory. Then say "ball," "flag," "tree"
clearly and slowly, allowing about one second for each. After you have said
all three words, ask the patient to repeat them. This first repetition determines
the score (0-3), but continue to say them (up to six trials) until the patient
can repeat all three words. If he does not eventually learn all three, recall
cannot be meaningfully tested.

"ball"............................... 11 ___
"flag"...............................12 ___
"tree"...............................13 ___

Number of trials: _____

iii. Attention and calculation (Maximum score: 5)
Ask the patient to begin at 100 and count backward by 7. Stop after five sub-
tractions (93, 86, 79, 72, 65). Score one point for each correct number.

"93"................................14 ___
"86"................................15 ___
"79"................................16 ___
"72"................................17 ___
"65"................................18 ___
or
Number of correctly
Placed letter.................... 19 ___

If the subject cannot or will not perform this task ask him to spell the word
"world" backward (D, L, R, O, W). Score one point for each correctly placed
letter, e.g. DLROW = 5, DLROW = 3,
Record how the patient spelled "world" backward: _____
                                                  D   L   R   O   W

iv. Recall (Maximum score: 3)
Ask the patient to recall the three words you previously asked him to
remember (learned in Registration).

"ball"...............................20 ___
"flag"...............................21 ___
"tree".............................. 22 ___

v. Language (Maximum score: 9)
Naming: Show the patient a wristwatch and ask "What is this?"
Repeat for a pencil. Score one point for each item named correctly.

Watch..............................23 ___
Pencil..............................24 ___

Repetition: Ask the patient to repeat: "No it's, and's or but's." Score one point
for correct repetition.

Repetition........................25 ___

Three-stage command: Give the patient a piece of blank paper and say
"Take the paper in your right hand, fold it in half and put it on the floor."
Score one point for each action performed correctly.

Takes in right hand ....26 ___
Folds in half ....27 ___
Puts on the floor ....28 ___

Reading: On a blank piece of paper, print the sentence "Close your eyes" in
letters large enough for the patient to see clearly. Ask the patient to read it
and do what it says. Score correct only if he actually closes his eyes.

Closes eyes ....29 ___

Writing: Give the patient a blank piece of paper and ask him to write a sentence.
It's to be written spontaneously. It must contain a subject and verb
and make sense. Correct grammar and punctuation are not necessary.

Writes sentence...............30 ___

Copying: On a clean piece of paper, draw intersecting pentagons as illustrated,
each side measuring about 1 inch, and ask the patient to copy it exactly
as it is. All 10 angles must be present and two must intersect to score 1 point.
Tremor and rotation are ignored.

Draws pentagons............. 31 ___

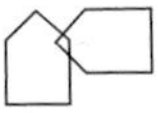

Score: Add number of correct responses, in Section 32: includes items 14 through
18 or item 19, not both, (Maximum total score: 30)
Cummings has suggested "apple", "table," "penny" for clarity — editor.
Level of consciousness: — coma — stupor — drowsy — alert.

Total score: _____

FIGURE 73–1. Mini-Mental State Examination. *It has become common practice to substitute "apple, table, penny" to
ease registration of the three words. (From J Psychiatr Res 1975;**12**:189.)

been extended; a well-educated person with definite progressive AD may score 100%! However, if there are abnormalities, the test provides quantitative confirmation of the cognitive domains often affected in any state of dementia.

a. The physician (or practice nurse) does not need to administer the test personally; a trained interviewer, maybe a medical assistant if available, can accurately record the MMSE. This takes some of the tension out of the examination, making it seem more like the acquisition of "vital signs." However, the patient should be informed that his or her memory is to be tested, and such questions should not be simply inserted into the patient interview. It is important to keep the original written record of the MMSE, as the scoring does not distinguish well between the less important aspects of orientation, for example, and major symptoms, such as memory.

b. If the results are equivocal, it may help to add tests of **symptoms not assessed by the MMSE.** Abstract thinking can be assessed by the ability to interpret proverbs (eg, "glass houses" where the typically concrete thinking of even quite early AD, for example, might create a response such as "the glass will break" when asked what the proverb means). A less culturally specific way of testing abstraction is to ask the patient to say what is similar about an arm and a leg, then (getting more complicated), asking the same question about laughing and crying or eating and sleeping. The range of the MMSE may also be enhanced by asking questions to test the retrieval of long-term memories, tested in category retrieval tests such as "Name all of the four-legged animals that you can think of in 30 seconds" (should be 10 or more.)

c. The **clock drawing test,** which some have attempted to standardize, can be done quite informally, with a paper and pencil. The patient is asked to "draw a clock." If necessary he or she is prompted to draw the circle, and then prompted/told to place the numbers "like a clock face." It is important to state that the hands "should point to 20 past 8" (see Table 73–11). Patients with abstract difficulties may well not be able to find the number that would represent "20 after." The clock does get progressively disorganized as the illness progresses. It is sometimes useful to show the clock to family members if one or several of them (as happens in disputing extended families at times) cannot accept that their parent's mind is failing. This is very hard for some family members to accept, and can lead to taking unnecessary risks, for example.

d. A comparable test of functional impairment is the **Functional Assessment Questionnaire** (FAQ) (Figure 73–2). This is currently the most widely recommended of many instruments that assess "instrumental activities of daily living," that is, the more complex daily activities that one does, not self-care skills, but those which are instrumental to daily life: balancing the checkbook, preparing a meal, following a television program, traveling alone, shopping, etc. The FAQ can be completed by family members if necessary, but is best done by having a staff person interview the family and fill in their responses. Each function is scored from three to zero, ranging from three, meaning that the person cannot perform the task at all (whereas they used to be able to), to zero, meaning that they have no difficulty or that it was something they never did. This test gives a measure of the functional impact and can be used to track its progression or stability. Results also give extra insight into the caregiver's role and burden.

e. Most clinicians working with AD would recommend repeating the MMSE and FAQ at intervals of 6–12 months in order to assess progress. Some spenders prefer this test to be done in order to justify the continuing expense of AChEIs.

3. **Assessing the severity or stage of the dementia.** It is necessary and helpful to the caregiving family members to assign an approximate stage to the dementing process. US Food and Drug Administration (FDA) approval for treatments at "mild or moderate" or "moderate to severe" stages of the dementia also necessitate this.

TABLE 73–11. CLOCK DRAWING TEST
_____

1. "Draw a clock."
2. "Put the numbers in."
3. "Put the hands at 20 after 8."
_____

Place a check mark under the column that best describes the patient's
ability to perform the tasks listed below:

	Completely unable to perform task (3 points)	Requires assistance (2 points)	Has difficulty but accomplishes task, or has never done, but the informant feels could do task with difficulty (1 point)	Normal performance, or has never done task, but the informant feels the patient could do the task if necessary (0 points)
1. Writing checks, paying bills, balancing a checkbook	_____	_____	_____	_____
2. Assembling tax records, business affairs, or papers	_____	_____	_____	_____
3. Shopping alone for clothes, household necessities, or groceries	_____	_____	_____	_____
4. Playing a game of skill, working on a hobby	_____	_____	_____	_____
5. Heating water, making a cup of coffee, turning off the stove	_____	_____	_____	_____
6. Preparing a balanced meal	_____	_____	_____	_____
7. Keeping track of current events	_____	_____	_____	_____
8. Paying attention to, understanding, discussing a TV show, book, or magazine	_____	_____	_____	_____
9. Remembering appointments, family occasions, holidays, medications	_____	_____	_____	_____
10. Traveling out of the neighborhood, driving, arranging to take buses	_____	_____	_____	_____
Points per column	_____	_____	_____	_____

Total points   _____

FIGURE 73–2. Functional Activities Questionnaire (FAQ). (Adapted and reprinted with permission from J Gerontol 1982;**37**:323–329.)

Although each patient is truly unique, Galasko's categorization into three stages, defined in terms of the most frequently reported problem areas in reported series of patients, is recommended for this purpose (Table 73–12). Note that the MMSE alone is not the criterion; a more global estimate, based on all three domains (cognitive, functional, and behavioral) is to be assessed by the primary care physician.
4. **What kind of dementia is it?** (Table 73–13).
    a. **Alzheimer's disease (AD).** In patients in their mid 70s and above, a very slowly progressive dementia, of insidious onset and with no abrupt declines (unless such an abrupt change can be fully explained by concurrent illness or injury, or relocation or some other disturbance), could appropriately lead to a "working" diagnosis of AD as the cause of the dementia. Features of the other primary dementing disorders can then be sought, at the initial visit, and at follow-ups.
        The next most frequent primarily dementing illnesses, both of them characterized by progressive decline, are dementia of Lewy body type (DLB) and vascular dementia (VaD).
    b. **Dementia of Lewy body type (DLB)** generally starts looking quite like AD in the early phases, but then complex visual hallucinations develop, with or without spontaneous parkinsonian signs (eg, bradykinesia, "pill rolling" tremor, flat faces, "cog wheel" rigidity, and the characteristic gait, with limited lifting of the feet while walking and a lack of spontaneous arm swing when doing so), which may be very subtle and should be specifically sought on observation and examination. Sometimes DLB starts looking much more like a depression, and frequently will be

TABLE 73–12. MILD, MODERATE, AND SEVERE DEMENTIA: COMMON CLINICAL FEATURES

Mild (MMSE typically 21–30)
Cognition:
  Recall/learning
  Word finding
  Problem solving
  Judgment
  Calculation
Function:
  Work
  Money/shopping
  Cooking
  Housekeeping
  Reading
  Writing
  Hobbies
Behavior:
  Apathy
  Withdrawal
  Depression
  Irritability

Moderate (MMSE typically 10–20)
Cognition:
  Recent memory
  Language (names, paraphasias)
  Insight
  Orientation
  Visuospatial ability
Function:
  Instrumental activities of daily living
  Misplacing things
  Getting lost
  Difficulty dressing (sequence and selection)

Behavior:
  Delusions
  Depression
  Wandering
  Insomnia
  Agitation
  Preserved social skills

Severe (MMSE typically <10)
Cognition:
  Attention
  Difficulty performing familiar activities
  Language
Function:
  Activities of daily living:
    Dressing
    Grooming
    Bathing
    Eating
    Continence
    Walking
  Motor slowing
Behavior:
  Agitation
    Verbal
    Physical
  Insomnia

Modified after Galasko D, et al: The Consortium to Establish a Registry for Alzheimer's Disease (CERAD): XI. Clinical milestones in patients with Alzheimer's disease followed for three years. Eurology 1995; **45**:1451.

treated as such, but then it becomes evident that there is cognitive decline as well, and then the hallucinatory or parkinsonian symptoms (or both) evolve. DLB patients are exquisitely sensitive to the extrapyramidal side effects of antipsychotic medications, even the more modern ones, with the possible exception of quetiapine (Seroquel). Experts on DLB recommend against using antipsychotics for the psychotic features of DLB, fearing long-term neurologic damage. Often, however, antipsychotics are used for psychotic features in a dementia, and only then are the extrapyramidal parkinsonian signs "revealed" clinically, but they can then persist after the initiating antipsychotic is discontinued. Whether the primary care physician makes the diagnosis or a neurologic consultation is sought, either approach is safe. Both DLB and AD respond to the AChEIs described below. (However, note that this is an "off label" comment; the FDA approval is for mild

TABLE 73–13. THE PRINCIPAL DEMENTIAS

Primary Progressive Dementias
- Alzheimer's disease (AD)
- Dementia of Lewy body type (DLB)
- Vascular dementia (VaD)
- Frontotemporal dementia (including Pick's)
- Huntington's disease
- Creutzfeldt-Jakob disease

Common Secondary Dementias
- Alcohol-associated
- Parkinson's-associated (subcortical)
- AIDS-associated
- Postanoxic encephalopathy
- Post-stroke
- Progressive supranuclear palsy

to moderate dementia "from AD"). Once DLB is recognized, antipsychotics are to be avoided, and a less predictable, rather more rapid course than is generally seen in AD is to be anticipated by physician and family alike.

c. **Vascular dementia (VaD),** once regarded as the cause of a high proportion of dementias, is a group of dementias attributable to vascular disease, and includes multi-infarct dementia, Binswanger's disease (due to small vessel changes) and post-stroke dementia. However, **mixed dementia** (AD and VaD together) is often seen, and anyway, as described elsewhere, stroke (and therefore possibly other manifestations of cerebrovascular disease) is a recognized risk factor for the development of AD. So VaD is probably a less-frequent primary cause of dementia than it was considered to be in years past. VaD is sometimes (inappropriately) diagnosed as a result of seeing vascular changes on a computerized tomography (CT) or magnetic resonance imaging (MRI) scan. Such findings are common in patients who at autopsy are shown to have AD. To diagnose VaD as the primary cause of a dementia requires a clear history of "stepwise" progression (not the smoothly inexorable progression of AD), especially if there is clinical (historical) as well as radiologic evidence of transient ischemic attacks (TIAs).

In practice, the primary care physician should always look for vascular risk factors in any patient with a progressive dementia and regard vascular changes on a CT or MRI scan simply as evidence of vascular disease and another cause of potential morbidity throughout the body. If there are vascular problems or risk factors, these must be addressed vigorously (control blood pressure, add aspirin, look for dysrhythmias—especially atrial fibrillation and heart block, sick sinus syndrome, and other bradycardic states—and listen for carotid bruits or request carotid ultrasound studies).

d. **Other, atypical dementias** are suspected because of features that are outside the range of symptoms characteristic of AD (eg, the striking family history found in Huntington's disease (autosomal dominant inheritance); the early, disinhibited, personality changes—sometimes overshadowing the memory deficits—of the frontal lobe dementias (such as Pick's disease). All of the "non-Alzheimer" dementias (Table 73–13), can look like AD at first. However, less harm results from mislabeling as AD a situation which evolves features suggesting, at follow-up, a more rare etiology than would result from failing to recognize and address an early AD.

e. **Major depressive disorder (MDE).** "The dementia syndrome of depression" is now the preferred term to characterize the way in which MDE can, particularly in an older person, exhibit so much cognitive impairment that it truly looks like a dementia. The term "pseudodementia" was previously used, but it does not express the actual diagnosis, which is a true depression. The history will be quite different from that of a dementia, if obtainable accurately, and the clinical features are subtly different on interview, including the way formal testing of mental status is answered by the patient (Table 73–14). However, MDE is more interconnected with AD than merely looking superficially like it: MDE is in fact yet another "risk factor" for the development of AD. The primary care physician should follow up on elderly patients who have sustained an MDE, even if it was successfully treated and appears to be largely resolved, since they are at increased risk of subsequently developing AD. (Whether this is because the depression is a sign of the brain's vulnerability or—more likely—that the depression itself is damaging to the aging brain has not been explained; the connection is strong enough to make this recommendation for primary care practice.)

f. **Differentiating delirium from dementia** may be a dilemma when a patient presents acutely without accompanying family members in an emergency situation. Delirium is an anticipated complication of dementia and may be the presenting symptom of a dementia. The greater moment-to-moment variability and the physiologic disturbance present in the patient with delirium helps the differentiation from dementia (Table 73–15). An acute change in mental status is an indication for urgent (even emergency) investigation because the acute delirium will, by definition, be a cerebral manifestation of some acute illness that may be a life-threatening one (eg, an evolving stroke, myocardial infarction, sepsis, pneumonia.)

TABLE 73-14. DEMENTIA VS. DEPRESSION

Dementia	Depression
Insidious onset (maybe months)	Abrupt onset (maybe days)
Long duration	Short duration
No psychiatric history	Often psychiatric history
Conceals disability (often unaware)	Highlights disabilities (complains)
Near-miss answers	"Don't know" answers
Day-to-day fluctuation in mood	Diurnal variation in mood, mood more consistent
Stable cognitive loss	Fluctuating cognitive loss
May try hard to perform, and be unconcerned about mistakes	Often does not try so hard, more distressed by mistakes
Memory loss greatest for recent events	Equal memory loss for recent and remote events
Memory loss first (before mood)	Depressed mood first (before cognition)
Associated with unsociability, uncooperativeness, hostility, emotional instability, confusion, disorientation, reduced alertness	Associated with depressed/anxious mood, sleep disturbance, changed appetite, suicidal thoughts

g. It is necessary to rule out the **reversible causes of dementia;** however, it is rare to find a true, "Alzheimer's like" progressive dementia that is entirely caused by some treatable physical illness. Such "causes" are generally in fact concurrent to the dementia under investigation and may well worsen the situation if untreated, but will not reverse the dementia when treated themselves. (This would apply to hypothyroidism, for example, which must always be ruled out.) This author has, over the years, modified the use of the well-known (anonymous) mnemonic "DEMENTIA" (Table 73–16) from being an aide-memoire for the "reversible causes of dementia" into its current version, a summary of the "aggravating factors of an apparent dementia," which form the basis for the work-up of a newly recognized dementia, or of an unexpected abrupt decline occurring in a person with known dementia.

C. Laboratory tests. The choices of investigations are driven by the differential diagnosis described above and by the aggravating factors that must be sought (Table 73–17).

    1. Brain imaging. It is customary US practice to always obtain a CT scan or MRI of the head in a probable dementia. A plain CT without contrast media is sufficient in most cases. The test is usually noncontributory. In some radiologists' hands, an MRI may be more sensitive to vascular changes, but the primary care physician must be wary of overinterpretation of vascular changes, since they are risk factors for AD, and are not confirmatory of VaD, the diagnosis of which is based on the history and sometimes neurologic findings, as outlined above. Some patients with advanced disease, presenting late in the illness with no suggestive history of trauma and no localizing neurologic signs, can forgo a scan. Some patients cannot tolerate either procedure; the risk/benefit of a long transfer from a remote area

TABLE 73-15. DELIRIUM COMPARED WITH DEMENTIA

Delirium	Dementia
Precise onset (identifiable date)	Gradual onset (cannot date)
Acute, days to weeks	Chronic, over years
Usually reversible, often completely	Generally irreversible, often chronically progressive
Disorientation early	Disorientation later (months or years)
Variability moment to moment, hour to hour	Slight daily variation
Prominent physiologic changes	Less physiologic changes
Clouded, altered, changing level of consciousness	Consciousness not clouded until terminal
Strikingly short attention span	Attention span not characteristically reduced
Disturbed sleep-wake cycle, hour-to-hour variation	Disturbed sleep-wake cycle, day-night reversal
Marked psychomotor changes	Psychomotor changes less dramatic

TABLE 73–16. CAUSES AND AGGRAVATIONS OF APPARENT DEMENTIA

D	Drugs
E	Emotional illness (including depression)
M	Metabolic/endocrine disorders
E	Eyes/ears/environment
N	Nutritional/neurologic
T	Tumors/trauma
I	Infections/impaction
A	Alcoholism/anemia/atherosclerosis
P	Pain ("postscript"!)

or sedation of the patient for the procedure may lead to a decision against a scan (although the family will need to know that the rare possibility of something intracranial has not been ruled out). Indeed, it must be clarified to the family that scans are only done to "rule out" space-occupying lesions such as an unsuspected brain tumor or metastases, an injury such as a subdural hematoma, or unsuspected cerebral infarction from stroke or TIAs.

The mere presence of cerebral atrophy on a scan should not be taken as evidence of the presence of a dementing process—atrophy can occur in individuals with no cognitive impairment. However, the fact that cerebral atrophy does occur in a proportion of elders makes a CT scan indicated in the emergency room when an elderly individual (especially a person with known dementia) has a head injury or is involved in a fairly high-speed auto accident, for the movement of the atrophic brain within the skull increases the risk of subdural bleeding as well as a heightened risk of "contra coup" brain contusion.

2. **Required blood tests** are pretty standard: a thyroid-stimulating hormone test, vitamin B_{12} and folate tests, and a screen for syphilis (RPR or VDRL), and if there is any clinical reason why the electrolytes or renal function should be impaired, tests for these should also be done. If the person has not been seen for some time, a complete blood count might be justified, and a urinalysis, but these are not specific to a dementia work-up (Table 73–17).

III. Treatment
   A. **Medications for the treatment of AD**
      1. **Acetylcholinesterase inhibitors (AChEIs).** These are the first type of medication to be approved by the FDA specifically for the symptomatic treatment of mild to moderate dementia caused by AD. The AChEIs are unfortunately severely underutilized in primary care practice, relative to the prevalence of AD, its terrible impact

TABLE 73–17. INVESTIGATIONS IN MEMORY DISORDERS

All:
Complete blood count
Basic metabolic panel
Thyroid and B_{12} stimulating hormone
Folate
RPR/VDRL

Most:
Computerized tomography or magnetic resonance imaging
Comprehensive metabolic panel

Some:
Neuropsychological testing
Erythrocyte sedimentation rate
Single photon emission computerized tomography or positron emission tomography
Electroencephalogram
Lumbar puncture
Human immunodeficiency virus

on families and economically and in other ways on society as a whole, and relative to the multiple double-blind, placebo-controlled trials in the United States (and internationally) that confirm that these medications, if given persistently, will postpone cognitive and functional decline and reduce the behavioral disturbances of AD. Patients on these treatments will generally have a period of relatively little decline, quite frequently almost a "plateau," and a very small proportion will actually improve (very exceptionally, and sometimes quite markedly and obviously for a time). However, families should not be led to expect improvement; rather, they should be counseled that a period of stability of the symptoms with "no change" in 6 months or a year should be regarded as a triumph in this otherwise inexorably progressive disease. They should also know that "slowed decline" is also a successful outcome of AChEI treatment. The cost of the medications is a consideration, since theoretically they should be given for at least several years. Therefore, the primary care physician should ensure that patients in need are made aware of the free programs that each of the companies manufacturing the three recommended medications offer.

    a. Outcomes. The data confirm that these medications are still keeping AD patients "ahead of the curve" at 3–5 years out (placebo-controlled, double-blind data) and even longer (up to 10 years: open-label, non–placebo-controlled data). Current trials in MCI (see description above) may tell us whether they should be begun in that virtually "predementia" phase.

    b. When to begin. At present, the "standard of care" is that the AChEIs should be started as soon as a dementia with a clinical history supporting the typical insidious onset and smooth progression of AD is shown to be present. It is no longer ethically acceptable to "watch and wait" for decline as "proof" of the presence of AD prior to starting treatment.

    c. Which one to choose. Of the four medications approved by the FDA, the first to be available, tacrine (Cognex) is virtually no longer used, in view of its frequent dosage and unacceptable side effects, plus its possible liver toxicity. The remaining three "second-generation" AChEIs (Table 73–18) are probably equally efficacious, although donepezil (Aricept), being given once daily, has a decided advantage in (by definition) forgetful patients. Rivastigmine (Exelon) is a little more complicated to give, being given twice daily, and since the starting dose is subtherapeutic, dose titration is always necessary. It also suffers from the FDA bolded warnings about its increased risk of gastrointestinal side effects, which are discouraging and uncomfortable for those patients so afflicted. Galantamine (Reminyl) has the same low side-effect profile as donepezil. Any patient already receiving any of these three medications should not be casually "swapped" to one of the others. Such swapping can result in gaps in therapeutic level and can even lead to permanent loss of the ground already gained by the previous period of AChEI treatment. Donepezil should not be stopped for longer than 3 weeks if at all possible. Somewhere between 2 or 3 and 6 weeks off donepezil treatment, some patients will so completely lose efficaciousness that the previously acquired level of function cannot be regained when treatment is restarted. The shorter half-lives of rivastigmine and galantamine may give even less leeway. So the rule is "don't stop and don't swap." The exceptions to not swapping might be the patient who genuinely cannot tolerate a particular AChEI (usually because of persistent gastrointestinal symptoms, which are rare, eg, diarrhea) and the patient who has continued to decline at the rate that would be expected

TABLE 73–18. ACETYLCHOLINESTERASE INHIBITORS: THE "SECOND GENERATION"

Name	Starting Dose	Titration Schedule	Recommended Dose Range
Donepezil (Aricept)	5 mg once daily	Increase to 10 mg after 4–6 weeks	5–10 mg/day
Rivastigmine (Exelon)	1.5 mg twice daily	Increase by 1.5 mg per twice daily dose every 2+ weeks to maximum 12 mg/day	6–12 mg/day
Galantamine (Reminyl)	4 mg twice daily	Increase by 4 mg per twice daily dose every 4+ weeks to maximum 24 mg/day	6–24 mg/day

without treatment (2–4 points on the MMSE per year in the mild to moderate stages), since theoretically the patient might respond to one medication in the group and not to another (although this has not been proved). In the latter case, it would be logical to swap to galantamine from rivastigmine or donepezil, or to donepezil or rivastigmine from galantamine, as galantamine works in a slightly different way from the other two, a relatively weak anticholinesterase with some direct cholinergic action. The only contraindication to the use of these medications is an unstable bradycardia syndrome or complete heart block. Occasionally patients who develop this and yet need an AChEI are justifiable candidates for a pacemaker. Also, since theoretically an existing peptic ulcer might be made worse by a cholinergic medication, questions about ulcer symptomatology should be asked, and should ulcer symptoms develop, they should be taken seriously and investigated and treated. In practice, such complications are extremely rare. Families should be warned that transient nausea or diarrhea may occur early on, particularly at increases of dosage during titration, and that either symptom generally resolves without stopping the AChEI. The characteristics of all four available AChEIs are summarized in Table 73–18.

2. **Memantine (Namenda)** has just (January 2004) been introduced to the United States. It is indicated as an additional medication, added on to one of the recommended AChEIs described above, when the person with AD reaches a moderate stage of dementia (Table 73–12) or first presents at a moderate or severe stage. The available data indicate that, whereas on average patients on memantine vs. placebo, or on memantine and donepezil vs. placebo and donepezil, do continue to decline in cognitive and functional (mostly activities of daily living [self-care] functions) parameters, the average decline is slowed significantly on memantine, with some patients actually improving. More US clinical experience and trials will clarify the precise place of memantine. Clearly it should be used whenever (as is usual) even a relatively slight improvement relative to the untreated course would significantly reduce the known enormous burden on caregivers and formal support services and personnel. Given the present evidence, an AChEI should overlap with the use of memantine, for at least the moderate phase of the dementia of AD. Trials have included patients with VaD, but no indication has been approved for VaD as yet for memantine (or the AChEIs), although the AChEIs are often used "off label" in probably vascular dementias by some experienced clinicians; at present this is justified by the slight diagnostic uncertainty, the frequency of "mixed" dementia (VaD and AD), and because benefit from enhancing cholinergic neuronal function in cognitively impaired patients is anyway probably not exclusive to AD.

B. **Behavioral management.** A major advantage of early diagnosis, with naming of the illness, is early training of the family members, the caregiver (spouse, daughter, son, or whomever), in how to handle the patient with AD, in order to improve the quality of life for caregiver and patient alike, and to reduce (or at least manage) the behavioral problems that will arise. The agency to teach all of this to the family is the Alzheimer's Association, many of whose chapters operate local instructional and support groups. The Alzheimer's Association itself can be accessed at its national headquarters toll-free (1-800-272-3900) or through their web site (www.alz.org).

1. Many popular books have been written about how to handle AD patients. The "classic" text is still "The 36-Hour Day" by Mace and Rabins. Family members should be advised to use it for reference. It describes all of the things that can go wrong and gives practical guidance to their resolution.

2. Many simple techniques have been evolved by caregivers and researchers to make life easier, to keep the patient more functional and able to enjoy life. Such techniques include:

   a. Making choices for the patient, but doing it subtly: choosing the right clothes for today's weather forecast and putting just those clothes in the patient's closet so he or she does not have to choose the clothes and can thus still dress without assistance; reducing choices of food presented to the patient, with the result that foods are eaten rather than the patient being overwhelmed by choices and eating nothing; organizing reminiscence, such as family photographs, or finding CDs and tapes of music and films that are evocative for the person. ("The Honeymooners" on video is perfect for the present cohort of elders!)

    b. Families should be counseled that the characteristic early apathy of AD and lack of organizational capacity means that their patient will not have the initiative to start things, but once started may well be able to continue unsupervised. The caregiver's role becomes, then, to "organize" reminiscence and activities, which the patient and family alike can then enjoy.

        Table 73–19 summarizes some common behavioral problems and the behavioral approaches that have been demonstrated to be useful.

IV. Management Strategies

A. Advance directives. As soon as a progressive dementia is diagnosed, the family should be given the appropriate paperwork to complete advance directives and a health care proxy, with or without a durable power of attorney for health care. Since the patient is likely to become confused as a result of any intercurrent illness, it is urgent to obtain this, so that the upsetting situation of trying to decide what the patient would have wanted in an extreme situation can be avoided. The family should realize that as long as the patient is competent, he or she will make the decisions, but once unable to do so, the health care proxy or the person holding the durable power of attorney for health care will have the power to make decisions "as the patient." They will be deciding what the patient would have wanted in the circumstances, not what they would personally choose. Advance directives and health care proxy documents can include details about desired and not desired aspects of medical management. This author advises against being too specific about such things, as medicine is continually advancing, and general attitudes (and people's own viewpoint) naturally change over time. Some patients will incorrectly specify "no tube feeding," failing to recognize that this technique may be life-saving if they are only temporarily unable to swallow (eg, following an incidental stroke). Embargos on antipsychotic drugs and intravenous therapy may be similarly unwise.

B. Nutrition is an issue that should be considered continually. Early in the disease patients will not eat if overwhelmed by choices. Later, they may need to be spoon-fed, as self-feeding becomes difficult. Later still, the issue comes up about maintenance with tube feeding. In most authorities' opinions, long-term tube feeding in the later stages of a dementing illness is inappropriate. However, individuals (or their families as surrogates) must make their own decisions; sometimes it may be reasonable to maintain an individual who has relatively early loss of appetite or dysphagia out of proportion to the degree of dementia.

C. Health maintenance activities will naturally not be sought by most patients with dementia. Depending on the progression and stage of the illness, preventive protocols should be somewhat modified (eg, in later dementia is it reasonable to keep doing mammograms and other cancer screens?). Maintenance of range of movement, of the ability to walk, of ears clear of wax, a comfortable mouth and painless feet represent more relevant health maintenance activities to a person with severe dementia.

D. Driving is a very difficult problem. Patients with early AD can drive, provided they do not have too many other problems such as impaired vision or hearing or inability to turn the head. Once an AD patient has had an auto accident to which they may have contributed, it is difficult to justify further driving. Absent such an incident, the best approach is a formal driving assessment in simulated conditions, but this is rarely available. Second best is to have a family member drive with the person on a regular basis, looking critically at driving performance. If no one in the family is willing to drive with the patient, you know that really the patient, sadly, needs to be off the road! If neighbors have warned the family that the person is not driving well, then this should be heeded. Otherwise sensible families sometimes take appalling risks. Sometimes a "co-pilot" truly increases safety, but the need to have one is a warning sign. Any older patient should

---

TABLE 73–19. EFFECTIVE BEHAVIORAL APPROACHES IN THE DEMENTIAS

- Counter cognitive deficits (notebook, calendar, reminders, notices, clocks, orientation)
- Improve function (limit choices, decide for the patient, simplify clothing, use finger foods, organize/start tasks, etc.)
- Create calming environment (the right lighting, the right noises, the right images)
- Stimulate reminiscence (photos, videos, music, audios, including of absent family)
- Organize pleasurable experiences (music, rides, pictures, conversations, social groups)

restrict their driving to quieter streets and daylight hours and should avoid driving in inclement weather. No patient with even early AD should drive alone; the co-driver needs to be able to take over. Emergency reactions can be required at anytime, even in the "quietest" streets.

E. **Depression** can complicate the early stages and later. If a dementia patient's condition declines rather abruptly, or over days, and the symptoms include characteristic MDE symptoms such as appetite change, loss of interest, worse mood in the morning, or characteristic insomnia, with even two such symptoms occurring concurrently, a trial of an antidepressant is justified (see Chapter 92). A selective serotonin reuptake inhibitor is first choice (Table 73–20). The dose should be started low, but should be raised to the normal therapeutic levels used in younger adults. Target symptoms for the family to observe and record should be defined. A trial is not over until at least 8 weeks at a normal therapeutic dose without the target symptoms relieved.

F. **Hallucinations and delusions** can occur, sometimes associated with intercurrent physical illness. Benign hallucinations are very frequent in the earliest stages of AD. They often involve children, and even if the patient realizes they are not quite "real," they are not particularly frightening, and therefore do not require treatment. However, if hallucinations become vivid and frightening, or directive, or start to foster a delusional system, then efforts should be made to ensure that the environment is not contributing to delusional activity (eg, patients may be misinterpreting noises they hear in the night, or lights they see on the drapes), yet frequently, treatment with an antipsychotic drug is also then justified. The more modern antipsychotic drugs should be used, to avoid the anticholinergic and extrapyramidal side-effect profiles of earlier antipsychotic drugs. Although generally associated with the "nursing home" stage of dementia care, such medications can occasionally control psychotic symptoms sufficiently to keep a person in their own home, or at an assisted-living level of care. Much lower doses than are recommended for schizophrenic patients should be used (eg, with risperidone [Risperdal], starting at even 0.25 mg a day may be reasonable, although the dose will often have to be increased from that). (See Tables 73–20 and 73–21.)

G. **Temporary sedation** for the purposes of dental care or other procedures is usually achieved with lorazepam (Ativan) or some other relatively short-acting benzodiazepine. For lorazepam an oral dose of 0.25 mg may suffice; it can be tried, on a weekend perhaps, prior to a procedure such as dental work, to judge the individual response. If used intravenously (or intramuscularly if necessary), the dose (0.5–1.0 mg would be appropriate) can be titrated or repeated according to the patient's individual response. In any event, all involved should be prepared for the possibility of more prolonged sedation than would be expected in younger patients, with the obvious dangers of falling or other harm from the patient's temporarily impaired attention. These drugs should be avoided for longer-term use in AD patients because of this impaired perception and increased to fall.

H. **Sundowning** is a phenomenon whereby psychotic features or near psychotic states occur in the night, often starting in the early evening, and possibly associated with primitive fears of the dark. Symptoms can thus be sometimes relieved by lighting, familiar music, warmth, security, and company, but when they are marked it is inhumane to withhold treatment with antipsychotic medications from such patients. Sedating a dementia patient at night does increase the risk of falling when up in the night for nocturia.

TABLE 73–20. PSYCHOTROPICS IN THE DEMENTIAS

Condition	Medications
Depression	SSRIs, bupropion
Agitation, aggressiveness	Divalproex, risperidone, quetiaprine, olanzapine, and haloperidol IM[1]
Psychosis with agitation	Risperidone, quetiapine, olanzapine, and haloperidol IM[1]
Anxiety	Lorazepam (short-term), buspirone
Agitation or anxiety with depression	SSRIs, consider initial lorazepam
Insomnia	Zolpidem and similar, trazodone, SSRI if insomnia from depression

[1] If intramuscular (IM) needed and only (very) short term.
SSRI, selective serotonin reuptake inhibitors.

TABLE 73–21. INDICATIONS FOR ANTIPSYCHOTICS IN DEMENTIAS

- Severe mental distress or fearfulness
- Agitation with aggressiveness
- Recurrent catastrophic reactions
- Sundowning syndrome, if psychotic
- Disturbing hallucinations
- Paranoia
- Frightening or directive delusions
- Aggression or restlessness if it prevents necessary management

I. **Level of care.** As an individual with dementia progresses, so increased services need to be made available in the home to assist the caregiver and relieve their burden. Unfortunately, most insurance does not pay for such services, and the cost must be found out of pocket by the family. The physician must counsel the family member or caregiver to spend wisely in order to relieve themselves of the burden and ensure that they can continue in the caregiving role for as long as they can reasonably continue.

1. **Assisted living facilities (ALFs)** are a rapid-growth industry for the accommodation of moderately impaired dementia patients who can yet manage self-care to a degree and yet need meal preparation, medication management, etc.

2. Once the patient needs skilled nursing care for a major portion of the day, it is generally necessary to consider placement in a nursing home, that is, a **skilled nursing facility (SNF).** Many facilities now have specific Alzheimer's units, or have modified their facility to be more "Alzheimer friendly." However, others truly have not and maintain an almost "hospital-like" environment, quite unsuitable for the needs of the AD patient, who requires reminders, familiarity, reminiscence, and calm, which cannot be achieved in the increasingly busy and noisy atmosphere of some nursing home settings, as they are challenged by having more and more medically complex patients. In practice, many SNF placements follow some setback such as hospitalization for pneumonia, or hip fracture, some complication that finally makes it clear that the person needs skilled care, at least in the short term. The SNF admission is then rather precipitate and choices are limited. It is also a "trial of rehabilitation" period; it generally becomes clear in a few weeks whether the patient will be able return home with increased services or stay on in the SNF in the long term.

3. **Nursing home care.** Once the dementia patient is in the nursing home, the environment and care is increasingly regulated. If not clarified before, advance directives and decisions about intensity of treatment in certain circumstances, and whether (or when) to hospitalize, as the terminal phase of the illness approaches, and whether to treat certain later complications (such as a relatively asymptomatic pneumonia) becomes a consideration. Many primary care physicians act as staff physicians in nursing homes. The physician/patient/family relationships are different from the long familiarity often achieved in office primary care. The nursing home primary care physician generally comes late into the management of patients who have been ill for a considerable time. It is thus important to get to know the family and their wishes and prejudices early on, to avoid conflict over the intensity of treatment. The physician must act as mentor and guide to doing enough, but not too much, recognizing that quality rather than quantity of life is important, particularly in the late-stage dementia patient. The physician should help families recognize when the patient's terminality is approaching, and appropriately involve the hospice, or at least hospice-type techniques of effective palliation, as the final months or year of the patient's life comes to pass. The issue of resuscitation must be addressed much earlier, because the outcomes of resuscitation of patients with dementia are much poorer than in nondemented individuals, because the brain in any dementia is so vulnerable to hypoxic damage.

V. **Prognosis.** Patients with AD are frequently diagnosed as much as 3–4 years after the onset of typical symptoms, and the range of duration from diagnosis to death in AD is from approximately 10–20 years, although some recent studies have suggested that the lifespan is relatively on the short side of that range. However, individual cases lasting a couple of decades or more have certainly been seen and it is difficult to prognosticate for the individual case.

REFERENCES

Alzheimer disease in the US population: Prevalence estimates using the 2000 census. Arch Neurol 2003;**60:**8.

American Psychiatric Association: Practice guidelines for the treatment of patients with Alzheimer's disease and other dementias of late life. Am J Psychiatry 1997;**154**(suppl):1.

Clinical Practice Guideline #19: Recognition and Initial Assessment of Alzheimer's Disease and Related Dementias. US Department of Health and Human Services; 1996.

Galasko D, et al: The Consortium to Establish a Registry for Alzheimer's Disease (CERAD): XI. Clinical milestones in patients with Alzheimer's disease followed for three years. Eurology 1995;**45:**1451.

Ham RJ: Dementias (and delirium). Chapter 17. In: Ham RJ, Sloane PD, Warshaw GA (editors): *Primary Care Geriatrics: A Case-Based Approach,* 4th ed. Mosby; 2002.

Mace NL, Rabins PV: *The 36-Hour Day,* 3rd ed. The Johns Hopkins University Press; 1999.

74   Diabetes Mellitus

Mark B. Mengel, MD, MPH

KEY POINTS

- The prevalence of type II diabetes mellitus (DM) is increasing as the prevalence of obesity increases.
- All adults older than 45 years should be screened every 3 years using a fasting plasma glucose test. The diagnosis of DM is made by 2 fasting plasma glucose values >126 mg/dL or one random >200 mg/dL.
- Instituting a healthy diet with just enough calories to maintain ideal body weight and engaging in regular exercise is the cornerstone of treatment for both type I and type II DM. Type I DM patients require insulin. Type II DM are usually started on an oral sulfonylureas, Glucotrol XL, 5 mg orally every day, or metformin, 500 mg, orally every day to twice daily if obese, with other oral agents added as needed.
- Hemoglobin A_{1C} is the best measure of diabetic control, should be checked every 3–6 months, and should be kept under 7% to minimize complications. Control of blood pressure and lipid levels and smoking cessation are also important to reduce the chance of macrovascular complications.
- Clinicians should also assess and reduce common barriers to care that prevent achievement of control goals, such as depression, family dysfunction, or lack of financial resources.

I. **Introduction**
  A. Diabetes mellitus (DM) is a heterogeneous group of disorders caused by a relative or absolute insulin deficiency, resulting in abnormalities of carbohydrate and fat metabolism. The two principal forms of diabetes mellitus, type I and type II, are the focus of this chapter.
  B. Type I DM, resulting from the destruction of pancreatic beta cells, occurs in roughly 10% of patients with DM, usually presenting between ages 10 and 15 years.
  C. Type II DM, resulting from insulin resistance, occurs in 90% of people with DM, usually presenting after age 40. As the prevalence of obesity has increased in this country over the past 20 years, so has the prevalence of type II DM. However, as the prevalence of obesity has increased in children and young adults, type II DM is increasingly being diagnosed in those populations as well. Major **risk factors** for type II DM include increasing age; being overweight; having a positive family history of DM; having a higher prediabetic fasting plasma glucose (FPG); being habitually physically inactive; and being a member of certain racial groups, specifically African Americans, Hispanics, Native Americans, Asian Americans, and Pacific Islanders.

II. **Diagnosis**
  A. **Symptoms and signs**
    1. **Type I DM.** Polyuria, polydipsia, weight loss, fatigue, and irritability are typical presenting complaints of patients with type I DM. Many type I DM patients are also in frank diabetic ketoacidosis at the time of diagnosis.

2. **Type II DM.** Many patients with type II DM are relatively asymptomatic initially. Physicians should suspect type II DM in patients with risk factors (see section I,C), recurrent infections, visual difficulties, unexplained peripheral neuropathy, and signs of other insulin-resistance states such as polycystic ovarian syndrome or the metabolic syndrome. Adults older than age 45, particularly those with a body mass index over 25, should be routinely screened every 3 years using an FPG.

B. **Laboratory tests**
  1. **Urinalysis.** Most patients with diabetes "spill" sugar into their urine at the time of diagnosis. Many substances, aging, and pregnancy affect the amount of glucose in the urine, however. Thus, urine testing for glycosuria is not useful in diagnosing and following up on patients with diabetes. Urine testing for ketones in patients with diabetes is still advisable; however, particularly when the patient becomes ill, to monitor for the onset of diabetic ketoacidosis.
  2. **Plasma glucose measurement.** This test is the preferred method of diagnosis. Meeting any one of the following criteria establishes the diagnosis in nonpregnant adults:
     a. One random plasma glucose measurement of >200 mg/dL (11.1 mmol/L) in a patient with classic diabetic signs and symptoms.
     b. Two fasting plasma glucose (FPG) levels of >126 mg/dL (7.0 mmol/L).
     c. A glucose tolerance test (75-g load) in which any blood glucose value between time zero and 2 hours exceeds 200 mg/dL.
     d. Those with non-normal FPG values that are not diagnostic for DM (110 mg/dL (6.1 mmol/L) < FPG <126 mg/dL (7.0 mmol/L)), or a post-load glucose tolerance test value of between 140 mg/dL (7.8 mmol/L) and 200 mg/dL (11.1 mmol/L) have impaired fasting glucose (if determined by a FPG), or impaired glucose tolerance (if diagnosed on an oral glucose tolerance test) and should be re-screened yearly.

III. **Treatment.** The goals of treatment are: (1) reduction of diabetic symptoms, (2) prevention of acute complications (eg, diabetic ketoacidosis, hyperosmolar nonketotic coma, hypoglycemia), (3) encouragement of normal growth and development in children with DM, and (4) prevention of chronic complications.

A. **Dietary therapy**
  1. Consultation with a dietitian is recommended for all patients with type I DM to achieve balance between food consumption and insulin administration. An appropriate-calorie, well-balanced meal plan combined with a high fiber intake actually improves diabetic control.
  2. In type II DM, dietary therapy is often ineffective in restoring glucose control, since few patients are able to maintain significant weight loss. Obesity contributes to the insulin resistance found in type II DM; 80% of patients with type II DM are overweight or obese. Even modest reductions in weigh can significantly improve diabetic control. Enrollment in behavior modification programs or support groups and involvement of the patient's family are necessary to increase the chances of weight-loss success.

B. **Exercise.** Although long-term, well-controlled studies of the effects of exercise on diabetic control are lacking, exercise does have a glucose-lowering effect and is recommended for the improvement of diabetic control. Patients with type II DM who engage in an exercise program that is integrated with dietary therapy may lose weight, with subsequent improvement in diabetic control. Guidelines for planning an exercise program include the following:
  1. An exercise program should begin at low intensity and increase gradually. Consultation with a clinician is recommended to integrate exercise with the other aspects of the therapeutic regimen. Patients with DM whose plasma glucose values are >300 mg/dL (16.7 mmol/L) should not exercise until their control has improved and their blood glucose levels have decreased. Self-monitoring of blood glucose (see section V,B) is useful during exercise.
  2. When possible, a patient with DM should exercise after meals to reduce postprandial hyperglycemia.
  3. Patients with DM should avoid exercise during peak insulin actions and should avoid exercising extremities in which insulin has recently been injected.

C. **Oral hypoglycemic agents** (Table 74–1). In patients with type II DM, oral hypoglycemic agents have become the mainstay of therapy, often using multiple oral agents as type II DM progresses. *These agents have no place in the treatment of patients with type I DM.*

TABLE 74-1. ORAL HYPOGLYCEMIC AGENTS

Drug	Starting Dose/Maximum Daily Dose	Side Effects and Notes	Cost[1]
Sulfonylureas—First generation			
Acetohexamide	500 mg po qd/1500 mg	Hypoglycemia, weight gain, rash, increased LFTs	$
Chlorpropamide (Diabinese)	100–250 mg po qd/750 mg	Hypoglycemia, weight gain, rash, increased LFTs, Disulfiram-like reaction, hyponatremia, extremely long half-life	$, (trade $$)
Tolazamide (Tolinase)	100–250 mg po qd/1000 mg	Hypoglycemia, weight gain, rash, increased LFTs	$, (trade $$)
Tolbutamide (Orinase, Tol-Tab)	250–500 mg po qd/3000 mg	Hypoglycemia, weight gain, rash, increased LFTs	$
Sulfonylureas—Second generation			
Glimepiride (Amaryl)	1–2 mg po qd/8 mg	Hypoglycemia, weight gain, rash, increased LFTs	$
Glipizide (Glucotrol and Glucotrol XL)	5 mg po qd/40 mg (20 mg for XL)	Hypoglycemia, weight gain, rash, increased LFTs	$
Glyburide (DiaBeta, Micronase)	1.25–2.5 mg po qd/20 mg	Hypoglycemia, weight gain, rash, increased LFTs	$, (trade $$)
Glyburide-micronized (Glynase PresTab)	1.5–3 mg po qd/12 mg	Hypoglycemia, weight gain, rash, increased LFTs	$
Alpha-Glucosidase inhibitors			
Acarbose (Precose)	25 mg tid before meals/300 mg	Bloating, flatulence, diarrhea/contraindicated in IBD	$$$
Miglitol (Glyset)	25 mg tid with meals/300 mg	Bloating, flatulence, diarrhea/contraindicated in IBD	$$$
Biguanides			
Metformin (Glucophage and Glucophage XR)	500 mg po qd–bid/2550 mg/day (2000 mg/day for XR)	Nausea, vomiting, diarrhea, lactic acidosis. Contraindicated if ethanol abuse, CHF, or renal insufficiency.	$$$
Metformin/Glyburide (Gluco Vance)	1.25/250 mg qd or bid with meals/10/2000 mg	Hypoglycemia, lactic acidosis, nausea, vomiting, diarrhea. Avoid if ethanol abuse, CHF, or renal failure.	$$$
Non-sulfonylureas secretagogues			
Nateglinide (Starlix)	60 mg tid before meals/360 mg	Hypoglycemia, weight gain, increased LFTs	$$$$
Repaglinide (Prandin)	0.5 mg tid before meals/16 mg	Hypoglycemia, weight gain, increased LFTs	$$$
Thiazolidinediones			
Pioglitazone (Actos)	15 mg po qd/45 mg	Hepatitis, edema. Monitor LFTs q 2 months for first year.	$$$$
Rosiglitazone (Avandia)	4 mg qd to bid/8 mg	Hepatitis, edema. Monitor LFTs q 2 month for first year.	$$$$

[1] Cost: $, AWP, $0–$10; $$, AWP, $10–25; $$$, AWP, $25–75; $$$$, AWP, $75–150.
AWP, average wholesale price; CHF, congestive heart failure; IBD, irritable bowel disease; LFTs, liver function tests.

1. **Oral sulfonylureas** act by enhancing insulin secretion. There is little cost difference among first-generation agents, although generic brands are less expensive.
2. **Second-generation oral sulfonylureas** are far more potent than first-generation agents, having a longer half-life allowing once- or twice-daily dosing, and thus these agents have become the drugs of choice for treating patients with type II DM. Second-generation agents lower hemoglobin A_{1C} levels by 1–2 percentage points on average, but can cause hypoglycemia and weight gain. All the sulfonylureas undergo hepatic metabolism and should be used with caution in patients with liver abnormalities. Glipizide is preferred in patients with renal abnormalities. Generic glipizide, glyburide, glimepiride (Amaryl), Glucotrol XL, and micronized glyburide are the most cost-effective agents in this class.
3. **Alpha-glucosidase inhibitors** inhibit the alpha-glucosidase enzyme that lines the brush border of the small intestine, delaying absorption of simple sugars. These drugs must be taken with each meal in order in order to lower postprandial glucose levels. On average, these agents lower hemoglobin A_{1C} by 0.5–percentage points. Patients taking these agents will have trouble treating hypoglycemic attacks with complex carbohydrates and so should have oral glucose tablets readily available. These agents are contraindicated in patients with bowel disease. These agents can be used in combination with other oral hypoglycemic agents.
4. **Metformin** (Glucophage) is a biguanide that acts by decreasing hepatic glucose output and increases utilization of glucose in peripheral tissues. Endogenous insulin is required for metformin to work. Metformin does not stimulate insulin secretion. Clinical trials suggest that metformin is as effective as other oral agents in the treatment of patients with type II DM, with less weight gain noted when compared with patients taking sulfonylureas. Metformin may be the agent of choice in type II DM patients who are obese or gain weight on other oral hypoglycemic agents. Adverse effects are mainly gastrointestinal and include nausea, vomiting, anorexia, diarrhea, and a metallic taste in the mouth. Lactic acidosis occurs rarely, but is potentially fatal. Since lactic acidosis usually occurs in the setting of renal failure, the drug should not be prescribed in patients with this condition. Metformin can be used with other oral hypoglycemic agents. Metformin has been used in patients with impaired glucose tolerance and shown to decrease the incidence of DM in that group (although a regimen of exercise and weight loss caused a greater decrease in the incidence of subsequent DM).
5. **Non-sulfonylureas secretagogues** rapid-acting agents that stimulate insulin release postprandially and thus must be taken before each meal. If a meal is missed, the drug should not be taken. Repaglinide is more effective than nateglinide, lowing hemoglobin A_{1C} by 1–2 percentage points on average. These drugs are more expensive than oral sulfonylureas but may prove useful in patients with renal impairment or patients who eat sporadically. These agents should be used cautiously in patients with liver abnormalities.
6. **Thiazolidinedione agents** enhance insulin action via direct stimulation of receptors in the nucleus of hepatic and skeletal muscle cells, thus directly increasing insulin sensitivity. On average, thiazolidinediones lower hemoglobin A_{1C} by 0.5–1.0 percentage points, at starting dosages. These agents can be used as monotherapy or in combination with other oral hypoglycemic agents. Only pioglitazone is currently approved by the US Food and Drug Administration for use with insulin. Liver function tests should be monitored every 2 months for the first 12 months in patients taking these agents and periodically thereafter. Weight gain due to fluid retention is also common and can lead to congestive heart failure.

D. **Insulin therapy**
   1. **Indications**
      a. **All patients with type I DM require insulin therapy.**
      b. Patients with type II DM may require insulin therapy if diet, exercise, and oral hypoglycemic agents do not control their DM sufficiently. Depending on the clinical situation, insulin may be added to oral hypoglycemics (for example, as a low dose of neutral protamine Hagedorn (NPH) insulin at bedtime [0.1 U/kg of body weight]), or oral hypoglycemics may be stopped and insulin started. Nocturnal insulin is then adjusted, based on the results of a morning FPG value. Insulin may also be indicated as initial therapy in patients with type II DM if the patient's initial fasting blood glucose value is >400 mg/dL, particularly in young, nonobese, symptomatic patients. As glucotoxicity is reduced, these patients may be able to

be switched to oral hypoglycemic agents. Premixed insulin preparations, such as Humulin or Novolin 70/30 (70% NPH, 30% regular), Humalog Mix 75/25 (75% insulin lispro protamine suspension and 25% lispro), and Novalog Mix 70/30 (70 insulin aspart protamine suspension and 30% insulin aspart), work particularly well in type II patients, with improvements in diabetic control due to decreased mixing errors. These premixed insulins are also appropriate to start as a single dose prior to dinner, rather than NPH insulin, when oral hypoglycemics cannot control the DM.

2. **Characteristics of insulin preparations.** Selection from available insulin preparation is based on **concentration** (usually U-100), **species source** (almost exclusively human insulin developed using recombinant DNA), **purity,** and **type** (Table 74–2). Recently rapid-acting insulins, insulin lispro and insulin aspart, have been developed and have been shown to be more effective than regular insulin in controlling postprandial blood sugar. Also, a long-acting insulin, insulin glargine, was recently released. Insulin glargine has no peak onset of action, mimicking basal insulin secretion. In patients with type I and type II DM, use of insulin glargine (rather than twice-a-day NPH), has been shown to be associated with less hypoglycemia, less weight gain, and better glucose control. Insulin glargine can be given once daily rather than twice a day.

3. **Initiating insulin therapy.** Patient newly diagnosed with type I DM either receive education and begin their insulin regimen while hospitalized or if not in ketoacidosis, can begin their insulin treatment as an outpatient. One injection of insulin per day rarely normalizes the glycemic response in such patients and often leaves type I DM patient hyperglycemic at night and in the morning. Therefore, patients with type I DM either typically receive a "split-dose" insulin regimen, consisting of a mixture of regular and NPH insulin before breakfast and in the late afternoon before supper, or now receive a once-daily shot of insulin glargine with shots of rapid-acting insulin prior to each meal. The amount of rapid-acting insulin given can be tailored to the amount of carbohydrate that will be eaten during the meal and the preprandial blood glucose value. Two methods are general used to initiate insulin therapy, as described below:

   a. Patients with type I DM may first receive preprandial and nighttime injections of either regular insulin or rapid-acting insulin based on preprandial blood glucose values shown in Table 74–3. When glucose values have stabilized, the daily insulin requirement is total. If "split-dose" insulin therapy is going to be used, then two thirds of the total amount of insulin is given in the morning and one third in the evening. The morning and evening dosages can then be split into 75% NPH and 25% regular insulin. If insulin glargine with rapid-acting insulin before each meal is used, then 40–50% of the total dose is given as insulin glargine first thing in the morning or at bedtime, with the other 50–60% split up and given as rapid-acting insulin prior to each meal based on preprandial glucose values.

   b. Alternatively, patients with type I DM can just begin "split-dose" therapy or therapy with insulin glargine and a rapid-acting insulin. Patients with type I DM should start with a total daily dose of 0.6 U/kg of body weight. Once again, if "split-dose"

TABLE 74–2. INSULIN TYPES

Type	Onset of Action (hr)	Maximum Action (hr)	Duration of Action (hr)
Rapid-acting			
Aspart (Lispro)	0.2–0.5	0.5–1	3–5
Short-acting			
Regular	0.5–1	2–3	4–12
Intermediate-acting			
Neutral protamine Hagedorn (NPH)	1–2	4–8	10–20
Lente	1–2	4–8	10–20
Long-acting			
Ultralente	2–4	8–20	24–32
Glargine	1–2	No peak	24

TABLE 74–3. TYPICAL SLIDING SCALE USED TO INITIATE INSULIN THERAPY

Blood Glucose Value (mg/dL)	Amount of Regular Insulin To Be Given (U)
150–200	6–8 U
200–250	8–12 U
250–300	12–16 U
>300	16–24 U

therapy is used, two thirds of that is given in the morning and one third in the evening. The morning and evening dosages are then split 75% NPH insulin and 25% regular insulin. If insulin glargine and rapid-acting insulin are used, 50% of the total daily dose is given as insulin glargine first thing in the morning, and the other 50% is given as rapid-acting insulin split up prior to each meal based on the results of preprandial glucose values. Self blood glucose monitoring (see section V,B) can then be used to adjust insulin therapy (Table 74–4).

4. **Intensive insulin therapy.** Three or more shots of insulin per day or the continuous subcutaneous insulin infusion (CSII) pump qualifies as intensive insulin therapy. Both methods require meticulous management including frequent self blood glucose monitoring in order to reduce the risk of hypoglycemic attacks and ensure good diabetic control. Although most primary care clinicians can manage three or more injections of insulin per day in their type I or type II DM patients, if four injections of insulin per day are not effective in achieving optimal glucose control, patients should be referred to an endocrinologist for consideration of CSII pump therapy.

5. **Honeymoon period.** Soon after insulin therapy is initiated, a "honeymoon period" of 12–18 months occurs in nearly all patients with type I or type II DM. During this time the patient's insulin requirements usually are drastically reduced. This phenomenon is thought secondary to reduced glucose toxicity. Therefore, patients should be encouraged to utilize self blood glucose monitoring, and the protocol should be designed so that they can reduce insulin therapy as their insulin requirements are reduced.

IV. **Management Strategies.** Achieving optimal diabetic control, near normal hemoglobin A_{1c} levels, while minimizing hypoglycemic episodes is the clear goal of treatment in patients with type I and type II DM. Achieving near normal hemoglobin A_{1c} levels in both type I and type II DM patients has been shown to reduce microvascular and macrovascular complications. Other risk factors for macrovascular complications, particularly in type II DM patients, should also be controlled, including blood pressure, cholesterol and triglyceride levels, and cessation of cigarette smoking. The American Diabetes Association (ADA) recommends that patients with DM strive for a hemoglobin A_{1c} of <7.0%, FPG of between 80 and 120 mg/dL, blood pressure <130/85 mm, a low-density lipoprotein cholesterol level <100 mg/dL, a high-density lipoprotein cholesterol level >40 mg/dL, triglycerides <150 mg/dL, and if smoking, patients should quit.

TABLE 74–4. ADJUSTMENT OF INSULIN DOSAGES BY SELF-MONITORING WITH A SPLIT-DOSE REGIMEN

Measurement Time	Dosage to Adjust if Blood Glucose Out of Target Range
0700	Afternoon NPH
1200	Morning regular
1700	Morning NPH
2200	Afternoon regular
0300	Afternoon NPH

Protocol for all insulin dosages
If blood glucose <60 mg/dL, decrease appropriate dose by 2 U
If 60 mg/dL < blood glucose <120 mg/dL, no adjustment
If 120 mg/dL < blood glucose <150 mg/dL, increase appropriate dose by 2 U
If 150 mg/dL < blood glucose <180 mg/dL, increase appropriate dose by 4 U
If blood glucose >180 mg/dL, increase appropriate dose by 6 U

NPH, neutral protamine Hagedorn.

A. **Hemoglobin A$_{1c}$ (glycosylated hemoglobin)** is one of several forms of hemoglobin A that result from the nonenzymatic attachment of glucose to hemoglobin A. Since the percentage of hemoglobin A$_{1c}$ depends on the average glucose concentration over the life of a red blood cell (approximately 120 days), hemoglobin A$_{1c}$ is a good measure of diabetic control over the previous 2–3 months. Hemoglobin A$_{1c}$ levels that are 1 percentage point above the upper range of normal for a particular reference laboratory indicate that the patient is not in optimal diabetic control and runs the risk of macrovascular and microvascular complications. Falsely elevated levels of hemoglobin A$_{1c}$ occur in the presence of uremia, fetal hemoglobin, alcoholism, and aspirin usage.

B. **Self-monitoring of blood glucose (SMBG).** This technique developed as the poor correlation between plasma glucose values and glycosuria became clear.

1. SMBG is a reliable technique, providing patients receive proper instruction in the procedure and potential problems.

2. Patients with diabetes who use SMBG determine their glucose values before meals, at bedtime, and occasionally in the middle of the night. They then adjust insulin dosages by using simple rules (Table 74–4). In addition, physicians can use the results of SMBG to adjust insulin dosages during regular follow-up visits. Patients with DM taking intensive insulin regimens must use SMBG to adjust dosages of preprandial insulin. SMBG is also helpful if patients with DM become ill, allowing adjustment of insulin dosages so that control is maintained during sickness.

3. Although the ADA recommends using SMBG at least twice daily in all patients with DM, because of cost, side effects, and recent epidemiologic studies that failed to show a correlation between frequency of SMBG use and diabetic control, most physicians compromise with their patients with type II DM. Patients with type II DM are typically asked to do SMBG only once daily but to vary the time so that over a 2- to 3-week period values have been obtained before all meals and at bedtime. Another option is to ask patients to do SMBG intensively four times daily for 3–5 days before seeing the physician.

C. **Reducing barriers to care.** Certain nonmedical factors are associated with poor diabetic control in patients with DM.

1. **Patient-centered care by the clinician.** Recent research has shown that encouraging the involvement of patients with DM in decisions regarding goal setting and management options improves glucose control. Excellent clinician-patient relationship and communication skills, particularly in the area of negotiation, also have been shown to be linked with improved control.

2. **Knowledge and self-management skills.** Patients with DM should be enrolled in an education program that discusses a wide range of topics pertinent to their care and encourages patient decision-making and self-management. A recent meta-analysis shows that such an approach increases knowledge about DM, increases the frequency and accuracy of SBMG, improves dietary habits, and improves glucose control.

3. **Psychosocial factors.** Clinicians should monitor for the following psychosocial factors that have been linked with poor diabetic control: pessimistic attitudes about DM, poor social support and social isolation, low self-efficacy skills, an external locus of control, excessive stress, being in precontemplation regarding necessary behavior change, and a passive pessimistic coping style. Screen all patients with DM periodically for depression and family dysfunction and recommend appropriate treatment. Determining use of complementary and alternative therapies by patients and discussing the efficacies of those therapies with patients has been shown to improve glucose control, as patients rely less on ineffective therapies.

4. **Health literacy.** Clinicians often use medical terminology that is not understood by patients. Patients rarely admit their ignorance, as that would cause embarrassment. Health illiteracy is commonplace and associated with decreased adherence to treatment regimens, inability to keep appointments, and not understanding instructions and education. If educational materials are used by clinicians, materials must be at a reading level and in a language understood by most patients.

5. **Financial.** Even with health insurance, the cost of medications and supplies for DM can be prohibitive. In those situations clinicians should make every attempt to use the most cost-effective treatment options available.

D. **Prevention and early detection of complications**

1. **Achieving near normal diabetic control.** Design of an effective treatment regimen and the assessment and correction of factors associated with poor diabetic

control and barriers to care constitute the first step in preventing the onset of both microvascular and macrovascular complications of DM. Risk factor reduction for macrovascular complications is essential, including smoking cessation, blood pressure control, and treatment of hyperlipidemia. Aspirin, 325 mg oral daily, to prevent macrovascular complications, is also indicated in all patients with type II DM.

   2. **Diagnosing complications as early as possible.** Period ophthalmologic, neurologic, vascular, renal (measurement of microalbuminuria), and foot examinations aid early diagnosis of diabetic complications. The exact frequency of examinations, except for annual ophthalmologic examinations and tests for microalbuminuria, has not been well studied; however, examining the feet of a diabetic patient at each visit has been associated with better diabetic control. Most clinicians follow up on patients with diabetes at least quarterly, with more frequent visits as necessary if diabetic control is poor.

   3. **Treating complications as they develop.** Once complications are diagnosed, risk-factor reduction and symptomatic treatment remain the mainstays of complication management. Painful peripheral neuropathies can often be treated with a low dose of a tricyclic antidepressant, such as amitriptyline, 50 mg orally at bedtime, whereas the progression of diabetic nephropathy can be slowed with an angiotensin-converting enzyme inhibitor (even if the patient is not hypertensive), such as captopril, 25–50 mg orally twice daily, or lisinopril, 10 mg orally daily.

E. **Office management.** An organized evidenced-based approach to the management of patients with DM in medical offices has been shown to improve diabetic control in patients visiting those offices. Use of multiple interventions has been associated with better control. Interventions include providing practitioner education through materials and meetings; developing a local consensus process regarding care protocols; auditing outcomes and providing that feedback to practitioners; using reminders for clinicians regarding when to conduct certain interventions, such as annual ophthalmologic examinations; enhancing the professional role of nurses in the office; and utilizing case management and disease management for patients who need that additional support. A multidisciplinary treatment team is needed for many patients, particularly those taking intensive insulin treatment regimens. Certain community-based interventions, such as diabetes self-management education in the community and self-management education programs in the home for children and adolescents with type I DM, have been shown to be effective. A recent study in the Oklahoma practice-based research network showed that exemplary clinicians, those with patients consistently in good glucose control and with good control of other risk factors for macrovascular complications, utilize the following successful strategies: **regularly scheduled follow-up visits,** a **chart label** identifying the patients with DM, **standard nurse/receptionist protocols,** a **diabetes registry,** use of a **limited number of consultants,** and a **chart documentation method** that reminded clinicians of activities they needed to do at each visit. More recently, the Kaiser Permanente System has popularized group visits for patients with DM. During these visits approximately 20 patients with DM receive a group educational session, discuss supportive strategies among themselves, and receive a brief visit from the clinician. Although the effects of these group visits have not been well studied, patients seem to be pleased with the camaraderie and social interaction.

V. **Prognosis.** The outcome of DM in a particular patient depends on several factors. These factors include the nature and severity of the disease in the patient, the simultaneous occurrence of other diseases, the presence of risk factors for diabetic complications (disease duration is the most important), genetic susceptibility to specific complications, and how well the patient responds to treatment. The patient's ability to adapt constructively to the disease also influences the course of the illness.

Patients with DM may experience acute complications, which develop over days to weeks and result in serious disturbances of fluid and electrolytes (diabetic ketoacidosis, nonketotic hyperosmolar coma, and hypoglycemia), and chronic complications, which develop gradually over months to years and involve nearly every organ system of the body, particularly the eyes, kidneys, vascular system, and nervous system.

A. **The mean survival** of patients with type I DM diagnosed before age 30 is currently 10–15 years less than that of the general population. Death usually results from end-stage renal disease (40–50%) or coronary artery disease, although ketoacidosis and hypoglycemic coma continue to cause significant mortality.

B. **Life expectancy** in type II DM patients is roughly one third less than that of age-matched nondiabetic patients. Cardiovascular disease accounts for 75% of the deaths in patients with type II DM after age 60. Except for ketoacidosis, all the complications associated with type I DM occur in patients with type II DM. Macrovascular complications are more common in type II DM patients, however. Hyperosmolar nonketotic coma, an acute complication, is seen almost exclusively in patients with non–insulin-dependent DM.

REFERENCES

American Diabetes Association: The Prevention or Delay of Type 2 Diabetes. Diabetes Care 2002; **25**(4):742.

Chaufan C: Patient compliance: In search of the real question in diabetes care. Am Fam Physician 2000;**61**(3):644.

DeWitt DE, Hirsch IB: Outpatient insulin therapy in type 1 and type 2 diabetes mellitus: Scientific review. JAMA 2003;**289**:2254.

Egede LE, Zheng D, Simpson K: Comorbid depression is associated with increased health care use and expenditures in individuals with diabetes. Diabetes Care 2002;**25**:464.

Huang ES, Meigs JB, Singer DE: The effect of interventions to prevent cardiovascular disease in patients with type 2 diabetes mellitus. Am J Med 2001;**111**(8):633.

Peterson KA, Hughes M: Readiness to change and clinical success in a diabetes educational program. J Am Board Fam Pract 2002;**15**(4):266.

Stratton IM, et al: Association of glycaemia with macrovascular and microvascular complications of type 2 diabetes (UKPDS 35): Prospective observational study. BMJ 2000;**321**:405.

---

75   Dyslipidemias

Michael A. Crouch, MD, MSPH

KEY POINTS

- One half of all American adults have **unhealthy blood lipid levels** (low-density lipoprotein [LDL] or high-density lipoprotein [HDL] cholesterol, or both, with or without triglycerides). Although higher cholesterol levels pose the greatest *relative* risk, over one half of all **myocardial infarctions** occur in those with suboptimal (100–129 mg/dL) or borderline (130–159 mg/dL) LDL cholesterol levels.
- Lowering intake of **dietary saturated fat, trans fats, and cholesterol** is the cornerstone for treating hypercholesterolemia and reducing risk for coronary heart disease. Other useful dietary measures include regular intake of fiber, fish, or fish oil (omega-3 fatty acids), nuts, soy protein, and plant sterols or stanols. Many patients with elevated LDL cholesterol require **medication** in addition to dietary modification to achieve **treatment target goals.** Weight loss and **exercise** raise HDL cholesterol and lower triglycerides but do not improve LDL cholesterol.
- **Dietary changes** maintained for 1 month lower LDL cholesterol all they are ever going to do. Prolonging dietary change yields no further reduction. It is not necessary to wait 6 months before initiating a trial of lipid medication. If 1 month of maintaining maximum achievable dietary change does not lower LDL cholesterol <130 mg/dL in a high-risk patient (>20% estimated 10-year coronary heart disease risk) or <160 in an intermediate-risk patient (10–20% estimated 10-year risk), it is appropriate to urge a trial of lipid medication. The most effective drugs for lowering LDL cholesterol are the HMG-CoA reductase inhibitors (**statins**). The usual daily starting dose is atorvastatin (Lipitor), 10 mg; rosuvastatin (Crestor), 5 mg; simvastatin (Zocor), 20 mg; pravastatin (Pravachol), 40 mg; lovastatin (Mevacor, Altocor), 40 mg; or fluvastatin (Lescol), 80 mg XL.
- The **goal** of hypercholesterolemia treatment is to reduce risk for **myocardial infarction** and **stroke** by one third or more, by lowering LDL cholesterol below **100 mg/dL** in those with diabetes or known coronary or carotid artery disease, or below **130 mg/dL** in high-risk patients not known to have diabetes or coronary or carotid artery disease.
- Long-term **compliance** with **statin therapy** is poor. Many patients are apprehensive about potential **adverse drug effects** and do not have a clear understanding of the **benefit/risk ratio.** Repetitive patient education in verbal, textual, and graphic formats, focused on specific patient concerns, may foster long-term statin compliance and maximize treatment benefit.

I. Introduction

A. Dyslipidemia is a broad term that includes several lipid disorders with primary genetic, secondary metabolic, lifestyle, and iatrogenic contributing factors.

1. Primary lipid disorders are **familial,** being transmitted across generations by both genetic factors and learned behaviors.

2. **Secondary** causes of dyslipidemias include diabetes mellitus, hypothyroidism, pregnancy, nephrotic syndrome, obstructive jaundice, chronic renal failure, dysgammaglobulinemia, anorexia nervosa, porphyria, and glycogen storage disease.

3. **Recommendations** for screening, diagnosis, and treatment are detailed in the **National Cholesterol Education Program (NCEP) Adult Treatment Panel (ATP) III guidelines (2001).**

B. Hyperlipidemia refers to elevated total blood cholesterol, low-density lipoprotein (LDL) cholesterol, or triglyceride (TG) levels (or both). **Familial combined (mixed) hyperlipidemia** is elevated LDL cholesterol and TGs.

C. Hypercholesterolemia is elevated total blood cholesterol (cutpoints below).

1. Familial heterozygous and homozygous hypercholesterolemia display Mendelian dominant inheritance, but most cases of hypercholesterolemia are polygenic.

2. The prevalence of hypercholesterolemia increases with age, peaking at age 55–65.

3. If 240 mg/dL (6.2 mmol/L) is used as the cutoff for elevated total cholesterol, about 10% of adults have hypercholesterolemia.

4. Given the designated cutoff value of 200 mg/dL (5.2 mmol/L) for borderline elevated total cholesterol, approximately 50% of adults in the United States have borderline elevated or high total cholesterol.

D. Hypertriglyceridemia is elevated fasting triglycerides.

1. High TG is >200 mg/dL or 1.7 mmol/L).

2. TGs of 150–199 mg/dL (1.3–1.7 mmol/L) are "borderline high."

3. Elevated TGs are seen in 20–25% of American adults.

4. Saturated fat and cholesterol are absorbed from the gut and packaged into TG-rich particles called chylomicrons. These chylomicrons are broken down into very low density lipoprotein (VLDL) particles that are rich in TGs.

5. Excessive **alcohol,** dietary **sugars,** and rapidly digested **starches** elevate TGs.

6. **Physical inactivity** or being **overweight** or **obese** elevates TGs and VLDL cholesterol.

E. Hyperbetalipoproteinemia is elevated LDL cholesterol. LDL cholesterol is one of the main risk factors for coronary artery disease (CAD).

1. High LDL cholesterol is >160 mg/dL (4.15 mmol/L).

2. "Borderline high" LDL cholesterol level is 130–159 mg/dL (3.35–4.15 mmol/L).

3. "Above optimal" LDL cholesterol is 100–129 mg/dL (2.6–3.35 mmol/L).

4. Optimal LDL cholesterol is <100 mg/dL (2.6 mmol/L).

5. CAD often occurs when LDL cholesterol stays in the 100–159 mg/dL range longterm, especially in the presence of diabetes, smoking, or multiple other major risk factors (Figure 75–1).

6. VLDL particles are metabolized (catalyzed by the enzyme lipoprotein lipase) into cholesterol-rich LDL particles. LDL particles attach to LDL receptors on cell membranes. Cholesterol from the LDL particles passes into cells. Influx of cholesterol into cells suppresses the activity of the rate-limiting enzyme in cholesterol synthesis, 3-hydroxy-3-methylglutaryl coenzyme A (HMG-CoA) reductase.

7. Excessive dietary intake of **saturated fat** raises LDL and total cholesterol more than does excessive cholesterol intake.

8. **Stress** and **coronary-prone (Type A) behavior** can markedly elevate LDL cholesterol and total blood cholesterol in susceptible persons.

9. **Iatrogenic** causes of lipid problems are common.

   a. **Diuretics** raise LDL cholesterol transiently but seldom have significant longterm effects.

   b. **Beta blockers** without intrinsic sympathomimetic activity (propranolol, etc) lower HDL cholesterol and may raise LDL cholesterol.

   c. **Chenodiol,** a gallstone dissolver, lowers both HDL cholesterol and LDL cholesterol.

   d. **Oral contraceptives** with strong androgen/progestin effect lower HDL cholesterol, raise TGs, and sometimes raise LDL cholesterol.

   e. High-dose **steroids** and **disulfiram** (Antabuse) raise TGs.

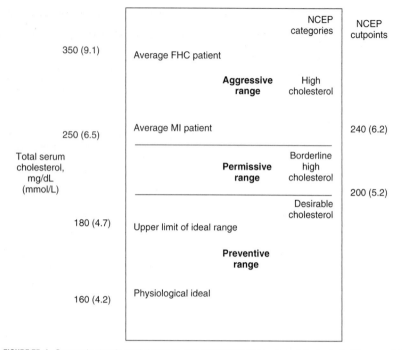

FIGURE 75–1. Prognostic range for total cholesterol. FHC, familial heterozygous hypercholesterolemia; MI, myocardial infarction; NCEP, National Cholesterol Education Program.

F. Hypoalphalipoproteinemia is low high-density lipoprotein (HDL) cholesterol.
   1. Low HDL cholesterol is <40 mg/dL or 1.0 mmol/L.
   2. Borderline low HDL cholesterol is 40–49 mg/dL (1.0–1.3 mmol/L).
   3. Five to 10% of adults have low HDL cholesterol, mostly on an inherited basis.
   4. HDL particles facilitate LDL metabolism, which results in cholesterol being carried back to the liver from peripheral tissues.
   5. Patients with low HDL cholesterol and elevated TGs tend to have smaller, more dense LDL particles that are more atherogenic.
   6. **Physical inactivity** or being **overweight** or **obese** decreases HDL_2 cholesterol.
   7. **Cigarette smoking** decreases HDL_2 cholesterol.
   8. **Alcohol** in moderation raises HDL_3 cholesterol, but not HDL_2 cholesterol.
G. Metabolic syndrome is a risk factor constellation seen in almost 25% of United States adults. It is associated with an extremely high risk for CHD. Metabolic syndrome is present if a patient has three or more of the following risk factors:
   1. Waist size greater than 40 in (102 cm) for men or greater than 35 in (89 cm) for women.
   2. Triglyceride level at or above 150 mg/dL (1.7 mmol/L).
   3. Blood pressure at or above 130/85 mm Hg.
   4. Fasting glucose value at or above 110 mg/dL (6.1 mmol/L).
   5. HDL-C level less than 40 mg/dL (1.0 mmol/L) for men or less than 50 mg/dL (1.3 mmol/L) for women.
II. Diagnosis
   A. Symptoms and signs. Lipid problems are usually asymptomatic for several decades.
      1. **Arcus senilis, xanthelasma, tendon xanthomas, and eruptive xanthomas** are late or uncommon physical signs of lipid problems.
      2. **Retinal arteriovenous crossing changes** signal atherosclerosis.

3. **Angina pectoris, intermittent claudication, and impotence** may develop as warning symptoms of advanced atherosclerosis.

4. **Myocardial infarction, cerebrovascular accident (stroke), or sudden death** is often the first sign of a lipid problem.

B. Laboratory tests

1. **Screening** is recommended by the National Cholesterol Education Program (NCEP) every 3–5 years for most adults younger than age 70. Adults with LDL cholesterol levels <130 mg/dL (3.35 mmol/L) and HDL levels >50 mg/dL (1.3 mmol/L) probably do not need to be rescreened this often unless they experience major changes in weight, diet, or physical activity. Children and adolescents with a family history of severe dyslipidemia or early atherosclerotic disease should also be screened.

   a. A **random or fasting lipid profile** (with total, LDL, and HDL cholesterol and TGs) should be obtained initially to detect elevated LDL cholesterol or TGs and low HDL cholesterol. The more convenient random lipid profile increases compliance with screening, and it gives useful information about the extent of postprandial hyperlipemia (considered to be a serious atherogenic factor).

   b. If a patient is at **high risk** for CAD and random LDL cholesterol levels are marginally or mildly elevated, a **fasting lipid profile** should be obtained to more accurately categorize the severity of elevated LDL cholesterol.

2. **Interpreting cholesterol results**

   a. Blood lipids change acutely in response to food intake. The TG level is lowest in the fasting state, rises by an average of 50 mg/dL postprandially, and peaks 3–6 hours after a meal. As the TG level rises, total and LDL cholesterol each fall by an average of 5–15 mg/dL. Thus total and LDL cholesterol tend to be higher when fasting. HDL cholesterol varies little between the fasting and postprandial states, averaging 45 mg/dL (1.16 mmol/L) for men and 55 mg/dL (1.42 mmol/L) for women.

   b. Blood lipids can fluctuate within minutes, days, or weeks in response to illness, emotional stress, or malnutrition.

   c. Blood lipid levels may fluctuate seasonally. In colder climates, cholesterol and TG levels tend to be somewhat higher in winter because of higher fat intake.

   d. Ranges of total blood cholesterol and LDL cholesterol that are preventive, permissive, or aggressive with respect to their risk for promoting atherosclerosis are shown in Figures 75–1 and 75–2.

3. **Diagnosing lipid disorders**

   a. If a screening lipid profile shows elevated LDL cholesterol, low HDL cholesterol, or high TGs, a **second lipid profile** should be obtained (fasting) before starting treatment, to confirm elevation and establish an accurate baseline.

   b. **Excluding secondary causes.** If symptoms or signs are suggestive, the physician should consider ordering thyroid, renal, or liver function tests to rule out secondary causes of dyslipidemia.

   c. **Prognosis categorization** identifies those patients at highest risk. **Lipid ratios** summarize two or more lipid values into one number that correlates strongly with long-term prognosis; however, these ratios (total cholesterol:HDL cholesterol or LDL cholesterol:HDL cholesterol) predict outcome only marginally better than absolute HDL cholesterol and LDL cholesterol values.

      (1) At **highest risk** are patients who **smoke** or have **diabetes mellitus, the metabolic syndrome, left ventricular hypertrophy,** or moderately elevated **C-reactive protein** levels.

      (2) Patients who have **low HDL** cholesterol levels are at some increased risk even if their LDL cholesterol levels are not elevated. Of the lipid values, HDL cholesterol is the best single predictor of adverse outcome. Above average or high HDL cholesterol levels (>60 mg/dL or 1.55 mmol/L) however, do not guarantee immunity from CAD. Recent research has identified a pro-inflammatory form of HDL in the blood of some patients who have HDL levels >80 mg/dL (2.1 mmol/L); this form of HDL greatly increases the risk for atherosclerosis.

      (3) Patients with markedly elevated LDL cholesterol levels (>190 mg/dL, or 4.9 mmol/L) are at increased risk even if they have HDL cholesterol levels at or above average.

      (4) Patients with high fasting TG levels are at increased risk, especially obese females with diabetes mellitus.

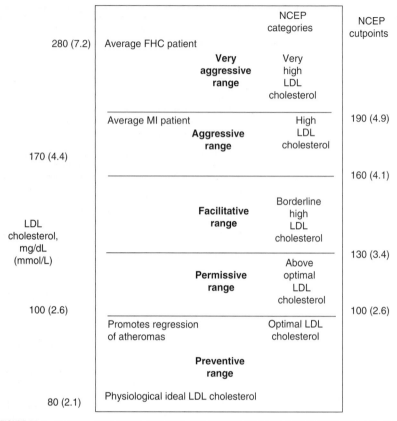

FIGURE 75–2. Prognostic range for LDL cholesterol. FHC, familial heterozygous hypercholesterolemia; LDL, low-density lipoprotein; MI, myocardial infarction; NCEP, National Cholesterol Education Program.

    d. Additional tests sometimes can be helpful to refine a patient's estimated risk and adjust the aggressiveness of treatment, especially in those a strong family history of CAD or stroke.

       (1) C-reactive protein (CRP) levels predict risk for myocardial infarction and stroke even better than LDL cholesterol levels do, when measured in healthy persons. CRP should be measured with the high-sensitivity cardiac method, not the older quantitative method. CRP is produced by the liver as an acute-phase reactant, quickly rising to exceed 10 mg/L with many acute infectious and inflammatory illnesses, and staying high with some chronic conditions (seen in about 5% of all patients screened). It falls rapidly to an individual's usual chronic level when illness resolves. About 25% of patients have high-risk levels of 3.0–10.0 mg/L (Table 75–1). About 50% of patients have "average risk" levels of 1.0–2.9 mg/dL, leaving 25% with low-risk levels <1.0 mg/dL. A CRP level of >10.0 mg/L usually indicates acute or chronic illness and should be repeated. A moderately elevated CRP should be repeated a few weeks later, at least once. It is unknown how often CRP should be retested for those with abnormal or normal results, and whether lowering CRP with aspirin or a statin is beneficial.

       (2) Homocysteine elevation predicts risk for myocardial infarction and stroke. Elevated homocysteine (>10.0 mg/L) is seen in about 5% of adults. No in-

TABLE 75–1. C-REACTIVE PROTEIN RISK PREDICTION RANGES

	C-Reactive Protein Level (mg/L)	Prevalence
Lowest risk	<1.00	25%
Average risk	1.00–2.99	45%
High risk	3.00–10.00	25%
Out of usual range	>10.00	5%

tervention outcome study results are available to evaluate the effects of lowering homocysteine with folate, pyridoxine, or vitamin B_{12}. (*Note: They are usually given together.*)

(3) **Apolipoprotein levels** predict outcome more accurately than does LDL cholesterol or HDL cholesterol, but their clinical usefulness has not been proved. Apolipoprotein levels can sometimes help the physician to decide how aggressively to treat patients with LDL cholesterol levels of 130–189 mg/dL (3.35–4.90 mmol/L) and patients with HDL cholesterol <40 mg/dL (1.0 mmol/L) whose LDL cholesterol is <130 mg/dL (3.35 mmol/L).

  (a) Prognosis is poor if the level of **apolipoprotein B,** the main apolipoprotein in LDL, is elevated.

  (b) A low level of **apolipoprotein A-I,** the main apolipoprotein in HDL, also indicates a poor prognosis.

(4) **Lipoprotein (a)** is a modified LDL moiety similar to plasminogen. Lipoprotein(a) elevation >50 mg/dL signals a bad prognosis, even if LDL cholesterol is <130 mg/dL (3.35 mmol/L). The test may be more useful than apolipoprotein levels for clarifying prognosis and adjusting treatment aggressiveness in marginal cases.

(5) **PLAC** is a newly available clinical test that measures the level of the enzyme **Lp-PLA2.** Lp-PLA2 combines with LDL and facilitates its movement into the arterial intima, where LDL becomes oxidized and accumulates in atheromatous plaque. Individuals with elevated Lp-PLA2 have a twofold increased CAD risk. Those with elevated Lp-PLA2 and CRP have a threefold increased risk.

(6) **Pro-inflammatory HDL** is measured by a test under development that may soon be available clinically. This test may help clarify the risk status of those with high HDL levels who also have strong family histories of CAD.

III. Treatment
  A. Treatment recommendations and treatment goals should be established based on the patient's clinical status, other risk factors (Table 75–2), and estimated 10-year risk for CHD (Table 75–3).
  B. The estimated 10-year risk for CHD is a key step in evaluating candidacy for statin therapy for patients not known to have diabetes, CHD, or CHD-equivalent.
    1. Ten-year CHD risk can be estimated manually using the NCEP risk calculator sheet (see section III,B,2,b, below).
    2. The 10-year risk for CHD can be estimated more quickly and easily by:
      a. Using any reliable Internet risk calculator online (http://hin.nhlbi.nih.gov/atpiii/calculator/.asp?usertype=prof).
      b. Downloading a risk calculator program for local use with a computer or personal digital assistant from a web site such as http://www.pdacortex.com/NCEP_ATPIII_CHD_Risk_Calculator_Download.htm
  C. With **clinical CAD** or CAD-equivalent (peripheral artery disease, abdominal aortic aneurysm, or symptomatic carotid artery disease, including transient ischemic attack and stroke), diabetes, or an estimated 10-year CHD risk above 20%, treatment goals are to lower LDL cholesterol to <**100** mg/dL (2.60 mmol/L). Treatment goals for other levels of risk are shown in Table 75–3.
  D. For all hyperlipidemic patients, the **TG goal** is to lower fasting TG to <**150** mg/dL (1.3 mmol/L).
  E. **Hygienic approaches** often improve lipid levels effectively. It is appropriate to encourage lifestyle changes in anyone with LDL cholesterol >130 mg/dL or HDL cholesterol

TABLE 75-2. OTHER RISK FACTORS FOR CORONARY ARTERY DISEASE

Factors cited by the National Cholesterol Education Program
Male gender
Cigarette smoking
Diabetes mellitus
Hypertension
Low HDL-cholesterol
Obesity
Personal history of atherosclerotic disease
Family history of lipid disorder
Family history of atherosclerotic disease (especially men <55 years and women <65 years)

Other factors (not cited by the National Cholesterol Education Program)
C-reactive protein elevation
Homocysteine elevation
Lipoprotein (a) elevation
Apolipoprotein B elevation
Low apolipoprotein A-I level
Postmenopausal status for females
Lp-PLA2 elevation
Small, dense low-density lipoprotein particles
Pro-inflammatory high-density lipoprotein
Coronary-prone (Type A) behavior or personality
Old age (risk rises with increasing age)

<40 mg/dL (1.0 mmol/L). Those with HDL cholesterol levels in the 40- to 49-mg/dL (1.03–1.16 mmol/L) range may also be appropriate candidates for exercise counseling.

1. **Dietary modification.** Depending on baseline diet, eating less saturated fat and cholesterol can often lower total blood cholesterol by 10–20%. Key dietary changes for lowering elevated cholesterol are listed below.
   a. Eat **less beef and pork** (especially fatty cuts).
   b. Eat **cold-water fish** twice a week (salmon, tuna, herring, mackerel). Fish that tend to have high mercury content (eg, swordfish) should be limited to once a month.
   c. Eat more **chicken** and **turkey** (white "skinless" meat).
   d. Eat 40–50 g of **soy protein** a day (tofu, soy burger, soy dog, soy milk).
   e. Drink **nonfat, ½%, or 1% fat milk,** instead of 2% or whole milk (3.5% fat). Eat minimal amounts of other whole-milk dairy products such as cheese, butter, ice cream, and sour cream.
   f. Use **polyunsaturated oil products** (safflower, corn, soybean) or **monounsaturated oil products** (olive) for margarine and cooking oil (desired ratio of polyunsaturated to saturated fat is >1.5:1). **Avoid hydrogenated oils** present in **stick margarines;** instead use **tub margarines** (preferably small amounts).
   g. Minimize intake of commercial **fried fast foods,** which are the main source of trans fats.

TABLE 75-3. LDL CHOLESTEROL TREATMENT GOALS

	Treatment Goal for LDL Cholesterol	
	2 or More CAD Risk Factors mg/dL (mmol/L)	<2 CAD RiskFactors mg/dL (mmol/L)
Known CAD or diabetes	<100 (<2.6)	<100 (<2.6)
No known CAD		
10-year risk = >20%	<100 (<2.6)	<100 (<2.6)
10-year risk = 10–20%	<130 (<3.35)	<160 (<4.2)
10-year risk = <10%	<160 (<4.2)	<190 (<4.9)

CAD, coronary artery disease; LDL, low-density lipoprotein.

   h. Eat **oat bran** as cereal or muffins, three to six servings per day. Oat bran can reduce total cholesterol and LDL cholesterol an average of 5–10% in some patients with elevated LDL cholesterol.
   i. Eat **nuts** (walnuts, pecans, almonds, peanuts, cashews) as a protein source, 1 oz a day. Nuts are high in alpha-linolenic acid, which is converted to omega-3 fatty acids in the body. Mounting evidence links nut intake with reduced risk for CAD events.
   j. **Fish oil** high in omega-3 fatty acids (ie, eicosapentaenoic [EPA] and docahexaenoic [DHA]) has been shown to be beneficial. Fish oils decrease secretion of TGs by the liver, and reduce hypertriglyceridaemia, but there is little or no effect on total blood cholesterol level and HDL-cholesterol. LDL-cholesterol level is unchanged or may increase with fish oil consumption. If regular intake of cold-water fish is ineffective or unacceptable, three capsules a day of fish oil provides close to the 1 g/day of EPA plus DHA that is recommended for preventive intake. To lower TGs, the recommended dose of is 2–4 g/day of EPA plus DHA daily.
   k. **Plant stanols** or **sterols** can be beneficial as dietary supplements. Plant stanols derived from soybeans and corn are available in over-the-counter products (eg, Benecol, Take Control). Stanols block absorption of dietary and biliary cholesterol in the intestine. Sterols work similarly but are absorbed more readily than stanols. Benecol costs about $5 per week when used as a food spread, like margarine. It has no significant medication interactions and no demonstrated side effects. At the recommended dose of 2–3 servings per day, plant stanols lower total cholesterol by 10–12% and reduce LDL-C by 14–17%.
   2. Exercise. Regular aerobic exercise, at least 30 minutes at a time, three or more times a week, raises HDL cholesterol by 5–15 mg/dL, lowers TG and VLDL cholesterol, and sometimes lowers LDL cholesterol. Walking daily for several miles has been shown to have smaller favorable effects on lipids.
   3. Weight loss lowers TG and VLDL cholesterol, raises HDL cholesterol by 5–10 mg/dL, but lowers LDL cholesterol only transiently during the weight reduction period.
   4. Smoking cessation increases HDL cholesterol by 5–10 mg/dL but does not affect LDL cholesterol, VLDL cholesterol, or TGs.
   5. Behavioral modification for coronary-prone (Type A) behavior may lower LDL cholesterol in the absence of other interventions.
F. Medications. The 2001 NCEP Adult Treatment Panel III recommends medical treatment if LDL cholesterol remains >190 mg/dL (4.9 mmol/L) despite hygienic management, regardless of the patient's clinical status and other CAD risk factors. If the patient has diabetes, coronary or carotid artery disease, or a 10-year estimated CHD risk over 20%, medication is recommended if LDL cholesterol stays >130 mg/dL (3.35 mmol/L). For these high-risk patients, medication is considered optional for the 100–129 mg/dL (2.6–3.35 mmol/L) range. The guidelines for drug therapy with other combinations of risk factors and LDL cholesterol levels are shown in Tables 75–4 to 75–7.
   1. Over-the-counter drugs are sometimes the preferred choice for medical treatment because they are inexpensive and relatively safe, and some are fairly effective (Table 75–4).
      a. Psyllium hydrophilic mucilloid (Metamucil and other brands). Psyllium, which lowers LDL cholesterol and total cholesterol an average of 5–10%, is a logical choice to treat mildly elevated LDL cholesterol (130–159 mg/dL) when HDL

TABLE 75–4. LDL CHOLESTEROL DRUG THERAPY LEVELS

Risk Category	10-Year Estimated Risk for CHD	LDL Level for Considering Drug Therapy
CHD or CHD risk equivalent (diabetes, stroke)	>20%	≥130 mg/dL (3.35 mmol/L) (100–129 mg/dL or 2.6 mmol/L: drug optional)
2+ risk factors	10–20% <10%	≥130 mg/dL (3.35 mmol/L) >160 mg/dL (4.2 mmol/L)
0–1 risk factors (not diabetes)	usually <10%	>190 mg/dL (4.9 mmol/L) (160–189 mg/dL or 4.2–4.9 **mmol/L: drug optional**)

TABLE 75-5. HOW TO RECOMMEND AND PRESCRIBE LIPID-ALTERING MEDICATIONS

Medication	Retail Cost[1]
Over-the-counter medications	
Psyllium hydrophilic mucilloid (PHM)	$7–10/mo unsweetened/with sugar;
Metamucil or equivalent	artificially sweetened $15–21/mo; orange/lemon-line
1 heaping tsp (tbsp if with sugar)	$11–21/mo
in 8 oz water/liquid, tid with meals	Metamucil Instant Mix $25/mo
Fiberall Fruit & Nut Fiber Wafer, 3.4-g	
1 to 2 wafers, tid with 8 oz+ liquid	$35–40/mo if sole PHM source
Niacin/nicotinic acid (OTC, regular release	$8–14 for 100 tab; max 3 g/d
500/750-mg tab)	
Sig: one to two 500-mg tab bid with meal	$10/20 mo for 1/2 g/d
One 750-mg tab bid with meal (med.)	$12/mo for 1.5 g/d
Niacin (Slo-Niacin), 500-mg or 750-mg ER	$35/25 for 180 tab of 500/750-mg
Initial dose: 1 tab bid	$15/10/mo
Increase to 2 tab bid in wk 2	$30/20/mo
Prescription medications	
Atorvastatin (Lipitor), 10/20/40/80-mg tab	$200/285/285/300 for 90 tab 10/20/40/80
Sig: 10 mg qd evening (usual start dose)	$65/mo
20 mg qd evening (medium dose)	$95/mo
40 mg qd evening (high dose)	$95/mo
80 mg qd evening (very high dose)	$1000/mo
Cholestyramine (generic/Questran), powder	$125/$215, 4 cans of cholestyramine powder or $150 for
(378 g/can or 4-g pks)	3 cartons (180 pks)
Sig: one 4-g scoop or pack bid (start dose)	$45/mo generic or $100/mo Questran
two 4-g scoops or packs bid (maint.)	$90/mo generic or $200/mo Questran
two 4-g scoops or packs tid (max dose)	$135/mo generic or $300/mo Questran
Cholestyramine (Questran Light or Prevalite),	$215, for 4 cans of generic or Questran Light or
powder (210 g/can; 1 pk = 4 g)	180 pks of Prevalite
Sig: one 4-g scoop or pack bid (start dose)	$55/mo
two 4-g scoops or packs bid (maint)	$175/mo
two 4-g scoops or packs tid (max dose)	$230/mo or $360/mo
Colesevelam (Welchol), 625 mg,	$440 for 540 tabs
Sig: 3 tabs, bid	$145/mo
Colestipol (Colestid), flavored granules,	$285 for three 450-g cans
Sig: 1 scoops (5 g) bid	$65/mo
2 scoops (10 g) bid	$130/mo
3 scoops (15 g) bid	$195/mo
Colestipol (Colestid), 1-g tab	$75 for 120 one-g tabs
Sig: 5 tabs, bid (start dose)	$190/mo
10 tabs, bid (medium dose)	$380/mo
15 tabs, bid (max. dose)	$570/mo
Colestipol (Colestid), 5-g powder pk	$165 for 90 five-g powder pks
Sig: 1 pk, bid (start dose)	$105/mo
2 pks, bid (medium dose)	$210/mo
3 pks, bid (max. dose)	$315/mo
Colestipol (Colestid), 7.5-g flavored gran. pk	$130 for 60 flavored granule pks
Sig: 1 pk bid (start dose)	$130/mo
2 pks bid (max dose)	$260/mo
Colestipol (Colestid), unflavored gran. can	$110 for 500 g unflavored granules
Sig: 1 scoop (5 g) bid (start dose)	$65/mo
2 scoops (10 g) bid (medium dose)	$130/mo
3 scoops (15 g) bid (max. dose)	$195/mo
Ezetimibe (Zetia), 10-mg tab	$210 for 90 tab
Sig: 1 tab, qd (usually taken with statin)	$70/mo
Fenofibrate (Tricor), 54/160-mg tab	$100/$300 for 90 tab
one tab qd (usual dose)	$33/100/mo
Fluvastatin (Lescol), 20/40/80-mg tab	$165/165/225 for 90 tab of 20/40/80 mg
Sig: 20 mg qd evening (low dose)	$60/mo
40 mg qd evening (medium dose)	$60/mo
80 mg SR, qd evening (usual dose)	$75/mo

(*continued*)

TABLE 75–5. (*Continued*)

Medication	Retail Cost[1]
Gemfibrozil (generic/Lopid), 600-mg tab	$60/245 for 180 tab
Sig: 1 tab bid with meals (usual dose)	$20/80/mo (generic/Lopid)
Lovastatin (generic), 10/20/40-mg tab	$90/165/300 for 90 tab of 10/20/40 mg
Sig: 10 mg qd evening (low dose)	$30/mo
20 mg qd evening (usual start dose)	$55/mo
40 mg qd evening (medium dose)	$100/mo
two 40-mg tabs qd evening (high dose)	$200/mo
Lovastatin (Mevacor), 10/20/40-mg tab	$115/200/360 for 90 tab of 10/20/40 mg
Sig: 10 mg qd evening (low dose)	$40/mo
20 mg qd evening (usual start dose)	$65/mo
40 mg qd evening (medium dose)	$120/mo
two 40-mg tabs qd evening (high dose)	$240/mo
Lovastatin (Altocor), 40/60-mg ER tab	$185/205 for 90 tab of 40/60 mg
Sig: 40 mg ER qd evening (low dose)	$60/mo
60 mg ER qd evening (high dose)	$70/mo
Lovastatin-niacin (Advicor),	$155/190/200 for 90 tab of 20–500/20–750/20–1000-mg
20–500/20–750/20–1000-mg tab	
Sig: 1 tab (20–500-mg), qd (low dose)	$50/mo
1 tab (20–500-mg or 20–750-mg), bid	$65/mo
1 tab (20–1000-mg), bid (high dose)	$65/mo
Niacin/nicotinic acid (Niaspan),	$230/300/375 for 180 tab of 500/750/1000-mg
500/750/1000-mg XR tab	
Sig: one 500-mg tab bid with meal (start)	$75/mo
One 750-mg tab bid with meal (med.)	$100/mo
one 1000-mg tab bid with meal (maint.)	$125/mo
Pravastatin (Pravachol), 10/20/40/80-mg tab	$255/255/375/375 for 90 of 10/20/40/80 mg
Sig: 10 mg qd evening (low dose)	$85/mo
20 mg qd evening (usual start dose)	$85/mo
40 mg qd evening (medium dose)	$125/mo
80 mg qd evening (high dose)	$125/mo
Rosuvastatin (Crestor), 5/10/20/40 mg tab	$210/210/210/210 for 90 of 5/10/20/40 mg
Sig: 5 mg qd evening (low dose)	$70/mo
10 mg qd evening (usual starting dose)	$70/mo
20 mg qd evening (medium dose)	$70/mo
40 mg qd evening (high dose)	$70/mo
Simvastatin (Zocor), 5/10/20/40/80 mg	$155/200/345/345/345 for 90 of 5/10/20/40/80 mg tabs
Sig: ½ a 10-mg or one 5-mg tab	
qpm (very low dose)	$35/50/mo
½ a 20-mg or one 10-mg tab qpm (low)	$60/115/mo
½ a 40-mg or one 20-mg tab qpm (start)	$60/115/mo
½ an 80-mg or one 40-mg tab qpm (med)	$60/115/mo
one 80-mg tab qd evening (high dose)	$115/mo

[1] Quoted by least expensive community pharmacy, December 200 survey, Houston, TX.
ER, extended release; Maint, maintenance dose; Start, starting dose.

cholesterol is >45 mg/dL, especially in elderly patients. It promotes bowel regularity and sometimes causes flatulence, but causes no serious adverse effects.

   b. Niacin. Niacin is a logical first choice for treating the healthy patient with moderately elevated LDL cholesterol who also has either low HDL cholesterol (<35 mg/dL) or high TGs. Niacin has demonstrated value for preventing myocardial infarction and CAD death.

   (1) When taken in a dose of 1–3 g/day, niacin lowers LDL cholesterol by 15–20%, markedly lowers elevated TGs, and raises HDL cholesterol by 5–15 mg/dL. Patients should begin with a low dose of 100–200 mg of the regular release form or 250–500 mg of the sustained-release form (Slo-Niacin); then the dose should be gradually increased to a maximum of 2–3 g/day based on patient tolerance.

   (2) Most patients experience minimal flushing and itching when taking sustained-release niacin. Patients who experience flushing and itching

TABLE 75–6. RETAIL COST[1] OF THERAPEUTIC EQUIVALENT DOSES OF HMG-CoA-REDUCTASE INHIBITORS (STATINS)*

Lovastatin	Fluvastatin	Simvastatin	Pravastatin			
generic	Lescol	Zocor	Pravachol			
20 mg	40 mg	10 mg	20 mg			
$55	$60	$65	$85			

Lovastatin-niacin	Lovastatin	Atorvastatin	Rosuvastatin	Fluvastatin	Simvastatin	Pravastatin
Advicor	Altocor	Lipitor	Crestor	Lescol	Zocor	Pravachol
20–500 mg	40 mg	10 mg	5 mg	80 mg	20 mg	40 mg
$50	$60	$65	$70	$75	$115	$125

Lovastatin-niacin	Lovastatin	Rosuvastatin	Atorvastatin	Simvastatin	Pravastatin
Advicor	Altocor	Crestor	Lipitor	Zocor	Pravachol
20–1000	60 mg	10 mg	20 mg	40 mg	80 mg
$65	$70	$70	$95	$115	$125

Rosuvastatin	Atorvastatin	Simvastatin
Crestor	Lipitor	Zocor
20 mg	40 mg	80 mg
$70	$95	$115

Rosuvastatin	Atorvastatin
Crestor	Lipitor
40 mg	80 mg
$70	$100

[1] Least expensive community pharmacy, December 2003 survey, Houston, TX, 3-Hydroxy-3-methylglutaryl coenzyme A (HMG-CoA) reductase inhibitors (statins).
*Based on taking whole tablets.

can block much of the adverse symptoms by taking 325 mg of aspirin daily before the first dose.

    (3) Although it is sometimes well tolerated and usually safe, niacin can worsen diabetic hyperglycemia, exacerbate gout, precipitate serious arrhythmias in patients with heart disease, or cause severe reversible liver toxicity.

2. Prescription drugs for modifying lipids all are relatively costly, especially higher doses (Table 75–5).

    a. Cholestyramine (Questran). This resin sequesters bile acids in the gut. It is available as a powder to be mixed with water or food. Questran Light may be more palatable for long-term compliance. Cholestyramine is a logical choice for the patient with moderate LDL cholesterol elevation and HDL cholesterol levels >45 mg/dL who will tolerate its inconvenient form.

    When two scoops or packs are taken two to three times a day, cholestyramine lowers LDL cholesterol and total cholesterol by 15–20%. Because over four doses a day causes severe constipation, the maximal dose of six scoops/packs a day is poorly tolerated.

    b. Colestipol (Colestid) is very similar to cholestyramine in form, dose, efficacy, high cost, and poor patient tolerance, with no advantages.

    c. Colesevelam (Welchol) is another resin binder similar to cholestyramine and colestipol, with no demonstrated advantages.

    d. Gemfibrozil (Lopid) changes the hepatic metabolism of lipoproteins. Gemfibrozil is a logical choice for the patient with low HDL cholesterol and moderately or severely elevated TGs who has not tolerated or responded well to niacin. The drug is well tolerated and appears to be relatively safe for long-term use.

    (1) Gemfibrozil lowers LDL cholesterol by 5–15%, markedly lowers TGs, and raises HDL cholesterol by 5–15 mg/dL. The usual dose is 600 mg twice a day; the maximum dose is 900 mg twice a day or 600 mg three times per day.

TABLE 75–7. COST-EFFECTIVE MEDICATION REGIMENS FOR TREATING ELEVATED LDL-CHOLESTEROL

Baseline LDL-C (mg/dL)	LDL-C Treatment Goal	
	<130 mg/dL	<100 mg/dL
130–159	Fluvastatin (Lescol), one-half a 40-mg tab qd, $30/mo, or lovastatin, generic, one 10-mg or one 20-mg qd, $30–55/mo, or simvastatin (Zocor), one-half a 10-mg or one-half a 20-mg tab qd, $35–60 mo, or lovastatin-niacin (Advicor), one 20–500-mg tab qd, $50/mo	Lovastatin-niacin (Advicor), one 20–500-mg tab qd, $50/mo, or lovastatin (Altocor), one 40-mg ER tab qd, $60/mo, or simvastatin (Zocor), one-half a 40-mg tab qd, $60/mo, or atorvastatin (Lipitor), one 10-mg tab qd, $65/mo, or rosuvastatin (Crestor), one 5-mg tab qd, $70/mo, or fluvastatin (Lescol XL), one 80-mg ER tab qd, $75/mo
160–189	Simvastatin (Zocor), one-half a 40-mg tab qd, $60/mo, or lovastatin (Altocor), one 40-mg ER tab qd, $60/mo, or atorvastatin (Lipitor), one 10-mg tab qd, $65/mo, or rosuvastatin (Crestor), one 5-mg tab qd, $70/mo, or fluvastatin (Lescol), one 80-mg ER tab qd, $75/mo	Simvastatin (Zocor), one-half to one 80 mg tab qd, $60–115/mo, or lovastatin-niacin (Advicor), one 20–1000-mg tab qd, $65/mo, or rosuvastatin (Crestor), one 10-mg tab qd, $70/mo, or lovastatin (Altocor), one 60-mg ER tab qd, $70/mo, or atorvastatin (Lipitor), one 20-mg tab qd, $95/mo
≥190	Simvastatin (Zocor), one-half an 80-mg tab qd, $60/mo, or lovastatin-niacin (Advicor), one 20–1000-mg tab qd, $65/mo, or rosuvastatin (Crestor), one 10-mg tab qd, $70/mo, or lovastatin (Altocor), one 60-mg ER tab qd, $70/mo, or atorvastatin, one 20-mg tab Lipitor $95/mo	Rosuvastatin (Crestor), one 20-mg or one 40-mg tab qd, $70/mo, or atorvastatin (Lipitor), one 40-mg or one 80-mg tab qd, $95–100/mo, or simvastatin (Zocor), one 80-mg tab qd, $115/mo, or simvastatin (Zocor), one-half a 40-mg tab qd, plus ezetemibe (Zetia), one 10-mg tab qd, $130/mo, or atorvastatin (Lipitor), one 10-mg tab qd, plus ezetemibe (Zetia), one 10-mg tab qd, $135/mo or rosuvastatin (Crestor), one 5-mg tab qd plus ezetemibe (Zetia), one 10-mg tab qd, $140/mo

LDL, low-density lipoprotein.

      (2) Gemfibrozil has been shown to lower CAD morbidity and mortality by 40% in patients with elevated LDL cholesterol, TGs, or both. It is most beneficial in patients with HDL cholesterol of <45 mg/dL. It may be used cautiously in combination with an HMG-CoA reductase inhibitor.

   e. **Fenofibrate** (Tricor) is similar to gemfibrozil and is appropriate for the same patients. Its long-term safety is unknown.

   f. **HMG-CoA reductase inhibitors (statins).** This category is the rational choice for patients with moderately or severely elevated LDL cholesterol and high-risk patients with any LDL elevation who do not reach target treatment levels with diet and other medications.

      (1) These agents lower LDL cholesterol by 30–60%—more than any other medication.

      (2) In controlled trials, statins have reduced heart attack, stroke, CHD death, and total mortality by 25–40%. Cost-effectiveness analyses of this class of agents have shown favorable cost–benefit ratios.

      (3) The cost-effectiveness of treatment can be greatly improved by prescribing twice the intended dose and having the patient take one half of a tablet; this works well for all statin tablets except atorvastatin, which is too crumbly to be reliably halved. Table 75–6 shows recommended medications and doses for cost-effectively treating patients with different baseline LDL-C levels and different treatment goals.

      (4) All statins are usually well tolerated, and serious **adverse effects** are uncommon.

(5) The most frequently reported side effects of statins are headache, flatulence, constipation, dyspepsia, and mild elevation of hepatic transaminases.

(6) Rare side effects of statin therapy include pruritus, rashes, myopathy, rhabdomyolysis, and lupus erythematosus.

(7) Statin use is contraindicated in patients with active **hepatic disease** or significantly elevated serum transaminase levels (>3 times normal upper limit). Because significant (but asymptomatic) elevation of alanine transferase (ALT) occurs in 1–2% and mildly elevated ALT (<3 times normal) occurs in about 5–10% of treated patients, it is prudent to obtain a baseline ALT level and to recheck ALT 6–12 wks after initiating treatment or after increasing the statin dose. It is not necessary to monitor aspartine transferase (AST) or other liver enzymes. No cases of serious or life-threatening liver toxicity have thus far been attributed to statin therapy.

(8) **Myalgias** or muscle weakness occur in about 10% of patients, either early on or after prolonged treatment. Muscle symptoms caused by statins usually resolve within a few days to weeks after drug discontinuation. **Myopathy** occurs rarely, sometimes leading to **rhabdomyolysis** and **acute renal failure.** Muscle toxicity occurs somewhat more often when statins are used along with niacin, gemfibrozil, fenofibrate, and other drugs (Table 75–8).

(9) Renal failure is a risk factor for muscle side effects only with pravastatin.

(10) Because they are metabolized differently from other statins, pravastatin and fluvastatin are least likely to cause drug interactions.

(11) Grapefruit juice interferes with the metabolism of simvastatin, atorvastatin, and lovastatin (but not pravastatin, fluvastatin, or rosuvastatin) and raises their blood level; thus, there is the risk of muscle toxicity.

(12) Supplemental intake of the antioxidant **vitamin E** does not appear to be advisable, since it interfered with the beneficial effects of statin therapy in the Heart Protection Study.

(13) Once started, statin therapy should be continued indefinitely, barring unacceptable side effects or allergic reactions. Two studies have suggested a short-term increase in risk for the first 6 months after statin therapy is discontinued.

(14) Perceived side effects from one statin can often be avoided by switching to a different statin. Pravastatin or fluvastatin may be least likely to cause side effects.

(15) Because of potential teratogenicity, statins should not be used in women of childbearing age unless contraception effectiveness is maximized and the potential benefits appear to exceed the risks.

(16) Statins are not approved by the US Food and Drug Administration for use in children younger than 14 years except for atorvastatin for homozygous familial hypercholesterolemia.

(17) **Statin choices**
    (a) **Lovastatin** (Mevacor) was the first available HMG-CoA reductase agent.
        (i) The 20-mg starting dose is well tolerated and often produces good results, lowering LDL cholesterol an average of 25–30%.

TABLE 75–8. DRUGS THAT INTERACT WITH HMG-CoA REDUCTASE INHIBITORS (STATINS)[1]

- Niacin—also called nicotinic acid (Slo-Niacin, Niacor, Niaspan, Nico-400, NIA delay, Endur-Acin)
- Gemfibrozil (Lopid)
- Femfibrate (Tricor)
- Itraconazole (Sporanox)
- Amlodipine (Norvasc)
- Diltiazem (Cardizem, Cartia, Dilacor, Diltia, Tiazac)
- Verapamil (Calan, Covera, Isoptin, Verelan)
- Amiodarone (Cordarone)
- Cimetidine (Tagamet)
- Erythromycin (EES, E-Mycin, EryC, PCE, Ery-Tab)
- Clarithromycin (Biaxin)
- Clindamycin (Cleocin)
- Cyclosporine
- Indinavir (Crixivan)
- Nelfinavir (Viracept)
- Ritonavir (Norvir)
- Saquinavir (Invirase)
- Tacrolimus (Prograf)

[1] Some statins (atorvastatin, simvastatin, and lovastatin, but not pravastatin, rosuvastatin, or fluvastatin) interact with other drugs metabolized by the cytochrome P-450 3A4 liver enzyme system.

    (ii) Newer formulations include generic (less expensive), sustained-release (Altocor), and in combination with niacin (Advicor).

(b) Pravastatin (Pravachol) is similar to lovastatin but is less costly.

    (i) The usual dose of 20–40 mg/day, taken 2–3 hours after the evening meal, lowers LDL cholesterol an average of 25–35%.

    (ii) Pravastatin has reduced CHD events by 24–40% in primary and secondary prevention trials.

    (iii) Pravastatin is the only statin with prominent renal excretion (about 50% renal), so it should be used with caution, if at all, with patients with renal insufficiency or renal failure.

(c) Simvastatin (Zocor) has a higher potency. (10 mg of simvastatin is equivalent to 20 mg of lovastatin or pravastatin.) It can be taken anytime in the evening.

    (i) Simvastatin, 20–80 mg/day, lowers LDL cholesterol by 35–50%.

    (ii) Simvastatin reduced acute myocardial infarction or death from CHD by 42% and reduced total deaths by 30% in a large secondary prevention trial.

    (iii) Simvastatin raises HDL-C somewhat more than other statins.

    (iv) Higher doses of simvastatin tend to be more expensive than other similar agents.

(d) Fluvastatin (Lescol) costs substantially less than the other agents.

    (i) Higher doses (40–80 mg/day) lower LDL cholesterol by 23–33% (Tables 75–3 and 75–5).

    (ii) Outcome studies for fluvastatin have shown benefits similar to the other statins.

(e) Atorvastatin (Lipitor) is the most effective "statin" for lowering elevated LDL cholesterol and the most cost-effective for those with severely elevated LDL cholesterol.

    (i) Atorvastatin in the usual dose of 10–20 mg/day lowers LDL cholesterol by an average of 38–45% and TGs by 20–35%.

    (ii) Higher doses of 40–80 mg lower LDL cholesterol an average of 50–55% and TGs by 35–50%.

    (iii) Atorvastatin outcome studies have demonstrated outcome efficacy similar to other statins.

(f) Rosuvastatin (Crestor), the newest statin on the market, was approved in 2003.

    (i) Rosuvastastin lowers LDL cholesterol and raises HDL cholesterol more than any currently available statin. Treatment goals are reached substantially more often by rosuvastatin (10 mg/day) than atorvastatin (10 mg/day) or simvastatin (20 mg/day).

    (ii) Rosuvastatin has a similar side effect profile and fewer drug interactions than some other statins (Table 75–8).

    (iii) Proteinuria occasionally occurs (usually at the 40-mg dose), so periodic urinalysis or spot microalbumin/creatine ratio testing may be advisable.

(g) Ezetemibe (Zetia), approved in 2002, lowers cholesterol by interfering with the absorption of cholesterol in the gut.

    (i) Used alone, ezetemibe lowers LDL cholesterol and triglycerides only modestly (15–20%).

    (ii) When ezetemibe is added to the usual starting dose of a statin, the combination lowers LDL cholesterol as much as the maximum statin dose.

    (iii) Since ezetemibe is minimally absorbed, its combined use with low-dose statin may produce less adverse effects than high-dose statin therapy.

    (iv) Adding ezetemibe usually costs more than higher doses of a statin (two copayments instead of one for managed care patients, higher retail cost for other patients).

G. Partial ileal bypass surgery, in conjunction with a low-fat diet, lowers LDL cholesterol by 40–50%. The operative and postoperative morbidity and mortality are low. This surgery is a reasonable option for patients with severely elevated LDL cholesterol that cannot be managed satisfactorily with any tolerable combination of lipid-altering medications.

IV. Management Strategies

  A. Long-term compliance with hygienic measures and lipid-altering medications is quite poor. Many patients are reluctant to take preventive medications for asymptomatic conditions. Fear of potential adverse effects from chronic medications appears to be a major deterrent to compliance. A customized informed consent process might improve compliance by using a combination of textual and graphic materials to communicate treatment benefits and risks more effectively, and to allay patient fears and bolster confidence in the safety of statin therapy.

  B. Patient education and discussions with key family members are vital in order to foster a thorough understanding of the importance of a lifelong commitment to hygienic and medical management of lipid problems. Explanations of important concepts need to be expressed in lay terms, accompanied by memory devices to help people remember them, such as drawing a "happy face" and characterizing HDL cholesterol as "healthy" cholesterol, and a "frown face" symbolizing LDL cholesterol as "lousy" or "lethal" cholesterol. Many good educational materials are available from the American Heart Association, the NCEP, and commercial sources.

  C. Family-oriented care entails screening as many family members as possible and educating nuclear and extended families who have a member with an identified lipid problem. It is particularly important to work with the persons who buy and prepare the family's food, so that they thoroughly understand how to select and prepare "heart-healthy" foods.

  D. Elderly patients are at a greatly increased risk for myocardial infarction or sudden death. Recent randomized controlled trials have shown that the identification and treatment of dyslipidemia in patients aged 65–85 years can decrease the risk of first and recurrent coronary events. Morbidity and mortality from cardiovascular disease was decreased by at least 29% in these studies. Data are limited for patients older than 85 years. The use of benign inexpensive medications such as psyllium seems prudent. Since outcome studies show similar benefits and no increase in adverse effects for elderly patients, the expense and small risk of statin therapy seems justified for those wishing to preserve their current quality of life as long as possible.

  E. Children and adolescents with dyslipidemias should receive ongoing family-oriented education about diet, exercise, and weight control, as indicated. Extreme low-fat diets should be avoided in children younger than 6 years because of the risk of essential fatty acid malnutrition having deleterious effects on nervous system development. No information is available on the cost-effectiveness and long-term safety of lipid-altering medication treatment in children and adolescents. Children and adolescents with severe dyslipidemias should be treated with lipid-altering medications only with considerable caution and preferably with written parental informed consent detailing the limitations of what is known about the benefits and risks.

  F. Secondary prevention focuses on identifying and treating persons who have already developed clinical atherosclerosis. Many times the lipid problems of these patients are ignored or discounted, based on the faulty logic of "it is too late now to prevent atherosclerosis complications by modifying lipids." Persons with atherosclerosis have clearly demonstrated their high vulnerability to CAD death. They are the **most** likely to benefit from treatment to prevent further atheroma progression, prevent atheroma rupture, and regress existing atheromas. The lowering of LDL cholesterol has clearly demonstrated substantial benefit in secondary prevention trials. Long-term compliance is improved when statin therapy is started **prior** to hospital discharge for patients admitted with acute myocardial infarction or unstable angina pectoris.

  G. Systematic follow-up at regular intervals is essential for effective long-term management of lipid problems. Initially monthly visits are advisable to monitor progress and sustain motivation. The interval can be gradually lengthened to every 6–12 months for dietary and medication management. A manual or computerized flowchart in the medical record documenting blood lipid results, dietary and exercise modifications, and medication regimens facilitates the evaluation and alteration of treatment for best results.

V. Prognosis. The clinical course of lipid problems depends on the type and severity of lipid disorder and on other risk factors for atherosclerosis, especially cigarette smoking, diabetes mellitus, and hypertension. Other detrimental factors include abnormal levels of C-reactive protein, lipoprotein(a), small dense oxidized LDL particles, homocysteine, and perhaps other factors yet to be discovered.

  A. Atherosclerotic disease. In childhood and adolescence, fatty streaks form on the lining of susceptible arteries and subsequently develop into atheromas. In adulthood, accumulation of cholesterol and fibrotic tissue causes atheromas to progress at variable rates. Atherosclerotic progression, plaque rupture, and thrombus formation may eventually block off crucial arteries, causing ischemic symptoms and necrosis in the tissue supplied by the arteries.

B. **Acute pancreatitis** can occur with severe TG elevation >1000 mg/dL (11 mmol/L). This serious lipid problem requires urgent treatment with intravenous heparin.

C. Other valuable measures for curtailing atherosclerosis or minimizing its damage include smoking cessation, good control of hypertension and diabetes, daily aspirin (81 or 325 mg, enteric coated), and perhaps supplemental folate and vitamin B_6 and B_{12} intake to lower elevated homocysteine levels. Some recent studies indicate that getting a flu shot annually may lower risk for CAD events.

REFERENCES

AHA Scientific Statement: Fish Consumption, Fish Oil, Omega-3 Fatty Acids and Cardiovascular Disease, #71-0241. Circulation 2002;**106**:2747.

Ballantyne CM: Current and future aims of lipid-lowering therapy: Changing paradigms and lessons from the Heart Protection Study on standards of efficacy and safety. Am J Cardiol 2003;**21**:92(4B):3K.

Food and Drug Administration. Mercury content of selected fish. U.S. Food and Drug Administration Center for Food Safety and Applied Nutrition, Office of Seafood. www.cfsan.fda.gov/~frf/sea-mehg.html, May 2001.

Heart Protection Study Collaborative Group. MRC/BHF Heart Protection Study of cholesterol lowering with simvastatin in 20,536 high risk individuals: A randomised placebo-controlled trial. Lancet 2002; **360**:7-22M.

Hu FB, Willett WC: Optimal diets for prevention of coronary heart disease. JAMA 2002;**288**:2569.

Jones PH, et al: Comparison of the efficacy and safety of rosuvastatin versus atorvastatin, simvastatin, and pravastatin across doses (STELLAR Trial). Am J Cardiol (July 15) 2003;**92**(2):152.

Summary of the third report of the National Cholesterol Education Program (NCEP) Expert Panel on Detection, Evaluation, and Treatment of High Blood Cholesterol in Adults (Adult Treatment Panel III). JAMA 2001;**285**:2486.

---

76   Hypertension

Charles B. Eaton MD, MS

KEY POINTS

- Multiple epidemiologic studies have shown a consistent, continuous, graded relationship between increasing systolic and diastolic blood pressure (BP) and cardiovascular disease risk. For each incremental increase of 20 mm Hg in systolic BP and 10 mm Hg in diastolic BP, across the entire spectrum of BPs (115/75 mm Hg to 185/115 mm Hg), the rates of stroke, myocardial infarction, congestive heart failure, and end-stage renal disease double.

- Taking these facts into account, the Seventh Report of the Joint National Committee (JNC 7) on Detection, Evaluation, and Treatment of High Blood Pressure has defined normal pressure as a systolic BP <120 mm Hg and diastolic BP <80 mm Hg; pre-hypertension as a systolic BP of 120–139 mm Hg or a diastolic BP of 80–89 mm Hg; and hypertension as a systolic BP ≥140 mm Hg or a diastolic BP ≥90 mm Hg. These results should be based on the average of two or more readings, taken at each of two or more visits, after initial screening.

- Recent studies have documented the benefits of lifestyle management (DASH, DASH-Sodium, PREMIER, TOPHS) in the treatment and prevention of hypertension and the importance of antihypertensive medications in controlling BP and improving outcomes for cardiovascular disease, including heart failure, myocardial infarction, and recurrent stroke (ALLHAT, CAPPP, STOP-2, NORDIL, INSIGHT).

- The most effective clinical strategy promoted by the JNC 7 recommendations is to assess risk factors, target-organ damage, and comorbidities and to tailor treatment accordingly (Figure 76–1). All hypertensive patients should be treated to a BP goal of <140/90 mm Hg or to a BP <130/80 mm Hg in patients with diabetes or chronic renal disease. Most patients will require two medications to reach the goal and will require lifelong therapy.

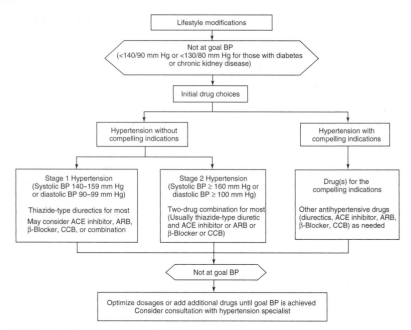

FIGURE 76–1. JNC 7 clinical strategies. ACE, angiotensin-converting enzyme; ARB, angiotensin-receptor blocker, BP, blood pressure; CCB, calcium channel blocker; JNC 7, Seventh Report of the Joint National Committee.

I. Introduction

A. **Epidemiology.** Hypertension affects approximately 50 million people in the United States, or approximately $\frac{1}{6}$ of Americans and $\frac{1}{4}$ of adults. According to recent surveys, 70% of Americans with hypertension are aware of the diagnosis, with 59% on treatment. However, only 34% of hypertensive patients are under good control, with a BP of <140/90 mm Hg (JNC 7). Recent estimates from the Framingham Heart Study suggest that the lifetime risk of developing hypertension is close to 90%. Those with prehypertension have twice the risk of developing hypertension as those with lower BP values.

B. **Primary (essential) hypertension.** Between 90% and 95% of individuals with hypertension do not have a known cause for their hypertension and are therefore labeled as having essential hypertension.

C. **Secondary, or identifiable, cause of hypertension.** About 5–10% of hypertension in the United States is due to a secondary cause. In order for physicians to treat cost-effectively, secondary causes should be evaluated only in patients whose age, history, severity of presentation, or initial laboratory work-up suggests a secondary cause. Patients with sudden onset of hypertension, those with poorly controlled BP, or those who were well controlled yet suddenly worsen should be evaluated for secondary causes.

Numerous independent processes are responsible for secondary causes of hypertension, including sleep apnea, drug-induced or related causes, renal (polycystic kidney disease, glomerular and interstitial disease) or renovascular disease, primary hyperaldosteronism (0.5%), increased intracranial pressure, chronic steroid therapy or Cushing's syndrome, pheochromocytoma, coarctation of the aorta, hyperthyroidism, or primary hyperparathyroidism. (With regard to renovascular disease, renal artery stenosis accounts for 1–2% of cases of hypertension.)

D. **Resistant hypertension.** Resistant hypertension is the failure to reach a BP goal in patients who are fully adherent to an appropriate three-drug regimen including a diuretic.

Common causes of resistant hypertension include improper BP measurement; excess dietary sodium; inadequate diuretic therapy; inadequate doses of medications; excess alcohol intake; and drug interactions such as use of nonsteroidal anti-inflammatory drugs, illicit drugs, oral contraceptives, sympathomimetics, herbal supplements, and over-the-counter preparations. Ruling out the secondary causes of hypertension mentioned above is crucial in evaluating resistant hypertension, if this has not already been done.

II. **Diagnosis.** The diagnostic work-up for hypertension should assess risk factors and comorbidities, reveal identifiable causes of hypertension, and assess presence of target-organ damage. This allows for appropriate risk stratification and tailoring of therapy. The major cardiovascular risk factors, besides hypertension, include cigarette smoking, obesity (body mass index >30), physical inactivity, dyslipidemia, diabetes mellitus, men older than 55 years, women older than 65 years, family history of premature cardiovascular disease, and microalbuminuria (or estimated glomerular filtration rate <60 mL/min). Target-organ damage includes the heart (left ventricular hypertrophy, angina or prior myocardial infarction, prior coronary revascularization or heart failure); the brain (stroke or transient ischemic attack); the kidneys (chronic kidney disease); the peripheral arteries (peripheral vascular disease); and the retina (retinopathy) (JNC 7).

A. **Symptoms.** Patients with hypertension usually remain asymptomatic, unless they have experienced severe BP elevations (eg, >220 mm Hg systolic BP or >130 mm Hg diastolic BP). Symptoms of hypertension can include fatigue, occipital and pulsating headaches in early morning, lightheadedness, flushing, epistaxis, chest pains, visual and speech disturbances, and dyspnea.

Specific symptoms of secondary causes can often aid in the diagnosis of hypertension: leg claudication from lower extremity ischemia (coarctation of the aorta); hirsutism; easy bruising (Cushing's syndrome); excessive perspiration; sustained or intermittent hypertension, paroxysmal headaches, palpitations, anxiety attacks, pallor, tremor, nausea or vomiting (pheochromocytoma); hypokalemia, muscle weakness, cramps, polyuria, paralysis, nocturia (primary hyperaldosteronism); and flank pain (renal or renovascular disease).

B. **Signs.** BP measurement should be performed while the patient is sitting or supine, and standing, on more than two occasions, to obtain an average for both systolic and diastolic readings. The patient should rest for 5 minutes prior to the reading and should not smoke tobacco or ingest caffeine for a minimum of 30 minutes before measurement. The BP cuff should be more than two thirds the circumference of the arm and placed at heart level. The cuff should be inflated 30 mm Hg above where the radial pulse can no longer be felt. The systolic reading is made at the onset of Korotkoff sounds (phase I), and the diastolic reading is taken when the sounds completely disappear (phase V). The BP should be measured in both arms; if there is a discrepancy in reading, the higher reading should be used.

C. **Ambulatory blood pressure monitoring.** Ambulatory BP monitoring provides BP readings during daily activities and sleep. Ambulatory BP measurements are usually lower than office readings. The level of BP using ambulatory measurements correlates with target-organ damage better than office measurements. Ambulatory BP measurements are indicated to evaluate "white-coat" hypertension in the absence of target-organ damage, resistant hypertension, and hypotensive episodes and for suspected autonomic dysfunction. Awake BP readings averaging >135/85 mm Hg or sleep BP readings averaging >120/75 mm Hg are consistent with the diagnosis of hypertension. Normally, there is a 15 mm Hg drop in the average systolic BP and a 10 mm Hg drop in the average diastolic BP between daytime ambulatory BP and sleeping ambulatory BP readings. Failure to find this "nocturnal dipping" suggests that a secondary cause of hypertension is more likely and is associated with an increased risk of cardiovascular disease (CVD) events. Besides aiding in the diagnosis, ambulatory BP monitoring allows for the measurement of overall BP load, percentage of readings that are hypertensive, and the extent of nocturnal dipping to be evaluated.

D. **Physical examination.** The initial physical examination of the hypertensive patient should include an assessment of target-organ damage, identification of signs suggesting a specific secondary cause, and evaluation of metabolic syndrome.

1. **Signs of target-organ damage.** Signs of target-organ damage include arteriolar narrowing, arteriovenous compression, hemorrhages, exudates, or papilledema

on funduscopic examination; carotid bruits and distended jugular veins in the neck; loud aortic second sound, precordial heave, arrhythmia, or early systolic click on cardiac examination; diminished or absent peripheral arterial pulses, peripheral edema of the extremities; aneurysm of the abdominal aorta; and abnormal neurologic assessment.

2. **Signs of secondary hypertension.** Signs suggestive of secondary hypertension include abdominal or flank masses (polycystic kidneys); absence of femoral pulses (aortic coarctation); tachycardia, diaphoresis, or orthostatic hypotension (pheochromocytoma); abdominal bruits (renovascular disease); truncal obesity, ecchymoses, or pigmented striae (Cushing's syndrome); and an enlarged or nodular thyroid gland (hyperthyroidism).

3. **Evaluation for metabolic syndrome.** Evaluation for metabolic syndrome is important in evaluating hypertension, since it is associated with an insulin-resistant state and increased cardiovascular risk. Metabolic syndrome is defined as the presence of three or more of the following risk factors: abdominal obesity (waist circumference >40 inches in men, >35 inches in women), BP >130/85 mm Hg, glucose intolerance (fasting plasma glucose >110 mg/dL), and dyslipidemia (triglycerides >150 mg/dL, or high-density lipoproteins (HDLs) <40 mg/dL in men or <50 mg/dL in women).

E. **Laboratory tests.** Baseline screening is important to assess target-organ damage, identify patients at high risk for developing cardiovascular complications, determine whether other cardiovascular risk factors exist, and screen for possible secondary causes of hypertension.

1. **Routine tests.** Routine tests on all newly diagnosed hypertensive patients include hemoglobin and hematocrit, potassium, creatinine, fasting glucose, calcium, a fasting lipid profile (consisting of total cholesterol, HDL cholesterol, low-density lipoprotein cholesterol, and triglycerides), urinalysis, and resting electrocardiogram. Obtaining a urinary microalbumin/creatinine ratio is optional. More extensive testing for identifiable causes is generally not indicated.

2. **Laboratory tests to identify secondary causes.** The following laboratory tests may be helpful when specific secondary causes are suspected, based on history, physiologic evaluation, and routine laboratory evaluation:

   a. Chest x-ray (coarctation of aorta)

   b. Captopril renal scan or magnetic resonance angiography of kidneys to evaluate for renal artery stenosis

   c. Urinary metanephrine and vanillylmandelic acid levels (pheochromocytoma)

   d. Plasma renin activity levels (primary aldosteronism or renovascular disease)

   e. Cardiac echocardiography to evaluate for LVH, evidence of asymptomatic systolic dysfunction, or previous myocardial infarction.

III. **Treatment**

A. **Goals of therapy.** Treatment of patients with elevated BP or pre-hypertension focuses on the prevention, or delay, of hypertension through lifestyle modification unless the patient has evidence of target-organ damage, in which case treatment with antihypertensive medications should begin immediately. If a patient has frank hypertension, then therapy is directed toward preventing cardiovascular and renal morbidity and mortality associated with hypertension. **Since most persons with hypertension will reach the diastolic BP goal once the systolic BP is at goal, the primary focus is to achieve a systolic BP goal.**

B. **Lifestyle modifications.** The lifestyle modifications are important in the treatment for all pre-hypertensive and hypertensive patients, no matter how severe the patient's hypertension. Lifestyle changes are not only effective but also reduce the number and dosage of medications needed to control hypertension. Evidence-based lifestyle modifications include weight reduction in those who are overweight, Dietary Approaches to Stop Hypertension (DASH) diet, dietary sodium reduction, physical activity, and moderate alcohol consumption (Table 76–1).

1. **Weight loss.** A 10% weight loss in patients with a body mass index >25 reduces systolic BP by 5–10 mm Hg. Weight loss is known to improve insulin sensitivity, decrease plasma norepinephrine and aldosterone levels, and decrease renin activity, which probably explains its benefits. Weight loss can be attained by a 500- to 1000-kcal dietary deficit, along with behavioral management that focuses on self-

TABLE 76–1. LIFESTYLE MODIFICATIONS TO MANAGE HYPERTENSION

Modification	Recommendation	Approximate Systolic BP Reduction, Range
Weight reduction	Maintain normal body weight (BMI, 18.5–24.9)	5–20 mm Hg/10-kg weight loss
Adopt DASH eating plan	Consume a diet rich in fruits, vegetables, and low-fat dairy products with a reduced content of saturated and total fat	8–14 mm Hg
Dietary sodium reduction	Reduce dietary sodium intake to no more than 100 mEq/L (2.4 g sodium or 6 g sodium chloride)	2–8 mm Hg
Physical activity	Engage in regular aerobic physical activity such as brisk walking (at least 30 minutes per day, most days of the week)	4–9 mm Hg
Moderation of alcohol consumption	Limit consumption to no more than 2 drinks per day (1 oz or 30 mL ethanol [eg, 24 oz beer, 10 oz wine, or 3 oz 80-proof whiskey]) in most men and no more than 1 drink per day in women and lighter-weight persons	2–4 mm Hg

[1] For overall cardiovascular risk reduction, stop smoking. The effects of implementing these modifications are dose and time dependent and could be higher for some individuals.
BMI, body mass index calculated as weight in kilograms divided by the square of height in meters; BP, blood pressure; DASH, Dietary Approaches to Stop Hypertension.

monitoring, goal setting, and positive reinforcement and promotes 30 minutes daily of moderate physical activity, such as walking.

2. **DASH-diet eating plan.** Diets high in potassium, calcium, and magnesium have been individually shown to have modest benefits in lowering BP. These minerals are found in abundance in fruits and vegetables. The recent landmark study, Dietary Approaches to Stop Hypertension (DASH), found that diets high in fruits and vegetables (8–10 servings) significantly decreased both systolic and diastolic BPs in patients with hypertension and yielded results in only 2 weeks. The DASH-diet eating plan is now recommended for most pre-hypertensive and hypertensive patients. Recipes and patient education materials are available at http://www.nhlbi.nih.gov/health/public/heart/hbp/dash/index.htm

3. **Sodium restriction.** Although previous epidemiologic studies have been inconsistent in their findings of the relationship between sodium and hypertension, new randomized trials have clearly shown the benefits of sodium restriction. The DASH-sodium study and the Trials of the Hypertension Prevention Collaborative have collectively shown that salt restriction successfully prevented hypertension in those with pre-hypertension and controlled BP in stage 1 hypertension. A salt restriction to 1500 mg per day, or ⅔ of a teaspoon, led to a 2–8 mm Hg reduction in systolic BP. The degree of BP lowering by sodium restriction appears to vary, with certain "salt-sensitive" individuals experiencing a significant effect and others receiving little apparent benefit. Therefore, if sodium restriction is burdensome for a patient, a trial of sodium restriction can be performed in order to tailor therapy.

4. **Physical activity.** A meta-analysis of trials has shown that physical activity is effective in lowering BP in normal-weight and overweight individuals and in those with pre-hypertension and hypertension (PREMIER). Aerobic exercise is associated with a 3–5 mm Hg reduction in systolic BP, and a 2–3 mm Hg reduction in diastolic BP. Sedentary and unfit people with normal BP have a 20–50% increased risk of developing hypertension when compared with physically active peers. The PREMIER study showed that increased physical activity could be successfully added to a DASH-sodium diet, with allowance for moderate alcohol consumption, to lower BP. All sedentary pre-hypertensive and hypertensive patients should be encouraged to participate in 30 minutes of moderate or vigorous physical activity between 5 and 7 days per week.

5. **Moderate alcohol consumption.** Fifteen randomized clinical trials have shown that reduction in alcohol consumption results in a modest reduction in systolic (3 mm Hg) and diastolic BP (2 mm Hg). All pre-hypertensive and hypertensive male patients should be encouraged to limit alcohol intake to two (2) drinks per day, with female patients encouraged to limit alcohol intake to one (1) drink per day; neither male nor female patients should consume more than five (5) drinks in any 24-hour period.

C. **Pharmacologic treatment.** In clinical trials, antihypertensive drug therapy is associated with a 35–40% reduction in stroke, 20–25% reduction in myocardial infarction, and 50% reduction in heart failure. Reducing systolic BP by 12 mm Hg in stage 1 hypertension will prevent 1 death for every 11 patients treated, whereas treating those with target-organ damage will prevent 1 death in every 9 patients treated (JNC 7).

1. **Initial drug therapy.** The recent ALLHAT study, and a meta-analysis of over 42 clinical trials, has demonstrated that low-dose diuretics are the most effective first-line treatment for preventing the occurrence of cardiovascular morbidity and mortality. The compelling reasons for use of alternative first-line antihypertensive drugs include existing systolic congestive heart failure, transmural myocardial infarction, diabetes mellitus, and chronic kidney disease. Table 76–2, adapted from the JNC 7, lists the indications and appropriate medications, based on evidence gathered from clinical trials. Clinicians should avoid the use of doxazosin for hypertension control, as the ALLHAT trial showed a higher rate of congestive heart failure and combined CVD events for doxazosin when compared to diuretic therapy.

2. **Drug regimens.** Drug regimens should be tailored based on multiple clinical factors, including age, cost, safety, effectiveness, disease severity, and general lifestyle (diet and exercise) patterns. Also to be taken into consideration are the impact on the patient's quality of life (physical state, emotional well-being, sexual and social functioning, and cognitive acuity), convenience, dosage frequency, possibility of other drug interactions, pathophysiologic mechanisms, concurrent risk factors and diseases, history of previous responses to other agents, and the potential use of the agent, or agents, for other medical problems. For instance, heart failure or hypertension complicated by diabetes mellitus with proteinuria can be treated with angiotensin-converting enzyme (ACE) inhibitors. Hypertensive patients with a myocardial infarction can be treated with beta blockers (non–intrinsic sympathomimetic activity), ACE inhibitors, or aldosterone antagonists; or all three, in the presence of systolic dysfunction. Table 76–3 provides a list of commonly prescribed antihypertensive agents by class and criteria.

3. **Effectiveness of drug regimens.** Even the most effective single agents are <70% effective on a long-term basis. However, 80% of compliant patients eventually achieve adequate control on one or two agents. Only a minority of patients require more than two pharmacologic agents. If the initial agent does not control BP sufficiently, a second agent of a different class may be added. Keeping both agents at low doses will decrease side effects. Combination treatment can be very effective, especially when a diuretic is added to monotherapy. For instance, the use of an ACE inhibitor with a diuretic can be effective for up to 85% of elderly patients. Common combinations include diuretic plus beta blocker, diuretic plus ACE inhibitor, diuretic plus calcium antagonist, calcium antagonist plus ACE inhibitor, and diuretic plus sympatholytic agent.

4. **Follow-up tests.** Serum potassium, sodium, blood urea nitrogen and creatinine, uric acid, and glucose levels should be measured periodically, especially if the patient has chronic renal disease or diabetes mellitus or is taking a diuretic agent. Fasting lipid profiles are indicated for most patients, given concomitant disease and the high prevalence of metabolic syndrome. The type and frequency of repeat laboratory tests should be based on the severity of target-organ damage and the effectiveness of treatment. A periodic urinalysis, or microalbumin/creatinine ratio, is also indicated to monitor for subclinical renal impairment.

IV. **Management Strategies.** Management strategies need to be individualized to take into consideration the severity of the patient's hypertension, the class, or classes, of pharmacologic agents being used for treatment, patient compliance, and cardiovascular risk factors or disease processes concurrent with hypertension. The three most common causes of uncontrolled hypertension are patient noncompliance (responsible for 50% of treatment failure), inadequate therapy, and inappropriate therapy.

TABLE 76–2. CLINICAL TRIAL AND GUIDELINE BASIS FOR COMPELLING INDICATIONS FOR INDIVIDUAL DRUG CLASSES

High-Risk Conditions with Compelling Indication[1]	Recommended Drugs						Clinical Trial Basis[2]
	Diuretic	β-Blocker	ACE Inhibitor	ARB	CCB	Aldosterone Antagonist	
Heart failure	•	•	•	•		•	ACC/AHA Heart Failure Guideline, MERIT-HF, COPERNICUS, CIBIS, SOLVD, AIRE, TRACE, ValHEFT, RALES
Post-myocardial infarction		•	•			•	ACC/AHA Post-MI Guideline, BHAT, SAVE, Capricorn, EPHESUS
High coronary disease risk	•	•	•		•		ALLHAT, HOPE, ANBP2, LIFE, CONVINCE
Diabetes	•	•	•	•	•		NKF-ADA Guideline, UKPDS, ALLHAT
Chronic kidney disease			•	•			NKF Guideline, Captopril Trial, RENAAL IDNT, REIN, AASK
Recurrent stroke prevention	•		•				PROGRESS

[1] Compelling indications for antihypertensive drugs are based on benefits from outcome studies or existing clinical guidelines; the compelling indication is managed in parallel with the blood pressure.

[2] Conditions for which clinical trials demonstrate benefit of specific classes of antihypertensive drugs.

AASK, African American Study of Kidney Disease and Hypertension; ACC/AHA, American College of Cardiology/American Heart Association; ACE, angiotensin converting enzyme; AIRE, Acute Infarction Ramipril Efficacy; ALLHAT, Antihypertensive and Lipid Lowering Treatment to Prevent Heart Attack Trial; ANBP2, Second Australian National Blood Pressure Study; ARB, angiotensin-receptor blocker; BHAT$_\beta$, Blocker Heart Attack Trial; CCB, calcium channel blocker; CIBIS, Cardiac Insufficiency Basoprolol Study; CONVINCE, Controlled Onset Verapamil Investigation of Cardiovascular End Points; COPERNICUS, Carvedilol Prospective Randomized Cumulative Survival Study; EPHESUS, Eplerenone Post-Acute Myocardial Infarction Heart Failure Efficacy and Survival Study; HOPE, Heart Outcomes Prevention Evaluation Study; IDNT, Inbesartan Diabetic Nephropathy Trial; LIFE, Losartan Intervention For Endpoint Reduction in Hypertension Study; MERIT-HF, Metoprolol CR/XL Randomized Intervention Trial in Congestive Heart Failure; NKF-ADA, National Kidney Foundation–American Diabetes Association; PROGRESS, Perindopril Protection Against Recurrent Stroke Study; RALES, Randomized Aldactone Evaluation Study; REIN, Ramipril Efficacy in Nephropathy Study; RENAAL, Reduction of Endpoints in Non-Insulin Dependent Diabetes Mellitus with the Angiotensin II Antagonist Losartan Study; SAVE, Survival and Ventricular Enlargement Study; SOLVD, Studies of Left Ventricular Dysfunction; TRACE, Trandolapril Cardiac Evaluation Study; UKPDS, United Kingdom Prospective Diabetes Study; ValHEFT, Valsartan Heart Failure Trial.

TABLE 76–3. ORAL ANTIHYPERTENSIVE DRUGS

Class	Drug (Trade Name)	Usual Dose, Range, mg/day	Daily Frequency
Thiazide diuretics	Chlorothiazide (Diuril)	125–500	1
	Chlorthalidone (generic)	12.5–25	1
	Hydrochlorothiazide (Microzide, HydroDIURIL)	12.5–50	1
	Polythiazide (Renese)	2–4	1
	Indapamide (Lozol)	1.25–2.5	1
	Metolazone (Mykrox)	0.5–1.0	1
	Metolazone (Zaroxolyn)	2.5–5	1
Loop diuretics	Bumetanide (Bumex)	0.5–2	2
	Furosemide (Lasix)	20–80	2
	Torsemide (Demadex)	2.5–10	1
Potassium-sparing diuretics	Amiloride (Midamor)	5–10	1–2
	Triamterene (Dyrenium)	50–100	1–2
Aldosterone-receptor blockers	Eplerenone (Inspra)	50–100	1–2
	Spironolactone (Aldactone)	25–50	1–2
β-Blockers	Atenolol (Tenormin)	25–100	1
	Betaxolol (Kerlone)	5–20	1
	Bisoprolol (Zebeta)	2.5–10	1
	Metoprolol (Lopressor)	50–100	1–2
	Metoprolol extended release (Toprol XL)	50–100	1
	Nadolol (Corgard)	40–120	1
	Propranolol (Inderal)	40–160	2
	Propranolol long-acting (Inderal LA)	60–180	1
	Timolol (Biocadren)	20–40	2
β-Blockers with intrinsic sympathomimetic activity	Acebutolol (Sectral)	200–800	2
	Penbutolol (Levatol)	10–40	1
	Pindolol (generic)	10–40	2
Combined α- and β-blockers	Carvedilol (Coreg)	12.5–50	2
	Labetalol (Normodyne, Trandate)	200–800	2
ACE inhibitors	Benazepril (Lotensin)	10–40	1–2
	Captopril (Capoten)	25–100	2
	Enalapril (Vasotec)	2.5–40	1–2
	Fosinopril (Monopril)	10–40	1
	Lisinopril (Prinivil, Zestril)	10–40	1
	Moexipril (Univasc)	7.5–30	1
	Perindopril (Aceon)	4–8	1–2
	Quinapril (Accupril)	10–40	1
	Ramipril (Altace)	2.5–20	1
	Trandolapril (Mavik)	1–4	1

A. **Patient education.** Patient education is an important part of the physician's management strategy. Education begins with the initial measurement of BP. For a patient who has elevated pressures after three readings, the diagnosis of hypertension should be explained clearly, concisely, and completely. The beliefs of the patient regarding hypertension should be identified with respect to the effectiveness of treatment, the seriousness of the disease (if left untreated), and personal susceptibility to complications that correspond to an increased risk of morbidity and mortality. Drug instructions should likewise be written clearly and succinctly. Lifestyle barriers to compliance should be identified as early as possible. Family education should be provided when appropriate. Patient education by itself has been shown to be inadequate for chronic disease management, including hypertension. It is important that the patient participates in the decision-making process when the goals of therapy are established and that strategies are delineated to reach these goals and achieve effective BP control. For individuals with high BP, the goal is a systolic BP consistently below 140/90 mm Hg, while the goal is 130/80 mm Hg for individuals with diabetes or chronic kidney disease.

B. Self-monitoring. Presently, only 34% of hypertensive patients are under good control. Recent studies have shown that this can be increased by self-monitoring. Having a record of BPs and receiving timely individualized feedback has been shown to enhance BP control significantly.

C. Initial follow-up. Monthly check-ups are recommended for the first 6 months of newly diagnosed hypertension and should include an interval history to identify symptoms that may have developed, a discussion of health concerns and compliance problems, an evaluation of drug effects and possible drug reactions, and measurement of BP and weight. Compliance can sometimes be improved by changing to an agent with a longer half-life, thereby reducing the number of doses. A memory-assist device, such as Medi-Set, is appropriate for patients receiving complex regimens or with a memory disturbance.

D. Early detection. Early detection of complications is an important management strategy to identify potential morbidity from hypertension (retinopathy, coronary artery disease, renal disease, cerebrovascular disease, or nephropathy). Furthermore, people with hypertension may be at increased risk of having vascular disease, target-organ damage, dyslipidemias, diabetes mellitus, obesity, arthritis, and problems affecting the liver or kidneys. Prevention, early identification, and treatment of these associated problems are important.

V. Prognosis. Natural history and prognosis are directly related to the effectiveness of treatment, patient compliance, the presence of coexisting diseases, the age of the patient at diagnosis, and the ability of the patient to follow adjunctive therapy recommendations to make lifestyle and behavioral changes. Studies completed prior to the discovery of antihypertensive drugs revealed that 70% of hypertensive patients died of congestive heart failure or coronary artery disease, 15% from cerebral hemorrhage, and 10% from uremia. Left ventricular hypertrophy (LVH) is a significant complication of hypertension. Progression of LVH can be prevented, and reversed, by good hypertension control. Development of LVH with strain is an ominous complication of hypertension, with a four- to eightfold increase in mortality. Within 5 years of the development of LVH with strain, one third of patients have a major cardiovascular event.

Patients with concurrent diabetes mellitus and hypertension are at greater risk for developing diabetic nephropathy. However, effective antihypertensive treatment (eg, ACE inhibitors) can reduce proteinuria and the rate of decline of the glomerular filtration rate, thus postponing end-stage renal failure. The likelihood of cardiovascular complications in elderly patients can best be predicted by systolic BP. Treatment has been shown to decrease cardiovascular events in patients up to the age of 80 years.

REFERENCES

ALLHAT Officers and Coordinators: Major cardiovascular events in hypertensive patients randomized to doxazosin vs chlorthalidone: The Antihypertensive and Lipid-Lowering Treatment to Prevent Heart Attack Trial (ALLHAT). JAMA 2000;**283:**1967.

ALLHAT Officers and Coordinators: Major outcomes in high-risk hypertensive patients randomized to angiotensin-converting enzyme inhibitor or calcium channel blocker vs diuretic: The Antihypertensive and Lipid-Lowering Treatment to Prevent Heart Attack Trial (ALLHAT). JAMA 2002;**288:**2981.

Appel LJ, et al: A clinical trial of dietary patterns on blood pressure (DASH). N Engl J Med 1997; **336:**1117.

Appel LJ, et al: Effects of Comprehensive Lifestyle Modification on Blood Pressure Control: Main Results of The PREMIER Clinical Trial. JAMA 2003;**289:**2083.

Chobanian AV, et al: The Seventh Report of the Joint National Committee on Prevention, Detection, Evaluation, and Treatment of High Blood Pressure: The JNC 7 report. JAMA 2003;**289:**2560.

Psaty BM, et al: Health outcomes associated with various antihypertensive therapies use as first-line agents: A network meta-analysis. JAMA 2003;**289:**2534.

Rogers MAM, et al: Home monitoring service improves mean arterial pressure in patients with essential hypertension: A randomized, controlled trial. Ann Intern Med 2001;**134:**1024.

Sacks FM, et al: Effects on blood pressure of reduced dietary sodium and the Dietary Approaches to Stop Hypertension (DASH) diet (DASH-Sodium). N Engl J Med 2001;**344:**3.

Vasan RS, et al: Impact of high-normal blood pressure on the risk of cardiovascular disease. N Engl J Med 2001;**345:**1291.

77   Ischemic Heart Disease

Jim Nuovo, MD, & Allen L. Hixon, MD

KEY POINTS

- The highest priority in the evaluation of patients with chest pain is distinguishing cardiac from noncardiac causes.
- The clinical history remains critical in the evaluation of each patient. A normal electrocardiogram result cannot be used to exclude ischemic heart disease.
- An exercise treadmill test remains the most valuable diagnostic tool for the diagnostic and prognostic information.
- Medical management includes risk factor modification, use of aspirin and antianginal drugs (eg, aspirin, 81 mg/day; atenolol, 25–50 mg/day; Isordil, 20 mg every 8–12 hours; or transderm nitropatch, 0.2 mg/hour on in the morning and off in the afternoon).
- Consensus guidelines should be used to determine management of patients with chronic angina or unstable angina.

I. **Introduction**
   A. **Definition. Ischemic heart disease (IHD)** results from the effects of atherosclerosis of the coronary arteries. Significant stenosis, along with newly discovered mechanisms that help regulate constriction and relaxation of the coronary arteries, often with superimposed coronary thrombosis, results in a variety of signs and symptoms. It is important for clinicians to recognize the many manifestations of this disease.
   B. **Epidemiology**
      1. Cardiovascular disease is the leading cause of death in both men and women, accounting for approximately 25% of all deaths. Eleven million people in the United States have coronary artery disease. Fifty percent of postmenopausal women die of coronary artery disease or its sequelae.
      2. IHD has an enormous impact on medical care in this country. The cost of treatment exceeds $56 billion annually and is expected to rise with the aging of the US population. In industrialized nations, economic loss, disability, and death from coronary artery disease exceeded any other cluster of illnesses.
   C. **Pathophysiology.** The heart muscle functions almost exclusively as an aerobic organ, with little capacity for anaerobic metabolism. At rest the heart extracts approximately 80% of the oxygen it receives, leaving it more susceptible to effects of decreased perfusion. Chest pain is the foremost manifestation of myocardial ischemia and results from a disparity between myocardial oxygen demand and coronary blood flow. The mechanisms for ischemia include coronary atherosclerosis (most common), vasoconstriction, and coronary thrombosis.
II. **Diagnosis.** Chest pain is one of the common reasons for patients to visit primary care physicians. The major diagnostic considerations for chest pain are addressed in Chapter 10. The highest priority is generally given to distinguishing cardiac from noncardiac chest pain. Studies have demonstrated that 10–30% of patients with chest pain who undergo coronary arteriography have no arterial abnormalities. Of the many noncardiac causes of chest pain, gastrointestinal (esophageal), bronchopulmonary, and psychiatric (panic attacks and major depression) are common. Less common causes include chest wall (herpes zoster, costochondritis), aortic dissection, and referred pain from the abdomen.
   A. **Risk factors.** Hyperlipidemia, cigarette smoking, hypertension, diabetes, older age, and male gender are commonly recognized risk factors for IHD. In addition, elevated homocysteine levels and C-reactive protein are independent risk factors for IHD.
   B. **Symptoms and signs**
      1. **Angina** is not simply one type of pain; it is a constellation of symptoms related to cardiac ischemia. The description of angina may fit several patterns.
         a. **Classic angina** presents as an ill-defined pressure, heaviness (feeling like a weight), or squeezing sensation brought on by exertion and relieved by rest.

The location of classic anginal pain is most often substernal and left-sided. It may radiate to the jaw, interscapular area, or down the arm. Angina usually begins gradually and lasts only a few minutes. It is important to appreciate that the qualitative description of pain may be greatly influenced by socioeconomic status, education, culture, and personality.

b. **Atypical angina.** The patient either experiences pain that is anginal in quality or has pain with exertional features. For example, this may be a sense of heaviness that is not consistently related to exertion or relieved by rest. Conversely, the pain may have an atypical character—sharp or stabbing—but the precipitating factors are anginal. This is the category of chest pain that is most prone to a diagnostic error. All presentations of chest pain should be taken seriously until proved to be benign.

c. **Anginal equivalent.** The sensation of dyspnea may be the sole or major manifestation.

d. **Nonanginal pain.** The pain has neither the quality nor precipitating characteristics of angina. Chest pain quality not consistent with IHD includes the following descriptive terms: needlelike, shooting, tingling, stabbing, jabbing, knifelike, and cutting.

e. **Diabetic patients.** IHD is the leading cause of death in adult diabetic patients. Hypertension, obesity, and hyperlipidemia cluster in patients with diabetes who have accelerated development of atherosclerotic vascular disease. Atypical clinical presentations have been thought to occur more frequently in diabetic patients; however, whether diabetic patients experience more "silent myocardial infarctions" (MIs) than the general population has recently been challenged.

f. **Women.** Women are twice as likely as men to present with angina and less likely to present with infarction or sudden death.

2. **Probability of IHD based on history.** Despite the well-known problems experienced in determining the cause of chest pain, the clinical history remains critical in the evaluation of each patient. From the information gathered in the history, the physician should strive to categorize the patient's symptoms as nonanginal, atypical angina, or typical angina. Table 77–1 provides a guideline as to the likelihood of whether a patient has significant IHD based on the history.

3. **Use of nitrate and response to nitroglycerin.** Response of the chest pain to sublingual nitroglycerin (NTG) may be used (with caution) as an adjunct for determining whether a patient's chest pain is from IHD. For example, a prompt response of <3 minutes increases the probability of IHD; however, esophageal spasm and biliary colic may also respond favorably to nitrate administration. Failure to respond to NTG should not be used to exclude the possibility of IHD.

4. **Signs.** There are no reliable, consistent physical signs found on examination for IHD. The main purpose of the examination is to assess the patient for evidence of complications from atherosclerotic disease (eg, peripheral vascular disease, cerebrovascular disease, congestive heart failure). The physician should pay attention

TABLE 77–1. LIKELIHOOD OF SIGNIFICANT IHD BASED ON SYMPTOMS

Age (yrs)	Nonanginal Chest Pain	Atypical Angina	Typical Angina
30–39	5% M 0.8% F	22% M 4% F	69% M 26% F
40–49	14% M 3% F	46% M 13% F	87% M 55% F
50–59	21% M 8% F	59% M 32%F	92% M 79% F
60–69	28% M 18% F	67% M 54% F	94% M 90% F

F, female; M, male.
Adapted from Diamond GA, Forrester JS: Analysis of probability as an aid in the clinical diagnosis of coronary-artery disease. N Engl J Med 1979;**300**:1350.

to the vascular examination, such as peripheral artery bruits, retinal arteriolar changes, and the presence of an S_3 or S_4, and for the consequences of diminished myocardial contractility, such as lower extremity edema.

C. Diagnostic tests

1. **12-Lead electrocardiogram (ECG)** and serial cardiac enzymes are frequently used to rule out an MI. Several new molecular markers and their sampling schedule are noted in Table 77–2.

2. The standard provocative test for IHD is the **exercise treadmill test (ETT).** In 1986, the American College of Cardiology and the American Heart Association Task Force on Assessment of Cardiovascular Procedures set guidelines for exercise treadmill testing. The recommendations are as follows:

   a. As a diagnostic test in patients with symptoms suggestive of IHD.
   b. To assist in identifying those patients with documented IHD who are at increased risk for higher-grade stenosis or degree of left ventricular dysfunction.
   c. To quantify a patient's functional capacity or response to therapies.
   d. To follow the natural course of the disease at appropriate intervals.

3. Many protocols exist; however, the **Bruce protocol has become the most widely used.** In the standard Bruce protocol, a patient is exercised on a motorized treadmill. Every 3 minutes the speed or elevation of the treadmill is increased. The patient is monitored for symptoms of chest pain, heart rate, and blood pressure response to exercise, arrhythmias, and ST-segment changes. A significant test includes an ST-segment depression of at least 1.0 mm below the baseline. A variety of factors may produce misleading results. Those that can produce false-positive results include the use of medications such as digoxin and estrogen and conditions such as hyperventilation, cardiomyopathy, and mitral valve prolapse. Factors leading to a false-negative result include the use of medications such as nitrates, beta blockers, and calcium channel blockers and the failure to attain a vigorous heart rate response to exercise. For example, approximately 20% of patients with an abnormal ETT have significant ST-segment changes occurring only at maximum or near-maximum heart rate changes. Therefore, if a family physician is reviewing the report of an ETT on a patient and the maximum predicted heart rate was <85%, the results should be interpreted more cautiously.

   There are patients who should not undergo the standard ETT for a number of reasons. These include the inability to exercise because of gait or instability problems and underlying ECG abnormalities that make the standard ETT unreadable, such as left ventricular hypertrophy with strain, left bundle branch block, and ST-segment baseline abnormalities in the lateral precordial leads. If the patient is able to exercise and has the noted ECG baseline abnormalities, a thallium ETT is preferred. If the patient is unable to exercise, a Persantine/thallium test or dobutamine echocardiogram is indicated. The sensitivity and specificity of ETT in women are less than for men. Although some advocate the use of a thallium/thallium or dobutamine echocardiography for women needing a diagnostic evaluation, these studies, which are not dependent on ECG interpretation, are limited by breast attenuation artifact and provide less functional data than an ETT. Women with a moderate probability of IHD based on age and type of symptoms who have a normal baseline ECG may undergo a standard ETT.

TABLE 77–2. MOLECULAR MARKERS USED OR PROPOSED FOR USE IN THE DIAGNOSIS OF ACUTE MYOCARDIAL INFARCTION

Marker	Range of Times to Initial Elevation (h)	Mean Time to Peak Elevations (Nonthrombolysis)	Time to Return to Normal Range	Most Common Sampling Schedule
Myoglobin	1–4	6–7 h	24 h	Frequent; 1–2 h after CP
CTnI	3–12	24 h	5–10 d	Once at least 12 h after CP
CTnT	3–12	12 h–2 d	5–14 d	Once at least 12 h after CP
MB-CK	3–12	24 h	48–72 h	Every 12 h × 3[1]

[1] Increased sensitivity can be achieved with sampling every 6–8 hours.
CP, chest pain; cTnI, cardiac troponin I; cTnT, cardiac troponin T; MB-CK, MB isoenzyme creatine kinase (CK).

4. **Prognostic value of an ETT.** In addition to the diagnostic implications of an ETT, there are prognostic implications. The following are considered to be parameters associated with a poor prognosis or increased disease severity: failure to complete stage II of a Bruce protocol, failure to achieve a heart rate >120 beats per minute (off beta blockers), onset of ST-segment depression at a heart rate of <120 beats per minute, ST-segment depression >2.0 mm, ST-segment depression lasting >6 minutes into recovery, ST-segment depression in multiple leads, poor systolic blood pressure response to exercise, angina with exercise, and exercise-induced ventricular tachycardia. Recently, heart rate recovery and the Duke treadmill exercise score have been determined to be independent predictors of mortality.

5. **Resting ECG.** A resting ECG, while important to do on all patients with suspected IHD, must be interpreted with caution. The ECG will be normal or show nonspecific changes in more than 50% of patients with IHD. A normal resting ECG may not be used to rule out IHD. The classic ECG changes of acute ischemia are peaked, hyperacute T waves, T-wave flattening or inversion with or without ST-segment depression, horizontal ST-segment depression, and ST-segment elevation.

6. **Ambulatory Holter monitoring.** Among patients with stable angina who undergo 24-hour Holter monitoring, 40–72% of the episodes are painless. For Holter monitoring when ST-segment changes that meet strict criteria are seen in a patient with known IHD, these episodes are generally considered to represent episodes of myocardial ischemia. Ischemic criteria include at least 1 mm of horizontal or downsloping ST-segment depression that lasts for at least 1 minute and is separated from other discrete episodes by at least 1 minute of normal baseline. This methodology has limitations, including difficulty reading ST-segment changes in patients with an abnormal baseline (left ventricular hypertrophy with strain) or in those with a left bundle branch block. This method is not thought to be superior to the ETT.

7. **Angiography.** Cardiac catheterization is not routinely recommended for initial evaluation of patients with stable angina. Patients who warrant such an evaluation are those who exhibit evidence of severe myocardial ischemia on noninvasive testing or who have symptoms that are refractory to antianginal medications. In patients who undergo catheterization, the most important determinant of survival is left ventricular function, followed by the number of diseased vessels. Patients with left main artery disease or three-vessel disease with diminished left ventricular function are candidates for a coronary artery bypass graft procedure. Others (those with one- or two-vessel disease) are managed medically or considered for percutaneous transluminal coronary angioplasty (PTCA) or stenting.

III. **Treatment**
A. **Stable angina.** Stable angina is characterized by no change in frequency, severity, duration, or precipitating factors for at least the past 2 months. The treatment of patients with stable angina includes identification and management of specific cardiovascular risk factors, low-dose aspirin, and antianginal drug therapy.

1. **Risk factor modification.** Dietary modification, smoking cessation, and physical conditioning programs should be instituted.

2. **Treatment of associated disease.** Thyroid disease, hypertension, anemia, diabetes, hyperlipidemia, congestive heart failure, valvular disease, and arrhythmias should be aggressively identified and managed.

3. **Aspirin.** Most experts recommend a range of 80–300 mg of aspirin per day to decrease platelet aggregability.

4. **Antianginal drug therapy.** The goals are to abolish or reduce anginal attacks and myocardial ischemia and to promote a more normal lifestyle. The three classes of antianginal drugs commonly used are nitrates, beta blockers, and calcium channel blockers (Table 77–3). Each reduces myocardial oxygen demand and may improve blood flow to ischemic areas. No greater efficacy in relieving chest pain or decreasing exercise-induced ischemia has been shown for one or another group of these drugs, although specific clinical indications may favor one over another (diastolic dysfunction, left ventricular hypertrophy, hypertension, asthma, depression, diabetes mellitus, etc).

a. **Nitrates.** The most significant issue for this class of drugs is tolerance. Most studies show that tolerance develops rapidly when long-acting nitrates are given. Tolerance can develop within 24 hours. When prescribing a patch, the usual initial dose of transdermal nitroglycerin is 0.2 mg/hour. It is important to have patch-free intervals of 10–12 hours to retain the antianginal effect. Oral

TABLE 77–3. ANTIANGINAL MEDICATIONS

Drug	Usual Starting Dosage	Maximum Daily Dosage	Cost	Common Adverse Effects	Comments
BETA BLOCKERS					
Noncardioselective					
Propranolol	20 mg qid 40 mg bid	320 mg	$	Fatigue (dose-related), exacerbation of bronchospasm, bradycardia, AV conduction defects, left ventricular failure.	Beta blockers are particularly useful in treating the following conditions that occur with IHD: hypertension, ventricular arrhythmia, supraventricular arrhythmias.
Nadolol	40 mg qd	240 mg	$$$	Raynaud's phenomenon, impotence, nightmares, mild increase in lipids; may block symptoms of hypoglycemia in diabetics.	There is no advantage in using a beta blocker with ISA or alpha$_1$-sympathomimetic blockade. Cardioselectivity will be overcome as the dose is raised. Abrupt discontinuation may exacerbate angina.
Cardioselective					
Atenolol	50 mg qd	200 mg	$		
Metoprolol	50 mg bid	400 mg	$		
Intrinsic Sympathomimetic Activity (ISA)					
Acebutolol	200 mg bid	1200 mg	$$		
Pindolol	5 mg bid	60 mg	$$		
Alpha, and beta blockade					
Labetalol	100 mg bid	2400 mg	$$		
CALCIUM CHANNEL BLOCKERS					
Diltiazem sustained-release	60 mg bid	360 mg	$$	Edema, headache, nausea, dizziness, constipation, left ventricular failure, AV conduction defects. Use caution with combined use of beta blockers or digitalis (may experience exacerbation of congestive heart failure or conduction delays). All calcium channel blockers have the potential to induce hypotension; it is important to titrate the dose especially in the elderly.	Calcium channel blockers are useful in treating the following conditions: IHD, hypertension, and supra-ventricular arrhythmias

Long-acting formulation			
Diltiazem	120 mg qd	$$$	
Nifedipine	30 mg qd	$$$	
Verapamil	120 mg bid	$$$	
SECOND-GENERATION CALCIUM CHANNEL BLOCKERS			
Amlodipine	2.5–5 mg qd	$$$	Edema, hypotension, flushing, headache.	Plasma T1/2 36 hours, little negative inotropic effect, may be useful in treatment of angina associated with hypertension.
NITRATES			
Short-acting nitroglycerin			
Nitrostat	0.4 mg q 5 min × 3-1/150 grain	$	Headache and hypotension. Potential for hypotension greater when used in combination with a calcium channel blocker.	Tolerance is the most significant issue in the use of nitrates. Oral nitrates are more effective given twice daily at a high dose than frequently at a low dose.
Nitrospray	1–2 sprays q 5 min × 3	$ $$		Nitroglycerin patches should be removed at night to prevent tolerance. Nitrates work well with either beta or calcium channel blockers.
Long-acting nitroglycerin			
Transderm NTG	0.2 mg/hr 0.8 mg/hr	$$		
ISOSORBIDE DINITRATE			
Immediate-release			
Isordil	5 mg qid 160 mg	$		Caution in patients taking medications for erectile dysfunction; potential hypotension
Longer-acting			
Isordil SR	40 mg bid–tid 240 mg	$		

AV, atrioventricular; IHD, ischemic heart disease.
$, least expensive; $$, moderately expensive; $$$, most expensive.

nitroglycerin (isosorbide dinitrate) in the sustained-release form is usually started at 40 mg every 8–12 hours.

   b. Beta blockers. All beta blockers, regardless of their selective properties, are equally effective in patients with angina. About 20% of patients do not respond to beta blockers. Those who do not are more likely to have severe IHD. The dose of the beta blocker should be adjusted to achieve a heart rate of 50–60 beats per minute. Examples of starting regimens include the following: propranolol, 20 mg four times daily or 40 mg twice daily; metoprolol, 50 mg twice daily; and atenolol, 50 mg every day.

   c. Calcium channel blockers. These are a diverse group of compounds that have different effects on the atrioventricular node, heart rate, coronary arteries, diastolic relaxation, cardiac contractility, systemic blood pressure, and afterload. Most studies show equal effects between beta blockers and calcium channel blockers. Calcium channel blockers may be preferred in patients with obstructive airway disease, peripheral vascular disease, or supraventricular tachycardia. The most troublesome side effects are constipation, edema, headache, and aggravation of congestive heart failure. Examples of starting regimens include the following: nifedipine sustained-release, 30 mg every day; and diltiazem sustained-release, 120 mg every day. A recent case-control study reported an increased rate of MI among a group of hypertensive patients treated with short-acting calcium channel blockers. There is no evidence of a similar effect with long-acting calcium antagonists.

   d. Angiotensin-converting enzyme (ACE) inhibitors. Information from studies such as the Heart Outcomes Prevention Evaluation (HOPE) study, have suggested that use of an ACE inhibitor substantially lowers the risk of death, MI, coronary revascularization, and heart failure in high-risk patients with pre-existing vascular disease. For dosage information, please see Chapter 76.

  5. Antioxidants. Oxidized low-density lipoprotein particles are implicated in the development and progression of atherosclerosis. In observational studies, vitamin E, 100–400 IU daily, has been associated with a decrease in coronary events and shown to slow progression of atherosclerotic lesions in patients who have undergone coronary artery bypass grafting. Further studies are under way to clarify the many questions that remain about the role of antioxidants.

  6. Vitamins B_6, B_{12}, and folate. Elevated homocysteine levels are associated with IHD. Although the mechanisms are not well understood, alteration in coagulation profile or endothelial damage is postulated to play a role. Supplementation with B_6, B_{12}, and folate reduce plasma homocysteine levels.

  7. Hormone replacement therapy. Recent studies including the Women's Health Initiative (WHI) and the Estrogen/Progestin Replacement Study helped to clarify the role of hormone replacement therapy (HRT) in relation to IHD. HRT led to an increase in IHD events by 29%. Based on these studies, and consistent with American Heart Association recommendations, HRT is not recommended for either primary or secondary prevention of IHD. The WHI trial of unopposed estrogen vs. placebo in women who have undergone hysterectomy showed no increase in heart disease, but showed an increase in stroke in the treatment group.

B. Unstable angina. Unstable angina manifests clinically as an abrupt onset of ischemic symptoms at rest or as an intensification or change in the pattern of ischemic symptoms as well as an increasing ease of provocation (symptoms at rest or with minimal effort). The most important recent development in the management of unstable angina has been the 1994 report of the Agency for Health Care Policy and Research (AHCPR). The guidelines allow physicians to consider outpatient management for a select group of patients, specifically, those who are felt to be low-risk for MI. Low-risk patients may be treated with aspirin, NTG, or beta blockers. Follow-up should be no later than 72 hours. High- or moderate-risk patients should be admitted for intensive medical management. Clinical features consistent with high-risk include the following:

  1. Prolonged rest pain (>20 minutes).
  2. Pulmonary edema.
  3. Angina with new or worsening mitral regurgitation murmurs.
  4. Rest angina with dynamic ST changes >1 mm.
  5. Angina with S_3 or rales.
  6. Angina with hypotension.

C. Percutaneous transluminal coronary angioplasty (PTCA) and stenting. Although there remains no consensus on definitive indications for PTCA, there has been a marked increase in its use. It is generally chosen for patients with angina who have failed maximum medical management. It is used for single- or double-vessel disease, excluding the proximal left anterior descending coronary artery. Among patients with unstable angina, PTCA is recommended for those who do not show an adequate response to medical treatment. Restenosis continues to be a complication; however, the long-term outcome after successful angioplasty has been reported to be excellent even when compared with patients undergoing bypass surgery. Further research is needed in the areas of long-term outcome for multiple lesions, extensive disease, and avoidance of complications. Stenting, particularly with antiproliferative agents (eg, paclitaxel-eluding stents) has become increasingly popular and compares favorably to minimally invasive bypass surgery.

D. Coronary artery bypass graft (CABG) surgery. Large randomized trials have shown that surgical revascularization is more effective than medical therapy for at least several years for controlling symptoms. Development of atherosclerosis in the graft resulting in angina generally occurs within 5–10 years. Improved survival with surgical vs. medical therapy is seen only in the "sicker" subset of patients who are older and have more severe symptoms, particularly left main coronary artery disease or left ventricular dysfunction.

IV. Management Strategies. It is important to maximize therapy with any one class of antianginal drug before considering it a failed trial. Generally, the drug classes complement each other. There is no literature to support one class of antianginal drugs as superior to another. It is a common practice to first use nitrates as needed for patients with infrequent symptoms. For more frequent symptoms, a long-acting beta blocker or calcium channel blocker in addition to the as-needed nitrate is often used. With increasingly frequent symptoms, combination or "triple therapy" (nitrate + beta blocker + calcium channel blocker) may be used. Calcium channel blockers and beta blockers should be used in combination with caution because of the greater risk of extreme bradycardia or heart block. Aggressive measures targeted at risk factor modification should be included for all patients with IHD.

V. Prognosis

A. The three major factors that determine the prognosis of patients with angina include the amount of viable but jeopardized left ventricular myocardium, the percentage of irreversibly scarred myocardium, and the severity of underlying coronary atherosclerosis. ETT has been used to establish the prognosis in patients with symptomatic IHD. The exercise parameters associated with poor outcome have been described above. Comparing medical management and PTCA, one randomized study of male patients with single-vessel disease found PTCA to be superior to medical management at 6 months, although 15% of patients required a second procedure. PTCA is superior to medical management in multivessel disease. Stenting with antiproliferative agents (eg, paclitaxel) may be as effective for isolated high-grade lesions as CABG. CABG is superior to both medical management or PTCA for proximal left anterior descending coronary artery lesions or multivessel disease.

B. Natural history. Based on current information, the following is known regarding the natural history and prognosis of IHD:

1. IHD is the leading cause of premature, permanent disability in the US labor force, accounting for 19% of disability, according to the Social Security Administration.
2. A substantial number of patients with IHD have moderate to severe limitations in their usual activities.
3. Unrecognized MIs are common and as lethal as symptomatic infarcts. At least 25% of MIs are silent and another 25% present with atypical chest pain. Only 20% of MIs are preceded by angina. Most MIs occur at rest and nearly as many occur during sleep as during heavy physical activity. Distressing life events reportedly occur with increased frequency in the months preceding an MI.

   Women are often overlooked as having significant IHD. Women older than 65 years are as vulnerable to IHD mortality as men. There is a precipitous increase in IHD in women after the menopause (whether natural or surgical).

REFERENCES

Braunwald E: *Heart Disease: A Textbook of Cardiovascular Medicine,* 6th ed. Saunders; 2001.

Ellestad MH: *Stress Testing: Principles and Practice,* 5th ed. Oxford Press; 2003.

Writing group for the women's health initiative investigators: Risks and benefits of estrogen plus progestin in healthy postmenopausal women: Principal results from the women's health initiative randomized controlled trial. JAMA 2002;**288:**321.

78   Menopause

Mark Mengel, MD, MPH

KEY POINTS

- Menopause usually presents with a progressive lengthening of the menstrual cycle with lighter menses, hot flashes, and flushes. Menopause can be diagnosed when no menses have occurred for 12 months.
- Diagnostic testing is rarely indicated in women who are at an age when menopause is expected; however, in younger menopausal women determination of a follicle-stimulating hormone (FSH) level is warranted. Menopausal status is indicated by an FSH level of >30 MIU/mL.
- Menopause is associated with changes in many organs including skin, the reproductive system, and bones. The high prevalence of osteoporosis in postmenopausal women, with its attendant increase in fractures, has led many clinicians prior to the recent publication of several recent trials to prescribe hormone replacement therapy for postmenopausal women.
- Publication of the WHI and HERS trials, revealing that synthetic estrogen/progesterone replacement therapy places women at greater risk for many significant illnesses, has resulted in a stunning reversal of the previous widespread use of hormone replacement therapy. In postmenopausal women with debilitating symptoms at menopause, short-term use of hormone replacement therapy is appropriate, but long-term use to prevent osteoporosis is no longer deemed acceptable.
- Certain other drugs (clonidine, gabapentin, venlafaxine, paroxetine, and megestrol) and herbal treatments such as black cohosh, soy protein, and isoflavones have been shown in some studies to be modestly effective in reducing menopausal symptoms. Some "anti-aging" proponents feel that bio-identical hormone replacement carries less risk than synthetic, although that issue has not been well studied.
- As women rapidly lose bone density once reproductive hormone secretion ceases, osteoporosis risk factor reduction, adequate intake of vitamin D and calcium, and routine use of bone density testing are indicated.

I. **Introduction**
   A. **Definition. Menopause** is the permanent cessation of menstruation caused by a loss of ovarian function. This condition can be diagnosed after no menses have occurred for 12 consecutive months. **Perimenopause** is the transitional period immediately prior to menopause. The **climacteric** is a term used to encompass the physiologic changes and symptoms surrounding the transition from reproductive to nonreproductive status. **Postmenopausal** is the label often applied to women if their last period has occurred more than a year ago.
   B. **Epidemiology**
      1. Between 0.2% and 1% of visits made to primary care physicians are for menopausal symptoms.
      2. The mean age of menopause is 51.4 years, with a range of 41–59. Risk factors associated with an earlier age of menopause are current smoking; lower educational attainment; being separated, widowed, or divorced; being unemployed; and having a history of heart disease. Risk factors for later age of menopause were increased parity, prior use of oral contraceptives, and Japanese race. By 55 years of age, 95% of women are menopausal.
      3. Disabling symptoms attributable to decline in estrogen production for which medical therapy is sought are estimated to occur in 10–15% of perimenopausal women Current smoking and high body mass index were risk factors associated with the onset of hot flashes.
   C. **Pathophysiology.** Menopause is associated with ovarian, hormonal, and target-organ changes. A progressive decrease in the number of ovarian follicles occurs from the

20th week of gestation in utero until the ovary is depleted of follicles at menopause. Levels of follicle-stimulating hormone (FSH) dramatically increase during the perimenopausal period, while levels of plasma estradiol (the principal ovarian estrogen) decline at rates corresponding to the rise in FSH levels. Other reproductive hormones, like testosterone, also decline. Many organs have specific receptors for particular circulating steroid. Many end-organ changes occur as a result of declining or absent circulating estrogen levels (Table 78–1).

II. Diagnosis

A. Symptoms and signs. Most women in their late 40s experience a progressive lengthening of the menstrual cycle with lighter menses. Irregular periods, caused by anovulation, are also common in the perimenopausal period.

1. **Vasomotor symptoms.** The hot flash and the flush are the two principal components of vasomotor symptomatology. Researchers believe that alterations in the hypothalamic set point due to estrogen withdrawal are responsible for the flush. Patients with such disorders as pheochromocytoma, hyperthyroidism, anxiety, excessive caffeine intake, hypoglycemia, and carcinoid syndrome usually present with vasomotor symptomatology in combination with other conditions, such as hypertension, tachycardia, and diarrhea. The presence of these conditions suggests a nonmenopausal origin.

   a. The **hot flash** is the sudden onset of warmth lasting 2–3 minutes. Experienced by 75–85% of menopausal women, the hot flash begins about 1 minute before the flush and lasts about 1 minute after its onset.

   b. The **flush** consists of visible redness of the upper chest, face, and neck and is followed by profuse sweating in these areas. The flush also lasts 2–3 minutes and is associated with a mean temperature elevation of 2.5 °C (4.5 °F). When left untreated, hot flushes are usually most severe in the first 1 or 2 years, after which severity gradually declines. Twenty-five percent of women report a duration of hot flushes of more than 5 years, and occasionally symptoms persist into the seventh or eighth decade.

TABLE 78–1. END-ORGAN CHANGES RESULTING FROM ESTROGEN DEFICIENCY

Target Organ	Change or Symptom
Neuroendocrine organs (hypothalamus)	Hot flushes, flashes, or both Atrophy, dryness, pruritus
Skin/mucous membranes	Dry hair or loss of hair Facial hirsutism Dry mouth
Skeleton	Osteoporosis with related fractures Backache
Vocal cords	Lower voice
Breasts	Reduced size Softer consistency Drooping (loss of ligamentous support)
Heart	Coronary artery disease
Vulva	Atrophy, dystrophy, or both Pruritus vulvae
Vagina	Dyspareunia Vaginitis
Uterus/pelvic floor	Uterovaginal prolapse
Bladder/urethra	Cystoureteritis Ectropion Frequency and/or urgency Stress incontinence

Adapted with permission from Utian WH: Overview on menopause. Am J Obstet Gynecol 1987;**156**:1280.

   c. Associated symptoms commonly reported with the above vasomotor phenomena are heart palpitations, headache, throbbing in the head or neck, and nausea.

  2. Psychological symptoms. The following symptoms all have been reported during the perimenopausal period: fatigue, insomnia, anxiety, and depression, although studies do not support menopause causing depression.

  3. Atrophy of the lower genital tract

   a. Vulvar pruritus is common, especially in fair-skinned women.

   b. Vaginitis and dyspareunia from atrophy of vaginal mucosa are experienced by about 10–20% of women. Symptoms include dryness, burning, leukorrhea, itching, and bleeding.

   c. Atrophy of the urethral mucosa, which leads to frank urethritis, dysuria, urgency, and frequency, is less common.

  4. Signs. The physical examination is usually normal during the early perimenopausal period, with characteristic findings evident after the onset of menopause.

   a. The **breasts** appear less firm and smaller, with a regression of glandular tissue and an increase in fibrous tissue.

   b. The **pelvic examination** is most revealing in the postmenopausal period.

    (1) The **labia majora** are smaller, and hair in the perivulvar area is thin.

    (2) The **vaginal epithelium** appears pale, thin, and dry, with a loss of rugae and secretions.

    (3) The **cervical os** is often smaller and may be stenotic. The cervical epithelium is thinner and more easily traumatized.

   c. Uterine size is diminished. Reduced collagen in the supporting ligamentous structures of the pelvis can lead to uterine prolapse and pelvic relaxation. This relaxation occurs especially when there is a history of multiparity, prior birth trauma, a family history of uterine prolapse or pelvic relaxation, or chronic pelvic stress from coughing, constipation, or heavy work.

   d. The **ovaries** should not be palpable on pelvic examination after menopause. Palpable ovarian enlargement in a menopausal woman suggests ovarian carcinoma until proven otherwise.

   e. Urethral prolapse can occur because of atrophy of the urethral mucosa. A prolapsed urethra or caruncle appears as a red, friable mass within the urethra itself.

   f. Dry, wrinkled, and more easily traumatized skin is attributable to both menopause and age. Thinning of scalp hair and increased facial hair (hirsutism) may also be evident.

 B. Laboratory tests. The presence of vasomotor symptoms, oligomenorrhea, and atrophy of the lower genital tract in women in their mid- to late 40s almost certainly confirms the onset of the perimenopausal period. Diagnostic testing (eg, circulating estrogen and gonadotropin levels) is rarely, if ever, indicated in this circumstance.

  Determination of FSH levels is warranted in any woman younger than age 35 experiencing signs and symptoms of menopause. Specific causes of premature ovarian failure include genetic abnormalities, autoimmune disorders, and rare hormonal defects (see Chapter 3). FSH levels are the most sensitive indicator of ovarian failure. Menopausal status is indicated by FSH level >30 mIU/mL. As FSH levels are highly variable in the perimenopause, high FSH levels should be confirmed by a second test 1–3 months after the first.

  Estrogen and progesterone are not reliably measured by single assays in perimenopausal women.

III. Treatment. The Women's Health Initiative (WHI) and the Heart and Estrogen/progestin Replacement Study (HERS) findings have dramatically changed the use of hormone replacement therapy in postmenopausal women. (The WHI is a primary prevention trial in postmenopausal women; the HERS is a secondary prevention trial in postmenopausal women with coronary artery disease.) Both studies showed that the risks of synthetic estrogen/progestin replacement therapy outweighed the benefit. Women on synthetic estrogen/progestin therapy were at greater risk for heart disease, strokes, invasive breast cancer, thromboembolic events, gallbladder disease, and dementia. Benefits included a reduction in fractures, osteoporosis, colorectal cancer, and diabetes. However, given that the average age of women in both of these trials was older than 60 years and that many had risk factors for coronary artery disease, it is likely that younger women without any risk factors would have less risk of harm. Therefore, in postmenopausal women with debilitating symptoms of menopause, short-term use of hormone replacement therapy is appropriate.

A. **Indications for estrogen replacement therapy**
   1. Moderate to severe hot flashes.
   2. Moderate to severe genital atrophy.
   3. Diminished moods secondary to menopause.
   4. Diminished quality of life secondary to menopausal symptoms.
   5. Osteoporosis prevention.

B. **Contraindications to estrogen replacement therapy** (Table 78–2).
   1. Absolute—estrogen-dependent neoplasia (breast or endometrium).
   2. Relative—endometrial hyperplasia.
   3. Relative—past history of thrombosis.
   4. Relative—cardiovascular risk factors such as hypertension, hyperlipemia, or diabetes mellitus.
   5. Relative—cholelithiasis.
   6. Relative—family history of estrogen-dependent neoplasia.

C. **Preparations available.** Estrogen is available as a pill, patch, vaginal ring, or cream.
   1. **Pills.** The most widely prescribed oral estrogen preparation is equine conjugated estrogen (Premarin), 0.30–2.5 mg orally every day. Synthetic conjugated estrogen (Cenestin), 0.625–1.25 mg orally every day, esterified estrogen (Estratab or Menest), 1.25–2.5 mg orally every day, and estropipate (Ogen or Ortho-Est), 0.625–5 mg orally every day, are also available. Many women prefer the nonequine varieties of estrogen, fearing the effects of the metabolic breakdown products of that preparation. A 28-day supply of these preparations typically costs $10–20, with generic micronized estradiol being the least expensive, at under $10 for a 28-day supply.
   2. **Patches.** Transdermal estradiol patches are available at a dose of 50–100 µg/day. Many preparations are available, including Alora (one patch two times per week), Climara (one patch weekly), Estraderm (one patch two times per week), and Vivelle (one patch twice weekly). Patches are typically more expensive, $20–30 for a 28-day supply. The advantage of patches is that they have a limited effect on hepatic function and thus they are thought to have less risk of clotting and lipid abnormalities associated with other estrogen preparations. Unfortunately, about 24% of women who use this method have some form of skin irritation, which often can be managed by site rotation.
   3. **Vaginal rings.** An estradiol acetate vaginal ring (Fem Ring) was recently approved by the US Food and Drug Administration at doses of 50–100 µg/day, lasting 90 days. Estring is a vaginal ring that provides 7.5 µg/day of estradiol, a very low dose, and is used only for treating vaginal symptoms.
   4. **Vaginal creams.** Vaginal creams are most useful for those women with severe symptoms of atopic vaginitis but have mild vasomotor symptoms. Intervaginal creams, such as conjugated estrogen (Premarin), 0.65 mg/g, and estropipate (Ogen), 1.5 mg/g, may be helpful. Daily administration of 1.2–2.4 g is typically recommended on days 1–21 of the month, although continuous therapy on weekdays only is increasingly popular. Intervaginal estrogen creams do achieve some systemic absorption.

      Vaginal pruritus responds poorly to topical estrogens. Regular application of a testosterone ointment, such as testosterone propionate cream, 2.5%, one application per day, will increase thickness of the vulvar epithelium, thereby relieving dryness and itching.

TABLE 78–2. CONTRAINDICATIONS TO ESTROGEN REPLACEMENT THERAPY

Absolute	Relative
Estrogen-dependent neoplasia (breast, endometrium)	Endometrial hyperplasia
	Past history of vaso-occlusive disease (thrombosis)
	Diabetes mellitus
	Hypertension
	Cholelithiasis
	Family history of estrogen-dependent neoplasia (breast, endometrium)

Adapted with permission from Whitehead MI: The menopause. Practitioner 1987;**231**:42.

D. **Progestins** have been shown to relieve vasomotor symptoms in postmenopausal patients either alone or in combination with estrogens. They are also useful in preventing endometrial hyperplasia in women on estrogen replacement therapy.
   1. **Progestin-only regimens.** Medroxyprogesterone acetate (Provera), 20 mg orally daily, is especially appealing for women for whom estrogen therapy is contraindicated or who have experienced intolerable side effects, such as breast tenderness, breakthrough bleeding, and nausea, on estrogen therapy. Other progesterone preparations include Micronor and Prometrium.
   2. **Combination estrogen and progestin therapy.** Estrogen replacement alone may lead to endometrial hyperplasia which, in a small group of women, progresses to endometrial carcinoma. Maximal protection against endometrial hyperplasia occurs when progestin is prescribed for at least 10 days of each calendar month. Because that regimen usually results in periods continuing, continuous daily combination therapy is often preferred. A low-dose version of Prempro, 0.45 mg of Premarin daily with 1.5 mg of Provera daily, will often relieve menopausal symptoms, and if not, stronger preparations are available.

      Progestin use for women who have had a hysterectomy and are receiving estrogen replacement therapy is not indicated given the results of the WHI and HERS trials.
E. **Effective nonhormonal treatments for menopausal symptoms.** Given the results of the WHI and HERS studies, nonhormonal treatments for menopausal symptoms have become more popular. Effective treatments include:
   1. Clonidine (Catapres), 0.1–0.2 mg orally twice daily.
   2. Gabapentin (Neurontin), 300 mg orally three times daily.
   3. Venlafaxine (Effexor), 37.5–75 mg orally every day.
   4. Paroxetine (Paxil), 20–60 mg orally every day.
   5. Megestrol (Megace), 20 mg orally twice daily.
F. **Selective estrogen-receptor modulators.** Raloxifene, 60 mg orally every day, a drug that has both estrogen-agonist effects on bone, liver, and heart and estrogen-antagonist effects on breast and uterus, has been shown to produce risks of breast cancer and decrease risk of osteoporosis in postmenopausal women. These effects make raloxifene an attractive alternative for those women concerned with estrogen's potential for cancer proliferation. Unfortunately, raloxifene has no effect on genital atrophy and may worsen the vasomotor symptoms of hot flashes and sweats. Like estrogen, the incidence of thrombophlebitis is increased compared with placebo. A 30-day supply costs $60–100.
G. **Complementary and alternative medicine treatments**
   1. Regular exercise has proven effective in one small trial.
   2. Soy proteins and isoflavones have proved modestly effective in some trials, although there are conflicting results.
   3. Herbal treatments such as black cohosh (Remifemin, 2 tablets orally twice daily (80 mg/day)), also appear modestly effective; however, these treatments may increase the risk for breast cancer just as estrogen does. Dong quai and ginseng appear not to work. Wild yams are promoted as a "natural" precursor to hormones, but are not converted to reproductive hormones in the human body and are not expected to work.
   4. Bio-identical hormone replacement. "Anti-aging" advocates promote the use of bio-identical or natural estrogen, progestin, and testosterone replacement, feeling that natural hormone replacement will lack the risks and side effects of synthetic hormone replacement. While not well studied, these compounded formulations are popular among a segment of the population. Natural estrogen is usually compounded into BIEST (80% estriol [E3] and 20% estradiol [E2]), 1.25–5 mg orally every day, or TRI-EST (70% E3, 20% E2, and 10% E1), 1.25–5 mg/day. Progesterone is often given in the form of a capsule, 100 mg orally twice daily; troche, 100 mg twice daily, or trichurite, 100 mg sublingual twice daily. Testosterone is often compounded into an 10 to 20-mg/g cream given at a dose of $\frac{1}{4}$ to $\frac{1}{2}$ g every night. Further studies of compounded bio-identical reproductive hormone replacement are needed before their widespread use can be advocated.
IV. **Management Strategies**
   A. **Patient education.** For many women, the worst thing about menopause is not knowing what to expect. Thorough evaluation of the woman's understanding of menopause and accurate education directed at identification of symptoms and management options

TABLE 78–3. KEY QUESTIONS TO UNCOVER SEXUAL PROBLEMS DURING THE PERIMENOPAUSAL AND POSTMENOPAUSAL PERIODS

1. Are you sexually active?
2. Do you have a partner at the present time?
3. Has there been any change in your interest in or desire for sexual activity?
4. Is intercourse pleasurable?
5. Do you experience any discomfort during intercourse?
6. Have you noticed any change in lubrication when you become aroused?
7. Do you reach orgasm satisfactorily?
8. Does your partner have any problems with your sexual relationship?

Adapted, with permission, from Iddenden DA: Sexuality during the menopause. Med Clin North Am 1987;**71**:87.

will greatly reduces anxiety in many postmenopausal women. Many myths surround menopause, including that menopause signals the end of a woman's sexual experience and that menopause is associated with a high incidence of mental health problems, cancer, and heart disease. Risk factor reduction for heart disease and cancer, a discussion of the patient's sexual interest and activities, and pertinent patient education are a good starting point (Table 78–3).

B. Patient follow-up
1. **Periodic follow-up visits,** at least yearly, are needed to monitor women on hormone replacement therapy. More frequent follow-up visits initially should be scheduled. Women should be specifically questioned on known side effects of hormone replacement therapy at every visit. Hormone replacement therapy should be reduced as symptoms abate and stopped as soon as possible. Current recommendations state that women should not be on hormone replacement therapy for longer than 5 years; although many women insist on continuing hormone replacement therapy past that time.
2. **Endometrial biopsy.** Vaginal bleeding in a women on hormone replacement therapy demands evaluation with either an endometrial biopsy or a vaginal ultrasound measuring the endometrial stripe. Biopsies every 2–3 years for women at particularly high risk for endometrial cancer, even if asymptomatic, have been suggested as prudent.
3. **Osteoporosis management.** Women rapidly lose bone density once reproductive hormone secretion ceases. Risk factor reduction, adequate intake of vitamin D and calcium, and routine use of bone density testing are all indicated (see Chapter 81 on osteoporosis).

REFERENCES

Apgar BS, Greenberg G: Using progestins in clinical practice. Am Fam Physician 2000;**62**:1839, 1849.
Bastian LA, Smith CM, Nanda K: Is this woman perimenopausal? JAMA 2003;**289**(7):895.
Hlatky MA, et al: Quality-of-life and depressive symptoms in postmenopausal women after receiving hormone therapy: Results from the Heart and Estrogen/Progestin Replacement Study (HERS) trial. JAMA 2002;**287**(5):591.
Kanaya AM, et al: Glycemic effects of postmenopausal hormone therapy: The Heart and Estrogen/Progestin Replacement Study. A randomized, double-blind, placebo-controlled trial. Ann Intern Med 2003;**138**(1):1.
Kligler B: Black cohosh. Am Fam Physician 2003;**68**:114.
Kronenberg F, Fugh-Berman A: Complementary and alternative medicine for menopausal symptoms: A review of randomized, controlled trials. Ann Intern Med 2002;**137**(10):805.
Nelson HD: Assessing benefits and harms of hormone replacement therapy: Clinical applications. JAMA 2002;**288**(7):882.
North American Menopause Society: Amended report from the NAMS Advisory Panel on Postmenopausal Hormone Therapy. Menopause 2003;**10**(1):6.
Rossouw JE, et al: Risks and benefits of estrogen plus progestin in healthy postmenopausal women: Principal results from the Women's Health Initiative randomized controlled trial. JAMA 2002; **288**(3):321.
U.S. Preventive Services Task Force: Postmenopausal hormone replacement therapy for the primary prevention of chronic conditions recommendations and rationale. Am Fam Physician 2003;**67**(2):358.
Whiteman MK, et al: Smoking, body mass, and hot flashes in midlife women. Obstet Gynecol 2003; **101**(2):264.

79   Obesity

Radhika R. Hariharan, MD, MRCP (UK), Brian C. Reed, MD, & Sarah R.
Edmonson, MD

KEY POINTS

- Obesity is diagnosed when the body mass index is ≥30 kg/m².
- The primary goal of treatment should be weight loss of at least 10% of initial body weight.
  Maintenance of this new weight is the next priority.
- Strategies for weight loss include a low-calorie diet, which is the cornerstone of management, along with exercise, behavioral therapies, and medications.
- Drug therapy is indicated when other therapies fail after 3 months of trial or when there is
  medical comorbidity indicating a need for more aggressive weight loss.
- Drug therapy should be viewed as long term and the risks should be carefully considered
  in the individual patient.
- Bariatric surgery is an appropriate alternative for those patients who have failed conventional therapy; long- and short-term risks should be considered carefully before considering surgery.

I. **Introduction**
   A. **Definitions**
      1. **Obesity** is a disorder that occurs when a person has such an excess amount of
         body fat that they become at risk for adverse health conditions.
      2. **Body mass index (BMI).** In 1997, the World Health Organization International
         Obesity Task Force recommended adoption of BMI as a standard for the assessment of body fat. BMI is calculated by dividing a person's weight in kilograms by
         one's height in meters squared. Based on these guidelines, one is considered
         overweight at a body mass index between 25.0 and 29.9 kg/m². A BMI ≥30 kg/m²
         meets the criteria for obesity (see Table 79–1).
   B. **Epidemiology**
      1. **Prevalence.** Over 97 million adults in the United States are overweight or obese.
         Data from the National Health and Nutrition Examination Survey conducted in 1999
         and 2000 reveal that the prevalence of obesity in the United States was 30.5%.
         The percentage of overweight adults in the United States is 64.5%.
      2. **Risk factors**
         a. **Race.** Higher percentages of non-Hispanic blacks and Mexican Americans
            were either obese or overweight when compared to similar non-Hispanic
            whites in similar age categories. Among non-Hispanic blacks, almost 70% of
            individuals older than age 20 met the criteria for being overweight and almost
            40% met the criteria for obesity. Of non-Hispanic whites older than 20 years,
            almost 63% met the criteria for being overweight and 28.7% met the criteria for
            being obese.
         b. **Age.** The prevalence of obesity increases with age and is particularly apparent
            between the ages of 20 and 40.
         c. **Inactivity.** The relative risk of obesity among children in the United States is
            5.3 times greater for children who watch television for 5 or more hours a day

TABLE 79–1. WORLD HEALTH ORGANIZATION CATEGORIZATION OF OBESITY

Body Mass Index	
Normal	Under 27 kg/m²
Overweight	27–29.9 kg/m²
Obesity Class I	30–34.9 kg/m²
Obesity Class II	35–39.9 kg/m²
Obesity Class III	over 40 kg/m²

compared with those who watched television for <2 hours. This was valid even after correcting for a wide range of socioeconomic variables.

   d. Socioeconomic status. In industrialized countries a higher prevalence is seen in those with lower educational levels and low income.

   e. Marital status. A tendency to increase weight after marriage and parity exists.

3. Current trends suggest that the prevalence of obesity will continue to increase.

C. **Etiology**

1. Obesity represents a heterogeneous group of conditions with multiple causes. By definition, it results from imbalance between energy intake and expenditure. Energy expenditure is primarily derived from the resting metabolic rate and physical activity.

2. **Environmental factors.** Migrant studies attest to the critical role of environment in the development of obesity. A marked change in BMI is frequently observed when populations with a common genetic heritage live under new circumstances of plentiful food and little exercise. Pima Indians in the United States, for example, are on average about 25 kg heavier than Pima Indians in Mexico.

3. **Genetic factors**

   a. Evidence from several twin and adoption studies shows a strong genetic predisposition in obesity. Recently, specific mutations causing human obesity have been found in those rare children with extreme obesity with clear evidence for monogenic inheritance. Genetic syndromes associated with severe obesity include Prader-Willi, Bardet-Biedl, Cohen, Alstrom, and Klinefelter's syndromes.

   b. The discovery of leptin, a novel adipocyte hormone, which is deficient in the obese ob/ob mouse, has significantly advanced the understanding of the neurobiology of obesity. Several mutations in leptin and leptin receptor have also been shown to cause monogenic human obesity.

   c. Genetic studies in the more common forms of obesity have shown a region of chromosome 2 that influences obesity-related phenotypes in several different racial groups. This region contains the pro-opiomelanocortin gene.

4. **Gene–environment interaction.** Body weight is determined by an interaction between genetic, environmental, and psychosocial factors. Although obesity runs in families, the influence of the genotype on the etiology may be modified by nongenetic factors. The genetic influences seem to operate through susceptibility genes, which increase the risk of developing obesity. The susceptible gene hypothesis is supported by findings from twin studies, in which pairs of twins were exposed to varying energy balance. The differences in the rate, proportion, and site of weight gain showed greater similarity within pairs than between pairs of twins.

5. **Other causes.** Medical conditions and some medications, such as long-term corticosteroid use, phenothiazines, and antidepressants, can also result in obesity, but such causes account for <1% of cases. Hypothyroidism and Cushing's syndrome are the most common diseases that cause obesity. Diseases of the hypothalamus can also result in obesity, but these are quite rare. Major depression, which usually results in weight loss, can occasionally present with weight gain. Consideration of these causes is particularly important when evaluating recent weight gain.

II. **Diagnosis**

A. **Assessment** of a patient's weight involves evaluation of **three key measures: BMI, waist circumference, and an individual's risk factors for diseases and conditions associated with obesity** (Table 79–2).

1. Assessing waist circumference is important because excess abdominal fat is an independent predictor of disease risk. Android obesity (excess fat located primarily in the abdomen or upper body) places an individual at greater risk for congestive heart disease, hypertension, lipid disorders, and type II diabetes mellitus. Gynoid obesity (excess fat located primarily in the lower extremities or hips) does not. A waist circumference of >40 inches in men and >35 inches in women signifies increased risk in those who have a BMI of 25–34.9.

2. Gross calculation of BMI is not an effective estimation of risk in the following subgroups:

   a. In children and adolescents, the appropriate ratio of weight to height differs from that for infants and toddlers; this ratio must be assessed on an age- and gender-specific table. Excessive calorie intake in children will usually manifest itself in additional height as well as excess weight. As such, children who demonstrate exceptional height should be evaluated for lifestyle factors that put them at risk for obesity.

TABLE 79–2. RISK ASSESSMENT IN OBESITY

	Normal/ Over-weight	Obesity Class I	Obesity Class II	Obesity Class III
Waist circumference <40 inches (male) or <35 inches (female)	Low risk	Moderate Risk		High risk
Waist circumference >40 inches (male) or >35 inches (female)	Moderate risk	Moderate Risk	High risk	
Presence of comorbidities such as osteoarthritis, gallstones, stress incontinence, and menstrual irregularities		High risk		
Presence of comorbidities such as established coronary artery disease, other atherosclerotic disease, type II diabetes mellitus, and sleep apnea	High risk			

    b. Individuals who are <4 feet tall, or >7 feet tall, cannot be evaluated with a BMI. For these individuals, secondary measures may be used, such as body fat analysis or fitness testing.

    c. Competitive athletes and body builders may have misleadingly high BMI levels. These patients often have low total body fat and excellent cardiovascular fitness. Although long-term survival data about this subgroup of patients is sparse, it seems likely that their excess muscle mass does not represent the same risk as in other overweight patients.

    d. Pregnant women should not use BMI to evaluate risk, particularly in the second or third trimester.

B. Screening for medical conditions that may promote obesity should be performed.

    1. Endocrine disorders that promote weight gain, such as thyroid disease, hyperandrogenism or polycystic ovarian syndrome, and hypercortisolism, are generally accompanied by global symptoms such as skin changes, hair loss and distribution changes, abnormal menstrual cycles, mood and energy derangement, gastrointestinal distress, and atypical fat distribution. In patients who demonstrate some or all of these symptoms, laboratory evaluation should precede weight loss efforts.

    2. Many medications are associated with weight gain, including corticosteroids, insulin or insulin secretagogues, antiepileptics, anxiolytics or antidepressants, and antipsychotics. Weight-loss plans are not necessarily contraindicated for patients on these drugs. However, changing therapy when possible will increase the patient's chance of successful weight loss.

    3. Assess the patient for the presence of comorbid **psychiatric disease** that could affect his or her ability to understand and follow a dietary plan.

C. Assess comorbidities

    1. Established coronary artery disease, other atherosclerotic disease, type II diabetes mellitus, and sleep apnea are considered to be very high-risk comorbidities. Patients with these conditions should be offered aggressive weight management.

    2. Osteoarthritis, gallstones, stress incontinence, and menstrual irregularities, while also associated with obesity, are less life-threatening.

    3. Other conditions that may increase mortality risk in association with obesity include hypertension, smoking, hyperlipidemia, elevated fasting glucose, and increased age.

D. Dietary history. Dietary history should include information about both typical daily intake and deviations from this routine. Information should be collected about family events, celebratory behavior, and binge eating behavior. The frequency and type of atypical behavior should be noted. Specifically inquire about high-calorie beverages, such as soda, juice, or milk. Alcohol intake should be noted and quantified.

    E. Exercise history should include type, intensity, duration, and frequency. Encourage the patient to list informal physical activity at work or home in addition to deliberate attempts to exercise.

    F. Laboratory evaluation. To rule out secondary causes and assess for comorbid conditions, an initial laboratory evaluation, including a fasting lipid profile, fasting chemistry panel including blood glucose, and a thyroid-stimulating hormone test, should be ordered.

III. Treatment. The aim of a treatment program should be to reduce weight and maintain lowered weight. The goals of treatment should be tailored to the individual. In general, the primary goal is a 10% reduction from the initial weight. Successful weight loss should be regarded as a loss of more than 5% of the initial weight while very successful weight loss would be that of greater than 20% of initial body weight. A loss of 10% of body weight is of major clinical benefit with associated changes such as lowered blood pressure, lowered total cholesterol and triglycerides, an increase in high-density lipoprotein (HDL) cholesterol, and a significant improvement in diabetic control. One appropriate treatment algorithm is described in Figure 79–1.

  A. Dietary interventions

    1. Diet control is the cornerstone of obesity management and its primary role should be emphasized to the patient. In order to successfully lose weight, one must create a deficit of 500–1000 kcal/day. There are several dietary approaches to achieve this goal.

      a. Low-calorie diets consisting of approximately 1000–1200 kilocalories/day have been successfully demonstrated to result in weight loss and decreases of abdominal fat.

      b. Very low calorie diets that only permit 400–500 kilocalories/day promote initial weight loss between 13–23 kg. However, randomized controlled trials have shown that very low calorie diets do not result in greater long-term weight loss when compared to low calorie diets.

    2. In addition to the total caloric intake, the patient may benefit from changes in the dietary composition.

      a. Lower-fat diets promote weight loss by limiting the percentage of daily calories from fat to 20–30%. Because dietary fat intake has been associated with cholesterol levels, heart disease, and increased risks for certain cancers, this approach may be desirable for patients with multiple comorbid conditions.

      b. Low-carbohydrate diets such as the Atkins diet are based upon the theory that overweight and obese people are efficient at converting excess carbohydrates into fat. Low-carbohydrate diets advocate restricting total daily carbohydrates to between 40 and 100 g/day. Currently there is insufficient evidence to make recommendations for or against such low-carbohydrate diets.

  B. Behavioral therapy

    1. Behavioral therapy refers to the application of psychological techniques to treatment of obesity and is now an accepted modality of treatment. Behavioral weight programs seek to alter lifestyle and environment in order to effect a change in weight. They encourage the patient to become more aware of eating behavior and physical activity, and to focus on changing the behaviors that influence them. The chief feature of this form of treatment is that it emphasizes personal responsibility for the initiation and maintenance of treatment.

    2. Behavior therapy is usually presented in an organized and comprehensive format and includes several components including stimulus control, self-reward, and cognitive restructuring.

    3. Although the degree of weight loss achieved with behavioral techniques alone is modest, averaging less than 10 kg in most studies, the advantages include the lack of side effects and the low attrition rate.

  C. Exercise. While exercise alone results in only modest weight loss, randomized controlled trials consistently show the maintenance of weight loss for 2 years. A combination of diet and exercise generally produces more weight loss than diet alone. Regular exercise results in reduction in blood pressure and improvements in lipid profiles, glycemic control, and cardiovascular fitness. Persuading an obese patient to participate and maintain an exercise program is difficult. Less vigorous forms of activity such as brisk walking and swimming may also provide significant improvement in metabolic profiles.

  D. Pharmacotherapy of obesity

    1. Indications

      a. For a minority of patients in whom there is considerable medical risk and who have failed nondrug treatments, medications may serve as useful long-term additions to behavioral therapy.

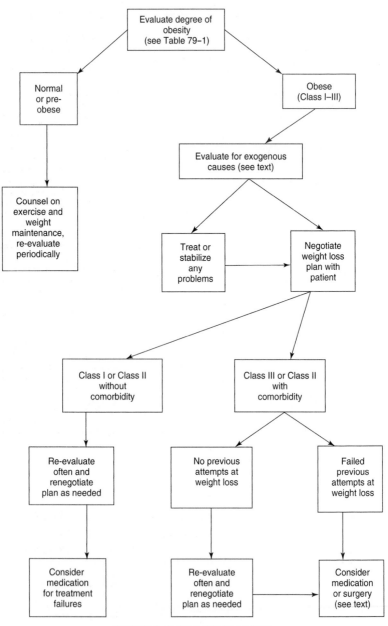

FIGURE 79–1. Treatment algorithm for obesity.

    b. Medications are currently regarded as appropriate for use in adults with a BMI of 27 or higher with obesity-related medical problems. It may also be appropriate to consider pharmaceutical treatment if the patient has failed a 3-month trial of diet, exercise, and behavior therapy and the BMI is >30 with weight loss being <10% of initial weight.

    c. Since weight loss with medications is maintained only for the duration of drug use, short-term use is generally unsuccessful. The long-term risks vs. benefits in the individual patient should be carefully weighed.

    d. At present, no medications have been approved for treatment of pediatric obesity.

2. Appetite suppressants (see Table 79–3 for starting doses). These act by decreasing appetite or increasing satiety. They work primarily by increasing the level of anorexigenic neurotransmitters such as norepinephrine, dopamine, and serotonin in the central nervous system.

    a. Noradrenergic agents that are approved for use include **phentermine, phendimetrazine, diethylpropion, and benzphetamine.** They are generally for short-term use only (generally presumed to be 3 months or less). Side effects are due to adrenergic stimulation, including insomnia, dry mouth, constipation, palpitations, and insomnia. Due to the potential for abuse, amphetamines are no longer recommended for routine use. Phenylpropanolamine, the only over-the-counter appetite suppressant approved for obesity management, was recently withdrawn due to concerns about its association with hemorrhagic stroke in women.

    b. Serotoninergic agents work by increasing levels of serotonin by increasing the release, inhibiting reuptake or a combination of both mechanisms. **Fenfluramine (Pondimin) and dexfenfluramine (Redux)** were both withdrawn in September 1997 following association with pulmonary hypertension and valvular heart disease. Some selective serotonin reuptake inhibitors, such as fluoxetine and sertraline, have been shown to induce weight loss in short-term studies. Long-term maintenance of weight loss has not been achieved in these patients.

    c. Sibutramine (Meridia) is a mixed noradrenergic and serotoninergic agent that is approved by the US Food and Drug Administration (FDA) for weight loss and maintenance along with a low-calorie diet. It also weakly inhibits dopamine reuptake. Weight loss is usually 5–8% of preintervention weight. The loss has been shown to be maintained for up to 1 year. Safety and efficacy beyond 1 year have not been clearly established. In addition to weight loss, other metabolic risk factors such as hyperlipidemia, hyperuricemia, glycemic control, and plasma insulin levels also improve. Unlike the pure serotoninergic agents, sibutramine does not induce serotonin release and has not been associated with valvular heart disease. Side effects of sibutramine include mild elevations of blood pressure and pulse, which may lead to discontinuation in up to 5% of patients. Other side effects, which tend to be self-limited, include dry mouth, insomnia, headache, and constipation.

TABLE 79–3. MEDICATIONS APPROVED FOR OBESITY TREATMENT

Generic Name	Trade Name	Cost	Dosage	Mechanism of Action
Benzphetamine	Didrex	$1–2/day	25–50 mg 1–3 times/day	Noradrenergic
Phendimetrazine	Bontril, Plegine	$1–5/day	17.5–70 mg 2–3 times/day OR 105 mg sustained-release/day	Noradrenergic
Phentermine	Adipex-P, Fastin	$1–2/day	18.75–37.5 mg/day	Noradrenergic
Diethylpropion	Tenuate, Tepanil	$1.75–2.00/day	25 mg 3 times/day OR 75 mg sustained-release/day	Noradrenergic
Sibutramine	Meridia	$2–4/day	5–15 mg/day	Mixed
Orlistat	Xenical	$3–4/day	120 mg 3 times/day with OR within 1 h of fatty meal	Inhibits fat absorption

3. **Agents that decrease nutrient absorption. Orlistat (Xenical)** is the only FDA-approved medication in this category. It acts by binding to gastrointestinal lipases in the gut lumen, thereby preventing hydrolysis of dietary triglycerides to absorbable free fatty acids and monoacylglycerols. Subjects who completed trials lasting 1 year lost about 9% of their preintervention weight. Orlistat has also been found to slow the rate of weight regain in the second year. Like sibutramine, orlistat has also been shown to improve metabolic parameters in addition to weight loss. These include modest decreases in fasting insulin levels, total cholesterol, low-density lipoproteins, and glycosylated hemoglobin. It was also associated with moderate decreases in blood pressure in long-term studies. Side effects are generally mild to moderate and decrease in frequency with continued use. They include flatulence, soft stools, fecal urgency, fecal incontinence, oily spotting, and steatorrhea. Fat-soluble vitamin absorption, primarily vitamin D, is decreased but may be counteracted by daily administration of a multivitamin.

4. **Combination therapy** in obesity treatment and maintenance is currently not recommended. While it is possible that safe combinations will eventually be developed, there are little data from large trials to support this at this time.

5. **Dietary supplements, nonprescription diet aids, and herbal agents**
   a. Agents such as chitosan, chromium picolinate, conjugated linoleic acid, and garcinia cambogia have been promoted for weight loss. Although some of these substances have mechanisms of action that could lead to weight loss, there are insufficient data at this time to indicate safety and efficacy.
   b. Short-term randomized double-blind, placebo-controlled studies with herbal products containing ephedra alkaloids and caffeine have indicated efficacy in promoting weight loss. Ephedrine, an adrenergic agent with thermogenic and appetite suppressant properties, has been found in controlled studies to promote weight loss. It is generally marketed in combination with caffeine, aspirin, or both.
   c. Dietary supplements with ephedra (ma huang) have unpredictable and unstandardized amounts of active ingredients and are not recommended. Side effects may be serious and include hypertension, arrhythmias, myocardial infarcts, seizures, stroke, and sudden death.
   d. Hormones have no place in the weight-loss regimen unless there are definite medical indications such as hypothyroidism. Injections of human growth hormone have not shown to be of benefit.

E. **Surgical treatment of obesity** may be very effective for a carefully selected group of morbidly obese adults. Recent advances have made these procedures safer and possibly more effective but very little data exists about the long-term safety and efficacy of bariatric surgeries. Recently developed laparoscopic approaches have reduced the complication rates of bariatric surgery, which has increased the popularity of these procedures in recent years.

1. **Secondary effects.** Bariatric surgery has been observed to improve insulin sensitivity, blood pressure, left ventricular ejection fraction, cholesterol and triglyceride levels, sleep apnea, fertility, menstrual irregularity, and urinary stress incontinence. These procedures have also been postulated to affect neuroendocrine feedback loops associated with satiety and food-seeking behavior as well as maintenance of metabolic rate, with variable results on long-term hunger levels and specific food cravings.

2. **Selection criteria**
   a. Bariatric surgery is indicated for the well-motivated, well-informed patient whose BMI is >40, or patients with a BMI of >35 who are experiencing significant obesity-related comorbid diseases such as type II diabetes mellitus. Patients should have failed at nonsurgical attempts at weight reduction.
   b. Bariatric surgery is contraindicated in patients with significant psychiatric disease or instability, alcohol or drug abuse, cardiac or other medical conditions that lead to high risk of intraoperative mortality, presence of endocrine disorders that promote obesity, inability to understand risks and benefits of surgery, children, and pregnant patients.

3. **Types of surgery**
   a. **Procedures that limit intake** include **gastric banding** and **stapled gastroplasty.** Stapled gastroplasty involves a partitioning of the stomach close to the gastroesophageal junction and creation of a small-caliber gastric outlet to the small intestine. In gastric banding, a diameter-limiting prosthetic device is places about the gastric body; this device may be adjustable in size through a

subcutaneous reservoir. Due to the reduced gastric capacity the patient reaches satiety earlier in the meal and presumably eats fewer calories.

    (1) Risks. Immediate postoperative complications may include surgical infection or wound dehiscence. Patients may develop severe gastroesophageal reflux or vomiting, chronic abdominal pain, obstructive disease, and incisional hernias. Up to 20% of patients may require reoperation for surgical correction of severe dysfunction, including stomal outlet stenosis. Gastric banding may cause foreign body reactions or gastric body erosions, leading to emergency surgery.

    (2) Outcomes. Early weight-loss results from these procedures can be up to 60% of the preoperative excess weight. Many patients regain a substantial proportion of their lost weight within 5 years of surgery. By the tenth year after surgery, a nearly 80% failure rate is reported.

  b. Procedures that promote malabsorption include gastric bypass procedures that not only reduce the size of the stomach pouch but also bypass a portion of the small intestine, causing variable amounts of caloric malabsorption. The most popular procedure is the Roux-en-Y bypass, in which a small stomach pouch is anastomosed to the mid-jejunum; the bypassed sections of duodenum and jejunum are all or partially left as a blind-ended pouch. More recent techniques vary the anatomical arrangement of bypassed sections in order to maximize caloric malabsorption while preserving absorption of important nutrients. Other gastric bypass techniques include the biliopancreatic bypass, the distal Roux-en-Y, and the duodenal switch.

    (1) Risks. Perioperative complications, such as pulmonary embolus and gastrointestinal leakage, may be as high as 15% with a 1% mortality rate. Long-term morbidity is strongly linked to malabsorptive syndromes, including anemia, fat-soluble vitamin deficiencies, and protein-calorie malnutrition. Diarrhea is typical after these surgeries. Some patients may develop dumping syndrome, an intense physiologic reaction when poorly digested food is deposited lower in the digestive tract. Dumping syndrome causes nausea, bloating, diarrhea, colic, lightheadedness, palpitations, and sweating.

    (2) Outcomes. Initial weight-loss results are excellent, with a mean loss of 75–80% of excess weight. Longer-term efficacy is less well established, but appears to be better than volume restriction procedures.

F. Complications of weight loss. Weight loss, particularly rapid loss, has been associated with a variety of medical sequelae. Clinically, we often emphasize the positive effects of weight loss, but our patients also should be advised of the medical risks of weight loss. These include:

  1. Biliary complications. Rapid weight loss is associated with an increased prevalence of gallstones and cholecystitis. This complication has been observed in both low- and high-fat diets. Dietary supplementation with ursodeoxycholic acid has been proposed as a preventative tactic for this problem, but very little data supports its efficacy.

  2. Ketosis. Insufficient carbohydrate intake can promote production of large numbers of ketone bodies in the bloodstream. The long-term health impact of this phenomenon is controversial; speculation centers on the potential for renal damage or kidney stone formation in people following ketotic diets. Such complications have been well documented in children placed on ketotic diets for epilepsy control.

  3. Dietary deficiencies. Caloric restriction can lead to insufficient intake of vitamins, minerals, essential fatty acids, or protein. Long term, this can cause protein-calorie malnutrition, vitamin deficiency, or osteoporosis.

  4. Cosmetic issues. Weight loss, particularly when rapid, may cause striae formation, which may be cosmetically offensive to the patient.

  5. Psychiatric changes. Slow or dramatic changes in body habitus may affect the patient's interaction with family, friends, and coworkers, as well as his own body image. Such changes are not always positive and may cause significant emotional distress.

IV. Management Strategies

  A. Obesity management should be an individually tailored approach.

  B. Although the goal of treatment is a 10% reduction from initial weight, weight loss of as little as 5% should be regarded as successful as there is consideration improvement in associated risk factors.

C. Weight maintenance after initial weight loss is often difficult and requires an ongoing program of diet, exercise, and behavioral therapy.

D. Regular physician contact is important to sustain maintenance efforts.

V. Prognosis. Obesity causes or exacerbates many disorders. It is, in particular, associated with the development of diabetes mellitus; coronary heart disease; congestive heart failure; obstructive sleep apnea; gallbladder disease; cancers such as breast, colon, and prostate; osteoarthritis of large and small joints; and premature death.

In the Framingham Heart Study, the risk of death within 26 years increased by 1% for each extra pound increase in weight between the ages of 30 and 42 years, and by 2% between 50 and 62 years.

REFERENCES

Capella JF, Capella RF: The weight reduction operation of choice: Vertical banded gastroplasty or gastric bypass? Am J Surg 1996;**171**:74.

Flegal KM, et al: Prevalence of obesity and trends in obesity among U.S. adults 1999—2000. JAMA 2002;**288**:1723.

Lyznicki JM, et al: Obesity: Assessment and management in primary care. Am Fam Physician 2001;**63**:2185.

National Institutes of Health: *The Practical Guide: Identification, Evaluation and Treatment of Overweight and Obesity in Adults.* NIH Publication No. 00-4084. National Institutes of Health, National Heart, Lung, and Blood Institute, and North American Association for the Study of Obesity, Bethesda, MD; 2000.

Yanovski SZ, Yanovski JA: Obesity. N Engl J Med 2002;**346**:591.

80   Osteoarthritis

Charles Kodner, MD

KEY POINTS

- Osteoarthritis is the most commonly encountered cause of joint pain and disability and will become increasingly common as the population ages.
- Osteoarthritis is no longer considered a normal process of aging and "wear and tear" on joints, but is a physiologically complex disorder involving physiologic and mechanical initiating events, joint and cartilage damage, synovial inflammation, and an imbalance of cartilage repair and destruction.
- Diagnosis is primarily on clinical grounds, emphasizing typical aching joint pain, crepitus, osteophyte formation, worsening pain with activity, and joint instability. Characteristic radiographic findings of joint space narrowing, osteophytes, irregular joint surfaces, and sclerosis of subchondral bone may assist in the diagnosis.
- Disease management should emphasize nonpharmacologic interventions, including regular exercise, physical therapy, weight loss, smoking cessation, physical pain relief modalities, gait support and other assistive devices, and patient education.
- Pharmacologic treatment should be initiated with adequate, scheduled doses of acetaminophen, starting at 500 mg twice daily up to 1 g four times daily.
- Other medication options include nonsteroidal anti-inflammatory drugs (NSAIDs), other analgesics such as tramadol, and narcotic analgesics. Details are available in Table 80–1, with a list of the most common medications and dosages below, including herbal compounds and other treatment options.
- Topical capsaicin, glucosamine, and chondroitin may also provide pain relief.
- Joint injection with corticosteroids or hyaluronic acid has been shown to be helpful in patients who have failed other treatment options or who are at risk of complications from NSAIDs or other therapy.
- Surgical joint replacement for hip or knee arthritis, or other surgical treatment options, should be considered for patients with disabling pain who have failed other treatment interventions.

TABLE 80–1. SELECTED ANTI-INFLAMMATORY ANALGESICS[1]

Drug Class	Generic Name (Trade Name)	Brand Name Cost[1]	Generic Cost[1]	Usual Effective Dose
Nonacetylated salicylates	Aspirin[2]		approx. $2.00	325–500 mg qd
	Diflunisal (Dolobid)	$68.06	$46.66	250–500 mg bid
	Salsalate (Disalcid)[3]	$39.51	$13.27	1500 mg bid
Propionic acids	Ibuprofen[2] (Motrin, Advil)	$18.48	$3.56	400–800 mg tid
	Naproxen (Naprosyn, Anaprox)	$50.16	$10.31	250–500 mg bid
	Ketoprofen (Orudis)	$103.96	$80.70	50 mg qid or 75 mg tid
	Oxaprozin (Daypro)[4]	$91.89	N/A	600–1200 mg qd
Acetic acids	Indomethacin (Indocin)	$33.65	$22.48	25–50 mg bid–tid
	Sulindac (Clinoril)	$70.10	$21.60	150 mg bid
	Diclofenac (Voltaren)	$76.99	$51.68	50 mg bid–tid
	Tolmetin (Tolectin)	$122.68	$62.06	200–600 mg tid
Fenamates	Mefenamic Acid (Ponstel)[4]	$37.46	N/A	250 mg qid
Oxicams	Piroxicam (Feldene)	$79.87	$17.89	20 mg once daily
	Meloxicam (Mobic)[4]	$59.40	N/A	7.5 mg qd–bid
Pyrrolizine Carboxylic acid	Ketorolac (Toradol)	$18.59 (5 days)	N/A	10 mg qid (not to exceed 5 days)
Naphthylalkanone	Nabumetone (Relafen)[4]	$72.66	N/A	1000 mg once daily
COX-2 Selective agents	Celecoxib (Celebrex)[4]	$72.60	N/A	100–200 mg qd (or 50–100 mg bid)
	Rofecoxib (Vioxx)[4]	$75.75	N/A	25–50 mg daily
	Valdecoxib (Bextra)	$87.45	N/A	10 mg qd–bid

[1] Costs are given for 30 days of therapy unless indicated otherwise.
[2] Available over-the-counter without prescription.
[3] The dose should be reduced in the elderly.
[4] Not available generically.

I. Introduction

A. Definition. Osteoarthritis (OA) is characterized by slowly progressive joint pain, cartilage destruction, and functional instability, with typical radiographic findings of osteophytes and other characteristic changes and a significant potential for disability and reduced quality of life. OA can be classified as primary (or idiopathic), involving the hands, feet, knees, hips, spine, and other joints; or secondary to trauma, obesity, congenital abnormalities affecting the limbs, other arthropathies (eg, tophaceous gout, rheumatoid arthritis, etc), metabolic disorders (eg, hemochromatosis), disorders of collagen, or other medical conditions.

B. Epidemiology. As of 1998, more than 20 million Americans had symptomatic OA; the prevalence increases with advancing age, and the prevalence of OA is expected to increase dramatically as the US population ages. Many more people have radiographic or clinical evidence of OA than have symptomatic disease, with radiographic changes of knee OA in approximately half of the population older than age 65.

C. Pathophysiology. OA is not simply due to expected "wear and tear" on aging joints related to activities, positioning, weight-related joint stresses, and other factors. Rather, OA is a complex disorder involving all joint structures, in which physical stresses act as disease initiating or aggravating factors, but the disorder primarily involves an imbalance between articular cartilage destructive and repair forces.

1. **Triggering factors** for OA appear to include excessive force applied to the joint, such as repetitive impact loading, or a genetic or metabolic defect in the articular cartilage or underlying subchondral bone. As a result of these triggering factors, chondrocytes multiply and become very metabolically active, initially overproducing articular cartilage to compensate for the triggering factors and maintain joint function. Over time, these factors lead to production of altered proteoglycans and collagen in the articular cartilage, which becomes subject to erosions, cracks, and other damage typical of OA.
2. **Synovial inflammation** appears to play an active role in the progression of OA and may lead to joint swelling and effusion, stiffness, pain, and other manifestations of OA. Established synovial inflammation eventually leads to production of cytokines and other agents that cause further degradation of articular cartilage.
3. **Metabolically active chondrocytes** appear to signal subchondral bone osteoblasts, which begin to form new bone tissue around the edges of the joints. The resulting "bone spurs" or osteophytes are characteristic clinical or radiographic findings and contribute to joint pain, instability, and loss of function as well as possible gross joint deformity in later stages of OA.

II. **Diagnosis.** In OA, the findings from the history and physical examination are key to the diagnosis and guide the intensity and nature of therapy. There is no "gold standard" for diagnosing OA, and clinical guidelines for diagnosis currently focus on typical pain symptoms, radiographic features, and no evidence of inflammatory arthropathies.

A. **Symptoms and signs**
   1. **History.** OA characteristically produces pain and stiffness in the joints, with the stiffness worsened by immobilization and resolving quickly with movement (generally in <30 minutes after arising in the morning). The pain is typically dull and aching in character and is aggravated by cold or damp weather and by increased activity. If activity-associated pain is present, it usually starts quickly when the joint is used but may last for hours after the activity has stopped. Often the history includes some minor injury leading to exacerbation of symptoms, though the true onset of OA symptoms is insidious in nature. Eventually, the pain becomes constant and wakes the patient from sleep.

   Many patients complain of instability or "giving way" in the case of OA involving the hips or knees and may have difficulty climbing or descending stairs. Some patients may actually fall as a result of knee or hip joint instability. Symptoms of crepitus—grinding, popping, catching, clicking—may also be present.
   2. **Physical examination.** Physical examination for OA should assess for features typical of OA, examine for evidence of other arthropathies, and assess the functional status of the joint. Specific findings to elicit include inspection for joint enlargement, including osteophytes or nodules; examination for signs of inflammation including erythema, warmth, or "bogginess" of the joint; crepitus with passive range of motion; focal tenderness; and stability with gait, squat-rise, or other movements.

   On examination of a normally mobile joint, crepitus may be noted when the joint is passively moved, and there may be localized tenderness. The range of movement of an osteoarthritic joint is limited. In testing the range of motion, the patient should move the joint actively first, because passive joint movement can be painful. In weight-bearing joints, it is important to assess joint stability and the status of the supporting musculature, which has therapeutic significance.
   3. **Joint-specific signs and symptoms.** In addition to the above general findings on history and physical examination, OA involving specific joints may have additional clinical findings.
      a. **Knees.** In the knees, crepitus may be marked, with limitation of flexion and extension. Patients may complain of pain in the thighs and calves related to compensatory muscle spasm. Osteophytes are sometimes actually palpable in the knee, and commonly there are effusions.

      American College of Rheumatology (ACR) criteria for the diagnosis of OA of the knees include typical knee pain plus osteophytes on radiographs, OR all of the following: morning stiffness <30 minutes, crepitus, and either age older than 40 years or synovial fluid suggestive of osteoarthritis (2 of 3: clear, viscous, and less than 2000 polymorphonuclear leukocytes/cc). These criteria have a 77% positive predictive value (PPV) for patient meeting these criteria, based on 30%

prevalence, and a 97% negative predictive value (NPV) for patients not meeting these criteria.

b. **Hips.** In the hip, manifestations include changed gait, with a characteristically flexed, externally rotated hip, with the gait "sparing" the painful side. There may well be limb shortening due to subluxation of the head of the femur. Note that the pain from OA of the hip is often referred, with pain being felt in the groin, the buttocks, or even the knee. The first sign of OA in the hip is loss of rotation (since the hip is a ball-and-socket joint); this loss should be tested for in all older patients. Ultimately, there is limitation of all movement of the joint.

ACR criteria for the diagnosis of OA of the hips include typical hip pain plus at least two of the following: erythrocyte sedimentation rate <20 mm/hour; femoral or acetabular osteophytes on radiographs; or joint space narrowing on radiographs (52% PPV, 99% NPV).

c. **Hands.** In the hands, typical joints affected by OA include the distal interphalangeal (DIP) joints, proximal interphalangeal (PIP) joints, and first carpometacarpal (CMC) joints. Heberden's nodes are a characteristic finding; these are firm, tender nodes on the dorsal aspect of the DIP joints, representing bony enlargement or osteophyte formation. Bouchard's nodes are similar lesions that occur over the PIP joints. Pain in the hands is worsened by fine motor or physical activities such as gardening, sports, hobbies, etc. Destructive joint changes are possible, but are not as common as in rheumatoid arthritis. ACR criteria for the diagnosis of OA of the hands include meeting all of the following: hand pain, aching, or stiffness; hard tissue enlargement of 2 or more of 10 selected joints (2nd and 3rd DIP joints, 2nd and 3rd PIP joints, and 1st CMC joints on both hands); metacarpophalangeal joint swelling in fewer than three joints; and hard tissue enlargement of 2 or more DIP joints OR deformity of 1 or more of the 10 selected joints (99% PPV, 86% NPV).

d. **Cervical spine.** Chronic neck pain from OA in the cervical spine may be related to work posture, repetitive athletic injuries, or other factors. Osteophytes in the spinal vertebrae can produce nerve root pressure, with radicular symptoms.

e. **Lumbar spine.** OA is common in the lumbar spine, but findings on examination or radiography do not correlate well with clinical symptoms. It is unclear where degenerative changes per se, facet joint changes, muscle spasm, disk herniation, soft tissue changes, or all of the above account primarily for lower back pain.

f. **Other joints.** A number of other joints can be affected by OA, including the joints of the feet and ankles, the temporomandibular joint (TMJ), the true joint of the shoulder as well as the acromioclavicular joint, and the sternoclavicular joints. OA should be included in the differential diagnosis of pain in these areas, though other diagnoses (TMJ dysfunction, rotator cuff tendinitis, etc.) need to be considered.

B. **Laboratory tests**

1. **Radiographic findings.** A number of radiographic features are common in OA, but especially in disease of the spine and hips, there may be relatively poor correlation between observed radiographic changes and symptoms. Approximately half of patients with radiographic changes of OA of the knees complain of persistent pain.

a. **Plain X-rays.** Typical findings consistent with OA on plain radiographs include joint space narrowing due to destruction of articular cartilage, including narrowed intravertebral disk space; osteophyte formation at the margins of affected joints; irregular joint surfaces; sclerosis of subchondral bone; and bony cysts.

b. **MRI and CT.** Computerized tomography (CT) and magnetic resonance imaging (MRI) are increasingly used, but have little role in diagnosing OA. These imaging modalities provide good visualization of soft tissues and subchondral bone changes, as well as of ligament and meniscal damage, and may be most useful to rule out other disorders causing joint pain, such as rotator cuff tear, knee ligament disruption, lumbar disc herniation, etc.

2. **Blood tests.** There are no specific blood tests to order as part of the routine diagnosis of OA. "Rheumatologic tests" such as erythrocyte sedimentation rate, rheumatoid factor, and antinuclear antibodies are frequently ordered in patients with arthralgias, but these tests have poor predictive value in patients where the clinical suspicion is low for systemic lupus erythematosus or other connective tissue disorders. These tests should not be ordered as a "screening panel" in patients with

arthralgias, and positive results in low-risk patients should be interpreted carefully. These tests should be ordered as confirmatory evidence in patients who are likely to have connective tissue disorders, rheumatoid arthritis, or similar conditions. Complete blood counts, uric acid levels, chemistry profiles, and other tests may be required to evaluate for septic arthritis, gout, renal osteodystrophy, or other disorders as the clinical picture dictates.

3. **Joint aspiration.** When joint effusion is present, joint aspiration is usually desirable in order to obtain a sample of fluid. Diagnostically, joint aspiration is typically indicated in a patient with a moderately inflamed, tender, and swollen joint with effusion, where it is important to definitively rule out septic arthritis, gout, pseudogout, or other disorders. Patients with septic arthritis may not present with characteristic findings of toxic appearance, fever, and marked joint tenderness and inflammation, but may only have focal joint inflammation early in the disease process.

4. **Arthroscopy.** Arthroscopy also has a place in the diagnosis of arthritis, particularly in a joint that is "locking." Through the arthroscope, fragments of tissue can be removed and the fibrillar changes in the cartilages, which can contribute to early symptoms, can be planed off. The arthroscopic procedure itself is temporarily disabling and should not be undertaken lightly.

III. **Treatment.** OA should be managed as any other chronic illness, with consideration of the patient's disease location and progression, the phase of the patient's illness, and attention to routine health maintenance and other medical comorbid conditions. Management of chronic pain can easily consume the time allotted to an outpatient office visit, and it is vital not to neglect these other management needs. The goals of therapy for OA include control pain; improve or maintain joint function and mobility; prevent destructive joint changes; minimize disability and preserve functionality; and improve overall quality of life. An additional therapeutic goals is to educate patients and their families about the illness and enlist them as active participants in their management.

A. **Physical interventions.** Nonpharmacologic interventions should be considered primary therapy in OA, to accomplish therapeutic objectives listed above.

1. **Exercise.** At-home or supervised exercise programs have been shown to provide benefits in pain control, functionality, overall well-being, and prevention of disability, primarily for OA of the knees and hips. Exercise of weight-bearing joints must be of low impact, with avoidance of torsion, prolonged standing, and kneeling. Patients can be instructed in performing appropriate exercise by their physician, or should be referred to a physical therapist for instruction or supervision. Types of exercise programs include range-of-motion and flexibility exercises; instructions in joint positioning and posture; aerobic exercises, especially aquatic aerobics; fitness walking; and strength training, especially quadriceps strengthening since quadriceps weakness is common in OA. Non-weight-bearing exercise is preferred, and impact on the knees can be spared by shoes and surfaces that cushion the limb while walking; an indoor skiing machine can be very helpful in OA of the knees.

2. **Physical therapy.** The physical therapist can be helpful in instructing patients in the above exercises, supervising their correct and safe performance of exercise, and monitoring their therapeutic response. Therapists can also be helpful to assess patients' muscle weakness and gait, assist with the use of pain-control modalities, and assess patients for assistive devices. Occupational therapy evaluation can also provide support or assist devices for activities of daily living for patients with OA of the hands.

3. **Gait assist devices.** The use of canes (held in the hand contralateral to the affected knee or hip joint), crutches, walkers, or other devices may be helpful for some patients but should not supplant the role of muscle-strength training, range-of-motion exercises, and other measures to improve functionality. Shoe orthotics may also be helpful to preserve joint positioning and help prevent joint damage.

4. **Pain control modalities.** Persistent pain, particularly nerve root pain, may be relieved from other pain-relieving methods such as transcutaneous electrical nerve stimulation (TENS), ultrasonography, and other physical therapy techniques.

5. **Knee braces.** Some patients find relief of pain and improvement of joint stability through the use of knee bracing, patellar taping, or other interventions. These can be helpful short-term, but also should not replace other measures to maintain joint function and muscle strength.

6. **Foot care.** When the feet are affected, attention to the shoes and to podiatric health is vital. Orthotic devices can be of considerable help in correcting chronic foot deformities, which predispose to other musculoskeletal pain, not only in the feet themselves but also in the knee, hip, or lumbar spine. The use of cushioned athletic shoes may be beneficial, though many older women have used high heels and moving rapidly to "flatties" (including sneakers) may produce Achilles' tendinitis and other problems.

7. **Activities of daily living.** In all forms of arthritis of the hand, it is important to pay attention to the patient's routine tasks. Devices can assist in opening containers that require torsion strength and grip, functions that can chronically exacerbate and acutely precipitate arthralgia. Other methods of reducing joint stress and improving functionality, such as a raised toilet seat, grab-bars, and tub seats or shower seats, can also reduce accidents.

B. **Behavioral interventions**

1. **Weight loss.** In the obese, weight must be reduced, if possible, where weight-bearing joints are involved. Patients should be enrolled in dedicated weight-loss programs where possible, or advised regarding diet, exercise, and the role of weight-loss interventions if such programs are not available. Simple topics to address regarding diet include limiting portion size, avoiding high-carbohydrate drinks and snacks, and increasing the fruit and vegetable content of the diet. Aquatic aerobic exercises can be valuable in obese patients in terms of limiting the weight applied to the knees.

2. **Smoking cessation.** Cessation of tobacco use is important in improving patients' overall sense of well-being, reducing the risks of NSAID-induced gastropathy, maintaining joint blood flow and tissue healing, and reducing the risk of cardiovascular disease and other comorbidities. Patients who smoke should specifically be counseled regarding cessation methods as part of the overall management of their OA.

C. **Medications.** Most patients with OA use pharmacologic treatment for pain relief, though there is no evidence that treatment alters the natural history of the disease. Medications should be seen as adjuncts to preventive and protective therapy, as above, rather than the primary focus of intervention.

1. **Analgesics.** Acetaminophen remains first-line therapy for OA, with efficacy comparable to NSAIDs in randomized trials, though some surveys and measures of quality-of-life scores indicate that patients prefer NSAIDs. The safety profile and low cost for acetaminophen support its use as initial therapy in patients with OA; patients should be instructed that pain is best managed with daily, scheduled dosing rather than as-needed administration, as is the case with most pain-control regimens. Treatment should be initiated at 1–2 g total daily dose divided twice daily, with a maximum dose of 4 g daily divided into four doses (1 g four times daily). Safety issues with acetaminophen include hepatotoxicity with overdose or in patients with liver disease, or prolongation of the half-life of warfarin.

   a. **Tramadol.** Other analgesic agents include tramadol hydrochloride, a synthetic opioid; tramadol is unscheduled, is approved for moderate to severe pain in OA, and may be equivalent to moderate-strength narcotics such as codeine. It may be particularly useful in older patients or other patients at high risk of NSAID toxicity. Typical dosages are 200–400 mg given as four divided doses; possible side effects include drowsiness, nausea, and constipation, with a low potential for addiction or tolerance. Seizures have been reported, but are rare and appear to have been in patients taking doses higher than recommended or in patients with epilepsy. Tramadol is marketed in formulations combined with acetaminophen.

2. **Anti-inflammatory medications.** A variety of anti-inflammatory medications can be used to treat pain in patients who do not respond adequately to acetaminophen. These agents are effective in pain relief and are preferred to acetaminophen by many patients, highlighting the role of inflammation in OA. Issues to consider in prescribing NSAIDs include medication selection, dosage, and prevention of side effects.

   a. **Selecting a medication.** Meta-analysis studies have not shown any consistent difference in efficacy among the many available NSAIDs, including older nonacetylated agents as well as newer selective COX-2 inhibitor agents. Selection of agents should therefore be based primarily on cost or availability, side effects, and ease of dosing. For unknown reasons, some patients seem to find relief with different classes of NSAIDs, whereas other agents are less effective; if patients find one NSAID ineffective, it may be appropriate to switch to a medication in a different class. A selection of anti-inflammatory agents by class, including typical dosing regimens and a cost summary, is provided in Table 80–1. For reasons of ease of administration, efficacy, low cost, and lack of proven differences in side effects, older NSAIDs such as ibuprofen are usually recommended for patients at low risk of gastrointestinal or other side effects.

b. **Dosage.** As with other analgesic regimens, it is appropriate to recommend that NSAIDs be dosed regularly to best affect the pain cycle rather than using these agents on an as-needed basis for a disorder that is chronic in nature. Dosing should therefore begin at low doses and titrate upward for therapeutic effect, given the high risk of toxicity with prolonged NSAID use.

c. **Preventing side effects.** The primary side effects for NSAIDs are gastrointestinal bleeding, potentiation of renal insufficiency, and inhibition of platelet aggregation with prolongation of bleeding times. For the latter two complications, it is important to minimize the use and dosage of NSAIDs as much as possible in older patients or those with other chronic medical conditions; specific risk factors for worsening renal function due to NSAIDs include age older than 65 years, hypertension, congestive heart failure, concomitant use of diuretics or angiotensin-converting enzyme inhibitors, or existing renal insufficiency. Hypersensitivity reactions and hepatotoxicity are also recognized NSAID side effects. However, the selection of agents is guided most by the effort to prevent gastrointestinal bleeding.

Among patients older than age 65, approximately 25% of hospitalizations and deaths due to peptic ulcer disease are attributable to NSAIDs. Factors that place patients at high risk of NSAID-induced gastropathy are listed in Table 80–2. In patients at low risk of NSAID-induced gastropathy, there is no proven difference in safety profiles among the various anti-inflammatory medications; in these patients, drug selection should be based on cost, efficacy, and other factors, and physicians should attempt to minimize the dose, use, and duration of NSAID therapy. All patients should be advised to take NSAIDs following a meal or a snack and to limit or cease use of alcohol and tobacco products.

In patients at high risk, options to limit the risk of adverse gastrointestinal events include the use of COX-2 specific agents or use of a gastroprotective medication. In high-risk patients, COX-2 specific medications have a significantly lower incidence of gastrointestinal complications. In patients requiring additional medications for prevention of ulcers or gastritis, proton pump inhibitors are the preferred agents, though histamine$_2$ receptor antagonists, misoprostol, or Carafate (cost may be prohibitive) are other options (see Chapter 82 for dosages).

3. **Narcotics.** Many patients with advanced OA do not respond adequately to acetaminophen, tramadol, or NSAIDs. Such patients can safely and effectively be treated with chronic opiates, including codeine, oxycodone, hydrocodone, and morphine (see Table 69–1). Some patients may require these agents only for short-term management of disease flares, though many will require chronic treatment with opioid

---

TABLE 80–2. RISK FACTORS FOR NSAID-INDUCED GASTROPATHY

Definite risk factors:
- Age older than 65 years
- Previous ulcer disease or upper gastrointestinal bleeding
- Use of multiple nonsteroidal anti-inflammatory drugs or use of high dosage of one of these drugs
- Concomitant oral corticosteroid therapy
- Concomitant anticoagulant therapy
- Duration of therapy (risk is higher in the first 3 months of therapy)

Possible risk factors:
- Tobacco abuse
- Alcohol abuse
- *Helicobacter pylori* infection

medications, possibly during medical management to defer joint replacement. Sedation, respiratory depression, nausea, and vomiting are possible complications of these agents, though these are more likely to be problems in cases of inadvertent or intentional overdose. Addiction is a possible complication, but is unlikely in patients who do not display other propensities to drug misuse or addiction. Physical dependence is common, requires careful patient education about the difference between dependence and addiction, and may require slow escalation in dosage over time. Constipation and obstipation are more common complications, and patients on long-term narcotic therapy should be treated with an appropriate bowel regimen including walking, fluid intake, fiber supplementation, regular use of a stool softener, and as-needed use of laxatives. Many opiates are marketed in formulation with acetaminophen or aspirin. It is important to monitor for appropriate medication use, drug addiction, and drug diversion as described below.

4. **Topical analgesics.** Capsaicin cream is more effective than placebo for pain relief, especially for disease localized to the knee or hand, but requires four-times-daily application, which may limit its continued use by patients.

5. **Herbal preparations.** Glucosamine (1500 mg/day in three divided doses) and chondroitin (800–1200 mg/day in three divided doses) appear to provide some pain relief in meta-analyses and should be considered as adjunctive medications that may help limit the dose of NSAIDs or narcotics required to reduce pain. Patients should be advised that these agents are available over-the-counter and that different formulations may use lower doses, which may be less effective. Patients may be reluctant to continue paying out of pocket for these agents for a long term, but a trial of therapy for efficacy may be appropriate. Other herbal agents that may have some benefit include *S*-adenosylmethionine (SAMe), 400–1200 mg/day; topical dimethyl sulfoxide 25% gel (DMSO); and avocado/soybean unsaponifiables, 300 mg/day.

D. **Joint injection.** In the presence of knee joint effusion and inflammation, corticosteroid injection has been shown to provide pain relief over 1–2 weeks but is not effective for long-term pain relief. Viscosupplementation via intra-articular injection of hyaluronic acid provides pain relief superior to placebo and may be an option for patients who do not respond appropriately to medical therapy or who are at high risk for NSAID-induced gastropathy, narcotic addiction or side effects, or other complications. Patients with persistent pain and functional limitations who are not surgical candidates may also benefit, though the ideal candidate for injection therapy has not been defined. Weekly injections are given for 3–5 weeks, and this regimen may be repeated only twice per year. The cost of these medications may be prohibitive in some patients (approximately $600 for a treatment course).

E. **Surgical management.** Surgical options for OA of the knee include arthroscopic debridement, distal femoral osteotomy, unicompartmental knee replacement or hemiarthroplasty, or total knee arthroplasty. Indications for surgical intervention include pain, instability, or disability uncontrolled with physical and medical management. Given the likelihood of prosthesis loosening and the need for subsequent reoperation after approximately 10 years, it is usually appropriate to defer surgical intervention using conservative measures until patients are older and have more limited activity requirements. Arthroscopic debridement was no better than placebo in a recent randomized trial.

IV. **Management Strategies.** It is very important for the family physician to manage the "whole patient" and not to focus solely on medications and formal physical therapy in treating OA. Patient-focused management includes educating the patient (and the caregiver if relevant) in the many techniques that can reduce symptoms by reducing the stress on diseased joints and addressing other social and medical dimensions of their care. These techniques thus reduce the impact of the arthritis on the patient's life and help address not only pain but total quality of life.

A. **Patient education and support.** Patients and families must be educated about the pathophysiology of OA and should be able to identify significant symptoms and recognize inflammatory phases and other symptoms that may necessitate modifications in management. An understanding of the disease process may be especially important in younger patients with OA, who are forced to begin management of a chronic illness. Patients and families should be directed toward such organizations as the Arthritis Foundation, which has local chapters and extensive educational and support activities.

In older patients, arthritis and its many consequences (which can be devastating to the patient's overall health and function) are often tolerated as "normal" accompaniments of aging, and patients should understand the nature of their illness and the breadth of management options available. Some patients may benefit from more frequent, scheduled visits than from "follow-up as needed" to continue patient education and address other aspects of disease management. Topics for anticipatory counseling should include sexuality, including sexual position; posture, including chair height and style; toileting and bathing needs; exercise and activity habits; and driving, including entering and exiting the car.

B. **Depression.** Depression often accompanies chronic joint pain and then interferes with motivation and compliance as well as increasing the patient's awareness of the pain itself. Good clinical management thus involves seeing patients and their families in the entire context of their lives, functionality, and the rest of their health, since movement and everyday activities are inevitably affected by these illnesses. Counseling and medical treatment for depression may be appropriate in depressed patients; use of tricyclic antidepressants, if otherwise appropriate, may provide additional benefit in terms of pain relief and help with sleep.

C. **Disability assessments.** Patients with chronic pain and self-assessed disability often request assistance from their physicians in applying for disability benefits. Assessing for true disability in terms of overall "whole patient" disability or isolated disabilities of specific limbs and joints is complex. Rational disability assessment is further complicated by issues of credibility, secondary gain, and effort on the part of the patient, and lack of expertise or familiarity on the part of the physician. Guidelines on disability determination are available, and consultation with a physician trained in occupational medicine is recommended. Patients in general should not be determined to be fully disabled without a more thorough assessment of their true functional capacity.

D. **Chronic narcotic therapy management.** Routine management of patients who are on chronic narcotic therapy includes the following: explanation of appropriate drug use and refill patterns (only obtain medications from one physician and one pharmacy; take medications as prescribed; no early refills on medications will be given; medications will be discontinued if there is evidence of substance abuse; and patients need to follow up with their physician as instructed); periodic urine drug testing to help evaluate for drug diversion; and assessment for "doctor-shopping" or other evidence of drug addiction or "drug-seeking." Many physicians prefer to refer to specialists in pain management or to use "narcotic contracts" signed by the patient to address these requirements. As above, physiologic tolerance or dependence is distinct from drug addiction, which is rare in patients with chronic pain who do not have a history of substance abuse.

E. **Referral criteria.** In general, patients with OA can be effectively managed by primary care physicians. Referral to physical therapists or occupational therapists is common, and joint management with therapists can be effective in overall patient care. Referral to rheumatologists should only be necessary to confirm the diagnosis of rheumatoid arthritis or other conditions, and referral to orthopedic surgeons should be undertaken when surgical intervention is required, or if the primary care physician is uncomfortable performing joint injections. Referral to pain management specialists, as above, may be helpful in patients requiring long-term narcotic therapy.

V. **Prognosis.** Symptoms of OA can be expected to worsen over time, although improving muscular support and general fitness and continual attention to mobility and range of motion can keep symptoms at bay for years. Major interventions in OA, such as joint replacement (particularly the knee or hip), can be seemingly "curative" of that particular joint, provided that the patient can fully collaborate in the necessary rehabilitative process.

REFERENCES

American College of Rheumatology: Recommendations for the medical management of osteoarthritis of the hip and knee: American College of Rheumatology Subcommittee on Osteoarthritis Guidelines. Arth & Rheum 2000;**43**(9):1905.

Easton BT: Evaluation and treatment of the patient with osteoarthritis. J Fam Pract 2001;**50**(9):791.

Manek NJ: Medical management of osteoarthritis. Mayo Clin Proc 2001;**76**(5):533.

Morelli V: Alternative therapies for traditional disease states: Osteoarthritis. Am Fam Physician 2003;**67**(2):339.

Moseley JB: A controlled trial of arthroscopic surgery for osteoarthritis of the knee. N Engl J Med 2002;**347**(2):81.

Nicholson B: Responsible prescribing of opioids for the management of chronic pain. Drugs 2003;**63**(1):17.

81   Osteoporosis

Richard O. Schamp, MD

KEY POINTS

- Consider candidates for osteoporosis therapy:
  - All postmenopausal women who present with vertebral, wrist, or hip fractures.
  - All women with bone mineral density T-scores below –2, in the absence of risk factors.
  - All women with T-scores below –1.5, if other risk factors are present.
- Adequate calcium intake is:
  - 1200 mg/day in men and all premenopausal (starting in the second or third decade) women.
  - 1500 mg/day in postmenopausal women.
  - Calcium carbonate is cheapest; maximum absorption occurs with 500-mg doses.
  - Calcium citrate has 3× better absorption and is preferred in patients with achlorhydria, constipation, or gas with calcium carbonate, or history of renal stones.
- Adequate vitamin D intake is:
  - 800 IU/day is the only dose shown to reduce fractures in at-risk patients.
  - Sunlight exposure and diet (eg, fortified milk) are important source of vitamin D, but are often impractical in the population at risk.
- Drug therapy (always in conjunction with adequate calcium and vitamin D)
  - All these drugs feature a high number needed to treat (NNT).
  - Alendronate (Fosamax), 10 mg every morning on an empty stomach or 70 mg once a week, sitting up for 30 minutes after dose to reduce risk of esophagitis.
  - Risedronate (Actonel), 5 mg every morning on an empty stomach, sitting up as above.
  - Calcitonin (Miacalcin nasal spray), 200 IU intranasally; one puff per day, alternating nostrils; or injectable calcitonin (Miacalcin), 100 IU subcutaneously every other day. (Calcitonin is alleged to reduce pain in acute compression fracture.)
  - Raloxifene (Evista), 60 mg every day, with relative contraindications of hot flashes and history of thromboembolic conditions.
  - Hormone replacement therapy has been associated with increased bone density in randomized controlled trials, fewer fractures in observational studies, and fewer fractures in a recent meta-analysis of randomized controlled trials, but is controversial due to risk-benefit ratio.
- Institutional care
  - Inpatient care may be needed for acute back pain, especially for new vertebral fractures (bed rest and analgesia) and for acute treatment of upper femoral and pelvic fractures.
  - Nursing home or home health care may be needed following fracture.
  - Start supplement/drug therapy as soon as a diagnosis is made, because this often is neglected when patients are discharged from acute treatment.
- Lifestyle changes
  - Use acute event or new diagnosis to assist patients' motivation in healthy lifestyle changes.
  - Both smoking cessation and avoiding excessive alcohol use reduce osteoporosis risk.
  - Weight-bearing exercise, such as walking 1 mile twice a day or dancing, is commonly recommended, but evidence is lacking to show fracture benefit, other than decreasing falls.
  - Patients should avoid maneuvers that increase compressive forces on the spine.

I. **Introduction**
   A. **Osteoporosis** is a heterogeneous group of metabolic bone diseases characterized by severe bone mineral loss, disruption of skeletal microarchitecture, and disturbed bone quality leading to enhanced bone fragility, chiefly manifested by atraumatic fractures of the vertebral column, upper femur, distal radius, proximal humerus, pubic rami, and ribs.

B. Osteoporosis is often defined (Table 81–1) as a bone mineral density (BMD) T-score >2.5 standard deviations (SDs) below mean or a fracture resulting from minimal trauma (fragility fracture). **Osteopenia** is simply bone on its way to osteoporosis, with a BMD T-score between −1 and −2.5. **Osteomalacia** is characterized by abnormal bone, and is a potentially treatable metabolic bone disorder caused, for example, by inadequate vitamin D.

C. Bone constantly remodels through the process of resorption and formation. This process occurs at age-related rates, ranging from complete renewal of all bones in the first year of life to renewal of 15–30% of the skeleton per year in adults. Loss of BMD alone explains only about 60–80% of the variation in bone strength. Trabecular bone architectural changes contribute significantly to fracture risk but are not easily assessed clinically.

D. Bone mass reaches a peak by age 35, with bone loss beginning by age 40 in both sexes. After menopause, the rate of bone resorption exceeds the rate of bone formation. Over her lifetime, a woman loses 35% of her cortical bone and 50% of her trabecular bone. Men lose only two thirds of the bone that women lose as muscle mass decreases.

E. Five types of osteoporosis are recognized:

1. **Postmenopausal (type I).** The most common form in Caucasian and Asian women, due to acceleration of trabecular bone resorption in the first decade or two following menopause.
2. **Involutional (type II).** Occurs in both sexes older than age 75 and is due to a subtle, prolonged imbalance between rates of bone resorption and formation. Type II weakens cortical bone more than type I. Mixtures of types I and II are common, with additive effects.
3. **Idiopathic.** A rare form of primary osteoporosis occurring in premenopausal women and in men younger than age 75. It is not related to secondary causes or risk factors predisposing to bone loss.
4. **Juvenile.** A rare form, with variable severity in prepubertal children and cessation of fractures at puberty.
5. **Secondary.** (Table 81–2). Although secondary factors can cause osteoporosis, consider them as additive risk factors and treatable.

F. Osteoporosis affects about 28 million people in the United States (>15 million symptomatic cases) and thus is commonly seen in adult primary care practices. Seven percent of ambulatory postmenopausal women older than 50 years have osteoporosis already, and a 50-year-old white woman has lifetime risks of fracture of the spine, hip, and distal radius of 32%, 16%, and 15%, respectively. These risks greatly exceed her risk of developing endometrial or breast cancer combined. Age is a strong predictor of osteoporosis, which is five times more common in women older than 65 years than in women younger than 65 years.

G. Risk factors for osteoporosis are listed in Table 81–3. Factors associated with decreased risk for osteoporosis included higher body mass index, African American heritage, estrogen use, thiazide diuretic use, moderate exercise, and moderate alcohol consumption. Clinical risk factors have poorly validated roles in predicting fractures and in determining who should have BMD measurement.

II. Diagnosis

A. Symptoms and signs, when present and not otherwise explained, indicate that significant bone loss, including fracture or microfracture, has already occurred, and thus establish the diagnosis of osteoporosis.

TABLE 81–1. BMD DEFINITIONS OF BONE DENSITY[1]

Bone Status	BMD Description
Normal	BMD value within 1 SD of the young adult reference mean (T >= −1.0)
Osteopenia	BMD value of more than 1 SD below the young adult mean but less than 2.5 SD below this value (−1.0 > T > −2.5)
Osteoporosis	BMD value of 2.5 SD or more below the adult mean value (T <= −2.5)
Established osteoporosis	BMD value of 2.5 SD or more below the adult mean value (T <= −2.5) in the presence of one or more fragility fractures

[1] As established by World Health Organization (WHO).
BMD, bone mineral density.

TABLE 81–2. CAUSES OF SECONDARY OSTEOPOROSIS

Sex hormone deficiency
  Gonadal failure (hypogonadism, including orchiectomy)
  Prolactin-secreting pituitary adenoma (prolactinoma)
  Smoking tobacco (decreases circulating estrogen)

Hormone excess
  Hyperthyroidism
  Hyperparathyroidism
  Corticosteroids, exogenous (not inhaled)
  Cushing's syndrome

Increased bone resorption/formation ratio
  Prolonged immobilization (localized osteoporosis)
  Space flight (lose 10% bone mass in 1 week)
  Long-term heparin use
  Cancers (eg, multiple myeloma, lymphoma, leukemia, breast cancer)
  Paget's disease
  Rheumatoid arthritis

Osteomalacia (defective bone mineralization)
  Vitamin D deficiency
  Anticonvulsants and chronic liver disease (25-hydroxylation of vitamin D)
  Malabsorption syndromes
  Eating disorders
  Alcoholism
  Calcium deficiency
  Renal calcium wasting (eg, distal renal tubular acidosis)

Genetic abnormalities
  Osteogenesis imperfecta
  Ehlers-Danlos syndrome
  Homocystinuria

1. **Back pain** may be caused by acute compression fractures or biomechanical changes resulting from previous fractures.
2. **Fractures** of vertebra, hip, and forearm produce pain and disability. Fractures may result from such minimal trauma as bending, lifting, or getting out of bed.
3. **Loss of height** is associated with loss of bone, and fractures of the vertebrae and may be accompanied by disfiguring cosmetic changes.
4. **Poor dentition** and premature tooth loss is associated with osteoporosis.

TABLE 81–3. RISK FACTORS FOR OSTEOPOROSIS

Nonmodifiable
  Most secondary causes (Table 81–2)
  Menopause (physiologic or surgical)
  Increasing age
  Female sex
  Family history of osteoporosis
  Personal history of fracture
  Caucasian, Hispanic, or Asian race
  Lean build, short stature, small bone, light weight

Modifiable
  Hyperathleticism
  Smoking
  Dietary excess of protein (>120 g/day) or vitamin A (retinol)
  Diet low in calcium, vitamin D, vitamin C, or magnesium
  Sedentary lifestyle or lack of exercise
  Alcohol excess

5. **Mechanical deformity** (kyphosis, or dowager's hump) caused by vertebral compression fracture may interfere with both respiration and abdominal processes and may cause early satiety, bloating, decreased exercise tolerance, constipation, and loss of self-esteem.

6. Observe for signs of **secondary causes** if osteoporosis is suspected (eg, moon faces, exophthalmos, etc)

B. Be wary of the distinction between diagnosis (identification of the cause of symptoms and signs) and screening (case finding in a population at risk). The evidence supporting one process may not support the other. The following recommendations are diagnostic interventions for the patient with suspected or established osteoporosis. Diagnostic tests are considered not only to confirm the diagnosis of osteoporosis but also to rule out associated conditions.

C. **Laboratory tests**

1. Testing healthy patients with osteoporosis may reveal bone and mineral metabolism disorders; retrospective chart review of 173 women in a referral population found 55 (32%) with previously undetected disorders including hypercalciuria, malabsorption, hyperparathyroidism, vitamin D deficiency, exogenous hyperthyroidism, Cushing's disease, and hypocalciuric hypercalcemia.

2. Order serum calcium, phosphate, alkaline phosphatase, creatinine, and thyroid-stimulating hormone (TSH) tests, which should be normal in primary osteoporosis.

3. Consider 25-hydroxyvitamin D, intact parathyroid hormone (iPTH), serum protein electrophoresis (SPEP), testosterone (men), estradiol (women) and 24-hour urinary calcium excretion tests to rule out other secondary causes.

4. Consider tests of bone metabolism in uncertain cases:
   a. **Urine calcium/creatinine** ratio.
   b. Tubular reabsorption of **phosphorus.**
   c. **NTx assay (Osteomark) or pyridinium crosslinks (Pyrilinks-D).** NTx and pyridinium crosslink assays are some type I collagen breakdown products in urine and serum and are used to assess osteoclast activity.

5. Bone biopsy is rarely needed and requires a nondecalcified bone specimen with tetracycline labeling and a specialized laboratory for interpretation.

6. Bone marrow aspiration and biopsy can rule out multiple myeloma, metastatic carcinoma, and lymphoma, if clinically indicated.

D. **Imaging studies**

1. **X-rays.** By the time osteoporosis is evident on x-ray, 20–40% of bone is lost. The following changes can be seen on plain x-ray of the vertebral column: increased lucency, cortical thinning, increased density of end plate, anterior wedging and biconcavity of vertebrae, and loss of horizontal trabeculae.

2. **Bone mineral density (BMD) testing.** The decision to order BMD testing in the patient with suspected or established osteoporosis entails several considerations.
   a. Chief among these is whether the results will change the treatment. Patients who are at sufficiently high risk for osteoporotic fracture (eg, those older than age 70 with multiple risk factors) will not likely benefit from BMD testing if treatment is indicated on clinical ground anyway.
   b. Deciding which patients to consider for BMD measurement requires weighing risk factors on an individual basis. Table 81–4 identifies indications for BMD testing.

TABLE 81–4. INDICATIONS FOR BONE MASS MEASUREMENT TO DIAGNOSE OSTEOPOROSIS[1]

Strong indications

Estrogen-deficient women to make treatment decisions based on bone mineral density
Patients receiving long-term steroids for treatment decisions
Patients with vertebral abnormalities or incidental osteopenia on x-ray
Patients with asymptomatic primary hyperparathyroidism or other disease associated with high risk of osteoporosis

Weaker indications

Patients who have lost height or sustained a probable osteoporotic fracture
Patients being treated for osteoporosis, to monitor changes

[1] Both males or females, unless stated.
Adapted from the National Osteoporosis Foundation.

    c. Some clinicians will order serial studies to follow the effects of treatment on BMD, but there is little evidence to support this, given the precision error of available techniques.

    d. Three imaging modalities are commonly available: dual-energy x-ray absorptiometry (DXA), quantitative computed tomography (QCT), and calcaneal ultrasonography.

    e. DXA is the most precise technique, is used most widely for measuring BMD, and correlates best with the World Health Organization criteria (Table 81–1). Measurements are typically taken from the lumbar spine, the proximal femur, and the distal forearm.

    f. QCT results are less likely to be affected by degenerative spinal changes than spine DXA scanning. Also, unlike DXA, QCT allows for selective assessment of trabecular bone, which may show metabolic changes earlier. QCT can predict spinal fracture similarly to DXA scanning, but the costs and radiation exposure are higher.

    g. Ultrasonography measures the speed of sound (related to bone density) and broadband ultrasonic attenuation (related to bone architecture) of the calcaneus, typically. Fracture risk prediction is equivalent to that of DXA, especially for hip fracture. Ultrasound is available for in-office use and is portable, making evaluation in the long-term care facility feasible. Lower precision makes this technique not recommended for serial measurements.

    h. Deciding which bone imaging modality depends upon availability, age, site of interest, and costs. For example, vertebral fractures are of greater concern than hip fractures in women who are within 15 years of menopause. Any of the imaging modalities may be appropriate, especially those that include imaging of the spine. In women older than 65 years, hip fractures become more of a concern, so DXA of the hip or calcaneal ultrasound might be appropriate.

III. Treatment

    A. The continuous distribution of BMD and current available evidence preclude an absolute "fracture risk threshold" to initiate treatment. Other factors, such as skeletal architecture (presently difficult to measure), fall risk, exercise patterns and the constellation of risk factors (Table 81–3), life expectancy, adverse side effects, and patient preferences, must be considered in a manner analogous to the management of hyperlipidemia, in which treatment thresholds may depend on other risk factors as well as lipid levels. An evidence-based, validated algorithm for the treatment of osteoporosis that includes patient-specific risk factors for fracture and BMD measure does not currently exist. Thus, current management has to be individualized.

    B. Primary prevention

        1. Lifestyle. Factors that can decrease calcium absorption, increase bone resorption, or impair bone formation, such as smoking, excessive alcohol intake, and medications associated with osteoporosis, should be avoided.

        2. Weight-bearing exercise. Exercise should be weight-bearing and skeletal-stressing. Prolonged low-to-moderate physical activity is associated with higher BMD than either sedentary lifestyle or endurance-trained athletic activity.

        3. Calcium supplements. The average American consumes <800 mg/day of calcium. Recommendations for calcium intake vary by age and a typical expert opinion is in Table 81–5. Calcium alone can prevent bone loss and fractures.

            a. Estimating calcium intake. An estimation of the patient's dietary intake can be made quickly and easily with Repka's rules of 300: the basal diet contains 300 mg of calcium, and each serving of dairy products, such as 8 oz milk, 8 oz yogurt, 1½ oz cheese, or 2 cups cottage cheese, provides 300 mg of calcium.

TABLE 81–5. DIETARY CALCIUM REQUIREMENTS

Children 4–8 years—800 mg/day
Children 9–18 years—1300 mg/day
Adults 19–50 years (including pregnant and lactating women)—1000 mg/day
Adults older than 50 years—1200 mg/day

Source: Institute of Medicine, 1997.

Excellent sources of nondairy calcium include sardines (372 mg in 3 oz) and pink salmon (167 mg in 3 oz).

b. General information. There is little evidence favoring specific calcium supplements for efficacy in preventing osteoporotic fractures. Absorption is improved with doses <500 mg and when taken with food. Calcium can interfere with absorption of other minerals and many drugs (eg, iron, zinc, quinolones, bisphosphonates, tetracycline). See Table 81–6 for typical supplements.

c. Calcium carbonate. Derived from oyster shells, this is the cheapest oral form of calcium supplement available and requires fewest tablets per day. It may cause more gastrointestinal upset (constipation, bloating, gas) than other preparations. Stomach acid is required for absorption, which may limit effectiveness in patients who are elderly, taking proton pump inhibitors, or have achlorhydria. Excess dosing can cause milk-alkali syndrome.

d. Calcium citrate is best absorbed, has fewest side effects, need not be taken with meals in order to maximize absorption, and costs more than calcium carbonate. If carbonate forms are poorly tolerated, this option can be helpful. Theoretically, lower doses may be as effective because three times as much is absorbed, but this has not been studied.

e. Absorption of all calcium products is improved with adequate vitamin D, with supplemental magnesium salts and with thiazide diuretics. Sodium restriction reduces urinary excretion of calcium, but has unclear effects on bones.

4. Vitamin D is traditionally recommended in supplemental form since intake or endogenous production is frequently suboptimal. This vitamin is manufactured variably in the skin following direct exposure to sunlight. Exposure of 10–15 minutes for the hands, arms, and face three times per week is enough. Vitamin D production is decreased by dark skin, sunscreen, window glass, clothing, air pollution, aging, and lack of sun exposure (northern latitude, homebound persons, or cultural dressing habits).

a. Typically recommended oral intake is 400 IU daily for adults (the usual amount in average multivitamin). This dose is not associated with fracture benefit; however, 800 IU daily is.

b. In combination with adequate calcium intake, 700–800 IU vitamin D can reduce fractures significantly, up to 50% in nursing home patients. Number needed to treat (NNT) = 45/year to prevent one fracture.

c. Potential (3–5%) for hypercalcemia exists with high doses of vitamin D.

d. Calcium and vitamin D together is strongly recommended for all patients taking long-term corticosteroids.

5. Secondary causes of osteoporosis should be sought and treated.

TABLE 81–6. COMPARISON OF TYPICAL CALCIUM SUPPLEMENTS

Calcium Supplement	Trade Name	Elemental Calcium (mg)	Vitamin D (IU)	Tablets per day	Relative Cost
Calcium carbonate	Generic	500	200	2	$
	Os-Cal 500 + D	500	200	2	$
	CalBurst	500	200	2	$
	Caltrate + D	600	200	2	$
	Tums 500	500	0	2	$
	Viactiv (chewable)	500	100	2	$
Calcium citrate	Calcium citrate + D	315	200	3	$$
	Osteo-Max (effervescent)	500	200	1	$$
Calcium lactate	Generic 650 mg	100	0	10	$$
Calcium glubionate liquid	NeoCalglucon	115/5 cc	0	45 cc	$$
Calcium complex (carbonate, lactate, gluconate)	Calcet	150	100	7	$$
Calcium phosphate	Posture-D 1500	600	125	2	$$
Calcium acetate	Phos-lo	667	169	6	$$
Calcium gluconate	Generic 650 mg	50	0	20	$$

    6. Risks factors for fracture, such as orthostatic hypotension, lower limb dysfunction, drug use, and visual impairment especially in the frail, elderly patient, should be sought and reduced. A home safety evaluation should be considered to prevent falls.

C. Secondary prevention attempts to detect disease early and minimize the risks in patients discovered to have asymptomatic osteoporosis, usually through screening or clinical suspicion. **Primary prevention strategies remain in force.** Drug therapy is often indicated and antiresorptive drugs include estrogen, raloxifene, bisphosphonates, and calcitonin. Agents shown to prevent vertebral fractures in postmenopausal women include alendronate, risedronate, and raloxifene, although only alendronate and risedronate also prevent hip fractures. Large trials with fracture outcomes are lacking regarding estrogen and calcitonin.

  1. Bisphosphonates inhibit bone resorption and have the best evidence for efficacy.

    a. Because calcium supplements or food taken at the same time as a bisphosphonate reduce already low (1%) absorption of the drug, it should be taken on an empty stomach (usually before breakfast) with a full glass of water and without eating or lying down for 30 minutes to avoid esophagitis.

    b. Alendronate (Fosamax), 10 mg orally every day or 70 mg orally once weekly, has an NNT of 45–140/year for symptomatic fracture prevention in women with known osteoporosis (previous vertebral fractures). Alendronate prevents bone density loss after discontinuation of hormone replacement therapy.

    c. Risedronate (Actonel), 5 mg orally every day or 35 mg orally weekly, has an NNT of 90/year for nonvertebral fracture prevention in women with preexisting vertebral fracture.

    d. Etidronate (Didronel) is not approved by the US Food and Drug Administration (FDA) for treatment of osteoporosis and has limited evidence that suggests a reduction in vertebral fractures but no effect on nonvertebral fractures.

    e. Zoledronic acid (Zometa) is a bisphosphonate with indications for use in myeloma and metastatic bone disease and hypercalcemia of malignancy. Infusions given at intervals of up to 1 year produce effects on bone turnover and bone density as great as other bisphosphonates, suggesting that an annual infusion of zoledronic acid might be an effective treatment for postmenopausal osteoporosis. More study is underway as the FDA does not yet approve it for treatment of osteoporosis.

  2. Raloxifene (Evista) is an example of a selective estrogen receptor modulator (SERM). These agents may provide the beneficial effects of estrogen replacement therapy without some of its potentially serious side effects.

    a. Raloxifene reduces risk of recurrent vertebral fracture in postmenopausal women with known osteoporosis (NNT 90/year for 60 mg/day; 64/year for 120 mg/day).

    b. The benefit of preventing hip fractures is yet unproven.

    c. Adverse effects include venous thromboembolism (NNH 440/year).

    d. No increase risk of heart disease or breast cancer mortality is found with raloxifene so far.

  3. Calcitonin (Miacalcin) intranasally one nasal puff (200 U) every day, alternating nostrils, is shown to reduce bone loss and decrease vertebral fracture risk (NNT 65/year).

    a. No studies are available on clinical or nonvertebral fractures.

    b. Calcitonin appears to preserve bone mass in steroid-induced osteoporosis, but fracture prevention is not established.

    c. The drug must be kept refrigerated.

    d. Decreased bone pain in acute vertebral fracture is reportedly due to the increase in endorphins stimulated by calcitonin.

    e. The intranasal form has largely replaced use of subcutaneous calcitonin 100–200 U 3×/week, although the subcutaneous form prevents more bone loss than intranasal calcitonin. The subcutaneous form is associated with nausea and occasional allergic reaction.

  4. Hormone replacement therapy (HRT). Estrogen alone or in combination with progestins has been prescribed routinely for prevention of postmenopausal osteoporosis for decades. Accumulated evidence is variable regarding the fracture benefits of this practice (NNT ranges from 132/year to 1429/year for vertebral fracture prevention and NNT 2000/year for hip fracture prevention). Further complicating the decision is the more clear evidence that the risks of estrogen supplementation are significant in regard to cancer, heart disease, and other conditions. When these products are being prescribed solely for the prevention of postmenopausal osteoporosis, approved nonestrogen treatments should be carefully considered. Estrogens and combined estrogen-progestin products should only be considered for women with significant risk of osteoporosis that outweighs the risks of the drug. The following options are available for osteoporosis treatment.

 a. Conjugated estrogens (eg, Premarin), 0.3–0.625 mg orally every day (days 1–25 of the month). Micronized estradiol (Estrace), 0.5–1 mg, is equivalent.

 b. A progestin such as medroxyprogesterone, 5–10 mg orally, should be added in a cyclical fashion in women with a uterus, to reduce the risk of endometrial cancer.

 c. Continuous HRT can be offered with a variety of products available that combine low-dose estrogen with progestin for daily dosing.

 d. Transdermal estrogen 0.025–0.1 mg/day reduces bone loss in hysterectomized women.

 e. Recent evidence concludes that BMD (but not fracture) benefits can be seen in 3 years of HRT and little is gained after that, nor is much lost if therapy concludes after 3 years.

 f. Combination HRT and alendronate improved BMD more than alendronate alone, which was more effective than HRT alone. However, fracture benefits are not proven yet.

5. Parathyroid hormone (PTH). Teriparatide (Forteo) is *N*-terminal fragment recombinant human PTH and the first FDA-approved agent that stimulates new bone formation for osteoporosis in postmenopausal women and men with primary or hypogonadal osteoporosis.

 a. Parathyroid hormone increases BMD.

 b. In high-risk patients with established osteoporosis, it prevents new vertebral fracture (NNT 10–11), new nonvertebral fractures (NNT 30) and new nonvertebral fragility fractures (NNT 35). So, PTH may be more effective than bisphosphonates.

 c. It is supplied as an injector pen with 750 µg/3 mL, given as 20 µg subcutaneously into the thigh or abdominal wall once daily.

 d. The black box warning states do not use if increased baseline risk for osteosarcoma, Paget's disease of bone, unexplained alkaline phosphatase elevations, open epiphyses, prior radiation therapy of skeleton, metastases, history of skeletal malignancies, metabolic bone diseases (other than osteoporosis), or preexisting hypercalcemia.

 e. Adverse effects include pain, arthralgia, asthenia, nausea, rhinitis, dizziness, headache, hypertension, increased cough, pharyngitis, constipation, diarrhea, dyspepsia, and poverty (>$500/mo).

6. Fluoride therapy is highly controversial.

 a. Fluoride can increase BMD in the lumbar spine but does not prevent vertebral fractures. Increasing doses of fluoride are associated with increased risk of nonvertebral fractures and gastrointestinal side effects.

 b. Sustained-release sodium fluoride prevented new vertebral fractures in two randomized trials.

 c. Most authorities are not recommending fluoride therapy currently. Some form of fluoride may have a role in osteoporosis therapy in the future.

7. Ipriflavone is a synthetic flavonoid (isoflavone) available over the counter (OTC). Ipriflavone promotes the incorporation of calcium into bone and inhibits bone resorption.

 a. Isoflavones are approved in European and Asian countries for osteoporosis prevention and treatment.

 b. It does not possess intrinsic estrogenic activity and behaves more like a SERM without significant adverse side effects.

 c. Studies are controversial regarding efficacy, but ipriflavone appears to prevent postmenopausal bone loss. No studies yet show a reduction in fracture rates.

 d. Unregulated manufacture of OTC products in the United States limits the reliability of OTC product purity and potency.

8. Hydrochlorothiazide in low doses (up to 25 mg/day) was associated with preservation of BMD in one randomized trial. In doses of 50 mg/day, thiazides may be beneficial in treating the high urine calcium of patients with idiopathic hypercalci-

uria via improving gastrointestinal absorption of calcium. Thiazides should be used only in conjunction with other therapies for osteoporosis.
9. **Secondary causes** of osteoporosis should be sought and treated.
10. **Risks factors for fracture,** such as orthostatic hypotension, lower limb dysfunction, drug use, and visual impairment especially in the frail, elderly patient, should be sought and reduced. A home safety evaluation should be considered to prevent falls.
D. **Tertiary prevention** involves the care of established symptomatic osteoporosis, with attempts made to restore to highest function, minimize the negative effects of disease, and prevent disease-related complications. Since the disease is now established, primary prevention activities may have been unsuccessful. Early detection through secondary prevention may have minimized the impact of the disease.
   1. **Pain relief** is of primary importance in the patient with acute fracture and often will require hospital or nursing home admission. The nature of the fracture will guide specific therapeutic options.
      a. Vertebral compression fractures are commonly treated with bed rest, prevention of further injury and, occasionally, spinal bracing.
      b. A long period of therapeutic exercises may be required to regain full function.
      c. Calcitonin may reduce pain acutely.
      d. Analgesics may be used liberally as the clinical situation dictates, and nonsteroidal anti-inflammatory drugs are often suitable if no contraindications exist. Beware the pitfalls of using analgesics in the elderly.
   2. **If bed rest** is prolonged, consider deep vein thrombosis prophylaxis.
   3. **Percutaneous procedures,** such as vertebroplasty, inject polymethylmethacrylate cement into the compressed vertebral body.
      a. Balloon kyphoplasty uses a balloon inflated inside the compressed vertebral body before the cement is injected.
      b. Vertebroplasty and kyphoplasty are associated with reduced pain and improved function in uncontrolled studies.
      c. These procedures, typically performed by orthopods, are not widely used yet, and long-term outcomes remain uncertain due to lack of good studies.
E. **Screening**
   1. The US Preventive Services Task Force (USPSTF) recommends that women aged 65 years and older be screened routinely for osteoporosis.
   2. The USPSTF recommends that routine screening begin at age 60 for women at increased risk for osteoporotic fractures.
   3. National Osteoporosis Foundation (NOF) urges bone density tests for all women older than 65 years + postmenopausal women with additional risk factor for osteoporotic fracture.
   4. The National Institutes of Health Osteoporosis Consensus Panel claims that there is no evidence that widespread screening will decrease important clinical outcomes (eg, fracture rates).
   5. Who should be screened? Current evidence suggests that measurement of BMD can predict fracture risk in populations but not in individuals. Four risk indices all performed well in identifying postmenopausal women with low bone density (T score < -2.5). Osteoporosis Self-assessment Tool (OST) is simplest since it is based on only age and weight: (weight in kilograms) minus (age in years) <10 in women or <3 in men suggests increased risk, thus a possible indication for screening.
   6. If one is going to screen, DXA scans of the femoral neck seem to be the best predictor of hip fracture. Since treatment of osteoporosis has been shown to decrease hip fractures, this indirectly supports the routine (every 2–3 years) screening of older women.
   7. Heel ultrasound has some utility in screening due to its portability and availability. Compared to DXA, a combination of risk factors or ultrasound had 90% sensitivity, 38% specificity, 22% positive predictive value, and 95% negative predictive value in detecting osteoporosis by BMD criteria.
IV. **Management Strategies**
A. **Patient education**
   1. **Counseling** should be offered to all women regarding universal preventive measures related to fracture risk, calcium and vitamin D intake, weight-bearing exercise, smoking cessation, avoidance of excess alcohol intake, and the risks and benefits of hormone replacement therapy.
   2. Hip protection pads and anchor rugs in the elderly decrease hip fractures.

3. The National Resource Center on Osteoporosis is a federally funded clearinghouse for the latest risks, prevention, and treatment of and information on osteoporosis. Phone (202) 223-0344. National Osteoporosis Foundation http://www.nof.org

B. **Compliance** with therapy (eg, HRT) is improved when women were given BMD testing. This may be due to the objectification of the disease when viewed as a laboratory report.

C. **Follow-up** after diagnosis or fracture includes the following:
   1. Schedule office visits bimonthly initially, then every 6 months.
   2. Promote periodic multiphasic screening, annual gynecologic examination, breast examination, and mammography.
   3. Every 2 or 3 years, obtain BMD using the same technique.
   4. Repeat x-rays for acute pain or suspected fractures.

V. **Prognosis**
   A. **Risk**
      1. 1 vertebral fracture at baseline = 5-fold risk of more vertebral fractures.
      2. >1 vertebral fracture at baseline = 12-fold risk of more vertebral fractures.
      3. 1 symptomatic vertebral fracture at baseline = 2-fold risk of hip fractures.
      4. 1 SD decrease in hip BMD = 2- to 3-fold increase in hip fracture.
      5. 1 SD in blood pressure = 1.5 increase in stroke mortality.
      6. 1 SD in cholesterol = 1.5 increase in coronary artery disease mortality.
   B. **Life expectancy**
      1. Hip fractures—50% of patients never fully recover; 25% require long-term care.

REFERENCES

Brunader R, Shelton D: Radiologic bone assessment in the evaluation of osteoporosis. Am Fam Physician 2002;**65**:1357.

Fitzpatrick LA: Secondary causes of osteoporosis. Mayo Clin Proc (May) 2002;**77**(5):453 (commentary in Mayo Clin Proc (September) 2002;**77**(9):1005).

Osteoporosis prevention, diagnosis, and therapy. NIH Consensus Statement 2000;**17**(1):1.

South-Paul JE, Osteoporosis: Part I. Evaluation and assessment. Am Fam Physician 2001; **63**:897–904, 908; and Osteoporosis: Part II. Nonpharmacologic and pharmacologic treatment. Am Fam Physician 2001;**63**:1121.)

Tannenbaum C, et al: Yield of laboratory testing to identify secondary contributors to osteoporosis in otherwise healthy women. J Clin Endocrinol Metab (October) 2002;**87**:4431; and Wagman RB, Marcus R: Beyond bone mineral density—navigating the laboratory assessment of patients with osteoporosis [editorial]. J Clin Endocrinol Metab (October) 2002;**87**:4429.

82	Peptic Ulcer Disease

Lesley D. Wilkinson, MD, Nancy Tyre, MD, & Carol Stewart, MD

KEY POINTS

- Peptic ulcer disease (PUD) is primarily caused by *Helicobacter pylori* infection or by non-steroidal anti-inflammatory drug (NSAID) use.
- Patients present complaining of epigastric pain. Most have gastroesophageal reflux disease (GERD) or functional dyspepsia; about 15% have PUD. Initial endoscopy is reserved for patients with "alarm" symptoms (weight loss, anemia, bleeding, dysphagia or odynophagia, prior PUD) suggesting bleeding, perforation, or cancer.
- All patients deserve a "test and treat" approach for *H pylori*. Rarely, one needs to consider more obscure causes such as Zollinger-Ellison syndrome.
- The first step in treatment is stopping any NSAIDs or aspirin, starting acid-blocking medication, and initiating treatment for *H pylori* if infection is present.

I. **Introduction**
   A. **Definition.** Peptic ulcer disease (PUD) is present when acid-peptic injury to the gastrointestinal mucosa results in defects (ulcerations) through the epithelial layer.

B. Pathophysiology. Peptic ulcer disease is due to one or both of two underlying causes: (1) *H pylori* infection or (2) use of NSAIDs. Less common causes are (3) idiopathic and (4) acid hypersecretory conditions (eg, Zollinger-Ellison syndrome). Infrequently, PUD is caused by Crohn's disease, systemic mastocytosis, alcoholism, malignancy, viral infections (herpes simplex, cytomegalovirus), and cocaine usage. Acid is necessary, but not sufficient by itself, to develop PUD lesions.

1. *H pylori* is a gram-negative microaerophilic, urease-producing bacterium that has adapted to the environment of the gastric mucosa. It causes persistent inflammation in the stomach with a vigorous immune response that rarely eliminates *H pylori*. (Children clear the infection up to 20% of the time.) *H pylori* gastritis is variable in clinical expression, and often asymptomatic. The lifetime risk of PUD in a patient infected with *H pylori* is 3% in the United States and 25% in Japan.

2. **NSAIDs** have a different mechanism of ulceration. They do not cause a diffuse gastritis. They primarily induce mucosal injury by disrupting prostaglandin-mediated cell protection and proliferation. Gastroprotective mechanisms that are disrupted include inhibition of acid secretion, bicarbonate production, gastric mucous production, and promotion of mucosal growth and repair. Many NSAIDs are also weak acids themselves and directly injure epithelial cells in the acid stomach environment.

C. Epidemiology. PUD affects 4 million patients per year in the United States, with a current lifetime prevalence of about 10% in men and 4% in women. US mortality due to PUD is about 5000 per year.

1. Patients usually present with dyspepsia (epigastric pain), not "PUD." Dyspepsia accounts for 2–5% of all symptomatic ambulatory care visits in the United States. Fifteen percent of patients with dyspepsia have PUD. Of the remainder, 1–2% have cancer, 6–24% have GERD, and over 60% have functional dyspepsia with normal endoscopies. Most patients with typical PUD symptoms do not have PUD.

2. The diagnosis and treatment of PUD have been transformed over the last 25 years by the development of medications that suppress acid formation and by the discovery that one of the primary etiologies of PUD is a curable infectious disease— *H pylori.*

   a. *H pylori* is extremely common in the developing world (prevalence over 80%), but rates in the industrialized world have been dropping as hygiene and public health have improved. Infection occurs almost exclusively before age 10 in the industrialized world, so current prevalence rates by age reflect a cohort effect. The adult infection rate is about 0.5% per year (Figure 82–1).

   b. *H pylori* is transmitted by fecal/oral or oral/oral routes. Its prevalence correlates strongly with socioeconomic conditions. Risk factors in the United States include birth in another country, older age, lower socioeconomic status, domestic crowding, and unsanitary conditions; these conditions are currently more common in nonwhite populations. US *H pylori* prevalence in individuals younger than 30 is <10%, so the incidence and etiology of PUD will be shifting in the future.

3. NSAIDs are a major cause of PUD, primarily due to the huge number of patients utilizing them. Thirty billion over-the-counter tablets and 70 million prescriptions for NSAIDs per year are purchased just in the United States. Nearly 40% of elderly Americans are prescribed NSAIDs each year, and NSAID use is gradually increasing due to the aging of the population and increasing use of aspirin prophylaxis. Since symptoms cannot reliably point to PUD with NSAIDs, it is important to be aware of preexisting risk factors for PUD when initiating NSAID treatment (Table 82–1).

II. Diagnosis

A. History. Epigastric distress is the most common presentation of PUD. Patients usually describe this as a midline gnawing discomfort or feeling of hunger. Sometimes it is painful with aching or burning, or a patient may have nausea with or without actual emesis. An acid taste is more common with GERD. The discomfort typically occurs 1–3 hours postprandially and overnight, classically 1–2 AM. Food, antacids, or vomiting may relieve the symptoms within minutes. Minor weight loss may occur in up to 50% of patients with benign gastric ulcers. Significant weight loss is a red flag for malignancy. Patients with duodenal ulcers who eat to control their pain are more likely to present with weight gain. **ALARM SYMPTOMS** may indicate complicating diagnoses (Table 82–2). The presence of alarm symptoms is an indication for immediate endoscopy in the dyspeptic patient.

B. Physical examination. The physical examination is usually nonspecific; epigastric tenderness is the most common finding.

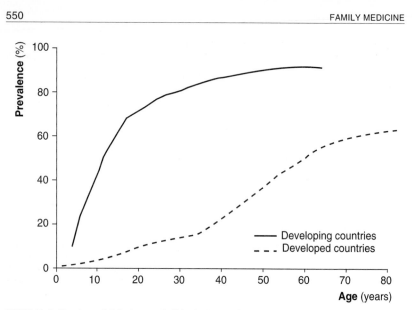

FIGURE 82–1. Prevalence of *Helicobacter pylori* infection by age. (From Logan RPH, Walker MM: ABC of the upper gastrointestinal tract: Epidemiology and diagnosis of *Helicobacter pylori* infection. BMJ 2001;**323**:920.)

C. Tests
1. Definitive diagnosis of PUD requires endoscopy. Barium studies can also confirm the diagnosis but do not allow for biopsy. Treatment with proton pump inhibitors (PPIs) significantly decreases the sensitivity of endoscopy. Ideally, endoscopy should take place prior to treatment, or PPIs should be discontinued for at least 4 weeks before endoscopy. Even cancer may partially heal with PPI treatment despite its malignant nature, and it can be deceptive even for skilled endoscopists.
2. Blood counts should be checked if there is any concern about a bleeding ulcer. Concerns about acute bleeding should prompt stool guaiacs and gastric aspiration.
3. Histology of tissue from at least two different sites remains the gold standard for diagnosis of *H pylori* infection, but many other methods are available (Table 82–3). Serology is the most common method used for diagnosis, but it is unsuitable for following up eradication. Stool antigen tests and urea breath tests generally revert to negative 1 month after effective treatment. Stool antigen tests are insensitive in the setting of PPI use.

D. Differential diagnosis. As noted above, most patients with PUD symptoms actually have functional dyspepsia or GERD. The differential does include serious illnesses that require a high index of suspicion to diagnose: bleeding ulcer, perforated ulcer, gastric or esophageal cancer (duodenal ulcer is almost never malignant), severe GERD with stricture, as well as pancreatitis, cholecystitis, and cardiac or pulmonary etiologies.

TABLE 82–1. RISK FACTORS FOR NSAID GASTROINTESTINAL COMPLICATIONS

- *Helicobacter pylori* infection, even if asymptomatic
- Older age, more risk with higher age
- History of peptic ulcer disease
- Alcoholism
- Female at advanced age
- Poor health
- Smoking
- Use of steroids, chemotherapy, anticoagulation, or alendronate
- High-dose or prolonged course of NSAID use, or both

NSAID, nonsteroidal anti-inflammatory drug.

TABLE 82–2. ALARM SYMPTOMS FOR PEPTIC ULCER DISEASE

1. Age older than approximately 45–50 years
   (*incidence of cancer increases with age,* <1% *younger than age 50*)
2. Unintentional weight loss
3. Anemia (*iron deficiency*)
4. Gastrointestinal bleeding (*either hematemesis or hematochezia*)
5. Dysphagia (*difficulty swallowing*)
6. Odynophagia (*pain on swallowing*)
7. Vomiting (*persistent*)
8. Epigastric mass
9. Prior gastric surgery or peptic ulcer disease
10. Family history of gastric cancer
11. Severe or penetrating pain, or both

III. **Treatment.** (Not directly applicable to geographic locations with high levels of *H pylori* infection.)

    A. **Test and treat.** There is a growing expert consensus that patients presenting with dyspepsia, but NO alarm symptoms, should first be managed with a "test and treat" approach, without obtaining a definitive diagnosis. Noninvasive testing for *H pylori* should be performed and treatment initiated if positive. If the patient is on an NSAID, it should be stopped if at all possible. Treatment with acid suppression should begin. If these treatments fail to control symptoms, then referral is indicated.

    B. **Acid suppression** promotes ulcer healing, and *H pylori* treatments require higher pH to be successful.

        1. PPIs are the most effective medications. They significantly raise gastric pH by disabling active hydrogen ("proton") pumps in the parietal cells. It takes 3–4 days to reach full activity because all of the pumps are not normally turned on at one time. All PPIs are similarly effective but differ somewhat in drug interactions (Table 82–4).

        2. H_2 receptor antagonists (H_2 blockers) quickly decrease acid secretion by blocking histamine stimulation of parietal cell activity (Table 82–5). They are effective, but tolerance develops, and they are not as potent as PPIs for acid suppression or healing. Although they work to an extent, they are not the primary treatment for PUD in the United States at this point.

        3. All other drugs are inferior at acid suppression and healing (Table 82–5). Patients can of course use antacids for symptom relief. Sucralfate is helpful but is inferior to H_2 blockers. Misoprostol (Cytotec) is fairly effective at preventing NSAID-induced ulceration but has a high (up to 30%) rate of diarrhea, is very expensive, and is inferior to PPIs.

    C. **Therapy for *H pylori***

        1. All diagnosed *H pylori* should be treated (even if PUD is ultimately ruled out). A drug regimen of at least two antibiotics and an acid suppressor is required (Table 82–6). Multiple regimens have been tried because none is ideal; all suffer from potential side effects, potential poor adherence, expense, and significant failure rates. (There is significant antibiotic resistance of approximately 40% to metronidazole and approximately 10% to clarithromycin.)

TABLE 82–3. DIAGNOSTIC TESTS FOR *HELICOBACTER PYLORI*

Diagnostic Tests	Sensitivity	Specificity
Histology (specialized stains)	93–96%	97–99%
Bacterial culture (of gastric contents)	80–94%	100%
Urea breath tests	90–96%	90–98%
Stool antigen tests	88–95%	90–98%
Rapid urease assays	88–95%	95–99%
Lab serology tests	85–94%	80–95%
Office whole blood tests	70–88%	75–90%

Data from Smoot DT, Go MF, Cryer B: Peptic ulcer disease. Primary Care; Clin Office Practice 2001;**28**(3):487.

TABLE 82–4. MEDICATIONS FOR TREATMENT OR PREVENTION OF PEPTIC ULCER DISEASE, PART I

Drug	Dose	Notes
Proton Pump Inhibitors (PPIs)		
Esomeprazole magnesium (Nexium)	20–40 mg qd	Maint: 20 mg qd ♀ (Pregnancy category) B
Lansoprazole (Prevacid)	DU: 15 mg qd GU: 30 mg qd	Maint: 15 mg qd for DU Hypersecretory conditions: 60 mg qd, adjust up to max 90 mg bid; ♀ B
Omeprazole (Prilosec)	DU: 20 mg qd GU: 40 mg qd OTC: 20 mg qd	Maint: 20 mg qd Hypersecretory conditions: 60 mg qd, adjust up to max 120 mg tid, Available OTC, ♀ C; more potential drug interactions than the other PPIs[1]
Pantoprazole sodium (Protonix)	40 mg qd	Maint: 40 mg qd Hypersecretory conditions: 40 mg bid, adjust up to max 240 qd; ♀ B
Rabeprazole sodium (Aciphex)	20 mg qd after morning meal	Maint: 20 mg qd Hypersecretory conditions: 60 mg qd, adjust up to max up to 100 mg qd or 60 mg bid, Swallow whole. Caution with severe hepatic impairment; ♀ B

[1] All PPIs have a risk rating of category D (consider therapy modification) for concomitant use with systemic antifungals (imida-zoles) and atazanavir. This is due to decreased absorption of these medications in a nonacidic environment. For category C (monitor therapy) interactions, omeprazole has more potential problems, especially with warfarin and benzodiazepines. All seizure medications, digoxin, statins, methotrexate, and their effects should be monitored if given with any PPI. Lansoprazole and rabeprazole are less effective if taken with St. John's wort.
DU, duodenal ulcer; GU, gastric ulcer; OTC, over the counter.
♀, Pregnancy class.

TABLE 82–5. MEDICATIONS FOR TREATMENT OR PREVENTION OF PEPTIC ULCER DISEASE, PART II

Drug	Dose	Notes
H₂ Blockers		
Cimetidine (Tagamet)	300 mg qid OR 400 mg bid OR 800 mg hs OTC 100 mg	Maint: 400 mg qhs Hypersecretory conditions: 300 mg qid up to 2400 mg qd. Many drug interactions; may induce confusional states, particularly in the elderly. ♀ B
Famotidine (Pepcid)	40 mg qhs OR 20 mg bid OTC 10 mg	Central nervous system adverse effects reported with moderate to severe renal insufficiency. Few drug interactions. ♀ B
Nizatidine (Axid)	300 mg qhs OR 150 mg bid OTC 75 mg	Maint: 150 mg qhs False-positive for urobilinogen with Multistix. ♀ C
Ranitidine (Zantac)	150 mg bid OR 300 mg qhs OTC 75 mg	Maint: 150 mg qhs Hypersecretory conditions: 150 mg bid Bradycardia reported with rapid infusion. Few drug interactions. ♀ B
Other Medications for PUD Treatment/Prevention		
Misoprostol (Cytotec)	200 μg qid, or if not tolerated, 100 μg qid	For prevention of NSAID-induced ulcers in patients at risk. ♀ X
Sucralfate (Carafate)	1 g qid ac and hs	Maint: 1 g bid on empty stomach, adheres to ulcer crater; ♀ B

OTC, over the counter; NSAID, nonsteroidal anti-inflammatory drug.
♀, pregnancy class.

TABLE 82-6. TREATMENT OPTIONS FOR *HELICOBACTER PYLORI*

Regimen	PPI	Antibiotic #1	Antibiotic #2	Bismuth	Number of Days	Efficacy
Triple therapy	PPI[1] bid	Amoxicillin 1 g bid OR tetracycline 500 mg bid	Clarithromycin 500 mg bid OR metronidazole 500 mg tid		10–14	80–95%
Quadruple therapy	PPI[1] bid	Amoxicillin 1 g qid OR tetracycline 500 mg qid	Clarithromycin 500 mg tid OR metronidazole 500 mg tid	Bismuth subsalicylate[2] 524 mg qid (Two 262-mg tabs)	10–14	90–99%
New regimen— Promising but not accepted standard	PPI[1] bid	Amoxicillin suspension 2 g qid	Metronidazole 500 mg qid	Bismuth subsalicylate[2] 524 mg qid (Two 262-mg tabs)	1 day	95%

[1] Any PPI can be used: omeprazole (Prilosec), 20 mg; esomeprazole (Nexium), 20 mg; lansoprazole (Prevacid), 30 mg; pantoprazole (Protonix), 40 mg; rabeprazole (AciPhex), 20 mg.
[2] Pepto-Bismol.
PPI, proton pump inhibitor.

2. To confirm eradication after *H pylori* treatment for PUD, the patient should be retested for active *H pylori* 4–8 weeks after treatment, with either the urea breath test or stool antigen test. Treatment failure requires a second regimen, generally quadruple therapy with alternative antibiotics. A second treatment failure requires specialty referral with endoscopy, and culture for sensitivities. (*Note:* It is fairly common for patients to resolve their *H pylori* and PUD but still require symptomatic PPI treatment for GERD or functional dyspepsia.)

D. **Therapy for NSAID-related ulcers.** The primary treatment is to stop the NSAID if at all possible and initiate acid suppression, usually with a PPI. Generally treatment is rapid and effective if the NSAID can be stopped. Unfortunately, many patients need continuing NSAID treatment or aspirin prophylaxis. Under those circumstances the NSAID dose should be minimized, and prophylaxis begun with a PPI. Alternatively, consideration can be given to COX-2-specific NSAIDs (Table 82–7). Their efficacy for pain control is identical to nonspecific NSAIDs, and their GI side effects, particularly for PUD, are close to placebo. COX-2-specific NSAIDs are, however, extremely expensive and their overall safety is not fully elucidated. Improved GI benefits may also be ameliorated if the patient needs aspirin for cardiac prophylaxis.

E. **Relapse.** If NSAIDs are discontinued and *H pylori* is cured but the patient clinically relapses, then referral to a specialist is indicated, and PPIs should be reinitiated. Consider unusual causes, particularly acid hypersecretory states. A fasting gastrin level is indicated for multiple ulcers, ulcers resistant to therapy, ulcer patients awaiting surgery, ulcers associated with severe esophagitis, and patients with a family history of similar ulcer problems or other endocrine tumors.

F. **Idiopathic PUD.** If all treatable etiologies for PUD are ruled out, then treatment focuses solely on acid suppression. Idiopathic ulcers are increasing as the percentage of all ulcers from *H pylori* is decreasing.

G. **Surgery.** Operative treatment is indicated for patients with acute complications or refractory PUD. Rates of surgery for PUD have plummeted.

IV. **Management Strategies.** The goal of ulcer therapy is complete healing without relapse. The most important aspects of management are reviewed in the Treatment section (section III). Prior to the appreciation of the role of *H pylori,* many lifestyle issues were thought to be important in the pathogenesis and treatment of PUD. Now, they are largely understood to be secondary or even unrelated.

A. **Smoking** does promote ulcerogenesis, at least in patients with *H pylori.* Smoking adversely affects ulcer development, healing, and complications. However, if *H pylori* is

TABLE 82–7. COX-2 INHIBITORS

Drug	Dose	Notes
Celecoxib (Celebrex)	OA: 200 mg qd or 100 mg bid RA: 100–200 mg bid Familial adenomatous polyposis: 400 mg bid w/food Acute pain/dysmenorrhea: 400 mg day 1, then 200 qd prn	Maint: 200 mg qd prn; reduce dose 50% for hepatic insufficiency. Contraindicated with sulfonamide hypersensitivity or with asthma, urticaria, or allergic-type reaction to ASA or NSAID. Check precautions and interactions before prescribing. ♀C (D 3rd trimester)
Rofecoxib (Vioxx)	Pain/dysmenorrhea 50 mg qd for up to 5 days. OA: 12.5 mg qd with max 25 mg qd RA: 25 mg qd	Caution with hepatic impairment, HTN, CHF, fluid retention. Check interactions and precautions before prescribing. ♀C (D 3rd trimester)
Valdecoxib (Bextra)	OA/RA: 10 mg qd Dysmenorrhea: 20 mg bid	Contraindicated with sulfonamide hypersensitivity or with asthma, urticaria, or allergic-type reaction to ASA or NSAIDs. Check interactions and precautions before prescribing. ♀C (D 3rd trimester)

ASA, acetylsalicylic acid; CHF, congestive heart failure; HTN, hypertension; NSAID, nonsteroidal anti-inflammatory drugs; OA, osteoarthritis; RA, rheumatoid arthritis.
♀, pregnancy class.

eradicated, smokers do not appear to be at continued increased PUD risk. It is considered appropriate to recommend smoking cessation to ulcer patients who smoke, but primary treatment remains that appropriate for the primary ulcer etiology (eg, *H pylori* or NSAIDs).

B. **Alcohol** has long been considered a cause of PUD. In fact, it is usually not a significant contributor. In large doses it does damage the stomach epithelium directly. In patients who drink more than 20 drinks a week, ulcer rates are significantly increased, especially in the presence of cirrhosis.

C. **Emotional stress** may affect ulcer frequency to some extent. Severe societal stressors (such as major earthquakes) cause an increase in PUD rates in the affected areas. Severe physiologic stressors (such as surgery or intensive care unit admissions) are well known to predispose patients to ulcers. Emotional stress may be one of the factors that causes patients exposed to *H pylori* or NSAIDs to become part of the small percentage that actually develop an ulcer. However, emotional strain does not interfere with treatment. Although conventional wisdom is that all ulcers are directly caused by "stress," reduction in stress is not necessary for adequate healing. Treatment should be directed at the primary etiology.

D. **Diet** does NOT contribute to PUD, nor are special diets needed during treatment. Patients may perceive diet as significant because it can affect symptoms of dyspepsia, but it does not affect ulcer healing.

E. **Alternative treatments** for PUD are unproven. Listed are a few of the most common strategies.
   1. Acupuncture may decrease epigastric pain, acid secretion, or both.
   2. Chinese herbal treatments include Xao Yao Wan at 8 tablets three times daily for soothing stress and gastric upset.
   3. Naturopathic remedies include aloe vera juice 1–2 tablespoons twice daily or "stomach formula" as directed.
   4. Homeopathic remedies are individualized by non-Western parameters.

V. **Prognosis.** The prognosis of PUD has improved dramatically. Although the mortality of acute upper GI bleed is about 5%, PUD can usually be cured or controlled for most of the patient population.

A. **NSAIDs.** Up to 4% of NSAID users develop serious complications such as frank PUD with bleeding or perforation each year. Between 5% and 20% of long-term NSAID users have peptic ulcers at any given time. Of NSAID users with PUD, there is a 400–500% increase in complications. However, even for patients who must continue NSAIDs, continuous treatment with PPIs causes relapse rates for PUD to decrease to 5%.

B. *H pylori.* Eradication of *H pylori* dramatically alters the natural history of PUD. Previously, the natural history of PUD was chronic and relapsing, with over 75% recurrence of ulcers. Now patients cured of *H pylori* often require no further treatment, with relapse rates for PUD decreased to 5%.

REFERENCES

Arents NLA, Thijs JC, Kleibeuker JH: A rational approach to uninvestigated dyspepsia in primary care: Review of the literature. Postgrad Med J 2002;**78**:707.

Malfertheiner P: Current concepts in the management of *Helicobacter pylori* infection—The Maastricht 2-2000 consensus report. Aliment Pharmacol Ther 2002;**16**(2):167.

Smoot DT, Go MF, Cryer B: Peptic ulcer disease. Primary Care; Clin Office Practice 2001;**28**(3):487.

Suerbaum S, Michetti P: *Helicobacter pylori* infection. N Engl J Med 2002;**347**(15):1175.

Talley NJ: Dyspepsia: Management guidelines for the millennium. Gut 2002;**50**:72.

---

83 Premenstrual Syndrome

Janice E. Daugherty, MD

KEY POINTS

- Premenstrual syndrome is a group of symptoms affecting many women of reproductive age. Sharing many features of depression and anxiety disorders, premenstrual syndrome represents a distinct entity characterized chiefly by its occurrence exclusively in the luteal phase of the menstrual cycle.
- Symptoms occur only within approximately 2 weeks before the onset of menses, and subside with the onset of bleeding. They may occur in either ovulatory or nonovulatory cycles.
- Symptoms usually include one or more of the following clusters:
  - Anxiety, irritability, or mood swings.
  - Weight gain, swelling, bloating, or breast tenderness.
  - Appetite change, food cravings, and fatigue.
  - Depression, sleep disturbance, or cognitive difficulty.
  - Pain, including headache and general muscular pains.
- Major depressive disorder with suicide risk must be ruled out, and hypothyroidism may present some of the same symptoms.
- Lifestyle modification includes the following:
  - Eating a low-fat diet that limits meat intake (see the Food Guide Pyramid www.eatright.org/pyramid/).
  - Supplementing the diet with magnesium, 200–400 mg; vitamin E, 400 mg; manganese, 6 mg; and calcium, 1000 mg daily.
  - Getting regular aerobic exercise.
  - Avoiding caffeine, tobacco, and excess alcohol intake.
- Education and cognitive therapy can also help.
- Medication, if necessary in addition to the above, starting approximately on day 12–14 of the menstrual cycle, can include:
  - A selective serotonin reuptake inhibitor. *The following have been studied and found effective for* premenstrual syndrome/*premenstrual dysphoric disorder:* fluoxetine, 20–60 mg daily; sertraline, 50–100 mg daily; citalopram, 10–20 mg daily; and paroxetine, 10–20 mg daily.
  - Consider buspirone, 30 mg daily in divided doses, if the selective serotonin reuptake inhibitor is not tolerated or if complaints are mostly anxiety-related or pain symptoms.

I. Introduction

A. Definition. Premenstrual syndrome (PMS) is the cyclic recurrence in the luteal phase of the menstrual cycle of a combination of distressing physical, psychological, and behavioral changes of severity that results in deterioration of interpersonal relationships or interference with normal activities.

B. Epidemiology. Most women report at least some minor physical and emotional symptoms in the postovulatory phase of the menstrual cycle. Thirty to 40% have symptoms of moderate intensity, and it is estimated that 3–5% of women of reproductive age have PMS of an intensity that is temporarily disabling.

    1. Age. Symptoms of PMS may occur at any age in the reproductive years; incidence of presenting for care peaks in the mid-30s. Some women experience cyclic symptoms even after menopause.

    2. Social class. No clinically useful differences have been defined.

    3. Race. PMS is reported to occur in all ethnic groups. Cultural variation in the prevalence rates and patterns of symptoms occur, but no clinically useful diagnostic or therapeutic differences have yet emerged.

    4. Reproductive factors. Women with regular (ovulatory) menstrual cycles, as well as those with longer cycles and heavier menstrual flow, report symptoms of swelling, mood swings, and depression more than other women. PMS may occur in spontaneous anovulatory cycles and following oophorectomy or hysterectomy. More than half of severe PMS patients have a history of pre-eclampsia or postnatal depression.

C. Pathophysiology. No single theory currently accounts for all the clinical and pathophysiologic features of PMS. The similarity of PMS to depressive illness, as well as its response to antidepressant therapy, suggests shared metabolic abnormalities. Metabolic differences between the two entities have been found, however. The interaction of several pathways may result in the development of PMS. Research seems to point toward an interaction of hormones, neurotransmitters, nutrients, and behavioral or environmental factors in the development of significant symptoms. Because of the differences in response to treatment for women with similar symptoms, subtypes of PMS have been postulated. It is likely that multiple physiologic alterations can coexist that yield the same symptomatic outcomes; correction of single abnormalities without normalizing others (as is likely to happen in a clinical trial) may explain the variability in reported effectiveness of various treatments in different studies.

II. Diagnosis. For the woman who presents with symptoms of PMS, beginning the diagnostic process with an open-ended inquiry will provide tremendously useful information. Symptoms commonly noted (Table 83–1) include depressed mood or feelings of hopelessness or self-deprecation; anxiety; affective lability; irritability; anger; feelings of difficulty concentrating; decreased energy; change in sleep, appetite, or both (increase or decrease); feelings of being out of control; and physical symptoms of bloating, breast tenderness, muscle or joint aches,

---

TABLE 83–1. RESEARCH CRITERIA FOR PREMENSTRUAL DYSPHORIC DISORDER

In most menstrual cycles during the past year, five (or more) of the following symptoms were present for most of the time during the last week of the luteal phase, began to remit within a few days after the onset of the follicular phase, and were absent in the week postmenses, with at least one of the symptoms being either (1), (2), (3), or (4):

(1) markedly depressed mood, feelings of hopelessness, or self-deprecating thoughts
(2) marked anxiety, tension, or feeling of being "keyed up" or "on edge"
(3) marked affective lability (eg, feeling suddenly sad or tearful or having increased sensitivity to rejection)
(4) persistent and marked anger or irritability or increased interpersonal conflicts
(5) decreased interest in usual activities (eg, work, friends, or hobbies)
(6) subjective sense of difficulty in concentrating
(7) lethargy, easy fatigability, or marked lack of energy
(8) marked change in appetite, overeating, or specific food cravings
(9) hypersomnia or insomnia
(10) a subjective sense of being overwhelmed or out of control
(11) other physical symptoms, such as breast tenderness or swelling, headaches, joint or muscle pain, a sensation of "bloating," or weight gain

The disturbance must seriously interfere with work or usual social activities or relationships, and not be merely an exacerbation of the symptoms of another disorder, such as major depression, panic disorder, dysthymia, or a personality disorder (although it may be superimposed on any of these).
The criteria must be confirmed by prospective, daily self-ratings during at least two cycles.

Adapted with permission from American Psychiatric Association (APA): *Diagnostic and Statistical Manual of Mental Disorders*, 4th ed. APA; 1994.

and headache. These symptoms must interfere with usual daily activities. The National Institute of Mental Health has recommended that, for a diagnosis of PMS, there must be a marked change in intensity (at least 30%) of symptoms measured from cycle days 5–10 compared to the 6-day interval prior to menses for at least two consecutive cycles.

In some studies, up to 50% of women presenting to PMS clinics did not meet diagnostic criteria for that disorder, but instead were assigned another diagnosis: most frequently, major depression, followed in frequency by dysthymia, anxiety disorder, menopause, or another gynecologic or medical disorder. "PMS" may be a diagnosis that is more acceptable to the patient than is depression or anxiety. By starting the evaluation in an unstructured manner, the clinician can avoid a premature (and possibly erroneous) diagnosis.

Once an overview of the symptoms has been obtained, the patient's symptoms can be rated to establish a baseline (Table 83–2), and other essential information can be requested, including: Is there a previous diagnosis of PMS? What criteria were used to make the diagnosis? Have the symptoms changed over time? What previous treatments have been successful or unsuccessful? Many patients will self-diagnose PMS from information found in the lay literature. Other important questions include the following.

A. **Is there a history of treatment for an affective disorder?** As many as 10% of women with PMS may report suicidal ideas and death wishes and thoughts.
   Are there vegetative symptoms of depression? (See Chapter 92.) Of women with major depression, over half will have exacerbation of symptoms in the premenstrual phase, including increased severity of usual symptoms or the appearance of new symptoms such as increased aggression, suicidal tendencies, or depersonalization.

B. **Is there seasonal variation of the depressive symptoms?** "Seasonal" and nonseasonal premenstrual dysphoric disorder (PDD) has been shown to improve with phototherapy.

C. **Does she consider her general health to be good, or is there chronic disease?** PMS must be differentiated from symptoms arising from other chronic disorders but which are exacerbated during the premenstrual phase of the cycle ("premenstrual magnification"). Some patients experience exacerbation or precipitation of other medical problems, such as asthma, migraine, epilepsy, or bipolar illness just prior to menstruation.

D. **Are her menses regular? Has she had pelvic inflammatory disease, surgery, or endometriosis? What contraceptive method does she use?** A primary complaint of pain may be related to gynecologic disease. By suppression of ovulation, oral contraceptives may provide relief of PMS, but studies have been inconsistent in this regard. Marked relief of symptoms was noted in a majority of women treated with depot medroxyprogesterone acetate in one study.

E. **Has she been pregnant? What was the outcome? Were her symptoms present during pregnancy? Did she have postpartum depression?** PMS is not present during pregnancy. Current affective symptoms could relate to a pregnancy outcome, such

---

TABLE 83–2. SHORTENED PREMENSTRUAL ASSESSMENT FORM

The patient is asked to consider the changes currently experienced with regard to her menstrual period:

Pain, tenderness, enlargement, or swelling of breasts
Feeling unable to cope or overwhelmed by ordinary demands
Feeling under stress
Outbursts of "irritability" or bad temper
Feeling sad or blue
Backaches, joint and muscle pain, or stiffness
Weight gain
Relatively steady abdominal heaviness, discomfort, or pain
Edema, swelling, puffiness, or "water retention"
Feeling bloated

Patients may rate each change on this list on a scale from 1 (not present or no change from usual)
   to 6 (extreme change, perhaps noticeable even to casual acquaintances)

Adapted with permission from Allen SS, McBride CM, Pirie PL: The shortened premenstrual assessment form. J Reprod Med 1991;**36**:769.

as abortion, other fetal loss, or abnormality. Postpartum depression is frequently found in patients with PDD.

F. Is the patient taking medications? Is she taking vitamin or mineral supplements, and on whose advice? What alternative therapies has she tried? Diuretic therapy can result in paradoxical water retention, especially in "idiopathic edema." Large amounts of dairy products may interfere with magnesium absorption, leading to chronic deficiency, which has been noted in PMS. High phosphate intake (eg, from colas) can cause relative deficiency of calcium, especially when coupled with low intake of dairy products. Some women will take large amounts (200 mg or more) of vitamin B_6 in an attempt to relieve PMS symptoms, without understanding the risk of peripheral neuropathy. However, some supplements, in the correct amounts, can be therapeutic for PMS. Women, in the search for PMS treatment, may have encountered clinicians who were less than empathetic toward their complaints. Many seek care from alternative practitioners, who may provide some relief of their symptoms, and this alternative treatment may be continued along with the traditional prescription obtained from the clinician. An understanding of all current treatments is necessary to avoid adverse interactions.

G. Is there a personal history of alcohol or drug abuse? Compared with the general population, women seeking treatment for PMS are more likely to have lifetime histories of depression, anxiety disorder, suicide attempts, panic disorder, and substance abuse.

H. Is there a history of smoking? Women who smoke are more likely to experience PMS symptoms.

I. Is there evidence of bulimia? Does she have food cravings? Does she follow any particular diet regimen? Electrolyte imbalances from frequent vomiting can yield behavioral symptoms, especially fatigue. Ingestion of large amounts of sugar can exacerbate symptoms in at least two ways: refined sugar increases the urinary excretion of magnesium (as do diuretics) and also interferes with renal clearance of sodium and water. In response to a large sugar load, the production of keto acids is suppressed by an insulin surge. The resulting impairment in excretion of sodium and water causes expansion of the extracellular fluid volume with resultant edema, bloating, and breast tenderness. This sodium retention is resistant to aldosterone inhibitors. Table salt enhances the intestinal absorption of glucose, which enhances this insulin response and contributes to the edema. Alcohol may play a role in reactive hypoglycemia of PMS.

J. Was there early victimization and trauma? Up to 40% of patients diagnosed with PMS have a history of sexual abuse.

K. Is there a family history of PMS, affective disorders, substance abuse, or alcoholism? Familial occurrence is documented.

L. Symptom clusters. PMS symptoms may fall into "clusters," which may be helpful in choosing therapy. Some women experience more anxiety, irritability, or mood swings. For some, the primary symptoms are weight gain, swelling, and bloating; for others changes in appetite or cravings, fatigue, and headache are most troublesome. Still others have depression, sleep disturbance, or cognitive difficulties. Some women experience any or all of these, with variations in severity and symptoms from cycle to cycle. Treatment success is not contingent upon identifying a particular symptom cluster.

M. Timing of symptoms. A calendar of symptoms experienced relative to phase of the menstrual cycle (Figure 83–1) can help confirm that they are indeed premenstrual; some women experience erratic symptom patterns and incorrectly attribute them to PMS. Basal temperature measurements can help rule out disorders of ovulation and provide further confirmation of the premenstrual timing of symptoms.

N. Physical examination. General physical and pelvic examinations are indicated to exclude rheumatologic disease, anemia, electrolyte imbalance, neoplasms, endometriosis, or menopause.

O. Laboratory tests. There are no specific laboratory tests for PMS at this time. Other laboratory or physiologic tests may be necessary in individual cases to rule out other potential causes of symptoms. Tests that are *not* likely to be useful in the diagnosis of PMS include follicle-stimulating hormone, luteinizing hormone, estrogen, progesterone, or testosterone unless other conditions are suspected.

1. **A complete blood cell count** if there is chronic fatigue or menorrhagia.
2. **SMA-18 chemistry profile** if there is chronic fatigue or suspicion of electrolyte disorder.
3. **Thyroid-stimulating hormone** (unless done within the last 3 months), as the prevalence of thyroid disease is high for women in this age group.

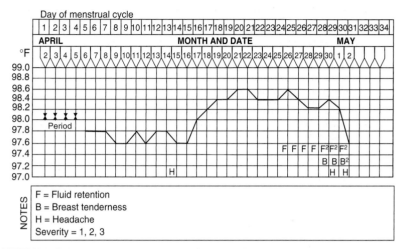

FIGURE 83–1. Premenstrual syndrome symptom diary. A minimum of two symptomatic cycles must be included to establish the diagnosis.

4. **Serum prolactin** in patients with galactorrhea, an irregular menstrual cycle, history of infertility, decreased libido, or atypical presentations of mastalgia.
5. **Chlamydia and gonorrhea testing** if there is high-risk behavior, cervicitis, or pain upon pelvic examination.

III. Treatment

A. **Patient education.** Patients are exposed to information about PMS from many medical and nonmedical sources and may have strong convictions about the condition and its treatment. Some express the fear that their symptoms represent an untreatable condition. Uncertainties about PMS causes in the literature notwithstanding, the likelihood of successful treatment of PMS is high, and reassurance of this fact is the first step to successful treatment. Empathy and affirmation are particularly useful in dealing with PMS.

Patient education alone may lead to a dramatic reduction in symptoms during the 3 months when the patient is completing the symptom diary. In addition, such general advice builds patient self-esteem and ability to cope with symptoms. In controlled trials of PMS treatment, the placebo response rate is typically greater than 20% and sometimes as high as 50%, emphasizing the significant therapeutic value of discussing symptoms with a caring clinician.

B. **Symptomatic treatments.** Encourage proper diet with adequate composition according to the current US Recommended Daily Allowances and Dietary Guidelines for healthy adults. Following the Food Guide Pyramid (http://www.nal.usda."gov/"fnic.html) with specific emphasis on avoiding salt and animal fats will often provide symptom relief and potentially confer general health benefits as well.

Supplementation may be necessary to assure adequate amounts of certain nutrients, including calcium (1000 mg of elemental calcium per day), vitamins (vitamin E, 400 IU/day), and trace minerals (magnesium, 200–400 mg/day; manganese, 6 mg/day). Regular aerobic exercise and elimination or reduction of adverse health habits, such as tobacco and alcohol use, may directly improve PMS through the pathophysiologic mechanisms previously described.

Teaching women to take control of symptoms through reduction of negative emotions by cognitive restructuring, improving problem-solving skills, and developing responsible assertiveness to deal with discomforts has been shown to provide significant relief of both physical and emotional symptoms. If there is suboptimal improvement after 2–3 months of the treatments described above or if symptoms are severe, secondary treatment modalities may be considered.

1. **Anxiety, irritability, and mood swings.** Several selective serotonin reuptake inhibitor (SSRI) antidepressants have been found effective for both the depressive as

well as the anxiety symptoms of PMS, including fluoxetine (20–40 mg daily); paroxetine (10–20 mg daily); sertraline (50–100 mg daily); and citalopram (10–20 mg
daily). If SSRIs are ineffective or cannot be used, buspirone, 30 mg/day (10 mg three
times a day) for 12 days prior to menses, is effective not only for social dysfunction
but also for fatigue, cramps, and general aches and pains. Clonidine, 0.1 mg twice
a day, and verapamil, 80 mg three times a day or one 240-mg sustained-release capsule once a day, have also been reported to have beneficial effects on mood in PMS.

2. **Weight gain, swelling, and bloating.** Spironolactone, 25 mg orally four times a
day, has produced relief of weight gain and abdominal bloating. Diuretic therapy
should only be prescribed after two or three cycles of restriction of intake of simple
sugars and salt, as the edema from these is diuretic-resistant, and other benefits
accrue from their restriction.

3. **Breast tenderness.** Vitamin E, 400 IU twice daily, may reduce mastodynia if lower
doses are ineffective. Treatment is usually continued for 4–6 months and resumed
if symptoms recur.

4. **Changes in appetite, cravings, and fatigue.** Adherence to dietary guidelines,
achievement of adequate sleep, and management of the environment to minimize
exposure to added stress may offer some mitigation of symptoms.

5. **Depression, sleep disturbance, and cognitive difficulty.** Antidepressant therapy with both tricyclic antidepressants (TCA) and SSRIs has been shown to be significantly more effective than placebo, with SSRIs preferred because of a lower
side effect profile. Several SSRI antidepressants have been found effective for
PMS, including fluoxetine (20–40 mg daily), paroxetine (10–20 mg daily), sertraline (50–100 mg daily), and citalopram (10–20 mg daily). Therapy during the luteal
phase only is often effective.

6. **Pain syndromes.** Isolated headaches and general muscular pains are best
treated with simple analgesics, such as acetaminophen and aspirin. Migraine
headaches occurring as part of PMS may be alleviated by daily treatment beginning approximately 10 days prior to menstruation. Possible preventive measures
and treatment of migraine attacks are described in Chapter 34.

C. **Treatments based on presumed hormonal cause**
1. **Progesterone.** Although progesterone therapy has been widely used, well-
controlled clinical trials have failed to prove consistent benefits, possibly because
of the dosing, measurement, and patient heterogeneity barriers noted above.

2. **Contraceptives.** Reports conflict, but generally an oral contraceptive low in estrogenic activity or a progestin-only pill is recommended. Relief may be found with
long-acting progestin contraceptives, but studies are few and side effects may be
significant.

3. **Gonadotropin-releasing hormone analogues.** Leuprolide has been shown to
be effective in reducing symptoms of PMS, but side effects are symptoms and
sequelae of menopause, which may be equal to or more troubling than PMS.

D. **Complementary and alternative therapies.** Massage therapy has been shown to decrease general pain symptoms in women with PMS or dysmenorrhea. In studies of depression, hypericin 300 mg three times a day (the principal active component of St. John's
wort) was found to be as effective as TCAs, with fewer side effects and at lower cost, but
with considerably slower onset. Photosensitivity may occur, and information about potential adverse interactions of hypericin with other medication is lacking. L-Tryptophan
(2 g three times daily with meals, from day 14 through day 3 of the cycle) has been a useful adjunct to antidepressant therapy. *Silix Donna,* a yeast-based dietary supplement, was
found effective in improving mood symptoms in mild to moderate PMS.

E. **Treatments likely NOT to be of help.** Several studies have documented improvement
in symptoms with alprazolam, but it has been shown to be associated with impairments
in cognitive performance and with worsening in mood during the follicular phase. A high
potential for dependence is another reason to avoid its use.

IV. **Management Strategies.** An approach to PMS management is diagrammed in Figure 83–2.

V. **Prognosis.** PMS ceases in most patients around the time of menopause. Many therapies
have been found to provide significant relief to a proportion of patients; therefore, the prognosis for improvement of symptoms in PMS is excellent. The medical team must be empathetic, creative, patient, and persistently willing to try different or multiple therapies. Other
comorbid conditions, such as memory of past trauma, may surface during treatment for
PMS and indicate the need for further treatment or referral.

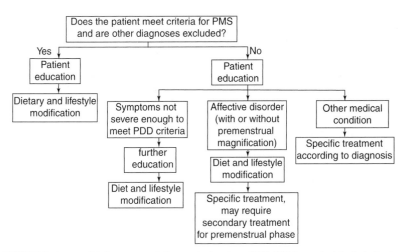

FIGURE 83–2. An approach to the management of premenstrual syndrome (PMS). PDD, Premenstrual dysphoric disorder.

REFERENCES

American Psychiatric Association (APA): *Diagnostic and Statistical Manual of Mental Disorders,* 4th ed. APA; 1994.

Daugherty JE: Treatment strategies for premenstrual syndrome. Am Fam Physician 1998;**58:**183.

Johnson WG, Carr-Nangle RE, Bergeron KC: Macronutrient intake, eating habits, and exercise as moderators of menstrual distress in healthy women. Psychosom Med 1995;**57:**324.

Wallin MS, Rissanen AM: Food and mood: Relationship between food, serotonin, and affective disorders. Acta Psychiatr Scand Suppl 1994;**377:**36.

---

84   Renal Failure

Terrence T. Truong, MD

KEY POINTS

- Prerenal disease may be distinguished from ischemic or nephrotoxic acute tubular necrosis by the recovery of renal function within 24–72 hours after fluid repletion.
- For patients with systolic heart failure, inotropic agents and vasodilator should be initiated when serum creatinine and blood urea nitrogen (BUN) rise with diuretic therapy. Calcium channel blocker or β-adrenergic blockers are indicated if diastolic heart failure is present.
- Treatment of hypertension in patients with polyarteritis nodosa and renal disease may require calcium channel blocker if angiotensin-converting enzyme (ACE) inhibitors worsen renal function.
- ACE inhibitors and angiotensin II receptor blockers are efficacious in treating hypertension and confer renal protection in patients with benign hypertensive nephrosclerosis. However, thiazide diuretics provide greater cardioprotective effects.
- Radiocontrast media–induced renal failure may be prevented by the use of lower dose low or iso-osmolal nonionic agents, maintenance of normovolemia, and avoidance of concomitant use of nonsteroidal anti-inflammatory drugs (NSAIDs).
- Bladder catheterization, performed to rule out bladder neck obstruction, may also be therapeutic in bladder and urethral obstruction.

I. Introduction

A. Definition. Renal failure is a syndrome describing disturbances in renal function resulting in impaired or loss of maintenance of extracellular homeostasis, systemic and renal hemodynamics, calcium and bone metabolism, and erythropoiesis. **Renal failure is defined as acute** when there is recent increase of serum creatinine concentration of at least 0.5 mg/dL with baseline concentration of <3.0 mg/dL, and at least 1.0 mg/dL when the baseline is higher. Acute failure may occur in patients with previously normal renal function or preexisting stable renal impairment.

B. Etiology. Renal diseases can be characterized by the anatomic location primarily affected by the underlying pathology.

1. **Prerenal disease** occurs with glomerular hypoperfusion secondary to entities that decrease circulating volume or cause relative hypotension, leading to acute decline of glomerular filtration rate. Etiologies include acute hemorrhage, gastrointestinal, urinary, or cutaneous fluid losses, congestive heart failure, hepatorenal syndrome, sepsis, and shock.

2. **Vascular disease** may cause acute or chronic renal failure. Malignant hypertension, thromboemboli, scleroderma, and systemic vasculitides cause acute disease while hypertensive nephrosclerosis and bilateral renal artery stenosis are the major causes of chronic renal failure.

3. **Glomerular disease** is caused by entities that result in focal nephritis, diffuse nephritis, or nephrosis. Overlap of these patterns may occur. Focal glomerulonephritis etiologies include postinfectious glomerulonephritis, Henoch-Schönlein purpura, IgA nephropathy, thin basement membrane disease, hereditary nephritis, mesangial proliferative glomerulonephritis, and systemic lupus erythematosus. Diffuse glomerulonephritis etiologies include postinfectious glomerulonephritis, membranoproliferative glomerulonephritis, rapidly progressive glomerulonephritis, vasculitides, and fibrillary glomerulonephritis. Nephrotic syndrome etiologies include diabetic nephropathy, IgA nephropathy, minimal change disease, focal glomerulosclerosis, mesangial proliferative glomerulonephritis, and membranous nephropathy.

4. **Tubular or interstitial disease** can lead to acute or chronic renal failure. Acute tubular necrosis, acute tubular nephritis, and cast nephropathy are the major causes of acute renal failure, while polycystic kidney disease, vesicoureteral reflux, autoimmune disorders, and analgesic abuse cause chronic disease.

5. **Obstructive uropathy** may occur secondary to urinary flow obstruction anywhere along the urinary tract. Prostatic disease, urinary calculus, and pelvic or retroperitoneal neoplasm are major causes in adults. Bilateral obstruction is obligatory to produce renal insufficiency in patients with otherwise normal renal functions. Urethral valves and strictures and ureterovesicular and ureteropelvic stenosis are major causes in children.

II. Diagnosis

A. Prerenal disease. Symptoms and signs are related to fluid loss, and the resultant electrolyte abnormalities. An elevated BUN to serum creatinine ratio, often greater than 20:1, occurs in the absence of increased urea production. However, a normal ratio may be observed with concomitant liver disease or decreased protein intake. Urinalysis is normal, though hyaline casts may be present. Urinary sodium concentration is typically <20 mEq/L, with fractional excretion of sodium <1% and urinary osmolality >500 mOsm/kg. Additionally, response to fluid administration with recovery of renal function within 24–72 hours is highly suggestive, though not diagnostic, of prerenal disease.

B. Vascular disease

1. **Acute.** Aside from characteristic systemic symptoms, systemic vasculitides produce renal function impairment and hypertension. Urinalysis reveals an active sediment with red cells, red cell and granular casts, and nonnephrotic range proteinuria. Classic polyarteritis nodosa, on the other hand, may only produce glomerular ischemia, and thus, a relatively normal urinalysis. Renal biopsy with histologic, immunofluorescence, and electron microscopic evaluation would be confirmatory. Patients with thromboemboli typically present with flank pain, nausea, vomiting, fever, and hypertension. Gross or microscopic hematuria occurs only in one third of patients. Serum lactate dehydrogenase levels are often elevated with no significant change of serum transaminases. Radioisotope renogram is confirmatory. Renal atheroemboli, in contrast, may present with acute marked renal impairment, pro-

gressive renal impairment interspersed with episodes of relatively stable function over periods of weeks, or chronic stable renal impairment. Typically, there is preceding aortic or other large artery manipulation. Urinalysis reveals few cells or casts. Proteinuria is usually in the nonnephrotic range. Eosinophilia, eosinophiluria, and hypocomplementemia may be present.

2. **Chronic.** Patients with benign hypertensive nephrosclerosis present with slowly progressive, worsening renal function and mild proteinuria with a history of pre-existing mild to moderate hypertension. Proteinuria is typically minimal unless an underlying renovascular disease is also present. Urinary sediments are relatively normal. Renal biopsy is rarely indicated, except in instances when there is no clear history of hypertension preceding the development of proteinuria and renal function impairment. Chronic renal failure secondary to bilateral artery stenosis should be considered in patients who have systemic atherosclerosis, hypertension that is severe or refractory, elevation of serum creatinine with ingestion of ACE inhibitor, or asymmetric renal size. Doppler ultrasonography may be confirmatory.

C. **Glomerular disease**

1. **Focal nephritic patients** have normal blood pressure and no edema. Urinalysis reveals red cells, occasionally red cell casts, and proteinuria <1.5 g/day. Renal function is preserved. Light microscopy reveals inflammatory lesions in less than half of the glomeruli.

2. **Diffuse nephritic patients** have hypertension, edema, and usually renal insufficiency. Urinalysis is similar to that of focal nephritic patients, although proteinuria may be in nephrotic range. Light microscopy reveals lesions in most or all of the glomeruli.

3. **Nephrotic syndrome,** by definition, requires the presence of proteinuria of ≥3 g/day, serum albumin <3.0 g/dL, and peripheral edema. Few cells or casts are observed in the urine. Hyperlipidemia and hyperlipiduria may also be present.

D. **Tubulointerstitial disease**

1. **Acute tubular necrosis,** secondary to ischemia or nephrotoxic drugs such as aminoglycoside antibiotic and radiocontrast media, can usually be distinguished from prerenal causes of acute renal failure by serial BUN and serum creatinine measurements. The BUN: serum creatinine ratio remains normal, with the rate of rise of serum creatinine >0.3–0.5 mg/dL per day. Additionally, urinary sodium concentration is >40 mEq/L. Fractional excretion of sodium is >2% in the absence of chronic prerenal states such as cirrhosis. Urine-to-serum creatinine concentration is <20. Muddy brown granular and epithelial cell casts and free epithelial cells are usually, though not universally, present on urinalysis. Urinary osmolality, usually <450 mOsm/kg, and urine flow rate are of limited value in distinguishing acute tubular necrosis from prerenal disease.

2. **Acute interstitial nephritis,** most commonly induced by medications such as NSAIDs, antibacterials, and sulfonamides, occurs within 3 days to months after exposure to the offending agent. Symptoms and signs include fever and skin rash associated with an acute rise in the serum creatinine concentration related to drug exposure. Eosinophilia and eosinophiluria are also present except in NSAID exposure in which there is no fever, rash, or eosinophilia. Urinalysis reveals pyuria, hematuria, and white cell casts. Minimal proteinuria, <1 g/day, is present except in the elderly, who can excrete up to 3 g/day, and NSAID exposure cases in which nephrotic syndrome can be concurrent. Additionally, signs of Fanconi syndrome may be observed. Renal biopsy is the only definitive diagnostic tool.

3. **Cast nephropathy** occurs with multiple myeloma secondary to tubular injury and intratubular cast formation and obstruction. Symptoms and signs, secondary to the underlying multiple myeloma, include weakness, bone pain, anemia, lytic bone lesions, and hypercalcemia. Renal failure can be acute or chronic. Radiocontrast media exposure may precipitate acute renal failure in this setting. Urinalysis reveals minimal or no albumin by dipstick, though is markedly positive with sulfasalicylic acid testing indicating the presence of light chains. Diagnosis is confirmed by bone marrow examination.

E. **Postrenal disease.** Obstructive uropathy may cause acute or chronic renal failure. Pain may or may not be present, depending on the location and rate of the developing obstruction. Normal urine volume is maintained except in complete bilateral obstruction and shock.

Hypertension may also be present. Urinalysis may be normal. Bladder catheterization should be performed to rule out bladder neck obstruction. Plain film x-ray of the abdomen, renal ultrasonography, or computerized tomography (CT) scanning is diagnostic in most cases. Intravenous pyelogram is of limited value except when staghorn calculus or multiple renal or parapelvic cysts are suspected, when CT cannot identify the level of obstruction, and when an obstructing calculus is suspected in the absence of collecting system dilatation.

F. **Laboratory tests**
   1. **Serum creatinine concentration** estimates glomerular filtration rate. A rise in serum creatinine concentration represents a reduction in glomerular filtration rate.
   2. **Creatinine clearance** is obtained from a 24-hour urine collection. It is more accurate than serum creatinine concentration in estimating glomerular filtration rate. Creatinine clearance may be estimated by the Cockcroft-Gault equation in patients with stable serum creatinine concentration.
   3. **Urinalysis** is an essential test to evaluate renal failure. Urinary sediment patterns may be indicative of the underlying renal disease.
      a. **Normal or near normal with few cells and little or no cast** indicates prerenal disease, obstruction, hypercalcemia, multiple myeloma, acute tubular necrosis, or vascular disease.
      b. **Hematuria with red cell casts and heavy proteinuria** indicates glomerular disease or vasculitis.
      c. **Renal tubular epithelial cells with granular and epithelial cell casts** indicate acute tubular necrosis.
      d. **Pyuria with white cell and granular or waxy casts and no or mild proteinuria** indicates tubular or interstitial disease or obstruction.
      e. **Hematuria and pyuria with no or variable casts or proteinuria** indicates glomerular disease, vasculitis, infection, obstruction, renal infarction, or acute, usually drug-induced, interstitial nephritis.
      f. **Hematuria alone** indicates vasculitis or obstruction.
   4. **Urinary sodium concentration** is useful in differentiating acute tubular necrosis from volume depletion as the cause of renal failure.
   5. **Fractional excretion of sodium** eliminates the effect of urine output on urinary sodium concentration.

III. **Treatment.** Careful history-taking and physical examination with judicious use of the laboratory will frequently identify the processes that require prompt intervention. Supportive measures are initiated to correct fluid balance and electrolyte abnormalities and to maintain optimum nutritional status. Medications are reviewed and withdrawn or adjusted accordingly. Dialysis is indicated when fluid overload, acidosis, or electrolyte imbalance develops despite medical therapy, or when uremia ensues.

A. **Prerenal disease**
   1. **Hypovolemia.** Fluid repletion is necessary to restore circulating volume. The tonicity of the fluid is dependent on the serum sodium concentration. Blood transfusion is required if the underlying abnormality is acute hemorrhage.
   2. **Hypotension.** As hypotension may occur with hypovolemia, cardiac dysfunction, or sepsis, treatment would be directed at the underlying entity. Additionally, hypotension may be the result of therapy of chronic severe hypertension. Unless an ACE inhibitor is given in the presence of underlying bilateral renal artery stenosis, renal function will improve without discontinuing the antihypertensive agent.
   3. **Heart failure.** Improvement of cardiac output will improve renal function. Diuretic therapy reduces pulmonary and peripheral edema, improving cardiac output. However, as serum creatinine and BUN levels increase with diuresis, inotropic agents and vasodilators should be started unless there is underlying diastolic dysfunction, in which case the non-dihydropyridine calcium channel blockers, verapamil and diltiazem, or β-adrenergic blockers would be indicated to improve ventricular filling (Table 84–1). Verapamil or diltiazem may be started at 120–240 mg orally every day or in divided doses. Atenolol or metoprolol may be initiated at 12.5–25 mg orally every day. Carvedilol, a nonselective β receptor and α_1 receptor antagonist with evidence of decreased cardiovascular mortality, is given 12.5 mg orally twice daily. Careful monitoring for hemodynamic compromise and drug accumulation is mandatory with titration.

TABLE 84–1. ANTIHYPERTENSIVE AGENTS: CALCIUM CHANNEL BLOCKERS AND BETA BLOCKERS

Agent Name	Starting/Max Dosage	Renal Impairment Dose	Side Effects/Benefits/Notes	Cost
Calcium channel blocker				
Amlodipine (Norvasc)	5 mg po qd/10 mg		Jaundice, elevated LFTs	$$
			2.5 mg po qd in hepatic dysfunction	
Diltiazem (Cardizem CD)	180 mg po qd/540 mg		Elevated LFTs	$$$
Felodipine (Plendil)	5 mg po qd/10 mg		Elevated level in elderly and hepatic dysfunction	$$$
Isradipine (DynaCirc CR)	5 mg po qd/20 mg		Elevated level in elderly and hepatic dysfunction	$$
			Elevated level in mild renal impairment	
Nicardipine (Cardene SR)	30 mg po bid/120 mg		Maximum BP effect 2–6 hrs after dose	$$$
Nifedipine (Procardia XL, Adalat CC)	30 mg po qd/120 mg		Giddiness, heat sensation, muscle tremor, Positive Coombs'	$$
Nisoldipine (Sular)	20 mg po qd/60 mg		Elevated level in elderly and hepatic dysfunction	$$
Verapamil (Calan SR)	180 mg po qd/480 mg		Elevated LFTs	$$$
β-adrenergic blocker				
Acebutolol (Sectral)	200 mg po bid/1200 mg	Total daily dosage reduction	Selective β₁-receptor blocker	$
			Reduce dose 50% when GFR <50, 75% GFR <25	
Atenolol (Tenormin)	50 mg po qd/100 mg	Max 50 mg/d GFR <35	Selective β-receptor blocker	$
		Max 25 mg/d GFR <15	Indicated for angina pectoris	
Carvedilol	6.5 mg po bid/50 mg		Decreased mortality with CHF, overall mortality	$$$$
Labetalol (Normodyne, Trandate)	100 mg po bid/2400 mg		Nonselective β- and α₁-receptor blocker	$$$
			Jaundice, elevated LFTs	
			Elevated levels in elderly and hepatic dysfunction	
Metoprolol (Lopressor, Toprol XL)	100 mg po qd/400 mg		Long-acting agent decreased mortality in CHF	$$
			Indicated for angina pectoris	
Nadolol (Corgard)	40 mg po qd/320 mg	Q36hr dose GFR ≤50	Nonselective β-receptor blocker	$
		Q48hr dose GFR ≤30	Indicated for angina pectoris	
		Q72hr dose GFR <10		
Propranolol (Inderal, Inderal LA)	80 mg po qd/640 mg		Nonselective β-receptor blocker	$$
			Reduction of CV mortality and reinfarction	
			Indicated for angina pectoris	
Timolol (Blocadren)	10 mg po bid/60 mg		Nonselective β-receptor blocker	$
			Reduction of CV mortality and reinfarction	

BP, blood pressure; CHF, congestive heart failure; CV, cardiovascular; GFR, glomerular filtration rate; LFTs, liver function tests.
$, least expensive; $$$$, most expensive.

4. **Cirrhosis.** Hepatorenal syndrome is most effectively treated with peritoneovenous shunting.
B. **Vascular disease**
  1. **Acute**
     a. **Vasculitides.** Corticosteroids and immunosuppressive agents are used in the treatment of the underlying disease. Treatment of hypertension in polyarteritis nodosa may require the use of a calcium channel blocker such as amlodipine, at 2.5–5 mg orally every day, if ACE inhibitors worsen renal functions (Table 84–1).
     b. **Thromboemboli.** Intravenous heparin and oral warfarin is the standard treatment. Thrombolytic therapy may be beneficial if treatment is instituted within 2 hours. Treatment of hypertension, which may be transient, can be effected with ACE inhibitors such as captopril at 12.5–25 mg orally twice daily; enalapril (5 mg) or lisinopril (10 mg) orally every day (Table 84–2). Monitoring for first-dose hypotension is advisable for patients who have not been previously exposed to ACE inhibitors or who are currently on diuretics.
     c. **Atheroemboli.** There is no effective medical therapy.
  2. **Chronic**
     a. **Hypertensive nephrosclerosis.** Blood pressure control is essential. ACE inhibitor and angiotensin II receptor blockers are drugs of choice for renal protection (Table 84–2). However, thiazide diuretics, such as hydrochlorothiazide (12.5–25 mg orally every day), may have greater cardioprotective effects.
     b. **Bilateral renal artery stenosis.** ACE inhibitors can control blood pressure in most patients. However, revascularization—whether by renal artery bypass grafting or percutaneous angioplasty—would be indicated with severe or refractive hypertension and progressive renal function decline.
C. **Glomerular disease.** Treatment involves corticosteroids and immunosuppressive agents directed at the underlying pathology.
D. **Tubulointerstitial disease**
  1. **Acute tubular necrosis.** As the process is short-lived, supportive measures are instituted and any offending agent is discontinued. Radiocontrast media–induced renal failure may be prevented by the use of lower-dose low or iso-osmolal nonionic agents, maintenance of normovolemia, and avoidance of concomitant use of NSAIDs. Treatment includes hydration with normal saline.
  2. **Acute interstitial nephritis.** Withdrawal of the responsible agent in drug-induced cases is the primary treatment. Corticosteroids may also be indicated.
  3. **Cast nephropathy.** Vigorous hydration, corticosteroids, and cyclophosphamide decrease light-chain production. Loop diuretics may be administered if hypercalcemia is present. Plasmapheresis and dialysis are other modalities that may be considered.
E. **Postrenal disease.** Treatment, directed at restoration of urinary flow by relieving the underlying obstruction, may include bladder catheterization, percutaneous nephrostomy, lithotripsy, ureteral stenting, and urethral stenting.
IV. **Management Strategies.** Effective management of renal failure begins with the evaluation and diagnosis of the underlying disease process. Proper management includes preventing, monitoring for, and treating complications. Nutritional support with protein restriction is maintained.
A. **Acute renal failure.** Prerenal disease and acute tubular necrosis are the most common etiologies in the inpatient setting. If there is difficulty in differentiating between the two, fluid replacement may be initiated, in the absence of heart failure and hepatorenal syndrome, and potentially offending agents are withheld while the work-up is ongoing. Recovery of renal function in the ensuing 24–72 hours would point to prerenal disease. Other acute causes will have their characteristic history, physical findings, or urinalysis findings. Their management would be specific to the underlying pathology.
B. **Chronic renal failure.** While treatments of chronic renal failure are determined by the primary diagnosis, supportive measures and treatment of hypertension are initiated to prevent in many instances further deterioration of renal function. Additionally, monitoring for, preventing and managing metabolic, fluid balance, hematologic, and nutritional complications are of paramount importance. Metabolic surveillance should include periodic assessment of serum potassium, calcium, phosphorus, albumin, and acidemia. Nephrology consultation is beneficial to assist in diagnosis of the renal disease, co-manage

TABLE 84–2. ANTIHYPERTENSIVE AGENTS: ANGIOTENSIN-CONVERTING ENZYME INHIBITORS (ACEI) AND ANGIOTENSIN RECEPTOR BLOCKERS (ARB)

Agent Name	Starting/Max Dosage	Renal Impairment Dose	Side Effects/Benefits/Notes	Cost
ACEI				
Benazepril (Lotensin)	10 mg po qd/40 mg	5 mg/day if CrCl <30 mL/min	Reduces progression to renal failure	$$
Captopril (Capoten)	25 mg po bid–tid/450 mg	Reduce initial dose	Neutropenia, nephritic syndrome, rash	$
			Reduces mortality in MI	
			Slows progression of diabetic nephropathy	
Enalapril (Vasotec)	5 mg po qd/40 mg	2.5 mg/day CrCl <30 mL/min	Reduces mortality in NYHA II–IV CHF	$
Fosinopril (Monopril)	10 mg po qd/80 mg	5 mg/day	Reduces renal function decline in type II diabetics	$$$
			Impaired LFT increases unchanged plasma level	
			Lower risk of MI, CVA than amlodipine	
Lisinopril (Prinivil, Zestril)	10 mg po qd/40 mg	5 mg/day CrCl 10–30 mL/min	Reduces mortality in MI	$
		2.5 mg/day CrCl <10 mL/min	Reduces renal function decline in type II diabetics	
Moexipril (Univasc)	7.5 mg po qd/40 mg	3.75 mg/day CrCl ≤30 mL/min	Food decreases bioavailability	$
			Dosage reduction in hepatic dysfunction	
Perindopril (Aceon)	4 mg po qd/16 mg	2 mg/day CrCl >30 mL/min	Safety not known CrCl <30 mL/min	$$
Quinapril (Accupril)	10 mg po qd/80 mg	5 mg/day CrCl 30–60 mL/min	Reduces tetracycline absorption	$$
		2.5 mg/day CrCl 10–30 mL/min	Not removed by dialysis	
Ramipril (Altace)	2.5 mg po qd/20 mg	1.25 mg/day CrCl <40 mL/min	Impaired LFT increases unchanged plasma level	$$$$
		5 mg/d maximum	Reduces mortality in MI with CHF; CVA, CVD,	
			MI and mortality in patients at high risk for CVD	
Trandolapril (Mavik)	1 mg po qd/4 mg	0.5 mg/day CrCl <30 mL/min	Reduce dosage to 0.5 mg/day in hepatic cirrhosis	$$$
			No data on removal by hemodialysis	
ARB				
Candesartan (Atacand)	16 mg po qd/32 mg		Reduces microalbuminemia in type II diabetes mellitus	$$$
Eprosartan (Teveten)	600 mg po qd/800 mg			$$$
Irbesartan (Avapro)	150 mg po qd/300 mg			$$$
Losartan (Cozaar)	50 mg po qd/100 mg			$$$
Olmesartan (Benicar)	20 mg po qd/40 mg		Decreased CHF morbidity and mortality	$$
Telmisartan (Micardis)	40 mg po qd/80 mg		Decreased CHF morbidity and mortality after MI	$$
Valsartan (Diovan)	80 mg po qd/320 mg			$$$

CHF, congestive heart failure; CrCl, creatine clearance; CVA, cerebrovascular accident; CVD, cardiovascular disease; LFT, left ventricular function; MI, myocardial infarction; NYHA, New York Heart Association. $, least expensive; $$$$, most expensive.

complications, initiate dialysis, and prepare the patient for kidney replacement as indicated. Comprehensive patient care consists of clear communication and concise coordination of care with the nephrologist and other specialists during the predialysis, dialysis, and transplantation period.

1. **Hypertension** is common once chronic renal failure develops. Often blood pressure responds well to ACE inhibitors or angiotensin II receptor blockers (Table 84–2). The goal blood pressure is <130/80. In the ACE inhibitor naïve or frail patient, captopril, with its short half-life and thus quicker clearance once discontinued should class-related side effects be detected, may be initiated at 6.25 mg orally two to three times daily and titrated up to 50 mg orally three times daily. Alternatively, longer-acting agents such as enalapril, 5 mg, or lisinopril, 10 mg orally every day, with titration up to 40 mg orally every day, would improve compliance without incurring significant cost. For patients who cannot tolerate an ACE inhibitor, losartan (50 mg) or irbesartan (150 mg) orally every day may also be used, with target doses of 100 mg and 300 mg orally every day, respectively. No dosage reduction for renal impairment is necessary. However, patient cost for these agents is approximately doubled. Up to a 35% increase in serum creatinine is acceptable in the course of therapy, unless hyperkalemia develops. Once glomerular filtration rate drops below 30 mL/min, increased doses of loop diuretics and the addition of other classes of medications are typically necessary to control blood pressure.

2. **Potassium metabolism**
    a. **Hyperkalemia** occurs commonly secondary to decreased tubular secretion, medications, volume depletion, dietary intake, and hypoinsulinemia. Specific treatments are dependent on the severity of hyperkalemia and may include removing offending medications, restoring fluid balance, maintaining a strict low-potassium dietary regimen, initiating thiazide or loop diuretics, and using sodium polystyrene, such as Kayexalate 15–30 g orally every 6 hours.
    b. **Hypokalemia** results from diuresis or renal disease itself. Each mEq/L decrease represents a 200-mEq reduction in total body potassium. Oral replacement with potassium chloride, 40–100 mEq/day, may be initiated for mild hypokalemia. Intravenous replacement is reserved for severe cases. Judicious replacement, 10 mEq/hour, is coupled with frequent assessment of serum levels.

3. **Calcium metabolism**
    a. **Hypocalcemia** is observed with renal disease when glomerular filtration rate is <30 mL/min or where there is secondary hypoparathyroidism or hypoalbuminemia. Serum ionized calcium and mathematical correction for hypoalbuminemia confirm hypocalcemia. 500 mg to 2 g of elemental calcium is given three to four times daily with meals. Replacement strategy, utilizing carbonate or acetate salt, is contingent on the presence of hyperphosphatemia. Calcium carbonate contains 40% elemental calcium. Though more expensive, calcium acetate, containing 25% elemental calcium, is preferred over calcium carbonate when serum phosphorus is >4.5 mg/dL.
    b. **Hypercalcemia** in renal failure occurs with multiple myeloma, malignancy, sarcoidosis, and calcium replacement therapy. Treatment is targeted at the underlying pathology. Calcium replacement is halted or decreased. When calcium × phosphate products exceeds 70, aluminum hydroxide, 300–600 mg orally three times daily with meals, can be used for no more than 10 days.

4. **Phosphorus metabolism** is impaired in renal failure. Phosphate retention leads to hyperphosphatemia and consequently secondary hyperparathyroidism. Treatment begins with dietary restriction of 0.8–1.2 g/day of phosphorus. Binders such as calcium carbonate or calcium acetate are then added if hyperphosphatemia persists. Aluminum hydroxide, 1.9–4.8 g orally two to four times daily, may also be used for short duration, though not concurrent with citrate-based binders.

5. **Serum albumin and prealbumin,** though limited in the presence of inflammation, can estimate nutritional status. Dialysis patient mortality rate increases with decreasing albumin levels.

6. **Metabolic acidosis** exists in renal failure secondary to accumulation of organic acids and impaired renal acidification. Treatment, aimed at raising serum bicarbonate level to 20 mEq/L, is effected by providing 0.5 mEq/kg/day of bicarbonate in divided doses. Each 650-mg tablet provides 7.6 mEq of bicarbonate.

7. **Volume overload** commonly occurs with chronic renal failure secondary to progressive renal impairment, excess salt load, inadequate diuresis, and medication side effects. Treatment initially includes weight monitoring and dietary salt restriction. A loop diuretic is then administered daily or twice daily if euvolemia is not achieved. A thiazide diuretic may be added if twice daily loop diuretic therapy is unsuccessful. Refractory volume overload is best treated with dialysis.

8. **Anemia** requires work-up when hemoglobin is <11 g/dL in premenopausal and prepubertal females and <12 g/dL in adult males and postmenopausal females. Evaluation should include iron studies, reticulocyte count, red blood cell indices, and occult stool blood test. Gastrointestinal blood loss is treated in consultation with a gastroenterologist. Oral iron replacement therapy, ferrous sulfate (325 mg orally three times daily without food or other medicines), begins when ferritin is <200 ng/mL and is maintained for 6 months or until iron deficiency anemia resolves. Intravenous iron, iron dextran, may be given if ferritin is <100 ng/mL or percent transferrin saturation is <20%. If hemoglobin remains <10 g/dL despite identification and adequate treatment of all causes of anemia, epoetin alfa should be considered. Treatment then should be coordinated with a hematologist/oncologist and a nephrologist. Red blood cell transfusions are necessary for patients with severe symptomatic anemia or those with epoetin resistance and chronic blood loss.

9. **Nutritional imbalance** is common in renal failure. Nutritionist consultation should be arranged early in the course of the disease. Assessment should include evaluation of general nutritional and energy status, electrolyte modification requirements, and lipid status. The daily caloric requirement is 35 kcal/kg body weight for patients younger than 60 years, and 30–35 kcal/kg body weight for those older than 60 years. A low-protein diet, 0.6 g/kg/day, may slow the progression of renal impairment. A very low protein diet, 0.3 g/kg, supplemented by 10 g/day of essential amino acids, is even more efficacious. However, compliance may be of issue. Additionally, this must be balanced with protein malnutrition that may result from adherence to a very low potassium-restricted diet in the treatment of persistent hyperkalemia.

10. **Dialysis** indications include metabolic derangement unresponsive to medical therapy, refractory volume overload, uremic symptoms unmanageable by dietary manipulation, or advanced uremia.

V. Prognosis. Generally, the prognosis for recovery of renal function depends on the underlying pathology, presence of coexisting diseases, and complications associated with renal failure.

A. **Prenal disease.** Recovery of renal function is generally expected when there is prompt resolution of glomerular hypoperfusion. Residual impairment may persist with prolonged ischemia. Patients with hepatorenal syndrome tend to have a poor prognosis overall.

B. **Vascular disease.** The prognosis is contingent on response to treatment of the underlying vascular disease. Patients with atheroembolic disease tend to have a very poor prognosis, though this may be related to the severity of the associated cardiac and vascular disease.

C. **Glomerular disease.** The prognosis depends on the underlying pathologic process. Children with post-streptococcal glomerulonephritis typically recover fully from the initial renal failure. Some, however, may develop hypertension, proteinuria, and renal insufficiency later in life.

D. **Tubulointerstitial disease**
   1. **Acute tubular necrosis.** Recovery of function occurs within 3 weeks except in those with preexisting renal disease and repeated ischemia or exposure to nephrotoxic agents.
   2. **Acute interstitial nephritis.** Though renal function may not return to baseline, most patients recover after withdrawal of the offending agent or treatment of the underlying infection.
   3. **Cast nephropathy.** The prognosis is dependent on tumor mass and light-chain production rate. Improvement is expected in treated individuals.

E. **Postrenal disease.** Recovery of renal function is inversely related to the severity and duration of the obstruction, as well as the presence of any preexisting renal disease and infection. Full recovery is expected in complete obstruction of <1 week's duration. It is much more variable in incomplete obstruction.

REFERENCES

Agrawal M, Swartz R: Acute renal failure. Am Fam Physician 2000;**61**(7):2077.

Alcazar JM, Rodicio JL: Ischemic nephropathy: Clinical characteristics and treatment. Am J Kidney Dis 2000;**36**(5):883.

ALLHAT Officers and Coordinators for the ALLHAT Collaborative Research Group: Major CV events in hypertensive patients randomized to doxazosin vs chlorthalidone: The antihypertensive and lipid-lowering treatment to prevent heart attack trial (ALLHAT). JAMA 2000;**283**(15):1967.

Chobanian AV, et al: The Seventh Report of the Joint National Committee on Prevention, Detection, Evaluation, and Treatment of High Blood Pressure: The JNC 7 Report. JAMA 2003;**289**(19);2560.

Palevsky PM: Acute renal failure. J Am Soc Nephrol 2003;**2**(2):41.

Veterans Health Administration, Department of Defense. VHA/DoD clinical practice guideline for the management of chronic kidney disease and pre-ESRD in the primary care setting. Department of Veterans Affairs (U.S.), Veterans Health Administration; May 2001.

---

85 Seizure Disorders

Shawn H. Blanchard, MD, & William L. Toffler, MD

KEY POINTS

- A seizure is a clinical sign of an underlying condition and does not necessarily warrant treatment acutely.
- Epilepsy is a condition of recurrent seizures requiring definitive diagnosis and treatment.
- Status epilepticus is an acute state of continued or frequent seizures without a return to consciousness or alertness and requires emergent treatment.
- Should the patient be seizing, ascertain the duration of the seizure, ensure airway, breathing, and circulation, and protect the patient from physical harm.
- A seizure continuing past 5 minutes warrants loading with 2–4 mg Ativan IV or 5–10 mg of Valium IV (see Table 85–3).
- Obtain a brief history from third-party witnesses shortly after the patient is stabilized so as to determine etiology. Follow with an examination and studies as predicated by presentation.

I. Introduction
 A. **Definition.** A seizure is a sudden change in cortical electrical activity, manifested through motor, sensory, or behavioral changes, with or without an alteration in consciousness. Seizures can be further divided into five categories:
  1. **Simple partial (focal) seizures** occur without loss of consciousness and involve one hemispheric eliptogenic focus. These may have motor, sensory, psychic, and autonomic characteristics and may progress toward a generalized seizure.
  2. **Complex partial seizures** cause loss of consciousness and maintain a hemispheric cerebral focus. This category includes absence (loss of consciousness or posture), myoclonic (repetitive muscle contractions), and tonic-clonic (a sustained contraction followed by rhythmic contractions of all four extremities).
  3. **Generalized seizures** involve alteration of consciousness, and both hemispheres of the cerebral cortex and have a nonfocal origin. These include absence seizures, tonic-clonic seizures, tonic seizures, and atonic seizures.
  4. **Febrile seizures** are one or more generalized seizures occurring between 3 months and 5 years of age associated with fever without evidence of any other defined cause.
  5. **Status epilepticus** is a neurologic emergency involving repetitive generalized seizures without return to consciousness between seizures.
 B. **Epidemiology**
  1. Four million people in the United States have had at least one seizure, 2 million people have had two or more seizures, and more than 200,000 people have more than one seizure per month despite receiving anticonvulsant therapy. The prevalence of

seizures in close relatives of seizure patients is three times that of the overall population. There is no significant difference in prevalence between genders.

2. About 1 in 15 children will have a seizure during their first 7 years of life. The prevalence of seizures in children delivered breech is 3.8% as compared with a prevalence of 2.2% in children delivered vertex.

3. Febrile seizures occur in 3–4% of all children. Fifty percent of febrile seizures occur during the second year of life and almost 90% before the third birthday. Most children with febrile seizures (64%) will have only one episode, but the earlier the age of onset, the more likely the child is to have more febrile seizures. No evidence exists that recurrent febrile seizures increase the risk of epilepsy.

4. The annual incidence of recurrent seizures is 54 in 100,000, excluding febrile convulsions, and 120 in 100,000, if all types of seizures are included. The prevalence of chronic, recurrent epilepsy is 10 in 100,000. The risk of recurrence after a single unprovoked seizure is about 35%.

5. More than 10,000 episodes of status epilepticus occur in the United States each year.

6. **The possible causes of a seizure** can be grouped into the following categories; the age of the patient may help find a cause (Table 85–1):

   a. **Focal brain disease,** including cerebrovascular events (eg, stroke), head trauma, and neoplasm.

TABLE 85–1. POSSIBLE CAUSES OF RECURRENT SEIZURES BASED ON AGE

Age at Onset (Yrs)	Most Likely Causes

Infancy (0–2)	Perinatal hypoxia
	Birth injury
	Congenital abnormality
	Metabolic
	    Hypoglycemia
	    Hypocalcemia
	    Hypomagnesemia
	    Vitamin B_{12} deficiency
	    Phenylketonuria
	Acute infection
	Febrile seizure
	Idiopathic

Childhood (2–10)	Acute infection Trauma Idiopathic
Adolescent (10–18)	Trauma Drug and alcohol withdrawal AV malformations Idiopathic
Early adulthood (18–25)	Drug and alcohol withdrawal Tumor
Middle age (25–60)	Drug and alcohol withdrawal Trauma Tumor Vascular disease

Late adulthood (over 60)	Vascular disease, AV
	Tumor
	Degenerative disease
	Metabolic
	    Hypoglycemia
	    Uremia
	    Hepatic failure
	    Electrolyte abnormality
	    Drug and alcohol withdrawal

AV, atrioventricular.

  b. Infection, such as meningitis, encephalitis, and abscess.
  c. Drug-related causes, such as cocaine, amphetamines, and alcohol withdrawal.
  d. Metabolic derangements, including uremia, hyponatremia, hypoglycemia, and deficiency states such as phenylketonuria.
  e. Subacute conditions, such as Creutzfeldt-Jakob disease and subacute sclerosing panencephalitis.
  f. Toxins, such as lead poisoning (especially in children) and mercury poisoning in adults.
  g. Conditions causing syncope, including vasovagal episodes, postural hypotension, and arrhythmias.
  h. Asphyxia from hypoxia, carbon monoxide poisoning, or birth injury.
  i. Idiopathic seizures, in which no clear etiology is found.
 C. Pathophysiologic abnormalities leading to seizures may be at the cellular level, such as with tumors, or at the subcellular level, such as with drug or alcohol withdrawal or febrile seizures. The exact mechanism by which a focal lesion creates seizure activity is not known.

II. Diagnosis
 A. Symptoms. The patient's history, often by a family member, detailing the episode including antecedent events, auras, progressing, duration, ictal period, and any prolonged neurologic impairment are vital toward an accurate diagnosis.
 B. Signs
  1. Fever may indicate an infectious cause such as meningitis or encephalitis, or it may directly trigger a febrile seizure.
  2. Focal neurologic findings may indicate a possible tumor or a localized injury to the brain.
  3. Papilledema indicates increased intracranial pressure that may be caused by an intracranial hemorrhage or tumor.
  4. Hemorrhagic eye grounds suggest underlying high blood pressure and may be a cause of seizure associated with hypertensive intercranial bleeding.
  5. Stiff neck (meningismus) may be present with inflamed meninges (meningitis).
  6. Headache is a nonspecific complaint compatible with infection or hemorrhage.
 C. Laboratory tests
  1. The following laboratory tests should be ordered for all patients with a new seizure and for those with recurrent seizures if indicated by the history and physical examination.
   a. Serum tests (glucose, sodium, potassium, calcium, phosphorus, magnesium, blood urea nitrogen, and ammonia levels) should be ordered in any clinical situations associated with dehydration, nausea, vomiting, alteration in consciousness, or drug ingestion.
   b. Anticonvulsant levels. The most common cause of recurrent seizures in children as well as many adults is subtherapeutic anticonvulsant drug levels. Drug levels should be obtained in all individuals already taking anticonvulsant medication who present with recurrence of their underlying seizure disorder.
   c. Drug and toxic screens, including a screen for alcohol, should be ordered, especially if an adequate history cannot be obtained.
   d. A complete blood count assists in the evaluation of a possible underlying infection.
   e. Brain imaging is useful unless the physician can confidently attribute the seizure to a metabolic cause.
    (1) Computerized tomography (CT). A head CT scan is indicated in the routine tonic-clonic seizure work-up.
    (2) Magnetic resonance imaging (MRI). A MRI of the head is superior to CT in evaluation of temporal lobe lesions.
  2. The following tests should be ordered only if the results might alter management.
   a. Electroencephalogram (EEG). The diagnosis of epilepsy is not made on the basis of EEG, unless the EEG captures a clinical seizure. The sensitivity, specificity, and predictive value of this test depend on the underlying cause and anatomic location of a seizure focus. EEG and video EEG are becoming increasingly valuable in diagnosing epilepsy, particularly in patients having difficulty with monotherapeutic control.

    (1) Delta waves (less than three waveforms per second) are an indication of a disturbance of cerebral function.

    (2) Generalized slowing is related to an acute disturbance such as encephalitis, encephalopathy, anoxia, or a metabolic disturbance. Generalized slowing may occur with hyperventilation, sleep, and drowsiness. Generalized slowing is age-dependent; it is more common in young patients.

    (3) Focal slowing implies acute local disturbance, such as contusion, stroke, local infection, or tumor. Focal slowing may occur as a postictal phenomenon that may last hours or days after a focal seizure. Slowing also varies with age and state of arousal.

    (4) Spikes generally represent an old disturbance seen after brain damage, but they may take years to develop. Spikes are less of an indication for further evaluation than focal slowing. A spike wave, defined as three spikes per second, is noted in absence seizures.

  b. 24-Hour ambulatory EEG may be very helpful in identifying "events" and is useful in separating true seizures from pseudoseizures or other paroxysmal behavior, especially when the two coexist.

  c. Video monitoring may be coupled with a continuous EEG. It may be useful in localizing seizures such as a frontal seizure or a temporal seizure, when the physician is considering surgical correction. This method may also be useful in evaluating suspected pseudoseizures, or psychogenic nonepileptic seizures (PNES) and other paroxysmal behaviors. The evaluation is generally performed with the patient as an inpatient.

  d. Skull x-rays are not usually helpful except in the evaluation of severe head trauma.

  e. Lumbar puncture is not routinely indicated in a child older than 12 months with a first febrile seizure. In infants younger than 12 months, it should be strongly considered because clinical seizures and symptoms of meningitis may be subtle.

  f. Positron emission tomography (PET) scans are used primarily in research but are becoming increasingly useful when recalcitrant epilepsy leads to surgical consideration.

III. Treatment

A. Acute treatment

1. The patient's airway must be protected (ABCs).
2. No medication is usually necessary.
3. If seizure activity persists longer than 5 minutes, intravenous medication may be given (Table 85–2).

B. Drug therapy

1. Only one drug should be prescribed. Drugs can be chosen from Table 85–3, where they are listed in order of effectiveness. A specific side effect (such as decreased cognitive function) might lead the physician to select a certain drug (such as phenobarbital over phenytoin) in certain circumstances.
2. Dosage should be increased as tolerated to achieve a therapeutic blood level. Clinical response is more reliable than blood levels, however.
3. Another drug can be substituted if therapy is ineffective. Only after failure of each single agent should combination therapy be considered.
4. Several newer agents—felbamate (Felbatol), gabapentin (Neurontin), lamotrigine (Lamictal), and phensuximide (Milontin)—have been approved primarily for partial seizures. Gabapentin has a relatively short half-life, necessitating multiple doses. Dosage adjustments are necessary with lamotrigine and felbamate when used with other anticonvulsants. Felbamate has been associated with aplastic anemia. Patients taking this medication should probably have it discontinued unless benefits clearly outweigh this potential complication.

C. Treatment during pregnancy

1. Drug metabolism may be drastically altered during pregnancy.
2. There is about a twofold risk of congenital malformation (predominantly facial cleft and neural tube defects) in mothers who take anticonvulsants to control seizures. Malformations are most strongly associated with trimethadione and valproic acid.

TABLE 85–2. DRUGS USED IN THE TREATMENT OF SEIZURE DISORDERS

Drug of Choice for Particular Type of Seizure	Adult Dose (mg/day)	Pediatric Dose (mg/kg/day)	Adult Starting Dose	Side Effects	Therapeutic Range (µg/mL)	Cost
Generalized—tonic-clonic						
Phenytoin (Dilantin)	300–400	4–7	100 mg bid-tid	Decrease in cognitive function, sedation, ataxia, diplopia, gingival hyperplasia	10–20	$
Phenobarbital	120–250	4–6	30–60 mg bid	Respiratory depression, hyperactivity, sedation	15–40	$
Carbamazepine (Tegretol)	600–1200	20–30	200 mg bid-qid	Sedation, diplopia, ataxia, aplastic anemia, hypo-osmolality	6–12	$
Valproic acid (Depakene)	1000–3000	10–60	250 mg tid	Sedation, nausea, vomiting, weight gain, hair loss, GI hematologic toxicity	50–100	$$$
Primidone (Mysoline)	750–1500	10–25	250 mg tid-qid	Sedation, vertigo, nausea, ataxia, change in behavior	6–12	$
Generalized—absence						
Ethosuximide (Zarontin)	250–1000	20–40	250 mg bid	Nausea, vomiting, lethargy, hiccups, headache blood dyscrasias	40–100	$$$
Valproic acid (Depakene)	1000–3000	10–60	250 mg tid	Sedation, nausea, vomiting, weight gain, hair loss, GI hematologic toxicity	50–100	$$$
Clonazepam (Klonopin)	1.5–20	0.01–0.3	0.5 mg tid	Drowsiness, ataxia, change in behavior	0.013–0.072	$$$
Generalized—myoclonic						
Valproic acid (Depakene)	1000–3000	10–60	250 mg tid	Sedation, nausea, vomiting, weight gain, hair loss, GI hematologic toxicity	50–100	$$$
Clonazepam (Klonopin)	1.5–20	0.01–0.3	0.5 mg tid	Drowsiness, ataxia, change in behavior	0.013–0.072	$$$
Phenytoin (Dilantin)	300–400	4–7	100 mg bid-tid	Decrease in cognitive function, sedation, ataxia, diplopia, gingival hyperplasia	10–20	$
Partial						
Carbamazepine (Tegretol)	600–1200	20–30	200 mg bid-qid	Sedation, diplopia, ataxia, aplastic anemia, hypo-osmolality	6–12	$
Phenobarbital (Dilantin)	120–250	4–6	30–60 mg bid	Respiratory depression, hyperactivity, sedation	15–40	$
Valproic acid (Depakene)	1000–3000	10–60	250 mg tid	Sedation, nausea, vomiting, weight gain, hair loss, GI hematologic toxicity	50–100	$$$$
Primidone (Mysoline)	750–1500	10–25	250 mg tid-qid	Sedation, vertigo, nausea, ataxia, change in behavior	6–12	$
Status epilepticus						
Lorazepam (Ativan)	0.05 mg/kg IV	0.05 mg/kg IV	2–4 mg q20–30 min	Respiratory depression, sedation	—	$$$
Diazepam (Valium)	0.25–0.5 mg/kg IV	0.25–0.5 mg/kg IV	5–10 mg q20–30 min	Respiratory depression, sedation	—	$
Phenytoin (Dilantin)	15–20 mg/kg IV drip at 30–50 mg/min	15–20 mg/kg IV drip at 0.5–1.6 mg/min	—	Decrease in cognitive function, sedation, ataxia, diplopia, gingival hyperplasia	10–20	$
Phenobarbital	300–800 mg IV drip at 25–50 mg/min	20 mg/kg IV drip at 25–50 mg/min	—	Respiratory depression, sedation	15–40	$

GI, gastrointestinal.
$, least expensive; $$$$, most expensive.

TABLE 85-3. STATUS EPILEPTICUS TREATMENT

1. Ensure airway—assist ventilation if necessary
2. IV with normal saline
3. Dextrostix, or give 50 mL of 50% dextrose solution
4. Diazepam IV, 0.25–0.4 mg/kg (up to 10 mg) at a maximum rate of 1 mg/min; may need to repeat in 20–30 min
5. If seizures continue, phenobarbital IV, 10–15 mg/kg; 20% of total dose every 5–10 min at a rate of less than 50 mg/min; preferred over phenytoin especially in very young children
6. Phenytoin, loading dose of 15 mg/kg, undiluted, at a rate of 0.5–1.5 mg/kg/min; an additional 5 mg/kg can be given after 12 hr
7. General anesthesia can be considered and given

    D. Converting from polytherapy to monotherapy
        1. The single agent most likely to be successful should be chosen. The dosage of the agent should be slowly increased while the undesirable drug is slowly withdrawn. Long-acting drugs should be discontinued slowly over 1–3 months by halving the dose once per week.
        2. The plan, including the alternatives and the risks, should be fully discussed with the patient. It should be modified if control of seizures is diminished.
    E. Febrile seizures
        1. In general, anticonvulsants are not indicated for a patient with febrile seizures. Anticonvulsant prophylaxis for febrile seizure should be considered, however, if the neurologic examination is abnormal, if the seizure activity lasts for more than 15 minutes, if a transient or permanent neurologic defect is present, or if there is a family history of nonfebrile seizures.
        2. Phenobarbital or other anticonvulsant therapy is effective in preventing recurrence of febrile seizures. Treatment does not affect the percentage of individuals who will develop epilepsy in the future, however.
IV. Management Strategies are dependent on the type of seizure the patient has experienced.
    A. Seizures beginning early in life may be caused by developmental defects, perfusion defects of the brain, intrauterine hypoxemia, or fetal infection. Assisting the patient with developmental problems such as learning deficits is as important as controlling the seizures.
    B. In 80% of childhood seizures, no clear cause is found despite an exhaustive work-up. If the seizures are controlled, normally no impairment in development occurs. If seizures are poorly controlled, difficulties with scholastic, emotional, and social development may arise.
    C. New onset of seizures in adolescence generally has no adverse effect on the patient's development as long as the seizures are controlled. Compliance with treatment is a significant problem in this age group, however.
    D. New onset of seizures in adults may indicate serious disease, including alcoholism or drug abuse. Patients in early adulthood or middle age must be screened carefully regarding the use of alcohol and "recreational" drugs, as well as the appropriate use of prescription drugs. Identification and intervention may prevent an extensive work-up.
    E. Onset of seizures late in life indicates possible cerebral vascular disease or tumor. If the cause of the seizures is not investigated, a potentially correctable problem may be missed and control of the seizures may be difficult to achieve.
V. Prognosis
    A. With time, seizure activity may become quiescent. Withdrawal of therapy should be considered after the patient has been seizure-free for 2 years. The relapse rate of patients who have been medication-free for 3 years is about 33%. Relapse is related to seizure type. Patients with complex partial seizures with generalization have the worst prognosis, and those with partial seizures without generalization have the best prognosis.
    B. Prognosis also is dependent on the cause of the seizure and whether the patient can change behavior, for example, alcohol abuse, that may cause or exacerbate seizures.

REFERENCES

American Academy of Pediatrics Provisional Committee on Quality Improvement, Subcommittee on Febrile Seizures: Practice parameter: The neurodiagnostic evaluation of the child with a first simple febrile seizure. Pediatrics 1996;**97**(5):769.

Gelb DJ: *Introduction to Clinical Neurology,* 2nd ed. Butterworth-Heinemann; 2000:129–151.

Hauser WA, et al: Risk of recurrent seizures after two unprovoked seizures. N Engl J Med 1998; **338**(7):429.

International League Against Epilepsy www.epilepsy.org

Marson AG, et al: The new antiepileptic drugs: A systematic review of their efficacy and tolerability. Epilepsia 1997;**38**(8):859.

Reuber M, Elger C: Psychogenic nonepileptic seizures: Review and update. Epilepsy Behav 2003; **4**(3):205.

Sadot B: Epilepsy: A progressive disease? Still no answer to the controversy over whether seizures beget more seizures. BMJ 1997;**314**(7078):391.

---

86   Stroke

Michael P. Temporal, MD

KEY POINTS

- Rapid evaluation (including noncontrast computerized tomography of the head) and use of intravenous recombinant tissue plasminogen activator (tPA) within 3 hours of onset of symptoms of ischemic stroke can improve outcome.
- Immediate stroke management should include management of fever, agitation, and glucose control. Aspirin (80–325 mg/day × 14 days) should be started 24 hours after tPA administration.
- Blood pressure control during the acute ischemic stroke syndrome may be detrimental and should be treated only if systolic blood pressure is >210 or diastolic blood pressure is >110. Aggressive treatment of blood pressure may be required in the setting of hemorrhagic stroke, post thrombolytic therapy, and postoperative carotid endarterectomy or subdural hematoma evacuation.
- Heparin in the acute setting should be used with caution as no clear benefit has been demonstrated. It may be helpful in the setting of crescendo transient ischemic attack, or progressive or posterior circulation stroke. Heparin is contraindicated in hemorrhagic stroke or immediately following tPA.
- Secondary prevention should be based on stroke etiology and may include warfarin (for cardiac embolic source or intracranial disease) or an antiplatelet agent (aspirin, 325 mg; ticlopidine, 250 mg twice daily; clopidogrel, 75 mg every day, or aspirin/dipyridamole twice daily) for stroke with an atherosclerotic etiology.
- Modifiable risk factors including smoking cessation, blood pressure control, reduction of elevated cholesterol, and diabetes management are important to decrease future stroke risk.

I. Introduction

A. **Stroke** is a clinical syndrome consisting of the sudden or rapid onset of a constellation of neurologic deficits that persist for more than 24 hours secondary to a vascular event. "Brain attack" is a term used to alert health care providers, patients, and their families and friends of the emergency condition that threatens the life and function of irreplaceable brain tissue.

B. Stroke and cerebrovascular disease is the third leading cause of death in the United States the most common cause of disability, and the most frequently cited reason for patients needing long-term care. Nearly 700,000 Americans have new (75%) or recurrent (25%) stroke each year. Although one third of stroke survivors will have permanent disability requiring help to care for themselves, up to one half of the 4.4 million survivors of stroke have no or little disability.

C. **Types of stroke.** In adults, 80% of strokes are **ischemic: atheroembolic/atherothrombotic stroke** (60–70% of strokes), **cerebral embolic,** and **lacunar (small vessel occlusive).** The rest of adult strokes are **hemorrhagic strokes.** Hemorrhagic strokes are classified by location: intracerebral or subarachnoid.

D. **Risk factors** have been classified by the American Heart Association (AHA) as **modifiable and not modifiable.**
   1. **Nonmodifiable risk factors for stroke include** age (risk doubles each decade beyond 55 years of age), family history of stroke, male gender, race (African American and Hispanic), and prior stroke. The approximate risk of recurrent stroke within the first year after an ischemic stroke is 12% and within 5 years is 50%.
   2. **Modifiable risk factors include** hypertension, cardiac disease, diabetes mellitus, cigarette smoking ("dose-related"), transient ischemic attack (TIA has a 10-fold increase in stroke risk), and polycythemia. Heavy alcohol use (binge or >5 drinks/day) predisposes one to stroke, whereas moderate consumption (<2 drinks/day) may have a protective effect. Use of oral contraceptives with cigarette smoking increases stroke risk as well. Nonvalvular atrial fibrillation, which leads to almost 50% of cardiogenic brain embolizations, carries an annual risk of embolus of about 5% if left untreated. While elevated cholesterol is a more significant risk factor for coronary artery disease than for occlusive cerebrovascular disease, high plasma homocysteine and Lp(a) lipoprotein levels may be equally important to both. Atherosclerotic vascular occlusive disease in other areas of the body (ie, coronary artery disease and peripheral arterial disease) may herald coexistent cerebrovascular disease.
   E. The **differential diagnosis for stroke** includes mass lesions (eg, subdural hematoma or neoplasm), metabolic abnormalities (eg, hypoglycemia, hyponatremia, or hypernatremia), infectious processes (eg, meningitis or cerebral abscess), inflammatory processes (eg, temporal arteritis), and idiopathic processes (eg, epilepsy). Illicit drug use may be a consideration.
II. **Diagnosis.** The presentation of stroke represents a continuum from TIA (with quickly resolving neurologic deficit) to acute stroke syndrome with progression (worsening deficits, most common with large vessel thrombosis, lacunes, or emboli) to completed stroke (static neurologic deficits). Early presentation, rapid imaging, and prompt treatment are key goals for health care providers and the communities they serve. The placid acceptance of the inevitable course of stroke of the past must become the vigorous battleground of active intervention to affect positively and dramatically the "brain attack" of today. This goal applies regardless of the age of the patient.
   A. **Symptoms** and **signs** of stroke reflect the cerebrovascular territory affected by the stroke process. The vessels most often involved are listed in Table 86–1. Sudden onset of weakness, numbness, or problems with speech or vision or the sudden development of dizziness, trouble walking, or headache are early warning signs of stroke. The initial history must document time of onset of symptoms, associated activities or trauma, other neurologic symptoms (headache, seizure, vomiting, alteration of consciousness) as well as present and past illnesses and surgeries, medications taken, illicit drug use, and allergies. Identifying stroke risk factors and contraindications to thrombolytic therapy are also essential.
   B. **Physical examination** must assess mental status and record level of alertness, test the ability to name objects, repeat spoken language, read, and write. Registration and recall of three words is a simple, reproducible test. Other aspects of neurologic examination (cranial nerves, muscle strength and tone, deep tendon reflexes, and cerebellar testing and sensation) are important baseline observations as well as cardiac examination (arrhythmia, blood pressure, murmurs, bruits).
   C. **Brain imaging studies** are used to detect the presence of hemorrhage and exclude other causes (tumor, abscess, or subdural hematoma). Advances in brain imaging promise early distinction of the core area of ischemic tissue with severely compromised cerebral blood flow (CBF) from the "penumbra," that is, the surrounding rim of moderately ischemic brain tissue with impaired electrical activity but preserved cellular metabolism and viability.
      1. **Computerized tomography (CT)** gives reliable differentiation of hemorrhagic from ischemic stroke with scanning obtained during the first 72 hours of the stroke. Most current tPA-administration protocols call for pretreatment noncontrast CT scan within 3 hours of onset of symptoms to rule out hemorrhagic events. CT will show a subarachnoid hemorrhage with 95% sensitivity if performed within 5 days of the event. Normal CT scans are frequently obtained in lacunar or brain-stem infarctions when the lesions are small. Early in the course of an ischemic infarction, plain CT scan results are usually negative unless edematous changes are present; however, various quantitative CBF imaging techniques with high sensitivity and

TABLE 86–1. CLINICAL PRESENTATION OF STROKE

Stroke Type/Artery or Site Involved	Clinical Presentation	Special Considerations
Atherothrombotic stroke Internal carotid artery (mostly extracranial) Vertebral artery (mostly intracranial) Basilar artery	Stuttering onset, can occur upon waking; cerebellar infarction causes severe edema/brain stem compression	Preceded by TIA in 50% of cases
Embolic stroke Middle cerebral artery Anterior cerebral artery Posterior cerebral artery	Sudden onset of maximal deficit	
Lacunar infarction **(penetrating arteries)** Middle cerebral perforator– lenticulostriate Posterior cerebral perforator Basilar artery perforating branches	Develops suddenly or over several hours; headache, loss of con- sciousness, and emesis do not occur	Lacunar syndromes: pure motor hemiparesis, pure sensory loss, crural paresis, and ataxia/dysarthria (clumsy hand syndrome)
Intracerebral hemorrhage Deep cerebral hemisphere (putamen) Subcortical white matter (lobar intracranial hemorrhage) Cerebellar Thalamic Midbrain	Smooth onset, although can be sudden; emesis and loss of consciousness do occur	Selective surgical clot evacuation; unpredictable course in cerebellar ICH; most midbrain ICHs improve with supportive care
Subarachnoid hemorrhage **(ruptured aneurysm)** Circle of Willis Internal carotid artery Anterior communicating artery Middle cerebral artery	Sudden onset ("brutal" headache, emesis, loss of consciousness then awakening with headache and stiff neck); **note:** aneurysms are rarely symp- tomatic before rupture	Complications: rerupture, obstruc- tion of spinal fluid flow (communi- cating hydrocephalus), vasospasm 3–14 days postevent

ICH, intracerebral hemorrhage; TIA, transient ischemic attack.

good spatial resolution have been demonstrated: xenon-enhanced CT as well as radiolabeled microsphere, 133Xe, and iodoantipyrine CBF techniques. The diagnostic yield of plain CT scanning in ischemia is greatest 7 days after the event.

2. **Magnetic resonance imaging (MRI)** is more sensitive than CT in detecting ischemic stroke. New MRI techniques for assessing acute cerebral infarction provide more functional information about the status of the brain on presentation of stroke symptoms: fluid-attenuating inversion recovery imaging, diffusion-weighted imaging (DWI), perfusion-weighted imaging (PWI), functional MRI, and magnetic resonance spectroscopy. These techniques promise ever-increasing delineation of infarcted (irreversibly damaged) tissue from "stunned" (at-risk, potentially reversibly ischemic) tissue. Abnormalities often appear within hours of stroke onset.

D. **Laboratory tests.** A **complete blood cell count** identifies anemia or polycythemia. The **coagulation profile** (ie, prothrombin time, activated thromboplastin time, and platelet count) provides baseline information for anticoagulation and thrombolysis. The International Normalized Ratio (INR) provides accurate monitoring of warfarin anticoagulation therapy. Evaluation of additional specific coagulation factors (eg, levels of coagulation factors such as proteins C and S and antithrombin III) identifies prothrombotic states. In young patients with progressive intracranial occlusion, such evaluation for prothrombotic states is warranted. Recent studies have shown tPA antigen levels and homocysteine levels to be elevated in patients at risk for stroke. Other measures of metabolic abnormalities identify potential aggravators of cerebral ischemia: **blood glucose, serum electrolytes, blood urea nitrogen,** and **creatinine.** Because a significant number of patients with carotid artery disease have concomitant asymptomatic coronary artery disease, cholesterol and lipid status is evaluated for treatment in the post-stroke patient.

E. **Additional studies**
1. **Imaging of the extracranial and intracranial vessels.** The initial evaluation of patients with symptoms of acute cerebrovascular ischemia includes **carotid noninvasive testing** (carotid duplex ultrasonography and color Doppler flow imaging), looking for significant lesions of the carotid arteries. **Transcranial Doppler ultrasonography (TCD)** detects middle cerebral and distal (intracranial) internal carotid artery stenosis with a sensitivity of 92% and a specificity of 100%. However, this technique is insufficient to detect stenosis or occlusion in the posterior circulation, and the middle cerebral artery cannot be seen in up to one fourth of patients. TCD is capable of detecting microembolic material of both gaseous and solid states within intracranial cerebral arteries. **Spiral computed tomographic angiography** provides definition of vascular lesions; however, the preferred technique for screening patients for extracranial carotid and intracranial artery disease (including the posterior circulation) is **magnetic resonance angiography. Cerebral angiography,** the "gold standard" of vascular imaging, is performed on a case-specific basis, primarily when surgical intervention is considered or when angiographic confirmation of stenosis detected by other techniques is required. **Digital subtraction angiography** is another technique. **Oculoplethysmography** offers an indirect measure of carotid arterial blockage by measuring arterial pulsations in the retinal artery.
2. **Echocardiography** (transthoracic or transesophageal) and **24-hour Holter monitoring** are performed when an embolic process is suspected, when surgical intervention is planned, or when the stroke patient has significant risk factors for emboli (eg, atrial fibrillation, suspected infective endocarditis, prosthetic heart valve, dilated cardiomyopathy, or recent anterior myocardial infarction).
3. A **lumbar puncture** is useful when brain imaging is normal and subarachnoid hemorrhage or meningitis is suspected. Although cerebrospinal fluid is usually bloody in ventricular extension of a hypertensive hemorrhage, vascular malformation, and ruptured aneurysm, a clear tap does not guarantee absence of hemorrhage. Leukocytosis in the cerebrospinal fluid suggests infection.
4. **Electroencephalography** may show slow waves in strokes involving the cortex and is performed when seizure activity has occurred or is suspected.

III. **Treatment.** Brain attack is a medical emergency. The first step is patient education directed at encouraging patients to seek medical care as soon as symptoms develop. Initiation of diagnosis and treatment within the first few hours of onset enhances the very real chances to minimize irreversible ischemic damage and thus improve outcomes. Care in specialized stroke units has been shown to improve outcomes. Attention to rehabilitation goals begins as soon as possible after the acute event.
1. **Stabilization of the patient** involves blood pressure (BP) control, arrhythmia detection and treatment, airway protection, and, if needed, ventilatory assistance and supplementary oxygenation. Proper positioning to avoid pressure sores, diligent correction of metabolic disturbances, and skilled monitoring of stroke progression via repeated neurologic examinations are important. Continuous cardiac monitoring during the first 24 hours is advised because of the high risk of cardiac arrhythmias.
2. **Blood pressure (BP) control.** The prevention of neurologic and cardiovascular compromise caused by the extremes of BP poses a unique clinical challenge in the stroke patient. Post-stroke BP elevation usually declines spontaneously by about 10% in the first 24 hours. In fact, elevated BP can be a physiologic response to acute brain ischemia. Normalization of BP often occurs when specific effects of stroke are controlled: pain, nausea, agitation, bladder distention, increased intracranial pressure, stress of stroke, and underlying hypertension. Data supporting specific BP guidelines for treatment of post-stroke hypertension are lacking, however. Furthermore, exaggerated responses to antihypertensive drugs can cause sudden drops in BP that compromise cerebral perfusion and thus worsen neurologic status. Thus, the National Stroke Association recommends pharmacologic therapy for hypertension associated with **ischemic stroke** only for specific indications (eg, myocardial infarction or arterial dissection) or for systolic BP >219 mm Hg or diastolic BP >119 mm Hg on repeated measurements over a 30- to 60-minute period. Oral therapy is preferred. In patients with extremely elevated BP (>130 mm Hg *mean*

or >200 mm Hg systolic), cautious administration of parenteral agents is recommended by the American Heart Association's Stroke Council. The approach to BP control must take into account whether the pre-event BP was known to be normotensive or not. Additionally, patients with **hemorrhagic stroke,** after **thrombolysis** and in the **postoperative period** (eg, carotid endarterectomy or hematoma removal) require more aggressive treatment of hypertension.

B. **Reverse ischemia**

1. **Reperfusion** therapy aimed at recanalization of the affected vessel(s) in the acute stroke is a very recent advancement. Pharmacologic, angioplastic, and surgical recanalization are the current options.

   a. **Pharmacologic agents** are infused during the initial 3 hours after onset of stroke symptoms. Streptokinase has serious adverse side effects with questionable efficacy in stroke. It has not been studied in the 3-hour window. Urokinase is primarily used in angioplasty. Recombinant tissue-type plasminogen activator (tPA) is approved by the US Food and Drug Administration (FDA) for treatment of CT-proved nonhemorrhagic stroke within the first 3 hours of onset of symptoms. Studies show the sooner the intervention, the greater the chance of a good outcome. While the guidelines for choice of optimal agent, dose, rate, and delivery mechanism are evolving, the advantages of reperfusion in selected patients are a well-proved reality. Intra-arterial administration of tPA is recommended for patients with occlusions of the internal carotid, main stem middle cerebral, and basilar arteries. Intravenous tPA is best for patients with intracranial circumferential branch artery occlusions. The greatest risk of thrombolysis in acute stroke is intracerebral hemorrhage (ICH). Intensive care unit monitoring after thrombolysis includes attention to signs of ICH: decreased consciousness, headache, nausea, vomiting, and increased neurologic focal deficits. The risk of ICH is decreased by close BP (treat for systolic >185 and diastolic >110). Neither aspirin nor anticoagulation is given for the initial 24 hours after thrombolysis, and neither is initiated after that until a repeat CT scan shows no hemorrhage. Inclusion and exclusion criteria for the use of tPA are included in Table 86–2.

   b. **Angioplasty** of extracranial and intracranial vessels is an emerging treatment modality. Increasing numbers of reports of successful angioplastic intervention in acute stroke are published. The advances in imaging and increased experience with angioplasty in acute stroke are expected to allow selection of appro-

---

TABLE 86–2. TISSUE PLASMINOGEN ACTIVATOR (tPA) USE IN PATIENTS WITH STROKE

Inclusion criteria
Stroke onset of <3 hours prior to drug administration
Patient age <75 years
Normal blood glucose
Normal coagulation assays

Exclusion criteria
Recent major surgery or trauma in past 14 days
Intra-arterial needle-sticks in noncompressible sites
Computerized tomography (CT) results showing involvement of more than
   one third of the distribution of the major carotid artery
Infective endocarditis
Seizure at onset of stroke
Any evidence of blood on CT imaging
Abnormal platelet counts (<100,000/mm^3)
Elevated International normalized ratio (>1.7) or partial thromboplastin time (PTT)
Administration of heparin in the past 24 hours
Chest compression
Gastrointestinal or urinary tract hemorrhage in past 21 days
Recent myocardial infarction
Recent lumbar puncture in past 7 days
Pregnancy
Uncontrolled hypertension: systolic >185 mm Hg; diastolic >110 mm Hg

priate angioplasty candidates based on evaluation of tissue reversibility and related risk factors. Randomized and controlled trials are desirable.

c. **Carotid endarterectomy (CEA)** for ipsilateral severe (70–99%) carotid artery stenosis in symptomatic patients with recent nondisabling carotid artery ischemic events (TIA or stroke) is clearly beneficial. Based on preliminary data, it appears that delay of CEA in such patients beyond 3 days after an event merely increases their risk of recurrent stroke. CEA, which is one of the most common surgical procedures performed, is not beneficial for symptomatic patients with <30% stenosis. The potential benefit of CEA for symptomatic patients with carotid artery stenosis of 30–69% is under investigation: NASCET (North American Symptomatic Carotid Endarterectomy Trial).

Recommendation for prophylactic CEA in **asymptomatic** patients based on the AHA Guidelines for CEA is related to surgical risk. The surgeon's specific morbidity and mortality statistics are a significant factor in estimating this risk. Patient selection and postoperative management of modifiable risk factors apply as well. For asymptomatic patients with a life expectancy of at least 5 years and a surgical risk <3% ipsilateral, CEA is considered a proven benefit when stenosis is greater than 59%, regardless of plaque characteristics (eg, ulceration), contralateral carotid status, or antiplatelet therapy. Unilateral CEA is acceptable at the time of indicated coronary artery bypass grafting in asymptomatic patients whose ipsilateral carotid artery stenosis is >59%. Those whose surgical risk is >3% have no proven indication.

2. **Anticoagulation.** There is no standard of care for the use of **heparin** in the acute phase of stroke. Its use in the acute phases of TIA and nonhemorrhagic stroke is based mainly on the historic observation that evolving stroke has a poor outcome. Preliminary studies from the International Stroke Trial indicate that excess major bleeding complications may negate any benefits. The use of heparin remains a matter of preference of the treating physician. Even for patients with recent cardioembolic stroke, the data regarding the safety and efficacy of heparin are inconclusive. Heparin anticoagulation is typically considered when patients are considered to have a high risk for recurrence: high stenosis in the affected vascular territory, current antiplatelet therapy (ie, failed antiplatelet therapy), cardioembolic cause, or crescendo TIA (ie, attacks occurring with increasing frequency). Small, stable brain ischemia with arterial or cardiac cause and a high risk of worsening because of recurrent embolization or thrombus extension is treated with anticoagulation. The risk of central nervous system hemorrhage is 4% in anticoagulated patients having TIA or acute or progressive stroke. Obvious contraindications are increased risk of worsening because of intraparenchymal bleeding, active bleeding elsewhere, and uncontrolled hypertension. Strokes with increased bleeding risk are large; they may be embolic and may reveal the hypodensity of hemorrhagic transformation on early CT. **Note that the heparin bolus is NOT given in patients with acute cardioembolic stroke because of the increased risk of hemorrhagic transformation. Furthermore, after initiation of heparin therapy for stroke/TIA, avoid additional boluses of heparin; instead, adjust the rate of infusion according to the goal of partial thromboplastin time of 50–60.**

Low–molecular weight heparin used within 48 hours of onset of stroke has been shown to decrease death and dependency during the first 6 months.

3. **Cerebral edema** is a leading cause of death in the first week of stroke. Treat or avoid conditions that tend to increase intracranial pressure (ICP): fever, pain, hypoxia, agitation, fluid overload, hypercarbia, and drugs that dilate intracranial vessels. Corticosteroids are ineffective in managing brain edema secondary to stroke. The two medical modalities used to treat cerebral edema are **osmotherapy** (eg, mannitol and glycerol) and **hyperventilation therapy** in patients with markedly increased ICP. Surgical intervention (eg, decompression hemicraniectomy) is sometimes necessary to control increasing ICP.

4. **Nimodipine** is a dihydropyridine calcium channel blocker that affects mainly the central nervous system vasculature. Approved for treating cerebral ischemia associated with subarachnoid hemorrhage, nimodipine is recommended at a dosage of 60 mg orally every 4 hours for 21 days (the period of time during which neurologic deficit from vasospasm is most likely).

C. **Prevention of stroke recurrence** through secondary risk reduction is key to continued reduction of morbidity and mortality of stroke.
   1. **Risk factor modification.** BP control (mean arterial BP goal of <100 mm Hg), smoking cessation, and cardiac disease treatment are essential. Most stroke and TIA patients succumb to cardiac disease.
   2. The role of **CEA** has been discussed (see section III,B,1,c).
   3. **Long-term anticoagulation therapy** with **coumadin** (warfarin sodium) is recommended on a case-specific basis. Warfarin therapy has been shown to decrease the risk of stroke in those with atrial fibrillation associated with rheumatic valvular disease, prosthetic valve disease, and, more recently, nonvalvular atrial fibrillation. High-risk subgroups of patients with atrial fibrillation include those with hypertension, previous embolic events, structural heart disease, and older age. Younger patients with lone atrial fibrillation have low embolic rates not warranting anticoagulation, although aspirin therapy is recommended.

      Anticoagulation also results in stroke reduction in those who have had a myocardial infarction. A smaller risk reduction is seen in those who are not candidates for long-term anticoagulation therapy and who take aspirin instead. Aspirin plus low-dose warfarin therapy and very low-intensity anticoagulation are under investigation. The American College of Chest Physicians has recommended long-term warfarin therapy with an INR of 2.0–3.0 for selected patients (ie, those with atrial fibrillation with associated cardiovascular disease, thyrotoxicosis, or age over 59 years).

      Survivors of stroke who have a definite cardiac–embolic cause and those TIA patients who have surgically inaccessible lesions and remain symptomatic when taking aspirin are considered candidates as well. Anticoagulation therapy is contraindicated when cerebral embolism is associated with subacute bacterial endocarditis, in which rapid treatment of the infection is indicated instead. Therapy should generally continue at least 6–12 months or even for the patient's lifetime.
   4. **Antiplatelet therapy**
      a. **Aspirin** is currently recommended for stroke and TIA patients whether or not CEA has been performed. Although the optimum dosage has not been established, daily dosage ranges of 50–1300 mg have been studied. Randomized, prospective studies comparing four dosages are under way at the NASCET centers. Recent data raised doubt about the effectiveness of low-dose aspirin. For now, 325 mg daily is the favored dosage. Those patients at high risk for cerebral hemorrhage would be excluded. The effect of intravenous acetylsalicylic acid (aspirin) on microemboli has been evaluated by TCD.
      b. **Clopidogrel bisulfate (Plavix)** is a potent, noncompetitive inhibitor of adenosine diphosphate–induced platelet aggregation. Its irreversible effect lasts the duration of platelet life (7–10 days). It inhibits activation of the GpIIa/IIIa receptor binding site for fibrinogen, thus blocking fibrinogen-linked platelet aggregation. The Clopidogrel versus Aspirin in Patients at Risk of Ischemic Events study showed clopidogrel to be marginally more effective than aspirin at reducing secondary stroke. A dosage of 75 mg daily is recommended and monitoring of complete blood cell counts is not necessary. Side effects include: skin eruption, diarrhea, and thrombotic thrombocytopenic purpura, which can be fatal.
      c. **Ticlopidine hydrochloride** (Ticlid), 250 mg orally twice a day, is currently indicated for use in patients who are intolerant of aspirin. It inhibits platelet aggregation by interfering with fibrinogen–platelet binding and subsequent platelet interaction. Side effects include diarrhea and skin eruptions. Reversible, absolute neutropenia is an uncommon but serious side effect of ticlopidine. Weekly monitoring of white blood cell counts is necessary within the first few months of starting ticlopidine. Ticlopidine offered a 21% relative risk reduction for recurrent stroke compared with aspirin at the end of 3 years in the Ticlopidine/Aspirin Stroke Study.
      d. **Dipyridamole** (Persantine) has been studied in a capsule form combined with aspirin twice daily (Aggrenox, 200 mg dipyridamole with 25 mg aspirin). In the European Stroke Prevention Study, the combined capsule was studied compared with aspirin alone and with dipyridamole alone for second stroke prevention in patients with recent completed ischemic stroke or TIA. The capsule showed an additive effect for marked reduction in re-stroke (37% decreased risk vs. aspirin (18%) or dipyridamole (16%)). FDA approval is expected for this

combination capsule. Dipyridamole prevents clot formation by inhibition of platelet activation and aggregation.

5. **A number of studies of cholesterol-lowering medications** have shown substantial reduction in incidence of stroke. Two statins have been approved by the FDA for prevention of first stroke or TIA in coronary artery disease. Pravastatin (Pravachol) is approved for patients with average cholesterol (<240) and a personal history of heart disease. Simvastatin (Zocor) is approved in patients with high cholesterol and coronary artery disease. (See Chapter 75 on dyslipidemias.)

6. **Blood pressure control** to <140/90 (or 130/85 in patients with renal insufficiency or heart failure; <130/80 in patients with diabetes mellitus) is another important treatment goal that impacts future stroke risk. While most hypertension treatment has focused on cardiac end points, trials have demonstrated secondary stroke risk reduction. The Heart Outcomes Prevention Evaluation (HOPE) demonstrated the benefit of angiotensin-converting enzyme inhibitors. The PROGRESS trial demonstrated the benefit of combination diuretics plus ACE. The losartan intervention for endpoint (LIFE) trial has found significant risk reduction with the use of angiotensin II receptor blockers.

7. **Antioxidant therapy** is under investigation for prevention and treatment of stroke (see discussion above).

IV. **Management Strategies.** Stroke indicates generalized vascular disease; it is one event in a prolonged and ongoing process. Management strategies center on prevention of further manifestations of the disease and maximization of post-stroke function during the three stages of stroke.

A. **Stage I.** The **acute stage** of stroke spans the first week. Attention to evaluation, maintenance, and return of function includes passive range of motion of extremities, proper positioning, frequent turning, and maintenance of good hygiene.

B. **Stage II.** The **subacute stage** of stroke usually lasts 3 months. Return of neurologic function is greatest during this interval. **Rehabilitation** involves interdisciplinary assessment and treatment by a team of nurses, physical therapists, occupational therapists, speech therapists, a dietitian, and the physician to maximize functional return and independence. Selection of the site of rehabilitation (eg, a formal rehabilitation unit, a skilled nursing home, the patient's home with home health care agency coordination, or outpatient facilities) depends on the patient's medical condition, the family situation (supports and weaknesses), financial considerations, and available resources. To benefit from any kind of rehabilitation, the patient must be able to communicate (verbally or nonverbally), follow a two- to three-step command, and remember what is learned. Rehabilitation units require that a patient's cardiopulmonary endurance allows 2–3 hours of intense therapy daily. Patients with marked dementia, severe chronic obstructive pulmonary disease, marked limitation of cardiovascular reserve, or severely debilitating multiple joint disease are not likely to benefit from acute inpatient rehabilitation, although such patients may receive benefit from skilled or subacute care in the immediate posthospitalization period.

C. **Stage III.** The **chronic stage** of stroke recovery begins after 3 months. Neurologic return may continue for as long as 1 year after an event and functional recovery can occur for as long as 2 years. Maintenance of the functional gains achieved in the subacute stage is important.

1. **Involvement of the family or caregiver** in the acute and intermediate phases of stroke care enhances their knowledge and expectations regarding the patient's condition. Careful coordination of patient and family involvement with discharge planning involves family or caregiver teaching sessions with the patient and with each of the patient's regular therapists and team nurse.

2. **Home health care agency involvement** allows for smooth transition and capable problem solving as the patient returns home.

3. **Monitoring of the patient by the physician** at regular intervals is important to assess and promote risk management strategies, identify and treat complicating illness (eg, depression), evaluate recurrence of symptoms, assess functional status (Barthel index [Table 86–3]), negotiate potential blocks to maintenance of function, and facilitate the patient's acceptance of disability.

V. **Prognosis.** Overall, the vast majority of initially alert patients survive the acute phase of stroke. Acute-phase deaths are generally due to cerebral causes related to irreversible failure of vital function of the brain stem. Pulmonary embolism and cardiac events contribute to

TABLE 86-3. BARTHEL INDEX

A score above 60 usually means that < 2 hours of personal care assistance is required each day. A score of 60 or less indicates that 4 or more hours of personal care assistance is needed daily. A score of 0 is given when a criterion cannot be met.

Functional activity
1. Feeding
   - 5 Dependent
   - 10 Independent
2. Transfer from bed to wheelchair, back to bed (includes sitting up in bed)
   - 5 Assisted out of bed only
   - 10 Needs some help/cueing
   - 15 Independent
3. Grooming (wash face; comb hair; shave, including preparing razor; clean teeth; and apply own make-up if worn)
   - 0 Dependent
   - 5 Independent
4. Toileting (transfer on/off toilet, handling clothing, wiping, and flushing)
   - 5 Dependent
   - 10 Independent
5. Bathing (tub, shower, or complete sponge bath)
   - 0 Dependent
   - 5 Independent
6. Ambulation, 50 yards, level surface
   - 0 Totally dependent
   - 5 Dependent on wheelchair but able to propel
   - 10 Able to walk with assistive device
   - 15 Able to walk without assistive device

Unable to walk (eg, wheeled walker or wheelchair required)
   - (5)
7. Ascending/descending stairs (mechanical assistive devices allowed)
   - 5 Dependent
   - 10 Independent
8. Dressing (includes tying shoes and donning assistive devices; excludes nonprescribed girdles or bras)
   - 5 Dependent
   - 10 Independent
9. Bowel continence (suppository, enema allowed)
   - 5 Dependent
   - 10 Independent
10. Urinary continence
   - 5 Dependent
   - 10 Independent

Modified with permission from Mahoney FI, Barthel DW: Functional evaluation: The Barthel index. Md Med J 1965;**14**:61.

early mortality in stroke patients. Systemic causes (eg, pneumonia, pulmonary embolism, ischemic heart disease, or recurrent stroke) are the usual causes of death in the subacute and chronic phases. The risk of recurrence of stroke is substantial. The major complications of stroke are aspiration, infection (eg, urinary tract infection or pneumonia), pressure sores, corneal abrasion, and depression. Third-nerve palsy (signaling uncal herniation), increased age of the patient, and hemorrhagic events are associated with grave immediate prognoses. In hemorrhagic events, the prognosis for total unilateral motor deficit and coma is poor. Brainstem infarctions such as pontine hemorrhages have an extremely poor prognosis. Lacunar infarctions involve subcortical small vessels and have the lowest mortality rate of all strokes.

REFERENCES

Albers GW, et al: Intravenous tissue-type plasminogen activator for treatment of acute stroke: The STARS study. JAMA 2000;**283**:1145.

Anderson CA: Evaluation and management of transient ischemic attack. Primary Care Case Reviews 2000;**3**:36.

Biller J, et al: Guidelines for carotid endarterectomy: A statement for health care professionals from a special writing group of The Stroke Council, American Heart Association. Stroke 1998;**29**:554.

Bravata DM, et al: Thrombolysis for acute stroke in routine clinical practice. Arch Neurol 2002;**162**:1994.

Goertler M, et al: Rapid decline of cerebral microemboli of arterial origin after intravenous acetylsalicylic acid. Stroke 1999;**30**:66.

Macko RF, et al: Elevated tissue plasminogen activator antigen and stroke risk: The stroke prevention in young women study. Stroke 1999;**30**:7.

Ueda T, et al: Angioplasty after intra-arterial thrombolysis for acute occlusion of intracranial arteries. Stroke 1998;**29**:2568.

ELECTRONIC RESOURCES

www.amhrt.org is the web site for the American Heart Association. Three times a year, STROKE, a publication of AHA, publishes a synopsis of the current ongoing multicenter trials related to stroke. www.ninds.nih.gov is the National Institute of Neurologic Disorders and Stroke (NIH) web site. www.stroke.org is the web site for the National Stroke Association.

---

87   Thyroid Disease

Stephen F. Wheeler, MEng, MD

KEY POINTS

- A sensitive thyroid-stimulating hormone assay (sTSH) is the best single screening test for both hypothyroidism and hyperthyroidism.
- Levothyroxine, usually begun at the full estimated replacement dose (average 125 µg/day) in patients younger than 50 years without cardiac disease, is the treatment of choice for hypothyroidism. In older patients and those with known or suspected cardiac disease, an initial dose of 12.5–50 µg/day is indicated.
- Radioactive iodine (^{123}I) uptake can help clarify hyperthyroidism of uncertain etiology.
- Oral radioactive iodine (^{131}I) is the treatment of choice for most patients with hyperthyroidism in the United States, but antithyroid drugs and surgery are appropriate in selected patients.
- The evaluation of a thyroid nodule usually begins with sTSH and a fine-needle aspiration biopsy.

I. Introduction

  A. Physiology. Thyrotropin-releasing hormone, secreted by the hypothalamus, stimulates the anterior pituitary to produce thyroid-stimulating hormone (TSH). The major hormone released by the thyroid gland in response to TSH is thyroxine (T_4), which is converted peripherally to triiodothyronine (T_3), a more potent hormone. T_4 and T_3 are both highly but reversibly bound to plasma thyroid-binding globulin (TBG) and, to a lesser extent, to albumin and prealbumin. Only the minute unbound (free) fractions are metabolically active. The most sensitive indicator of thyroid status is the level of TSH, which is controlled in classic negative-feedback fashion by the concentration of unbound thyroid hormones.

  B. Laboratory tests. Diagnosis of thyroid disease depends on symptoms, clinical signs, and laboratory tests, and thyroid function tests are most accurately interpreted in conjunction with appropriate clinical data.

   1. Sensitive TSH (sTSH). The inverse log/linear relationship between sTSH and unbound T_4 (free T_4) means that sTSH will always be more sensitive than free T_4 at indicating thyroid function. Thus, a normal sTSH, except in rare instances, excludes both hypothyroidism and hyperthyroidism. Clinically useful sensitive assays for TSH reliably measure concentrations of 0.02 mIU/L or less.

   a. In addition to hyperthyroidism, sTSH may be **suppressed** by severe nonthyroidal illness, use of dopamine, and glucocorticoid therapy. Also, sTSH may be suppressed in some euthyroid elderly patients.

   b. sTSH may be mildly **elevated** during recovery from severe nonthyroidal illness, by various drugs, including lithium and amphetamines, and in some euthyroid elderly patients.

2. **Serum total T_4 (T_4) and total T_3 (T_3).** These tests measure both protein-bound and free hormone by radioimmunoassay and are affected by changes in the concentration of thyroid-binding proteins.
3. **T_3 resin uptake (T_3 RU).** A laboratory assessment of the protein binding of both T_4 and T_3, T_3 RU is **not** a measure of circulating T_3 levels. Rather, it is inversely proportional to the unsaturated hormone binding sites on TBG and is most useful in helping to interpret a given level of T_4.
4. **Free thyroxine index (FTI)** is the product of T_4 and T_3 RU and provides an **estimate** of free T_4 by adjusting for variations in total hormone concentration secondary to altered protein binding.
5. **Free T_4,** measured directly and reliably, is now commonly used for the routine diagnostic evaluation of thyroid disease. Severe or chronic nonthyroidal illness, which affects other types of free T_4 assays, has historically been the major indication for this test. Direct measurement of free T_3 is also available.

C. **Diagnostic evaluation versus screening**
1. Table 87–1 lists the most common symptoms and signs of hypothyroidism according to frequency.

TABLE 87–1. SYMPTOMS AND SIGNS OF HYPOTHYROIDISM

Symptom or Sign	Percent of Cases
Weakness	99
Dry skin	97
Coarse skin	97
Lethargy	91
Slow speech	91
Edema of eyelids	90
Sensation of cold	89
Decreased sweating	89
Cold skin	83
Thick tongue	82
Edema of face	79
Coarseness of hair	76
Cardiac enlargement (x-ray)	68
Pallor of skin	67
Memory impairment	66
Constipation	61
Gain in weight	59
Loss of hair	57
Pallor of lips	57
Dyspnea	55
Peripheral edema	55
Hoarseness	52
Anorexia	45
Nervousness	35
Menorrhagia	32[1]
Palpitation	31
Deafness	30
Poor heart sounds	30
Precordial pain	25
Poor vision	24
Fundus oculi changes	20
Dysmenorrhea	18[1]
Loss of weight	13
Atrophic tongue	12
Emotional instability	11
Choking sensation	9
Fineness of hair	9
Cyanosis	7
Dysphagia	3

[1] In 41 premenopausal women.
Adapted from DeGroot LJ: *The Thyroid and Its Diseases.* John Wiley & Sons; 1984.

2. Table 87–2 lists the most common clinical findings of hyperthyroidism according to frequency.
3. **Diagnostic evaluation** of patients with signs and symptoms suggestive of thyroid dysfunction often requires multiple specific tests, beginning with sTSH and free T_4. Further work-up depends on the clinical situation and the initial laboratory results.
4. **Screening** patients at low risk of having thyroid disease is controversial. However, certain populations are at higher risk of having overt but unrecognized illness. **Suspect populations** include newborns; postpartum women 4–8 weeks after delivery; persons with a family history of thyroid disease; patients with dyslipidemias; women older than 50 years; and patients with immunologically mediated diseases such as Addison's disease, insulin-dependent diabetes mellitus, and rheumatoid arthritis. The initial screening test of choice is sTSH, with follow-up of abnormal values using free T_4 and other tests as indicated.

II. Hypothyroidism

A. Introduction. Hypothyroidism results from insufficient production of thyroid hormones. Overt hypothyroidism is found in 1–3% of the general population. It is at least twice as common in females as in males and prevalence increases progressively with age.

1. **Primary hypothyroidism,** most commonly from chronic autoimmune (Hashimoto's) thyroiditis, radioactive iodine therapy, or surgery, accounts for the overwhelming majority of hypothyroidism cases. A high sTSH and a low free T_4 are indicative of primary hypothyroidism.
2. **Secondary hypothyroidism** results from decreased pituitary secretion of TSH. This condition is usually accompanied by other manifestations of pituitary hyposecretion. Causes include postpartum pituitary necrosis (Sheehan's syndrome) and pituitary tumors.

B. Diagnosis

1. In a patient with suggestive signs and symptoms, a high sTSH (>15 μU/mL) and a low free T_4 are diagnostic of primary hypothyroidism. When autoimmune thyroiditis

TABLE 87–2. SYMPTOMS AND SIGNS OF HYPERTHYROIDISM

Symptom or Sign	Percent of Cases
Goiter	87
Dyspnea on exertion	81
Tiredness	80
Hot hands	76
Palpitation	75
Preference for cold	73
Hands sweating	72
Excessive sweating	68
Regular pulse rate: over 90 bpm	68
Finger tremor	66
Lid lag	62
Nervousness	59
Weight loss	52
Goiter, diffuse enlargement of thyroid gland	49
Hyperkinesis	39
Exophthalmos	34
Goiter, nodular	32
Increased appetite	32
Auricular fibrillation	19
Scant menses	18
Constipation	15
Diminished appetite	13
Diarrhea	8
Weight gain	4
Goiter, single adenoma	4
Excessive menses	3

Adapted from Wayne EJ: The diagnosis of thyrotoxicosis. Br Med J 1954;**1**:411.

is the presumptive cause, confirmation with a serum antithyroid peroxidase level (formerly called antimicrosomal antibody) may be helpful.

2. In the setting of overt hypothyroidism, a sTSH that is normal or only mildly elevated suggests secondary hypothyroidism. Concurrent amenorrhea, galactorrhea, postural hypotension, loss of axillary and pubic hair, and visual field deficits may be present.

C. **Treatment**

1. **Levothyroxine** is preferred for routine replacement therapy. Interchangeability studies of levothyroxine products have not shown significant fluctuations in hormone levels when switching among name-brand or generic preparations. Current evidence does not support the use of combinations of levothyroxine and T_3 for replacement therapy.

2. Adults require approximately 1.7 µg/kg/day for full replacement, with an average maintenance dose of 125 µg/day. Older patients may need <1 µg/kg/day. Therapy is usually initiated with the full replacement dose in patients younger than 50 years. In patients older than 50 years, or in younger patients with known or suspected cardiac disease, a lower initial dose of 12.5–50 µg/day is indicated.

3. Clinical and biochemical **re-evaluation** at 6- to 8-week intervals is necessary until the levothyroxine dose has been titrated to produce a normalized sTSH. Subsequently, an interim history and physical examination pertinent to thyroid status and a sTSH should be performed at least annually.

4. **Drugs** such as cholestyramine, ferrous sulfate, sucralfate, and antacids containing aluminum hydroxide may interfere with levothyroxine absorption. Other drugs, such as phenytoin, carbamazepine, and rifampin, may accelerate levothyroxine metabolism, necessitating higher replacement doses.

D. **Subclinical hypothyroidism**

1. **Introduction.** Subclinical hypothyroidism is distinguished by an elevated sTSH, a normal free T_4, and few, if any, hypothyroid symptoms. As many as 15% of geriatric patients, as well as many younger adults, meet these criteria. Generally, women show a higher prevalence than men.

2. **Clinical course.** Subclinical hypothyroidism does not always progress to overt hypothyroidism. Risk factors for progression include the presence of thyroid autoantibodies, age older than 65 years, female gender, and a higher sTSH level ($\geq$10 µU/mL). Patients who do not progress are considered to be euthyroid with a reset thyrostat, probably because of a subtle insult to the thyroid gland.

3. **Treatment** must be individualized, based on risk factors for progression and the presence of subtle symptoms and signs, including elevated lipids. In some patients, levothyroxine may ameliorate vague symptoms or those attributed to other sources. Patients **not treated** should be monitored clinically and biochemically at yearly intervals for evidence of progressive thyroid dysfunction.

III. **Hyperthyroidism**

A. **Introduction.** Hyperthyroidism results from elevated levels of thyroid hormones.

Hyperthyroidism is less common than hypothyroidism in the general population. Community-based studies have found prevalences of 1.9% in women and 0.16% in men. Approximately 15% of cases occur in persons older than 60 years. Graves' disease, which accounts for about 90% of hyperthyroidism in those younger than 40 years, demonstrates a familial predisposition.

Hyperthyroidism encompasses a heterogeneous group of disorders.

1. **Graves' disease** is an autoimmune disease that results from the action of thyroid-stimulating immunoglobulin G antibody (TS Ab) on thyroid gland TSH receptors.

2. **Toxic multinodular goiter (Plummer's disease),** the most common cause of hyperthyroidism in those older than 40 years, occurs when a patient with nontoxic multinodular goiter develops one or more autonomous hyperfunctioning nodules.

3. **Toxic adenoma,** the least common cause of hyperthyroidism, is produced by one or more hyperfunctioning thyroid adenomas capable of functioning independently of TSH or other thyroid stimulators.

4. **Thyroiditis** may produce transient hyperthyroidism as hormone leaks from an inflamed gland. Transient hypothyroidism often follows as the intrathyroidal stores of hormone are depleted.

B. **Diagnosis**

1. In a patient with suggestive signs and symptoms, a suppressed sTSH and an elevated free T_4 level are diagnostic of hyperthyroidism. In a clinically hyperthyroid

patient with a suppressed sTSH and a normal free T_4 level, T_3 or free T_3 should be measured to evaluate for possible T_3 thyrotoxicosis.

2. The **history** and the **physical examination** are critical to distinguish among the causes of hyperthyroidism (Table 87–3).

3. **Radioactive iodine (^{123}I) uptake** can help clarify hyperthyroidism of uncertain origin. Diffuse increase in ^{123}I uptake is consistent with Graves' disease, whereas nodular concentration indicates toxic adenoma or multinodular goiter. If ^{123}I uptake is decreased, a serum **thyroglobulin** measurement can distinguish between exogenous (factitious) hyperthyroxinemia (thyroglobulin decreased) and thyroiditis, iodine-induced thyrotoxicosis, or struma ovarii (thyroglobulin increased).

C. **Therapeutic modalities**

1. The **antithyroid drugs (ATDs)** methimazole and propylthiouracil (PTU) inhibit thyroid hormone synthesis. PTU also inhibits peripheral conversion of T_4 to T_3. ATDs suppress thyroid autoantibodies, decrease TS Ab, and lead to remission in 37–70% of patients with Graves' disease treated for 1–2 years. The addition of levothyroxine to ATD therapy has not been shown to improve remission rates.

   a. The usual starting doses are 10–30 mg/day for methimazole and 100–150 mg three times daily for PTU. If there is no decrease in free T_4 in 4–8 weeks, the dose should be increased. Doses as high as 60–90 mg/day of methimazole and 300 mg three or four times daily of PTU may be required to normalize thyroid function. TSH may remain suppressed for several months after thyroid hormone levels normalize.

   b. Once euthyroidism is achieved (usually within 6–8 weeks), the dose can be titrated down to maintain euthyroidism. Typical maintenance doses are 100–200 mg PTU or 10–20 mg methimazole daily.

   c. Most clinicians treat patients for 12–24 months before attempting to withdraw antithyroid therapy. ATDs more commonly induce long-lasting remissions in older patients with mild disease and small goiters. Males, patients younger than 40 years, and those with ophthalmopathy or high serum TS Ab concentrations at the time of diagnosis are less likely to permanently remit. Overall, 33–50% of those who respond will relapse.

   d. Adverse reactions, which are encountered in 1–5% of patients taking ATDs, include rash, itching, fever, arthralgias, and hepatic abnormalities. The most serious reaction to ATDs is agranulocytosis, which occurs in up to 0.3% of patients. Onset is usually within 2 months and rarely after 4 months. Most physicians do not obtain routine leukocyte counts, but this is controversial. Certainly, all patients developing fever, chills, jaundice, sore throat, or bleeding gums should stop taking the drug immediately and contact their physician for appropriate evaluation, including a complete blood count with differential.

2. **Radioactive iodine (RAI, ^{131}I),** usually administered orally, concentrates in the thyroid gland, where it destroys follicular cells. It is the hyperthyroidism treatment of choice for most patients in the United States.

   a. A single dose permanently controls hyperthyroidism in about 90% of patients. If symptomatic hyperthyroidism persists 3–6 months after therapy, a second ^{131}I treatment is given.

TABLE 87–3. DIAGNOSIS OF HYPERTHYROIDISM

Gland Size	Nodule	Tender	Other Findings	Suggested Diagnosis
I	0	NT	Proptosis; pretibial myxedema; thyroid bruit in 50%	Graves' disease
I	0	T	Recent viral illness in many	Subacute thyroiditis
Modest I	0	NT	Some postpartum	Silent thyroiditis (consider Hashimoto's thyroiditis)
I	Multiple	NT		Toxic multinodular goiter (consider Hashimoto's thyroiditis)
D	0	NT		Consider extrathyroid source
D	Single	NT		Toxic adenoma

D, decreased; I, increased; NT, nontender; T, tender.

      b. RAI exerts its full effect over a 2- to 3-month period. Follow-up at 4- to 6-week intervals to measure free T_4 and assess clinical response is appropriate until thyroid function stabilizes within the normal range or hypothyroidism ensues.

      c. The most common complication of therapy is the early or late development of hypothyroidism. Thyroid replacement therapy should be initiated as the free T_4 and sTSH pass from normal into the hypothyroid range. The end point of replacement is a normal sTSH.

      d. RAI is contraindicated during pregnancy, and it is usually advised that pregnancy be postponed 4–6 months following therapy. Treatment with ^{131}I does not cause cancer or infertility and has not been shown to produce ill effects in subsequent children of those so treated.

   3. Surgery for hyperthyroidism has declined in popularity because of the effectiveness of ATDs and [131]I.

      a. Specific indications include patients unwilling or unable to take ATDs or to be treated with ^{131}I, as well as those with neck obstruction, very large goiters that may be relatively resistant to ^{131}I, or cosmetic concerns.

      b. Any patient undergoing surgery for hyperthyroidism should be pretreated with methimazole until euthyroid status is attained. Iodides are added in the week prior to surgery in Graves' disease patients to reduce thyroid vascularity. Alternative regimens using various combinations of methimazole, potassium iodide, and a β-adrenergic antagonist are also effective at reducing postoperative thyrotoxic crisis.

      c. Complications of surgery depend on the skill and experience of the surgical and anesthesiology teams. Potential complications are transient hypocalcemia, transient hypothyroidism, thyroid crisis, permanent hypoparathyroidism, recurrent laryngeal nerve damage, and postoperative hemorrhage. The mortality rate for elective surgery is close to 0%, and the rate of complications is reported to be less than 4%.

      d. Recurrent hyperthyroidism occurs in at least 10% of patients who are treated surgically. Permanent hypothyroidism occurs in 5% of patients within the first year, and subsequently in 1–2% of patients per year. Up to 50% of patients are hypothyroid 25 years after surgery.

   4. Adjunctive medical therapies are useful for relieving symptoms in patients undergoing definitive therapy with other agents or in those with transient forms of hyperthyroidism.

      a. β-Adrenergic antagonists provide prompt symptomatic relief of the hyperadrenergic manifestations of hyperthyroidism. Propranolol is the most widely used beta blocker for this purpose. Initial doses of 10–20 mg four times daily are adjusted to control tachycardia and symptoms. In most cases, a dose of 80–320 mg/day is sufficient. Hyperthyroid patients relatively resistant to the effects of beta blockers may require higher and more frequent doses.

      b. Calcium channel blockers such as diltiazem or verapamil may be used in patients who cannot tolerate, or have contraindications to, beta-blockers.

D. Choice of therapy

   1. Graves' disease

      a. RAI is the treatment of choice for most elderly patients.

      b. For children and adolescents, ATDs have commonly been recommended for initial therapy, with surgery or RAI reserved for patients who either fail ATD therapy or experience complications. However, the high failure rate of ATDs and the efficacy and apparent safety of RAI have prompted increasing use of RAI in this age group.

      c. The treatment of young adults is also controversial. Specific patient characteristics, along with the risks and benefits of each treatment, should be considered. In young women with this condition who are anticipating pregnancy, RAI is often preferred to obviate future concern about ATDs causing fetal goiter or hypothyroidism.

      d. RAI therapy may exacerbate **ophthalmopathy** in Graves' disease, especially in smokers. This exacerbation is often transient and can be prevented by prednisone (40 mg/day, with the dose tapered to zero over a period of 3 months). Usually, however, only simple measures (avoidance of bright light and dust, sleeping with head raised, artificial tears, eye ointment at night) are needed to treat mild to moderate ophthalmopathy. Although it is controversial, some physicians substitute ATDs for RAI in patients with active eye disease, until pertinent signs and symptoms stabilize. Avoidance of clinical hypothyroidism after therapy may also be important in minimizing subsequent eye abnormalities. Aggressive treatment with high-dose glucocorticoids, in consultation with an ophthalmologist experienced in the treatment of orbital disease, can also be considered for progressive and severe ophthalmopathy.

2. **Toxic multinodular goiter.** There are no spontaneous remissions of hyperthyroidism resulting from nodular thyroid disease. RAI is usually the treatment of choice. Surgery may be appropriate for very large goiters, if there is concern about thyroid cancer, or in children, adolescents, or young adults. ATDs are valuable as pretreatment before thyroid surgery and before or after RAI in elderly patients and those with concurrent health problems.

3. **Toxic adenoma.** RAI is usually the treatment of choice. Surgical removal may be appropriate in young patients.

4. **Thyroiditis** produces only transient hyperthyroidism, so treatment focuses on symptom control with beta blockers and other adjunctive medical therapies. Mild inflammatory symptoms and pain can usually be controlled with nonsteroidal anti-inflammatory drugs or salicylates. Severe symptoms respond to prednisone, 20–40 mg/day. Transient hypothyroidism may follow the initial hyperthyroid phase and may be symptomatic enough to warrant levothyroxine therapy.

E. **Subclinical hyperthyroidism**
   1. **Introduction.** Subclinical hyperthyroidism is distinguished by a low or undetectable sTSH and normal free T_4, T_3, and free T_3 in an asymptomatic person.
      a. Subclinical hyperthyroidism is more common than overt hyperthyroidism among the elderly. Various studies have shown a prevalence of 4–12%. Excluding patients receiving thyroid hormone therapy, 0.9–1.9% of older persons meet these criteria.
      b. Excessive thyroid hormone replacement is the most common cause. Other important causes include nodular thyroid disease, subclinical Graves' disease, and thyroiditis.
      c. Factors that can suppress sTSH levels, such as severe illness, high-dose glucocorticoids, dopamine, and pituitary dysfunction, should be excluded.
      d. Laboratory findings consistent with subclinical hyperthyroidism can be a normal variant in the elderly.
   2. **Clinical course.** Subclinical hyperthyroidism often disappears, and progression to overt hyperthyroidism is uncommon. However, it does increase the risk for atrial fibrillation and may increase the risk for other atrial arrhythmias, left ventricular hypertrophy, muscle weakness, neuropsychological dysfunction, and accelerated bone loss.
   3. **Treatment**
      a. If excessive hormone replacement is the cause, the dose should be reduced.
      b. If subclinical hyperthyroidism is associated with nodular thyroid disease, subclinical Graves' disease, arrhythmias, other cardiac disorders, or accelerated bone loss, antithyroid treatment should be seriously considered.
      c. In patients not meeting the above criteria, careful follow-up is acceptable.

IV. **Thyroid nodules**
A. **Introduction**
   1. Palpable nodules are present in 4–7% of adults. However, physical examination is relatively insensitive, and up to 50% of patients demonstrate thyroid nodules by ultrasonography or at autopsy. Prevalence is four to nine times greater in women than in men. Approximately 5% of all solitary nodules are carcinomas.
   2. Prior radiation exposure increases the rate of development of both benign and malignant new nodules to about 2% per year. Peak incidence is 15–25 years after exposure.
   3. Up to 35% of glands examined at surgery or autopsy contain tiny, clinically unimportant papillary carcinomas.
   4. Since similar frequencies of cancer have been found in patients who have solitary or multiple nodules on palpation, dominant nodules in multinodular glands should also be considered for diagnostic evaluation.
B. **Thyroid cancer risk factors**
   1. **Family history** of familial goiter, medullary or papillary cancer, or familial polyposis.
   2. **Personal history** of prior head and neck radiation exposure. Childhood exposures increase thyroid cancer risk 10-fold.

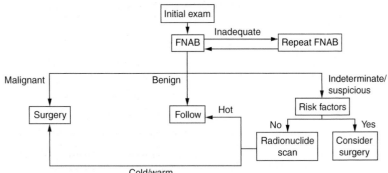

FIGURE 87-1. Treatment of a solitary or dominant thyroid nodule. FNAB, Fine-needle aspiration biopsy.

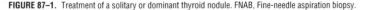

3. **Physical findings** suggestive of cancer are nodule size > than 4 cm, recurrence of cystic nodules after aspiration, progressive or rapid growth, firmness, fixation to surrounding structures, local lymphadenopathy, and hoarseness.

4. **Other risk factors** include age younger than 20 years or older than 60 years and male gender.

C. **Diagnostic and management strategies**

1. A thorough **history** and **physical examination** should focus on thyroid cancer risk factors.

2. Serum **sTSH** identifies patients with unsuspected thyroid dysfunction. Other tests may be beneficial in specific settings: free T$_4$ if sTSH is abnormal; serum antithyroid peroxidase if sTSH is elevated; basal serum calcitonin if there is a family history of medullary thyroid cancer or multiple endocrine neoplasia, type II.

3. **Fine-needle aspiration biopsy (FNAB)** should be the initial test in most patients. It is safe and inexpensive and more effectively selects patients for surgery than any other test. FNAB has reduced the number of patients undergoing thyroid surgery by 25–50%, increased the yield of carcinoma in those who do have surgery from 15% to 30–40%, and decreased the cost of care by 25%.

4. An algorithm for the evaluation and management of nodular thyroid disease is displayed in Figure 87-1. Follow-up of thyroid nodules not surgically explored should include clinical examination with palpation and consideration of repeat FNAB. Thyroid ultrasonography and sTSH may also be helpful in following selected patients.

5. **Thyroid hormone suppression** has been used routinely in the past in both the diagnosis and treatment of thyroid nodules. Recent controlled trials have not shown it to be efficacious for these purposes. If suppressive therapy is considered, the risks associated with subclinical hyperthyroidism must be included in the risk–benefit analysis.

REFERENCES

American Association of Clinical Endocrinologists (AACE) Thyroid Task Force: *AACE Medical Guidelines for Clinical Practice for the Evaluation and Treatment of Hyperthyroidism and Hypothyroidism.* Endocr Pract 2002;**8:**457.

American Association of Clinical Endocrinologists (AACE) and American College of Endocrinology: *AACE Clinical Practice Guidelines for the Diagnosis and Management of Thyroid Nodules.* Endocr Pract 1996;**2:**78.

Hefland M, Redfern CC: Screening for thyroid disease: An update. Ann Intern Med 1998;**129:**144.

Landerson PW, et al: American Thyroid Association guidelines for detection of thyroid dysfunction. Arch Intern Med 2000;**160:**1573.

Singer PA, et al: Treatment guidelines for patients with thyroid nodules and well-differentiated thyroid cancer. Arch Intern Med 1996;**156:**2165.

Woeber KA: Update on the management of hyperthyroidism and hypothyroidism. Arch Intern Med 2000;**160:**1067.

SECTION III. Psychiatric Disorders

88 Alcohol & Drug Abuse

Robert Mallin, MD

KEY POINTS

- The diagnosis of substance use disorders is most typically begun with a screening test that identifies a user at risk. The CAGE questionnaire (Table 88–1) is perhaps the most widely used screening tool for the identification of patients at risk for substance use disorders. When answering yes to two or more questions on the CAGE, the sensitivity is 60–90% and the specificity 40–60% for substance use disorders. Because a screening test is more predictive when applied to a population more likely to have a disease, clinical clues (Table 88–2) to substance use disorders may be useful to determine whom to screen. Once the patient screens positive for a substance use problem, the question becomes, Is it abuse or dependence?
- Substance abuse is a pattern of misuse during which the patient maintains control, whereas in substance dependence, control over use is lost. Physiologic dependence, evidenced by a withdrawal syndrome, may exist in either state (see Tables 88–3 and 88–4 for the diagnostic criteria for substance abuse and dependence). The primary means by which the diagnosis of substance abuse or dependence is made, then, is a careful history. Although substance-disordered patients may be consciously less than truthful in their history, more often the defense mechanism of denial is what prevents the patient from seeing the connection between substance use and consequences.
- Biochemical markers may help support the diagnostic criteria gathered in the history, or can be used as a screening mechanism to consider patients for further evaluation (Table 88–5).
- There is a strong relationship between the time and intensity spent in alcohol and drug treatment and success at remaining abstinent.
- The prognosis for professionals who participate in a monitoring program after treatment is better than nonprofessionals.

I. Introduction

A. The prevalence of alcohol and drug disorders in primary care outpatients is between 23% and 37%. The high prevalence of these disorders in primary care outpatients suggests that family physicians are confronted with these problems daily. These disorders rarely present overtly, however. Patients in denial about the connection between their substance use and the consequences caused by it frequently minimize the amount of their use and often do not seek assistance for their substance problem.

B. The epidemiology of alcohol and drug disorders has been well studied and is most often reported from data of the National Institute of Mental Health Epidemiologic Catchment Area Program (ECA). Lifetime prevalence rates for alcohol disorders from the ECA survey data were 13.5%. For men, the lifetime prevalence was found to be 23.8%, and for women, 4.7%. The National Comorbidity Survey revealed lifetime prevalence of alcohol abuse without dependence to be 12.5% for males and 6.4% for females. For alcohol dependence, males' lifetime prevalence as 20.1% and females', 8.2%. The ECA data yield an overall prevalence of drug use disorders to be 6.2%. As with alcohol use disorders, drug use disorders occur more frequently in men (lifetime prevalence 7.7%) than in women (4.8%). Characteristics known to influence the epidemiology of substance use disorders include gender, age, family history, marital status, employment status, and occupation/educational status. Males have a higher risk than females, substance use disorders become less frequent with age, the risk of alcoholism for the child of an alcoholic is approximately 50%, single persons have a higher risk than married, and the unemployed and less educated have a higher risk.

C. The difference between abuse and dependence is an important one. With substance abuse, the patient retains control of their use. This control may be affected by poor judgment and social and environmental factors and mitigated by the consequences of their

TABLE 88–1. CAGE QUESTIONS ADAPTED TO INCLUDE DRUGS

1. Have you felt you ought to **C**ut down on your drinking or drug use?
2. Have people **A**nnoyed you by criticizing your drinking or drug use?
3. Have you felt **G**uilty about your drinking or drug use?
4. Have you ever had a drink, or used drugs first thing in the morning to steady your nerves or to get rid of a hangover or to get the day started? (**E**ye-opener)

Two or more yes answers indicates a need for a more in-depth assessment. Even one positive response should raise a red flag about problem drinking or drug use.
Adapted from Schulz JE, Parran T Jr: Principles of identification and intervention. In: Graham AW, Shultz TK (editors). *Principles of Addiction Medicine*, 2nd ed. American Society of Addiction Medicine; 1998:249.

TABLE 88–2. CLINICAL CLUES TO ALCOHOL AND DRUG PROBLEMS

Social history
Arrest for driving under the influence
Loss of job or sent home from work for alcohol or drug reasons
Domestic violence
Child abuse/neglect
Family instability (divorce, separation)
Frequent, unplanned absences
Personal isolation
Problems at work/school
Mood swings

Medical history
History of addiction to any drug
Withdrawal syndrome
Depression
Anxiety disorder
Recurrent pancreatitis
Recurrent hepatitis
Hepatomegaly
Peripheral neuropathy
Myocardial infarction <age 30 (cocaine)
Blood alcohol level >300 or >100 without impairment
Alcohol on breath or intoxicated at office visit
Tremor
Mild hypertension
Estrogen mediated signs (telangiectasias, spider angiomas, palmer erythema, muscle atrophy)
Gastrointestinal complaints
Sleep disturbances
Eating disorders
Sexual dysfunction

TABLE 88–3. DSM-IV CRITERIA FOR SUBSTANCE ABUSE

A maladaptive pattern of substance use, leading to clinically significant impairment or distress, as manifested by one (or more), of the following occurring at any time within 12-month period:
1. Recurrent substance use resulting in failure to fulfill major role obligations at work, school, or home (eg, repeated absences or poor work performance related to substance use; substance-related absences, suspensions, or expulsions from school; neglect of children or household.)
2. Recurrent substance use in situations in which it is physically hazardous (eg, driving an automobile or operating a machine when impaired by substance use)
3. Recurrent substance-related legal problems (eg, arrests for substance-related disorderly conduct)
4. Continued substance use despite having persistent social or interpersonal problems caused or exacerbated by the effects of the substance (eg, arguments with spouse about consequences of intoxication, physical fights)

The symptoms have never met the criteria for Substance Dependence for this class of substance.

Modified from American Psychiatric Association *Diagnostic and Statistical Manual of Mental Disorders IV*. American Psychiatric Press; 1994:182.

TABLE 88-4. DSM-IV CRITERIA FOR SUBSTANCE DEPENDENCE

A maladaptive pattern of substance use, leading to clinically significant impairment or distress, as manifested by three (or more) of the following occurring at any time in the same 12-month period:
1. Tolerance as defined by either of the following:
   a. A need for markedly increased amounts of the substance to achieve intoxication or the desired effect.
   b. Markedly diminished effect with continued use of the same amount of the substance
2. Withdrawal, as manifested by either of the following:
   a. The characteristic withdrawal syndrome for the substance
   b. The same (or closely related) substance is taken to relieve or avoid withdrawal symptoms
3. The substance is often taken in larger amounts or over a longer period than was intended
4. There is a persistent desire or unsuccessful efforts to cut down or control substance use
5. A great deal of time is spent in activities necessary to obtain the substance, use the substance, or recover from its effects
6. Important social, occupational, or recreational activities are given up or reduced because of substance use
7. The substance use is continued despite knowledge of having a persistent or recurrent physical or psychological problem that is likely to have been caused or exacerbated by the substance

Modified from American Psychiatric Association *Diagnostic and Statistical Manual of Mental Disorders IV*. American Psychiatric Press; 1994:181.

use. When patients become dependent (addicted), they no longer have full control of their drug use. The brain has been "hijacked by a substance that affects the mechanism of control over the use of that substance." This addiction is far more that physical dependence. The need to use the drug becomes as powerful as the drives of thirst and hunger. The evidence that the brains of addicted individuals are different than those of nonaddicted persons is enormous. Many of these abnormalities predate the use of the substance and are thought to be inherited. In genetically predisposed individuals, substances of abuse cause changes in the dopaminergic mesolimbic system that result in a loss of control over substance use. These changes are mediated by a number of neurotransmitters: dopamine, γ-aminobutyric-acid (GABA), glutamate, serotonin, and endorphins. The different classes of substances of abuse act through one or more of these neurotransmitters, ultimately affecting the level of dopamine in the mesolimbic system, otherwise known as the reward pathway. These changes in the brain are permanent and are the primary reason for relapse in the addicted patient trying to maintain abstinence, or control of use.

II. **Diagnosis**
   A. **Differential diagnosis.** Because substance abuse is a behavioral disorder, when one thinks of a differential diagnosis, psychiatric disorders often come to mind. There is a high comorbidity of substance use disorders with psychiatric disorders. Patients with psychiatric disorders have a high rate of substance abuse. Approximately 50% of psychiatric patients have a substance use disorder. When one looks at patients with addictions, however, the rates of psychiatric disorders are similar to those in the general population. Problems such as substance-induced mood disorders (frequently noted in alcohol, opiate, and stimulant abuse) and substance-induced psychotic disorders (most frequently associated with stimulant abuse), complicate differentiating the primary psychiatric disorders from those that are primarily substance use disorders. Most clinicians agree that psychiatric disorders cannot be reliably assessed for patients who are currently or recently intoxicated. Thus detoxification and a period of abstinence are necessary before evaluation for other psychiatric disorders may effectively be done.
   B. **Symptoms and signs.** The signs and symptoms of substance abuse are varied and often subtle. Most patients do not recognize their substance use as the cause of their problems and are often quite resistant to that interpretation. Signs, such as those

TABLE 88-5. BIOCHEMICAL MARKERS OF SUBSTANCE USE DISORDERS

Marker	Substance	Sensitivity	Specificity	Predictive Value
Mean corpuscular volume (MCV)	Alcohol	24%	96%	63%
γ-glutamyltransferase (GGT)	Alcohol	42%	76%	61%
Carbohydrate-deficient transferrin (CDT)	Alcohol	67%	97%	84%

described in Table 88–2 as potential clues to substance abuse, should lead the clinician to obtain a full substance use history (Table 88–6) from the patient. While physical dependence is not always seen with substance abuse, its presence suggests abuse unless the patient is on long-term, prescribed addictive medicines.

C. Symptoms and signs of withdrawal. In dealing with sedative hypnotic, alcohol, or opiate withdrawal, assessment of the degree of withdrawal is important to determine appropriate use and dose of medication to both reduce symptoms and, in the case of sedative

TABLE 88–6. ELEMENTS OF THE SUBSTANCE USE HISTORY

1. Determine the type, frequency, route of administration, and amount of substance use
  a. Alcohol
  b. Tobacco
  c. Other drugs
    i. cocaine
    ii. marijuana
    iii. others

2. Determine consequences of substance use; ask about
  a. Legal problems
    i. arrests (driving under the influence, public intoxication, disorderly conduct, etc)
    ii. Civil suits for financial problems, bankruptcy, etc
  b. Social problems
    i. social isolation
  c. Family problems
    i. marital problems
    ii. parenting problems
    iii. domestic violence
    iv. family members with depression
    v. divorce
  d. Work or school problems
    i. frequent absences
    ii. poor performance
    iii. frequent job changes
  e. Financial problems
    i. significant debt
    ii. selling personal possessions
    iii. stealing and selling possessions of others
  f. Psychological problems
    i. agitation
    ii. irritability
    iii. anxiety
    iv. panic attacks
    v. mood swings
    vi. hostility
    vii. violence
    viii. sleep disturbance
    ix. sexual dysfunction
    x. depression
    xi. blackouts
  g. Medical problems
    i. gastritis
    ii. peptic ulcer
    iii. abdominal pain
    iv. hypertension
    v. peripheral neuropathy
    vi. nasal septum perforation
    vii. vasospasm
    viii. dysrhythmias
    ix. weight loss
    x. HIV
    xi. Skin abscesses
    xii. trauma

hypnotic drugs or alcohol, prevent seizure and mortality. The Clinical Institute Withdrawal Assessment Scale (Table 88–7) allows quantification of the signs and symptoms of withdrawal in a predictable fashion that allows clinicians to discuss the severity of withdrawal for a given patient and thus choose intervention strategies that are effective and safe.

TABLE 88–7. CLINICAL INSTITUTE WITHDRAWAL ASSESSMENT SCALE

Patient _____ Date _____ Time _____ BP __/__

Age ____ Race/Sex ____ Drugs of choice (Primary) _____ Other _____

1. Autonomic hyperactivity
   Pulse rate/minute
   - 0   <80
   - 1   81–100
   - 2   101–110
   - 3   111–120
   - 4   121–130
   - 5   131–140
   - 6   141–150
   - 7   >150

   Sweating (observation)
   - 0   No sweating
   - 1   Barely perceptible sweating, palms moist
   - 2
   - 3
   - 4   Beads of sweat obvious on forehead
   - 5
   - 6
   - 7   Drenching sweats

2. Hand tremor: arms extended and fingers spread apart:
   Observation
   - 0   No tremor
   - 1   Not visible
   - 2
   - 3
   - 4   Moderate with patients arms extended
   - 5
   - 6
   - 7   Severe, even with arms not extended

3. Anxiety: Ask, "Do you feel nervous or anxious?"
   Observation
   - 0   No anxiety, at ease
   - 1   Mildly anxious
   - 2
   - 3
   - 4   Moderately anxious
   - 5
   - 6
   - 7   Severe equivalent to panic

Total Score _____   Max Score = 56

Rater's initials _____

4. Transient tactile auditory or visual disturbances: Ask, "Have you any itching, pins and needle sensations, any burning or numbness, or do you feel bugs crawling on or under your skin" Are you more aware of sounds around you and are they harsh? Are you hearing things that you know are not there? Does the light appear to bright? Does it hurt your eyes? Are you seeing anything that is disturbing to you?"
   Observation
   - 0   Not present
   - 1   Present but minimal
   - 2
   - 3   Moderate
   - 4   Frequent
   - 5
   - 6
   - 7   Hallucinations almost continuous

5. Agitation:
   Observation
   - 0   Normal activity
   - 1   Somewhat more than normal activity
   - 2
   - 3
   - 4   Moderately fidgety and restless
   - 5
   - 6
   - 7   Paces back and forth during most of the interview, or constantly thrashes about

6. Nausea or vomiting: Ask, "Do you feel sick to your stomach or have you vomited?" Include recorded vomiting since last observation
   Observation
   - 0   Not present
   - 1   Very mild
   - 2
   - 3
   - 4   Moderate
   - 5
   - 6
   - 7   Severe

7. Headache: Ask, "Does your head feel full? Does it feel like there is a band around your head?" Don't rate for lightheadedness. Otherwise rate severity
   - 0   Not present
   - 1   Very mild
   - 2
   - 3
   - 4   Moderate
   - 5
   - 6
   - 7   Severe

D. Laboratory tests

1. **γ-Glutamyl transferase (GGT).** GGT is an enzyme produced in the liver and induced by heavy alcohol consumption. In addition, damage to the hepatic cells during chronic heavy alcohol consumption results in leakage of GGT into the serum. It has a sensitivity that is higher than mean corpuscular volume, but its specificity remains low secondary to nonalcoholic liver disease, diabetes, pancreatitis, hyperthyroidism, heart failure, and anticonvulsant and anticoagulant use, all of which may cause it to be elevated.

2. Other liver functions that may be elevated during heavy alcohol consumption include aspartate aminotransferase (AST) and alanine aminotransferase (ALT). These markers are also elevated as the result of hepatic cellular damage due to heavy alcohol consumption. Sensitivity of these markers is low, because there must be significant liver damage before these markers rise. Specificity is compromised because nonalcoholic liver disease also causes increases. Differences in the ratio of AST/ALT may help to distinguish between alcohol and non–alcohol-related liver disease. A ratio of >2 is highly suggestive of alcohol-related liver disease.

3. **Carbohydrate-deficient transferrin (CDT).** CDT has recently become available in clinical settings to screen for excessive alcohol consumption. Consumption of four to seven drinks daily for at least a week results in a decrease in the carbohydrate content of transferrin. Sensitivity and specificity of CDT is high with regard to differentiating heavy drinkers from those who drink very little or not at all. When used in larger, more heterogeneous populations, it appears less sensitive, and is less sensitive in females than in males.

   Urine drug screening is a sensitive test for common substances of abuse. Knowledge of drug half-life and the importance of confirmation of positive tests by gas chromatography is essential for interpretation of results.

III. Treatment. Many substance use disorders resolve spontaneously, or with brief interventions on the part of physicians or other authority figures in the workplace, legal system, family, or society. This resolution occurs because the patient with a substance abuse disorder continues to maintain control over their use, and when the consequences of that use outweigh the benefits of the drug, they choose to quit. Patients with substance dependence disorders, on the other hand, have impaired control by definition. They rarely get better without assistance.

Substance use disorders can be treated successfully. Brief interventions and outpatient, inpatient, and residential treatment programs reduce morbidity and mortality associated with substance abuse and dependence. Detoxification, patient education, identification of defenses, overcoming denial, relapse prevention, orientation to 12 step recovery programs, and family services are the goals of substance abuse treatment.

A. Formal process. The traditional intervention for alcohol or drug addiction is a formal process, best accomplished by an addictions specialist trained in this process. This approach is often effective, resulting in positive results in about 80% of cases. Although effective, the traditional, formal model of intervention is often less than ideal for the primary care provider. Specialist involvement and orchestration of significant relationships of the patient is sometimes difficult to achieve. In addition, if the intervention fails, the physician's relationship with the patient may become difficult if not impossible to continue.

B. Brief interventions. This highly effective approach to intervention is based on the work of Miller and Rollnick on motivational interviewing and Prochaska and DiClementi's work on stages of change. Presenting the diagnosis of a substance use disorder by itself may be viewed as a brief intervention. As many as 70% of patients are in the precontemplation or contemplation stage when presented with the diagnosis. The resistance associated with these stages tends to force the clinician into one of two modalities, that of avoiding the diagnosis, or confronting and arguing with the patient, generally both futile approaches. One approach in presenting the diagnosis is to use the SOAPE glossary (Table 88–8) for positive suggestions to use when talking to patients about their addiction.

Even when the patient is in the precontemplative stage at presentation of the diagnosis, continued use of the brief intervention strategy, will ultimately at least reduce the amount of drug use if not result in abstinence. Brief interventions should include some

TABLE 88–8. SOAPE GLOSSARY FOR PRESENTING THE DIAGNOSIS

Support: Use phrases such as "We need to work together on this," "I am concerned about you and will follow-up closely with you," and "As with all medical illnesses, the more people you work with, the better you will feel." These words reinforce your physician-patient relationship, strengthen the collaborative model of chronic illness management, and help to convince the patient that the physician will not just present the diagnosis and leave.

Optimism: Most patients have controlled their alcohol or drug use at times and may have quit for periods of time. They may expect failure. By giving a strong optimistic message, such as "You can get well," "Treatment works," and "You can expect to see improvements in many areas of your life," the physician can motivate the patient.

Absolution: By describing addiction as a disease and telling the patient that they are not responsible for having an illness, but that now only they can take responsibility for their recovery, the physician can lessen the burden of guilt and shame that often is a barrier to recovery.

Plan: Having a plan is important to the acceptance of the illness. Using readiness to change categories can help you design a plan that takes the patient's willingness to move ahead. Indicating that abstinence is desirable, but recognizing that all patients will not be able to commit to that goal immediately, can help prevent a sense of failure early in the process. Ask "What do you think you will be able to do at this point?"

Explanatory model: Understanding your patient's beliefs about addiction may be important. Many patients believe this is a moral weakness and that they lack willpower. An explanation that willpower cannot resolve physical illnesses like diabetes mellitus, hypertension, or alcoholism may go a long way to reassure the patient that recovery is possible.

Modified from Clark WD: Alcoholism: Blocks to diagnosis and treatment. Am J Med 1981;**71:**285.

of the elements of motivational interviewing. These elements include offering empathetic, objective feedback of data, meeting patient expectations, working with ambivalence, assessing barriers and strengths, reinterpreting past experience in light of current medical consequences, negotiating a follow-up plan, and providing hope.

C. **Detoxification.** Detoxification, treatment of withdrawal, and any medical complications must have first priority. Alcohol and other sedative hypnotic drugs share the same neurobiological withdrawal process. Chronic use of this class of drugs results in downregulation of the GABA receptors throughout the central nervous system (GABA is an inhibitory neurotransmitter). Abrupt cessation of sedative hypnotic drug use results in an upregulation of GABA receptors and a relative paucity of GABA for inhibition. The result is stimulation of the autonomic nervous system.

   1. **Withdrawal seizures** are a common manifestation of sedative hypnotic withdrawal. They have been described to occur in 11–33% of patients withdrawing from alcohol. Alcohol withdrawal seizures are best treated with benzodiazepines and by addressing the withdrawal process. Lorazepam is a good choice because it can be given intravenously or intramuscularly, 2–4 mg every 1–4 hours as needed for seizure activity. Patients should be on a cardiac monitor and may need to be intubated to protect their airway if seizure activity is persistent. Long-term treatment for alcohol withdrawal seizures is not recommended, and phenytoin should not be used to treat seizures associated with alcohol withdrawal.

   2. **Other withdrawal symptoms.** The cornerstones of treatment for alcohol withdrawal syndrome are the benzodiazepines. All drugs that provide cross-tolerance with alcohol are effective in reducing the symptoms and sequelae of alcohol withdrawal, but none have the safety profile and evidence of efficacy of the benzodiazepines (see Table 88–9 for recommendations in the treatment of alcohol withdrawal).

   3. **Opiate withdrawal** may not be life-threatening, but the symptoms are significant enough that without supportive treatment most patients will not remain in treatment (see Table 88–10 for recommendations for the treatment of opiate withdrawal). The symptoms of cocaine and other stimulant withdrawal are somewhat less predictable and much harder to improve. Despite multiple studies with many different drug classes, no medications have been shown to reliably reduce the symptoms and craving associated with cocaine withdrawal.

D. **Patient education.** Patient knowledge and understanding of the nature of substance use disorders is key to recovery. For patients still in control of their use, education about

TABLE 88–9. TREATMENT REGIMENS FOR ALCOHOL WITHDRAWAL

Using the Clinical Institute Withdrawal Assessment (CIWA) for monitoring
Do CIWA scale every 4 hours until score is below 8 for 24 hours
For CIWA >10
Give Chlordiazepoxide 50–100 mg
or   Diazepam 10–20 mg
or   Oxazepam 30–60 mg
or   Lorazepam 2–4 mg
Repeat CIWA 1 hour after dose to assess need for further medication.

Non–symptom-driven regimens
For patients likely to experience withdrawal:
Chlordiazepoxide, 50 mg every 6 hours for 4 doses, followed by 50 mg every 8 hours for 3 doses, followed by 50 mg
   every 12 hours for two doses, and finally by 50 mg at bedtime for one dose.
Other benzodiazepines may be substituted at equivalent doses.

Patients on a predetermined dosing schedule should be monitored frequently both for breakthrough withdrawal symptoms as well as for excessive sedation.

---

appropriate substance use will help them to choose responsibly if they continue to use. For patients who meet the criteria for substance dependence (addiction), abstinence is the only safe option. Once having made the transition to addiction, one can never use addictive substances reliably again. The neurobiologic changes in the brain are permanent, so loss of control may occur at any time when the brain is presented with an addictive substance. Unfortunately, this occurrence of loss of control can be unpredictable. Consequently, the addicted patient may find that they can use for a variable period of time with control. This sense of control gives them the false impression that they were never addicted in the first place, or perhaps that they have been cured. Invariably if they continue to use addictive substances they will lose control of their use and begin to experience consequences at or above the level that they did before. Understanding addiction as a chronic disorder for which there is remission but not cure becomes essential. The question then becomes not if one should remain abstinent, but rather how one remains abstinent.

E. **Identification of defenses/overcoming denial.** During this phase of treatment, patients typically work in a group therapy setting and are encouraged to look at the defenses that have prevented them from seeking help sooner. Denial can best be defined as the inability to see the causal relationship between drug use and its consequences. Thus the patient who believes he drank because he lost his job may be encouraged to consider that he lost his job because he drank.

TABLE 88–10. TREATMENT FOR OPIOID WITHDRAWAL

Methadone: A pure opioid agonist restricted by federal legislation to inpatient treatment or specialized outpatient drug
   treatment programs. Methodone 15–20 mg for 2–3 days then tapered by 10–15% reductions daily, guided by
   patient's symptoms and clinical findings.

Clonidine: An α-adrenergic blocker, 0.2 mg every 4 hours to relieve symptoms of withdrawal, may be effective.
   Hypotension is a risk and sometimes limits the dose. It can be continued for 10–14 days and tapered by the third day
   by 0.2 mg daily.

Buprenorphine: This partial mu receptor agonist can be administered oral or sublingually, in doses of 2, 4, or 8 mg
   every 4 hours for the management of opioid withdrawal symptoms.

Naltrexone/clonidine: A rapid form of opioid detoxification involves pretreatment with 0.2–0.3 mg of clonidine followed by 12.5 mg of naltrexone (a pure opioid antagonist). Naltrexone is increased to 25 mg on the second day,
   50 mg on day three, and 100 mg on day 4, with clonidine given at 0.1–0.3 mg three times daily.

F. Pharmacologic treatment of addiction

   1. These drugs attempt to have an impact on drug use by one of several mechanisms: (1) sensitizing the body's response to result in a negative reaction to ingesting the drug, causing an aversion reaction, such as with disulfiram and alcohol; (2) reducing the reinforcing effects of a drug, such as the use of naltrexone, or acamprosate in alcoholism; (3) blocking the effects of a drug by binding to the receptor site, such as the use of naltrexone for opiates; (4) saturating the receptor sites by agonists, such as the use of methadone in opioid maintenance therapy; and (5) using unique approaches, such as the creation of an immunization to cocaine. Drug therapy for addiction holds promise. As our understanding of the neurobiology of addiction improves, so does the chance that we can intervene at a molecular level to prevent relapse. At the current level, however, pharmacotherapy to prevent relapse must be relegated to an adjunctive position. No drug alone has provided sufficient power to prevent relapse to addictive behavior. Still, in some patients the use of appropriate medication may give them the edge necessary to move closer to recovery.

   2. Disulfiram is a drug that is not often initiated by family physicians but is frequently continued and monitored in the primary care setting. The usual dose of this medication is 250–500 mg every morning. It works as a deterrent to drinking alcohol. When a patient who is taking disulfiram ingests alcohol (in any form), a severe negative reaction occurs that is manifested by flushing, nausea, and vomiting. Disulfiram's record in achieving abstinence is mixed and is enhanced by taking the medication in an observed fashion. It must be avoided in patients who are hypersensitive to its use, those who have drunk alcohol in the past 12 hours, or those with psychosis or severe coronary artery disease. The cost is about $40/month retail.

   3. Naltrexone, an opiate antagonist, has been shown to be effective in reducing the craving to drink in alcoholics. At doses of 50 mg daily this medication may reduce the patient's desire to drink. It is contraindicated with opiate use, liver failure, or acute hepatitis. Its cost is considerable—$147.20/month. This medication is less effective when not accompanied by a comprehensive recovery program.

IV. Management Strategies

   A. Relapse prevention. Once patients are educated to the nature of their disease and have identified destructive defense mechanisms, relapse prevention becomes the primary goal. Identification of triggers for alcohol and drug use, plans to prevent opportunities to relapse, and new ways to deal with problems help patients to maintain their abstinence. In most treatment programs a relapse prevention plan will be developed and individualized for each patient. The most effective way that the family physician can support relapse prevention is to be aware of the relapse prevention plan that the patient has developed in treatment and reinforce its application. For example it is useful, when seeing a patient who is new to recovery, to ask them about their 12-step meeting attendance, sponsor contacts, and whether they have been able to remain abstinent since your last meeting. For patients who have not had the benefit of treatment, identification of triggers followed by cognitive strategies to avoid these triggers may enhance their recovery. These are usually relatively simple to create. For example, for patients who report that they drink after an argument with their spouse, consideration of alternative means of coping, such as calling a friend, exercising, or engaging in relaxation techniques, may be helpful.

   B. Orientation to 12-Step Recovery. Despite millions of dollars in research, and the efforts of a large segment of the scientific community, there has been no treatment, medication, or psychotherapy that has taken the place of the 12 steps of Alcoholics Anonymous (see Table 88–11).

   Important other 12-step programs for patients with substance use disorders include Al-Anon, for friends and family of alcoholics; Narcotics Anonymous, for those with drug problems other than alcohol; and Cocaine Anonymous, for those with cocaine addiction.

   At the heart of each of these fellowships is the program of recovery outlined in the 12 steps. AA and related 12-step programs are spiritual, not religious, in nature. No one is told they must believe in anything, including God. Agnostics and atheists are welcome in AA and are not asked to convert to any religious belief. Newcomers in AA are encouraged to go to meetings regularly (daily is wise initially), get a sponsor, and begin work on the 12 steps. A sponsor is someone of the same sex who is in stable recovery

TABLE 88–11. THE TWELVE STEPS OF ALCOHOLICS ANONYMOUS

We:

1. Admitted we were powerless over alcohol—that our lives had become unmanageable;
2. Came to believe that a Power greater than ourselves could restore us to sanity;
3. Made a decision to turn our will and our lives over to the care of God *as we understood Him;*
4. Made a searching and fearless moral inventory of ourselves;
5. Admitted to ourselves, and to another human being the exact nature of our wrongs;
6. Were entirely ready to have God remove all these defects of character;
7. Humbly asked Him to remove our shortcomings;
8. Made a list of all persons we had harmed, and became willing to make amends to them all;
9. Made direct amends to such people wherever possible, except when to do so would injure them or others;
10. Continued to take personal inventory and when we were wrong promptly admitted it;
11. Sought through prayer and meditation to improve our conscious contact with God *as we understand Him,* praying only for knowledge of His will for us and the power to carry that out;
12. Having had a spiritual awakening as the result of these steps, we tried to carry this message to alcoholics, and to practice these principles in all our affairs.

From Alcoholics Anonymous World Service.

and has worked the steps. The sponsor helps guide the newcomer through the steps and provides a source of information and encouragement. At meetings members share their experience, strength, and hope around topics of their recovery. In this fashion, storytelling often becomes the means by which information about strategies for recovery is relayed. AA meetings vary in their composition and structure, given that one of the traditions of AA is that each group is autonomous. Consequently, if a patient feels uncomfortable at one meeting, another may be more acceptable. There are meetings for women or men only, for young people, and for doctors or lawyers; virtually any special-interest group is represented in large cities.

There is often a great deal of confusion about what AA does and does not do. AA is not treatment. Despite the close connection many treatment programs have with 12-step recovery fellowships, these fellowships are not affiliated with treatment centers by design.

C. **Effectiveness of AA.** From multiple sources, it appears clear that AA and other 12-step recovery programs are among the most effective tools we have to combat substance disorders. About 6–10% of the population have been to an AA meeting during their lives. This number doubles for those with alcohol problems. Although one half of those who come to AA leave, of those who stay for a year 67% stay sober; of those who stay for 2 years, 85% stay sober; and of those who stay sober for 5 years, 90% remain sober indefinitely. Outcome studies of 8087 patients treated in 57 different inpatient and outpatient treatment programs showed that those attending AA at 1 year were 50% more likely to be abstinent than those not attending. Adolescents studied were found to be four times more likely to be abstinent if they attended AA/Narcotics Anonymous, when compared to those who did not. Finally, in an effort to identify what groups in AA did better than others, studies of involvement in AA (defined as service work, having a sponsor, leading meetings, etc) found that those who were involved, as compared to those just attending meetings, did better in maintaining abstinence.

D. **Contacts.** Having a list of AA members willing to escort potential new members to meetings is a powerful tool for physicians to help patients into recovery. Generally in every AA district, there is a person identified as the chair of the Cooperation with Professional Community Committee who can help physicians identify people willing to perform this service. Al-Anon and Narcotics Anonymous have similar contacts. The telephone numbers for most of these 12-step groups can be found in the phone book. These contacts can often supply the physician with relevant literature to help dispel some of the myths patients may hold regarding 12-step recovery. Patients will often use these myths as excuses for why AA will not work for them.

V. **Prognosis.** Alcohol causes approximately 100,000 deaths yearly and is associated with motor vehicle accidents, other accidents, homicides, cirrhosis of the liver, and suicide. Injection drug use is responsible for the fastest-growing population of human immuno-

TABLE 88–12. MEDICAL COMPLICATIONS OF SUBSTANCE ABUSE

Drug	Medical Complication
Alcohol	Trauma
	Hypertension
	Cardiomyopathy
	Dysrhythmias
	Ischemic heart disease
	Hemorrhagic stroke
	Esophageal reflux
	Barrett's esophagus
	Mallory-Weiss tears
	Esophageal cancer
	Acute gastritis
	Pancreatitis
	Chronic diarrhea malabsorption
	Alcoholic hepatitis
	Cirrhosis
	Hepatic failure
	Hepatic carcinoma
	Nasopharyngeal cancer
	Headache
	Sleep disorders
	Memory impairment
	Dementia
	Peripheral neuropathy
	Fetal alcohol syndrome
	Sexual dysfunction
	Substance-induced mood disorders
	Substance-induced psychotic disorders
	Immune dysfunction
Cocaine (other stimulants)	Chest pain
	Congestive heart failure
	Cardiac dysrhythmias
	Cardiovascular collapse
	Seizures
	Cerebrovascular accidents
	Headache
	Spontaneous pneumothorax
	Noncardiogenic pulmonary edema
	Nasal septal perforations
Injection drug use	Hepatitis C, B
	HIV infection
	Subacute endocarditis
	Soft tissue abscesses

deficiency virus infection. See Table 88–12 for common medical complications from substance abuse.

REFERENCES

Enoch MA, Goldman D: Problem drinking and alcoholism: Diagnosis and treatment. [summary for patients in Am Fam Physician 2002;**65**(3):449; PMID: 11858628]. [Journal article] Am Fam Physician 2002;**65**(3):441.

Friedmann PD, Saitz R, Samet JH: Management of adults recovering from alcohol or other drug problems: Relapse prevention in primary care. JAMA 1998;**279**:1227.

Mallin R, Tumblin M: Addiction treatment in family medicine. *Home Study Self-Assessment Program.* Monograph, Edition No. 249. American Academy of Family Physicians; February 2000.

McLellan T, et al: Drug dependence, a chronic medical illness: Implications for treatment, insurance, and outcomes evaluation. JAMA 2000;**284**:1689.

89 Anxiety

John C. Rogers, MD, MPH

KEY POINTS

- More than 19 million adult Americans aged 18–54 years have anxiety disorders. Anxiety disorders encompass several clinical conditions:
  - Generalized anxiety disorder: Exaggerated worry and tension over everyday events and decisions.
  - Panic disorder: Feelings of extreme fear and dread strike unexpectedly and repeatedly for no apparent reason, accompanied by intense physical symptoms.
  - Phobias: Fear of an object or situation or fear of extreme embarrassment.
  - Post-traumatic stress disorder: Reaction to a terrifying event that keeps returning in the form of frightening, intrusive memories and brings on hypervigilance and deadening of normal emotions.
- There is extensive evidence that cognitive-behavioral therapies are useful treatments for a majority of patients with anxiety disorders. The hallmarks of cognitive-behavioral therapies are evaluating apparent cause-and-effect relationships between thoughts, feelings, and behaviors as well as implementing relatively straightforward strategies to lessen symptoms and reduce avoidant behavior.
- Medications typically used to treat patients with anxiety disorders are benzodiazepines, antidepressants, and buspirone (See Table 89–5 for drug-prescribing information.)
  - Four benzodiazepines widely prescribed for treatment of anxiety disorders are diazepam (starting dose, 2 mg twice to four times daily); lorazepam (1 mg twice or three times daily); clonazepam (0.25 mg twice daily); and alprazolam (0.25 mg three times daily). Each is now available in generic formulations. Benzodiazepines have the potential for producing drug dependence (ie, physiologic or behavioral symptoms after discontinuation of use). Shorter-acting compounds have somewhat greater liability because of more rapid and abrupt onset of withdrawal symptoms.
  - Most antidepressant medications have substantial antianxiety and antipanic effects in addition to their antidepressant action. Current practice guidelines rank the tricyclic antidepressants below the selective serotonin reuptake inhibitors (SSRIs) for treatment of anxiety disorders because of the SSRIs' more favorable tolerability and safety profiles. When effective in treating anxiety, antidepressants should be maintained for at least 4–6 months, then tapered slowly to avoid discontinuation-emergent activation of anxiety symptoms. (Starting doses: sertraline, 25 mg every day; paroxetine, 10 mg every day; escitalopram, 10 mg every day.)
  - Buspirone is most useful for treatment of generalized anxiety disorder, and it is now frequently used as an adjunct to SSRIs. Buspirone (starting dose, 5 mg three times daily) takes 4–6 weeks to exert therapeutic effects, like antidepressants, and it has little value for patients when taken on an "as-needed" basis.

I. Introduction

A. One or more fearful experiences prime a person to respond excessively to situations where most people would experience no fear or only moderate nervousness. Deeply etched memory results in hypervigilance, making it hard to focus, leading to feelings of anxiety in many situations.

B. Recent research suggests that anxiety disorders may be associated with activation of the amygdala.

1. Studies suggest that memories stored in the amygdala are relatively indelible. Research aims to develop therapies that increase cognitive control over the amygdala so that the "act now, think later" response can be interrupted.

2. Cognitive factors play a significant role in the onset of anxiety disorders. People at risk tend to be overly responsive to potentially threatening stimuli.

3. Research evidence points to genetics as a factor in the origin of anxiety disorders. Studies of twins found that genes play a role in panic disorder and social phobia.

C. **Generalized anxiety disorder** is a syndrome of excessive or unrealistic anxiety or worry about two or more life circumstances for 6 months or longer.

1. Generalized anxiety disorder is the fourth most common mental disorder, following substance abuse, major depressive disorder, and phobias. Two to 5% of the US population exhibits this disorder in any given year.

   a. The mean age at onset of symptoms is in the mid-20s, with most cases developing between the ages of 16 and 40. The mean duration of symptoms before treatment is about 5 years.

   b. In the general medical care setting, the female–male ratio is 2–3:1, but among psychiatric patients, the sex ratio is 1:1. First- and second-degree relatives of a person affected by generalized anxiety disorder have at least a threefold increased risk of being affected.

   c. Comorbidity with depression is frequent (just over 50% of depressed patients have concurrent generalized anxiety disorder).

D. **Panic disorder** is the recurrence of episodic periods of intense fear or apprehension accompanied by at least four somatic symptoms, such as diaphoresis, dyspnea, faintness, paresthesias, or flushing.

1. Panic disorder occurs in 1.4% of the US population.

   a. The mean age at presentation is 25 years, with onset generally between ages 17 and 30 years.

   b. The female–male ratio is 2.5–3:1. This disorder has a familial tendency, with first-degree relatives having a twofold increased risk of being affected compared to control subjects.

   c. Comorbidity with depression occurs (nearly 10% of depressed patients have panic disorder) and leads to more frequent and severe symptoms.

E. **A phobia** is a persistent fear of an object, activity, or situation that is out of proportion to the objective danger.

1. Phobia is the most common anxiety disorder. Fifteen to 20% of the population may be affected by phobias.

   a. Social phobia usually begins during the early to late teens. Simple phobias can begin at any age, however, depending on typical exposure to the object or situation. The most common objects of simple phobia are, in descending order and frequency, animals, storms, heights, illness, and death.

   b. Social phobia is reportedly more frequent in males than in females, whereas simple phobias are more frequent in females than in males.

   c. Comorbidity with depression is common (over 20% of depressed patients have concurrent phobia).

F. **Post-traumatic stress disorder** develops after an individual experiences emotionally or physically distressing events that are outside the range of usual human experience and would be extremely traumatic for virtually any person. Examples include combat experience, natural catastrophes, assault, rape, serious threat or harm to one's family members, or sudden destruction of one's home or community.

1. The cause of this disorder is related to the severity of stressor, the social environment of the victim and availability of social supports, the personality traits of the victim, and the victim's premorbid biologic vulnerability.

2. Post-traumatic stress disorder affects 0.5% of men and 1.2% of women in the general population. Onset may be at any age, but because of the types of precipitating situations that are most common, this disorder is most common in young adults. The initiating trauma for men is usually combat experience. The initiating trauma for women is most often assault or rape.

II. **Diagnosis**

A. **Generalized anxiety disorder.** Diagnostic criteria are specified in Table 89–1. Diagnoses that must be ruled out include medical disorders and diagnosable mental disorders.

1. **Biomedical disorders** may include thyrotoxicosis, paroxysmal atrial tachycardia, mitral valve prolapse, hyperventilation, caffeine intoxication, stimulant abuse, alcohol withdrawal, and sedative or hypnotic withdrawal.

2. **Mental disorders** may include panic disorder, phobias, obsessive–compulsive disorder, adjustment disorder with anxious mood, depression, dysthymia, somatization disorder, and schizophrenia.

B. **Panic disorder.** Diagnostic criteria are displayed in Table 89–2. Panic attacks, which are spontaneous, unexpected episodes that occur in the absence of any apparent

TABLE 89–1. DIAGNOSTIC CRITERIA FOR GENERALIZED ANXIETY DISORDER

A. Excessive anxiety and worry (apprehensive expectation), occurring more days than not for at least 6 months, about a number of events or activities (eg, work or school performance)
B. The person finds it difficult to control the worry
C. The anxiety and worry are associated with three or more of the following six symptoms (with at least some symptoms present for more days than not for the past 6 months). **Note:** Only one item is required in children
    (1) Restlessness or feeling keyed up or on edge
    (2) Being easily fatigued
    (3) Difficulty concentrating or mind going blank
    (4) Irritability
    (5) Muscle tension
    (6) Sleep disturbance (difficulty falling or staying asleep, or restless unsatisfying sleep)
D. The focus of the anxiety and worry is not confined to features of an axis I disorder; for example, the anxiety or worry is not about having a panic attack (as in panic disorder), being embarrassed in public (as in social phobia), being contaminated (as in obsessive–compulsive disorder), being away from home or close relatives (as in separation anxiety disorder), gaining weight (as in anorexia nervosa), having multiple physical complaints (as in somatization disorder), or having a serious illness (as in hypochondriasis), and the anxiety and worry do not occur exclusively during post-traumatic stress disorder
E. The anxiety, worry, or physical symptoms cause clinically significant distress or impairment in social, occupational, or other important areas of functioning
F. The disturbance is not due to the direct physiologic effects of a substance (eg, a drug of abuse or a medication) or a general medical condition (eg, hyperthyroidism) and does not occur exclusively during a mood disorder, psychotic disorder, or pervasive developmental disorder

Adapted with permission from American Psychiatric Association (APA): *Diagnostic and Statistical Manual of Mental Disorders,* 4th ed. APA; 1994.

TABLE 89–2. DIAGNOSTIC CRITERIA FOR PANIC DISORDER WITHOUT AGORAPHOBIA

A. Both (1) and (2):
    (1) Recurrent, unexpected panic attacks (see below)
    (2) At least one of the attacks has been followed by 1 month (or more) of one or more of the following:
        (a) Persistent concern about having additional attacks
        (b) Worry about the implications of the attack or its consequences (eg, losing control, having a heart attack, or "going crazy")
        (c) A significant change in behavior related to the attacks
B. Absence of agoraphobia
C. The panic attacks are not caused by the direct physiologic effects of a substance (eg, a drug of abuse or a medication) or a general medical condition (eg, hyperthyroidism)
D. The panic attacks are not better accounted for by another mental disorder, such as social phobia (eg, occurring upon exposure to feared social situations), specific phobia (eg, on exposure to a specific phobic situation), obsessive–compulsive disorder (eg, upon exposure to dirt in someone with an obsession about contamination), post-traumatic stress disorder (eg, in response to stimuli associated with a severe stressor), or separation anxiety disorder (eg, in response to being away from home or close relatives)
E. Criteria for panic attack: A discrete period of intense fear or discomfort, in which four or more of the following symptoms developed abruptly and reached a peak within 10 minutes
    (1) Palpitations, pounding heart, or accelerated heart rate
    (2) Sweating
    (3) Trembling or shaking
    (4) Sensations of shortness of breath or smothering
    (5) Feeling of choking
    (6) Chest pain or discomfort
    (7) Nausea or abdominal distress
    (8) Feeling dizzy, unsteady, lightheaded, or faint
    (9) Derealization (feelings of unreality) or depersonalization (being detached from oneself)
    (10) Fear of losing control or going crazy
    (11) Fear of dying
    (12) Paresthesia (numbness or tingling sensations)
    (13) Chills or hot flushes

Adapted with permission from American Psychiatric Association (APA): *Diagnostic and Statistical Manual of Mental Disorders,* 4th ed. APA; 1994.

precipitant, generally last no more than 20–30 minutes, with attacks of 1 hour being rare. Fear without any apparent source and an impending sense of death and doom are characteristic. Such mental thoughts are associated with somatic symptoms, typically tachycardia, palpitations, dyspnea, and sweating. As many as 20% of patients may experience syncope during panic attacks.

  C. Phobia. Diagnostic criteria are listed in Table 89–3.
  1. The most common biomedical disorders are intoxication with hallucinogens, sympathomimetics, and other drugs of abuse; small cerebral tumor; and cerebrovascular accidents.
  2. The most common mental disorders in the differential diagnoses are depression, schizophrenia, obsessive–compulsive disorder, and personality disorders (schizoid, avoidance, or paranoid).

  D. Post-traumatic stress disorder. Diagnostic criteria are specified in Table 89–4.
  1. Biomedical conditions to be ruled out include head injury and alcohol and drug abuse.
  2. Psychiatric conditions include generalized anxiety disorder, panic disorder, depression, adjustment reaction, factitious disorder, malingering, borderline personality disorder, and schizophrenia.

III. Treatment

  A. Generalized anxiety disorder treatment is directed toward reduction in symptoms so that patients can function in relationships and work. To achieve this goal, the physician must provide patience, realistic reassurance, education about the condition, and encouragement to socialize and assume work and family responsibilities.
  1. Elimination of caffeine and other stimulants and regular exercise may help reduce symptoms.
  2. **Pharmacologic therapy**
    a. Benzodiazepines have been the mainstay of pharmacologic treatment of this disorder. The pharmacologic properties of common benzodiazepines are displayed in Table 89–5. Patients respond best to anxiolytic agents with short half-lives. Use of rapid-acting benzodiazepines as needed may be superior to routine dosing. The problems with the use of these drugs are that 20–30% of patients fail to respond to these agents, tolerance and dependence may occur, and impaired alertness and increased risk of accidents are possible.

TABLE 89–3. DIAGNOSTIC CRITERIA FOR SPECIFIC PHOBIA

A. Marked and persistent fear that is excessive or unreasonable, cued by the presence or anticipation of a specific object or situation (eg, flying, heights, animals, receiving an injection, or seeing blood).

B. Exposure to the phobic stimulus almost invariably provokes an immediate anxiety response, which may take the form of a situationally bound or situationally predisposed panic attack. **Note:** In children, the anxiety may be expressed by crying, tantrums, freezing, or clinging.

C. The person recognizes that the fear is excessive or unreasonable. **Note:** In children, this feature may be absent.

D. The phobic situation(s) is avoided or else is endured with intense anxiety or distress.

E. The avoidance, anxious anticipation, or distress in the feared situation(s) interferes significantly with the person's normal routine, occupational (or academic) functioning, or social activities or relationships, or there is marked distress about having the phobia.

F. In individuals under age 18 years, the duration is at least 6 months.

G. The anxiety panic attacks, or phobic avoidance associated with the specific object or situation, are not better accounted for by another mental disorder, such as obsessive–compulsive disorder (eg, fear of dirt in someone with an obsession about contamination), post-traumatic stress disorder (eg, avoidance of stimuli associated with a severe stressor), separation anxiety disorder (eg, avoidance of school), social phobia (eg, avoidance of social situations because of fear of embarrassment), panic disorder with agoraphobia, or agoraphobia without history of panic disorder. Specify type.
  (1) Animal type
  (2) Natural environment type (eg, heights, storms, or water)
  (3) Blood–injection–injury type
  (4) Situational type (eg, airplanes, elevators, or enclosed places)
  (5) Other type (eg, phobic avoidance of situations that may lead to choking, vomiting, or contracting an illness; in children, avoidance of loud sounds or costumed characters).

Adapted with permission from American Psychiatric Association (APA): *Diagnostic and Statistical Manual of Mental Disorders*, 4th ed. APA; 1994.

TABLE 89–4. DIAGNOSTIC CRITERIA FOR POST-TRAUMATIC STRESS DISORDER

A. The person has been exposed to a traumatic event in which both of the following were present:
   (1) The person experienced, witnessed, or was confronted with an event or events that involved actual or threatened death or serious injury, or a threat to the physical integrity of self or others
   (2) The person's response involved intense fear, helplessness, or horror. **Note:** In children, this may be expressed instead by disorganized or agitated behavior
B. The traumatic event is persistently re-experienced in one or more of the following ways:
   (1) Recurrent and intrusive distressing recollections of the event, including images, thoughts, or perceptions.
       Note: In young children, repetitive play may occur in which themes or aspects of the trauma are expressed
   (2) Recurrent distressing dreams of the event. **Note:** In children, there may be frightening dreams without recognizable content
   (3) Acting or feeling as if the traumatic event were recurring (includes a sense of reliving the experience, illusions, hallucinations, and dissociative flashback episodes, including those that occur upon awakening or when intoxicated). **Note:** In young children, trauma-specific re-enactment may occur
   (4) Intense psychological distress at exposure to internal or external cues that symbolize or resemble an aspect of the traumatic event
   (5) Physiologic reactivity upon exposure to internal or external cues that symbolize or resemble an aspect of the traumatic event
C. Persistent avoidance of stimuli associated with the trauma and numbing of general responsiveness (not present before the trauma), as indicated by at least three or more of the following:
   (1) Efforts to avoid thoughts, feelings, or conversations associated with the trauma
   (2) Efforts to avoid activities, places, or people that arouse recollections of the trauma
   (3) Inability to recall an important aspect of the trauma
   (4) Markedly diminished interest or participation in significant activities
   (5) Feeling of detachment or estrangement from others
   (6) Restricted range of affect (eg, unable to have loving feelings)
   (7) Sense of a foreshortened future (eg, does not expect to have a career, marriage, children, or normal life span)
D. Persistent symptoms of increased arousal (not present before the trauma), as indicated by two or more of the following:
   (1) Difficulty falling or staying asleep
   (2) Irritability or outbursts of anger
   (3) Difficulty concentrating
   (4) Hypervigilance
   (5) Exaggerated startle response
E. Duration of the disturbance (symptoms in B, C, and D) is more than 1 month.
F. The disturbance causes clinically significant distress or impairment in social, occupational, or other important areas of functioning. Specify if:

   Acute: if duration of symptoms is less than 3 months
   Chronic: if duration of symptoms is 3 months or more

   Specify if:
   With delayed onset: if onset of symptoms is at least 6 months after the stressor

Adapted with permission from American Psychiatric Association (APA): *Diagnostic and Statistical Manual of Mental Disorders,* 4th ed. APA; 1994.

   b. Antidepressants such as imipramine are being used more frequently to treat this disorder. Imipramine starts at 50–75 mg/day and is increased every 2 weeks, depending on response, to a maximum of 150 mg/day in divided doses. The efficacy of monoamine oxidase (MAO) inhibitors is unknown. SSRIs have shown comparable efficacy to benzodiazepines in acute treatment of generalized anxiety disorder and are appropriate for patients with concurrent depression.
   c. Beta blockers are used to treat peripheral somatic symptoms such as tremor or palpitation. Propranolol can be started at 60–80 mg/day in divided doses and gradually increased to optimum response or a maximum dose of 240 mg/day. Combination of a beta blocker and a benzodiazepine is more effective than a benzodiazepine alone.
   d. Azepirones act on the serotoninergic system. These drugs do not act through the γ-aminobutyric acid–benzodiazepine receptor complex, so problems of tolerance, dependence, and impaired alertness are avoided. Buspirone should be started at 5 mg three times a day for 3–7 days and then increased to 10 mg

TABLE 89–5. DRUG TREATMENT OF ANXIETY DISORDERS

Drug	Starting Dosage (mg)	Usual Daily Dosage (mg)	Maximum Daily Dosage (mg)	Rate of Onset	Half-life (hr)	Common Side Effects
Benzodiazepines						
Alprazolam (Xanax)	0.25 tid	0.5–4	10	Intermediate	12–15	Transient drowsiness, alexia, confusion, depression
Chlordiazepoxide (Librium, Lipoxide, Mitran, etc)	5 tid or qid	15–80	100	Intermediate	5–30	Withdrawal symptoms upon abrupt discontinuation
Clonazepam (Klonopin)	0.25 tid	0.5–1.5	4	Rapid	18–50	Withdrawal symptoms upon abrupt discontinuation
Clorazepate (Tranxene)	7.5 qd or bid	15–30	60	Rapid	30–100	
Diazepam (Valium, Vazepam)	2 bid–qid	4–40	40	Very rapid	20–80	
Halazepam (Paxipam)	20 tid or qid	60–160	160	Intermediate to slow	14	
Lorazepam (Alzapam, Ativan)	1 bid or tid	2–4	10	Intermediate	10–20	
Oxazepam (Serax)	10–15 tid or qid	30–90	120	Intermediate to slow	5–20	
Prazepam (Centrax)	20 hs	20–40	60	Slow	30–100	
Azepirone						
Buspirone (BuSpar)	5 tid	20–30	60	Delayed	2–3	Dizziness, nervousness, nausea, headache
Tricyclic antidepressants						
Imipramine (Tofranil, Janimine)	75 qd or hs	50–150	200	Delayed	11–25	Sedation, anticholinergic effects, orthostatic hypertension
Desipramine (Norpramin, Pertofrane)	50 qd	100–200	300	Delayed	12–24	
Monoamine oxidase inhibitor						
Phenelzine (Nardil)	15 tid	45–60	90	Delayed	NA	Orthostatic hypotension, dizziness, jitteriness, overstimulation
Beta blocks						
Propranolol (Inderal)	40 bid	80–120	320	Rapid	3–5	Bradycardia, dizziness, fatigue, depression, impotence
Selective Serotonin Reuptake Inhibitors						
Fluoxetine (Prozac)	5 mg qd	10–20	40	Delayed	Days	Insomnia, agitation, anorgasmia
Sertraline (Zoloft)	25 mg qd	50–100	200	Delayed	26	Insomnia, nausea, sexual dysfunction
Paroxetine (Paxil)	10 mg qd	20–40	50	Delayed	21	Drowsiness, fatigue, delayed ejaculation
Fluvoxamine (Luvox)	25 mg bid	100–150	300	Delayed	15	Drowsiness, nausea, anorgasmia
Escitalopram (Lexapro)	10 mg qd	10–20	20	Delayed	27–32	Nausea, insomnia, delayed ejaculation, somnolence, increased sweating, fatigue
Citalopram (Celexa)	20 mg qd	20–60	60	Delayed	35	Nausea, dry mouth, somnolence, increased sweating

twice or three times daily, the usual maintenance dose. The dose should not exceed 60 mg/day.

B. Panic disorder treatment is directed toward control of symptoms so that the patient may be as functional as possible.

1. **Selective serotonin reuptake inhibitors (SSRIs)** are considered the first-line pharmacologic treatment: they are as effective as benzodiazepines in improving anxiety, have fewer side effects than the alternatives, have no interference with cognitive behavioral therapy, and provide treatment of concurrent depression. Fluoxetine, 5–40 mg/day, is recommended as a single morning dose. The starting dose is 5 mg (2 mg if there is significant insomnia or agitation) with increases each week. The dose for sertraline is 25 mg/day to start, with a maximum of 200 mg/day. The starting dose for paroxetine is 10 mg/day, with 50 mg/day maximum. Fluvoxamine starts at 25 mg twice a day, with a maximum of 150 mg twice a day. The dose of escitalopram is most often 10 mg/day with 20 mg/day used infrequently. The starting dose of citalopram is 20 mg/day, with a maximum of 60 mg/day. Full response occurs after 4 weeks, and perhaps 8–12 weeks. Treatment should continue for 12–24 months with slow discontinuation over 4–6 months.

2. **Tricyclic antidepressants.** Imipramine and desipramine are effective agents. Imipramine, 150–300 mg/day, is recommended as a single bedtime dose. The starting dose is 50–100 mg/day, which can be increased every 2 weeks until an optimum response or maximum dose is reached. Desipramine is sometimes better tolerated by patients than is imipramine.

3. **MAO inhibitors.** Phenelzine, 45–90 mg/day, and iproniazid, up to 150 mg/day, are effective in controlling symptoms. Administration of MAO inhibitors may be either divided equally three times a day or given according to whether an activating or sedating effect occurs in the patient, in which case a morning dose (activating effect) or an evening dose (sedating effect) is prescribed to blend with the patient's sleep routines. The possibility of a serious reaction such as a hypertensive crisis or intracranial bleeding must be kept in mind, and patients must be warned to avoid certain foods and beverages.

4. **Benzodiazepines.** Alprazolam is as effective as imipramine and phenelzine in treating this disorder. Clonazepam and lorazepam also appear to be effective. High-dose diazepam (mean of 30 mg/day) can also markedly decrease panic attacks. The disadvantages of using benzodiazepines are that nearly half of patients with panic disorder have concurrent major depression that is not helped by benzodiazepines, abuse can be a potential problem, and benzodiazepines are more difficult to taper than are tricyclic antidepressants or MAO inhibitors.

C. Treatment of phobia requires commitment on the part of the patient and clear identification of the phobic object or situation.

1. **Behavioral treatment techniques** are the most effective, with systematic desensitization being used more frequently. A cognitive strategy of suggesting new ways of thinking about the phobic object or situation may be used in addition to muscle relaxation techniques.

2. **Pharmacologic therapy**
   a. Beta blockers such as propranolol may be useful just prior to direct challenge by the phobic situation. Propranolol, 10–20 mg 1 hour before exposure to the phobic object, or up to 40 mg, should be effective.
   b. Tricyclic antidepressants, MAO inhibitors, and SSRIs (fluvoxamine and sertraline) may be of use, particularly in patients with social phobia.

D. Post-traumatic stress disorder treatment consists primarily of psychotherapy. Pharmacotherapy is used most often when the patient has symptoms of depression or a panic-like disorder.

1. Time-limited psychotherapy uses cognitive and supportive approaches to minimize the risk of dependency and chronicity. The patient is encouraged to garner support from friends and relatives; to review emotional feelings associated with the event; to consciously re-enact the event through imagination, words, or actions; and to plan for future recovery. Group and family therapies have been particularly effective.

2. Drug therapy may include tricyclic antidepressants (amitriptyline and imipramine), MAO inhibitors (phenelzine), benzodiazepines, propranolol, lithium, anticonvulsants, or antipsychotic medications, such as chlorpromazine, trifluoperazine, or mesoridazine.

IV. **Management Strategies**
  A. **Generalized anxiety disorder.** Physician time and involvement need not be extensive. Education of the patient about the disorder and the scheduling of frequent, short office visits are the physician's primary responsibilities. Listening carefully to the patient's account of problems is very beneficial. Specific management techniques include being supportive of patient choices, expanding coping strategies, normalizing symptoms through reassurance, encouraging confrontation of anxiety-provoking situations, and being available for brief clinical encounters.
  B. **Panic disorder.** Patients with panic disorder should be reassured that they have a treatable condition. The patient's somatic symptoms should be discussed in such a way as to avoid the attachment of any stigma to the patient. Eliciting the patient's explanation of the symptoms and goals for treatment is crucial. Panic-focused cognitive behavioral therapy and medications are effective treatments for panic disorder. There is no evidence that one is superior to the other, so the choice between psychotherapy and pharmacotherapy depends on the efficacy, benefits, risks, and the patient's personal preferences.
  C. **Phobias.** The goal of therapy is for the affected person to discover that the feared situation is not as much of a threat as previously thought. Avoidance should be discouraged, and behavioral techniques should be used until the phobic object or situation has been fully confronted. Hypnosis may be used as an adjunct method of relaxation and as a method of offering alternative cognitive appraisals of the phobic object. Family therapy may be particularly useful in this condition.
  D. **Post-traumatic stress disorder.** Physicians caring for patients with this disorder must deal effectively with suspicion, paranoia, and mistrust on the part of the patient. Gentle confrontation is necessary to overcome the patient's denial of the traumatic event and to encourage the individual to remain in the treatment program of therapy and medications. Groups of individuals suffering similar events, such as assault self-help groups, may also be useful. Hospitalization may be necessary if the patient is suicidal or a danger to others.
V. **Prognosis**
  A. **Generalized anxiety disorder** is a chronic condition with a typical duration of illness just over 10 years. Affected individuals usually respond to treatment, but relapse after withdrawal of treatment may occur in as many as 80% of patients, nearly 25% of whom may go on to develop panic disorder.
  B. **Panic disorder** is a chronic, remitting, and relapsing condition that is often precipitated by stressful life events. In one study, at 5-year follow-up, 30% of affected patients were moderately to severely impaired and 50% were mildly impaired; at 20-year follow-up, 15% had moderate to severe symptoms, and 70% had mild symptoms with no disability. Between 30% and 70% of patients experience a major depressive disorder subsequent to the onset of the panic attacks. These individuals are at increased risk for suicide, alcohol and drug dependence, and obsessive–compulsive disorder. Once an effective drug dose is achieved, the medication should be continued unchanged for 6–12 months. At that time, the medication is slowly tapered. Drug treatment should be reinstituted if symptoms return. Patients with good function prior to development of symptoms of brief duration tend to have a better prognosis.
  C. **Phobias** beginning in childhood may resolve without treatment, but others may become chronic. Those that are chronic in nature seem to increase after middle age. Most affected individuals experience little disability, since the phobic object or situation can usually be easily avoided.
  D. **Post-traumatic stress disorder.** The full syndrome usually develops sometime after the traumatic event, and delay can be from 1 week to as long as 30 years. Symptoms fluctuate with exacerbations during periods of stress. Individuals with a good prognosis usually have rapid onset of symptoms, symptoms of less than 6 months' duration, good functioning before the onset of the syndrome, strong social support, and the absence of any other medical or emotional disorders. Over time, 10% of affected patients remain unchanged or become worse, 20% have moderate symptoms, 40% have mild symptoms, and 30% recover.

REFERENCES

American Psychiatric Association (APA): *Diagnostic and Statistical Manual of Mental Disorders,* 4th ed. APA; 1994.
Borkovec TD, Newman MG, Castonguay LG: Cognitive-behavioral therapy for generalized anxiety disorder with integrations from interpersonal and experiential therapies. CNS Spectr 2003;**8**(5):382.

Bruce S, et al: Are benzodiazepines still the medication of choice for patients with panic disorder with or without agoraphobia? Am J Psychiatry 2003;**160**(8):1432.

Hambrick JP, et al: Cognitive-behavioral therapy for social anxiety disorder: Supporting evidence and future directions. CNS SPectr 2003;**8**(5):373.

Kapczinski F, et al: Antidepressants for generalized anxiety disorder. Cochrane Database Syst Rev 2003;(2):CD003592.

Lepola U, et al: Sertraline versus imipramine treatment of comorbid panic disorder and major depressive disorder. J Clin Psychiatry 2003;**64**(6):654.

Mavissalkalian MR, Perel JM: Long-term maintenance and discontinuation of imipramine therapy in panic disorder with agoraphobia. Arch Gen Psychiatry 1999;**56**(6):821.

Pollack MH: New advances in the management of anxiety disorders. Psychopharmacol Bull 2002; **36**(4 Suppl 3):79.

Quilty LC, et al: Quality of life and the anxiety disorders. J Anxiety Disord 2003;**17**(4):405.

Rayburn NR, Otto MW: Cognitive-behavioral therapy for panic disorder: A review of treatment elements, strategies, and outcomes. CNS Spectr 2003;**8**(5):356.

Resick AP, Nishith P, Griffin MG: How well does cognitive-behavioral therapy treat symptoms of complex PTSD? An examination of child sexual abuse survivors within a clinical trial. CNS Spectr 2003; **8**(5):240.

Solvason HB, Ernst H, Roth W: Predictors of response in anxiety disorders. Psychiatr Clin North Am 2003;**26**(2):411.

Stein DJ: Algorithm for the pharmacotherapy of anxiety disorders. Curr Psychiatry Rep 2003;**5**(4):282.

CLINICAL GUIDELINES

American Psychiatric Association (APA). Practice guideline for the treatment of patients with panic disorder. American Psychiatric Press; 1998. 86 p. [273 references]

Institute For Clinical Systems Improvement (ICSI). Major depression, panic disorder and generalized anxiety disorder in adults in primary care. Institute For Clinical Systems Improvement (ICSI) (Bloomington, Minnesota); (May) 2002; 55 p. [108 references]

Practice guideline for the treatment of patients with panic disorder. Work Group on Panic Disorder. American Psychiatric Association (APA). Am J Psychiatry (May) 1998;**155**(5 suppl):1–34. [273 references]

WEB SITES

http://www.nlm.nih.gov/medlineplus/anxiety.html
http://www.nlm.nih.gov/medlineplus/panicdisorder.html
http://www.nlm.nih.gov/medlineplus/phobias.html
http://www.nlm.nih.gov/medlineplus/posttraumaticstressdisorder.html
http://www.surgeongeneral.gov/library/mentalhealth/chapter4/sec2.html
http://www.nimh.nih.gov/anxiety/anxiety.cfm#anx2
http://www.nimh.nih.gov/publicat/anxresfact.cfm

90   Attention-Deficit/Hyperactivity Disorder

H. Russell Searight, PhD, MPH, Jennifer Gafford, PhD, & Stephanie L. Evans, Pharm D, BCPS

KEY POINTS

- Attention-deficit/hyperactivity disorder (ADHD) has three core symptom clusters: inattention, hyperactivity, and impulsivity.
- Among US children, current prevalence rates are 6–8%.
- Approximately 70% of children diagnosed with ADHD continue to manifest symptoms in adolescence, with 50–60% exhibiting symptoms in adulthood.
- Common comorbid psychiatric conditions include oppositional defiant and conduct disorder.
- Evaluating suspected ADHD includes a history and physical, detailed clinical interview, behavioral ratings, and on occasion, referral for specialized assessment.
- Stimulant pharmacotherapy continues to be the most common treatment. However, there are several nonstimulant medication options.

I. Introduction

A. Overview of condition. Attention-deficit/hyperactivity disorder (ADHD) is a common neurobehavioral disorder that begins in childhood, typically continues through adulthood, and is characterized by a chronic, pervasive pattern of inattention, hyperactivity-impulsivity, or both that is inconsistent with the child's developmental level and affects cognitive, academic, behavioral, emotional, and social functioning.

1. The initial diagnosis is typically made between the ages of 6 and 10 years, when symptoms of hyperactivity, impulsivity, and inattention tend to peak.

2. Although children may begin to develop symptoms of ADHD as early as age 3, diagnoses of ADHD made during preschool tend to be less reliable. Approximately 50% of these individuals will no longer meet criteria by later childhood.

3. Approximately 50–75% of children with ADHD continue to exhibit symptoms into adulthood.

4. ADHD is often comorbid with other conditions, including learning disabilities, speech and language disorders, oppositional defiant disorder, conduct disorder, mood disorders, anxiety disorders, and Tourette syndrome.

5. Additionally, ADHD is often associated with substantial impairments such as low self-esteem, poor family and peer relationships, school difficulties, and academic underachievement.

B. Etiology. The etiology of ADHD is not entirely clear but is thought to be influenced primarily by genetic factors, particularly heredity. A number of other contributing factors have been proposed as well, such as neurologic factors, psychophysiologic variables, and psychosocial factors. The influence of allergens and environmental toxins has been studied, but they do not appear to play a role in the development of the disorder.

C. Risk factors. A number of risk factors have been identified for the development of ADHD.

1. Family history of ADHD is a major risk factor for the development of the disorder. Family studies have reported rates of ADHD as high as 30% in siblings of individuals with ADHD, 15–20% in mothers, 20–30% in fathers, and 50% in at least one parent.

2. The emergence of difficult temperament in the preschool years also appears to be associated with increased risk for the development of ADHD.

3. Children with ADHD who are very active and demanding, coupled with maternal psychological distress and family dysfunction, exhibit symptoms of ADHD that are more persistent into later childhood and often comorbid with oppositional behaviors.

II. Diagnosis

A. Primary features of ADHD include inattention, hyperactivity, and impulsivity (behavioral disinhibition). Deficient rule-governed behavior and variability in task performance may be considered core features as well.

1. Inattention refers to problems with alertness, arousal, selectivity, sustained attention, and distractibility, which tend to be most evident in situations in which the children are required to sustain attention to tasks that are repetitive and monotonous. Children with attentional problems are commonly described by parents and teachers as "not listening to instructions," "not finishing assigned work," "daydreaming," and "becoming bored easily." In addition, they may be perceived as forgetful, careless, or lazy because of failing to follow through on tasks, losing things, or making mistakes.

2. Hyperactivity across multiple settings is the most classic, distinguishing feature of ADHD. Described by parents and teachers as "in constant motion," "always on the go," "driven by a motor," and "talks excessively," ADHD children are thought to be deficient in their ability to regulate their activity level to the particular setting or task demands. They tend to be more active, restless, and fidgety than normal children throughout the day and even during sleep. In addition to heightened motor activity, ADHD children are characterized by excessive speech and commentary. Because of the disruption these behaviors typically cause in situations such as the classroom, hyperactivity tends to be the most socially problematic of the primary features for children with ADHD.

3. Impulsivity, or behavioral disinhibition, is also socially problematic for ADHD children, especially in situations in which cooperation, sharing, and restraint with peers is required. Clinically, these children appear to respond quickly to situations without waiting for instructions or considering consequences. They are

characterized by poor delay of gratification, poor behavioral inhibition, and high risk-taking behavior.

B. Other core features

1. Difficulty with rule-governed behavior may be another primary deficit of children with ADHD. Failing to follow through with instructions or to comply with rules is a common problem for ADHD children, particularly in situations in which directions are not repeated or when there is no adult present. ADHD children do not necessarily refuse to follow rules and directions; it is more a problem of behavioral self-regulation, or sustaining response to rules or commands.

2. Children with ADHD also tend to show high variability in task performance. While all children display a certain amount of behavioral inconsistency, children with ADHD exhibit this fluctuation to a much greater degree.

C. ADHD tends to be associated with a variety of other problems in addition to the primary features of inattention, hyperactivity, and impulsivity.

1. Children with ADHD often experience behavior problems such as noncompliance, argumentativeness, and temper outbursts.

2. Peer relations are also problematic for many children with ADHD. Because of their inability to control their behavior in social situations, ADHD children may have difficulty in forming and maintaining friendships.

3. Emotional functioning tends to be impaired in children with ADHD, including low self-esteem, reduced tolerance for frustration, and symptoms of depression or anxiety (or both).

4. Academic performance and cognitive and language abilities represent other areas of difficulty for these children. They are typically underachievers in school and frequently exhibit learning disabilities and language problems. As a whole, children with ADHD score lower on standardized intelligence tests as compared to normal controls and exhibit more difficulty on complex problem solving tasks.

5. Children with ADHD tend to experience medical and health problems more commonly than normal controls. These include physical injuries, minor physical anomalies, sleep disturbances, and ear and respiratory infections.

D. DSM-IV criteria for ADHD require that six or more symptoms of inattention, hyperactivity-impulsivity, or both are present for at least 6 months, and that the symptoms are severe, maladaptive, and inconsistent with the child's developmental level. By definition, some symptoms must have been present before the age of 7 years. Additionally, symptoms must be present in two or more settings and result in clinically significant impairment in social, academic, or occupational functioning. The symptoms do not occur exclusively during the course of a pervasive developmental disorder, schizophrenia, or other psychotic disorder and are not better accounted for by another mental disorder (eg, mood disorder, anxiety disorder, dissociative disorder, or a personality disorder).

1. **Inattention**
   a. Fails to give close attention to details or makes careless mistakes in schoolwork, work, or other activities.
   b. Has difficulty sustaining attention in tasks or play activities.
   c. Does not seem to listen when spoken to directly.
   d. Does not follow through on instructions and fails to finish schoolwork, chores, or duties in the workplace (not due to oppositional behavior or failure to understand instructions).
   e. Has difficulty organizing tasks and activities.
   f. Avoids, dislikes, or is reluctant to engage in tasks that require sustained mental effort (such a schoolwork or homework).
   g. Loses things necessary for tasks or activities (eg, toys, school assignments, pencils, books, or tools).
   h. Is easily distracted by extraneous stimuli.
   i. Is forgetful in daily activities.

2. **Hyperactivity-impulsivity**
   a. Fidgets with hands or feet or squirms in seat.
   b. Leaves seat in classroom or in other situations in which remaining seated is expected.
   c. Runs about or climbs excessively in situations in which it is inappropriate (in adolescents or adults, may be limited to subjective feelings of restlessness).

    d. Has difficulty playing or engaging in leisure activities quietly.
    e. Is "on the go" or often acts as if "driven by a motor."
    f. Talks excessively.
    g. Blurts out answers before questions have been completed.
    h. Has difficulty awaiting his or her turn.
    i. Interrupts or intrudes on others (eg, butts into conversations or games).
E. **The DSM-IV describes three different subtypes,** to distinguish between individuals who display symptoms of primarily inattention, primarily hyperactivity-impulsivity, or both.

    1. **Attention-deficit/hyperactivity disorder, combined type** represents the most common diagnosis of the three subtypes and includes features of both inattention and hyperactivity-impulsivity. Children with this subtype are commonly diagnosed at 6–7 years of age when symptoms of hyperactivity and impulsivity begin to peak.

    2. A diagnosis of **attention-deficit/hyperactivity disorder, predominantly hyperactive type** is indicated when the individual exhibits symptoms of hyperactivity and impulsivity without meeting criteria for inattention. Children with this subtype are also often diagnosed at approximately 6–7 years of age.

    3. A diagnosis of **attention-deficit/hyperactivity disorder, predominantly inattentive type** is appropriate when symptoms of inattention are present without associated hyperactivity and impulsivity. This initial diagnosis is often made somewhat later, at the age of 9 or 10 years, when symptoms of inattention typically become more noticeable.

F. **Limitations of DSM-IV criteria**

    1. A major difficulty with the criteria is that they are most applicable to children between the ages of 7 and 12. Applying the criteria to young children, adolescents, and adults can be problematic due to developmental variations in which inattention, hyperactivity, and impulsivity are exhibited across the lifespan.

    2. There is little evidence supporting the requirement of six symptoms for a diagnosis. Authors have suggested that developmentally sensitive criteria would require more than six symptoms to be present for a diagnosis in preschool, and fewer symptoms for a diagnosis in adolescence and adulthood.

    3. Determining whether symptoms are present in two or more settings is often difficult because the behavioral characteristics specified in the definition are often interpreted differently by different observers. Interrater agreement coefficients for behavior ratings between parents and teachers, for example, are often less than 0.50. Ratings between parents differ as well, with coefficients typically less than 0.6 or 0.7.

    4. Finally, the symptoms of ADHD overlap many other disorders, making it often difficult to determine whether symptoms of other disorders are mimicking ADHD or comorbid with ADHD.

G. **Epidemiology.** ADHD is among the leading reasons school-age children in the United States are referred to mental health practitioners. As one of the most widespread childhood psychiatric disorders, the rate of ADHD in the general population is estimated to be 9% of males and 3% females. Rates vary, however, depending on the population studied, the geographic region under investigation, the definition of ADHD employed, and the degree of agreement required among parents, teachers, and professionals. In fact, prevalence estimates range from between 1% and 20% depending on these factors.

    1. ADHD occurs two to four times more commonly in boys than girls for the predominantly inattentive and predominantly hyperactive-impulsive subtypes, respectively. In clinical populations, the ratio of males to females is estimated to be as high as 9:1 due to referral biases.

    2. Based on current childhood rates, it appears that between 1% and 7% of the adult population experiences ADHD symptoms.

    3. Rates of ADHD appear to vary as a function of socioeconomic status (SES), although the differences are relatively minor. Women from lower-SES groups tend to have a higher incidence of ADHD in their offspring. This may be due to prenatal and postnatal factors in their development; higher rates of instability in these families, exacerbating marginal cases of ADHD; or to "social drift." Social drift theories suggest that individuals with psychopathology tend to "drift" into lower SES levels as a function of their disorder. For example, a child with ADHD may grow up to

have less education than his or her peers, drift into a lower financial level of employment, and therefore occupy a lower SES level.
  H. Variations in symptoms presentation through the lifespan. Symptoms of inattention, hyperactivity, and impulsivity peak at different ages, decline with age at different rates, and manifest differently depending on the individual's level of development. As a result, ADHD presents differently from preschool through adulthood.
    1. **Preschool.** Many children begin to exhibit symptoms of ADHD in preschool, as early as 3–4 years of age. However, it is often difficult to differentiate ADHD in preschool children from other discipline problems at this age; some children have simply never learned limits, rules of behavior, or empathy. Preschool children with ADHD tend to show predominantly features of hyperactivity and impulsivity. Developmentally, these are the first ADHD symptoms to appear before reaching their peak at the age of 7 or 8. Symptoms of inattention tend to peak several years later and are less apparent during the preschool years.
    2. **Late childhood/adolescence.** By adolescence, features of hyperactivity have declined steadily while symptoms of inattention and impulsivity continue to be problematic. Individuals with the predominantly inattentive subtype may have only recently been diagnosed with ADHD, because symptoms of inattention are typically not apparent until the child is at least 8 or 9 years of age. Comorbidity increases dramatically in adolescents with ADHD, to the extent that "pure" ADHD may be the exception rather than the rule by this age. Problems that tend to be associated with ADHD include poor academic performance; over half of adolescents with ADHD have repeated a grade by the end of high school. Affective disorders, school suspensions, expulsions, cigarette and alcohol use, illicit drug use, aggressive behavior, and conduct problems are also not uncommon. Adolescents with ADHD who are untreated, poorly supervised, and in an environment in which alcohol and other illicit substances are readily available appear to be at highest risk for negative outcome.
    3. **Adults.** The symptom picture is likely to be more subtle in adults than in children. The "hyperactivity" of childhood may be replaced by experiences of restlessness, difficulty relaxing, and feeling chronically "on edge." Patients with impulsivity, or behavioral disinhibition, may be unable to prevent immediate responding and have deficits in their capacity for monitoring their behavior and controlling the display of emotions. They may appear socially inappropriate at times by, for example, blurting out thoughts that are rude or insulting. Impulsive adults may also find themselves with higher rates of financial mismanagement related to impulsive buying. Deficits in sustained attention and concentration are more likely to remain from early adolescence and may become more apparent as responsibilities increase. Appointments, social commitments, as well as school and work deadlines, are frequently forgotten. Tasks and appointments may be written on lists, calendars, or Post-it notes, but these are also forgotten. Completed work is frequently misplaced amid clutter. Prioritizing is a common source of frustration. Important tasks are not completed while trivial distractions receive inordinate time.
  I. **Differential diagnosis**
    1. **Medical conditions.** While psychiatric conditions are more common differential diagnoses, some medical conditions may present with ADHD-like symptoms. Vision and hearing should be routinely screened among children. Elevated lead levels may be associated with cognitive impairment and hyperactivity. An audiologic condition that may appear similar to the inattentive subtype of ADHD–inattentive type is auditory processing disorder (APD). **APD,** typically diagnosed by audiologists, is a deficit in comprehending or tracking information presented through auditory channels despite normal hearing. APD may arise from deficits in underlying functions such as auditory discrimination, pattern recognition, and management of competing input. Cognitive deficits may also be attributable to mental retardation and fetal alcohol or drug syndrome. Thyroid disturbance may affect activity and secondarily, attention and concentration. Cognition and motor activity may also be altered pharmacologically. For example, anabolic steroids commonly used by athletes are associated with impulsive aggression while the anticonvulsant, phenytoin, often results in cognitive inefficiency. Among adolescents and adults, obstructive sleep apnea may impair attention, concentration, and short-term recall. Seizure dis-

orders, particularly convulsive status epilepticus, produces cognitive impairment similar to the inattention seen in ADHD.

2. **Psychiatric conditions.** Many pediatric and adult psychiatric conditions feature impulsivity and impaired attention, concentration, and short-term memory as commonly associated symptoms. The diagnosis of ADHD is complicated by conditions appearing similar to ADHD that also are part of the differential diagnosis. These psychiatric disorders are challenging because they are often comorbid with ADHD. Pediatric and adult patients will be discussed separately.

   a. **Pediatric conditions.** Table 90–1 summarizes common psychiatric conditions that are part of the differential diagnosis of childhood ADHD, including features shared with ADHD as well as distinguishing symptoms.

   Childhood ADHD is a risk factor for developing other psychiatric conditions. Over 40% of children with ADHD have at least one other disorder, with about 30% having two comorbid psychiatric conditions. Developmentally, rates of comorbidity increase with age. For example, up to half of ADHD adolescents may also have oppositional–defiant disorder.

   b. **Adult conditions.** While the differential diagnosis of adult ADHD includes some of the same conditions as in childhood, symptoms of both ADHD and other psychiatric syndromes vary with age. Adult ADHD symptoms are more subtle than those in children. While some ADHD adults will have an established diagnosis from early childhood, many patients will be seeking assistance for the first time as adults. Up to two thirds of adults self-referred for inattention, distractibility, and impulsivity actually have a different primary psychiatric condition (Table 90–2.)

J. **Process of diagnosis in primary care** (Table 90–3)

   1. **Thorough diagnostic interview.** Parents should be encouraged to describe their concerns about their child in an open-ended manner. Physicians should carefully listen for core symptoms of ADHD vs. those of other psychiatric conditions. Examples of specific behavior concerns should be elicited. The duration and degree of functional impairment should also be assessed. In order to meet DSM-IV criteria, the patient should be exhibiting significant deficits in at least two life domains (school, work, family relationships). Parents should be asked when they initially noticed symptoms. Fluctuation or variability symptoms according to time of day or setting should also be noted. A detailed developmental history is also important, with particular attention to specific milestones and the initial appearance and course of ADHD symptoms.

   2. **Medical history and physical examination.** A history of ADHD symptoms in all biological relatives should be elicited. During the physical examination the physician may note multiple scars and abrasions among ADHD children due to their impulsivity.

TABLE 90–1. DIFFERENTIAL DIAGNOSIS OF PEDIATRIC ADHD

Condition	Commonly Shared Features	Distinctive Features
Conduct disorder	Disruptive, impulsive behavior	Severe rule violations; illegal acts; significant aggression
Oppositional–defiant disorder	Disruptive behavior annoying to others; noncompliant with adult requests	Argumentative; negativistic; irritable
Learning disabilities	Poor academic performance; may appear "off task" in classroom.	Academic skills significantly below level expected for IQ.
Major depression	Impaired attention and concentration; initial insomnia	Hypersomnia/terminal insomnia; a ppetite/weight disturbance; pervasive dysphoric/irritable mood; suicidal ideation
Bipolar disorder	High activity level; distractibility	Delusions, pronounced insomnia, cyclic mood variation

TABLE 90–2. DIFFERENTIAL DIAGNOSIS OF ADULT ADHD

Condition	Commonly Shared Features	Distinctive Features
Major depression	Subjective report of poor concentration, attention, and memory (often not supported by objective data); difficulty with task completion	Enduring dysphoric mood or anhedonia; sleep and appetite disturbance
Bipolar disorder	Hyperactivity, difficulty with maintaining attention; distractibility	Enduring dysphoric or euphoric mood; insomnia; delusions
General anxiety	Fidgetiness; difficulty concentrating	Exaggerated apprehension and worry; somatic symptoms of anxiety
Substance abuse or dependence	Difficulties with attention, concentration, and memory; mood swings	Pathologic pattern of substance use with social consequences; physiologic and psychologic tolerance and withdrawal
Personality disorders, particularly borderline and antisocial personality	Impulsivity; affective lability	Arrest history (antisocial personality); repeated self-injurious or suicidal behavior (borderline personality); lack of recognition that behavior is self-defeating

Adapted from Searight HR, Burke JM, Rottnek F: Adult AD/HD: Evaluation and treatment in family medicine. Am Fam Physician 2000; 62:2077, 2091

3. **Laboratory tests.** Blood chemistry should be obtained with particular attention to abnormal thyroid function and elevated serum lead levels. While most ADHD children do not exhibit abnormal laboratory values, these tests can exclude other causes of symptoms.
4. **Behavioral rating forms.** Standardized behavioral rating forms should be given to the parents and teachers to complete. Commonly used pediatric scales are classified into broad-band measures, assessing a number of psychiatric conditions, vs. narrow-band instruments, assessing only externalizing behavioral problems such as ADHD, oppositional–defiant disorder, and conduct disorder. The Child Behavior Check List (CBCL) and the longer Connors Parent and Teacher Rating Scales assess a wide range of psychiatric symptoms. More narrowly focused instruments include the Connors-Short Forms, the Disruptive Behavior Disorder (DBD) Scale, and the NICHQ Vanderbilt Assessment Scale. The Vanderbilt Scale is included in the National Initiative for Children's Healthcare Quality (NICHQ) ADHD toolkit and includes depressive symptoms along with externalizing behaviors.

With adults, the Brown and the Connors Adult ADHD Rating (CAARS) are used to assess current symptoms. Both the CAARS and the Brown scales are self-report measures but can also be administered to a collateral informant such as a spouse,

TABLE 90–3. EVALUATION PROCESS FOR SUSPECTED ADHD

Typically at initial office visit
1. Diagnostic interview
2. Medical history and physical examination
3. Any indicated laboratory tests
4. Behavioral rating forms to teachers, parents, other collateral informants, and with adults, to patients themselves
5. Review of behavior ratings and other relevant documents (eg, report cards)

Typically at follow-up office visit
6. Mental status evaluation (possible continuous performance testing)
7. If indicated, referral for specialized psychological or educational testing
8. If ADHD, institute treatment
9. If other conditions are present, refer for mental health or educational intervention (or both)

parent, or close friend. Brown's Scale is based on five dimensions: organization/ activation, attention and concentration, sustained energy and effort, management of emotionality, and working memory/access to previously learned material. The CAARS assesses hyperactivity, impulsivity, emotional lability, attention/memory, and self-concept. The Wender Utah Rating Scale (WURS) features retrospective items regarding the patient's functioning during childhood. In conjunction with other sources, the WURS may be helpful in establishing a long-standing history of symptoms.

In reviewing completed rating scales, the physician should distinguish core symptoms of ADHD such as inattention, distractibility, and impulsivity from other problem behaviors. Extreme ratings—particularly when they suggest significant levels of broad-band symptomatology—should be viewed with caution. While these extreme profiles suggest a significant degree of disruptive behavior, they may have limited value in making a specific diagnosis. Comparing teacher and parent rating is also valuable. In general, when parent ratings suggest high levels of perceived problems at home with few symptoms reported at school, a diagnosis of ADHD is less likely. (Sources for scales are provided at the end of the reference section. Most of those instruments are proprietary.)

5. **Office mental status examination.** Brief cognitive screening conducted in the office, focusing on short-term memory and attention and concentration, while not adequate for diagnosis, does provide useful clinical data. Immediate recall and attention may be assessed by orally presenting progressively longer strings of random digits and asking the patient to repeat them. Attention may also be assessed through vigilance tasks such as asking the patient to hold up a finger whenever the physician says the letter "A" in a series of random letters. A slightly more demanding task involving a higher level of concentration and attentional focus is asking patients to repeat digits in reverse order. Both children and adults may be asked to remember four words and queried about their recall at 5, 10, and possibly 15 minutes. Adolescents' and adults' short-term recall may be further assessed by reading them a short paragraph and asking them to verbally present it back to the examiner.

6. **Continuous performance tasks.** There are several computer-based tests of attention, concentration, and ability to manage distractions such as the Gordon Diagnostic System, the Test of Variable Attention (TOVA), and the Conners Continuous Performance Task. These tests are brief and provide a useful source of data that can be obtained in a standard office visit. Qualitatively, it is often helpful to observe children performing these tasks to determine their ability to maintain focused attention, the amount of time spent in "off task" behavior, and level of undirected motor activity. While these tests are promising, there is no single task that is diagnostic of ADHD.

7. **Diagnosis and referral.** The evaluation process typically leads to one of four outcomes:
   a. **ADHD is not present.** Symptoms are attributable to another medical or psychiatric condition.
   b. **Clear, unequivocal evidence of ADHD.** Pharmacotherapy will likely be instituted.
   c. **Diagnosis of ADHD and a comorbid condition.** The physician may initiate pharmacotherapy for ADHD and refer the patient to a mental health provider for further assessment and treatment of comorbid conditions, such as oppositional–defiant disorder or learning disability.
   d. **Diagnosis remains unclear.** In cases of an ambiguous diagnostic picture, the patient may be referred for more in-depth testing. For example, when a learning disability is suspected, the physician may refer the patient to the school district for a psychoeducational evaluation. Concerns about auditory processing disorder would lead to referral to a clinical audiologist. The results of these consultations may lead the physician to exclude ADHD or diagnose ADHD with a comorbid condition or ADHD alone.

III. **Treatment.** Treatment aims to decrease the core symptoms of ADHD-inattentiveness, hyperactivity, and impulsiveness—without causing adverse effects.
   A. **Pharmacotherapy** (Table 90–4). Stimulant medications (ie, methylphenidate [MPH], D-amphetamine, D,L-amphetamine) are first-line pharmacologic agents in conjunction with behavioral techniques, if appropriate. If a patient does not respond to stimulant

TABLE 90-4. DOSE AND TITRATION OF MEDICATIONS USED IN ADHD

Medication	How Supplied	Usual Initial Dose	Titration Schedule	Maximum Dose/Day	Dosage Schedule	Duration
Stimulant						
Methylphenidate						
Rapid onset, short duration						
Ritalin, Methylin[1]	Tablet: 5, 10, and 20 mg	5 mg bid	Increase 5–10 mg weekly	80 mg	bid–tid 30 minutes before breakfast and lunch; after school, if needed	3–6 h
Slower onset, longer duration						
Metadate ER[1]	Tablet: 10, 20 mg	10 mg qd	Increase by 10 mg at weekly intervals	60 mg	qd–bid	5–8 h
Ritalin SR[1]	Tablet: 20 mg	20 mg qd	Increase by 20 mg at weekly intervals	80 mg	qd–bid	5–8 h
Rapid onset, longer duration						
Metadate CD	Capsule: 20 mg	20 mg qd	Increase by 20 mg at weekly intervals until target of 1–2 mg/kg/day is reached	60 mg	qd	8 h
Ritalin-LA	Capsule: 20, 30, and 40 mg	Younger child or adolescent: 30 mg qd Older child or adolescent: 30 mg qd	Increase 10 mg weekly until target of 1–2 mg/kg/day is reached	60 mg	qd	8 h
Concerta	Tablet: 18, 27, 36, and 54 mg	Younger child: 18 mg qd Older child and adolescent: 36 mg qd	Increase weekly until target range of 1–2 mg/kg/day is reached	54 mg	qd	12 h

Amphetamine

Rapid, onset, short duration

	Formulation	Starting dose	Titration	Max dose	Frequency	Duration
Dexedrine[1] (dextroamphetamine)	Capsule: 5, 10, and 15 mg; Tablet: 5, 10, and 15 mg	2.5 mg bid	Increase 5–10 mg weekly	40 mg	bid–tid	4–6 h
DextroStat[1] (dextroamphetamine)	Tablet: 5 and 10 mg	2.5 mg bid	Increase 5–10 mg weekly	40 mg	bid–tid	4–6 h

Slower onset, longer duration

Dexedrine Spansules[1] (dextroamphetamine)	Capsule: 5, 10, and 15 mg	5 mg each morning	Increase 5–10 mg weekly	40 mg	qd–bid	6–10 h

Rapid onset, longer duration

Adderall[1] (dextroamphetamine/ amphetamine)	Tablet: 5, 7.5, 10, 12.5, 15, 20, and 30 mg	2.5 mg	Increase 5 to 10 mg weekly	40 mg	qd–bid	6–8 h
Adderall XR (dextroamphetamine/ amphetamine)	Capsules: 5, 10, 20, and 30 mg	Younger child: 10 mg qd Older child or adolescent: 20 mg qd	Increase weekly until target range of 0.5–1 mg/kg/day is reached	30 mg	qd	10–12 h

Miscellaneous

Slower onset, longer duration

Pemoline[1] (Cylert)	Tablet: 18.75, 37.5, and 75 mg Chewable tablet: 37.5 mg	18.75 mg each morning	Increase 18.75 or 37.5 mg increments every 3 days	112.5 mg	qd–bid	6–10 h

(continued)

TABLE 90–4. DOSE AND TITRATION OF MEDICATIONS USED IN ADHD (*Continued*)

Medication	How Supplied	Usual Initial Dose	Titration Schedule	Maximum dose/day	Dosage Schedule	Duration
Nonstimulant						
Atomoxetine (Strattera)	Capsule: 10, 18, 25, 40, 60 mg	<70 kg—0.5 mg/kg/day >70 kg—40 mg qd	Increase to 1.2 mg/kg/day after 3 days Increase to 80 mg after 3 days; may increase to 100 mg after 2–4 weeks	1.4 mg/kg/day or 100 mg (whichever is less)	qd–bid	
Bupropion[1] (Wellbutrin)	IR Tablet: 75 mg and 100 mg	50 mg bid	Increase 50 to 100 mg every 7–10 days	450 mg qd	qd–tid (Separate doses by at least 6 hours)	
Clonidine[1] (Catapres)	Tablet: 0.1, 0.2, 0.3 mg	0.05 mg qd	Increased in increments of 0.05 or 0.1 mg per dose, usually starting with hs dose		bid–qid (unless dosing at hs to decrease insomnia)	
Guanfacine[1] (Tenex)	Tablet: 1, 2 mg	Children: 0.5 mg qd Adolescents: 1 mg qd	Increased every 3 or 4 days in increments of 0.5 to 1 mg until benefit noted	4 mg	qd	
Imipramine[1] (Tofranil)	Tablet: 10, 25, and 50 mg	Younger children: 10 mg bid Older children: 20 mg bid Adolescents: 25 mg bid	Increase every 7–10 days by 10, 20, or 25 mg increments until improvement noted	300 mg qd	bid (to prevent excess sedation)	
Wellbutrin SR	SR Tablet: 100, 150, 200 mg	100 mg bid			bid (Separate doses by at least 8 hours)	

[1] Generic available.

medications or there are contraindications, then alternative nonstimulant medications such as atomoxetine, antidepressants (tricyclics and bupropion), or antihypertensives (clonidine and guanfacine) may be used.

1. **Stimulants** reduce symptoms of hyperactivity, impulsivity, and inattentiveness. Inhibition of dopamine and norepinephrine reuptake is the principal mechanism. Children and adolescents can see a response rate of approximately 70% for a specific stimulant, and approximately 90% respond to at least one stimulant. Careful dose titration reduces adverse effects. One stimulant agent is not preferred over another, but if a child does not respond to one stimulant medication, then another one may be tried. A positive response to a stimulant is not diagnostic of ADHD since children with comorbid conditions such as narcolepsy and depression may show a positive response as well. Additionally, children and adults without ADHD who ingest stimulants demonstrate improvement in attention, concentration, and memory tasks.

   a. **Adverse effects.** Common adverse effects include anorexia or appetite disturbance (80%), sleep disturbances (3–85%), and weight loss (10–15%). Less common side effects include headaches, social withdrawal, nervousness, and irritability. In controlled studies, MPH has not been shown to worsen motor tics in Tourette's syndrome and has shown no increase in motor tics in children without Tourette's syndrome. Studies have shown stimulants to have no effect on growth suppression during treatment or on ultimate adult height.

   b. **Contraindications.** Concomitant use of monoamine oxidase (MAO) inhibitors, psychosis, glaucoma, history of recent stimulant drug abuse or dependence, existing liver disorder, or abnormal liver functions tests (pemoline).

   c. **Drug interactions.** Stimulants should not be used in combination with MAO inhibitors because of the risk for developing serotonin syndrome.

      (1) **Methylphenidate** is available in various dosages and delivery systems. Immediate release (IR) forms (ie, Ritalin, Methylin) should be dosed two to three times daily. A third dose may be added after school to help children on homework and after-school activities. Metadate CD and Ritalin LA are extended-release capsules with a bimodal release profile. Metadate CD's 20-mg capsules contain a mixture of IR and extended-release (ER) beads in a 70:30 ratio; whereas Ritalin LA's capsules are in a 50:50 ratio. Both capsules' contents may be emptied and sprinkled over a spoonful of applesauce. Ritalin SR is composed of a wax matrix that provides a sustained release (SR) of MPH. It is not widely used by clinicians because of its erratic absorption, delayed onset of action and lower plasma peak concentrations. Concerta is dosed once daily and uses osmotic pressure to deliver MPH at a constant rate. Table 90–5 includes conversions of IR MPH to Ritalin LA and Concerta.

      (2) **D-Amphetamine** is also available in IR and ER forms. It is as effective as MPH, but may be preferred for those who do not tolerate or do not respond to MPH. The IR formulation, Dexedrine, is dosed two to three times a day, with a third optimal dose in late afternoon. Dexedrine spansule is a SR preparation that lasts for 8–10 hours and is consistently absorbed.

      (3) **D,L-Amphetamine (Adderall)** has a longer half-life than IR MPH, but not as long as the Dexedrine spansule. Adderall XR is a capsule composed of IR and delayed-release beads in a ratio of 50:50 and may be sprinkled over food.

      (4) **Pemoline** has a 12-hour half-life, thus allowing it to be dosed once to twice daily. Pemoline can cause life-threatening hepatotoxity, and therefore should not be used unless (1) a child has failed treatment with two stimulants and one antidepressant, (2) parents have signed a consent form stating that the child is at risk for hepatotoxicity and death with this medication and that biweekly liver functions tests must be performed, and (3) baseline liver function tests are normal. The manufacturer recommends that if the child does not respond after 3 weeks, then the medication should be discontinued. If the alanine aminotransferase is greater than two times the normal limit, pemoline must be discontinued.

      (5) **Miscellaneous.** When writing a prescription for multiple daily doses, it is helpful to write for a separate labeled bottle that may be taken to school

TABLE 90–5. CONVERSION OF IMMEDIATE-RELEASE TO SUSTAINED-RELEASE PREPARATIONS

Previous Methylphenidate (MPH) Dose	Recommended Dose
5 mg IR MPH bid	Concerta 18 mg qam
5 mg IR MPH tid	
MPH-SR 20 mg qd	
MPH IR 10 mg bid	Concerta 36 mg qam
MPH IR 10 mg tid	
MPH-SR 40 mg qd	
MPH IR 15 mg bid	Concerta 54 mg qam
MPH IR 15 mg tid	
MPH-SR 60 mg qd	
MPH IR 10 mg bid	Ritalin LA 20 mg qd
MPH-SR 20 mg qd	
MPH IR 15 mg bid	Ritalin LA 30 mg qd
MPH IR 20 mg bid	Ritalin LA 40 mg qd
MPH-SR 40 mg qd	
MPH IR 30 mg bid	Ritalin LA 60 mg qd
MPH-SR 60 mg qd	
MPH IR 10 mg bid	Metadate CD 20 mg qd
MPH IR 20 mg bid	Metadate CD 40 mg qd

by the child that only has the school dose on it. Sustained-release preparations may be used to help increase compliance since many children may be uncomfortable taking a dose at school or may forget the second or third daily doses.

2. **Nonstimulant medications,** such as atomoxetine, antidepressants, and antihypertensives, should be considered when stimulants have failed or patients have contraindications or significant adverse effects to stimulants. Except for atomoxetine, nonstimulant medications usually do not demonstrate benefit for all three core ADHD symptoms—hyperactivity, inattention, or impulsivity. The antidepressants, tricyclics and bupropion, decrease hyperactivity and inattention; however, they do not reduce impulsivity. Antihypertensives, such as the α_2 agonists, are effective in decreasing impulsivity and hyperactivity but do not improve attentiveness. These alternative medications require closer patient monitoring than stimulants but may be dosed less frequently.

   a. **Atomoxetine** is the first nonstimulant medication to be approved by the US Food and Drug Administration for treatment of both pediatric and adult ADHD. Similar to stimulants, atomoxetine inhibits norepinephrine reuptake. Advantages of atomoxetine include little, if any, cardiovascular toxicity; no known adverse effects on tic disorders; and no growth suppression. The manufacturer recommends using atomoxetine with caution in patients with hypertension, tachycardia, or cardiovascular or cerebrovascular disease. However, in clinical trials, increased blood pressure (BP) (2 mm Hg diastolic BP and 3 mm Hg systolic BP) and pulse (8 beats per minute) were clinically insignificant. These increases plateau during therapy but normalize once treatment is discontinued. During clinical trials, the most common reasons for discontinuation trials were decreased appetite, sleep disturbances, and anxiety or nervousness.

      (1) **Adverse effects.** These included decreased appetite (14%), vomiting (11%), dizziness (6%), fatigue (4%), nausea and dyspepsia (4%), and mood swings (2%).

      (2) **Contraindications.** Use with MAO inhibitors or narrow angle glaucoma.

      (3) **Drug interactions.** Atomoxetine is a CYP-2D6 substrate; therefore, its levels may increase when used with CYP-2D6 inhibitors such as fluoxetine and paroxetine. For patients using atomoxetine concomitantly with strong CYP-2D6 inhibitors, atomoxetine should only be increased up to 1.2 mg/kg/day after 4 weeks if the patient weighs <70 kg and only increased to 80 mg/day after 4 weeks if the patient weighs >70 kg. Concomitant use with albuterol can increase heart rate.

b. Antidepressants
   (1) Tricyclic antidepressants (TCAs) inhibit the reuptake of norepinephrine and serotonin. When using TCAs, blood pressure, pulse, complete blood count, electrocardiograms (ECGs), and serum blood levels should be carefully monitored. There have been several case reports of sudden cardiac death in young adolescents. While there is no clear explanation for these events, it is recommended that ECGs should be performed every 3–6 months. Blood pressure should not exceed 140/90 mm Hg and resting pulse should not be >130 beats per minute. Serum blood levels do not correlate with the therapeutic effect in the treatment of ADHD, but rather with the incidence of adverse effects. Serum levels should be routinely monitored for toxicity. Serum levels for depressin for imipramine are 180–240 ng/mL; for desipramine, 100–300 ng/mL; and for nortriptyline, 50–150 ng/mL. (Nortriptyline is the least sedating of the three, while imipramine is the most sedating.) Routine serum levels to determine efficacy are not recommended, but may be drawn if adverse effects are noticed.
      (a) Adverse effects. Dry mouth, constipation, blurred vision, and sedation.
      (b) Contraindications. Concomitant use with an MAO inhibitor. Use with extreme caution in children with cardiac conduction abnormalities.
      (c) Drug interactions. TCAs should not be used in combination with MAO inhibitors because of the risk for developing serotonin syndrome.
   (2) Bupropion inhibits reuptake of dopamine and norepinephrine. Although safety has not been formally established in children younger than age 18, bupropion has been studied in children and adolescents. Results were better in adolescents than in children. Bupropion appears to be particularly beneficial in adolescents with comorbid psychiatric conditions.
      (a) Adverse effects. These include nausea, headache, and insomnia.
      (b) Contraindications. These include a history of seizure disorder or history of anorexia/bulimia.
      (c) Drug interactions. Avoid concomitant use of other drugs that increase dopamine levels.
   (3) MAO inhibitors, while an effective alternative treatment, are limited by food and drug interactions.
   (4) SSRIs have not been found to reduce the symptoms associated with ADHD, but may be used in combination with stimulants to treat with comorbid depression.
   (5) Venlafaxine possesses both noradrenergic and serotonergic properties. Several studies have shown promising results, but further investigation is needed.
c. Antihypertensives—α_2 agonists, such as **clonidine** and **guanfacine**—can be useful in children not responding to MPH alone, or those with post-traumatic stress disorder or significant aggression. Clonidine, while not as effective as stimulant medications, has been shown to reduce hyperactivity and impulsivity but not improve attention span. Guanfacine, on the other hand, may improve inattentiveness. Sedation may limit the use of these drugs, but a bedtime dose of clonidine may be beneficial in children with sleep disturbances. α_2 Agonists do not worsen tics. Guanfacine is preferred by many practitioners over clonidine because of its longer duration of action, possibly fewer sedative effects, and reduced likelihood of inducing hypotension. α_2 Agonists should not be used in children with pre-existing cardiac or vascular disease without consultation with a cardiologist. Blood pressure and pulse should be measured when initiating clonidine, increasing the dose, and periodically while taking the medication. Clonidine should be tapered over 7–14 days to avoid rebound hypertension. Adverse effects include sedation and dry mouth.

B. Discussing pharmacotherapy with patients
   1. Listen to the parents' concerns and dispel any myths that may arise. Reassure parents that the child will not become addicted to the stimulant medication, final adult height will not be affected, and that stimulant safety and efficacy have been demonstrated in numerous studies and years of clinical practice. Set realistic behavioral goals with the parent and child. Emphasize the benefits of treatment, such as decreased hyperactivity, improved concentration, control of impulses, and decreased

disruptive behavior. Educate the parents about the potential consequences of untreated ADHD, such as poor school performance, relationship difficulty, disorganization, and inability to complete tasks.

2. Parents should be educated that the most common adverse effects of stimulants include appetite suppression (with weight loss), sleep difficulties, and rebound moodiness and irritability. Parents should periodically assess their child's nutritional status. It may be helpful to have the child eat breakfast before taking their morning dose. If the child's appetite seems to be decreased at lunch, the child will usually eat a hearty snack in the afternoon as their medication is wearing off. Difficulty falling asleep may be addressed by delaying the child's bedtime to after 9 PM or adding a sedating medication such as clonidine. Rebound moodiness and irritability may manifest after school for about 30–60 minutes as the medication is wearing off. The addition of a small, short-acting dose immediately after school or allowing the child some quiet time before beginning homework may help alleviate these symptoms.

3. It is reported that 30–66% of individuals diagnosed with ADHD as a child will continue to have symptoms persisting into adulthood. As in other chronic health conditions, pharmacotherapy may be lifelong.

4. Although drug holidays have been advocated in the past, many children will require drug therapy year-round to maintain attention and decrease hyperactivity—symptoms that frequently disrupt family, recreational, and social activities.

5. Children who have been responding well to medication treatment for many months may return to the physician with complaints by parents and teachers that the medication is no longer "working." While adjustments of medication dosages may be indicated, other causes should be considered. The physician should very specifically inquire about the types of behavior that are of concern. Issues such as lying, talking back, and angry outbursts may reflect development comorbid conditions. Adults' point of reference for ADHD child may have unconsciously shifted over time. Initially, children treated with medication are compared with themselves prior to medication initiation. However, over time this reference point may change and the ADHD child may be implicitly compared to school-aged peers or siblings. Most ADHD children continue to manifest some symptoms of the disorder even when on an optimal regimen of medication. When questions of medication effectiveness arise, a new set of behavioral ratings may clarify the clinical picture.

C. **Special issues in pharmacotherapy with adults.** To date, atomoxetine is the only medication formally approved by the FDA for the treatment of adult ADHD. Stimulants are effective in adults, but must be used with caution in patients with a history of drug abuse. Even though patients will not become "high" from oral MPH because of its slow release to the brain, patients can become "high" from injecting a liquid form of MPH. This "high" is similar to that of cocaine. For adults who do not respond to stimulants or have contraindications for their use, bupropion, TCAs, and atomoxetine are suitable alternatives. Bupropion and TCAs are used more often in adults and may be beneficial in patients with comorbid psychiatric conditions.

D. **Nonpharmacologic treatment for children and adolescents with ADHD**

1. Pharmacotherapy is clearly the treatment of choice for ADHD and is beneficial for the vast majority of patients. Studies investigating the efficacy of adjunctive psychosocial treatments suggest that the core features of ADHD do not significantly improve with the combined interventions. However, comorbid conditions and associated features of the disorder may improve with psychological and psychosocial treatments, and therefore are often important adjuncts to treating a patient with ADHD. The American Academy of Pediatrics, American Medical Association, and American Academy of Child and Adolescent Psychiatry all recommend the use of multimodal treatments.

2. Psychosocial interventions include psychoeducation, parent/family-focused strategies, child interventions, and school interventions.

   a. Psychoeducation provides the child, parents, family, and school with information about ADHD, its treatment, and its impact on learning, behavior, self-esteem, social skills, and family functioning. Educating the family also allows the physician an opportunity to correct misperceptions. For example, the child may feel that s/he is "dumb," or the parents may fear that the child is going to become a "drug addict" as a result of the stimulant medication. Patient education is also likely to facilitate treatment planning, including the identification of specific behavioral goals, follow-up activities, and monitoring. Family physicians should inform families of appropriate sources for ADHD information, such as Children and Adults with Attention Deficit/Hyperactivity Disorder (CHADD) (www.chadd.org), The Society for Developmental and Behavioral Pediatrics (www.dbpeds.org/handouts), and the American Academy of Child and Adolescent Psychiatry (AACAP) (www.aacap.org/publications/factsfam/noattent.htm).

b. Parent- or family-focused strategies may include support groups, advocacy groups, and behavior therapy focused on parent skills training.

   (1) The content of parent training programs for children with ADHD typically includes components such as an overview of the disorder, review of behavior management principles, the use of positive reinforcement, extinction, response cost, and the development of a reward-oriented behavioral system.

   (2) The MTA Cooperative Group (1999) represents the largest and best-designed study published to date regarding the efficacy of pharmacotherapy, behavioral parent training, child-focused treatment, and school-based intervention in the treatment of ADHD. Compared to wait-list controls, children with ADHD receiving adjunctive parent training displayed significant changes in several areas of psychosocial functioning immediately after the treatment and during a 2-month follow-up.

c. Child interventions for ADHD such as social skills training, cognitive behavioral therapy, and study/organizational skills do not have solid empirical support for the treatment of ADHD, and the gains achieved in the treatment setting typically do not transfer into the classroom or home settings. Again, however, child interventions may be indicated when there are comorbid disorders, particularly internalizing symptoms, that are also the focus of treatment.

d. School interventions such as classroom accommodations, ongoing collaboration and communication between teacher and primary care providers, and special education services are often important in the treatment and monitoring of ADHD symptoms.

   (1) ADHD is included as a disability under the Individuals with Disabilities Education Act (IDEA [PL-101-476]). Therefore, children with ADHD may qualify for special education services or appropriate accommodations within the regular classroom setting under Section 504 of the Rehabilitation Act of 1973. Patients may also be eligible for reasonable accommodations in secular private schools and postsecondary education under The Americans with Disabilities Act.

   (2) Classroom accommodations may include changes in the child's educational programming, including tutoring, resource room support, extended time to complete tasks, or decreased workload. Additional modification may be helpful, such as providing increased structure for assignments and behavioral expectations, having assignments written on the blackboard, and placing the child in the front of the classroom or close to the teacher.

   (3) Collaboration with the school may include the identification of appropriate behavioral goals that should guide treatment. No more than three target behaviors should be monitored at once, and goals should be realistic, attainable, and measurable. The teacher's completion of a daily report card facilitates the monitoring of symptoms and the need for changes in the treatment plan.

E. Organizational skills and environmental modification for the ADHD adult. While there is little empirical research on nonpharmacologic treatment of adult ADHD, these suggestions are helpful:

1. To foster **self-management skills,** organizers such as calendars, day planners, and Palm Pilots when consistently employed may prompt recall and improve personal organizational skills.

2. **Reducing distractions in the workplace** is helpful. For ADHD adults with flexible work times, going into work before most coworkers arrive is helpful. This "quiet time" may help the ADHD adult get organized and accomplish tasks before there are increased distractions. Similarly, this strategy of early awakening is also useful in managing a household. The patient's immediate workplace itself should be free of clutter and other distractions such as family photos and personal mementos.

3. For adults in an ongoing relationship, conjoint counseling can address **communication issues** and help educate both spouses about the impact of ADHD in their daily lives. Formal documentation of an ADHD diagnosis is typically required.

4. For adults involved in a formal educational program such as college or professional school, accommodations may be available. Examples include **extended time for tests and the option of taking tests alone** in a special resource room rather than in a traditional classroom with other students.

F. **Complementary and alternative medicines.** Complementary and alternative treatments may be sought by parents who are looking for a more "natural" remedy for ADHD or who are fearful about their children taking stimulants. While some of the alternative complementary and alternative treatments have been evaluated in placebo-controlled trials, most of the evidence is from anecdotal reports. Neurofeedback, iron supplements, diet, homeopathy, herbal medicines, and dietary supplements have all been used in the treatment of ADHD.

1. **Neurofeedback** is believed to improve attentiveness and impulsivity. While it may have some success in reducing symptoms, the long-term effects are not known.

2. **Iron supplements** are based on the belief that children with ADHD have an iron deficiency. If iron-deficiency is suspected, hematologic testing should be performed; otherwise, routine use of iron supplementation should not be used in non-deficient children.

3. **Diet** for children has been altered in several different ways to decrease the symptoms of ADHD. Despite popular myths, sugar does not exacerbate or cause hyperactivity. Elimination of food dye from food and drinks has yielded inconclusive evidence.

4. **Homeopathic** treatments such as Cina and Hyoscyamus niger have been used to decrease symptoms. Despite potential use for these products, additional evaluation is needed to determine efficacy and place in therapy.

5. **Herbal medicines,** such as ginkgo, evening primrose, valerian, lemon balm, and more have been used to decrease symptoms of hyperactivity. Parents should be reminded that herbal medications are not regulated by the FDA and may not contain standardized doses.

6. **Dietary supplements.** There is no evidence to support that ADHD children benefit from megadoses of vitamins.

Until more controlled studies are done to determine efficacy of complementary and alternative treatments, proven pharmacological therapies should remain first line.

IV. **Prognosis.** ADHD is a chronic neurologically based condition with at least some symptoms persisting into adolescence and adulthood in up to 70% of diagnosed children. Developmentally, specific symptoms may change, with marked reductions in hyperactivity and impulsivity beginning at age 9. However, inattention typically persists through adolescence and into adulthood.

The relatively few prospective ADHD studies suggest that adolescents and adults with ADHD histories are at risk for legal problems, traffic accidents, noncompletion of formal education, substance abuse, and other psychiatric disorders. However, in counseling parents about the prognosis for ADHD children, available ADHD research has several limitations. Diagnostic standards have changed during the past 15 years, with current DSM-IV criteria identifying milder forms of ADHD than previously. These changing diagnostic criteria are likely to be a major factor in recent increased ADHD prevalence rates than previously reported. Adults with ADHD, if diagnosed as children, were likely to have had particularly severe symptoms.

ADHD's longitudinal course is further complicated by increased comorbidity through the lifespan. Comorbidity rises to at least 50% during adolescence and may be as high as 70% in adulthood. A consistent research finding is the particularly poor psychiatric and legal outcomes for ADHD with comorbid conduct disorder. Significant attrition in prospective studies limits knowledge of ADHD's independent prognosis.

With these caveats, adolescents with an ADHD history are two to four times more likely to be arrested, two to four times more likely to be diagnosed with antisocial personality, and four times more likely to have nonalcohol substance abuse problems. While severity of substance use is greater for ADHD with comorbid conduct disorder, young adults with ADHD alone are more likely than non-ADHD controls to smoke cigarettes. Primary care risk counseling should be particularly thorough with ADHD teenagers.

Among adults, an ADHD history is associated with a greater likelihood of receiving both inpatient and outpatient psychiatric treatment. These adults are more likely to be fired from or quit jobs and have lower SES than non-ADHD adults. ADHD is also a risk factor for relationship conflict, including separation and divorce.

While data are scarce, ADHD treatment during childhood appears to reduce the incidence of later adverse outcomes. A common parental fear is that stimulant pharmacotherapy during childhood may lead to substance abuse. A recent meta-analysis concluded that stimulant treatment actually protected against later adolescent and young adult drug and alcohol abuse.

REFERENCES

Barkley RA: *Attention Deficit Hyperactivity Disorder: A Handbook for Diagnosis and Treatment,* 2nd ed. Guilford; 1998.

Biederman J: Practical considerations in stimulant drug selection for the attention-deficit/hyperactivity disorder patient—efficacy, potency and titration. Today's Therapeutic Trend 2002;**20**(4):311.

Biederman J, Mick E, Faraone SV: Age-dependent decline of symptoms of Attention-Deficit/Hyperactivity Disorder. Impact of remission definition and symptom type. Am J Psychiatry 2000;**157**:816.

Clinical Practice Guideline: Treatment of school-aged child with Attention-Deficit/Hyperactivity Disorder. Pediatrics 2001;**108**(4):1033.

Greydanus DE, Sloan MA, Rappley MD: Psychopharmacology of ADHD in adolescents. Adolesc Med 2002;**13**(3):599.

Practice Parameters for the Use of Stimulant Medications in the Treatment of Children, Adolescents, and Adults. J Am Acad Child Adolesc Psychiatry 2002;**41**(suppl 2):26S.

Searight HR, Burke JM, Rottnek F: Adult AD/HD: Evaluation and treatment in family medicine. Am Fam Physician 2000;**62**:2077, 2091.

Subcommittee on Attention-Deficit/Hyperactivity Disorder, Committee on Quality Improvement: Clinical practice guideline: Treatment of the school-aged child with attention-deficit/hyperactivity disorder. Pediatrics 2001:**108**(4):1033.

Weckerly J: Pediatric bipolar mood disorder: Developmental and behavioral pediatrics. 2002;**23**:42.

Wilens TE, et al: Does stimulant therapy of Attention-Deficit/Hyperactivity Disorder beget later substance abuse? A meta-analytic review of the literature. Pediatrics 2003;**111**:179.

Zametkin AJ, Ernst M: Problems in the management of attention deficit hyperactivity disorder. N Engl J Med 1999:**340**(1):40.

SOURCES FOR RATING SCALES

Achenbach System of Empirically Based Assessment (www.asbca.org)

Brown Attention Deficit—Disorder Scales for Adolescents and Adults. The Psychological Corporation. (www.marketplace.psychcorp.com)

Child Behavior Checklist (CBCL). (www.asbca.org)

Connors Ratings Scales. Wide Range Inc. (www.widerange.com)

Disruptive Behavior Disorders Rating Scale. Comprehensive Treatment for Attention Deficit Disorder. (www.13dd.com/ctadd/)

National Initiative for Children's Healthcare Quality. Vanderbilt Parent and Teacher Scales. American Academy of Pediatrics (www.aap.org/bookstore)

Wender Utah Rating Scale. Paul Wender, MD (www.add-pediatrics.com/add/wender)

---

91   Family Violence: Child, Intimate Partner, & Elder Abuse

F. David Schneider, MD, MSPH, Nancy D. Kellogg, MD, & Melissa A. Talamantes, MS

KEY POINTS

- Know the laws in your state regarding mandatory reporting of family violence, including child abuse, intimate partner violence, and elder abuse. Most states have mandatory reporting laws for both those younger than 18 years and older than 64 years.
- Ask about family violence as a routine part of your history taking. This gives patients permission to talk about it when they feel comfortable.
- Assess the situation for lethality—use of guns or knives by the perpetrator or escalating violence may require immediate intervention by police.
- Learn about your community resources for support of victims of family violence, and use them when appropriate with your patients.

I. Child Abuse and Neglect

A. Definitions

1. **Child physical abuse** is any intentional injury resulting in tissue damage, including bruises, burns, lacerations, fractures, and organ or blood vessel rupture. In addition, any inflicted injury that lasts more than 24 hours constitutes significant injury. Physical abuse comprises approximately 25% of the four types of abuse and neglect.

2. **Child sexual abuse** encompasses a variety of interactions that adults or adolescents use to take advantage of vulnerable children in a sexual manner, including both sexual contact and exploitation for pornography or prostitution. Another form of sexual abuse involves solicitation through the computer; almost one in five children who go "online" regularly is approached by strangers for sex. Approximately 15% of abuse and neglect is sexual abuse.

3. **Neglect** is the inadequate nutrition, shelter, or care (or all of these) necessary to meet the basic needs of a child, allowing him to grow and develop. Medical neglect occurs when the caretaker ignores important medical or dental treatment plans. Neglect is most common of the four types and comprises 50% of the total.

4. **Emotional abuse** includes rejecting a child's worth or needs, constant berating or belittlement, or making the child engage in destructive behavior. While accounting for 10% of all types, emotional abuse commonly accompanies physical abuse, sexual abuse, and neglect.

B. Epidemiology.
There are 3 million reported cases of child abuse and neglect in United States annually; 2000–4000 children die of abuse or neglect each year. Eighty percent of child abuse fatalities occur in children younger than age 5, and 40% occur during a child's first year of life. Neglect most often involves preverbal children, whereas sexual abuse is reported during school-age and adolescent years. Despite large numbers of reported cases, child abuse and neglect remains an underdetected and underreported problem. It has been estimated that 20% of children will sustain an abusive injury during childhood, and 14–40% of females will be sexually abused before reaching adulthood.

C. Diagnosis

1. **Barriers to diagnosis.** Since child abuse only recently became a mandated component of primary care residency training, many physicians lack the knowledge and training to recognize the signs and symptoms of abuse and neglect. Detection is also compromised by the following: the child or family may attribute injuries to discipline rather than abuse; physicians typically rely on a caretaker's history, which may be untruthful if abuse has occurred; victims may be preverbal and unable to provide important information; verbal victims may be reluctant to disclose abuse out of fear, guilt, or shame; and injuries may be old, indistinct, or nonexistent. In addition, the physician must have an index of suspicion in order to make the diagnosis.

2. **Physical abuse.** The diagnosis of physical abuse and neglect typically begins with "what you see." Bruises are the most common manifestation of physical abuse, yet most bruises of childhood are accidental rather than inflicted. Patterned bruises, and location of bruises (such as buttocks, neck, and side of face) help distinguish nonaccidental from accidental causes. In addition, any unexplained injury in a younger child is suspicious for abuse; as one study suggests, "if you don't cruise (developmental milestone achieved around 8 months of age), you don't bruise." Table 91–1 lists injuries and conditions that are suspicious for abuse and neglect.

   a. **Explanation consistency.** Once a suspicious injury or condition is identified, the physician must establish whether the explanation is consistent with the characteristics of the injury or condition. Vague or no explanation for a severe injury is suspicious for nonaccidental trauma or criminal neglect. An explanation that is inconsistent with the severity, age, or pattern of the injury(s) constitutes a suspicion of abuse. The physician should listen carefully and respectfully to the caretaker's statements, maintain a nonjudgmental demeanor, and document all explanations, including discrepancies. Caretakers should be interviewed separately, gathering detailed information about the child's injury, developmental capabilities, food intake, and behavior and activity prior to the injury or deterioration in condition. If the child is 4 years or older, the physician may question the child out of the presence of the parent. The physician must

TABLE 91–1. INJURIES (BRUISES, BURNS, FRACTURES) THAT SHOULD BE CAREFULLY EVALUATED FOR PHYSICAL ABUSE

1. Age 0–6 months: *Any injury.*
2. Age 6 months or older:
   a. Bruises, lacerations, or burns to protected, fleshy, or flexor surfaces—*for example,* inner thighs, abdomen, neck, face (other than frontal prominence), pinna, genitalia.
   b. Bruises, lacerations, or burns showing an object pattern—*for example,* belt loop, cigarette burn, curling iron.
   c. Oral injuries, *especially* frenulum and palate lacerations.
   d. Third-degree burns or large second-degree burns, *especially* scald burns.
   e. Fractures, *especially* metaphyseal fractures, complex or wide skull fractures, rib fractures, spiral fractures of humerus or femur, scapula fractures.
   f. Significant head injury, *especially* subdural hematoma, retinal hemorrhage, subgaleal hematoma, avulsed hair, complex or wide skull fracture. Head injury should be considered whenever a child presents with vomiting or altered consciousness, or bloody spinal fluid is found on lumbar puncture, but an infectious process cannot be readily diagnosed.
   g. Intra-abdominal injury, *especially* rupture or hematoma of internal organ.
3. Age 0–10 years: Positive urine or blood screen for alcohol or drugs of abuse.

Findings that should be carefully evaluated for *sexual abuse:*
1. Any injury to the genitalia (*especially* to the hymen or vestibule in girls) or anus.
2. Identification of an STD: Chlamydia, gonorrhea, HSV, HPV, HIV, HBV, HCV, *Trichomonas,* syphilis.
3. Positive pregnancy test.
4. Any history or statement or witnessed incident consistent with sexual abuse.

Findings that should be carefully evaluated for *neglect:*
1. Growth parameters below expected for age.
2. Lack of medical care for a significant health problem—*for example,* no medications for asthma, diabetes; no care of severe dental caries.
3. Lack of normal bonding with parent/guardian.
4. Disregard of one or more basic child care needs—*for example,* soft drink in baby bottle, child found in street, failure to place child in auto safety seat or belt.

Note: A child may have findings suggesting more than one form of abuse or neglect.
HBV, hepatitis B virus; HCV, hepatitis C virus; HIV, human immunodeficiency virus; HPV, human papilloma virus; HSV, herpes simplex virus; STD, sexually transmitted disease.
Excerpted from the Texas Pediatric Society Committee on Child Abuse "Clinical Practice Resource for Hospitals and Emergency Departments."

remain unbiased, and ask questions that are not leading or suggestive. For example, "What happened to your arm?" is preferable to "Who hurt your arm?" or "Did Daddy hurt you?" Physicians should remain emotionally neutral, and strive to earn, not assume, the child's trust.

   b. **Tests.** Serious injuries warrant further laboratory and radiologic testing to rule out blood disorders that may mimic abuse and assess for occult liver (liver function tests), bone (skeletal survey), and intracranial (magnetic resonance imaging or computerized tomography of the head) injuries. In addition, a dilated ophthalmologic examination is indicated to look for retinal hemorrhages, which may be attributable to abusive head trauma. In evaluating suspected neglect, complete electrolyte and hematologic profiles may establish the severity and chronicity of malnutrition.

3. **Sexual and emotional abuse.** These forms of abuse begin with "what you hear." Over 90% of child sexual abuse is first discovered when the child tells someone about the abuse. Emotional abuse is typically detected when a child's behavioral or emotional state causes concern and questioning confirms the diagnosis. The diagnosis of sexual abuse is based on the history from the child. Forensic evidence, genital or anal injury, and sexually transmitted diseases are each detected in fewer than 15% of sexual abuse or assault victims. While forensic evidence is recovered in approximately 25% of victims, few children present within 72 hours of their assault, the time frame within which such evidence is recoverable. Injuries due to acute sexual assault occur less than 25% of the time and are most likely to heal completely within a week. While most examinations are normal, "normal" does not

mean "nothing happened." Documentation of the child's history, preferably in quotes, is critically important, and may be read during civil or criminal court proceedings. In addition, photo-documentation of physical or sexual abuse injuries, as well as visible signs of neglect, is a standard of care for abuse evaluations.

D. Management strategies. Once a physician has established that the child may have been abused, laws in all 50 states require that the physician report to Child Protective Services or law enforcement. Centralized or local reporting procedures are established in each state. The physician is not required to prove that abuse has occurred in order to report; failure to report suspected abuse is a criminal offense. The decision to inform the family of reporting depends on whether sharing such information could potentially jeopardize the child's safety until reporting agencies can intervene.

Many areas have established specialized child abuse assessment programs that include trained medical professionals. A primary care physician may opt to conduct a limited medical assessment once abuse is suspected and refer such cases to specialized child abuse programs, when available. Children's Advocacy Centers are located in most states and can provide assistance to physicians regarding resources, services, and assessments for abused children.

E. Prognosis. Abused children are at greater risk for psychiatric disorders, both in child and adulthood, learning disabilities, eating disorders, and low school functioning. Abused and neglected children are also more likely to become teenage mothers, substance abusers, runaways, and delinquents. Affective, anxiety, and personality disorders often persist into adulthood. Obesity, anxiety disorders, post-traumatic stress disorder, and chronic pelvic pain are frequently seen in adult survivors of child sexual abuse. Child abuse and neglect clearly compromise children's abilities to become productive, healthy members of society.

Without effective intervention, child abuse becomes an intergenerational cycle. An abused child is more likely to become an abuser, an adult partner of a child abuser, or an abused adult.

II. Intimate Partner Violence

A. Definition. *Wife or spouse abuse* is often used interchangeably with *domestic violence* or **intimate partner violence (IPV).** IPV is used more often today because it is more inclusive of all kinds of intimate relationships, including dating, sex partners, and same-sex relationships. IPV includes verbal harassment or threats, sexual assault, financial or physical isolation of the victim, and physical attacks. The battering syndrome, which includes all of these forms of abusive behavior, is used to gain control of the victim's behavior. Examples of these forms of abuse include the following:

1. **Verbal abuse,** which ranges from repeated insults or insinuations up to threats to hurt or kill the victim or loved ones.
2. **Sexual assault,** which includes any form of nonconsensual sexual activity, occurs in about 35–40% of battered women.
3. **Isolation** of the victim from family, friends, and financial resources serves to give the abuser complete control over the victim's environment, make the victim dependent on the perpetrator, and often to conceal any physical abuse.
4. **Physical abuse,** in its extreme, includes punching, kicking, choking, and use of a knife or a gun.

B. Epidemiology. A minimum of 2 to 4 million women are abused annually by their male partners. More than 1.8 million of these women are seriously assaulted. The abuse can become lethal; domestic violence causes one third of the female murders in the United States. Ninety percent of these cases are the result of males' violently assaulting their female partners. Although mutual battering exists, studies have shown that men are more likely than women to perform more severe acts of violence. Men who admit to acts of violence often cite a desire to control or alter their victim's behavior. On the other hand, women who admit to violence indicate that they are responding to a perceived threat.

C. Cyclic pattern of violence. Within an abusive relationship, there is usually a typical pattern of tension building, violence, and reconciliation. Over the duration of an abusive relationship, this cycle recurs many times, often with the violence increasing in severity.

1. Tension building is characterized by frequent hostile verbal attacks, heightened surveillance of the victim, and escalating demands. This part of the cycle is actually the most destructive to the woman's ego and self-esteem.

2. Violence occurs after a build-up of days or months of increasing tension. This can be precipitated by a particular event or can come without warning. Some women have been awakened by beatings.
3. The reconciliation phase quickly follows. The attacker is often remorseful and promises never to be physically abusive again.

D. **Diagnosis**
1. **Awareness.** The key to identification by the primary care physician is the realization that anyone could be a battered woman. Stereotypes regarding poor, uneducated, minority women or the woman who somehow "provokes" her partner to attack her must be dispelled. A heightened awareness is necessary to consider battering when evaluating women. Victims of abuse commonly present with multiple somatic complaints, including headache, abdominal pain, muscle aches, joint pain, fatigue, vaginal or pelvic complaints, anxiety disorders, or depression. Battered women often go from doctor to doctor and are frequently identified as "difficult patients." Feelings of guilt, shame, and low self-esteem are the primary reasons that many battered women are hesitant to discuss the abuse.
2. **Screening** for abuse should be done routinely as part of any history and physical examination. By asking about abuse, the physician lets the patient know that he or she is approachable and willing to help. Battered women who do not reveal abuse at an initial visit may discuss it later if they feel safe and that their doctor is receptive. A nonjudgmental statement such as "I often see depression in women who have been hurt by someone close to them. Has this ever happened to you?" is a good screening question for partner abuse. This statement lets the patient know that her physician is willing and able to help. Additionally, literature in a safe place, such as the restroom, gives the patient the knowledge that their physician is open to discussing IPV.

E. **Management strategies.** Physicians are often reluctant to elicit a history of abuse because they are unsure about how to proceed if abuse is reported. Consider the following in offering treatment to victims of domestic violence:
1. The therapeutic process has already begun when the patient can talk to the physician about the abuse. The physician needs to convey the fact that there are many women who have had similar experiences, that it is not their fault, that abuse is wrong, and that they are not crazy. It is normal for them to feel overwhelmed and in need of support. It is also important that the patient understands that her symptoms are a reaction to the abuse. Reassurance helps decrease the sense of isolation and helplessness.
2. The level of continuing danger must be assessed. If there is imminent danger of serious harm or death, arrangements for a shelter should be made before the patient leaves the office. If children are involved in the abuse, by law this must be reported to your state's child protection agency. Every physician should be aware of your state's laws concerning child and elder abuse. If there is no shelter in your area, encourage the patient to report the abuse to the police. Most police agencies have a Victims Assistance Unit or equivalent.
3. The patient needs to know what resources are available, even if she is not yet ready to leave an abusive relationship. Group sessions with women who have had similar experiences are especially helpful. The patient should be given the telephone number of a women's shelter or other resources in the area before she leaves the office. If you are not familiar with your area's resources for victims of domestic violence, contact your local police department and ask.
4. Documentation including as many details as possible in the history and physical examination is very helpful. Drawing figures or diagrams, depicting exact areas of ecchymoses, swelling, lacerations, etc, further documents the abuse. Taking photographs may contribute evidence if this were to go to court and is helpful to the victim.
5. The physician may feel frustrated because the patient cannot or will not leave an abusive relationship. The physician cannot make this decision for the patient. The role of physician is that of facilitator, helping the woman work through the process of recovery.

F. **Prognosis.** Effects on the victim vary, but certain emotional and behavioral sequelae are commonly seen in an abused partner.

1. Depression is one of the most common manifestations suffered by battered women. Depression can come from anger at the abuser turned inward, and feelings of guilt or self-blame for "allowing the abuse to happen." Additionally, survivors of abusive relationships often end up lacking financial resources, which adds to their depression. Suicide attempts are not uncommon. Depression can persist after the victim has left the abusive relationship.

2. Living in an abusive relationship produces high levels of anxiety, and even after the relationship has terminated, many women will still have environmental triggers that can provoke panic attacks. Anxiety, post-traumatic stress disorder, and depression are common ways battered women will present to the primary care physician. Victims and survivors are often substance abusers, self-treating their undiagnosed psychiatric disorders. Other self-destructive behavior is common and can manifest itself as smoking, or failure to use safety items such as seat belts.

III. **Elder Abuse.** Abuse is a symptom of underlying family dysfunction. Treatment must include the family unit as well as the victim of abuse. The physician cannot treat elder abuse alone; a team approach, using social workers, mental health professionals, and lawyers, is more likely to be successful.

   A. **Definitions.** The term *elder abuse* is used interchangeably with *elder mistreatment* and includes many types of abuse against older adults. The National Aging Resource Center on Elder Abuse (NARCEA) has developed working definitions for elder abuse and neglect. The types of elder abuse include physical, psychological, and sexual abuse; psychological and physical neglect; violation of rights; and financial or material abuse. Neglect and physical and psychological abuse may also be self-inflicted.

   1. **Physical abuse** is the act of causing physical pain or injury resulting in bruising, fractures, dislocations, abrasions, burns, welts, lacerations, and other multiple injuries. Physical abuse can be intentional or unintentional and includes at least one act of violence including beating, slapping, burning, cutting, inappropriate use of physical restraints, and intentional overmedicating.

   2. **Physical neglect** is the failure of a caregiver to meet care obligations such as providing goods and services such as food, clothing, shelter, and medical and personal care. Indicators of neglect may include malnutrition, dehydration, decubitus ulcers, poor hygiene, and lack of caregiver compliance with medical regimens.

   3. **Psychological neglect** is the failure of a caregiver to provide a dependent elder with meaningful social contact or stimulation. Examples of this type of neglect include isolating or ignoring the elder for long periods. This commonly results in depression, extreme withdrawal, or agitation.

   4. **Psychological abuse** includes the infliction of mental anguish through intimidation, threats, verbal assaults, berating, deprivation, infantilization (treating the older adult like an infant), humiliation, or the provocation of internal fear. The end result of this type of abuse is similar to that of psychological abuse in which the elder is depressed, withdrawn, or fearful, and can present with symptoms of "failure to thrive."

   5. **Sexual abuse** is defined as molestation or forced sexual activity. Although this type of abuse is the most underreported, it may occur more often than previously suspected.

   6. **Violation of personal rights** includes preventing elders from making their own decisions regarding housing arrangements, financial matters, and personal decisions such as marriage, divorce, and medical treatment. Physicians can observe for signs of violation of personal rights through observation of the caregiver–elder interaction. Does the caregiver insist on being present for the examination? Does the caregiver interrupt the elder's conversation, never allowing the elder to respond to the physician's questions? Does the caregiver deny the elder the right to make health care decisions?

   7. **Material or financial abuse** refers to the illegal exploitation of monetary or material assets. This type of abuse includes control of the elder's income and assets by the caregiver; coercion in signing contracts or making changes in a will or durable power of attorney; or the theft of money or property. Specific indicators include a caregiver's refusal to release funds to purchase needed care or patient complaints that they have inadequate funds to buy medication.

   B. **Epidemiology**

   1. **Prevalence and incidence.** The NARCEA estimates that between 1.5 and 2 million older adults in the United States suffer from physical abuse or neglect annu-

ally. Elder abuse occurs in all communities, regardless of gender, ethnicity or race, socioeconomic status, or religious affiliation. Because of the variation in state reporting requirements, it is difficult to determine the actual rate of elder abuse; however, the majority of state adult protective and regulatory agencies responsible for the identification, investigation, and prevention of elder abuse report an increase in reported cases over the last decade. In Boston, 3.2% of elders reported experiencing some form of physical or psychological abuse or neglect. A longitudinal study in Connecticut found that mistreated older adults reported to Adult Protective Services were more likely to die within the 13-year follow-up study period than older adults who experienced self-neglect or those who were not reported to Adult Protective Services.

2. **Identity and background of the perpetrators.** Physical abuse is perpetrated most often by spouses with acute or chronic health problems or responsibilities for providing companionship, financial resources, or property maintenance for their dependent spouse. Adult children tend to psychologically abuse and neglect their parents as well as financially exploit them. These children are often financially dependent on the parent and have a history of mental illness or substance abuse. Pillemer and Suitor found that 64% of abusers were financially dependent on their victims and 55% were dependent on them for housing needs.

3. **Risk factors for abuse.** Increased life expectancy, functional or psychological dependency, learned helplessness, poor physical health, and stress and burnout experienced by the caregiver are primary risk factors for abuse. Other risk factors include living arrangements, caregivers with mental illness or substance abuse, or a family history of violence. Lachs et al found that mistreated elders were likely to live with someone and have fewer social networks. Potential predictors of elder mistreatment include poverty, race, and cognitive impairment.

C. **Diagnosis.** A comprehensive biopsychosocial assessment of the elderly patient is important to determine whether there are clinical findings to support abuse or neglect. Table 91–2 outlines the clinical procedures for detecting abuse.

TABLE 91–2. ASSESSMENT GUIDELINES FOR DETECTING ELDER MISTREATMENT

Area	Recommendation/Assessment
Patient history	Interview patient and suspected perpetrator separately and alone; ask specific questions about neglect and physical violence and record details regarding frequency; assess patient's functional status (ADLs and IADLs) and psychosocial stressors (illness, widowhood, finances)
Social/community support	Assess other family or caregiver availability, social support through friends, churches, other relatives; and whether the patient feels safe to return to their current situation
Finances	Assess the financial resources that patient has for their care provision
Behavior (patient and caregiver)	Assess demeanor of patient (withdrawn, fearful, anxious); is the caregiver controlling interview or infantilizing the patient?
Physical examination	
General appearance	Hygiene, mannerisms, appropriate attire
Skin, mucous membranes	Bruises, skin lesions/lacerations, abrasions; skin turgor, dehydration, decubitus ulcers
Head and neck	Trauma, traumatic alopecia, scalp hematomas, lacerations
Chest, abdomen, back	Bruising, lacerations, welts, burns, rib fractures
Musculoskeletal system	Occult fracture, extremities (wrist or ankle lesions), gait, immersion, cigarette or other pattern burns
Genitourinary tract	Vaginal or rectal bleeding or both, decubitus ulcers, infestations
Neurologic/psychiatric	Assess mental status and cognitive impairment through use of a formal mental status questionnaire; assess focality, depressive symptoms, anxiety, and other psychiatric symptoms such as delusions, hallucinations
Laboratory and other tests	As indicated from clinical examination, albumin, blood urea nitrogen, creatinine levels, toxicologic screening

ADLs, activities of daily living; IADLs, instrumental activities of daily living.
Adapted from Lachs MS, Pillemer K: Abuse and neglect of elderly persons. N Engl J Med 1995;**332**:437.

D. Management. The American Medical Association (AMA) recommends that all physicians ask their patients about family violence regardless of whether there is clinical evidence or suspicion of abuse or neglect. If the elderly patient is not cognitively impaired, a thorough interview, separate from the caregiver, should occur to assess whether the patient is safe. Non-threatening questions should be asked, such as (1) "Do you feel safe in your home?," (2) "Who helps you with your personal care, such as bathing, taking your medications, preparing your meals?," (3) "What happens if your family member becomes tired or cannot help you?," (4) "What happens if you have a disagreement?," and (5) "Who helps you pay your bills?" If the patient has cognitive impairment, history and screening questions must be obtained from the caregiver or family member if available.

If the elder does not feel safe and accepts physician intervention, hospitalization should be considered. If hospitalization is not an option, the physician should discuss other placement options with Adult Protective Services (APS). APS has several emergency, court-ordered options available and can facilitate this process. The following approach with the caregiver facilitates the interview process and reduces some of the tension that may exist: "It must be very difficult to care for your mother with this type of illness. Do you find yourself feeling tired, frustrated, and unable to deal with the situation?" Advising the family member that you will be making a report to APS in order to help reduce some of the stress that the caregiver may be experiencing may be less threatening to the caregiver. The caregiver should be informed of available resources such as adult day care, respite care, home health care, senior companion programs, caregiver support groups, and individual counseling.

E. Ethical and legal obligations. Physicians play a critical role in the assessment of elder abuse and neglect, as well as in the intervention process. In long-term physician-patient relationships in which trust has been established, the process may be easier to facilitate.

Physicians have a legal responsibility to report suspected cases of abuse or neglect. Mandatory reporting laws exist in most states. Designated state agencies are responsible for conducting investigations and interventions. APS is the agency assigned to investigate and intervene with elder abuse cases. Persons who are licensed, registered, or certified to provide health care, education, and social, mental health, and other human services are required to report abuse. Anonymous reports can be made. Physicians usually are granted immunity from civil suits in reporting cases of suspected abuse or neglect. Failure to report suspected abuse can result in civil liability and fines for any subsequent damages that may occur. Failure to follow state guidelines for reporting abuse may result in criminal prosecution, professional delicensure, or other penalties.

REFERENCES

Adams JA: Evolution of a classification scale: Medical evaluation of suspected child sexual abuse. Child Maltreatment 2001;**6**:31.

Campbell JC, Lewandowski LA: Mental and physical health effects of intimate partner violence on women and children. Psychiatric Clin North Am 1997;**20**:353.

Christian CW, et al: Forensic evidence findings in prepubertal victims of sexual assault. Pediatrics 2000;**106**(1):100.

Ferris LE, et al: Guidelines for managing domestic abuse when male and female partners are patients of the same physician. JAMA 1997;**278**:851.

Hamberger LK, et al: *Violence Issues For Health Care Educators and Providers.* Haworth Maltreatment and Trauma Press, 1997.

Kellogg ND, Hoffman TJ: Child sexual revictimization by multiple perpetrators. Child Abuse & Neglect 1997;**21**(10):953.

Kini N, Lazortiz S: Evaluation for possible physical or sexual abuse. Pediatr Clin North Am 1998;**45**:205.

Lachs MS, Pillemer K: Abuse and neglect of elderly persons. N Engl J Med 1995;**332**:437.

Lachs MS, et al: The mortality of elder mistreatment. JAMA 1998;**280**:5.

Lachs MS, et al: Risk factors for reported elder abuse and neglect: A nine year observational cohort study. Gerontologist 1997;**37**:4.

Melvin SY, Rhyne MC: Domestic Violence. Adv Intern Med 1998;**43**:1.

Mitchell KJ, Finkelhor D, Wolan J: Risk factors for and impact of online sexual solicitation of youth. JAMA 2001;**285**:3011.

Taliaferro E: Screening and identification of intimate partner violence. Clin Fam Pract 2003;**5**:89.

92   Depression

Rhonda A. Faulkner, PhD, & Martin S. Lipsky, MD

KEY POINTS

- Depression is the most common psychological disorder that primary care practitioners will encounter. According to recent studies, depression is more common than any other disorder (with the exception of hypertension) and is the seventh most common outpatient diagnosis in family medicine. The point prevalence of major depressive disorder (MDD) in Western industrialized nations is 2.3–3.2% for men and 4.5–9.3% for women. The risk of developing MDD over one's lifetime is 7–12% for men and 20–25% for women. The point prevalence of MDD in primary care patients is 4.8–8.6%; 14.6% of adult medical inpatients meet criteria for MDD.
- In 2002, The US Preventive Services Task Force (USPSTF) made a grade B recommendation for all clinicians to routinely screen adults for depression. They recommend asking the following two simple questions regarding mood and anhedonia: (1) "Over the past 2 weeks, have you felt down, depressed, or hopeless?" and (2) "Over the past 2 weeks, have you felt little interest or pleasure in doing things?"
- There are several types of depressive illnesses classified by diagnosable symptoms as defined by the American Psychological Association's *Diagnostic and Statistical Manual of Mental Disorders* (DSM-IV; Table 92–1). It is recommended that primary care providers be familiar with the distinctive classifications of depression. In particular, since approximately 1% of patients with depression may have bipolar disease, the family physician should be alert for manic episodes that might be precipitated by treatment with an antidepressant.
- Physicians have a variety of treatment options for depression. Among the choices, selective serotonin reuptake inhibitors (SSRIs) offer simpler dosing schedules and fewer side effects than some of the older antidepressants (Table 92–2). *The combination of antidepressant medications with psychotherapy has proven to demonstrate the best outcomes in treatment of depression.* Patients starting a course of antidepressant therapy should be advised that symptoms will not subside for 2–6 weeks, with a trial of 6–8 weeks at maximum dose necessary to confirm treatment success or failure. In order to prevent the risk of relapse, a treatment period of 6–9 months is recommended.
- The prognosis for patients who receive treatment for depression is generally favorable. Most antidepressants are effective in about 50–60% of patients with MDD. Patients who do not respond to one particular type of medication may respond well to another. At least 80% of patients will respond to at least one antidepressant medication. Studies show that patients respond best when antidepressant medications are combined with counseling.

I. Introduction
A. Definitions

1. **Major depressive disorder (MDD),** the most severe form of depression, is a mood disorder characterized by at least 2 weeks of five or more of the following symptoms: (1) depressed mood; (2) loss of interest or pleasure in daily activities; (3) weight loss or gain; (4) insomnia or hypersomnia; (5) psychomotor agitation or retardation; (6) fatigue or loss of energy; (7) feelings of guilt or worthlessness; (8) inability to concentrate; and (9) thoughts of death or suicidal ideation.

2. **Dysthymia** is a milder, chronic disorder that is diagnosed when patients experience depressed mood and at least two other DSM-IV criteria of depression for at least 2 years. Patients with dysthymia may be thought of as having a depressive personality or character style. Although depressive symptoms in dysthymia are not as severe as those of major affective disorder, they are too prolonged to be thought of as adjustment responses.

3. **Adjustment disorder with depressed mood** is a type of mood disorder readily attributable to a recent psychosocial stressor such as a loss of a loved one or employment and should resolve as the stressor decreases. It is distinguished from

TABLE 92–1. DSM-IV CRITERIA FOR MAJOR DEPRESSIVE EPISODE

Five (or more) of the following symptoms have been present during the same 2-week period and represent a change from previous functioning; at least one of the symptoms is either (1) depressed mood or (2) loss of interest or pleasure.

Note: Do not include symptoms that clearly result from a general medical condition or mood-incongruent delusions or hallucinations.

(1) Depressed mood most of the day, nearly every day, as indicated by either subjective report (eg, feels sad or empty) or observation made by others (eg, appears tearful). **Note:** In children and adolescents, can be irritable mood
(2) Markedly diminished interest or pleasure in all, or almost all, activities most of the day, nearly every day (as indicated by either subjective account or observation made by others)
(3) Significant weight loss when not dieting or weight gain (eg, a change of >5% of body weight in a month) or decrease or increase in appetite nearly every day. **Note:** In children, consider failure to make expected weight gains
(4) Insomnia or hypersomnia nearly every day
(5) Psychomotor agitation or retardation nearly every day (observable by others, not merely subjective feelings of restlessness or being slowed down)
(6) Fatigue or loss of energy nearly every day
(7) Feelings of worthlessness or excessive or inappropriate guilt (which may be delusional) nearly every day (not merely self-reproach or guilt about being sick)
(8) Diminished ability to think or concentrate, or indecisiveness, nearly every day (either by subjective account or as observed by others)
(9) Recurrent thoughts of death (not just fear of flying), recurrent suicidal ideation without a specific plan, or a suicide attempt or a specific plan for committing suicide

Reprinted with permission from American Psychiatric Association (APA): *Diagnostic and Statistical Manual of Mental Disorders,* 4th ed (DSM-IV). APA; 1994.

an MDD by its milder severity and shorter time course. Some bereaved patients manifest primarily psychological symptoms and seek counseling, while others develop somatic symptoms and seek medical attention. Unfortunately, many individuals with MDD have stressors that may be identified as the cause of their depression, and thus their illness may be overlooked.

4. **Depressive disorder not otherwise specified (NOS)** is a depressive illness that lasts longer than 6 months. This diagnosis is used to describe mixed states of anxiety and depression that do not meet the criteria for other anxiety or depressive diagnoses.
5. **Mood disorder due to a general medical condition (or substance).** This condition is diagnosed when a prominent mood disturbance can be attributed to a direct physiological consequence of a general medical condition (ie, hypothyroidism, AIDS), substance abuse (ie, alcohol withdrawal), or medication (ie, beta blockers, levodopa, steroids, reserpine, and oral contraceptives).
6. **Bipolar disorder** (also known as manic-depressive illness), a condition with a strong genetic predisposition, occurs in approximately 1% of the population. These patients experience symptoms of depression along with mania.
7. **Other psychiatric disorders.** Depressive symptoms may also be present in other psychiatric disorders, although they are not predominant. In particular, depression and anxiety are highly comorbid conditions. Therefore, the evaluation of depressive symptoms should include a psychiatric history and a brief review of systems, looking for psychotic features, phobias, panic attacks, somatization, and personality disorders.

B. **Epidemiology.** At any one time, at least 3% of the US population suffers from chronic depression. More than 17% of the population have had a major depressive episode in their lifetime, and more than 10% have experienced an episode within the past 12 months. Epidemiologic studies indicate that a lifetime prevalence of major depression in 7–12% of men and 20–25% of women. Studies report a 5–10% prevalence of major depression in primary care settings with 20–40% prevalence in patients with coexisting medical problems.

1. A depressive disorder may begin at any age, but the average age at onset is the late 20s. Psychosocial events or stressors may play a significant role in precipitating the first or second episode of MDD, but may play little or no role in subsequent episodes.
2. Multiple studies support the finding that major depression is more common in women than in men. This gender difference is found in community samples and is

TABLE 92–2. ANTIDEPRESSANTS

Drug	Starting Dose	Therapeutic Daily Dose	Cost	Adverse Effects					
				Sedation	Anticholinergic	Orthostatic Hypotension	Cardiac Conduction	Insomnia
Tricyclics								
Amitriptyline (Elavil)	50 mg qhs[1]	75–300 mg	$	High	High	High	High	Very low
Doxepin (Sinequan)	50 mg qhs[1]	75–300 mg	$	High	Moderate	Moderate	Moderate	Low
Imipramine (Tofranil)	50 mg qd[1]	75–300 mg	$	Moderate	Moderate	High	High	Very low
Nortryptiline (Pamelor)	25 mg qd[1,2]	40–200 mg	$$	Low	Low	Low	Moderate	Low
Heterocyclics								
Bupropion (Wellbutrin)	100 mg bid[3]	200–450 mg	$$	Low	Very low	Very low	Very low	Moderate
Trazodone (Desyrel)	150 mg qhs[1]	75–300 mg	$$	High	Very low	Moderate	Very low	Very low
Selective serotonin reuptake inhibitors								
Citalopram (Celexa)	20 mg qd	20–60 mg qd	$$$	Low	Very low	Very low	Very low	Very low
Escitalopram (Lexapro)	10 mg	20 mg qd	$$$	Very low	Very low	Very low	Very low	Very low
Fluoxetine (Prozac)	10–20 mg qam	10–80 mg	$$$	Very low	Very low	Very low	Very low	High
Paroxetine (Paxil)	10–20 mg qd	10–60 mg	$$$	Low	Low	Very low	Very low	Low
Sertraline (Zoloft)	50 mg qd	50–200 mg	$$$	Very low	Low	Very low	Very low	Low
Serotonin/norepinephrine reuptake inhibitor								
Venlataxine (Effexor)	37.5 mg bid	75–300 mg	$$	Low	Low	Very low	Low	Low
Other antidepressants								
Mirtazapine (Remeron)	7.5–15 mg qhs	30–45 mg qhs	$$$	High	Low	Low	Low	Low
Nefazodone (Serzone)	50–100 mg bid	100–300 mg bid	$$$	High	Low	Low	Low	Low
Trazodone (Desyrel)	50 mg qhs	100–300 mg bid	$	High	Low	Moderate	Low	Low

[1] May be better tolerated if given in divided doses.
[2] Begin at lower dose in the elderly, titrate to serum level of 50–150 ng/mL.
[3] Not to exceed 150 mg/dose to minimize seizure risk.
$, least expensive; $$, moderately expensive; $$$, most expensive.

not the result of higher rates of help-seeking behavior by women. Recent studies have disproved the belief that the incidence of depression in women increases during the climacteric. Prevalence rates for MDD are unrelated to race, education, or income.

   3. Certain individuals are at increased risk for depression, including alcohol and drug abusers, hypochondriacs, patients with a life-threatening disease such as a stroke or myocardial infarction, individuals recovering from major surgery, women in the postpartum state, and patients with a family history of depression. Screening for postpartum depression is particularly important, as recent data demonstrates that between 50% and 80% of women experience this "normal" reaction within 1–5 days after childbirth, lasting up to 1 week. This condition should be distinguished from postpartum psychosis, which occurs in 0.5–2% of women, with symptoms beginning 2–3 days after delivery.

C. **Etiology**
   1. **Genetic factors.** A combination of biological and environmental factors causes depression. Multiple lines of research point to a genetic or inherited predisposition for MDD that may be activated or precipitated by psychosocial or physiologic stressors. The general understanding of how these stressors interact with a genetic predisposition to produce clinical depression is limited.
   2. **Psychosocial factors.** Psychosocial stressors such as death of a spouse, divorce, or developmental life course transitions (eg, empty nest syndrome) may make patients more vulnerable to experiencing depression. The presence of social support is a mitigating factor for depression; therefore, primary care providers should assess social support and facilitate mobilization of these resources.
   3. The interaction among these environmental and genetic factors is postulated to culminate in the final common pathway of limbic–hypothalamic dysfunction, which is clinically manifested as a depressive illness. It was originally believed that a depletion of neurotransmitters, including norepinephrine, serotonin, and γ-aminobutyric acid, in hypothalamic centers of the brain contributed to the symptom complex of depression. More recent studies suggest a dysregulation hypothesis rather than depletion of a single neurotransmitter.

II. **Diagnosis.** Recent studies have documented improvements in the recognition and treatment of MDD in primary care settings, with two thirds of patients recognized and nearly half prescribed antidepressants.

A. **Symptoms and signs**
   1. The clinical diagnosis of depression depends on recognition of an identifiable cluster of signs and symptoms suggesting the disorder. See Table 92–1 for a list of criteria for diagnosing MDD according to the DSM-IV. Any of the symptoms listed may represent the leading edge of a cluster of depressive symptoms. For example, a recent study found that 80% of patients with the chief complaint of fatigue go on to be diagnosed with an affective disorder. The DSM-IV requires that five or more symptoms be present during the same 2-week period and that at least one be either a depressed mood or loss of interest or pleasure. It is important to note that the DSM-IV includes a loss of interest in all, or almost all, activities as an alternative to depressed mood as the primary symptom. It is not uncommon for a depressed patient to deny feeling sad, but instead admit to "not caring anymore."
   2. Although the DSM-IV is useful in evaluating the possibility of depression in a patient, it was designed primarily by and for psychiatric researchers and was validated on a psychiatric population. DSM-IV criteria may not be as applicable to a primary care population.
   3. The wide application of the term *depression* often leads to confusion about its diagnosis. The following guidelines are suggested to distinguish bereavement or dysphoric symptoms from clinical depression.
      a. Patients with established clinical depression usually need more treatment than positive changes in the psychosocial environment.
      b. Clinical depression is usually incapacitating and interferes with work performance and relationships.
      c. Diurnal variation of symptoms, which become worse in the morning, is more common with clinical depression.
      d. Psychomotor retardation, which may be associated with depression, is almost never observed with bereavement.

     e. Recurrence is especially characteristic of a mood disorder. A prior history of a similar episode is strong evidence for clinical depression. More than half of all patients with depression will experience a recurrence in their lifetime and therefore should be advised of this risk.

     f. Finally, a positive family history of a similar disorder is characteristic of a primary mood disorder.

   4. Age-specific features in the diagnosis of depression.

     a. Elderly patients with psychomotor retardation, slow thinking, and indecisiveness may be misdiagnosed as having dementia (see Chapter 73).

     b. Prepubertal children often present with somatic complaints, irritable mood, or a psychomotor agitation that may manifest itself as a marked drop in school performance.

     c. In adolescents, similar findings may occur. Antisocial behavior, restlessness, agitation, **substance abuse,** aggression, poor school performance, withdrawal from social activities, and increased emotional sensitivity are also common. Children and adolescents are often unable to recognize these changes or to associate them with depression.

     d. Patients with depression may present with vague physical symptoms without organic diseases or with symptoms out of proportion to the physical examination. Complaints such as fatigue and dizziness that result in multiple visits without a specific diagnosis should alert the clinician to consider depression.

B. Laboratory tests

   1. The clinical interview remains the most effective method for detecting depression. No reliable biochemical markers for depression exist. Only a limited number of laboratory tests should be conducted to detect potential general medical causes of depressive symptoms. No standard "screening" work-up can be used to rule out potential underlying organic causes for depressive symptoms. The evaluation should be directed by demographic and historical clues. For example, hypothyroidism should be considered in an older patient who presents with depressive symptomatology. Medications known to be associated with depressive symptoms should be stopped, especially if recently prescribed.

   2. Several **self-administered questionnaires and depression screening tools** are available for use across the lifespan and are designed to help identify patients with depressive symptomatology. (Please see the following website for access to screening tools: http://www.aafp.org/afp/20020915/1001.html.) These tests, which are more useful as case-finding instruments than as screening tests, possess sensitivities in the 70% range and specificities in the 80% range. They are easily administered and well accepted by patients. Widely used tests include the following.

     a. Beck Depression Inventory, including the short-form version with 13 items.

     b. The National Institute of Mental Health (NIMH) Center for Epidemiologic Studies Depression Scale (CES-D), which has 20 items.

     c. The Zung Self-Rating Depression Scale (SDS), which also has 20 items.

III. Treatment. Primary care physicians, not mental health professionals, treat most patients with symptoms of depression. The objectives of treatment are (1) to resolve all signs and symptoms of the depressive syndrome, (2) to restore occupational and psychosocial functioning to baseline, and (3) to reduce the likelihood of relapse and recurrence. Treatment may be divided into three phases: acute, continuation, and maintenance.

  A. Acute phase treatment. In primary care, the most common acute treatment modalities are medication, psychotherapy or counseling, or a combination of medication and psychotherapy.

   1. Medication

     a. Medications have been shown to be effective in all forms of MDD and should be considered first-line therapy in moderate to severe MDD.

     b. Medication selection should be based on side effect profiles; history of prior response; and patient symptoms, concurrent medical conditions, and concurrently prescribed medications (Table 92–2). Although there are no clinically significant differences in the effectiveness of antidepressant medications, selective serotonin reuptake inhibitors (SSRIs) are often preferred over tricyclic antidepressants (TCAs) and monoamine oxidase inhibitors (MAOIs) due to more simple dosing schedules and fewer side effects. No single medication results in remission for all patients.

c. In order to be proficient in the treatment of depression, the primary care physician should learn how to use at least three or four antidepressants well and become familiar with dosages, side effects, and serum levels. The chosen medications should have varying side effect profiles and be applicable to different types of presenting symptomatologies.

d. Suggested guidelines for selection include the following:

    (1) If the patient has insomnia and early morning awakening, a more sedating medication, such as a TCA such as amitriptyline or imipramine, should be chosen.

    (2) If patient's symptoms are characterized by an excessive need for sleep, then a more stimulating and less sedating medication should be selected. Patients with hypersomnia and motor retardation may benefit from bupropion or venlafaxine and should avoid using nefazodone and mirtazapine.

    (3) If anxiety is a major component of the symptom complex, then a medication with a lower index of insomnia or agitation side effects is recommended. For patients with generalized anxiety and insomnia, nefazodone and mirtazapine are good choices.

    (4) For patients in whom weight gain is a goal, mirtazapine is a good choice.

    (5) For patients in whom smoking cessation is also a goal, bupropion is a good medication of choice.

    (6) Elderly patients are especially sensitive to the orthostatic and anticholinergic side effects of some antidepressants. As a result, the SSRIs have replaced TCAs as first-line therapy in the elderly. Careful observation of cardiac function, vital signs, cognitive functioning, and physical complaints will often help identify potential problems early.

    (7) If the medication is relatively sedating, compliance can be improved by having the patient take the entire dosage either at bedtime or a few hours before.

e. Contraindications for specific antidepressants:

    (1) Nefazodone should not be used in patients with liver disease.

    (2) Bupropion is contraindicated for patients with seizure disorder.

    (3) For patients who have experienced sexual dysfunction prior to depression, SSRIs **should** be avoided.

    (4) Hypertension is a relative contraindication to venlafaxine.

    (5) Patients experiencing hypersomnia and motor retardation should avoid nefazodone and mirtazapine.

    (6) For patients experiencing agitation and insomnia, bupropion and venlafaxine should be avoided.

    (7) Mirtazapine and TCAs are **less** preferred for patients with obesity.

2. Psychotherapy

a. Studies have shown that the combination of medication with psychotherapy provides a better response than either form of treatment used alone.

b. Depression rarely occurs independent of psychosocial issues. It is vital that the patient begin to address these issues if true recovery is to occur. If relationships within the family, such as a poor marital relationship, prove to be a precipitating factor, then involvement of other family members in counseling may be important.

c. Psychotherapy alone may be preferable in patients with milder forms of MDD who do not desire medication, who have unacceptable side effects to medication, and who have medical conditions limiting medication options.

d. Physicians may find it useful to use the **BATHE** technique in order help focus the counseling encounter. The acronym "BATHE" stands for the following: B = *background:* "What is going on in your life?"; A = *affect:* "How do you feel about that?"; T = *trouble:* "What about this situation or problem troubles you the most?"; H = *handling:* "How are you handling that?"; and E = *empathy:* "That must be very difficult for you."

    (1) Often, the patient needs only a sympathetic listener to be able to work through the conflicts he or she is experiencing.

    (2) Encounters need not be lengthy. Ten or 15 minutes is enough time to allow the patient to explore problems in a therapeutic way, with the physician facilitating this process by asking open-ended questions.

(3) It is not important that the physician produce a final answer to all of the patient's questions, doubts, or problems, but help the patient's to set goals and decrease negative thoughts about their life.

e. Many physicians establish a good working relationship with a local psychiatrist, psychologist, or family therapist to whom they can refer patients for counseling or psychotherapy.

3. **Patient education**

a. A key element in acute phase treatment is the provision of adequate information to both the patient and his or her family about the condition. In addition, the provision of support, advice, reassurance, and hope is critical for depressed patients who are experiencing fatigue, low mood, and poor concentration. Several studies have found that patient education improves adherence to treatment in depressed outpatients.

b. An important point to make with many patients is that antidepressant medication is not habit-forming or addictive. Many patients are fearful of "nerve pills" because of friends or relatives who may have developed a drug dependence.

c. Nearly half of all patients will stop taking their antidepressant medication within the first month of treatment. Patients should be educated in advance about the side effects of the medications, such as dry mouth, constipation, sexual side effects, and sedation. Patients should be reassured that most will resolve with time.

d. Patients should be told not to expect overnight results. It often takes 4–6 weeks for noticeable improvement to occur. It is often helpful to remind patients that their symptoms developed over a similar, if not longer, time interval.

4. **Herbal products.** Many patients may attempt to use herbal remedies, such as St. John's wort (*Hypericum perforatum*), for treatment of their depression without consulting their physician. In a recent multisite, large-scale clinical trial of St. John's wort, The National Institutes of Health found that St. John's wort is no more effective for treating major depression of moderate severity than placebo.

B. **Continuation and maintenance treatment**

1. The goal of continuation treatment is to decrease the likelihood of relapse (a return of the current episode of depression).

a. Patients who respond well to acute treatment should be continued on the same dosage for at least 6–12 months after they have resolved their depressive symptoms. There is very strong evidence that continuation of treatment for this time interval is effective at preventing relapse and recurrence.

b. Those patients who experience a second episode of depression will have an 80% chance of additional recurrences and should continue with antidepressant medications for 1–2 years. Patients experiencing a third episode of depression have a 90% chance for recurrence and will require indefinite treatment maintenance.

IV. **Management Strategies**

A. **Overcoming patient resistance**

1. **Depression** is often difficult for the primary care physician to treat because the diagnosis itself is often socially unacceptable and culturally invalid for many patients. A survey of 350 family practice physicians revealed that the major obstacle to treatment of depressed patients was patient resistance to the diagnosis.

2. Many physicians find it useful to approach an explanation of the illness in terms that are better understood by the patient.

a. Such an explanation often begins by explaining how the human body responds to stress and then defining the illness as an imbalance of chemical messengers in the nervous system.

b. Patients are often more accepting of the diagnosis of depression and more willing to address the psychosocial precipitants, as well as use medication properly, when such an explanation is given.

3. It is often useful, if not crucial, to involve the family in such an explanation, since their support is vital to a successful outcome.

B. **Suicide.** Suicide potential and prevention must always be considered when the diagnosis of depression is made.

1. Many physicians are leery of asking about suicide out of fear that it may precipitate a suicide attempt. Such fears are unfounded. The evidence to date suggests that

patients appreciate the concern demonstrated by such questioning. Many physicians find it useful to ask a patient who has considered suicide to form a suicide pact or agreement. The patient agrees to call the physician or another health provider before taking any action. No studies exist to support the efficacy of this arrangement, however.

2. Those individuals at highest risk for suicide attempt are young females. These attempts are usually gestures and are often not successful. Medication overdose is a common method of suicide in females. If suicide is judged to be a risk, it is prudent to limit the amount of medication prescribed to <1500 mg of an antidepressant at any one time.

3. Those persons at highest risk for successful suicide are middle-aged to older men. Other high-risk factors include social isolation and substance abuse.

C. **Referral or hospitalization.** Even though most depressed patients who present to primary care settings can be managed as outpatients, some will need hospitalization in an inpatient psychiatric unit or referral to a psychiatrist. General recommendations are given below.

1. The patient who presents with suicide ideation and specific suicide plans is at serious risk, and hospitalization should be strongly considered.

2. The patient whose depression is severe enough to interfere with activities of daily living, such as dressing and feeding, should probably be hospitalized.

3. Referral should be considered if the patient has a history suggestive of bipolar disorder.

4. Referral should be sought if evidence of a thought disorder or psychotic features of the depression itself, such as fixed delusions, are present.

5. If the patient fails to respond to treatment after 3 months, referral to a psychiatrist should be considered.

D. **Frequency of office visits**

1. Follow-up should be scheduled at 2 weeks after the initial diagnosis for most mild to moderate depression. Patients with more severe forms of MDD should be seen weekly for the first 4–6 weeks of treatment. Subsequent visits may be scheduled at 4- to 12-week intervals, depending on the degree of response and the need for office counseling.

2. Therapeutic blood levels of antidepressant drugs have been established. Nortriptyline, imipramine, and amitriptyline have well-established minimal therapeutic blood levels. Drug levels should be obtained in the following instances.

   a. **When an adequate response is not achieved on full therapeutic doses.** Nonresponsiveness to a medication cannot be established unless the steady-state serum level is within the therapeutic range for 2–4 weeks.

   b. **When serious side effects occur at normal doses.** Similarities exist between depressive and toxic symptoms in patients who are clinically deteriorating.

E. **Screening.** The US Preventive Services Task Force (USPSTF) recently found evidence that screening improves the accurate identification of depressed patients in primary care settings and that treatment of depressed adults identified in primary care settings decreases clinical morbidity. Based on these findings, the USPSTF made a grade B recommendation that primary care practitioners routinely screen their adult patients for depression. *There was insufficient evidence to support a recommendation for routine screening of child and adolescent patients, although primary care physicians should use their clinical judgment about screening their younger patients.* They recommend asking the following two simple questions regarding mood and anhedonia: (1) "Over the past 2 weeks, have you felt down, depressed, or hopeless?" and (2) "Over the past 2 weeks, have you felt little interest or pleasure in doing things?"

V. **Prognosis**

A. **Prognosis without treatment**

1. An untreated episode of depression typically lasts 6 months or more. A remission of symptoms then occurs, and functioning often returns to the premorbid level.

2. Of those patients with recurrent episodes, 5% will have a manic attack at a later date, resulting in a change in their diagnosis to a bipolar mood disorder.

3. The toll in lives lost is high; half of all suicide victims are thought to have had a major depression. Suicide occurs in 1% of patients with an acute episode of depression and in 25% of patients with a chronic depression.

B. **Prognosis with treatment**
  1. Most antidepressants are effective in about 50–60% of patients with MDD. Patients who do not respond to one particular type of medication may respond well to another. At least 80% of patients will respond to at least one antidepressant medication.
  2. In severe cases of MDD, electroconvulsive therapy has a high rate of therapeutic success, including speed and safety. However, this is not administered as a first-line treatment and patients requiring this form of treatment should be referred for psychiatrist consultation.

REFERENCES

Feldman MD, Christensen JF: *Behavioral medicine in primary care: A practical guide,* 2nd ed. McGraw-Hill; 2003.

Gillette RD: Diagnosis and management of depression. Am Fam Physician 2000; Monograph: 1–24.

Hypericum Depression Trial Study Group: Effect of *hypericum perforatum* (St. John's wort) in major depressive disorder: A randomized, controlled trial. JAMA 2002;**287:**1807.

Sharp LK, Lipsky MS: Screening for depression across the lifespan: A review of measures for use in primary care settings. Am Fam Physician 2002;**66:**1001.

Stuart MR, Lieberman JA: *The Fifteen Minute Hour: Practical Therapeutic Interventions in Primary Care,* 3rd ed. Saunders; 2002.

Sutherland JE, Sutherland SJ, Hoehns JD: Achieving the best outcome in treatment of depression. J Fam Pract 2003;**52:**201.

U.S. Preventive Services Task Force: Screening for depression: Recommendations and rationale. Ann Intern Med 2002;**136:**760.

Whooley MA, Simon GE: Managing depression in medical outpatients. N Engl J Med 2000;**343:**1942.

---

93   Eating Disorders

Brian C. Reed, MD

KEY POINTS

- Individuals with anorexia nervosa or bulimia nervosa have altered perceptions of their body weight or shape and often engage in food restriction or purging.
- Weight and cardiac status are the most important components of the physical examination of individuals with eating disorders.
- Psychotherapy and nutritional rehabilitation are essential components in the treatment of eating disorders. Adjunctive treatment with antidepressants may provide additional benefit during the weight maintenance phase of treatment of patients with anorexia nervosa and may decrease binge eating behavior in patients with bulimia nervosa. Examples of medication doses are as follows:
  - **Fluoxetine (Prozac).** This drug is typically dosed at 40 mg/day during the weight-maintenance phase of anorexia or 60–80 mg/day in the treatment of bulimia nervosa.
  - **Tricyclic antidepressants.** These drugs are typically dosed at the same levels for the management of depression. Doses are imipramine (Tofranil), between 50–300 mg/day; amitriptyline (Elavil, Endep), 50–300 mg/day; or nortriptyline (Pamelor, Aventyl), 50–150 mg/day.
  - **Monoamine oxidase inhibitors (MAOIs).** Phenelzine or isocarboxazid dosed between 30 and 45 mg/day reduces binge eating behavior in patients with bulimia.

I. **Introduction**
  A. **Definition.** Eating disorders are psychological disorders characterized by an altered perception of body weight or shape and serious disturbances in eating behavior.
  1. **Anorexia nervosa** (Table 93–1). Individuals may have anorexia nervosa if they concurrently exhibit the following behaviors or characteristics:
    a. **Criterion A.** Shows a refusal to maintain a minimally normal body weight. As a guideline, an individual fails to maintain a minimally normal weight if he or she

TABLE 93–1. DIAGNOSTIC CRITERIA FOR EATING DISORDERS

Anorexia nervosa

A. Refusal to maintain body weight at or above a minimally normal weight for age and height (eg, weight loss leading to maintenance of body weight less than 85% of that expected; or failure to make expected weight gain during period of growth, leading to body weight less than 85% of that expected).

B. Intense fear of gaining weight or becoming overweight, even though the patient is underweight.

C. Disturbance in the way in which one's body weight or shape is experienced, undue influence of body weight or shape on self-evaluation, or denial of the seriousness of the current low body weight.

D. Amenorrhea in postmenopausal females (ie, the absence of at least three consecutive menstrual cycles. A woman is considered to have amenorrhea if her periods occur only with hormone administration.)

E. Type

    1. Restricting type: During the current episode, the patient has not regularly engaged in binge eating or purging (ie, self-induced vomiting or the misuse of laxatives, diuretics, or enemas).

    2. Binge eating/purging type: During the current episode, the patient has regularly engaged in binge eating or purging.

Bulimia nervosa

A. Recurrent episodes of binge eating. An episode of binge eating is characterized by both of the following:

    1. In a discrete period of time (eg, within any 2-hour period), eating an amount of food that is larger than what most people would eat during a similar period of time and under similar circumstances.

    2. A sense of lack of control over eating during the episode.

B. Recurrent inappropriate compensatory behaviors in order to prevent weight gain, such as self-induced vomiting; misuse of laxatives, diuretics, enemas, or other medications; fasting; or exercising excessively.

C. The binge eating and inappropriate compensatory behaviors both occur, on average, at least twice a week for 3 months.

D. Self-evaluation is unduly influenced by body shape and weight.

E. The episode does not occur exclusively during episodes of anorexia nervosa.

F. Specify type

    1. Purging type: During the current episode, the patient has regularly engaged in self-induced vomiting or the misuse of laxatives, diuretics, or enemas.

    2. Nonpurging type: During the current episode, the patient has used inappropriate compensatory behaviors, such as fasting or exercising excessively, but has not regularly engaged in self-induced vomiting or the use of laxatives, diuretics, or enemas.

Reprinted from the American Psychiatric Association's *Diagnostic and Statistical Manual of Mental Disorders*, 4th ed, text revision. American Psychiatric Association; 2000:589, 594.

weighs <85% of the weight that is considered normal for that individual's age and height based on published Metropolitan Life Insurance Tables or pediatric growth charts. The use of a body mass index equal to or below 17.5 kg/m² serves as alternative guideline in determining when an individual is underweight.

    b. **Criterion B.** Has an intense fear of gaining weight or becoming fat.

    c. **Criterion C.** Possesses a distorted perception of body weight and shape.

    d. **Criterion D.** Has amenorrhea if the individual is a postmenarcheal female.

    e. Two subtypes of anorexia nervosa exist: restricting type and binge eating/ purging type. An individual with the restricting type of anorexia nervosa accomplishes weight loss through dieting, fasting, or excessive exercise. An individual who has the binge eating type of anorexia nervosa regularly engages in binge eating and purging.

2. **Bulimia nervosa** (Table 93–1). An individual may have bulimia nervosa if they concurrently display the following behaviors or characteristics:

    a. **Criterion A.** Has recurrent episodes of binge eating.

    b. **Criterion B.** Shows recurrent use of inappropriate compensatory behaviors to prevent weight gain.

    c. **Criterion C.** Performs these binge eating and inappropriate compensatory behaviors at least twice a week for the duration of 3 months.

    d. **Criterion D.** Possesses a distorted perception of body weight or shape.

    e. **Criterion E.** Displays these behaviors not exclusively during an episode of anorexia nervosa.

    f. Like anorexia nervosa, two subtypes of bulimia nervosa exist: purging type and nonpurging type. Individuals with the purging subtype regularly engage in self-

induced vomiting, laxative abuse, and misuse of diuretics and enemas. A person with the nonpurging type of bulimia nervosa employs fasting or excessive exercise as a means of compensating for an episode of binge eating.
3. **Eating disorder not otherwise specified.** This category describes disorders of eating that fail to meet the criteria for either anorexia nervosa or bulimia nervosa. Examples include females who display all of the behaviors consistent with anorexia nervosa except that they have regular menstruation or someone who engages in binge eating and inappropriate compensatory behaviors at a frequency of less than twice a week for 3 months. Two other conditions are:
   a. **Binge eating disorder**
      (1) Binge eating disorder features recurrent episodes of binge eating similar to bulimia nervosa.
      (2) Since individuals with binge eating disorder do not regularly employ inappropriate compensatory behaviors such as purging or fasting, this disorder differs from bulimia nervosa.
   b. **Female athlete triad**
      (1) When associated with athletic training, the combination of disordered eating, amenorrhea, and osteoporosis is known as the female athlete triad.
      (2) Usually these athletes do not meet the criteria for anorexia nervosa.
      (3) Amenorrhea in female athletes results from intense training, fluctuations in weight, and low levels of estrogen.
      (4) Prolonged low levels of estrogen may lead to osteoporosis and fractures.
B. **Epidemiology**
   1. **Anorexia nervosa**
      a. **Prevalence.** Studies estimate that the lifetime prevalence of anorexia nervosa ranges between 0.5% and 3.7% of women. Among men, the prevalence of anorexia nervosa is approximately one tenth that among females. Over 90% of the individuals with anorexia nervosa are women.
      b. Due to the typical age of onset, anorexia nervosa is most commonly encountered in adolescents and young women.
      c. When comparing women of different ethnic origins, anorexia nervosa is more common among Caucasians and Hispanic women in the United States.
   2. **Bulimia nervosa**
      a. **Prevalence.** The lifetime prevalence of bulimia nervosa ranges between 1.1% and 4.2% among women. Like the prevalence of anorexia nervosa, the prevalence of bulimia nervosa among men is one tenth that of women.
      b. When comparing women of different ethnic origins, bulimia nervosa is most common among Caucasians. However, studies reveal that African American women are more likely to develop bulimia nervosa than anorexia nervosa and are much more likely to engage in purging with laxatives instead of vomiting.
   3. **Risk factors**
      a. **Cultural factors.** Women and adolescents who are preoccupied with their weight and experience social pressure to be thin are at an increased risk for developing an eating disorder. Such societal pressures are found more commonly in industrialized nations such as the United States, Canada, Western Europe, and Japan.
      b. **Familial factors.** Studies reveal that a hereditary component in the development of eating disorders, especially anorexia nervosa, may exist.
         (1) First-degree female relatives of individuals with anorexia nervosa have higher rates of both anorexia nervosa and bulimia nervosa.
         (2) Studies of the identical twin siblings of individuals who have anorexia nervosa or bulimia nervosa reveal that they have higher prevalence of eating disorders.
         (3) However, the studies of first-degree relatives of patients with bulimia nervosa do not conclusively demonstrate a hereditary transmission of bulimia nervosa.
      c. **History of sexual abuse.** Between 25% and 50% of individuals with anorexia nervosa and bulimia nervosa have been victims of sexual abuse.
      d. **Psychiatric illness.** High rates of comorbid psychiatric illness, such as major depression or dysthymia, have been reported to exist among 50–75% of individuals with anorexia nervosa and bulimia nervosa.

   C. Pathophysiology. Although a conclusive origin of eating disorders has yet to be discovered, several theories exist regarding their etiology of anorexia nervosa and bulimia nervosa.
   1. Some studies suggest a neuroendocrine etiology in anorexia nervosa and bulimia nervosa. Some researchers have noted impaired serotonin transmission among individuals with eating disorders. Other studies have observed alterations in serum leptin levels, an important regulator of weight gain and loss.
   2. A genetic etiology has been postulated. Refer to section I,B,3,b for further detail.
   3. Cultural influences and a history of dieting are also thought to be a component in the development of eating disorders.
II. **Diagnosis.** One must meet the diagnostic criteria mentioned in section I,A in order to have either anorexia nervosa or bulimia nervosa. See Table 93–2 for a suggested medical evaluation.
   A. **Symptoms and signs**
       1. Anorexia nervosa usually begins in mid to late adolescence (age 14–18 years). The disorder rarely occurs in women older than 40 years. Bulimia nervosa usually begins in late adolescence or early adulthood.
       2. Patients with eating disorders may **present with nonspecific complaints** such as fatigue, dizziness and general lack of energy. Additional complaints include symptoms associated with starvation or purging behaviors such as abdominal pain, constipation, amenorrhea, sore throat, and palpitations. Since patients with anorexia rarely possess insight into their illness, they rarely present with complaints about weight loss. Concerned family members and friends may bring patients with eating disorders.

TABLE 93-2. SUGGESTED MEDICAL EVALUATION OF PATIENTS WITH EATING DISORDERS

	Anorexia Nervosa		Bulimia Nervosa	
Evaluation	Restricting Type	Binge/Purge Type	Purging Type	Nonpurging Type
Weight for height	X	X	X	X
Temperature, pulse, blood pressure	X	X	X	X
Physical examination	X	X	X	X
Dental examination		X	X	
Electrocardiogram	X	X	X	
Complete blood cell count	X	X	X	X
Urinalysis	X	X	X	X
Blood urea nitrogen Creatinine	X	X	X	X[1]
Amylase		X[1]	X[1]	X[1]
Electrolytes	X	X	X	X[1]
Magnesium	X	X	X[1]	
Calcium	X	X	X[1]	
Phosphate	X		X	X[1]
Albumin	X	X	X[1]	
Bone mineral densitometry[2]	X[1]	X[1]	X[1]	X[1]
LH/FSH/estradiol[2]	X[1]	X[1]	X[1]	X[1]
Liver enzymes	X	X	X	
TSH, T_4	X	X	X	X
Cholesterol	X	X	X	X
Glucose	X	X	X	X
Blood/urine screen for drugs/alcohol, laxatives/ diuretics	X[1]	X[1]	X[1]	X[1]

[1] May be indicated, depending on the patient's clinical circumstances.
[2] In patients with long-standing amenorrhea.
FSH, follicle-stimulating hormone; LH, luteinizing hormone; TSH, thyroid-stimulating hormone.

3. When obtaining a history, it is important to **establish rapport and obtain a thorough diet history.** Questions should include inquiries about number of diets used within the past year and questions about the patient's perception of their weight.

4. Weight and cardiac status are the most important components of the physical examination of individuals with eating disorders.

5. During treatment, one must closely monitor the weight of patients. Patients with eating disorders may wear extra layers of clothing, place weights in their pockets, and drink extra fluids prior to being weighed.

6. Early in the disorder, the physical examination may be normal.

7. As the severity of the eating disorder worsens, complications may cause several abnormal findings on physical examination. Listed below are some physical examination findings:

   a. **Cardiac.** Bradycardia, orthostatic hypotension, and acrocyanosis are among the cardiac abnormalities.

   b. **Dental.** Erosion of dental enamel and salivary gland enlargement are signs of purging behavior.

   c. **Gastrointestinal.** Patients may have significant abdominal distention secondary to decreased bowel motility.

   d. **Skin.** Patients may develop lanugo, dry skin, or loss of subcutaneous fat. Repeated induction of vomiting may cause calluses or scarring on the dorsum of the hand (Russell's sign).

B. **Laboratory findings**

1. Among individuals with eating disorders, laboratory testing may be normal until complications develop.

2. Due to complications, testing may reveal abnormal electrolytes, renal functioning, complete blood cell counts, thyroid function test abnormalities, and osteopenia. See section V,A (medical complications) for further detail.

C. **Differential diagnosis**

1. **General medical conditions.** When evaluating an individual for anorexia nervosa or bulimia nervosa, one must consider other possible causes of weight loss and binge eating.

   a. Gastrointestinal disorders, endocrine diseases, occult malignancies, and acquired immunodeficiency syndrome (AIDS) are among the medical conditions that should be considered.

   b. Individuals with the neurologic disorder Kleine-Levin syndrome may experience binge eating similar to a person with bulimia nervosa.

   c. However, patients who experience weight loss due to a medical condition usually do not experience the distortion of body image that individuals with anorexia nervosa display.

2. **Psychiatric disorders.** Several psychiatric disorders can cause severe weight loss.

   a. **Major depressive disorder** may cause decreased appetite and weight loss.

   b. Patients with **schizophrenia** may display odd eating behaviors and experience weight loss.

   c. **Social phobia** may provoke feelings of humiliation or embarrassment while eating in public.

   d. **Body dysmorphic disorder** can cause altered perception of body image.

   e. Some individuals with **obsessive–compulsive disorder** may experience obsessions and compulsions related to food.

III. **Treatment**

A. **Goals**

1. **Anorexia nervosa.** Goals in the treatment of anorexia nervosa include the restoration of a healthy weight, management of physical complications, restoration of healthy eating patterns, correction of maladaptive thoughts regarding food and treatment of comorbid psychiatric conditions, building of a support network, and prevention of relapse.

2. **Bulimia nervosa.** A reduction in binge eating and purging are the primary goals in the treatment of bulimia nervosa. Since most individuals with bulimia nervosa have a normal body weight, weight restoration is not a primary goal.

B. **Treatment location** (Table 93–3). Weight and cardiac and metabolic status are the most important physical parameters in the determination of treatment location.

TABLE 93–3. LEVEL-OF-CARE CRITERIA FOR PATIENTS WITH EATING DISORDERS

Characteristic	Level 1: Outpatient	Level 2: Intensive Outpatient	Level 3: Full-day Outpatient	Level 4: Residential Treatment Center	Level 5: Inpatient Hospitalization
Medical complications	Medically stable to the extent that more extensive monitoring as defined in Levels 4 and 5 is not required			Medically stable (not requiring NG feeds, IV fluids, or multiple daily laboratories)	Adults: HR <40 beats per minute, BP <90/60 mm Hg; glucose <60 mg/dL (3.3 mmol/L); K⁺ <3 mg/dL (0.8 mmol/L); temperature <36.1°C (97°F); dehydration; renal, cardiovascular, or hepatic compromise. Children and adolescents: HR <50 beats per minute; BP <80/50, orthostatic BP, hypokalemia, hypophosphatemia.
Suicidality	No intent or plan			Possible plan but no intent	Intent and plan
Weight, as percent of healthy body weight	>85%	>80%	>70%	<85%	Adults <75%. Children and adolescents: acute weight decline with food refusal.
Motivation to recover (cooperativeness, insight, ability to control obsessive thoughts)	Good to fair	Fair	Partial, preoccupied with ego-syntonic thoughts more than 3 hours/day; cooperative	Fair to poor; preoccupied with ego-syntonic thoughts 4–6 hours/day; cooperative with highly structured environment.	Poor to very poor; preoccupied with ego-syntonic thoughts, uncooperative with treatment or cooperative only with with highly structured environment.

Comorbid disorders (substance abuse, depression, anxiety)	Presence of comorbid condition may influence choice of level of care			Any existing psychiatric disorder that would require hospitalization.
Structure needed for eating/gaining weight	Self-sufficient	Needs structure to gain weight	Needs supervision at all meals or will restrict eating	Needs supervision during and after all meals, or NG/special feeding
Impairment and ability to care for self, ability to control exercise	Able to exercise for fitness; fitness; able to control obsessive exercise	Structure required to prevent excessive exercise	Complete role impairment, cannot eat and gain weight by self; structure required to prevent patient from compulsive exercise	
Purging behavior	Can greatly reduce purging in nonstructured settings; no significant medical complications such as ECG abnormalities or others suggesting the need for hospitalization		Can ask for and use support or skills if desires to purge	Needs supervision during and after all meals
Environmental stress	Others able to provide adequate emotional and practical support	Others able to provide at least limited support and structure	Severe family conflict, problems or absence so as unable to provide structured treatment in home, or lives alone without adequate support system and structure	
Treatment availability/ living situation	Lives near treatment setting			Too distant to live at home

BP, blood pressure; ECG, electrocardiogram; HR, heart rate; IV, intravenous; K⁻, potassium level; NG, nasogastric.
Adapted from Practice guideline for the treatment of patients with eating disorders (revision) American Psychiatric Association Work Group on Eating Disorders. Am J Psychiatry 2000;**157** (suppl 1):20.

1. **Inpatient hospitalization**
   a. Indications for immediate hospitalization are marked orthostatic hypotension with an increase in pulse of >20 mm Hg or drop in blood pressure >20 mm Hg/minute standing, bradycardia <40 beats per minute, tachycardia >110 beats per minute, or inability to sustain body core temperature.
   b. Severely underweight individuals (usually those patients who weigh <75% of their individually estimated healthy weights), physiologically unstable individuals, and adolescents and children with rapid weight loss will also require 24-hour hospitalization.
   c. Partial hospitalization and day hospital programs are being increasingly used in the treatment of eating disorders.
   d. Failure of outpatient treatment, persistent weight loss and declines in oral intake despite participation in outpatient treatment programs, and the presence of additional stressors such as concurrent viral illnesses are indications for inpatient treatment.

2. **Outpatient treatment**
   a. Highly structured outpatient programs are often necessary for individuals with anorexia nervosa who weigh <85% of their individually estimated healthy weight.
   b. Most patients with uncomplicated bulimia do not require inpatient hospitalization.

C. **Nutritional rehabilitation**
   1. A program of nutritional rehabilitation should be established for those who are markedly underweight.
   2. **Typical goals for weight gain are 2–3 lbs per week for patients in the inpatient setting and 0.5–1 lb per week in the outpatient setting.** Initial intake levels should begin at 30–40 kcal/kg/day and should be gradually advanced. During the weight-gain phase, daily food intake may be increased 70–100 kcal/kg/day.
   3. During refeeding, solid foods are preferable to liquid diets.
   4. In life-threatening situations, nasogastric feeding and parenteral feedings may be necessary.
   5. During nutritional rehabilitation or refeeding, medical monitoring of vital signs, electrolytes, edema, and volume overload is essential.
   6. Since many patients with bulimia nervosa have a normal weight, restoration of weight is often not necessary. In these patients, nutritional counseling should focus on reducing dysfunctional eating behaviors and correcting nutritional deficiencies.

D. **Psychosocial interventions**
   1. For patients with anorexia nervosa, the goals of treatment are to encourage patient cooperation during their physical and nutritional rehabilitation, change dysfunctional behaviors related to their eating disorder, address comorbid psychopathology, and improve their social functioning.
   2. Systematic trials, case series, and expert opinions suggest that a well-conducted regimen of psychotherapy helps to improve symptoms of anorexia nervosa and prevent relapse. One meta-analysis that compared behavioral psychotherapy programs to treatment with medication alone revealed that behavioral therapy resulted in more consistent weight gain and shorter hospital stays. Clinical consensus favors individual psychotherapy during the acute phase of treatment for anorexia nervosa.
   3. Structured inpatient and partial hospitalization programs have been demonstrated to produce good short-term therapeutic effects. These behavioral programs often employ nonpunitive reinforcers such as empathic praise and privileges for achieving weight goals.
   4. Individual psychotherapy and family psychotherapy have been proved to be helpful in the management of anorexia nervosa.
   5. Cognitive behavioral therapy has been proved to be effective in the treatment of bulimia nervosa.
   6. Additionally, studies have demonstrated that group treatment, family therapy, and individual psychotherapy have been proved helpful in the treatment of bulimia nervosa.

E. **Medications**
   1. **Antidepressants.** Antidepressants have been demonstrated to be effective in the weight maintenance phase of treatment plans for individuals with anorexia ner-

vosa. Additionally, antidepressants have been proved to be effective in the acute treatment of bulimia nervosa. Studies have demonstrated 50–75% reductions in binge eating and vomiting with antidepressant medications. Selective serotonin reuptake inhibitors, or SSRIs, such as fluoxetine are commonly considered for patients with anorexia nervosa who have depressive, obsessive, and compulsive symptoms. Presently, fluoxetine (Prozac) is the only medication to be approved by the US Food and Drug Administration for the treatment of eating disorders. Fluoxetine is typically dosed at 40 mg/day in the weight-maintenance phase of anorexia. Similarly, a 60- to 80-mg daily dose of fluoxetine has been proved beneficial in the treatment of bulimia nervosa. Additionally, tricyclic antidepressants, bupropion, and monoamine oxidase inhibitors (MAOIs) have been demonstrated to be effective in the treatment of bulimia nervosa. The MAOIs phenelzine or isocarboxazid dosed between 30 and 45 mg/day may reduce binge eating behavior in patients with bulimia. Dosing of the tricyclic antidepressants usually starts at 50 mg/day.

   2. **Psychotropic medications.** Thus far, controlled studies have yet to demonstrate efficacy of psychotropic medications such as neuroleptics in the treatment of anorexia nervosa or bulimia nervosa.
   3. **Other medications**
      a. **Treatment of osteoporosis.** Calcium (500 mg two to three tablets daily), estrogen replacement, and bisphosphonates have been used in the treatment of patients with anorexia nervosa to prevent osteopenia and osteoporosis. Usually oral contraceptives are used as a means of hormone replacement and restoration of menstruation. Presently, no evidence has proved the effectiveness of these interventions.
      b. **Management of abdominal pains.** Metoclopramide, 10 mg with meals, has been used in the treatment of gastroparesis and early satiety.

IV. **Management Strategies**
   A. **Establish a therapeutic relationship.** The idea of gaining weight for an individual with an eating disorder or discontinuing binge eating patterns can be anxiety provoking. Without patients having a trusting relationship with their physician, such goals will never be achieved.
   B. **Collaborate with other health professionals.** Nutritional counseling, group psychotherapy, and medical consultation with specialists may be necessary to fully restore the health of an individual with bulimia nervosa or anorexia nervosa.
   C. **Monitor dysfunctional eating behaviors.** The careful assessment of a patient's perceived food intake and the anxiety provoked by eating is necessary. Having a meal with a patient may allow the clinician further insight into the patient's disordered patterns of eating.
   D. **Monitor the patient's general medical condition and psychiatric status.**
   E. **Assess the family and provide treatment.** Parents often struggle with denial, feelings of guilt, anger, and feelings of rejection. Family assessment and family therapy is usually a significant part of comprehensive care.

V. **Prognosis**
   A. **Medical complications.** Patients with anorexia nervosa and bulimia nervosa are susceptible to serious medical complications as a result of starvation and purging.
      1. **Cardiovascular complications.** Cardiovascular complications include orthostatic hypotension, palpitations, and arrhythmias such as bradycardia. Cardiomyopathy may result from low weight or syrup of ipecac abuse. Additionally, severe electrolyte imbalances may lead to sudden cardiac death.
      2. **Dental complications.** Multiple dental caries and dental enamel erosions can occur after several years of induced vomiting in anorexia nervosa. Patients may also develop enlarged salivary glands.
      3. **Gastrointestinal complications.** Vomiting related to the compensatory purging behavior in patients with anorexia nervosa and bulimia nervosa may eventually cause gastritis, esophagitis, or Mallory-Weiss tears. Patients may develop esophageal dysmotility disorders like gastroesophageal reflux. Individuals who repeatedly use laxatives as a means of purging may develop melanosis coli and other problems with colonic motility. Chronic constipation and bloating may

occur in laxative abusers. Cases of rectal prolapse have been reported in the literature.

4. **Endocrine complications.** Patients with anorexia nervosa may develop elevated serum cortisol levels and decreased levels of serum thyroxine (T_4) and triiodothyronine (T_3).

5. **Hematologic complications.** Nutritional deficits and changes associated with starvation may cause normochromic normocytic anemia, neutropenia, and thrombocytopenia. Rarely patients with anorexia nervosa may experience clotting disorders.

6. **Metabolic complications.** Due to starvation and purging, patients may develop serious electrolyte imbalances. Laxative abusers may develop a metabolic acidosis, hypomagnesemia, and hypophosphatemia. Metabolic alkalosis (elevated serum bicarbonate levels, hypochloremia, and hypokalemia) and hyperamylasemia can result from repeated induced vomiting.

7. **Musculoskeletal complications.** Musculoskeletal complications include osteoporosis and arrested skeletal growth. Young female athletes with amenorrhea and altered eating behaviors are particularly at risk for the development of stress fractures. Bone mineral density testing for osteoporosis and osteopenia should be considered in patients with chronic amenorrhea.

8. **Renal complications.** Renal abnormalities are seen in up to 70% of patients with anorexia nervosa. Complications include decreased glomerular filtration rate, increased blood urea nitrogen, and pitting edema. Monitoring of renal function during treatment is strongly recommended.

9. **Reproductive complications.** Reproductive complications include amenorrhea and infertility. Amenorrhea occurs in women secondary to low estrogen levels. Males with anorexia nervosa may have low serum testosterone levels. Both males and females with eating disorders may have loss of libido and infertility. Adolescents and young women may experience arrest of sexual development or regression of secondary sexual characteristics.

10. **Skin complications.** Repeated manual stimulation of the gag reflex to induce vomiting may cause callus development and scarring on the dorsum of the hand. This is known as Russell's sign.

11. **Suicide.** Suicide is a major cause of death among patients with anorexia nervosa.

B. **Outcomes**
   1. **Anorexia nervosa**
      a. Approximately 44% of patients with anorexia nervosa fully recover and successfully restore their weight to within 15% of recommended weight for height. About 24% of patients never restore their weight and between 2.5% and 5% of patients with anorexia nervosa die.
      b. Worse prognosis is associated with lower minimum weight, earlier age of onset, and disturbed family relationships.
      c. Follow-up studies conducted over 10–15 years reveal that it may take between 57 and 79 months to achieve full recovery.
   2. **Bulimia nervosa**
      a. Approximately 25–30% of patients with bulimia demonstrate spontaneous improvement within a 1- to 2-year period.
      b. With interventions such as medication and psychosocial intervention, between 50% and 70% of patients have some significant reductions in binge eating and purging.

REFERENCES

American Psychiatric Association. *Diagnostic and Statistical Manual of Mental Disorders,* 4th ed., text revision. American Psychiatric Association; 2000:583–595.

Hobart JA, Smucker DR: The female athlete triad. Am Fam Physician 2000;**61:**3357, 3367.

The McKnight Investigators. Risk factors for the onset of eating disorders in adolescent girls: Results of the McKnight Longitudinal Risk Factor Study. Am J Psychiatry 2003;**160:**248.

Practice guideline for treatment of patients with eating disorders (revision). American Psychiatric Association Work Group on Eating Disorders. Am J Psychiatry 2000;**157**(suppl 1):1.

Pritts SD, Susman J: Diagnosis of eating disorders in primary care. Am Fam Physician 2003;**67:**297, 311.

94 Somatization

John L. Coulehan, MD, MPH

KEY POINTS

- Somatization is frequent among primary care patients.
- Diagnosis involves the application of positive criteria (Table 94–6), as well as ruling out specific diseases.
- Treatment is multifaceted but relies heavily on active listening and developing a therapeutic contract that includes both supportive care and setting limits.

I. **Introduction**
   A. **Definition.** Somatization is a process by which persons experience and express emotional discomfort or psychosocial stress using physical symptoms.
   B. **Epidemiology**
      1. **Prevalence**
         a. Between 60% and 80% of healthy persons experience somatic symptoms in any given week. About one third of all primary care patients have ill-defined symptoms not attributable to physical disease, and 70% of those with emotional disorders present a somatic complaint as the reason for their office visit.
         b. The prevalence of **somatization disorder,** as defined in the *Diagnostic and Statistical Manual of Mental Disorders,* 4th edition (DSM-IV) (Table 94–1), is less than 1% in community-based studies, 5% among primary care outpatients, and 9% among hospitalized medical and surgical patients. The great majority of these patients are female. Clinical somatization is more common than these percentages suggest. For example, a diagnosis of **abridged somatization disorder** requires fewer and less diverse unexplained symptoms (6 in women or 4 in men) than are needed for diagnosing somatization disorder and has a reported prevalence of between 8% and 37% in primary care practice. These patients have utilization patterns, clinical features, and outcomes similar to those with somatization disorder.
         c. The prevalence of **psychogenic pain disorder** is unknown, but the disorder appears to be quite common in medical settings.

TABLE 94–1. DIAGNOSTIC CRITERIA FOR SOMATIZATION DISORDER

A. A history of many physical complaints beginning before the age of 30, occurring over a period of several years and resulting in treatment being sought or significant impairment in social or occupational functioning

B. Each of the following criteria must have been met at some time during the course of the disorder. To count a symptom as significant, it must not be fully explained by a known general medical condition, or the resulting complaints or impairment is in excess of what would be expected from the history, physical examination, or laboratory findings
   1. Four pain symptoms: a history of pain related to at least four different sites or functions (eg, head, abdomen, back, joints, extremities, chest, rectum, during sexual intercourse, during menstruation, or during urination)
   2. Two gastrointestinal symptoms: a history of at least two gastrointestinal symptoms other than pain (eg, nausea, diarrhea, bloating, vomiting other than during pregnancy, or intolerance of several different foods)
   3. One sexual symptom: a history of at least one sexual or reproductive symptom other than pain (eg, sexual indifference, erectile or ejaculatory dysfunction, irregular menses, excessive menstrual bleeding, or vomiting throughout pregnancy)
   4. One pseudoneurologic symptom: a history of at least one symptom or deficit suggesting a neurologic disorder not limited to pain (conversion symptoms such as blindness, double vision, deafness, loss of touch or pain sensation, hallucinations, aphonia, impaired coordination or balance, paralysis or localized weakness, difficulty swallowing, difficulty breathing, urinary retention, or seizures; dissociative symptoms such as amnesia or loss of consciousness other than fainting)

    d. In primary care practice, the prevalence of **hypochondriasis,** a preoccupation with the fear or belief that one has serious illness, may be as high as 10%. Full-blown somatization disorder is rare in men, but hypochondriasis appears in both sexes with equal frequency.

    e. Conversion symptoms (eg, sudden blindness or paralysis), while apparently common several decades ago, are now infrequent.

  2. Risk factors

    a. Personal characteristics associated with somatization include female gender, older age, currently unmarried state, lower level of education, lower socioeconomic class, and urban residence.

    b. Cultural factors. Somatization occurs throughout the world but is more prevalent in cultures in which emotional distress is generally couched in nonpsychological terms. In the United States, somatization appears to be particularly frequent among Hispanic and Asian populations.

C. Pathophysiology. Multiple theories have been proposed to explain somatization (Table 94–2). These are not mutually exclusive, and it is likely that somatization is a complex phenomenon with multiple risk factors playing a role in its causation.

II. Diagnosis. Somatization is a complex, multifactorial process. Rather than considering its variants as separate entities, it is perhaps best to think of somatization as a spectrum that ranges from occasional functional somatic symptoms to full-blown DSM-IV somatoform disorders.

A. Differential diagnosis

  1. Poorly understood conditions in which somatization might play a role or which might be confused with somatization include **fibromyalgia** or **fibromyositis, chronic fatigue syndrome, multiple chemical sensitivity,** and **temporomandibular joint dysfunction.** Other disorders with vague, multiple, and confusing symptoms (eg, hypothyroidism, multiple sclerosis, porphyria, systemic lupus erythematosus, or musculoskeletal and neuropsychiatric manifestations of Lyme disease) must also be considered, although, except for hypothyroidism, the prevalence of these conditions in the primary care setting is quite low.

  2. Amplified symptoms of underlying organic disease may also be involved in somatization.

  3. Psychiatric disorders in which somatization is not the primary process may be "masked" by an array of somatic complaints. These disorders include **major depression** (see Chapter 92), **alcohol and substance abuse** (see Chapter 88), and **generalized anxiety** and **panic disorders** (see Chapter 89). Physician recognition of psychiatric distress is decreased when patients present with high levels of somatization. Among somatizers in one primary care study, 24% had major depression, 17% had dysthymia, and 22% had generalized anxiety disorder.

  4. Somatoform disorders

    a. Somatization disorder (Table 94–1).

    b. Conversion reaction (Table 94–3)

    c. Hypochondriasis (Table 94–4).

    d. Psychogenic pain disorder (Table 94–5).

  5. Factitious disease occurs when a patient consciously reports nonexistent symptoms for secondary gain. Some patients with "disability neurosis" may have factitious symptoms, but they more likely suffer from true somatization in which secondary gain serves as a maintaining factor. Less than 5% of patients referred to psychiatrists for evaluation of unexplained somatic symptoms have factitious disease. Patients who persistently report factitious disease have **Munchausen syn-**

TABLE 94–2. THEORIES OF SOMATIZATION ETIOLOGY

1. **Neurobiological.** Abnormal central nervous system regulation of incoming sensory information leads to an impairment in attentional processing.
2. **Psychodynamic.** Somatization is a defense mechanism.
3. **Behavioral.** Somatization is a learned behavior in which environmental reinforcers maintain abnormal illness behavior.
4. **Sociocultural.** "Correct" ways of dealing with emotions and feelings are culturally determined.

TABLE 94–3. DIAGNOSTIC CRITERIA FOR CONVERSION DISORDER

A. One or more symptoms or deficits affect voluntary motor or sensory function, suggesting a neurologic or general medical condition
B. Psychological factors are judged to be associated with the symptom or deficit because the initiation or exacerbation of the symptom or deficit is preceded by conflicts or other stressors
C. The symptom or deficit is not intentionally produced or feigned (as in factitious disorder or malingering)
D. The symptom or deficit cannot, after appropriate investigation, be fully explained by a neurological or general medical condition and is not a culturally sanctioned behavior or experience
E. The symptom or deficit causes clinically significant distress or impairment in social, occupational, or other important areas of functioning or warrants medical evaluation
F. The symptom or deficit is not limited to pain or sexual dysfunction, does not occur exclusively during the course of somatization disorder, and is not better accounted for by another mental disorder

TABLE 94–4. DIAGNOSTIC CRITERIA FOR HYPOCHONDRIASIS

A. Preoccupation with fears of having, or the idea that one has, a serious disease based on the person's misinterpretation of bodily symptoms
B. The preoccupation persists despite appropriate medical evaluation and reassurance
C. The belief in A is not of delusional intensity (as in delusional disorder, somatic type) and is not restricted to a circumscribed concern about appearance (as in body dysmorphic disorder)
D. The preoccupation causes clinically significant distress or impairment in social, occupational, or other important areas of functioning
E. The duration of the disturbance is at least 6 months
F. The preoccupation does not occur exclusively during the course of generalized anxiety disorder, obsessive–compulsive disorder, panic disorder, a major depressive episode, separation anxiety, or another somatoform disorder

TABLE 94–5. DIAGNOSTIC CRITERIA FOR PSYCHOGENIC PAIN DISORDER

A. Pain in one or more anatomic sites is the predominant focus of the clinical presentation and is of sufficient severity to warrant clinical attention
B. The pain causes clinically significant distress or impairment in social, occupational, or other important areas of functioning
C. Psychological factors are judged to have an important role in the onset, severity, exacerbation, or maintenance of the pain
D. The pain is not better accounted for by a mood, anxiety, or psychotic disorder and does not meet criteria for dyspareunia

drome. Diagnostic tests and medical interventions often lead to additional symptoms (eg, drug side effects), clinical findings (eg, surgical scars), and dysfunction (eg, intestinal adhesions) in these patients.

B. **Symptoms and signs**

1. Symptoms favoring somatization are presented in Table 94–6. The presence of several of these characteristics strongly suggests somatization, even though evidence of organic disease may also be present.

2. **Pain** is the most frequent single complaint, present in over 80% of patients with somatization.

3. **Three symptom clusters suggestive of somatization secondary to depression, anxiety, or panic disorder are described below.**

   a. Atypical chest pain, palpitations, tachycardia, or difficulty catching one's breath (sighing, not true dyspnea), or all of these.

   b. Headache, dizziness, lightheadedness, presyncope, or paresthesias.

   c. Dyspepsia, heartburn, "gas," flatulence, or other gastrointestinal symptoms, or all of these.

4. **Globus hystericus,** the sensation of a lump in the throat that interferes with swallowing, is a frequent symptom of anxiety or conversion.

TABLE 94–6. POSITIVE CRITERIA FOR DIAGNOSIS OF PSYCHOGENIC SYMPTOMS

1. The patient's descriptions of symptoms are vague, inconsistent, or bizarre.
2. Symptoms are in excess of objective findings.
3. There are multiple symptoms in different organ systems.
4. Symptoms persist despite apparently adequate medical therapy.
5. The illness began in the context of a psychologically meaningful setting (eg, death of relative, conflict with spouse, work injury, or job promotion).
6. The patient denies that any emotional distress or psychological factors play a role in symptom development.
7. The patient has visited several physicians or has had several operations.
8. There is evidence of an associated psychiatric disorder.
9. Discussion reveals that the patient attributes an idiosyncratic meaning to symptom.
10. Alexithymia (ie, difficulty describing emotions or inner processes in words) is present.

    C. Laboratory tests. Laboratory and imaging studies serve only to rule out organic disease, although evidence of a disease entity does not exclude the diagnosis of somatization. Moreover, abnormalities unrelated to the patient's symptoms may be discovered with sophisticated diagnostic technology. For example, the presence of minimal mitral valve prolapse on echocardiography cannot explain an array of somatic symptoms.

III. Treatment. Appropriate treatment for the underlying problem is the first priority. Additionally, treatment is not likely to be effective unless maintaining factors are addressed and minimized.

    A. Basic treatment principles

        1. The patient's problem should be considered as deserving of attention. This requires attentive listening, empathic responses, and avoidance of statements that the patient might construe to mean "There's nothing wrong with you" or "It's all in your head."

        2. Clear explanations of symptoms should be presented in functional or physiologic terms. The physician should describe the problem in terms the patient can understand and in a way that fits in with his or her belief system about health and illness. Disease labels should be avoided as much as possible. When you do not understand and cannot explain a symptom, tell the patient in unambiguous terms.

        3. A well-defined treatment program should be initiated. Even if treatment consists only of explanation, reassurance, observation, and symptomatic measures, the physician should provide relatively definite information about how to proceed, how long the symptoms might last, and what to do next. Ambiguity increases anxiety.

        4. It is important to engage the patient's active participation in treatment by behavioral means, such as by keeping a diary to identify factors that influence symptoms, which may serve to make the problem appear less unpredictable and out of control. General behavior change techniques also may be initiated. For example, an exercise program to enhance "muscle tone" or a diet for weight reduction, if successful, generally enhances the patient's sense of control and self-mastery.

    B. Multifaceted treatment approach required by primary chronic somatization

        1. Pharmacotherapy. There are no adequate clinical trials of drug treatment for primary somatization per se. However, drugs may be effective in the following situations.

            a. Specific intractable symptoms such as headaches, myalgias, and other forms of chronic pain may be ameliorated by **selective serotonin reuptake inhibitors** or **tricyclic antidepressants** (see Chapter 92, page 639, for starting dosages).

            b. Even when DSM-IV criteria for depression are not present, patients who demonstrate somatic symptoms of depression often benefit from adequate doses of serotonin reuptake inhibitors. Likewise, anxious patients may experience relief of somatic symptoms in response to **benzodiazepine therapy,** even though they do not fulfill DSM-IV criteria for panic or anxiety disorders (see Chapter 89, page 609, for starting dosages).

            c. Because patients who somatize often have a low tolerance for the side effects of medications, symptomatic medications (eg, analgesics or antispasmodics) should be used sparingly and in the minimal effective doses.

            d. There is rarely, if ever, a place for opioids in treating somatization symptoms.

        2. Psychiatric consultation has been shown over the short term (ie, 1 year) to be effective in reducing hospitalizations and overall medical costs of patients with somatization disorder. In one study, a single consultation report to the primary physician was associated with a 12% reduction in costs. The physician should refer the patient to a consultation–liaison service or to a psychiatrist comfortable with somatizing patients. Such a consultation may lead to short-term psychotherapy, in addition to the recommended management strategies for the primary care physician. A course of cognitive behavioral therapy has been associated with improvements in functioning and decreases in health care utilization for up to 18 months. However, most patients with somatization disorder do not respond well to open-ended referral for psychiatric care.

   3. Patients with severe chronic somatization may benefit from comprehensive inpatient treatment programs that include individual, group, and family therapy; educational programs; physical and occupational therapy; biofeedback; and vocational rehabilitation.

IV. Management Strategies. Optimal management of somatizing patients requires relief of symptoms, treatment of underlying medical or psychiatric disorders, and avoidance of the pathologic cycle of intervention (medical treatment, temporary improvement, renewal of symptoms, disappointment, patient and physician anger).

   A. The **therapeutic contract** should be emphasized and its parameters defined. While recognizing the reality of the patient's symptoms, one should attempt to develop a broader framework for physician–patient interaction by following the guidelines described below.

   1. Tolerate symptoms and scale down the goals of therapy. Speak in terms of reduction, lessening, and coping, rather than complete symptom alleviation. Evaluate new symptoms as they occur, but do so conservatively in a stepwise fashion. Openly discuss the risks of medication side effects and the possibility of complications with invasive procedures.

   2. Discuss psychiatric or psychosocial issues not as direct causes of symptoms, but rather as possible aggravating factors or as unfortunate results of physical symptoms.

   3. Promote stability in the physician–patient relationship by scheduling office visits at regular intervals (usually ranging from 2 to 4 weeks, depending on patient and physician tolerance), thereby diminishing the patient's need for a "ticket of admission." Increase the length of office visits to allow relatively unrushed attention. Schedule visits at times when interruptions will be minimal, not on "emergency-prone" days such as Mondays or Fridays.

   4. Explicitly discourage dependent behaviors, such as unscheduled phone calls or drop-in visits. Prearranged follow-up phone calls may allow a reduction in the frequency of office visits. Ask the patient not to "doctor shop" or to seek specialist care without consulting the primary care physician.

   B. Somatization may be a sign of **family dysfunction** in which the identified patient's symptoms may serve to stabilize a pathologic family situation. It may be necessary to enlist family members in behavioral strategies to "wean" the patient from secondary gain (eg, using somatization to avoid household tasks, to require special meals, or to excuse irritability and angry outbursts).

   C. While remaining supportive of the symptomatic person, the physician should attempt to avoid certifying the person as **permanently and totally disabled.** The label of *disability* can be viewed as another "medical intervention" with adverse consequences as well as benefits. Nonetheless, the physician should realize that severe and chronic somatization is a disabling condition. Chronic pain syndrome, for example, may qualify under Medicare guidelines as a cause of total disability. While perhaps not desirable in terms of "curing" the somatization, disability may, in certain cases, for economic and social reasons be the best palliative option.

   D. Physicians develop a great deal of **anger** and **frustration** when treating patients who somatize. To maintain equanimity, the physician may use the following strategies.

   1. Make the diagnosis of somatization and modify treatment objectives accordingly, rather than wallowing in frustration over the absence of objective findings of disease.

   2. Set up firm and explicit guidelines as described above, and review them frequently with the patient. Arrange office appointments so that somatizers are not clustered together.

   3. Develop an informal relationship with a psychiatrist or a psychologist to whom feelings about these patients can be ventilated and with whom treatment problems can

be discussed. More structured group experiences (eg, Balint groups) for providers are also quite effective.
V. **Prognosis**
   A. A large proportion of patients with functional somatic symptoms recover without specific intervention. Favorable prognostic factors include acute onset and short duration of symptoms, younger age, higher socioeconomic class, absence of organic disease, and absence of personality disorder.
   B. The long-term prognosis for patients with somatization disorder is guarded, and usually lifelong supportive treatment is required. If somatization is a mask for another psychiatric disorder, its prognosis depends on that of the primary problem. In one study of patients with psychiatric disorders presenting with a recent onset of physical symptoms, 40% subsequently developed chronic somatoform disorders.
   C. If hypochondriasis is conceptualized as an "amplifying somatic style," patients who exhibit this condition are likely to have recurrent physical complaints and require frequent medical intervention. Appropriate treatment for somatization should minimize these complaints by providing education and reassurance, by reducing anxiety, and by enhancing the patient's coping skills.
   D. Discrete conversion symptoms have a better prognosis. They may resolve spontaneously when no longer "required" or may respond to specific psychotherapy.

REFERENCES

Coulehan JL, Block MR: Seal up the mouth of outrage: Interactive problems in interviewing. Chapter 12. In: The *Medical Interview: Mastering Skills for Clinical Practice.* Davis; 2001:195–219.

Dickinson WP, et al: The somatization in primary care study: A tale of three diagnoses. Gen Hosp Psychiatry 2003;**25:**1.

Escobar JI, Hoyos-Nervi C, Gara M: Medically unexplained symptoms in medical practice: A psychiatric perspective. Environ Health Perspect 2002;**110**(suppl 4):631.

Hiller W, Fichter MM, Riet W: A controlled treatment study of somatoform disorders including analysis of healthcare utilization and cost-effectiveness. J Psychosomatic Res 2003;**54:**369.

Maynard CK: Assess and manage somatization. Nurse Pract 2003;**28:**20.

Stanley IM, Peters S, Salmon P: A primary care perspective on prevailing assumptions about persistent medically unexplained physical symptoms. Int J Psychiatry Med 2002;**32:**125.

Kathleen C. Amyot, MD

KEY POINTS

- There is an enormous demand for contraception in the United States.
- Knowledge of contraceptive efficacy, risks, and benefits allows the provider to "match" the contraceptive method to the needs and desires of the patient.
- Condoms are the only method that offers some protection against sexually transmitted diseases.
- Hormonal methods of birth control are the most commonly used.

I. **Introduction**
   A. The demand for birth control is great; an estimated 41 million women in the United States are sexually active.
   B. Three million women in this country between the ages of 15 and 44 years do not use contraception, however. Half of all pregnancies in the United States are unintentional, as are 92% of pregnancies in adolescents aged 15–19 years. They occur either because contraceptives are not use or because they are used sporadically or incorrectly.
   C. Other nonusers who are at risk for unintended pregnancy are women who have no prior sexual experience, those who have lost partners due to separation or death, and those who believe they are protected because they are postpartum or nursing. Age, socioeconomic status, and level of education are inversely correlated with the failure rate of contraceptives.
   D. Numerous contraceptive options are available, so the choice of a particular option should take place after a review of the risk and benefits of all choices and through education on the option chosen so correct use is assured.

II. **Choosing a Birth Control Method.** The only 100% effective method of birth control is abstinence. Correct use of any contraceptive device does not guarantee protection. Up to 20% of women who experienced unintended pregnancy used their selected methods consistently and properly. Consideration of the following factors will help patients and physicians make the best possible choices. Desirable properties of contraceptives are a high rate of effectiveness, prolonged duration of action, rapid reversibility, privacy of use, protection against sexually transmitted diseases (STDs), and easy accessibility.
   A. **Theoretical efficacy rates** are defined as the number of unintended pregnancies per 100 women that occur during the first year of use of a given contraceptive method (if the method is used correctly). **Actual efficacy rates** reflect the percentage of women who become pregnant during the first year of contraceptive use. The efficacy of a given contraceptive method is influenced by the fertility, individual motivation, and risk-taking attitude of each partner; the frequency of intercourse; the ability of the patient to master the method; and the theoretical efficacy rate of the method. Using two forms of contraception at once significantly lowers the risk of accidental pregnancy.

   Patient education and physician understanding promote increased efficacy of a birth control method by minimizing discontinuation of a particular method or switching to another form without guidance. Too often, women quit using a method in frustration or due to side effects and then conceive; for example, 50% of oral contraceptive users stopped taking the pills in the first year. When discussing the possible side effects and use of a particular method of birth control with patients, the physician should explain how problems can be minimized and point out the benefit and risks of the method. When a patient reports breakthrough bleeding while taking the pill, use this as an opportunity to see if she is taking the pill daily, since spotting may reflect missed pills.
   B. **Safety concerns** include risks of morbidity and mortality as well as noncontraceptive safety benefits, such as protection from STDs or the resolution of menstrual problems.

  C. Acceptability of a method depends on a number of factors.
    1. Cost. This includes the financial cost of the product, as well as the cost of time and money in physician visits and necessary medical testing.
    2. Individual preferences. The effect of a birth control method on subsequent fertility should be considered as well as ease of use of the method and ethical or religious concerns regarding birth control. See Table 95–1 for questions women should ask themselves before selecting a contraceptive method.
III. Hormonal Contraception. This method works by suppressing ovulation, changing cervical mucus so that sperm are less effective, and making the endometrium less receptive to implantation. When used as "emergency contraception" it causes alteration of the transport of sperm or ova and inhibition or delay of ovulation and may create a deficient luteal phase having some endometrial effect. Some women may be uncomfortable with the possible abortifacient effect if ovulation and conception occur, but the conceptus is unable to implant in an unfavorable endometrium.
  A. Oral contraceptives. This birth control method, used by 18 million women, is the most popular reversible form of contraception in the United States. Except for the progestin-only pills, all oral contraceptive pills have different doses of two types of estrogen and nine types of progestin. Biphasic and triphasic oral contraceptives contain different amounts of hormone throughout the menstrual cycle in an attempt to more closely mimic natural hormone production. Choosing among the many oral contraceptives can be done on the basis of characteristics of both the patient and the contraceptive. Low-dose pills (30–35 μg of estrogen) may be used initially, and the dosage may be altered as needed (see Table 95–2 for suggestions).
    1. The **failure rate** for the ideal user is 0.1% for combined pills and 0.5% for progestin-only pills. Actual failure rates are 5% for both types of contraceptives.
    2. Contraindications
      a. Women older than age 35 who smoke. Healthy women who do not smoke can safely use oral contraceptives until menopause if they desire.
      b. Women **with cardiovascular problems,** such as a history of thromboembolic disease, cerebrovascular disease, and ischemic heart disease. Other conditions, such as breast cancer, liver tumor, or undiagnosed vaginal bleeding, preclude oral contraceptive use.
      c. Lactating women <6 weeks postpartum because oral contraceptives can diminish breast milk production. Progesterone-only pills are acceptable (see Table 95–2 for dosage information).
    3. Side effects are much less of a problem than they were in the past because the amounts of estrogen and progestin in oral contraceptives have decreased. In the United States, it is safer for women to use oral contraceptives than to deliver a baby. Many of the side effects are temporary. If the woman can tolerate spotting, acne, breast tenderness, and nausea, these conditions often improve after 3 months. Continued spotting may be a symptom indicating that a woman is not taking her pills every day.

TABLE 95–1. QUESTIONS A WOMAN SHOULD ASK BEFORE SELECTING A BIRTH CONTROL METHOD

1. Am I afraid of using this method?
2. Would I rather not use this method?
3. Will I have trouble remembering to use this method?
4. What are my chances of becoming pregnant using this method?
5. Will I have trouble using this method carefully?
6. Do I have unanswered questions about this method?
7. Does this method cost more than I can afford?
8. Could this method ever cause me serious health problems?
9. Do I object to this method because of religious beliefs?
10. What problems can I expect?
11. Is my partner opposed to this method?
12. Am I using this method without my partner's knowledge?
13. Will using this method embarrass me or my partner?
14. Will I enjoy intercourse less because of this method?
15. Will this method interrupt my lovemaking?

Modified from Hatcher RA, et al: *Contraceptive Technology 1994–1995,* 16th ed. Irvington; 1994.

TABLE 95–2. CHOOSING AMONG ORAL CONTRACEPTIVES (OCPS)

Characteristic	Oral Contraceptive	Comment
Nursing women	Ovrette Micronor	Progesterone-only pills will not interrupt blood supply
Nausea or breast tenderness when taking OCPs	Ovrette Micronor	Progesterone-only or lower estrogenic activity pills
No prior use of OCPs	Ortho Novum 1/35 Tri-Norinyl Ortho Novum 7/7/7 Ortho Tri-cyclen Ortho cyclen Alesse Loestrin 1/20	Lower-dose pills minimize side effects
Acne, hirsutism, or obesity	Demulen Desogen/Ortho-Cept Ovcon 35 Ortho Tri-Cyclen	Less androgenic activity pills
Hypertension, hyperlipidemia, or diabetes mellitus	Desogen/Ortho-Cept Ortho Cyclen Ortho Tri-cyclen Ovocon-35	All produce favorable cholesterol pattern
Scanty or absent withdrawal bleeding	Increase estrogen component or lower progestin	Build up endometrium
Spotting (over 3 months)	Increase estrogen and progestin in monophasic combinations	Stabilize endometrium
Minimize risk of thrombosis	Loestrin 1/20 Alesse	Less estrogen
Use of rifampin or dilantin	Ovral Ovcon 50 Demulen Ortho-Novum/Norinyl 1/50	Increase estrogen

a. **Breast cancer.** Results of studies conflict, but the US Food and Drug Administration currently considers evidence suggesting that long-term use of oral contraceptives increases the risk of breast cancer to be insufficient.
b. **Cervical neoplasia** rates are higher in women who use oral contraceptives, but studies have not determined whether oral contraceptives or other factors are responsible.
c. **Lactation** can be interrupted because estrogen inhibits milk production. Nursing mothers who want to use oral contraceptives should use progestin-only pills.
d. **Gallbladder disease** symptoms may be precipitated by oral contraceptives that contain estrogen, although the incidence of gallbladder disease is not itself increased.
e. **Normal menses and fertility** may be slightly delayed, but most women have no trouble conceiving within the first year after oral contraceptives are discontinued. Ninety-nine percent of women resume regular menses within the first 6 months after they stop taking contraceptive pills.
f. **Estrogen-related effects** such as nausea, breast tenderness, cyclic weight gain, headaches, and growth of fibroids may occur. Progestin-related effects include increased appetite, weight gain, depression, fatigue, decreased libido, acne, decreased glucose tolerance, headaches, and increased levels of low-density lipoprotein (LDL) cholesterol and decreased levels of high-density lipoprotein (HDL) cholesterol.
g. **Mild mood swings and depression** have been described by women using oral contraceptives. Contraceptive pills deplete vitamin B_6 (pyridoxine) levels.

Symptomatic women should receive supplements. Pyridoxine, 50 mg/day, is the usual dose.

    h. Low-dose oral contraceptive pills do not impact glucose metabolism adversely. Some progestins do decrease HDL cholesterol and increase LDL cholesterol (see Table 95–2 to choose wisely).

  4. Noncontraceptive benefits of low-dose estrogen oral contraceptives (≥50 µg)
   a. **Protection from endometrial cancer** after 1 year of use.
   b. **Reduction in the risk of ovarian cancer** after 6 months of use.
   c. **More regular** and *less painful* menstrual periods with less bleeding and iron deficiency anemia. Premenstrual syndrome is less common and less severe in women using oral contraceptives, as are benign breast disease and benign ovarian cysts, endometriosis, acne, hirsutism, and anovulatory bleeding.
   d. **Pelvic inflammatory disease (PID)** caused by *Chlamydia* occurs less often because of the effects oral contraceptives have on the menses, cervix, and mucus.

  5. Acceptability of oral contraceptives may be limited if remembering a pill daily is difficult. The cost is $100–130 per year for generic pills and $200–400 per year for nongeneric pills.

  6. Evaluation and follow-up. Monitoring includes yearly Pap smears and blood pressure monitoring.

B. Injectable hormones. Depo-Provera (depo-medroxyprogesterone acetate) has been used safely by over 10 million women worldwide. It has been approved in over 90 countries, including the United States. It is given as a deep intramuscular injection of 150 mg every 12 weeks.

  1. The **failure rate** is very low—only 0.3% failure in ideal and actual cases. Low body weight decreases the efficacy.

  2. Contraindications. This method should not be used in women who are at significant risk for breast cancer or who have been treated for this type of cancer.

  3. Side effects
   a. **Breast cancer** is most feared because of data from animal studies, but recent studies have not supported this association in humans, nor has the large experience worldwide.
   b. **Menstrual irregularities** occur, with more time elapsing between menses the longer Depo-Provera is used. After 6 months (two injections), one half of the women are amenorrheic, and most women are without menses after 1 year of therapy. Normal menses and fertility will not return immediately upon stopping the drug and may take more than 1 year to normalize. The average time to conception after the last injection is 8–9 months. If menses do not resume within 1 year of discontinuation, a work-up for amenorrhea is necessary.
   c. **Headache** is experienced by 1–3% of women.
   d. **Weight gain** resulting from an increase in appetite averages 5 lbs in the first year and up to 14 lbs by year four of treatment.

  4. Noncontraceptive benefits
   a. **Amenorrhea** is a consequence that many women enjoy. Baseline luteinizing hormone and follicle-stimulating hormone levels do not change, so these women have no symptoms of estrogen deficiency.
   b. **Lactation** is not adversely affected if the hormone is given immediately postpartum; trace amounts are detectable in breast milk without adverse outcome to infants.
   c. **Women with epilepsy** have fewer seizures.

  5. Acceptability is high for women who need or want very effective birth control that is not coitally dependent and who prefer or do not mind amenorrhea.

  6. Administration. Give Depo-Provera, 150 mg intramuscularly, every 3 months. The first injection should be given immediately postpartum or within the first 5 days of a woman's menses.

C. Norplant consists of six flexible silicone rubber rods, each of which is 1.3 inches long and contains 36 mg of levonorgestrel. Inserted subdermally at the inside of the upper arm, the rods continuously release a low dose of this progestin, which inhibits ovulation and causes thickening of the cervical mucus, preventing conception for up to 5 years. Norplant was voluntarily pulled from the market by the manufacturer in 2002.

D. Ortho Evra is a combination contraceptive that is provided in a transdermal system. Patches containing 6.00 mg norelgestromin and 0.75 mg ethinyl estradiol are placed on the skin of the buttocks, abdomen, and upper torso or upper outer arms weekly.

Each patch releases 150 µg of norelgestromin and 20 micrograms of ethinyl estradiol daily. It functions in the same manner as combination oral contraceptives, but is more convenient for some women in a transdermal route.

1. The **failure rate** is <1% per year, but the patch may be less effective in women who weigh over 198 lbs. In clinical trials 2–6% of women had at least one patch detach. If the patch is off for >24 hours, alternative birth control must be used for a week after the new patch is placed.
2. **Contraindications** are the same as those for oral contraceptives.
3. **Side effects** are also similar to those of oral contraceptives. (See section III,A.). Some women have mild skin irritation.
4. **Noncontraceptive benefits** are the same as for oral contraceptives.
5. **Acceptability** is enhanced over that of oral contraceptives because of the weekly transdermal route of administration.

E. **Nuvaring** is another newer alternative route of administration for combination hormonal contraceptives. It is a flexible ring impregnated with etonogestrel and ethinyl estradiol. It delivers 0.120 mg of etonogestrel and 0.015 mg ethinyl estradiol daily. The ring is placed weekly in the posterior fornix of the vagina. Because of the "local" administration of hormones, lower doses can be used.

1. The **failure rate** is 1–2% per year.
2. **Contraindications** are the same as those for oral contraceptives, as well as undiagnosed vaginal bleeding.
3. **Side effects** again are similar to combination oral contraceptives as well as vaginal discharge or irritation. Some patients are aware of the ring during intercourse or at random times. Ninety percent of couples did not find this to be a problem. The ring can be accidentally expelled during straining or removal of a tampon. If this occurs, it should be rinsed with cool water and replaced. If the ring remains out of the vagina for more than 3 hours, contraceptive effectiveness may be reduced and an alternative contraceptive method should be used.
4. **Noncontraceptive benefits** include regulation of cycles as in oral contraceptives.
5. **Acceptability** is good for women who want a method of birth control that is not coitally dependent and have difficulty remembering daily pills. It is also a good choice for women who desire a lower dose of hormones.

F. **Emergency contraception (ECP)** using oral contraceptive pills containing ethinyl estradiol and norgestrel or levonorgestrel reduces the risk of pregnancy after unprotected intercourse. The precise mechanisms are unknown; however, the hormones appear to inhibit ovulation if it has not occurred. They also may impact gamete transport, function of the corpus luteum, and implantation of a conceptus. It is essential to check a pregnancy test as well as to discuss future contraception plans and whether the woman is at high risk for STDs and to counsel her about risk-reduction activities. It is an important opportunity to educate women about use of precoital methods of birth control, because the failure rate of ECP accumulates over time.

1. When used within 72 hours of unprotected intercourse, ECP prevents three of four pregnancies that would have occurred. The earlier the method is used, the more effective it is.
2. Pregnancy is the only **contraindication** to its use.
3. **Side effects** include nausea in 30–50% of women and vomiting in 15–25%, as well as fatigue, breast tenderness, abdominal pain, headache, and dizziness for a day or two. Antiemetic medication given prior to the first dose of ECP helps with the nausea. Progestin-only forms of ECP cause less nausea and vomiting.
4. The **availability** of ECP is important to discuss at health maintenance visits for reproductive-age women as well as precoital methods of contraception in case of contraceptive failure. It is also an essential part of the treatment for victims of sexual assault. There is currently debate regarding offering ECP as an over-the-counter medication.
5. ECP is gaining acceptability as it becomes more commonly used, although concerns about its possible abortifacient effect (if life begins at conception) are also becoming more prevalent. ECP is not recommended for routine use because it is less effective than other forms of birth control.
6. **Administration.** All forms of ECP are administered as the first dose, then the second identical dose is given 12 hours later. There are two specific ECP formulations on the market—Preven (two blue pills) and Plan B (one white pill). Alternatively, other oral contraceptives can be used as emergency contraceptives, and women can then

use the rest of the pills in the pack as their birth control method. Nordette comes in four light orange pills; Ovral, in two white pills per dose; Triphasil, in four yellow pills; Alesse, in five pink pills; and Lo/Ovral, in four white pills. Women should expect their menses within 3 weeks of taking ECP; otherwise, they need a pregnancy test.

IV. **Barrier Methods.** These methods prevent contraception by providing a mechanical barrier to sperm. If such methods are used with a spermicidal, sperm inactivation results. Avoid using oil-based lubricants and medications (Femstat, Monistat, estrogen, and Vagisil creams), because they cause the latex in condoms to deteriorate.

A. **Condoms** are made of latex, the cecum of lambs ("skins"), or polyurethane (for latex-sensitive individuals). Most condoms have a shelf life of 5 years if stored properly in a cool place. Condoms for women offer increased coverage of the external genitalia and line the vagina entirely. They can be inserted 8 hours before intercourse. Acceptance has been limited because of the condom's bulkiness. Female and male condoms should not be used together because they can adhere, causing one or both to slip out of position.

1. **Failure rates** for the ideal user are 3%. For the actual user, they are 14%. Latex condoms with spermicide are the most effective.
2. **Contraindications.** Condoms should not be used if one or both partners are allergic to them.
3. **Side effects** are limited to allergy to latex or the spermicidal.
4. **Noncontraceptive benefits** include protection from STDs (including human immunodeficiency virus [HIV]) for latex and polyurethane condoms; skin condoms are too porous. Protection from infertility and from cervical intraepithelial neoplasia also occurs. Seventy-five percent of men agree that using condoms "shows you are a caring person," while 32% agree that using a condom "makes sex last longer."
5. **Acceptability** is limited if a couple finds using condoms distracting or embarrassing. Expense is minimal, although specialty items are more costly. Condoms are available over the counter. No office visit is required. Patient instructions are given by the manufacturer. At least 25% of men are still embarrassed to buy condoms and may not know how to negotiate condom use with partners.

B. **Diaphragms** are dome-shaped, rubber cups with arching or coiled rims. They must be left in place for at least 6 hours and not more than 24 hours after intercourse. Additional spermicide must be inserted before each coital act.

1. **Failure rate.** The failure rate is 3% ideally and 18% actually. Efficacy improves as patient age and duration of use increase.
2. **Contraindications.** If a woman has a cystocele, is allergic to latex or spermicide, has a history of toxic shock syndrome, or is <12 weeks postpartum, or is too squeamish to use a diaphragm properly, another birth control method should be chosen.
3. **Side effects.** Spermicide sensitivity is the most common problem. Allergic reactions to latex may also occur.

V. **Chemical Methods.** These methods **inactivate** the sperm by interfering with motility. Spermicides are available in the form of gels, creams, foams, suppositories, and film. The two most widely used are nonoxynol 9 and octoxynol 9. Douching is not a reliable contraceptive even when women put spermicide in the solution, because it is too late to inactivate the sperm. Women who routinely douche have an increased risk of PID and ectopic pregnancy.

A. **Failure rate.** The failure rate is 3% ideally and 21% actually. Using a barrier method with a chemical method together increases efficacy.
B. **Contraindications.** Spermicides should not be used if either partner has an allergy to the spermicidal agents.
C. **Side effects.** Side effects are limited to allergy. There is no increased risk of congenital malformation if conception occurs while using spermicides. There is some question if frequent daily use of nonoxynol 9 may increase the rate of HIV infection because of its disruptive effect on the vaginal epithelium and cervix. Studies are ongoing.
D. **Noncontraceptive benefits** (see section III,D,4).
E. **Acceptability.** Acceptability is high for those individuals or couples who like nonprescription, fairly inexpensive protection, but low for people who find this method to be messy.

VI. **Intrauterine Devices (IUDs).** IUDs immobilize sperm, prevent implantation of the fertilized ovum, and dislodge the blastocyst from the endometrium. Both IUDs that are available are T-shaped; the ParaGard T380A has copper wound around the base, and the Progestasert is impregnated with progesterone. Both have fine, nylon tails that hang through the cervix, which allows women to check for the presence of the IUD.

A. Failure rates. The failure rates are 0.5% for the first year and 1.9% after 4 years of use.
B. Contraindications
   1. Women who are not in mutually monogamous relationships, who are at risk of acquiring STDs for other reasons, or who have acute pelvic infections should not use IUDs.
   2. It is not wise to insert an IUD in a nulliparous woman because of the concern about infertility.
   3. Pregnancy is a contraindication.
   4. Pre-existing severe dysmenorrhea will become worse with the copper IUD.
   5. To women with valvular heart disease, some physicians give prophylactic antibiotics before IUD insertion. Some practitioners will not use IUDs in such cases.
   6. Copper allergy or Wilson's disease precludes the use of the T380A IUD.
C. Side effects
   1. Salpingitis with subsequent infertility and ectopic pregnancy are the most feared problems. If PID occurs, the IUD should be removed and another form of birth control can be used. The patient should wait 3 months before having the IUD replaced.
   2. Perforation of the uterus at insertion or at a later time occurs with 1 in 2500 users.
   3. Menometrorrhagia and dysmenorrhea are problems for some women with the copper IUD. Iron deficiency anemia may also result.
   4. If pregnancy occurs with an IUD in place, spontaneous abortions are more likely. If left in place, 50% of intrauterine pregnancies will spontaneously abort. If the IUD is removed, the rate is only 25%.
   5. Spotting may occur.
   6. Expulsion of the IUD, which often goes undetected, occurs in 5–8% of users the first year. This rate is highest for women who are parous.
D. Noncontraceptive benefits. The Progestasert decreases the volume of menstrual blood and dysmenorrhea in symptomatic women.
E. Acceptability. Acceptability is high for women who want a reversible, safe method of contraception when they are fairly sure their family is complete. Expense and availability can be a problem, since not all health insurance policies cover costs. An IUD costs at least $150. Some women are very uncomfortable with the idea of the IUD inside them, and other women dislike the idea that conception is not prevented, but the potentially fertilized egg cannot implant. Yearly replacement of the device, which is required for the Progestasert IUD, is not accepted by some women.
F. Insertion and removal. Always read the manufacturer's instructions for the specific kind of IUD to be used. The insertion and removal of an IUD are office procedures. A consent form must be signed. Both types of IUDs come with lengthy forms that take considerable time for women to complete.
   1. One size of both IUDs discussed above fits all women.
   2. One dose of a nonsteroidal anti-inflammatory drug such as Anaprox or Motrin is helpful if taken 1 hour prior to insertion or removal.
   3. Insertion is easiest during menses because the cervix is slightly dilated, although the incidence of expulsion and infection is slightly higher if the IUD is inserted at this time. Any time during the cycle is acceptable for insertion. The preferred time for removal is at the menses, both for comfort and to insure that recent exposure will not result in pregnancy.
   4. Leave a tail of at least 4 cm to allow the patient to check for expulsion of her IUD and to allow for easy removal. Let her feel the remnant of string so that she knows what to feel for monthly after her menses.
   5. The Lippes Loop, which was available from 1974 to 1986, is the only IUD that can stay in place until menopause. All other IUDs may stay in place for a maximum of 4 years. The Progestasert must be replaced yearly.
VII. Natural Family Planning
A. Periodic abstinence depends on avoidance of coitus during fertile days. These can be determined by many different methods. The Billings method of family planning relies on changes in cervical mucus. Other methods use the length of past menstrual cycles or a combination of basal body temperature and cervical mucus changes (symptothermal method). These methods rely heavily on motivated patients, but can enhance awareness of a woman's body and cycles. Two newer methods are the Creighton model NaProEducation system and the newer Standard Days Method from Georgetown

method. Abstinence is usually required for 6–9 days during the cycle. Some couples use barrier methods during the fertile time.

1. The theoretical failure rate is 1% with an actual failure rate quoted from 5–20%. The failure rate is less if barrier methods are used during fertile times. More recent studies using the Creighton and standard days methods show actual failure rates of 94.8–97.4% and >95%, respectively.
2. There are no contraindications to the use of natural family planning. The calendar method alone should not be used in women with irregular menstrual cycles (as in lactating or nearing menopause).
3. There are no side effects.
4. Noncontraceptive benefits include self-knowledge of a woman's cycles, which can be helpful if desiring pregnancy as well. This information also enhances both partners' awareness and involvement in family planning.
5. Acceptability is limited by the period of abstinence required and the need to keep track of cervical mucus, temperature changes, or both. This method works well for some couples because of the lack of side effects and affordability and acceptance by all religions. Many couples engage in noncoital sexual activities to make this method work for them.
6. Patient instructions are complex initially and take some time to master. A course with a trained instructor is necessary. More information is available through Natural Family Planning Practitioners, Couple to Couple League, or Georgetown University Institute for Reproductive Health.

B. **Lactational Amenorrhea Method (LAM)** is based on the normal time of infertility after pregnancy. If a woman breast-feeds exclusively, the average length of infertility is 14 months. If a woman has given birth in the past 6 months, is exclusively breast-feeding (no solids, water, juice, or pacifier) and has not yet menstruated, she has approximately 98% effectiveness for breast-feeding alone. The longest time between feedings is the strongest factor leading to the return of fertility. Few women nurse exclusively on demand; thus, this is rarely effective or used in the western world today.

C. **Coitus interruptus**, or the withdrawal method, depends on withdrawal of the penis from the vagina before ejaculation occurs.

VIII. **Sterilization.** Sterilization is a permanent form of birth control resulting from obstruction of the vas deferens in males (vasectomy) or the fallopian tubes in females (tubal ligation). It is the most widely relied-on form of birth control in the United States. It is used by about one third of women to prevent pregnancy.

A. **Failure rate.** The theoretical failure rate is 0.15%, and the actual rate is <3% for a vasectomy.

B. **Contraindications.** Sterilization is contraindicated if any doubt about wanting permanent sterilization exists, since reversal of either a vasectomy or a tubal ligation is not always successful.

C. **Side effects**
1. **Vasectomy**
   a. Swelling, bruising, and pain are common. Hematomas occur in <2% of cases, and infections, including epididymitis, result <3% of the time.
   b. The risk of cardiovascular problems does not increase, as was once believed.
   c. The mortality rate in the United States is essentially 0%.
2. **Tubal ligation**
   a. Women often report a change in their menses, including menorrhagia and dysmenorrhea and "post-tubal syndrome," although studies do not clearly support this. Some women may notice a change after discontinuing oral contraceptives prior to the ligation.
   b. Infection and hemorrhage are infrequent.
   c. Mortality is low, with 3 deaths per 1000,000 cases in the United States. It is even lower if general anesthesia is not used.
   d. Ectopic pregnancy must be ruled out if signs of pregnancy occur. Failure rates are approximately 1% after tubal occlusion, of which 30–40% were tubal pregnancies.

D. **Noncontraceptive benefits** are limited to a diminished rate of PID in women who have had tubal ligations.

E. **Acceptability** is high for individuals who desire a permanent, effective birth control method. The cost is high initially if it is not covered by insurance, particularly for tubal ligations, but the expense is reasonable if five or more potential childbearing years remain. Vasectomy is an office procedure that takes about 20 minutes to perform. These patients return to work in a few days, depending on the nature of their job. Tubal ligation requires at least outpatient surgery and has a longer recovery period, depending on the method used and the surgeon.

F. **Patient instructions**
1. Informed consent is critical for either procedure and must describe the methods as irreversible, yet acknowledge a small risk of failure and pregnancy (possibly ectopic for the tubal ligation).
2. It is important for patients to think carefully about whether any change such as death or separation from a partner or from a child would make them regret the choice. A good question to ask is "If anything were to happen to your current spouse and children, would you want to have another child?"

REFERENCES

Hatcher RA, et al: *Contraceptive Technology,* 17th ed. Ardent Media; 1998.
Hatcher RA, et al: *Managing Contraception.* Bridging the Gap Foundation (Tiger, Georgia); 2002.
Kippley JF, Kippley SK: *The Art of Natural Family Planning,* 4th ed. Couple to Couple League International; 2000.
Wertheimer RE: Emergency postcoital contraception. Am Fam Physician (November 15) 2000;**62**:2287.

96 Infertility

Keith A. Frey, MD, MBA, & Ketan S. Patel, MD

KEY POINTS

- Infertility is a common disorder seen by the primary care physician.
- A thorough evaluation of both partners is necessary, as 25% of couples have more than one etiologic factor.
- Emotional support for the couple is an important aspect of their care.

I. **Introduction**
A. **Definition.** Infertility is defined as 1 year of unprotected intercourse in which a pregnancy has not been achieved. Fifteen percent of couples in the United States are infertile.
B. **Common diagnoses.** The causes of infertility include abnormalities of any portion of the male or female reproductive system. Although infertility results from a single cause in the majority of couples, more than one factor contributes to infertility in as many as 25% of couples. "Unexplained" infertility, in which no specific cause is identified, occurs in approximately 20% of infertile couples. The following causes of infertility have been identified.
1. **Male factors** (40% of infertile couples).
2. **Ovulatory dysfunction** (25% of infertile couples).
3. **Tubal and pelvic pathology** (35% of infertile couples).
4. **Unusual problems** (5% of infertile couples).
C. **Pathophysiology**
1. **Male factors.** The most commonly encountered cause of male infertility is a varicocele. Other causes include oligospermia or azoospermia, disorders of sperm function or motility (asthenospermia), and abnormalities of sperm morphology (teratospermia). Male infertility associated with antisperm antibodies is quite rare.
2. **Ovulatory dysfunction.** The possible causes of anovulation may be grouped into four major categories.
a. **Hypothalamic anovulation** (psychogenic trauma, anorexia nervosa, pseudocyesis, pharmacologic agents, anatomic defects, or congenital defects).
b. **Pituitary anovulation** (pituitary tumors or ischemia).

    c. Ovarian anovulation (ovarian dysgenesis, premature ovarian failure, or ovarian tumors).

    d. Integrative anovulation (polycystic ovarian syndrome or nonpsychogenic weight disturbances).

  3. Tubal and pelvic pathology. Infertility may be associated with tubal damage or adnexal adhesions. Tubal obstruction may result from acute salpingitis, although many cases of tubal occlusion are encountered in which no episodes of salpingitis are recalled. Anatomic distortion of adnexal structures may also be caused by endometriosis. The chronic inflammation associated with endometriosis may disrupt normal conception by causing tubal damage or by secretion of toxic substances.

  4. Unusual problems. Cervical mucus abnormalities occur if at the time of ovulation the mucus is either insufficient in quantity or poor in quality. Factors contributing to the formation of such "hostile" (unreceptive) cervical mucus include cervical infections, previous cervical surgery or cautery, and clomiphene therapy.

II. Diagnosis. The physician should arrange a meeting with the couple early in the diagnostic work-up. This provides an important opportunity to review reproductive biology and the rationale for subsequent laboratory test results.

  A. Signs and symptoms. Since infertility may arise from one or more areas of the reproductive system, it requires a comprehensive diagnostic evaluation. The initial assessment of both the male and the female partner consists of a thorough history and physical examination. Specific areas requiring extra attention are noted in Table 96–1.

  B. Laboratory tests (Tables 96–2 and 96–3). In addition to a comprehensive history and physical examination, each couple must be evaluated by a series of routine laboratory tests and appropriately timed studies to evaluate each major reproductive factor that may be the cause of infertility. This comprehensive diagnostic survey can and should be completed for most couples in 6–12 months. Each couple's evaluation must be individualized based on the findings of the history and the physical examination. However, an initial survey of each major reproductive factor is necessary in *all* couples and can be coordinated by the primary care physician.

    1. Male factors. Evidence of oligospermia after two or more semen analyses will require further diagnostic evaluation. The initial evaluation includes blood levels for follicle-stimulating hormone (FSH) and testosterone. If the testosterone level is low, a pituitary etiology may be evaluated by luteinizing hormone (LH) and prolactin levels. Testicular biopsy may be required, particularly if azoospermia is discovered.

    2. Tubal factors. The female partner must undergo an evaluation for tubal patency. If the history or the physical examination shows no clear evidence of tubal dam-

TABLE 96–1. THE INFERTILITY WORK-UP IN OUTLINE: HISTORY (MALE, FEMALE, OR BOTH)

Marriage	Occupation and habits	Review of systems
Duration of infertility	Exposure to radiation, chemicals,	Focus on endocrine conditions
Fertility in previous relationships	excessive heat (saunas, hot	(diabetes, thyroid disorders)
Frequency of intercourse	tubs, etc)	
Sexual potency and techniques		**Gynecology**
Use of coital lubricants	**Childhood illness**	Coital frequency and techniques
	Cryptorchidism	Contraceptive use
Adult illnesses	Timing of puberty	Diethylstilbestrol use by mother
Acute viral or febrile illness in		Douche and lubricant use
past 3 months	**Surgery**	Exposure to radiation and
Mumps orchitis	Herniorrhaphy	chemicals
Renal disease	Retroperitoneal surgery	Fertility in previous relationships
Radiation therapy	Vasectomy	Menarche
Sexually transmitted disease	Female pelvic surgery	Menses (regularity and flow)
Stress and fatigue		Mittelschmerz
Tuberculosis	**Drug use**	
	Alcohol, tobacco, marijuana, and	**Genetic diseases**
	cocaine	Cystic fibrosis
	Alkylating agents	Tay–Sachs
	Anabolic steroids	Others
	Nitrofurantoin	
	Sulfasalazine	
	Cimetidine	

TABLE 96–2. THE INFERTILITY WORK-UP IN OUTLINE: PHYSICAL EXAM/ROUTINE LABORATORY TESTS (MALE AND FEMALE)

Male		Female	
Physical Examination	Routine Laboratory Tests	Physical Examination	Routine Laboratory Tests
Hair pattern	**CBC**	**Breast formation**	**CBC, RPR, Rubella titer**
Genitalia	**Semen analysis**	**Distribution of body fat**	**Pap smear**
Meatus size and location	Abstinence of 2–8 days	**Galactorrhea**	**Urinalysis and urine culture if indicated**
Prostate and seminal vesicles	Masturbation into sterile vessel	**Hair pattern (virilization)**	**Day 3 FSH and Estradiol (for age ≥ 30 years)**
Scrotum	To laboratory (warm) within 1 hour	**Height and weight**	**TSH and Prolactin (if oligoovulation or anovulation)**
Testicular size (≥4 cm in long axis)	Results	**Neurology**	**At-home test**
Varicocele (standing and Valsalva's	Volume: 2–5 mL	Anosmia	
maneuver)	Liquelaction: complete within 30 minutes	Visual fields	**Basal body temperature**
	Sperm count: >20 million/mL	**Pelvis**	Measure temperature for 5–10 minutes orally before arising
Neurology	Sperm motility: 50%	External genitalia	Measure temperatures throughout evaluation and treatment
Anosmia	Morphology: 50% normal forms	Retrovaginal area (endometriosis)	Bring chart on each visit
Visual fields	Repeat testing if azoospermia or severe	Uterus and adnexa	
	oligospermia	Vagina and cervix	
	Urinalysis and urine culture if indicated		
	RPR		

CBC, complete blood cell count; RPR, rapid plasma reagin; TSH, thyroid-stimulating hormone.

TABLE 96–3. THE INFERTILITY WORK-UP IN OUTLINE: FURTHER DIAGNOSTIC TESTS

Postcoital (Sims–Huhner) test
Determines the number and condition of sperm and their ability to penetrate cervical mucus
Performed around the time of ovulation
Poorly correlated to pregnancy rates

Hysterosalpingography
Preferred test of tubal patency
Performed 2–6 days after cessation of menstrual flow
May enhance fertility temporarily

Laparoscopy
Performed if hysterosalpingography is unproductive
Permits examination of pelvic contents

Endometrial biopsy
Determines whether luteal phase defect exists
Performed 2–3 days before expected menses
Informed consent required
Requires histologic dating

Serum progesterone
May be an alternative to endometrial biopsy
Sample drawn 5–7 days after supposed ovulation
Serum level >3 ng/mL is compatible with ovulation

---

age, proceed with a hysterosalpingogram; otherwise, refer the patient for laparoscopy (especially if there are other indications for laparoscopy, such as possible endometriosis).

3. **Ovulatory dysfunction.** Anovulation or inconsistent ovulation may be diagnosed by the history (irregular menses), a nonbiphasic basal body temperature pattern, abnormally low serum progesterone levels, or endometrial biopsy.

4. **Cervical mucus factors.** When a significant number of white blood cells is noted on cervical mucus samples at the time of expected ovulation (ie, during the postcoital test), a specific bacteriologic diagnosis should be sought. See Chapter 51 and 64 for specific recommendations.

III. **Treatment.** Generally, treatment should not be initiated until the diagnostic evaluation is completed. The male and female partners should be treated as a couple whenever possible. Therapy should proceed at a rate that the couple finds comfortable.

A. **Male factors.** Specific antibiotics are used to treat infections such as prostatitis and epididymitis (see Chapter 61). Consultation with a urologist will generally be required to complete the evaluation and coordinate treatment.

B. **Ovulatory dysfunction.** If anovulation is diagnosed, consider treatment with clomiphene.

1. **Clomiphene treatment.** A careful evaluation for galactorrhea and a prolactin level should precede treatment. Chronic anovulation and unexplained infertility patients attempting to conceive are among the patients best suited for clomiphene. Patients with other causes of anovulation generally respond best to specific therapy, such as surgery for a pituitary tumor. The usual starting dose is 50 mg/day orally on days 5–9 of the menstrual cycle. The dose may be increased by 50 mg/day in the second and third cycles.

Common side effects include vasomotor flushes (10%), abdominal or pelvic discomfort (5.5%), nausea (2.2%), and breast tenderness (2%).

2. **Expected results.** Ovulation should be expected 5–10 days after the treatment ends; this should be confirmed by biphasic basal body temperature (BBT) and an elevated level of serum progesterone on day 21. If ovulation does not occur despite clomiphene therapy, consultation with a reproductive endocrinologist is recommended.

C. **Tubal and pelvic pathology.** Tubal blockage or deformity may necessitate surgical correction. The management of endometriosis in a woman desiring to achieve pregnancy depends on the degree and location of endometrial deposits. Conservative surgical treatment may enhance fertility potential by destroying endometrial implants and endometriomas. Laparoscopic conservative surgical treatment should be considered as a treatment option for mild endometriosis-associated infertility. For patients with more severe tubal and pelvic pathology, referral for assisted reproductive technologies is warranted.

D. Unusual problems. For cervical mucus abnormalities, antibiotics should be used to treat the specific bacterial cause of the problem. Low-dose estrogens can be used for poor cervical mucus that does not result from infectious causes. However, intrauterine insemination (IUI) is the best treatment option for a cervical factor.

IV. Management Strategies. The work-up, diagnosis, and treatment of infertility can precipitate intense emotional reactions. The sensitive physician should discuss such emotions as anger, guilt, self-doubt, depression, and grief with the couple. The actions described below may also prove beneficial.

A. Help the couple understand their motives for parenting, which may include desires (1) to parent, (2) to experience a pregnancy, (3) to meet the expectations of others, and (4) to promote genetic continuity.

B. Assist the couple in the development of mutual support and an adaptive "couple-coping" style. Discuss sexual issues, and encourage the couple to nurture their intimacy; they will need its strength to deal with the problems associated with infertility. Periodic meetings with the couple to review diagnostic progress provide further opportunity to reinforce coping skills.

C. Help the couple broaden their support systems, including self-help groups, such as Resolve, Inc.

V. Prognosis. The exact prognosis of infertility is difficult to define because of the multiple potential causes. For most of these, conception will not be achieved without specific treatment. However, with specific therapy, subsequent pregnancy rates have been studied and the results are favorable. "Unexplained" infertility is the persistent inability to conceive after a comprehensive diagnostic assessment of the couple fails to establish a specific diagnosis. If a comprehensive diagnostic work-up fails to identify a cause, or if the appropriate treatment is unsuccessful, the physician should discuss adoption options with the couple.

REFERENCES

Kolettis PN: Evaluation of the subfertile man. Am Fam Physician 2003;**67**:2165.

Petrie K, Frey KA: *Preconception Care/Infertility.* Monograph, Edition No. 234, Home Study Self-Assessment program. American Academy of Family Physicians; November 1998.

Speroff L, Glass RH, Kase NG: *Clinical Gynecologic Endocrinology and Infertility,* 6th ed. Williams & Wilkins; 1999.

ELECTRONIC RESOURCES

RESOLVE National Home Page. http://www.resolve.org

---

97   Preconception & Prenatal Care

Megeen Parker, MD

KEY POINTS

- Preconception care that offers smoking cessation, folic acid supplementation, excellent glycemic control in patients with diabetes mellitus, monotherapy for seizures and avoidance of phenytoin and valeric acid, immunization against rubella, and alcohol cessation has been shown to improve subsequent pregnancy outcome.
- Comprehensive prenatal care, particularly if begun early in pregnancy, has been shown to improve pregnancy outcomes. Clinicians should follow specific evidence-based protocols and monitor women for signs of obstetric emergencies, particularly late in pregnancy. Women older than age 35 should be offered genetic counseling and testing. To prepare for labor and delivery, all women and their partners should be enrolled in prenatal classes. A great majority of women deliver in hospitals utilizing family-centered birthing, focusing on safety for the mom and child, and fostering a positive experience for the woman and her family.

I. **Introduction**
  A. **Antenatal care** refers to a comprehensive approach to medical care and psychosocial support of the family that ideally begins prior to conception and ends with the onset of labor.
  B. **Preconception care** is the physical and mental preparation of both parents for pregnancy and childbearing prior to conception in order to improve pregnancy outcomes.
  C. **Prenatal care** formally begins with the initial diagnosis of pregnancy and includes ongoing risk assessment, education, and counseling to promote health as well as identification and management of problems.
II. **Preconception care**
  A. **Medical history.** All women of childbearing age are potential candidates for preconception evaluation. Identifying conditions and risks that could adversely affect a future pregnancy, followed by appropriate interventions and counseling to improve the outcome of pregnancy, are the primary tasks of the preconception evaluation.
    1. **Chronic medical conditions** should be evaluated both for potential effects on pregnancy and for effects that pregnancy may have on the medical condition. Significant chronic illnesses include diabetes mellitus, hypertension, thyroid disorders, anemias, coagulopathies, seizure disorders, asthma, human immunodeficiency virus (HIV)/acquired immunodeficiency syndrome, and cardiovascular diseases. Also notable are a past history of recurrent urinary tract infections and phlebitis.
    2. Note **previous surgeries,** particularly abdominal and pelvic procedures.
    3. A thorough review of **prescription and over-the-counter medications** currently being taken is helpful to anticipate and minimize adverse effects, particularly during the period of organogenesis from the fourth to the tenth weeks of gestation. The US Food and Drug Administration's Pregnancy Categories and other reviews such as the Teris classifications are useful in determining risk vs. benefit and teratogenic risk. Drugs clearly proved to have significant teratogenic risk in humans include alcohol, chemotherapeutic agents, anticonvulsants, androgens, warfarin, lithium, and isotretinoin.
    4. Note **allergies and sensitivities** to medications and anesthetics.
    5. **Current methods of contraception.** Ideally, methods should be discontinued several menstrual cycles prior to conception to assist with accurate dating.
    6. **Genetic risk assessment** performed in the preconception period, as opposed to the prenatal period, allows women and their partners to consider a greater number of options in family planning. The background incidence of congenital malformations is approximately 3%. Genetic causes account for about 20% of anomalies. Genetic counseling and further testing may be beneficial when the following conditions are identified: advanced maternal (older than 35 years) or paternal (older than 55 years) age; family history of or previous child with neural tube defect (NTD), congenital heart disease, hemophilia, thalassemia, sickle cell disease, Tay–Sachs disease, cystic fibrosis, Huntington's chorea, muscular dystrophy, mental retardation, Down syndrome, or other inherited disorders; maternal metabolic disorders; recurrent pregnancy loss (three or more); use of alcohol, recreational drugs, and medications; and environmental or occupational exposures.
    7. **Obstetric and menstrual history.** Review the number, date, length, and outcome of prior pregnancies. Record any history of significant pregnancy-related health concerns, such as gestational diabetes, intrauterine growth retardation, preterm labor, or hemorrhage. Make note of any complications during labor and delivery. A detailed menstrual history is helpful, paying particular attention to irregular menses and infertility.
  B. **Psychosocial history.** This is a critical area of the history, since significant risks may be identified that may be addressed prior to pregnancy. A potential pregnancy may also serve as an incentive to the patient to alter certain unhealthy habits. Unhealthy habits include tobacco use, alcohol consumption, illicit drug use, and poor nutrition. Psychosocial risks include a past history of mental illness, inadequate personal supports and coping skills, high stress, exposure to domestic violence or abuse, single marital status, inadequate housing, low income, and less than high school education.
  C. **Immunization history.** Rubella, varicella, and hepatitis B immunity are best addressed prior to conception.

D. Physical examination
1. **Height and weight.** Patients who weigh >200 lbs or <90 lbs may be at greater risk for problems in pregnancy.
2. **Blood pressure**
3. **Breast examination**
4. **Pelvic examination,** including clinical pelvimetry (although pelvimetry is unlikely to affect the outcome of the pregnancy).

E. Laboratory tests
1. **Recommended laboratory tests** include hemoglobin or hematocrit, rubella titer, urine dipstick for protein and glucose, Pap smear, screening for gonorrhea and *Chlamydia,* hepatitis B surface antigen, and syphilis serology. Counseling regarding HIV testing should occur with all patients.
2. Additional screening may be appropriate for women with the following, who are identified to be at greater risk: tuberculosis, toxoplasmosis, cytomegalovirus, herpes simplex, varicella, and hemoglobinopathies.

F. Health promotion
1. Optimize management of pre-existing medical conditions such as diabetes mellitus and hypertension.
2. Administer appropriate immunizations (see Chapter 101).
3. The US Public Health Service recommends that all women of childbearing age should consume 0.4 mg of folic acid per day to reduce the risk of NTDs.
4. Provide counsel and educate regarding the following topics.
   a. **Pregnancy planning.** Accurate recording of menstrual cycles is helpful. Oral contraceptives should be discontinued and a barrier method should be used to establish regular cycles prior to attempting pregnancy.
   b. **Nutrition and weight correction, if necessary.**
   c. **Smoking cessation and avoidance of alcohol and illicit drugs.**
   d. **Genetic risks, if any.**
   e. **Avoidance of teratogens, including prescription and nonprescription medications, and occupational and environmental exposures.**
   f. **Preparation of the family for pregnancy and enhancement of social support.**
   g. **Proper exercise.**

III. Prenatal Care
A. Initial diagnosis of pregnancy
1. **Symptoms** include cessation of menses, breast tenderness and enlargement, nausea, fatigue, and frequent urination.
2. **Signs** such as uterine enlargement and a dark bluish coloring of the cervix and vaginal mucosa (Chadwick's sign) are present.
3. **Urinary tests for elevated levels of β-human chorionic gonadotropin (β-hCG)** are generally positive at about the time of the first missed menses and have a sensitivity of 98% and a specificity of 99%.

B. The **first prenatal visit** should occur before 8 weeks' gestation, as it is critical for determining an accurate delivery date, evaluating risk status, and providing essential patient education. The visit may be abbreviated if a recent preconceptual visit has occurred.
1. **Patient history** (see section II). A detailed menstrual history as well as the last contraceptive method used is important for establishing dates. The estimated date of delivery (EDD) should be established before 20 weeks' gestation, when techniques for dating are most accurate. The date of the start of the last menstrual period is the most accurate predictor for EDD, with adjustments made for cycle length. A first-trimester ultrasound can confirm gestational age within ±4 days, although routine use for dating is controversial. In addition, a history of illnesses, medications, and exposures since the last menstrual period (LMP) should be obtained. A patient's questions concerning common symptoms in early pregnancy can be answered at this time.
2. **Complete physical examination.** This should include evaluation of fetal heart tones (usually heard by hand-held Doppler between 11 and 13 weeks).
3. **Routine laboratory work.** In addition to testing recommended during the preconception visit (see section II,E), blood and Rh type, antibody screen, microscopic urinalysis, and urine culture are recommended.

4. **Patient education** early in pregnancy is critical. Important issues to be addressed are described below.

   a. **High-risk behaviors**

      (1) **Smoking** has been associated with intrauterine growth retardation (IUGR), prematurity, placenta previa, placental abruption, and preterm rupture of membranes.

      (2) **Alcohol use** is linked to fetal alcohol syndrome (craniofacial abnormalities, limb and cardiovascular defects, growth and mental retardation) and other childhood behavioral problems such as learning disabilities and attention-deficit/hyperactivity disorder.

      (3) **Cocaine** is associated with increases in spontaneous abortions, placental abruption, preterm labor and delivery, low birth weight, neonatal withdrawal syndromes, and central nervous system damage.

      (4) **Opiates** may cause IUGR, preterm delivery, and an increased rate of intrauterine hypoxemia and fetal distress.

      (5) Daily consumption of more than 300 mg of **caffeine** (about three cups of coffee) has been associated with an increased risk of IUGR and low birth weight.

   b. **Nutrition and weight gain.** Total weight gain of 25–35 lbs is recommended for women at an appropriate weight at the time of conception. Women at <90% or >120% of ideal body weight (IBW) should gain 30–35 pounds or 18–20 pounds to minimize risks. A weight gain of <10 lbs at 20 weeks' gestation is associated with increased complications.

      (1) The average pregnant woman needs approximately 1900–2750 kcal/day (300 kcal more than nonpregnant patients). The best clue to adequate caloric intake is maternal weight gain.

      (2) The diet should include increased amounts of calcium (1200 mg daily, equivalent to 3–4 milk servings), iron (30 mg essential iron), vitamins C and D, and folic acid (0.4–0.8 mg daily) and consist of 50–60% complex carbohydrate, up to 20% protein, and no more than 30% fat. A prenatal multivitamin and mineral supplement is recommended when dietary intake is inadequate. Vegetarians require additional iron, vitamin B_{12}, and zinc. Excessive doses of vitamins, particularly vitamins A, C, and D, can be harmful to the fetus.

   c. **Patient expectations,** the benefits of childbirth education classes, and family issues should be discussed.

   d. **Sexual intercourse** during pregnancy is contraindicated only for patients with placenta previa and for those at risk for abortions or premature labor.

   e. **Physical activity** should not be significantly increased during pregnancy; however, regular, low-intensity exercise (walking, swimming, bicycling) should be encouraged. Contact sports, activities requiring repeated Valsalva's maneuvers or rapid changes in direction, or those involving unpredictable risk should be discouraged.

   f. **Symptoms for which patients need to promptly contact their physician** should be clearly outlined. These include any vaginal bleeding or escape of fluids from the vagina, swelling of the face and fingers, severe continuous headache, dimness or blurring of vision, abdominal pain, persistent vomiting, chills or fever, dysuria, and change in frequency or intensity of fetal movements.

C. **Common symptoms**

   1. **Nausea and vomiting,** which usually begin at about 6 weeks and disappear by 14–16 weeks, are commonly worse in the morning and occur in up to 70% of pregnant women. Nonpharmacologic therapies include having frequent, small meals; avoiding greasy, spicy foods; having a protein snack at bedtime; eating dry crackers before getting out of bed in the morning; and avoiding drinking liquids on an empty stomach. Purposeful stimulation of the P6 (Neiguan) acupuncture point located three fingerbreadths proximal to the distal wrist crease and between the two central flexor tendons of the forearm, via pressing firmly with the fingers for 5 minutes every 4 hours while awake or via use of Seabands, can be quite helpful. Pharmacologic measures include antiemetics such as meclizine (12.5–25 mg every 8–12 hours) or metoclopramide (5–10 mg every 6–8 hours), or pyridoxine (vitamin B_6) 25 mg two or three times daily or in combination with 10 mg of doxy-

lamine found in Unisom. Sipping red raspberry, German chamomile, or peppermint tea can also be helpful. Reassurance that symptoms may be related to higher levels of maternal estrogens and an associated improved pregnancy outcome may also be useful.

2. **Headache** is common before 20 weeks' gestation and is usually benign, although in most cases no specific cause can be found. This symptom may be safely treated with acetaminophen. Relaxation and use of warm compresses may help. The pattern of migraine may change during pregnancy. The physician must consider preeclampsia, particularly later in pregnancy.

3. **Gastrointestinal symptoms common during pregnancy**

    a. Heartburn occurs in about one half of pregnant women at some time. This condition has been attributed to a number of factors, including decreased tone in the lower esophageal sphincter, displacement and compression of the stomach by the uterus, and decreased gastric motility. Treatment consists of having frequent small meals and avoiding bending over or lying flat soon after eating. Low-sodium liquid antacids are helpful and safe; however, those agents that contain magnesium or aluminum hydroxides impair absorption of iron. Over-the-counter H_2-blockers such as ranitidine are also considered safe for use in the second and third trimesters.

    b. Constipation is common in pregnancy because of steroid-induced changes in bowel transit time. Dietary measures are the mainstay of treatment and include high-fiber foods, liberal consumption of water and other liquids, and regular, low-intensity exercise. Mild laxatives, such as milk of magnesia, stool softeners, and bulk laxatives, are safe and effective.

    c. Abdominal pain may occur in pregnancy and warrants evaluation. The physician should consider the same causes for abdominal pain that occur in the nonpregnant state. However, these conditions may present differently in pregnant patients. Types of abdominal pain specific to pregnancy are described below.

       (1) Ectopic pregnancy should be ruled out in women with lower abdominal or pelvic pain early in pregnancy (see Chapter 51).

       (2) Pre-eclampsia may be associated with upper abdominal pains in the epigastrium or the right upper quadrant.

       (3) Placental abruption should be considered when pain is associated with bleeding, particularly in the third trimester.

       (4) Urinary tract infections (see Chapter 21).

       (5) Other, less significant causes include round ligament or broad ligament discomfort, which results from increased tension on these structures as the uterus enlarges.

4. **Urinary complaints,** such as increasing frequency and stress incontinence, are often noted, especially during the first and third trimesters, because of uterine pressure on the bladder. Decreasing nighttime fluid intake (without any overall restrictions) and Kegel's exercises can be helpful. Infection, however, is common and should be considered when frequency is associated with dysuria.

5. Increased **vaginal discharge (leukorrhea)** is common, often with no pathologic cause. This physiologic discharge is related to increased estrogen. Infectious causes should be ruled out (see Chapter 64) in the presence of associated symptoms of itching, burning, foul odor, or labial swelling.

6. **Vaginal bleeding** may occur at any time during pregnancy and should always be considered significant enough to warrant further evaluation, including pelvic examination, appropriate cultures, and pelvic ultrasound.

    a. Bleeding in the first trimester is a relatively frequent occurrence. Causes range from physiologic bleeding as a result of implantation to life-threatening conditions. Extrauterine pregnancy should be considered when bleeding occurs during this time, even in the absence of pain. Any bleeding occurring in the first half of pregnancy, particularly with cramping, may be associated with spontaneous abortion.

    b. Bleeding in the latter half of pregnancy occurs less frequently and may be associated with cervical trauma during coitus. Painless bleeding may suggest placenta or vasa previa, whereas painful bleeding is classically associated with placental abruption.

7. **Edema in the feet and the ankles** is common, particularly during the third trimester. This edema is secondary to sodium and water retention combined with increased lower extremity venous pressure. Edema should raise concerns of preeclampsia when it is accompanied by hypertension and proteinuria. Benign edema normally responds to leg elevation, avoidance of long periods of sitting or standing, and use of support stockings.

8. **Backache** is relatively common during pregnancy and is partially related to increased joint laxity as well as compensatory postural changes that occur as the uterus enlarges. Avoiding excessive weight gain, wearing flat or low-heeled shoes, and improving posture may provide some relief. Chiropractic care may be effective and is safe during pregnancy.

9. **Varicose veins** are aggravated by pregnancy, prolonged standing, and advancing age. This condition usually worsens as pregnancy advances, because of increased femoral pressure. Treatment is limited to periodic rest with leg elevation and elastic stockings; more definitive treatment is delayed until after pregnancy.

10. **Hemorrhoids** are the result of increased pressure on hemorrhoidal veins by the uterus and by the tendency toward constipation during pregnancy. Effective treatments include sitz baths with warm water for 20 minutes and followed by local application of witch hazel, topically applied anesthetics, and stool softeners (see Chapter 52).

D. **Additional prenatal care.** Traditionally, prenatal visits should occur every 4 weeks through the 28th week of pregnancy, every 2–3 weeks through the 36th week, and then weekly until delivery. The frequency of visits may be altered based on the risk status of the patient. Measurement of weight, blood pressure, and fundal height; assessment of edema; check of a urine dipstick for protein and glucose; and documentation of fetal heart rate should occur at every visit. Other tests and interventions may be needed at specific times during pregnancy, as noted below.

1. **Care prior to 14 weeks (first trimester).** Initial care during the first trimester can prepare both clinician and patient for a healthy pregnancy.
   a. Review initial laboratory work and define maternal risk status more precisely.
   b. Counsel patients regarding the initial troubling symptoms of pregnancy, such as nausea, fatigue, and emotional changes. Encourage good nutrition. Review signs of miscarriage. Inquire about the partner's adjustment.
   c. Offer early prenatal diagnostic studies to all patients with genetic risk factors (see section II,A,6). Chorionic villus sampling (CVS) is performed between 9 and 12 weeks' gestation, which allows for earlier termination of pregnancy with less maternal morbidity. Amniocentesis is usually performed after 15 weeks, but can be done as early as 13 weeks' gestation. Unlike amniocentesis, CVS cannot be used for prenatal diagnosis of NTDs and may be associated with limb reduction defects. Amniocentesis carries a 0.5–1% risk of fetal loss. The risk from CVS is slightly higher. A detailed ultrasound scan performed in the second trimester can also assist in the evaluation of fetal anomalies but is not recommended as a screening test.
   d. Fetal heart tones are first heard with Doppler ultrasound between 11 and 13 weeks' gestation and sometimes as early as 8 weeks in multigravidas.

2. **Care between 14 and 28 weeks' gestation (second trimester).** An obviously pregnant body and the first sensations of fetal movement often lead to an increased appreciation of being pregnant. The second trimester is an excellent time to schedule a joint visit with the patient and her partner to discuss expectations about parenting.
   a. **Confirmation of the estimated date of delivery.** At approximately 20 weeks' gestation, the uterine fundus is at the level of the umbilicus, and fetal heart tones can usually be heard with a fetoscope. The sensation of fetal movement (quickening), which may first be a fluttering sensation, is usually felt at 16–20 weeks.
   b. **Routine prenatal screening for neural tube defects and chromosomal abnormalities** such as Down syndrome (trisomy 21) are offered during this time. NTDs occur in 4 per 10,000 live births. Screening involves measuring the **maternal serum α-fetoprotein (MSAFP)** between 16 and 18 weeks' gestation. Approximately 50 of 1000 women will have an elevated (>2.5 multiples of the

median) MSAFP, indicating the possibility of an NTD. Most will be falsely positive, resulting from inaccurate dating, multiple gestation, or other anomalies. A targeted anatomic ultrasound to confirm dates can detect 90–95% of NTDs. An amniocentesis is more accurate in detecting NTD but carries a small but discrete risk of fetal loss (0.5–1%).

Reduced levels of MSAFP (<0.7 multiples of the median) indicate an increased risk of Down syndrome. An association with reduced levels of estradiol and elevated levels of hCG and inhibin-A (the more recently available "**quadscreen**") has a false-positive rate of 5% and will identify approximately 76% of cases. (The older "triple screen" has a similar false-positive rate but a lower detection rate of 60–69%.) Amniocentesis offers the only definitive diagnosis, once dating is confirmed by ultrasound. Parents should be carefully advised of the benefits and risks of these screening tests, with documentation of the discussion and their decision recorded in the chart.

   c. Despite growing controversy that **screening for gestational diabetes** is not proved to positively alter outcomes for either mother or infant, universal screening between 24 and 28 weeks is widely recommended and practiced. Measurement of plasma blood glucose 1 hour after ingesting a 50-g oral glucose load is most commonly done, and fasting is not required. Levels >140 mg/dL require further evaluation with a 3-hour oral glucose tolerance test. Women with borderline levels between 130 and 140 may benefit from repeat testing in several weeks. Some physicians advocate earlier screening (prior to 24 weeks) when conditions increasing risk for gestational diabetics are present. Such conditions include a past history of gestational diabetes or a macrosomic infant (>4000 g), family history of type II diabetes, or a maternal weight >200 lbs.

   d. The hemoglobin or hematocrit can be repeated at the same time as screening for diabetes, along with antibody screening for D (Rh)-negative women.

   e. **D (Rh)-negative** women should be given D (Rh) immune globulin at 28 weeks' gestation if the antibody screening is negative. D (Rh) immune globulin should be given earlier if an event has occurred exposing the patient to fetal blood (eg, CVS, amniocentesis, or significant trauma). A repeat dose given within 72 hours after delivery is also necessary.

3. **Care beyond 28 weeks of gestation (third trimester).** This is often a period of increasing discomfort for the patient, with sleep disturbances, dyspnea, urinary frequency, and fatigue being common. The incidence of complications such as pre-eclampsia, maternal hypertension, and malposition of the fetus lead to a need for more frequent and intensive monitoring. Allow time to discuss expectations and wishes regarding labor and delivery, and review indications for calling the office.

   a. **Blood pressure** should be carefully monitored. Systolic blood pressures ≥140 mm Hg or diastolic blood pressures ≥90 mm Hg are diagnostic of gestational hypertension and warrant further evaluation for pre-eclampsia, particularly when associated with proteinuria.

   b. **Fetal position** should be regularly assessed. Most babies are vertex by the final month of pregnancy. For other presentations, external version is often successful and increases the chances of a vaginal delivery.

   c. Testing for **sexually transmitted diseases** in high-risk women, if appropriate, should be repeated at 36–38 weeks' gestation. Testing allows for treatment prior to delivery.

   d. The Centers for Disease Control and Prevention (CDC) revised guidelines for **screening for group B streptococcal (GBS) infection** in 2002, based on findings that universal screening was >50% more effective in preventing GBS infection in newborns than basing treatment on risk factors. The CDC now recommends that all pregnant women (except for those with a history of GBS bacteriuria or a past history of an infant with invasive GBS disease) be screened with vaginal and rectal swabs for GBS between 35 and 37 weeks' estimated gestational age. Intrapartum antibiotic prophylaxis is then offered to all women who test positive, as well as to those women with a history of GBS bacteriuria in the current pregnancy or a past history of an infant with invasive GBS disease. Antepartum prophylaxis is not recommended.

E. Medications in pregnancy. Most drugs should be used only when benefits clearly outweigh risks, particularly in the first trimester. Patients need to understand that taking any medication during pregnancy involves some small degree of risk.

1. **Antihistamines** are generally acceptable when used in normal therapeutic doses, with the possible exception of brompheniramine.

2. **Antiemetics** may be used safely if other conservative measures are not effective.

3. **Decongestants.** Pseudoephedrine (30 mg every 6 hours) is relatively safe to use for limited periods, but large doses should be avoided, as they may negatively influence uterine perfusion. Decongestants are contraindicated when uteroplacental insufficiency is suspected. Try recommending the substitution of saline nose spray or irrigation or judicious use of topical decongestants.

4. **Oral analgesics and anti-inflammatory agents**
   a. Acetaminophen is the drug of choice for mild analgesia and antipyresis. Continuous high doses may cause maternal anemia and fatal kidney disease in the newborn.
   b. Low-dose aspirin has been used to lower the risk of pre-eclampsia in high-risk women. Although there is no clear consensus regarding the benefits related to pre-eclampsia, aspirin has proved to be a relatively safe drug, although there does seem to be an increased risk of placental abruption. Caution should be used in the second half of pregnancy.
   c. Nonsteroidal anti-inflammatory drugs, such as ibuprofen and naproxen, have a theoretical risk of prenatal closure of the ductus arteriosus when used near term. Indomethacin, if used after 34 weeks' gestation, may lead to persistent pulmonary hypertension of the newborn, inhibition of labor, and prolongation of pregnancy. There is no evidence of adverse effects in the first half of pregnancy.
   d. Codeine is not absolutely contraindicated, although association with malformations has been reported. Neonatal withdrawal has been documented. Hydrocodone–acetaminophen combinations (Vicodin) may be safer in pregnancy than codeine.

5. **Antibiotics**
   a. Penicillins (with or without clavulanate) and cephalosporins are among the most effective and least toxic of available antibiotics and can be used at any time during pregnancy.
   b. Erythromycin has not been reported to be of harm to the fetus, except as the estolate salt, which is contraindicated in pregnancy.
   c. Tetracyclines and quinolones are contraindicated in pregnancy because of adverse effects on developing teeth and bones.
   d. Sulfonamides may be used in the first two trimesters. Use near term and during nursing should be avoided, since sulfonamides may cause significant jaundice or hemolytic anemia in the newborn.
   e. Oral metronidazole is contraindicated in the first trimester, since it may result in fetal malformations. Topical metronidazole is safe throughout pregnancy.
   f. Nitrofurantoin should be used with care in late pregnancy since it has the ability to induce hemolysis in neonatal red blood cells.

6. **Antidepressants and benzodiazepines**
   a. Tricyclic antidepressants should be used with caution, as no extensive studies of their use in the first trimester are available.
   b. Selective serotonin reuptake inhibitors, particularly fluoxetine, have generally been proved to be relatively safe during pregnancy. Several recent studies found no increased teratogenesis, pregnancy loss, or childhood developmental abnormalities. Use in the third trimester may require caution, however, as there is some evidence of increased rate of preterm births.
   c. Lithium is contraindicated during pregnancy.
   d. Benzodiazepines should be used cautiously, if at all, as there is some evidence of an increased risk of cleft palate or cleft lip.

IV. **Preterm Labor (PTL)** is defined as regular uterine contractions accompanied by descent of the presenting part and progressive dilatation and effacement of the cervix occurring before 37 weeks from the first day of the LMP. PTL complicates only 8–10% of pregnancies but is responsible for over 60% of all perinatal morbidity and mortality. Risk factors include occult maternal genitourinary tract infections, maternal smoking, high levels of stress, low socioeconomic status, maternal age younger than 18 years or older than 35 years, cervical dilatation >1 cm or cervical effacement >30% between 26 and 34 weeks' gestation, and uterine anomalies. Risk factors most likely are synergistic.

A. Diagnosis. Early diagnosis is crucial, as tocolysis is most effective before 3 cm of cervical dilatation or 50% effacement. Symptoms suggestive of regular uterine contractions should be evaluated with serial examinations for cervical change and by external monitoring of uterine activity. Vaginal ultrasound to assess cervical length, along with fetal fibronectin measurements, may be helpful in predicting the likelihood of preterm birth.

B. Treatment. The risks of preterm delivery must outweigh the risks of tocolysis. Advancing gestational age clearly improves the preterm infant's prognosis until approximately 35 weeks, when delaying delivery has less effect overall. Survival increases to 90% at 29 weeks; mortality then decreases about 1% per week. The acuteness and severity of preterm labor suggest the type of treatment.

    1. Uterine irritability without significant cervical change may benefit from rest at home, intake of fluids, and treatment of causative factors, such as urinary tract infection, if present.

    2. Tocolytic therapy is indicated in preterm labor if no contraindications, such as severe pre-eclampsia or chorioamnionitis, exist. All tocolytics have potentially severe side effects for both mother and fetus. Choices include β-sympathomimetics, magnesium sulfate, nifedipine, and indomethacin.

    3. Evaluation for possible triggers, particularly occult urinary tract infection, is indicated. Randomized controlled trials have found no clear benefit to the use of antibiotics in PTL with intact membranes on prolonging gestation or improving neonatal morbidity or mortality. Treatment with antenatal corticosteroids given before 34 weeks' gestation and >24 hours but <7 days prior to delivery has been shown to be of benefit in reducing the incidence and severity of respiratory distress syndrome and improves neonatal survival rates.

V. Fetal Assessment and Postdates Pregnancy

A. Fetal assessment. Several methods have been developed to assess the well-being of the fetus when risk factors exist. Fetal assessment begins between 34 and 36 weeks' gestation or whenever the risk develops. Major indications for antenatal testing include diabetes mellitus, hypertensive disorders, maternal substance abuse, third-trimester bleeding, IUGR, previously unexplained stillbirth, D (Rh) sensitization, oligohydramnios, multiple gestation, and decreased fetal movement as perceived by the mother. Fetal assessment techniques also are routinely applied when a pregnancy becomes postdates (42 weeks from the LMP).

    1. Fetal movement counts. A quantitative method of counting fetal movements has been developed as a means of fetal assessment near term. The patient is asked to count fetal movements during a 2-hour period each day and report less than 10 movements during that period. A positive test (fewer than 10 movements) is an indication for additional fetal assessment. The advantages of this test are its low cost and maternal involvement.

    2. Fetal heart rate testing

        a. The nonstress test (NST) is a noninvasive method based on the premise that in a healthy fetus, acceleration of the heart rate occurs during fetal movement. An external monitor is used to record the fetal heart rate while the mother reports fetal movement. A reactive or normal test has two or more accelerations of more than 15 beats per minute, each lasting for 15 seconds, in a 20-minute period and in the absence of decelerations. If fetal movement does not occur in 20 minutes, abdominal palpation or vibro-acoustic stimulation may be applied to awaken a sleeping fetus. A reactive NST accurately identifies a healthy fetus 98% of the time.

        Evaluation of a nonreactive NST should include extending the testing period to 60–90 minutes when possible. Nonreactive NSTs and variable decelerations on reactive NSTs must be followed by a contraction stress test.

        b. The contraction stress test (CST) is a test of the fetal heart rate in response to uterine contractions. The uterus may be stimulated to contract through intermittent stimulation of one breast nipple or through intravenous infusion of low-dose oxytocin. A satisfactory test requires at least three contractions in 10 minutes. The test is interpreted as negative, or normal, if there are no decelerations and positive, or abnormal, if late decelerations follow 50% or more of contractions. A nonreactive, positive CST is highly suggestive of fetal distress and must be treated immediately with oxygen, positional changes, labor induction, or cesarean section. Equivocal results occur with occasional late decelerations and should be repeated in 24 hours.

3. An **amniotic fluid index** is used to complement fetal heart rate testing. Ultrasonography is used for estimating amniotic fluid volume, which is an indirect measure of placental function. The largest anteroposterior fluid depths in each of four quadrants of the uterus is measured. The sum should exceed 5 cm.

4. The **biophysical profile** is a quantitative score that combines the NST with ultrasonic observation of the fetus for up to 30 minutes and measurement of the amniotic fluid index. A score of 2 is given **for each normal result** (fetal breathing movements, gross body movements, tone, amniotic fluid index, and NST) and 0 for an abnormal condition. A total score of 8–10 is reassuring, 6 is equivocal, and 4 or less is worrisome. A combination of NST and amniotic fluid evaluation is considered comparable to the biophysical profile in assessing fetal well-being.

B. **Postdates pregnancy.** Defined as lasting longer than 42 weeks from the beginning of the LMP, approximately 3.5–12% of pregnancies are postdates. Prolonged pregnancy is one lasting longer than 41 weeks. Accurate dating is essential to avoid mislabeling a pregnancy as postdates.

1. Chronic uteroplacental insufficiency leading to fetal compromise occurs in up to 20% of postdates pregnancies. Additional complications include oligohydramnios, meconium passage, and macrosomia, which may contribute to a higher cesarean section rate.

2. **Evaluation.** Fetal assessment testing should be performed in all postdates pregnancies, and some nonrandomized studies suggest that beginning noninvasive fetal assessment at 41 weeks with a biweekly NST may lower the rate of stillbirths and intrapartum fetal distress.

3. **Management.** International randomized controlled clinical trials have shown a clear benefit to induction of labor at 41–42 weeks' gestation. The fetal mortality rate of 2 per 1000 at this gestational age is lowered to virtually zero, and cesarean rates are lowered. Elective induction with Pitocin, using prostaglandins for cervical ripening, is relatively safe and effective.

VI. **Normal Labor and Delivery.** Signs of labor include passage of the mucus plug, bloody show (small amount of blood-tinged mucoid vaginal discharge), regular uterine contractions, and spontaneous rupture of membranes. In the general population, about 90% of women should be able to have a healthy birth outcome without medical intervention. The great majority of women deliver in the hospital utilizing family-centered birthing focusing on safety for the mother and child and fostering a positive experience for the woman, her partner, and family.

REFERENCES

American Academy of Pediatrics and The American College of Obstetricians and Gynecologists: *Guidelines for Perinatal Care,* 5th ed. American Academy of Pediatrics; 2002.

Briggs GG, Freeman RK, Yaffe SJ: *Drugs in Pregnancy and Lactation: A Reference Guide to Fetal and Neonatal Risk,* 6th ed. Williams & Wilkins; 2001.

Centers for Disease Control and Prevention. Prevention of Group B streptococcal disease. MMWR 2002;**51**(No. RR-11):1.

Cochrane Pregnancy and Childbirth Group. Cochrane Database of Systematic Reviews (available in the Cochrane Library). The Cochrane Collaboration, Issue 1, 2003. Available from BMJ Publishing Group.

Muchowski K, Paladine H: An ounce of prevention: The evidence supporting periconception health care. J Fam Pract 2004;**53**:126.

Ratcliffe SD, et al (editors): *Family Practice Obstetrics,* 2nd ed. Hanley and Belfus; 2001.

US Preventive Services Task Force: *Guide to Clinical Preventive Services: Report of the US Preventive Services Task Force,* 3rd ed. 2003. Available through the Agency for Healthcare Research and Quality (http://www.ahcrp.gov).

98 Postpartum Care

Jeannette E. South-Paul, MD

KEY POINTS

- Puerperal infections usually occur 2–5 days postpartum. Presenting symptoms include malaise, anorexia, abdominal pain, and fever. The most common puerperal infections are endometritis, perineal infections, and toxic shock syndrome. Intravenous antibiotics are used to treat these infections initially. First-line treatments are clindamycin, 2.4–2.7 g/day, divided four times daily; and gentamicin, 2 mg/kg loading dose followed by 1.5 mg/kg every 8 hours; or cefoxitin, 1 g (2 g if severe) every 8 hours.
- The most common nonpuerperal infections that can occur in the postpartum period are urinary tract infections or pyelonephritis, which usually present with fever, dysuria, frequency, and urgency, and mastitis, which usually presents with a sore, tender breast. Amoxicillin (500 mg orally three times daily for 10–14 days) is a good first choice for urinary tract infections, while mastitis is usually treated with an antistaphylococcal antibiotic like dicloxacillin, 500 mg orally four times daily for 10 days.
- Other common postpartum complication include thromboembolic disease, which requires heparin when deep disease is present; postpartum hemorrhage, which requires oxytocin, 10 U intramuscularly every 4 hours until bleeding stops; and postpartum depression, which requires supportive care or antidepressants.
- Discharge instructions should include daily rest, sitz baths, instructions on when to resume sexual activity, encouragement of breast-feeding (and continuation of prenatal vitamins if doing so), and when to return for the postpartum examination (6–8 weeks after birth).

I. Introduction

A. Definition. The postpartum period, or puerperium, is that period of time that begins with the delivery of the placenta and ends with the resumption of ovulatory menstrual cycles, which, in nonlactating women, usually occurs 6–8 weeks after delivery.

B. Pathophysiology and epidemiological data

1. **Uterus.** The uterus decreases in size dramatically following delivery (involution); it weighs only about 500 g at the end of the first week and lies again in the true pelvis. This change is accompanied by a high level of uterine activity (contractions, afterpains) that diminishes smoothly and progressively after the first 2 hours postpartum. The placental implantation site sheds organized thrombi and obliterated arteries in order to prevent scar formation and preserve normal endometrial tissue.

2. **Cervix.** The cervical os admits two fingers for the first 4–6 days postpartum, but constricts thereafter and admits only a small banjo curette by the end of the second week.

3. **Vagina.** Large and smooth-walled following delivery, the vagina begins to develop rugae by the end of the fourth week. It regains its nonpregnant size by the end of the sixth to eighth week.

4. **Lochia.** The uterine discharge, which is bright red at delivery, changes within a few days to the reddish-brown lochia rubra, composed of blood and decidual and trophoblastic debris. Lochia serosa, a more serous combination of old blood, serum, leukocytes, and tissue debris, appear 1 week postpartum and last for a few days. Lochia alba, a whitish-yellow discharge that contains serum leukocytes, decidua, epithelial cells, mucus, and bacteria, then begins and continues until approximately 2–4 weeks postpartum. Lochia rubra that lasts >4 weeks suggests the presence of retained secundines or the formation of placental polyps, organized placental fragments.

5. **Urinary tract.** Passage of the infant through the pelvis traumatizes the bladder, and its wall may be edematous. Trauma or conduction analgesia may also cause the bladder to be insensitive to changes in intravesicular pressure, resulting in an impaired urge to urinate. Symptoms of urinary incontinence increase with parity.

Practice of pelvic muscle exercise by primiparas has resulted in fewer urinary incontinence symptoms during late pregnancy and the puerperium. The glomerular filtration rate remains elevated during the first postpartum week. Urinary output, which often reaches 3 liters in a 24-hour period, exceeds fluid intake. This output, combined with insensible losses, accounts for the approximately 12-lb weight loss seen during this period. The pregnancy-induced dilation of the ureters and renal pelves subsides to normal within 6 weeks.

6. **Abdominal wall.** The abdominal wall begins to resume a nonparous condition in about 6–7 weeks. The skin remains lax, but the muscles regain substantial tone with proper exercise.

7. **Cardiovascular changes.** Cardiac output decreases to nonpregnant levels within 2–3 weeks postpartum. Lower-extremity varicosities and pelvic varices regress during this period. Plasma volume decreases more rapidly than do cellular components initially, so that the hematocrit increases slightly during the first 72 hours postpartum.

8. **Weight change.** Weight gain during the first 20 weeks of pregnancy predicts postpartum retained weight. The influence of lactation on weight loss postpartum is unclear. Women lose approximately half of the average weight gain of pregnancy (25 lbs) in the first 2 weeks after delivery. The remainder is lost during the following weeks. Women should return to their nonparous weight in approximately 8 weeks.

9. **Breasts.** Milk production and engorgement begin within 3 days postpartum, following the decrease in estrogen and the increase in prolactin produced by suckling. Suckling is the single most important stimulus for the maintenance of milk production. A mother wishing to stop breast-feeding need only discontinue suckling. The accumulation of milk in the alveoli and major ducts leads to increased intraalveolar and intraductal pressure, resulting in the cessation of milk formation. The historical practice of breast binding is thought to work by the same mechanism, but is being discouraged. Recent studies suggest that women who use breast-binding techniques postpartum experience greater breast tenderness and breast leakage and require more analgesia than those who only use a firm bra.

10. **Hypothalamic–pituitary–ovarian function.** Forty percent of nonlactating women will resume menstruation within 6 weeks following delivery, 65% within 12 weeks, and 90% within 24 weeks. Approximately 50% of the first cycles are ovulatory. In nursing mothers, menstruation is resumed within 6 weeks in only 15% and within 12 weeks in only 45%. In 80% of these women, the first ovulatory cycle is preceded by one or more anovulatory cycles. Rapid decreases in blood levels of estrogen, progesterone, human placental lactogen, and insulin occur following delivery.

II. **Diagnosis and Treatment** (see Table 98–1 for a summary).

A. **Abnormalities of the puerperium**

1. **Puerperal infections.** *Puerperal infection* is defined as infection of the genital tract that sometimes extends to other organ systems. Onset is insidious and may occur 2–5 days postpartum. Nonspecific symptoms are malaise, anorexia, and fever. In many cases, a temperature of 38 °C (100.4 °F) or higher on any 2 of the first 10 days postpartum, exclusive of the first 24 hours, indicates a puerperal infection. Extragenital infections and noninfectious causes of fever must be excluded. The differential diagnosis includes urinary tract infections (UTIs), mastitis, and thrombophlebitis, as well as other causes of fever unrelated to the postpartum state. Onset of fever after the tenth postpartum day is usually of a nonobstetric nature. Puerperal infections that are usually polymicrobial in origin are caused predominantly by anaerobes and sometimes by aerobes. *Escherichia coli* and group B streptococci are very common. Multiple bacteria of low virulence, common in the genitourinary tract, may become pathogenic as a result of hematomas and devitalized tissue. Cultures are of limited usefulness, since the same organisms are identified in patients with or without infections.

a. **Predisposing factors**

(1) **Antepartum.** Premature or prolonged rupture of membranes, malnourishment, and anemia increase the likelihood of puerperal infections.

(2) **Intrapartum.** Soft tissue trauma, residual devitalized tissue, prolonged labor, and hemorrhage are also risk factors.

(3) **Late-onset indolent metritis** has been attributed to antepartum *Chlamydia trachomatis* cervical infection, but this organism has not been isolated at the time these infections developed postpartum.

TABLE 98–1. POSTPARTUM COMPLICATIONS REQUIRING TREATMENT

Complications	Symptoms	Etiology	Predisposing Factors	Treatment
Puerperal infection	2–5 days postpartum, T>100.4 °F, anorexia	Polymicrobial—anaerobes and aerobes; *Escherichia coli;* Group B streptococci	Prolonged ROM; malnutrition; hemorrhage/anemia; soft tissue trauma	Clindamycin 2.4–2.7 g/day in 3–4 doses + gentamicin 2 mg/kg load, then 1.5 mg/kg q 8 hours IV OR ampicillin 2 g IV + sulbactam 1 g IV q 6 hours OR cefoxitin or moxalactam
Endometritis/parametritis	Lethargy; T >100.4 °F; lower abdominal pain	Polymicrobial	Prolonged labor and ROM; prior gynecologic infections; hematomas; devitalized tissue; maternal age younger than 17 years	Same as above
Urinary tract infections	Fever; abdominal pain; ± dysuria	Polymicrobial	Trauma-induced bladder hypotonicity; frequent catheterizations	Amoxicillin 500 mg PO tid × 10–14 days
Deep vein thrombosis	Deep vein tenderness; Homan's sign; extremity swelling	Sluggish circulation; estrogen-induced hypercoagulability	Trauma to pelvic veins	Heparin 5000–10,000 U load to get PTT at 2× normal or Enoxaparin 1 mg/kg SC bid followed by warfarin PO to maintain INR 2.0–3.0
Superficial thrombophlebitis	Palpable cords in lower extremities; tenderness; skin warmth		High estrogen state	Elastic support stockings; walking; leg elevation at rest; moist local heat
Pelvic vein thrombosis (right ovarian syndrome)	Abdominal pain, fever, tender, sausage-shaped mass in right mid abdomen		High estrogen state	Heparin anticoagulation (as above)
Necrotizing fasciitis	3–5 days postpartum; symptoms as in other puerperal infections	Polymicrobial, especially anaerobes	Diabetes; immunocompromised state; status post C-section	Clindamycin 2.4 g/kg in 4 doses + gentamicin 1.5 mg/kg q 8 hours IV; surgical debridement
Toxic shock syndrome	T >102 °F; macular erythematous rash, especially on palms and soles	*Staphylococcus aureus* exotoxin-1	Prolonged tampon use	Hospitalization; fluid; electrolytes; PRBCs; coagulation factors; oxacillin or nafcillin or methicillin 1 g IV q 4 hours or vancomycin 100 mg q 6 hours

INR, international normalized ratio; PRBCs, packed red blood cells; PTT, partial thromboplastin time; ROM, rupture of membranes; T, temperature.

b. Specific puerperal infections

(1) Endometritis. This term describes inflammatory involvement, especially leukocytic infiltration, of the superficial layers of the endometrium or decidual layer. When severe, endometritis may be accompanied by chills, extreme lethargy, lower abdominal pain, and fever. Temperature spikes to 40 °C (104 °F) usually indicate associated sepsis. It is not necessarily associated with significant uterine tenderness by abdominal or vaginal palpation. The prevalence of this type of infection, which is relatively uncommon following uncomplicated vaginal delivery, has decreased from 2.5%–1.3% in the last 15 years. This prevalence approaches 6%, however, in high-risk women: those with protracted labor and prolonged rupture of membranes, prior history of gynecologic infections, hematomas or devitalized tissue, postpartum anemia, maternal age younger than 17 years, and where there is manual removal of the placenta. Prior to the common use of perioperative antimicrobials for women undergoing cesarean section, these women had an extraordinarily high risk of developing endometritis. The reported overall prevalence of postoperative uterine infection was 13–50%, depending on the socioeconomic group of the parturient.

The polymicrobial cause of endometritis necessitates broad-spectrum therapy. A combination of clindamycin and gentamicin has been used traditionally. Clindamycin is administered intravenously in a dose of 2.4–2.7 g/ day in three or four divided doses. Gentamicin is given in a loading dose of 2 mg/kg and then 1.5 mg/kg every 8 hours thereafter. Other treatment regimens have been evaluated recently, but the number of subjects studied has been small. Regimens reported to be as effective as clindamycin plus gentamicin include cefoxitin, moxalactam, cefoperazone, cefotaxime, piperacillin, cefotetan, and clindamycin plus aztreonam. Evidence now suggests that ampicillin (2 g) and sulbactam (1 g) intravenously every 6 hours is equally as effective as the clindamycin/gentamicin regimen for clinical cure, bacterial eradication, and incidence of adverse experiences. In all cases, intravenous therapy should be continued until the patient has been free of symptoms for approximately 48 hours.

(2) Parametritis. This infection involves the broad ligament adjacent to the uterus. Parametritis is usually associated with endometritis. In its most isolated mild form, it may follow cesarean section. Treatment is the same as for endometritis.

(3) Perineal infection. Such an infection is more likely in the presence of a small, unnoticed hematoma. Examination of the perineum reveals an edematous, erythematous lesion with purulent drainage. Sutures must be removed to enhance drainage.

(4) Mastitis (see Chapter 8).

2. Nonpuerperal complications

a. Urinary tract infections (UTIs). The high incidence of UTIs during the postpartum period is usually attributed to trauma-induced hypotonicity of the bladder and frequent catheterization. Most patients with cystitis have had a negative result on initial screening culture and no urologic abnormalities. A 10- to 14-day course of antibiotics (amoxicillin, 500 mg orally three times daily for 10–14 days) is begun before cultures are ready (see Chapter 21). For a penicillin-allergic patient, refer to the alternative medications noted in Chapter 21, Table 21–1. Cystitis usually results in local symptoms without fever. In contrast, the symptoms of pyelonephritis are more severe: flank pain, shaking chills, and fever to 40 °C (104 °F) are frequent accompaniments.

b. Thrombophlebitis and thromboembolic disease. These conditions occur in fewer than 1% of all parturients, but occur significantly more often in the parturient than in the nonpregnant woman.

(1) Disorders of the deep veins in the postpartum period have been attributed to sluggish circulation, trauma to pelvic veins secondary to pressure from the fetal head, estrogen-induced hypercoagulability, and pelvic infection. Deep vein thrombophlebitis is characterized by fever, deep vein tenderness, Homan's sign, and extremity swelling secondary to venous obstruction. A useful, reliable diagnostic procedure is venography. The accuracy of Doppler ultrasonography depends on the skill of the technician (see Chapter 42).

    (2) Superficial thrombophlebitis usually involves the saphenous system and is palpable on physical examination. Tenderness and increased skin warmth are also evident. Treatment methods include **elastic support stockings, walking, elevation of the legs at rest, a combination of analgesic drugs,** and **application of moist local heat** to the area. To prevent this form of thrombophlebitis, women should remain active and refrain from taking estrogens to suppress lactation or oral contraceptives, since these agents increase the risk of hypercoagulation. They should also avoid anti-inflammatory agents during pregnancy and lactation because of risk of premature closure of the fetal ductus arteriosus.

    (3) *Right ovarian vein syndrome,* or **pelvic thrombophlebitis,** is the term used to describe thrombophlebitis occurring in the ovarian veins and other pelvic vessels. The patient often complains of abdominal pain and fever. If no evidence of pelvic abscess exists, and appropriate antibiotic therapy has resulted in no improvement in 72 hours in a patient with suspected endometritis, the diagnosis of ovarian vein syndrome should be considered. A sausage-shaped, tender mass may be palpated in the right midabdomen. Dramatic improvement usually results once **anticoagulation with heparin** is initiated, but defervescence may only occur after 4–5 days of heparin therapy, in doses similar to those used for the treatment of pulmonary embolism (see Chapter 23). Currently available imaging studies (computerized tomography scan and ultrasound) are poor in diagnosing this entity, so clinical suspicion is important.

    (4) Massive pulmonary embolism is characterized by the sudden onset of pleuritic chest pain, cough (with or without hemoptysis), fever, apprehension, and tachycardia. Friction rub, signs of pleural effusion and atelectasis, hypotension, diaphoresis, electrocardiographic signs of right heart strain, and increasing central venous pressure may all be present in severe cases (see Chapter 20).

  c. Parametrial phlegmon. A phlegmon, a three-dimensional mass that is palpable adjacent to the uterus on pelvic examination, develops most frequently when appropriate antimicrobial therapy has been delayed following evaluation of a postcesarean fever. A parametrial phlegmon is an intense area of induration within the leaves of the broad ligament occurring when endometritis and accompanying parametrial cellulitis follow cesarean delivery. The infection can be localized in the retroperitoneal area and presents with symptoms of peritonitis, such as an adynamic ileus. Treatment includes **bed rest, hydration with intravenous fluids, decompression of the bowel,** and **maintenance of electrolyte balance.** Clinical response occurs following intravenous antimicrobial therapy (the same antibiotics as are used for endometritis), although not usually until 5–7 days after initiation of treatment.

  d. Toxic shock syndrome (TSS). Toxic shock syndrome toxin-1, an exotoxin produced by *Staphylococcus aureus,* causes TSS by provoking severe endothelial injury. Nearly 10% of pregnant women have been found to be colonized vaginally by *S aureus,* and TSS has been reported in parturients. The syndrome most commonly occurs in young menstruating women who are using tampons. This severe, multisystem, acute febrile illness is characterized by a fever of 38.9 °C (102 °F) or higher; a macular erythematous rash, especially on the palms and the soles, that desquamates 1–2 weeks after onset of illness; hypotension, <90 mm Hg systolic, or orthostatic syncope; and involvement of three or more of the following organ systems: gastrointestinal, muscular, mucous membrane, renal, hepatic, hematologic, or central nervous.

    Initial management includes hospitalization, fluid and electrolyte resuscitation (up to 12 L/day), and administration of packed red blood cells and coagulation factors as necessary. In addition to baseline laboratory studies, blood and vaginal cultures of *S aureus* should be obtained promptly. Treatment with a β-lactamase–resistant antibiotic, such as nafcillin, oxacillin, or methicillin, is indicated; the dosage is 1 g intravenously every 4 hours. Vancomycin, 100 mg every 6 hours, is effective if the patient is allergic to penicillin.

  e. Necrotizing fasciitis. This deep, soft tissue infection that involves muscle and fascia may develop adjacent to myofascial edges, including surgical incisions and other wounds. Such infections rarely develop during the postpartum period in healthy women, but are seen in diabetic and immunocompromised women. Symptoms most commonly occur 3–5 days following delivery. The microbes implicated in these perineal infections are similar to those causing other pelvic infections, but anaerobes predominate. A high index of suspicion is necessary with rapid surgical exploration if the diagnosis is probable. Therapy consists of **broad-spectrum antibiotics** (eg, clindamycin, 2.4 g/kg in four divided doses) plus gentamicin (1.5 mg/kg every 8 hours), or others as noted above, as well as vigorous surgical **debridement.**

3. **Postpartum hemorrhage**
   a. **Uterine atony.** This condition, which is the most common cause of postpartum hemorrhage, can result from excessive uterine stretching secondary to polyhydramnios, multiple gestation, multiparity, prolonged labor, and certain general anesthetic agents. Initial management includes **fundal massage, removal of any remaining placental fragments,** and **oxytocin** (10 U intramuscularly every 4 hours, or 10–40 U intravenously diluted in 1000 mL of 0.5 normal saline titrated intravenously) to control atony. Methylergonovine maleate (0.2 mg intramuscularly every 4 hours for 48 hours) may be used instead of oxytocin.
   b. **Lacerations.** Routine inspection of the cervix, vagina, and perineum immediately following delivery affords the opportunity for timely repair of extensions to the episiotomy or lacerations.
   c. **Hematomas.** Perineal pain and noticeable mass suggest hematomas, which usually occur at the sites of lacerations or episiotomy repair. If managed within the first 24 hours after delivery with incision, drainage, and ligation of bleeding vessels, the cavity can be closed with a figure-of-eight suture.
   d. **Less common causes** of postpartum hemorrhage are placenta accreta, inverted uterus, coagulation defects (eg, associated with amniotic fluid embolism or pre-eclampsia–eclampsia), retained placental fragments, or uterine rupture. Digital examination of the uterus and lower uterine segment upon delivery is necessary to detect uterine rupture, especially after a vaginal delivery following prior cesarean section.

4. **Postpartum emotional disorders**
   a. **"Baby blues,"** or **"postpartum blues."** This transient depression, which is encountered in 70–80% of women during the first week postpartum, usually on the second or third day following delivery, can be accompanied by tearfulness. This self-limited disorder usually resolves within 3–7 days. Twelve percent of women will present with clinically relevant depressive disorders within 6 weeks postpartum, but 90% of these cases are associated with a situational or longstanding problem. Postpartum depression, occurring between 2 weeks and 12 months postpartum, may relate to employment factors in the working parturient, such as work hours and duration of maternity leave, maternal fatigue, and quality of prenatal social support. If the symptoms are severe enough to interfere with the new mother's ability to cope with ordinary daily tasks and activities, counseling and pharmacotherapy are advisable (see Chapter 92).
   b. **Psychiatric disorders.** If the patient exhibits excessive or no tearfulness, lack of interest in the baby, or excessive concern with the problems that will be encountered upon returning home that persist more than 24 hours while still in the hospital, or does not respond to counseling about problems developing subsequently, psychiatric evaluation is needed. Not only can major affective disorders appear during this time, but also the stress of gestation and parturition are nonspecific factors that may contribute to the development of various psychotic disorders.

III. **Management Strategies**
   A. **Immunizations**
      1. Nonisoimmunized D-negative women who deliver a D-positive infant should be given 300 mg of anti-D immune globulin (RhoGAM) shortly after delivery.
      2. The postpartum hospitalization period is also an appropriate time for vaccination of women not already immune to rubella. Some hospitals also give a tetanus toxoid booster injection prior to discharge unless it is contraindicated.
   B. **Discharge instructions**
      1. Periods of rest during the day are advisable for the **first month postpartum.** All parturients, especially those who have been sedentary during pregnancy, become

detrained during the third trimester and the postpartum period and should begin exercising at a baseline level. If vaginal bleeding increases upon resumption of exercise, parturients should stop for 2–3 days to allow further uterine involution and then resume activity. The parturient may gradually increase her activity and exercise level as soon as 2 weeks following an uncomplicated delivery. Only half of women seem to regain their usual level of energy by 6 weeks postpartum, however.

2. **Sitz baths,** basins designed to fit over the toilet seat and be filled with warm water and 1 oz of Betadine solution, or tub baths for 30 minutes two to three times daily, are helpful for painful episiotomies or lacerations.

3. **Sexual intercourse**
   a. For some time, **abstinence** has been recommended in the 6 weeks following delivery. The most common complaint is concern about dyspareunia during this period, which can be minimized by careful episiotomy. This period of discomfort can be shortened safely if no episiotomy is needed or if episiotomy repair is done meticulously so that healing occurs rapidly and comfortably. If tender areas in the episiotomy scar or in the vaginal wall persist after healing, a 1:1 steroid–lidocaine (1–2 mL of 1% Xylocaine without epinephrine and 1–2 mL of triamcinolone acetonide, 10 mg/mL) injection to the painful area can be used for relief.
   b. Otherwise, **sexual intercourse** can be resumed between the second and third postpartum weeks. The parturient can be encouraged to resume sexual activity when bleeding slows and when acceptable contraception has been provided. Contraception should be discussed and a method should be selected prior to discharge from the hospital (see Chapter 95). Intrauterine devices, diaphragms, sponges, and foams are not advised until after the puerperium.

4. **Breast-feeding**
   a. **Components of milk**
      (1) **Colostrum.** This liquid is secreted by the breasts for the first 5 days of parturition. It contains more protein, mostly globulin, and minerals and less sugar and fat than the more mature milk that is ultimately secreted. Host resistance factors, such as complement components, macrophages, lymphocytes, lactoferrin, lactoperoxidase, and lysozyme, as well as immunoglobulin, are present in colostrum and milk.
      (2) **Milk.** The major components are proteins (α-lactalbumin, β-lactoglobin, and casein), lactose, water, and fat. All vitamins except vitamin K are present in human milk in variable amounts. Iron is present in low concentrations, and iron levels in breast milk do not seem to be influenced by maternal iron stores. The predominant antibody present is secretory immunoglobulin A. These antibodies are thought to act locally within the infant's gastrointestinal tract.
   b. **Nursing**
      (1) **Advantages**
         (a) Accelerates involution of the uterus via oxytocin release.
         (b) **Gives ideal nourishment.** Breast milk meets the nutritional needs of the infant.
         (c) **Provides immunologic advantage.** In addition, breast-fed babies are less prone to respiratory and enteric infections than are bottle-fed babies.
         (d) **Contributes to bonding.** Nursing is generally well tolerated by infants.
         (e) **Delays ovulation**
      (2) **Disadvantages**
         (a) Privacy is needed for frequent feedings.
         (b) Contraindications include concurrent usage of certain drugs (eg, chloramphenicol, streptomycin, metronidazole, sulfa drugs, antithyroid drugs, some anticancer agents, certain anticonvulsants, some diuretics, and radioactive agents). Women with certain maternal illnesses (eg, active hepatitis A or B or tuberculosis) should not engage in breast-feeding.
         (c) Nursing can be an additional stressor in an already stressed mother.
   c. **Breast care.** Cleanliness and attention to fissures on the nipples are important. Water and mild soap can be used to cleanse the areolae before and after nursing. Lanolin-containing cream is recommended for nipple protection during the

initial weeks of breast-feeding to deter chapping and cracking of the nipples. Should severe irritation of the nipples occur, a nipple shield can be used for 24 hours or more.

5. **Suppression of lactation.** Women who do not wish to breast-feed should avoid all breast stimulation, suckling, manipulation, and showers, and should use a firm bra (rather than breast binding), and analgesia for 1 week. Minor symptoms of tenderness and a sense of fullness are common. Otherwise, there are no risks or side effects. Neither parenteral Deladumone nor oral bromocriptine is currently recommended. Following the use of Deladumone, rebound symptoms are common; in 25% of cases, there is an associated risk of thromboembolism, and use of the medication rarely results in substantial decrease in lactation. Rebound symptoms affect approximately 25% of women using bromocriptine as well. Furthermore, additional risks include hypotension, nausea, headache, dizziness, strokes, and early ovulation.

6. **Postpartum examination.** The postpartum visit is usually scheduled for 6–8 weeks after delivery, since most of the systemic signs of pregnancy have resolved by this time. Recent research evaluating optimal timing of the postpartum examination demonstrates that scheduling the Pap smear at least 8 weeks following delivery, rather than at 4–6 weeks, results in an approximately 30% decrease in the number of abnormal smears requiring follow-up or colposcopic examination. Following normal labor and puerperium, the postpartum evaluation should consist of blood pressure and weight determinations, palpation of the thyroid gland, a breast examination, a pelvic examination with cytologic examination of the cervix, evaluation of rectal sphincter tone, examination of abdominal wall tone, and urinalysis. Routine postpartum hematocrits are unnecessary in clinically stable patients with an estimated blood loss of <500 cc.

REFERENCES

Ely JW, et al: Benign fever following vaginal delivery. J Fam Pract 1996;**43:**146.

Gall S, Koukol DH: Ampicillin/sulbactam vs clindamycin/gentamicin in the treatment of postpartum endometritis. J Reprod Med 1996;**41:**575.

Sampselle CM, et al: Effect of pelvic muscle exercise on transient incontinence during pregnancy and after birth. Obstet Gynecol 1998;**91:**406.

South-Paul JE, Deuster PA: Physical activity during pregnancy. Clin Consult Obstet Gynecol 1993;**5:**245.

Spitz M, Lee NC, Peterson HB: Treatment for lactation suppression: Little progress in one hundred years. Am J Obstet Gynecol 1998;**179:**(6 Pt 1):1485.

Swift K, Janke J: Breast binding . . . is it all that it's wrapped up to be? J Obstet Gynecol Neonatal Nurs 2003;**32:**(3):332.

Witlin AG, et al: Septic pelvic thrombophlebitis or refractory postpartum fever of undetermined etiology. J Matern Fetal Med 1996;**5:**355.

---

99   Sexual Dysfunction

John G. Halvorsen, MD, MS

KEY POINTS

- Interference with their sexual response affects most people at some time in their sexual relationships.
- A simple question like, "How are things going for you sexually?" is important in helping physicians to discover patients' sexual concerns, since research indicates that patients are willing to talk with their physicians about their sexuality but hesitant to raise the subject themselves.
- Sexual dysfunction (eg, erectile dysfunction in men and arousal disorder in women) may be the presenting sign or symptom of another serious underlying disorder (eg, diabetes, hyperlipidemia, atherosclerosis, depression, tobacco, or drug abuse). Therefore, a thorough organic and psychological diagnostic evaluation performed by the primary physician is a necessary part of comprehensive management.
- Multiple treatment options can help to manage each one of the sexual dysfunctions.

I. **Introduction**
   A. **Definition.** The sexual dysfunctions represent disturbances in sexual desire and in the psychophysiologic changes that characterize the sexual response cycle.
   B. **Common diagnoses.** The *Diagnostic and Statistical Manual of Mental Disorders,* 4th edition (DSM-IV-TR), classifies the dysfunctions according to the following system. All must be "persistent or recurrent," "cause marked distress or interpersonal difficulty," and not be "better accounted for by another Axis I disorder" or "due exclusively to the direct psychophysiologic effects of a substance (eg, a drug of abuse, a medication) or a general medical condition." All disorders are further classified by subtype to indicate their onset (lifelong type or acquired type), the context (generalized type or situational type), and causative factors (caused by psychological factors or by combined factors) associated with each dysfunction.
   1. **Sexual desire disorders (SDDs)**
      a. **Hypoactive sexual desire disorder (HSDD):** deficient (or absent) sexual fantasies and desire for sexual activity. In the National Health and Social Life Survey (NHSLS), a large, randomly chosen, representative national sample, 15% of men and 33% of women indicated that they lacked interest in sex for at least 1 of the past 12 months. Problems in a couple's relationship are the most common cause of **SDD.**
      b. **Sexual aversion disorder:** extreme aversion to, and avoidance of, genital contact with a sexual partner. A rare desire disorder, sexual aversion is sometimes associated with vaginismus or dyspareunia. Patients commonly relate a history of sexual abuse accompanied by negative but unexpressed feelings about the partner relationship.
   2. **Sexual arousal disorders**
      a. **Male erectile disorder (ED):** inability to attain or maintain an adequate erection until sexual activity is completed.
         Epidemiological surveys indicate that over 10 million men in the United States experience ED and that 4–9% of all men and 25% of men older than 65 years have organic etiologies. In a large cross-sectional, random sample survey of men aged 40–70 years, the prevalence of **minimal ED** was 17%; of **moderate ED,** 25%; and of **complete ED,** 10%. Multiple organic and psychogenic risk factors are implicated (Table 99–1).
      b. **Female sexual arousal disorder (FSAD):** inability to attain or maintain an adequate lubrication–swelling response of sexual excitement until sexual activity is completed.
         Estimates of arousal disorders in women range from 20% to 48%. Causative factors in women are less well known, but are presumed to include many of the same factors implicated in ED.
   3. **Orgasmic disorders**
      a. **Female orgasmic disorder (FOD):** delayed or absent orgasm following normal sexual excitement.
         Surveys suggest that **anorgasmia** affects 5–25% of women and that 20–48% report problems lubricating or reaching orgasm. Underlying psychogenic factors include fears of pregnancy, vaginal damage, or rejection by a sexual partner; hostility toward men; and guilt feelings associated with sexual impulses. Some women equate orgasm with losing control or with aggressive, destructive, or violent behavior. These women may express their associated fear through inhibited arousal or orgasm. Cultural expectations and societal restrictions on women may also contribute.
      b. **Male orgasmic disorder (MOD):** delayed or absent orgasm following normal sexual excitement.
         Recent studies indicate a prevalence of 4–10%. Many men with this disorder were raised in rigid, puritanical families that considered sex sinful and the genitalia "dirty." These men also experience problems with closeness in relationships. Orgasmic disorders are more common in men with obsessive–compulsive personality disorders and in those with unexpressed hostility toward women.
      c. **Premature ejaculation (PE):** ejaculation with minimal stimulation before it is wanted, before, on, or shortly after penetration.
         Thirty-five to 40% of men treated for sexual dysfunction experience PE. The community prevalence rate in one recent study was 36–38%. In the NHSLS, 28% of men reported climaxing too early.

TABLE 99–1. COMMON ORGANIC AND PSYCHOGENIC FACTORS ASSOCIATED WITH SEXUAL DYSFUNCTION

Organic Factors

1. Chronic illness
   a. Congenital illness or malformation
   b. Endocrine disease (eg, diabetes mellitus; gonadal dysfunction; pituitary, adrenal, or thyroid disorders)
   c. Neurologic disorders (eg, multiple sclerosis, spinal cord injury)
   d. Vaginal or pelvic pathology (eg, vaginal atrophy, infections, endometriosis, childbirth injury)
   e. Genital trauma
   f. Cardiovascular and peripheral vascular disease
   g. Postsurgical complications (eg, after prostatectomy, abdominal vascular surgery, sympathectomy, gynecologic procedures)

2. Pregnancy (especially in the first and last trimesters)

3. Pharmacologic agents

	Primarily Affects			
	Desire	**Arousal**	**Orgasm**	**Hormones**
a. Anticholinergics		+		
b. Antidepressants	+	+	+	
c. Antihistamines	+	+		
d. Antihypertensives	+	+	+	+
e. Antipsychotics	+	+	+	+
f. Anxiolytics	+		+	
g. Narcotics	+	+	+	+
h. Sedative–hypnotics	+	+	+	
i. Other drugs				
Cimetidine	+	+		+
Clofibrate	+	+		
Digitalis	+	+		
Ethinyl estradiol		+		+
Levodopa			+	
Lithium		+		
Ketoconazole	+	+		
Niacin		+		
Norethindrone	+	+		+
Phenytoin		+	+	
Primidone	+			
4. Drugs of abuse				
a. Alcohol	+	+	+	+
b. Amphetamines	+	+	+	
c. Cocaine		+	+	
d. Heroin	+	+	+	
e. Marijuana	+			
f. MDMA	+	+	+	
g. Methadone	+	+	+	
h. Phencyclidine (PCP)	+		+	
i. Tobacco		+		

Psychogenic Factors

1. General psychogenic factors
   a. Personal problems (eg, depression, anxiety, diminished self-esteem, intrapsychic conflict)
   b. Relationship problems (eg, poor communication, unrealistic marital expectations, unresolved conflict, lost trust, poor relationship models, family system distress, sex role conflicts, divergent sexual values)
   c. Psychosexual factors (eg, prior sexual failure, chronic performance inconsistency, negative learning and attitudes about sex, prior sexual trauma, sexual performance anxiety, gender identity conflict, paraphilias)

2. Remote versus immediate factors
   a. Remote factors have historical origins (eg, negative sexual learning in childhood, dysthymic depression, prior relationship failures)
   b. Immediate factors occur during sexual activity (eg, sexual anxiety, denial of erotic feelings, ineffective sexual behaviors, failure to communicate desires and feelings)

Sexual Enactment Factors

Skill and knowledge deficits (eg, inadequate penile stimulation, inadequate stimulation for vaginal lubrication, unfavorable pelvic position for intercourse)

MDMA, S-methoxy-3,4-methyleredioxy amphetamine.

Most men with PE ejaculate prior to or within 1–2 minutes after vaginal intromission. PE is more common in college-educated men and may relate to an excessive concern for their partner's satisfaction. It also relates to anxiety about the sex act, societal conditioning about men's sex roles, and stressful marriage relationships. Recent data indicate that men with PE come from families where other men experience rapid ejaculation and that this may result from disturbed or maladaptive serotonin receptors in specific brain loci.

4. **Sexual pain disorders**

   a. **Dyspareunia:** genital pain in either men or women associated with sexual intercourse.

   As many as 30% of surgical procedures on a woman's genital tract result in temporary **dyspareunia**, and 30–40% of the women seen in sex therapy clinics for dyspareunia demonstrate pelvic disease. In the NHSLS, 5% of men and 15% of women reported dyspareunia in the past 12 months.

   Many medical conditions may cause **dyspareunia in women**—inadequate vaginal lubrication, pelvic or urinary tract infections, vaginal or hymenal scar tissue, endometriosis, estrogen deprivation, allergic reactions, and gastrointestinal conditions.

   Structural abnormalities in the penis, Peyronie's disease, priapism, urethral stricture, prior genital surgery, or genital infections may cause **dyspareunia in men.**

   Psychogenic theories for dyspareunia and vaginismus are similar and may involve a host of intrapsychic conflicts, faulty learning, or negative conditioning.

   b. **Vaginismus:** involuntary muscular spasm of the outer third of the vagina that interferes with sexual intercourse.

   Incidence estimates for **vaginismus** arising from sexual dysfunction clinics range widely, from 7.8% to 42%. It most often occurs in more educated women from higher socioeconomic groups.

   Most vaginismus is psychogenic. Risk factors include sexual trauma (eg, rape or incest), a strict religious background that associates sex with sin, unexpressed negative feelings toward a sexual partner or other important men, and phobia about the sexual response or intercourse.

5. **Sexual dysfunction due to a general medical condition:** sexual dysfunction that is fully explained by the direct physiologic effects of a defined medical condition.

6. **Substance-induced sexual dysfunction:** sexual dysfunction that develops during or within 1 month of substance intoxication or when medication use is causally related.

II. Diagnosis

A. **Symptoms.** Physicians should include a brief query about sexual relationships during routine clinical encounters. They may bridge their conversation about the medical history to the sexual history with a statement such as, "Your sexual functioning is just as important to me as the rest of your body's functioning, so as a part of a complete history, I always ask a few questions about how things are going sexually."

   General case-finding questions include queries such as "How are things going for you sexually?" "What questions or concerns do you have about your sexuality at this time?" or "How satisfying is your sex life for you?" Questions like these give patients "permission" to discuss their sexuality with the physician if they wish.

   Specific questions that inquire into problems with various phases of the sexual response cycle are also appropriate.

   1. **Present history.** Define the sexual problem better by collecting the following data: date and mode of onset; problem duration (lifelong, recent, episodic); situational context (generalized to all encounters or only to specific ones); current sexual interactions of the couple, including frequency of intercourse or sex play, frequency that the patient and the partner would prefer, time of day for lovemaking, presence of fatigue during lovemaking, difficulties with privacy, verbal and nonverbal communication of desires, type and pleasurability of sex play that precedes intercourse, arousal level during intercourse, orgasm frequency, thoughts, visualizations, and fantasies during sex, pain felt during intercourse (this symptom itself must be pursued in more detail), any exacerbations or remissions of the problem; effects of any attempted treatment; the presence of any associated symptoms in other body systems; the level of personal distress caused by the problem; and what the patient believes might be causing the difficulty.

2. **Sexual history.** Explore early experiences, emotional reactions, attitudes toward sexuality, sexual knowledge, frequency and types of past sexual practices, acceptance of cultural myths, the onset and development of the current sexual relationship, self-pleasuring practices and fantasies, homosexual experiences, any past negative sexual experiences (eg, incest or sexual assault), personal body image, and sexual developmental history.

3. **Developmental and family history.** Discuss the family-of-origin's attitudes toward sexuality, parental modeling, religious influences, relationships with parents and siblings, family violence, and the level of function in the couple's families of origin.

4. **Nature of the current relationship.** Focus on the development and stability of the current relationship, changes in feeling toward the partner, the presence of unresolved conflict, loss of trust or fidelity, and communication problems (eg, failures to listen and understand, hidden agendas, or using sex for power in the relationship).

5. **Current stressors.** Inquire about stresses that are both intrafamilial (eg, death, illness, or problems with children) and extrafamilial (eg, financial, occupational, or legal). Focus both on stresses and strains that normally occur as the individual and family progress through their life cycle stages and on stresses and strains that arise unexpectedly.

6. **Past medical history.** Identify any acute or chronic disease, injury, or surgery that could affect sexual functioning. Inquire specifically about those organic factors included in Table 99–1.

   Many commonly used drugs may contribute to sexual dysfunction (Table 99–1). Drug effects vary by individual, depending on age, absorption, body weight, dosage, duration of use, rates of metabolism and excretion, presence of other drugs, underlying disorders, patient compliance, and suggestibility.

7. **Habits.** See Table 99–1 for the types of sexual dysfunctions associated with the common drugs of abuse.

8. **Questionnaires.** The **International Index of Erectile Function (IIEF)** is a 15-item inventory designed to assess erectile function, orgasmic function, sexual desire, intercourse satisfaction, and overall sexual satisfaction. It demonstrates test reliability, construct validity, and treatment responsiveness. A shortened 5-item version, the **IIEF-5,** is a useful screening instrument for ED, with a sensitivity of 98% and specificity of 88%. The **Female Sexual Function Index (FSFI)** is a 19-item questionnaire designed to assess desire, subjective arousal, lubrication, orgasm, satisfaction, and pain in women. It demonstrates discriminant validity between normal women and those with FSAD, FOD, and HSDD.

   These tools are brief, reliable, and valid measures that can help the busy physician focus the history-taking process.

B. **Signs.** A comprehensive physical examination will help identify any concurrent acute or chronic illness and any associated physical conditions that could affect sexual functioning or treatment.

   1. **Focus special attention on the following.**

      a. **General:** obesity, cachexia, vital signs, secondary sex characteristics, gynecomastia in men, and galactorrhea in women.

      b. **Cardiovascular:** bruits (especially femoral), peripheral pulses, evidence of venous stasis, arterial insufficiency (especially in the lower extremities), and a pulsatile epigastric mass.

      c. **Abdominal:** pain, tenderness, mass, guarding, tympany, and bowel activity.

      d. **Neurologic:** gait, coordination, deep tendon reflexes, pathologic reflexes, sensation, motor strength, integrity of the sacral reflex arc (S_2–S_4) with perineal sensation, anal sphincter tone, and bulbocavernosus reflex (clinically present in 70% of normal men). Test penile temperature sensation with alcohol swabs and penile vibration perception threshold with a tuning fork placed sequentially on the glans and the midshaft.

   2. Observe the **male genitalia** for testicular size and consistency, penile size, malformations, and structural lesions. A normal flaccid adult penis is >6 cm in length and >3 cm in width.

      Obtaining **penile blood pressure** measurements on any man with **ED** can help to diagnose arterial insufficiency. Place and inflate a 3-cm pediatric blood pressure cuff around the base of the penis and auscultate the central artery of the corpora cavernosa with a 9.5–MHz Doppler stethoscope as the cuff is deflated. The penile systolic pressure is the pressure at which one first hears the arterial pulse. The ratio between the penile systolic pressure and the brachial systolic pressure, the **penile brachial index (PBI),** should exceed 0.75. If it is below 0.60, significant penile vascular insufficiency likely exists. The **PBI** is most predictive in patients with evidence for peripheral vascular disease but without other risk factors like diabetes or a pharmacologic agent that could affect erectile function.

3. **Female pelvic examination.** Focus on the following:
   a. **External genitalia:** dermatitis, vulvar inflammation, episiotomy or other scars, clitoral inflammation, and adhesions.
   b. **Introitus:** hymenal rigidity, tags, or fibrosis; urethral carbuncle; and Bartholin's gland inflammation.
   c. **Vagina:** spasm of the vaginal sphincter and adduction of the thighs with attempted vaginal examination, atrophy, discharge, inflammation, stenosis, relaxation of supporting ligaments, and tenderness along the vaginal urethra or posterior bladder wall.
   d. **Bimanual examination:** cul-de-sac masses or tenderness; adnexal mass or tenderness; and position, size, mobility, and tenderness of the uterus.
   e. **Rectovaginal examination:** hemorrhoids, fissures, constipation, tenderness, and a stool specimen positive for occult blood.

C. **Laboratory tests**
   1. **Evaluation for systemic disease. Baseline studies** include a complete blood cell count, fasting blood sugar level, urinalysis, tests for sexually transmitted diseases, lipid profiles, and tests of thyroid, liver, and renal function.
   2. **Evaluation for specific disorders**
      a. **SDDs.** Obtain a morning **serum bioavailable testosterone** level in men with **SDDs.** If levels are low or borderline, or if the low desire is associated with little or no masturbation history, obtain a **serum prolactin** level. Correlation between **sexual desire** and **levels of follicle-stimulating hormone (FSH), androstenedione, luteinizing hormone (LH),** and **estradiol is presently inconclusive.**
      b. **FSAD.** Experimental techniques for measuring nocturnal vaginal blood flow using a specially designed vaginal probe demonstrate that vaginal engorgement cycles occur in women during rapid eye movement (REM) sleep with the same frequency that erectile cycles occur in men.
      c. **ED**
         (1) **Serum tests.** Obtain a morning **serum bioavailable testosterone** level to screen for hypogonadism. If the level is low, obtain **FSH, LH,** and **prolactin** levels. If FSH and LH are low and prolactin is normal, then the diagnosis is pituitary or hypothalamic failure. If FSH and LH are high and prolactin is normal, then the diagnosis is testicular failure. If FSH and LH are low, but prolactin is high, then there is a 25–40% chance that the patient has a pituitary adenoma. In this case request a **computerized tomographic** scan or **magnetic resonance imaging** scan of the sella turcica.
         (2) **Nocturnal penile tumescence (NPT) evaluation.** Because sleep eliminates the psychological factors that inhibit arousal, NPT evaluation helps to differentiate psychological from organic **ED.** Normally, three or four erections occur each night during REM sleep with a total night erection time >90 minutes. Organic interference persists during sleep, disturbing erections. Psychogenic interference should not persist and erections will occur. Several techniques evaluate and quantify NPT.

         The **snap gauge** (Timm Medical Technologies, Eden Prairie, MN) is a ring of opposing Velcro straps that are connected by three plastic strips. The man wraps the ring around the penis before sleep. During a normal rigid nocturnal erection, all bands break. By noting whether no, one, two, or three bands break, one can estimate the maximum erectile response during sleep. The three elements break at degrees of tension corresponding to intracorporeal pressures of approximately 80, 100, and 120 mm Hg. This is a useful screening tool, since it is inexpensive, is simple, and can be performed at home. False-negative results occur if it is not applied tightly enough. False positives occur if bands break while turning during sleep. This method only detects the maximal erectile event during sleep and does not measure erection duration, maximum number, or actual rigidity. Furthermore, one cannot correlate erections with REM sleep cycles. More sophisticated tests, including the **RigiScan** (Timm Medical Technologies), the **NEVA System** (Urometrics, Inc., St. Paul, MN), and **NPT monitoring** performed in a sleep laboratory are also available.

(3) **Pharmaco-penile duplex ultrasonographic scanning** provides high-resolution real-time ultrasonographic imaging and pulse Doppler analysis of the actual blood flow in the cavernous arteries before and after injection of a vasodilator. Normal vessels should double in size with an initial peak systolic flow velocity of 0.30 cm/sec.

(4) **Pudendal angiography.** Selective internal pudendal angiograms can determine whether an arterial block exists that could be corrected by penile revascularization. This procedure is used most commonly in younger patients with clinical and noninvasive findings that suggest an arterial cause for their **ED** and who are candidates for reconstructive surgery.

(5) **Dynamic infusion cavernosometry and cavernosography** evaluate the veno-occlusive mechanisms of the corpus cavernosum. Through a butterfly needle inserted into the corpus cavernosum, the procedural physician first infuses a vasoactive agent (45–60 mg papaverine with 1–2.5 mg phentolamine or 20 μg of PGE_1), then heparinized saline and finally radiographic contrast. X-rays are taken to identify leaks in specific veins and to evaluate for glans or spongeosal leaks. These procedures are performed less frequently now since surgical procedures designed to correct venous leaks are less successful than anticipated.

(6) **Bulbocavernosus reflex latency tests** measure the integrity of the sacral reflex arc (S_2–S_4). When the glans penis is stimulated with a pinch or a squeeze, electromyographic needles in the bulbocavernosus muscle record muscle contraction. The time delay from stimulation to contraction is calculated. Longer times suggest a neurologic cause for **ED** and can help document suspected sacral nerve root, cauda equina, or conus medullaris lesions caused by multiple sclerosis, spinal cord trauma, spinal cord tumors, and herniated intervertebral disks.

(7) **Pudendal nerve somatosensory evoked potentials** record waveforms over the sacrum (conus medullaris) and the parietal cortex in response to dorsal penile nerve stimulation, and can therefore help localize neurologic lesions to peripheral, sacral, or suprasacral locations.

(8) **Vibration perception threshold** screens for abnormalities within the penile sensory afferent pathway. A portable handheld electromagnetic vibration device with a fixed vibration frequency and variable amplitude is placed against the penile shaft. A loss or decrease in sensation suggests a peripheral neuropathy.

(9) **Perineal electromyography** identifies problems in pudendal motor pathways that may relate to metabolic or toxic disorders such as diabetes and alcoholism.

(10) **Summary of evaluation for ED.** After conducting a comprehensive history, physical examination, and laboratory screening, one must form a "most probable" hypothesis for the man's **ED.** Is it psychological or organic? If it is organic, is the cause likely neurologic, vascular, endocrine, or a combination of these factors?

If one cannot separate psychological from organic factors, consider an **NPT evaluation.** If the hypothesis is "organic: neurologic or vascular," consider a therapeutic trial of one of the noninvasive agents used to treat **ED.** If the trial succeeds, continue therapy. If it fails, consider further specific procedural evaluation for neurologic or vascular causes.

If the hypothesis is "organic: endocrine," then obtain a **serum bioavailable testosterone** level. If this is low, then obtain **FSH, LH,** and **prolactin** serum levels. If the serum testosterone is normal, revise the hypothesis and consider a therapeutic trial with a noninvasive agent.

d. **Sexual pain disorders.** Laboratory evaluation, guided by the clinical evaluation, helps to detect associated organic factors.

(1) **Office laboratory procedures** include saline and potassium hydroxide wet mounts of vaginal secretions to diagnose vaginitis or vaginosis; urinalysis, urine culture, and examination of prostatic secretions to diagnose associate genitourinary infections; and tests to diagnose chlamydial, herpes simplex, and gonococcal infections (see Chapters 21, 51, 61, and 64).

(2) **Colposcopy** may be useful in diagnosing specific vaginal or cervical disease such as human papillomavirus infections.

(3) **Pelvic ultrasonography** can help diagnose adnexal, uterine, or cul-de-sac problems.

(4) **Laparoscopy** can help diagnose, and in some cases treat, adnexal or intraperitoneal disease.

(5) **Anoscopy or sigmoidoscopy** is used to identify associated colorectal problems (see Chapter 52).

III. Treatment

A. Therapeutic strategies. Physicians can relate to patients with a sexual problem at one of five levels.

1. **Level 1: Case finding.** Ask the initial sexual history question, but then refer to another professional for evaluation and treatment.

2. **Level 2: Evaluate the chief complaint.** Collect the basic sexual history during routine visits and provide basic education about normal anatomy, physiology, and sexual functioning. When patients raise sexual concerns, obtain a "history of present illness" with appropriate symptom pursuit and perform a focused physical examination. Refer to another professional if treatment involves more than reassurance or basic education.

3. **Level 3: Comprehensive evaluation.** Obtain a detailed sexual history that includes both the psychosocial and medical history. Perform a comprehensive physical examination and evaluate for organic causes with appropriate laboratory tests and diagnostic procedures.

4. **Level 4: Manage organic problems and refer for psychosexual therapy.** Treat any organic problems or coordinate care with another physician if a special procedure such as a penile implant is required. Continue to provide psychological support, but refer psychosexual therapy to a sexual therapist.

5. **Level 5: Manage both organic and psychosexual therapy.** Before primary physicians determine which role to play, they must ascertain their own interest in sexual concerns and the care they wish to provide. They must also build a professional referral network to provide care that is beyond their own competence or interest. Membership in or certification by one or more of the following organizations is one indication of a sexual therapist's competence: Society for Sex Therapy and Research (SSTAR); American Association for Sex Education, Counseling and Therapy (AASECT); and Society for Scientific Study of Sex (SSSS).

B. Psychosexual therapy

1. **Standard principles.** Several basic principles undergird current psychosexual therapy.

   a. People are responsible for their own sexuality.

   b. Growth in sexual attitudes, performance, and feelings results from behavioral change.

   c. Every person deserves sexual health.

   d. Physiologic relaxation creates the foundation for sexual excitement.

   e. Boundaries between the sexual and the nonsexual aspects of sexual dysfunction (eg, career stress or marital problems) must exist.

2. **Cognitive–behavioral therapy** that incorporates behavioral therapy into other treatments is the treatment of choice for managing most sexual dysfunctions. Behavior therapists assume that sexual dysfunction is learned maladaptive behavior that causes patients to fear sexual interaction. During treatment, the therapist establishes a hierarchy of anxiety-provoking situations for the patient and then helps him or her master the anxiety through systematic desensitization. This process inhibits the learned anxious response by encouraging antianxiety behaviors.

3. **Masters and Johnson dual-sex therapy** requires that a man–woman co-therapy team work with couples. It acknowledges that men and women differ in sexual

experiences and roles and establishes the therapeutic importance of gender fairness and balance. Few centers currently use dual-gender treatment teams, since other models are successful and less expensive.

4. **Sensate focus.** The original behavioral tasks developed by Masters and Johnson are termed "sensate focus" exercises, since they heighten sensory awareness to touch, sight, sound, and smell. As patients focus on their own sensations, they often relax and overcome barriers that impede natural physiologic responses. Partners first learn to enjoy touching, stroking, exploring, massaging, and fondling all the contours of each other's bodies except for their genitals. When both partners are adept and comfortable exchanging nongenital caresses, they add genital stroking exercises. Erogenous stroking progresses to vaginal penile containment, first without genital thrusting and then to full intercourse with orgasm. Couples learn to use fantasies to distract them from obsessive performance concerns and to communicate mutual needs verbally and nonverbally.

5. **Hypnotherapy** begins with a series of nonhypnotic sessions to build a secure doctor–patient relationship and to establish treatment goals. Therapy focuses on removing symptoms and altering attitudes. Patients begin to use relaxation techniques before a sexual encounter, and they also learn alternative ways to deal with anxiety-provoking sexual situations.

6. **Group therapy** methods can examine patients' intrapsychic and interpersonal problems within a strong support system that can counteract sexual myths, correct misconceptions, and provide accurate information about sexual anatomy, physiology, and varieties of behavior. Groups composed of sexually dysfunctional married couples are particularly effective in validating individual preferences and in enhancing self-esteem and self-acceptance.

7. **Traditional marital therapy** is also important, since marital or relationship problems that generate stress, fatigue, and dysphoria commonly underlie the sexual dysfunctions. Therapy helps the couple develop communication skills, establish realistic marital expectations, resolve conflict, and build trust.

C. **Specific sexual therapy techniques**

1. **Directed masturbation** is the most effective treatment program to date for primary orgasmic dysfunction in women. Beginning with basic education in sexual anatomy and physiology, women progress through the stages of tactile and visual self-exploration, manual stimulation to areas of pleasurable sensation, sexual fantasy and image development, sensate focus exercises alone and then with a partner, and finally sharing effective masturbation techniques with a partner.

2. The **stop–start, or squeeze, technique.** The stop–start technique of Semans and the squeeze technique modification of Masters and Johnson are used to treat **PE.** The technique begins as the couple embrace and caress one another until the man's penis is erect. He then lies on his back, his partner begins stimulating his penis, and he concentrates on his arousal sensations. Just before he reaches the point of imminent ejaculation, he tells his partner to stop stimulation. At this point, Masters and Johnson direct the woman to squeeze the penis firmly between her thumb and forefinger, under the corona of the glans. Most current therapists now suggest that the man apply the squeeze himself. When the woman applies the squeeze, it paradoxically suggests that control over erections is hers rather than the man's. With or without the squeeze, the couple wait for several minutes until arousal sensations dissipate. This process of stimulation and stopping repeats several times before the man ejaculates.

After four or five successful stimulation–stopping sessions, the couple tries the stop–start process with the penis in the vagina. The woman assumes the woman-superior position and the man glides her slowly up and down the shaft of his penis. As he again almost reaches the point of ejaculation, he ceases moving his partner until the need subsides. This process is also repeated several times before he ejaculates.

When the man can control ejaculation with this level of stimulation, his partner begins to stimulate the penis with vaginal thrusting until the man begins to feel the need to ejaculate. At this point, he tells her to stop stimulation until arousal wanes. This sequence is also repeated several times before he ejaculates.

The couple completes a start–stop sequence at least weekly until they learn to use it automatically during intercourse. Eventually, they use the method with other sexual positions. Most men, however, experience the greatest difficulty controlling ejaculation in the man-superior position. The couple-on-their-side often becomes the favored position for intercourse.

3. **Systematic desensitization** is a technique that treats both dyspareunia and vaginismus. The pelvic examination is the first step in the treatment process and must be conducted with care, reassurance, and proper education. The examination confirms the absence of pelvic disease, demonstrates that vaginal comfort is possible, confirms that vaginal events are under the woman's control, allows the woman to see the psychophysiologic components of the dysfunction (eg, involuntary introital contractions can be seen with a mirror, allowing the woman to visualize the relationship between psychological conditioning and a physical event), and allows the physician to reassure the woman about her normality and to teach her specific techniques to help her overcome the disorder. During the examination, the physician also educates the partner in anatomy and psychosomatic physiology. It is important that he observes the process of successful vaginal containment.

The first desensitization step after examination is to assure the woman that she is in complete control. When she says "Stop!," the examination stops. It may take several sessions to demonstrate painless vaginal insertion. The woman is given a handheld mirror to use throughout the examination so that the physician can teach vulvar and vaginal anatomy and so that she can visualize her own muscle contractions. She is taught to contract and relax her abdominal, medial thigh, and vaginal introital muscles sequentially. By identifying and contracting these muscles, she will have an easier time relaxing them.

The woman is then taught to "bear down and pull in" while contracting her introital muscles (Kegel exercises). When she can do this easily, the physician (with the patient's permission) places the tip of his or her index finger at the introitus and asks the woman to bear down and push the finger away. When this process is repeated several times, the fingertip will enter the vagina spontaneously. The woman often feels that instead of penetrating the vagina, the finger is "captured" by it. She learns that she can actively control what enters her vagina and that it can be painless.

When the woman comfortably contains the physician's fingertip, she repeats the same process first using her own fingertip and then her partner's. As she contracts and relaxes her vaginal muscles around a finger, she learns that she can control penetration and experience painless vaginal containment.

After the woman is comfortable with these exercises, she progresses through small steps to initiate intercourse. She inserts her partner's penis into her vagina after she is sufficiently aroused. Both partners must understand that the woman always controls the amount of contraction, relaxation, and penetration that occurs during intercourse and that she will not experience vaginal pain.

D. HSDD

1. **Testosterone** does not benefit men with normal serum levels. In fact, it can compound the problem in men with **ED** who have normal levels by increasing sexual desire without concomitantly increasing arousal. In hypogonadal men with testosterone values <100 ng/dL, intramuscular testosterone enanthate or cypionate (100–200 mg every 2–4 weeks) is the preferred treatment. Transdermal systems are also effective methods for replacing testosterone (Androderm, 2.5–7.5 mg daily, or Androgel, 50–100 mg daily). Oral agents are less effective and may cause hepatic disorders (eg, cholestatic jaundice). Potential hazards of testosterone therapy include increased prostate-specific antigen levels and increased prostatic volume. These may increase the risk for prostatic cancer, and men should be screened for cancer at regular intervals.

   One well-designed study demonstrated that testosterone in doses of 300 μg per day increased sexual desire and orgasm pleasure in women following a hysterectomy. A 2% testosterone vaginal cream has also been used to enhance desire in women, but its use is not supported by convincing evidence.

2. **Dopaminergic agents** have been associated with increased libido, including apomorphine (see section III,F), bromocriptine, pergolide, levodopa, and cabergoline.

   Bromocriptine mesylate (Parlodel) specifically treats hyperprolactinemia. Doses begin at 1.25 mg/day and increase by 1.25 mg every 3–7 days until the serum prolactin level is normal. The usual treatment dose is 2.5 mg twice daily.

3. Some studies indicate that **antidepressants** from several classes can increase libido. These agents include bupropion, nomifensine, trazodone, venlafaxine, and fenfluramine. See Chapter 92 on depression for dosing information.

E. **Sexual aversion. Psychosexual therapy** that includes cognitive–behavioral techniques, desensitization, and resolving past abuses in combined individual and couples therapy is the most effective management strategy for sexual aversion.

F. **ED**

1. **Systemic agents**

   a. **Testosterone** is used in hypogonadal men, as described for **HSDD.**

   b. **Sildenafil** is an orally active inhibitor of the type-V cyclic guanosine monophosphate-specific phosphodiesterase (the predominant isoenzyme in the human corpus cavernosum). It increases levels of nitrous oxide, which relaxes the endothelial muscles, increasing blood flow into the corpora cavernosa. It effectively treats **ED** of organic, psychogenic, and mixed etiology. It enhances the erectile mechanism with sexual stimulation and does not work without stimulation. A man takes a single oral dose of 50–100 mg about an hour before intercourse. Sildenafil's activity begins in 30 minutes and lasts up to 4 hours. The most common adverse effects are headache (16%), flushing (10%), dyspepsia (7%), nasal congestion (4%), urinary tract infection (3%), visual effects (3%), and diarrhea (3%). Drug levels are increased by other drugs that are metabolized by or that inhibit the cytochrome P450 system. Sildenafil also potentiates the hypotensive effects of nitrates and is **absolutely contraindicated** in patients using organic nitrates in any form. More specific phosphodiesterase type-V inhibitors are now being developed and tested.

   c. **Yohimbine** is an α_2-adrenoceptor antagonist that theoretically enhances penile erections by restricting penile venous outflow and by increasing libido through a central nervous system effect. The dosage is 6 mg orally three times daily. To date, few double-blind, placebo-controlled studies have been performed to document its efficacy. The American Urological Association now states that it "should not be recommended as a treatment for the standard patient" based on lack of proven effectiveness. Some studies indicated that it may be effective in treating selective serotonin reuptake inhibitor (SSRI)-induced sexual dysfunctions and that it may have a synergistic effect when administered with trazodone (100–200 mg at bedtime).

   d. **Phentolamine mesylate (Vasomax)** is an oral adrenergic receptor antagonist that causes erections by relaxing smooth muscle tissue and dilating arteries. It has been studied in men with minimal **ED** of broad-spectrum etiology. A man takes 20–80 mg about 15 minutes prior to intercourse. Side effects include headache, facial flushing, and nasal congestion. The drug appears safe and effective for treatment of mild **ED.**

   e. **Apomorphine** is believed to cause erections through its effect as a dopaminergic agonist that lowers the response threshold for erectile and ejaculatory reflexes. It has also been studied on men with minimal or insignificant organic disease. It is taken as a transbuccal tablet in dosage strengths of 2 mg, 4 mg, or 6 mg. The main adverse effect is nausea. Other observed adverse effects include persistent yawning, vomiting, and hypotension.

   f. **Naltrexone** is a long-acting opioid antagonist that reportedly promotes erectile function in doses of 25–50 mg daily. It may also act synergistically when combined with yohimbine.

2. **Topical agents**

   a. **Nitroglycerine** has a local effect on penile smooth muscle, causing relaxation and subsequent engorgement. Although controlled studies that support its effectiveness are sparse, men with mild vascular, neurologic, or mixed arousal dysfunction may benefit from a therapeutic trial with nitroglycerin before starting more invasive therapies. Men apply 0.5–1 inch of 2% ointment to the penile shaft just prior to intercourse, using a condom during intercourse to avoid mucosal absorption of the nitroglycerin and adverse systemic effects in their partners. A transdermal nitroglycerin patch applied 1–2 hours prior to intercourse also reportedly improves erections.

   b. Several studies indicate that men can also apply topical 2% **minoxidil** solution to the glans to produce erections, and that it may be even more effective than nitroglycerin.

3. **Intracavernosal injections.** Patients may inject either **papaverine** or **PGE₁** into a corpus cavernosum with a 27-gauge needle to induce an erection. This technique is quite successful in men with neurogenic disorders, mild vascular problems, or combined neurogenic and vascular disorder, and in selected men with psychogenic causes for whom psychosexual treatment has failed. Therapy begins with a low dose of either drug, gradually titrating the dose to provide an adequate erection that lasts 1–2 hours. This usually requires 10–80 mg of papaverine or 10–40 μg of PGE₁. Injections are limited to three times per week and 10 times per month. Complications include priapism (0.33%), cavernous tissue fibrosis (2.8%), hematoma, cavernositis, pain, and changes in blood pressure (usually orthostatic hypotension). Erections that last more than 4 hours should be reversed by irrigating the corpora cavernosum with diluted phenylephrine.

   VIP 0.025 mg mixed with phentolamine 2.0 mg is an investigational agent that comes as a prefilled, ready-to-use autoinjector and demonstrates a reported overall efficacy of 80% and a 70% efficacy in men who failed other intracavernosal therapy. The most common adverse reaction is transient facial flushing (53%). The incidence of priapism, fibrosis, and pain occurs less frequently than with other injection therapies.

   Intracavernosal injections may be used to treat **PE** as well as **ED**. In the case of PE, they may allow sexual activity to continue despite the man's premature climax.

4. **Intraurethral PGE₁** therapy requires a man to insert a PGE₁ medicated pellet into his urethra with an applicator following urination. When absorbed through the mucosa, the PGE₁ relaxes smooth muscles and dilates arteries. Following insertion, the man must manually stimulate the penis for 10 seconds and then walk around for another 10 minutes to promote erection. The maximal response occurs in 20–25 minutes. Pellets are available in 125-, 250-, 500-, and 1000-μg dosage strengths. Adverse effects include penile pain (32%), urethral burning (12%), minor urethral bleeding (5%), testicular pain (5%), hypotension (3%), and dizziness (2%).

5. **Surgical procedures**
   a. **Arterial revascularization.** Successful surgery for proximal artery occlusion (eg, endarterectomy, transluminal balloon angioplasty, or graft placement) reportedly improves blood flow through the hypogastric vessels. Success depends on whether the distal vessels are disease free and can accept the increased flow and whether surgery damages the autonomic nerves that course over the vessels. Many other surgical techniques can revascularize the corpora when distal vessels (internal pudendal and penile arteries) are occluded.
   b. **Venous surgery.** Surgical procedures vary, depending on where venous incompetence occurs. If a shunt is found from the corpus to the deep dorsal vein, the surgeon ligates the vein, any accessory veins, and all the circumflex and emissary veins that join the dorsal vein, thus providing added resistance to venous outflow. These procedures are now performed much less frequently, since their long-term success rates have not reached expectations.
   c. **Penile prosthesis.** The penile prosthesis is the most reliable surgical option in the United States, with the inflatable prosthesis implanted most frequently. Manufacturers now provide reliable protheses consisting of cylinders that expand in both girth and length, a single scrotal pump, and an abdominal reservoir. To decrease the chance of mechanical failure in multicomponent devices and to mimic natural erection, self-contained inflatable devices have also been designed that include an inflation chamber, reservoir, and pump mechanism in a self-contained cylinder. Prosthesis implantation is relatively uncomplicated, but most devices require replacement after 48–60 months. Potential complications include mechanical failure (0–3.2%), infection (1.9–8.3%), erosion, penile gangrene, improper sizing, and silicone shedding.

6. **Mechanical therapy**
   a. **Vacuum pump.** Penile vacuum pumps can also aid erections. The man places a lubricated cylinder over his penis, and using an attached handheld pump to withdraw air, he creates a vacuum that draws blood into the corpora cavernosum. When his penis is erect, he maintains engorgement by applying an elastic band around the penile base and removes the cylinder. Potential complications include penile edema, decreased penile sensation, impaired ejaculation, subcutaneous bleeding, and penile necrosis. These devices no longer require a physician's prescription.

     b. Constriction rings are usually packaged with the vacuum pump, but may be the only devices needed to manage erectile dysfunction in men with mild to moderate venous leakage and no arterial insufficiency. The **Soft Touch** ring (Mission Pharmacal Co., San Antonio, TX) has the advantage of easy removal without entangling pubic hair, and the **Pressure Point** ring (Osbon, Augusta, GA) includes a V-shaped ventral section to reduce urethral obstruction, thereby enhancing seminal flow.

G. FSAD

  1. Treating comorbid conditions and underlying disease is the first step for managing **FSAD**. It rarely occurs as an isolated disorder but frequently accompanies a concurrent condition that preceded the arousal problem. If genital pain, anorgasmia, or a chronic organic illness exist, those problems should be addressed and treated before attending specifically to arousal as a separate entity.

  2. Systemic

     a. Sildenafil (50–100 mg) can increase blood flow to the clitoral corpus cavernosum. Clinical studies evaluating its effectiveness in treating **FSAD** are still in progress.

     b. Phentolamine mesylate enhanced vaginal blood flow and improved subjective arousal in one study.

  3. Mechanical. Eros Therapy (UroMetrics) is a small, handheld device composed of a soft plastic cup that is connected to a small vacuum pump. The woman places the cup over her clitoris and the pump creates a gentle vacuum that increases genital blood flow and subsequent clitoral engorgement. Increasing blood flow into the clitoris reportedly also increases vaginal lubrication and enhances the woman's ability to achieve orgasm.

H. FOD

  1. Psychosexual therapy. Sensate focus, systematic desensitization, and directed masturbation consistently show the highest rates of improvement for orgasmic dysfunction in many controlled treatment outcome studies.

  2. Systemic. Bupropion in doses of 150–300 mg/day demonstrated significant improvement in orgasmic ability in one sample of nondepressed women.

  3. Mechanical. Eros Therapy (discussed under section III,G,3, treatment for **FSAD**) reportedly increases a woman's orgasmic capacity when used regularly (three or four times per week).

I. MOD. The most common cause for anorgasmia in men is using an antidepressant drug that interferes with orgasm. Strategies for managing antidepressant-related sexual disorders (SDs) are discussed below in section III,L, antidepressant-associated SDs.

J. PE

  1. Psychosexual therapy. The **start–stop–squeeze technique** (see section III,C, specific sexual therapy techniques) was the standard therapy for **PE** before pharmacologic agents became available. It is now used most frequently in combination with pharmacologic agents (see the next section) for men who do not respond optimally to the drugs alone.

  2. Systemic

     a. Clomipramine at doses of 25–50 mg, taken 12–24 hours prior to intercourse, effectively prolonged intravaginal intercourse to at least 2 minutes in 70% of men with **PE** in one study. In another study, it prolonged ejaculatory latency from 2 to 8 minutes. The minimum time between drug ingestion and the maximum ejaculatory control is not yet known. The shortest studied interval was 4–6 hours.

     b. Paroxetine. Paroxetine demonstrates increased ejaculatory latency when administered following several different protocols: as 20 mg 3–4 hours prior to intercourse as needed; as 10 mg once-daily chronic administration; and as 10 mg once daily with an additional 20 mg taken as needed 3–4 hours prior to intercourse. All methods increased ejaculatory latency, with the 10 mg daily plus 20 mg as needed protocol showing the greatest improvement. Another study demonstrated that one could achieve further benefit by adding 50 mg of sildenafil 1 hour prior to intercourse to this last protocol.

     c. Sertraline also delays ejaculation through its serotonergic effects. The usual dose is 50–100 mg taken 3–5 hours prior to sexual activity. The most common side effect is drowsiness.

     d. Fluoxetine is also used to treat **PE** at doses of 20–60 mg.

e. **Tricyclic antidepressants** may help treat **PE** because they inhibit the cholinergic component of ejaculation. Men take a low initial dose (eg, 25 mg of amitriptyline) 3–5 hours prior to sexual activity, increasing subsequent doses until they experience ejaculatory control, have side effects, or reach the maximal recommended dose.

f. **Thioridazine,** at standard antidepressant doses, may also benefit men with **PE.** It is the most potent anticholinergic and α-adrenergic blocking agent in its class and presumably delays ejaculation through these effects.

g. **Phenoxybenzamine (PBZ)** is an α-adrenergic blocker indicated for treating hypertension. Used by men with **PE** in daily doses of 20–30 mg, PBZ benefits ejaculation and erection with minimal side effects. It is best used by men who do not wish to procreate, since PBZ inhibits seminal emission.

3. **Topical agents.** A lidocaine–prilocaine cream can help to prevent **PE.** In pilot studies men applied 2.5 g to the glans and penile shaft at least 30 minutes before sexual contact, and then covered the penis with a condom. Analgesia reaches its maximum at 2–3 hours.

K. **Dyspareunia and vaginismus.** All physical causes should be treated in women who experience pain with intercourse. For persistent dyspareunia, and for vaginismus, programs of **systematic desensitization** (see section III,C, specific sexual therapy techniques) are the most effective management.

L. **Antidepressant-associated SD.** Antidepressants commonly cause sexual dysfunction, with 40–70% of patients taking SSRIs reporting problems with sexual functioning. One must effectively manage these treatment-emergent dysfunctions so that patients will maintain therapeutic antidepressant treatment and thereby prevent relapse and recurrence of serious depression. Five treatment options are available to manage these troublesome side effects.

1. **Prescribe drugs that counter the side effects.** Various receptor agonists, partial agonists, or antagonist agents have been tried, but they lack well-designed placebo-controlled, double-blind studies to support their effectiveness. Limited studies with cyproheptadine, buspirone, amantadine, and granisetron do not demonstrate a response rate that significantly exceeds placebo.

2. **Select an antidepressant less likely to cause SD.** When initiating antidepressant treatment, choose an agent such as nefazodone, mirtazapine, or bupropion that produces sexual dysfunction less frequently.

3. **Augment or substitute with another antidepressant.** Bupropion is used most in this context, and prescribed in one of three ways: 75–150 mg as needed 1–2 hours prior to sexual activity, as daily add-on therapy in conjunction with an SSRI, or as an initial daily full dose add-on to relieve the SD, followed by a taper and discontinuation of the initial SSRI.

4. **Adaptation.** Some patients develop spontaneous remission, or tolerance to treatment-emergent SD side effects. Controversy exists, however, about whether this occurs at a clinically significant rate. Since better management options exist, this wait-and-see approach has less support.

5. **Sildenafil.** Evidence shows that sildenafil significantly improves ejaculation and orgasm in men with **ED** who are also taking SSRIs. Furthermore, depressed men with ED respond to sildenafil as well as any other subgroup of men. Study doses ranged from 25 to 200 mg taken 1 hour prior to anticipated sexual activity. Using sildenafil allows men to continue therapeutic doses of an effective antidepressant.

In both open-label and double-blind, placebo-controlled studies, sildenafil, dosed at 50–100 mg prior to intercourse, also reversed treatment-emergent SD in women with an efficacy that compared to its use in men.

IV. **Prognosis**

A. **SDDs.** The few published studies indicate that **SDDs** for both men and women resist sustained behavioral change. Following therapy, one study noted initial improvement that was sustained at 3 months but that had regressed to below pretherapy levels by 3 years. Prognosis is better if the problem is secondary, the partners are younger, the symptoms are present <1 year, the marital relationship is stable, the partners are emotionally calm and motivated toward intervention, both partners view each other as loving and attractive, both partners find pleasure in sexual behavior, neither partner has a different sexual orientation or major psychopathology, and the couple complies with homework assignments during therapy.

B. ED. The natural history and prognosis of ED depend on many variables, most particularly the underlying problem. Most data on **psychosexual treatment** success were obtained before recent diagnostic advances permitted better differentiation between organic and psychogenic causes. Reported success rates range from 50% to 90%. Treatment success for **surgical implants** is 85–95% in achieving effective erections, with long-term patient satisfaction rates approaching 80% and partner satisfaction rates between 60% and 80%. Success with **intracavernosal injections** varies from 60% to 92%, but only 50–80% of men who start on self-injections continue to use them long-term. Satisfaction with the **vacuum-constriction** device is 68–92%, with 60% of men who are able to apply it successfully continuing to use it long-term. Reported success rates with **intraurethral PGE₁** are approximately 40%. Oral agents also vary in success. From 70% to 85% of men using **sildenafil** achieve erections firm enough for intercourse. Men with diabetes, and some of those with neurologic dysfunction, spinal cord injuries, prostatic surgery, and pelvic irradiation, report lower response rates, between 35% and 67%. In men with mild ED, **phentolamine** has a response rate of 37% at the 40-mg dose and 45% at the 80-mg level. Reported success with **apomorphine** in mild ED is 46% with 2 mg, 52% with 4 mg, and 60% with 6 mg.

C. FOD. The natural history of untreated **FOD** is unknown. Women whose orgasmic disorder is primary respond rapidly to treatment with a high success rate when therapy focuses specifically on sexual matters. Women with secondary orgasmic disorders do better when traditional marital therapy is combined with sexual therapy. Masters and Johnson report success rates of 83% for primary disorders and 77% for secondary disorders using **dual-gender therapy. Directed masturbation** training to treat primary disorders is successful in helping women reach orgasm 90% of the time during masturbation and 75% of the time with a partner. As new pharmacologic agents and Eros Therapy become integrated into treatment, these outcome figures may improve even more.

D. MOD. Outcome studies on treatment for MOD are limited by its relative rarity. Reported success rates range from 46% to 82%.

E. PE. Masters and Johnson report 95% success rates with the **start–stop–squeeze technique.** Others report rates around 60%. Long-term successes, however, are disappointing. In one study, men treated for PE showed immediate post-treatment gains in foreplay length, sexual relationship satisfaction, male acceptance, and intercourse duration. By 3 years post-treatment, however, frequency and desire for sexual contact, intercourse duration, and marital satisfaction all regressed, with marital satisfaction and intercourse duration dropping to pretreatment levels.

The best data on **pharmacologic management** are available for clomipramine, sertraline, fluoxetine, and paroxetine. Sexual satisfaction rates are reported at 53% for **clomipramine** along with a statistically significant increase in ejaculation latency time. For **sertraline,** sexual satisfaction rates range from 42% to 87%, with significantly increased ejaculation latency. The data on **fluoxetine's** success are variable. Some studies indicate a significant increase in ejaculation latency, but others suggest that it is no better than placebo. When men use **paroxetine,** they report as much as a 75% improvement in the quality of their sexual activity. When they **add sildenafil to paroxetine,** they can further prolong ejaculatory latency and the quality of overall sexual activity increases to 87.5%. In the pilot sample used to study **topical lidocaine–prilocaine,** 80% graded the result as "excellent" or "better."

F. Dyspareunia. Prognosis depends on the nature of any associated organic problems and the success with which they are treated. Women with a pure psychogenic basis for their problem report treatment success rates of around 95%.

G. Vaginismus is very amenable to treatment. In one group of women who were followed up for 4 years, 95% achieved and maintained sexual functioning. A desire for childbearing, a husband-initiated consultation, and a couple's perception that the problem was psychogenic predicted successful outcomes. Unsuccessful outcomes were associated with a firm belief that the problem was organic, experience with a previous anatomic problem, abundant sexual misinformation, a negative attitude toward genitalia, fear of sexually transmitted disease, and negative parental attitudes toward sex.

GENERAL REFERENCES

Halvorsen JG: The clinical evaluation of common sexual concerns. CNS Spectrums 2003;**8**(3):217.
Heimann JR, Meston CM: Evaluating sexual dysfunction in women. Clin Obstet Gynecol 1997;**40**(3):616.

Kandeel FR, Koussa VKT, Swerdloff RS: Male sexual function and its disorders: Physiology, patho-physiology, clinical investigation, and treatment. Endocrine Rev 2001;**22**(3):342.
Laumann EO, Paik A, Rosen RC: Sexual dysfunction in the United States: Prevalence and predictors. JAMA 1999;**281**:537.
Meston CM, Frohlich PF: The neurobiology of sexual function. Arch Gen Psychiatry 2000;**57**(11):1012.

REFERENCES FOR QUESTIONNAIRES

Rosen RC, et al: The International Index of Erectile Function (IIEF): A multidimensional scale for assessment of erectile dysfunction. Urology 1997;**49**:822.
Rosen RC, et al: Development and evaluation of an abridged, 5-item version of the International Index of Erectile Function (IIEF-5) as a diagnostic tool for erectile dysfunction. Int J Impotence Res 1999;**11**(6):319. http://www.viagra.com/consumer/aboutED/findOutShim.asp
Rosen R, et al: The female sexual function index (FSFI): A multidimensional self-report instrument for the assessment of female sexual function. J Sex Marital Therapy 2000;**26**:191. http://www.fsfi-questionnaire.com/default.htm

SECTION V. Preventive Medicine & Health Promotion

100   Counseling

Angela D. Mickalide, PhD, CHES

Patient education and counseling is one of the most effective prevention strategies available to primary care providers. The Institute of Medicine recommends that schools of medicine incorporate into their core curriculum basic screening techniques for adverse health habits and nonpharmacologic preventive strategies. Efforts by clinicians to influence such behaviors as tobacco use, exercise, nutrition, and alcohol and other drug abuse are more likely to decrease illness and premature death than are many other types of clinical preventive interventions. Forty to 70% of the 12 million years of productive life lost annually in the United States is preventable by adopting healthier lifestyles. Although a study of state trends in the delivery of clinical preventive services reveals some improvements over the past decade, physicians, in general, continue to counsel patients too infrequently. Sparse financial remuneration, lack of behavioral education skills, and organizational constraints are among the factors accounting for low rates of physician counseling.

I. Behavioral Risk Factors Amenable to Counseling

A. Tobacco use. The effectiveness of clinician counseling in prevention of tobacco use is well documented, particularly when multiple intervention strategies are used, including face-to-face counseling, scheduled reinforcement, behavioral contracts, self-help materials, referral to community programs, and drug therapy (Table 100–1). A prescription for nicotine patches or gum is recommended for certain patients.

1. Cigarette, cigar, pipe, and smokeless tobacco cessation counseling should be offered to patients who use such products and to nonusers at risk for beginning this habit, for example, adolescents, who should be advised not to start.

2. The detrimental effects of tobacco use and secondhand smoke on unborn and young children should be discussed with all pregnant women and parents.

B. Nutrition. Clinicians have several roles in nutritional counseling: taking a complete and accurate dietary history, working with patients to identify the obstacles to changing dietary patterns, and providing advice on food selection and preparation. Physicians who lack the time or skills to assist patients with their nutritional knowledge and behaviors should involve registered dietitians, nutritionists, and other trained staff.

1. Dietary intake of calories, fat (especially trans fat and saturated fat), cholesterol, complex carbohydrates, fiber, and sodium is among the nutritional topics that clinicians should discuss routinely with patients. Caloric intake should be balanced with energy expenditures through a well-balanced diet and regular exercise.

2. An ideal diet consists of the Food Guide Pyramid's five major food groups, which together meet nutritional requirements. These are (1) breads, cereals, and grains; (2) fruits; (3) vegetables; (4) milk, yogurt, and cheese; and (5) meats and proteins. Patients should consume fats, oils, and sweets sparingly. An individual's age, gender, and physical activity can help determine the number of servings needed to maintain a well-balanced diet.

3. Adolescent and adult females should be alerted to the importance of dietary calcium and iron intake.

4. Pregnant women should be advised of their special nutritional needs, and parents should be counseled about the dietary requirements of infants and young children.

C. Exercise. Clinicians should advise all patients, especially women, ethnic minorities, adults with lower educational attainment, and older adults, to engage in regular moderate-intensity physical activity. Recommendations for regular physical activity should be tailored to the health status and lifestyle of each patient.

1. Every American adult should accumulate 30 minutes or more of moderate-intensity physical activity over the course of most days of the week. Activities that can contribute to the 30-minute total include walking, gardening, dancing, or washing windows or floors, as well as planned exercise such as jogging, swimming, and bicycling (Table 100–2).

2. Patients should be given instructions on the safe performance of exercise, and those at increased risk of injury or medical complications should be advised about

TABLE 100–1. SYNOPSIS FOR PRIMARY CARE PROVIDERS: HOW TO HELP YOUR PATIENTS STOP USING TOBACCO

1. Ask about tobacco use at every opportunity
2. Advise all tobacco users to stop
3. Assist the patient in stopping
   a. Help set a quit date
   b. Provide self-help materials
   c. Recommend nicotine gum or prescription drugs for tobacco cessation, especially for highly addicted patients (those who smoke one pack a day or more; those who smoke their first cigarette within 30 minutes of waking; or those who use other tobacco products several times daily)
   d. Consider signing a stop-tobacco contract with the patient
4. Arrange follow-up visits

Modified with permission from Glynn TJ, Manley MW: *How to Help Your Patients Stop Smoking: A National Cancer Institute Manual for Physicians.* National Cancer Institute; April 1990. Publication No. DHHS (PHS) 90-3064.

appropriate physical activity. Clinicians who lack the skills or time to design effective exercise programs for patients should rely on the expertise of accredited fitness centers and exercise specialists.

D. **Intentional injuries**
   1. **Suicide**
      a. Clinicians should be alert to suicidal ideation among patients at high risk as a result of recent divorce, separation, unemployment, depression, alcohol and other drug abuse, major medical illnesses, living alone, and recent bereavement. Adolescents are at particular risk for suicide; risk factors include declines in school performance or attendance, isolation or changes in peer relations,

TABLE 100–2. EXAMPLES OF MODERATE AMOUNTS OF PHYSICAL ACTIVITY

Activity[1,2]	Relationship of Time Spent and Intensity of Effort
	Less Vigorous, More Time
Washing and waxing a car for 45–60 minutes	
Washing windows or floors for 45–60 minutes	
Playing volleyball for 45 minutes	
Playing touch football for 30–45 minutes	
Gardening for 30–45 minutes	
Wheeling self in wheelchair for 30–40 minutes	
Walking 1¾ miles in 35 minutes (20 min/mile)	
Basketball (shooting baskets) for 30 minutes	
Bicycling 5 miles in 30 minutes	
Dancing fast (social) for 30 minutes	
Pushing a stroller 1½ miles in 30 minutes	
Raking leaves for 30 minutes	
Walking 2 miles in 30 minutes (15 min/mile)	
Water aerobics for 30 minutes	
Swimming laps for 20 minutes	
Wheelchair basketball for 20 minutes	
Basketball (playing a game) for 15–20 minutes	
Bicycling 4 miles in 15 minutes	
Jumping rope for 15 minutes	
Running 1½ miles in 15 minutes (10 min/mile)	
Shoveling snow for 15 minutes	
Stairwalking for 15 minutes	
	More Vigorous, Less Time

[1] A moderate amount of physical activity is roughly equivalent to physical activity that uses approximately 150 Calories (kcal) of energy per day, or 1000 Calories per week.
[2] Some activities can be performed at various intensities; the suggested durations correspond to expected intensity of effort.
From Centers for Disease Control and Prevention, National Center for Chronic Disease Prevention and Health Promotion, Division of Nutrition and Physical Activity; 1996.

and excessive anger or fighting behavior. Older adults are also at excess suicide risk.

  b. Patients with suicidal ideations should be questioned about the extent of their plans (eg, distribution of possessions, obtaining a weapon, writing a suicide note). If suicidal intent is serious, clinicians should make immediate referrals to mental health professionals and consider possible hospitalization. Persons with suicidal thoughts should also be alerted to community resources such as local mental health agencies and crisis intervention centers.

2. Violence

  a. Both the history (discussion of previous violent experiences and current risk factors, such as weapons in the home and discord in the peer group and community) and the physical examination (detection of burns, bruises, and other traumatic injuries) can be used to identify victims of abuse or neglect. Clinicians who suspect violence among patients should refer both the victims and the perpetrators to mental health professionals and other community resources to prevent future episodes.

  b. Certain physical, behavioral, and medical signs indicate child neglect and abuse (see Chapter 91). Physicians must report probable cases of such abuse to local child protective service agencies. In addition, clinicians should be alert to risk signs for adolescent violence such as fighting, bullying, chronic victimization, weapon-carrying, history of domestic violence, and changes in peer relations.

E. Unintentional injuries

1. **Motor vehicle-related injuries.** Physicians should urge all patients to use federally approved occupant restraints (eg, safety belts and child safety seats), to wear safety helmets when riding motorcycles and bicycles, and to avoid driving while under the influence of alcohol or other psychoactive drugs. Clinician counseling is particularly urged for individuals at increased risk of motor vehicle injury, such as adolescents and young adults, alcohol and other drug users, and patients with certain medical conditions that affect safety. These individuals should be encouraged to discuss with their families transportation alternatives for social activities in which any drugs are being used.

2. **Environmental and household injuries.** Although passive interventions (eg, child-resistant containers to prevent poisoning) are the most effective measures to control injuries, clinician counseling may help patients reduce their risks of household and environmental injuries (eg, falls, drowning, fire, poisoning, suffocation, and firearm mishaps).

  a. Patients should be advised to abstain from alcohol or other psychoactive drug use when participating in potentially dangerous activities (eg, swimming, boating, bicycling, driving, or handling firearms).

  b. Smokers should be advised against smoking near upholstery or in bed.

  c. Patients should be urged to install, and check monthly, smoke detectors in their homes and to set hot-water heaters at 48.4 °C (120 °F).

  d. Patients with **children in the home** should be counseled to lock all medications, toxic substances, matches, and firearms out of the reach of children; to have a 1-oz bottle of syrup of ipecac available; and to display emergency numbers prominently near telephones (eg, the police department, the fire department, 911, the local Poison Control Center, and toll-free number [1-(800) 222-1222]).

    To prevent falls, adults should be advised to place collapsible gates or other barriers at stairway entrances, to install four-sided fencing with self-latching and self-closing gates around swimming pools and spas, and to install window guards on all windows not designated as emergency fire exits.

    Bicyclists and parents of children who ride bicycles should be made aware of the importance of wearing safety helmets and avoiding riding in motor vehicle traffic.

  e. To prevent falls among **older patients,** clinicians should suggest modifications to their home environments, for example, tacking down carpets and arranging furniture so that pathways are not cluttered; testing their visual acuity periodically; and closely monitoring their use of drugs that can increase the risk of falls. Older patients should receive instructions on appropriate physical exercises to maintain and improve flexibility and mobility. Patients with medical conditions affecting mobility should receive special counseling on measures to prevent falls.

F. Sexual behavior
   1. Sexually transmitted diseases (STDs)
   a. Clinicians should take a complete sexual and drug use history of all adolescent and adult patients and offer STD screening according to recommended guidelines (see Chapter 102). Clinicians should discuss sexual behavior with respect, compassion, and confidentiality.
   b. Sexually active patients should be counseled that the most effective strategy to prevent infection with human immunodeficiency virus (HIV) or other STDs is to abstain from sex or maintain a mutually monogamous sexual relationship with a partner known to be uninfected. Patients should be counseled to engage in routine screening since many STDs are asymptomatic. Sexual activity with persons of uncertain infection status should be discouraged. Clinicians should counsel women of childbearing age on the dangers of HIV and STD infection during pregnancy.
   c. Patients should be alerted that a nonreactive HIV test does not rule out infection if the sexual partner has engaged in sexual intercourse during the 6 months prior to testing. Safe (or "safer") sexual practices (eg, massage, hugging, or dry kissing [Table 100–3]) should be encouraged. Reducing the number of sexual partners and consistent and proper use of condoms should be discussed with patients who have multiple sexual partners (see Chapter 95).
   d. Intravenous drug users should be urged to participate in drug treatment programs, warned against sharing and using unsterilized drug paraphernalia, and directed to community programs making uncontaminated equipment available.
   2. Unintended pregnancy. Clinicians should discuss the efficacy, limitations, and proper use of available contraceptive techniques (see Chapter 95). Clinicians

---

TABLE 100–3. "SAFER SEX" PRACTICES SUGGESTED FOR REDUCING THE RISK OF SEXUALLY TRANSMITTED DISEASES

The most effective strategies are sexual abstinence or the maintenance of a mutually monogamous sexual relationship. In other cases, the following practices should be observed

_____ Always use a latex condom during sexual intercourse. The application of spermicides and the use of diaphragms by women may also decrease risk

_____ Avoid multiple partners, anonymous partners, prostitutes, persons with multiple partners, persons who use intravenous drugs, and those not known to be seronegative for human immunodeficiency virus (HIV)

_____ Avoid sexual contact with persons who have a genital discharge, genital warts, genital herpes lesions, or evidence of hepatitis B surface antigen

_____ Do not practice anal intercourse. Avoid all sexual activities that could cause cuts or tears in the lining of the rectum, vagina, or penis

_____ Avoid oral–anal sex to prevent enteric lesions

_____ Avoid genital contact with oral herpetic lesions

_____ Persons at increased risk should be especially careful to avoid mouth contact with the penis, vagina, or rectum

_____ Persons who use intravenous drugs should receive treatment and should never use unsterilized or shared injection equipment

_____ Persons at increased risk should have a periodic examination for sexually transmitted diseases

Safe sexual activities
Massage
Hugging
Body rubbing (dry)
Kissing (dry)
Masturbation (on healthy skin)
Hand-to-genital touching or mutual masturbation

Possibly safe sexual activities (these activities are completely safe if both partners are known to be uninfected)
Kissing (wet)
Oral sex on men wearing latex condoms
Oral sex on women (who are not menstruating or experiencing a vaginal infection with discharge)

Data from Novello A: *Surgeon General's Report on Acquired Immune Deficiency Syndrome.* Office of the Surgeon General, US Department of Health and Human Services, Public Health Service; 1993.
Additional data adapted from Sexually transmitted diseases treatment guidelines, September 1993. MMWR 1993;**42**:RR-14.

should review the menstrual cycle with patients, as appropriate, so that they better understand their contraceptive options and their own fecundity.

G. Dental disease
  1. Clinicians should counsel patients to visit a dentist regularly, to brush their teeth daily with a fluoride-containing toothpaste, and to use dental floss daily to clean between teeth. Young children should have their first dental visit by age 2. Children, particularly those younger than age 6, should be taught to spit out rather than swallow toothpaste containing fluoride, to prevent dental fluorosis. Patients with dental abnormalities found through visual examination (eg, nursing bottle tooth decay, crowding or malalignment of teeth, dental caries, or periodontal infections) should be referred to their dentist for further evaluation.
  2. Patients should be advised to limit their intake of foods containing refined sugar, particularly between-meal snacks. To reduce the risk of early childhood caries, infants should not be put to bed with a bottle. If a bedtime bottle is necessary, only those filled with water should be used.
  3. Children living in areas with inadequate fluoride in their drinking water should be prescribed daily fluoride drops or tablets according to recommended guidelines (Table 100–4). Clinicians prescribing fluoride supplements for children must know the concentration of fluoride in the child's drinking water.
  4. Clinicians should urge patients to reduce their risk of oral cancer by eliminating tobacco use and limiting alcoholic beverage consumption. All patients who smoke cigarettes, pipes, or cigars or who use spit tobacco should be counseled to stop, and those who do not use tobacco, especially adolescents and young adults, should be encouraged to resist pressure to start.

H. Alcohol and other drugs
  1. The routine history for all adolescents and adults should include questions about the quantity, frequency, and other patterns of use of wine, beer, liquor, or other drugs. Questionnaires are available for more systematic detection of problem drinking, but there are limitations in either their accuracy or their suitability for routine use in busy practices.
  2. Clinicians should provide substance-abusing patients with information about chemical dependence, the effects of the drug, and its effect on health. Intravenous drug users should be referred for treatment and warned against the use of contaminated or shared needles, which can transmit HIV, hepatitis B virus, and other organisms. Treatment plans should be tailored to the drug of abuse and the individual needs of the patient and his or her family (see Chapter 88).

I. Self-examination. Although widely practiced, self-examination of the breast, testes, skin, and other sites has not been conclusively proved to be an effective maneuver for reducing cancer mortality. The teaching of self-examination is neither specifically recommended nor discouraged.

J. Exposure to ultraviolet light
  1. To prevent skin cancer, clinicians should advise all patients of effective techniques to reduce outdoor exposure to ultraviolet (UV) light. Patients with increased occupational or recreational exposure to sunlight as well as those who live in tropical climates should be counseled to regularly apply broad-spectrum sunscreen with

TABLE 100–4. DIETARY FLUORIDE SUPPLEMENT DOSAGE SCHEDULE

| Age of Child | Fluoride Ion Level in Drinking Water (ppm)[1] | | |
	<0.3 ppm	0.3–0.6 ppm	>0.6 ppm
Birth–6 mo	None	None	None
6 mo–3 yr	0.25 mg/day[2]	None	None
3–6 yr	0.50 mg/day	0.25 mg/day	None
6–16 yr	1 mg/day	0.50 mg/day	None

[1] 1 ppm = 1 mg/L.
[2] 2.2 mg of sodium fluoride contains 1 mg of fluoride ion.
From American Dental Association: Council on Scientific Affairs, association report on dietary fluoride supplements. JADA 1995; **126:**19-S.

UVA/UVB protection. They should also be advised to wear protective clothing, such as wide-brimmed hats and long-sleeved shirts and slacks and to try to reduce outdoor activity between 10 AM and 3 PM.

   2. Parents should also be reminded to limit their children's exposure to ultraviolet light through similar measures.

II. Techniques for Counseling. The Counseling and Behavioral Interventions Work Group of the United States Preventive Services Task Force has developed a broad range of counseling strategies, referred to as the Five A's construct, applicable across a variety of risk behaviors. The minimal contact interventions provided by clinical staff in a primary care setting are as follows:

- **Assess:** Ask about/assess behavioral health risk(s) and factors affecting choice of behavior change goals/methods.
- **Advise:** Give clear, specific, and personalized behavior change advice, including information about personal health harms and benefits.
- **Agree:** Collaboratively select appropriate treatment goals and methods based on the patient's interest in and willingness to change behavior.
- **Assist:** Using behavior change techniques (self-help, counseling, or both), aid the patient in achieving agreed-upon goals by acquiring the skills, confidence, and social/environmental supports for behavior change, supplemented with adjunctive medical treatments when appropriate (eg, pharmacotherapy for tobacco dependence, contraceptive drugs/devices).
- **Arrange:** Schedule follow-up contacts (in person or by telephone) to provide ongoing assistance/support and to adjust the treatment plan as needed, including referral to more intensive or specialized treatment.

REFERENCES

Gebbie K, Rosenstock L, Hernandez LM: *Who Will Keep the Public Healthy? Educating Public Health Professionals for the 21st Century.* Institute of Medicine of the National Academies; 2003.

Healthy People 2010. US Department of Health and Human Services (Conference Edition, in two volumes). US Department of Health and Human Services; January 2000.

Jones DA, et al: Moderate leisure-time physical activity: Who is meeting the public health recommendations? A national cross-sectional study. Arch Fam Med May/June 1998;**7**:285.

McGinnis JM: Health in America—The sum of its parts. JAMA (May 22/29) 2002;**287**(20):2711.

O'Donnell GO, Mickalide AD: *SAFE KIDS at Home, At Play & On the Way: A Report to the Nation on Unintentional Childhood Injury.* National SAFE KIDS Campaign; April 1998.

US Centers for Disease Control and Prevention: HIV prevention through early detection and treatment of other sexually transmitted diseases: United States. MMWR July 1998; vol 47.

US Preventive Services Task Force: *Guide to Clinical Preventive Services,* 2nd ed. Williams & Wilkins; 1996, and *Guide to Clinical Preventive Services,* 3rd ed. 2000–2003. http://www.ahrq.gov/clinic/cps3dix.htm.

Wallis AL, Cody BE, Mickalide AD: *Report to the Nation: Trends in Unintentional Childhood Injury Mortality, 1987–2000.* National SAFE KIDS Campaign, May 2003.

Whitlock EP, et al: Evaluating primary care behavioral counseling interventions. Am J Prev Med 2002;**22**(4):267.

---

101   Immunization

William E. Cayley, Jr., MD, MDiv, & Cynthia Haq, MD

I. Introduction. Immunizations are among the most cost-effective preventive health measures, having significantly reduced the rates of infectious disease among children, adolescents, and adults. Nevertheless, vaccine coverage of the general population is less than optimal due to missed opportunities or to misconceptions by parents and clinicians. Furthermore, since no vaccine is completely safe or completely effective, administration of vaccines requires an understanding of the risks and benefits involved—the benefits to the individual and to society at large, weighed against the risks to the individual. Additional immunization resources, as well as updates on vaccine shortages and other important issues, can be found on the centers for Disease Control and Prevention (CDC) web site at: http://www.cdc.gov/nip/

A. Timing. Every health care visit is an opportunity to update a patient's immunization status. Current recommendations for vaccinations are available on the CDC web site and should be followed as closely as possible. Childhood schedules are updated annually in January, and schedules for adolescents and adults are revised as needed. Recommendations are based on immunizing the youngest age group at risk of disease in whom the vaccine is safe and effective. Doses administered too closely together may lead to inadequate immune response. Since delays in dosing do not reduce final antibody response, catch-up doses are not needed. Administering multiple vaccines at the same visit is both safe and effective; but while inactivated vaccines can be given any time before or after other live or inactivated vaccines, live vaccines not administered at the same time should be separated by at least 4 weeks. Interruptions or delays in a vaccination series do not require restarting that series, but if past records cannot be located, the patient should be considered nonimmune and started on the appropriate schedule of doses.

B. Administration. Routes of administration are recommended by the manufacturer of each vaccine. Subcutaneous (SC) injections are administered at a 45-degree angle into the thigh of infants 12 months or younger, and into the upper-outer triceps of older patients. Intramuscular (IM) injections are given at a 90-degree angle into the deep muscle mass of the anterolateral thigh (for infants) or the deltoid (for older children and adults). IM injections should not be given into the buttock, due to risk of injury to the sciatic nerve. Intradermal (ID) injections are usually given on the volar aspect of the forearm, with the needle inserted parallel to the long axis of the arm with the bevel facing up so that the entire bevel penetrates the skin and the injected solution raises a small bleb. If two or more vaccinations are given, each should be given at a different anatomic site. The location of each injection should be documented in the medical record.

C. Cautions. The only contraindication applying to all vaccines is that patients with a history of severe allergic response to a vaccine or one of its components should not receive further doses of that vaccine. Mild illnesses, such as upper respiratory tract infections, otitis media, or diarrhea, are not contraindications to vaccination, and research has generally demonstrated adequate antibody response to vaccinations given at the time of mild illness. Patients with more severe illness should be immunized once the acute phase of the illness is over, to avoid confusing effects of the illness with vaccine side effects. Routine examinations and temperature measurements are not prerequisites for immunizing children—an appropriate procedure is to ask the parent if the child is ill, and then postpone vaccination only for those with moderate or severe illnesses. Live vaccines may pose some risk for immunosuppressed family members, and in this context an inactivated vaccine may be preferred.

II. Childhood Immunizations. Immunizations should be given according to the annually updated schedule published on the CDC web site. For the 2004 recommendations, see Table 101–1.

A. Hepatitis B (HBV)

1. **Overview.** Each year approximately 4000 people in the United States die of sequelae of hepatitis B infection such as chronic liver disease and primary hepatocellular carcinoma. In 1991, the CDC advocated universal immunization of infants against hepatitis B in order to protect children younger than 5 years, who are at higher risk of chronic disease if they become infected, and in order to increase immunity among the general population, since targeted immunization of high-risk groups had been ineffective at lowering the incidence of new infection. Hepatitis B vaccines are manufactured using recombinant DNA technology.

2. **Timing and administration.** Three doses of vaccine are required for adequate immunity. Infants born to mothers who are hepatitis B surface antigen (HBsAg) negative should receive a first dose of single-antigen hepatitis B vaccine between birth and age 8 weeks (ideally, at birth). If the infant's mother is HBsAg positive or her HBsAg status is unknown, a first dose single-antigen hepatitis B vaccine should be given in the first 12 hours of life, along with 0.5 cc of hepatitis B immune globulin (HBIG) injected IM at another site. The series is always started with a single-antigen HBV such as Recombivax or Engerix-B (dosing for both is 0.5 cc IM for ages 0–19 years), and may be completed with either a single-antigen vaccine or with a combination vaccine such as Pediarix (HBV–diphtheria–tetanus–acelluar pertussis [DtaP]-inactivated poliovirus vaccine [IPV]) or COMVAX (HBV–*Haemophilus influenza* type B [Hib]). For the recommended dosing schedules, see Table 101–2.

TABLE 101-1. RECOMMENDED CHILDHOOD AND ADOLESCENT IMMUNIZATION SCHEDULE—UNITED STATES, JANUARY–JUNE 2004

Vaccine ▼ / Age ►	Birth	1 mo	2 mo	4 mo	6 mo	12 mo	15 mo	18 mo	24 mo	4–6 y	11–12 y	13–18 y
Hepatitis B[1]	HepB #1	only if mother HBsAg (-)	HepB #2		HepB #3						HepB series	
Diphtheria, Tetanus, Pertussis[2]			DTaP	DTaP	DTaP		DTaP			DTaP	Td	Td
Haemophilus Influenzae Type b[3]			Hib	Hib	Hib[3]	Hib						
Inactivated Poliovirus			IPV	IPV	IPV		IPV			IPV		
Measles, Mumps, Rubella[4]						MMR #1				MMR #2	MMR #2	
Varicella[5]						Varicella					Varicella	
Pneumococcal[6]			PCV	PCV	PCV	PCV	PCV		PCV	PCV	PPV	
Hepatitis A[7]										Hepatitis A series		
Influenza[8]					Influenza (yearly)							

Vaccines below this line are for selected populations

This schedule indicates the recommended ages for routine administration of currently licensed childhood vaccines, as of December 1, 2003, for children through age 18 years. Any dose not given at the recommended age should be given at any subsequent visit when indicated and feasible. ■ indicates age groups that warrant special effort to administer those vaccines not previously given. Additional vaccines may be licensed and recommended during the year. Licensed combination vaccines may be used whenever any components of the combination are indicated and the vaccine's other components are not contraindicated. Providers should consult the manufacturers' package inserts for detailed recommendations. Clinically significant adverse events that follow immunization should be reported to the Vaccine Adverse Event Reporting System (VAERS). Guidance about how to obtain and complete a VAERS form can be found on the Internet: http://www.vaers.org/ or by calling 1-800-822-7967.

From the Advisory Committee on Immunization Practices, Centers for Disease Control and Prevention. Department of Health and Human Services, 2004

Approved by the Advisory Committee on Immunization Practices (www.cdc.gov/nip/acip), the American Academy of Pediatrics (www.aap.org), and the American Academy of Family Physicians (www.aafp.org).

1. Hepatitis B (HepB) vaccine. All infants should receive the first dose of hepatitis B vaccine soon after birth and before hospital discharge; the first dose may also be given by age 2 months if the infant's mother is hepatitis B surface antigen (HBsAg) negative. Only monovalent HepB can be used for the birth dose. Monovalent or combination vaccine containing HepB may be used to complete the series. Four doses of vaccine may be administered when a birth dose is given. The second dose should be given at least 4 weeks after the first dose, except for combination vaccines which cannot be administered before age 6 weeks. The third dose should be given at least 16 weeks after the first dose and at least 8 weeks after the second dose. The last dose in the vaccination series (third or fourth dose) should not be administered before age 24 weeks.

Infants born to HBsAg-positive mothers should receive HepB and 0.5 mL of Hepatitis B Immune Globulin (HBIG) within 12 hours of birth at separate sites. The second dose is recommended at age 1 to 2 months. The last dose in the immunization series should not be administered before age 24 weeks. These infants should be tested for HBsAg and antibody to HBsAg (anti-HBs) at age 9 to 15 months.

Infants born to mothers whose HBsAg status is unknown should receive the first dose of the HepB series within 12 hours of birth. Maternal blood should be drawn as soon as possible to determine the mother's HBsAg status; if the HBsAg test is positive, the infant should receive HBIG as soon as possible (no later than age 1 week). The second dose is recommended at age 1 to 2 months. The last dose in the immunization series should not be administered before age 24 weeks.

2. Diphtheria and tetanus toxoids and acellular pertussis (DTaP) vaccine. The fourth dose of DTaP may be administered as early as age 12 months, provided 6 months have elapsed since the third dose and the child is unlikely to return at age 15 to 18 months. The final dose in the series should be given at age ≥4 years. **Tetanus and diphtheria toxoids (Td)** is recommended at age 11 to 12 years if at least 5 years have elapsed since the last dose of tetanus and diphtheria toxoid-containing vaccine. Subsequent routine Td boosters are recommended every 10 years.

3. Haemophilus influenzae type b (Hib) conjugate vaccine. Three Hib conjugate vaccines are licensed for infant use. If PRP-OMP (PedvaxHIB or ComVax [Merck]) is administered at ages 2 and 4 months, a dose at age 6 months is not required. DTaP/Hib combination products should not be used for primary im-

munization in infants at ages 2, 4 or 6 months but can be used as boosters following any Hib vaccine. The final dose in the series should be given at age ≥12 months.

4. Measles, mumps, and rubella vaccine (MMR). The second dose of MMR is recommended routinely at age 4 to 6 years but may be administered during any visit, provided at least 4 weeks have elapsed since the first dose and both doses are administered beginning at or after age 12 months. Those who have not previously received the second dose should complete the schedule by the 11- to 12-year-old visit.

5. Varicella vaccine. Varicella vaccine is recommended at any visit at or after age 12 months for susceptible children (i.e., those who lack a reliable history of chickenpox). Susceptible persons age ≥13 years should receive 2 doses, given at least 4 weeks apart.

6. Pneumococcal vaccine. The heptavalent **pneumococcal conjugate vaccine (PCV)** is recommended for all children age 2 to 23 months. It is also recommended for certain children age 24 to 59 months. The final dose in the series should be given at age ≥12 months. **Pneumococcal polysaccharide vaccine (PPV)** is recommended in addition to PCV for certain high-risk groups. See *MMWR* 2000;49(RR-9):1–38.

7. Hepatitis A vaccine. Hepatitis A vaccine is recommended for children and adolescents in selected states and regions and for certain high-risk groups; consult your local public health authority. Children and adolescents in these states, regions, and high-risk groups who have not been immunized against hepatitis A can begin the hepatitis A immunization series during any visit. The 2 doses in the series should be administered at least 6 months apart. See *MMWR* 1999;48(RR-12):1–37.

8. Influenza vaccine. Influenza vaccine is recommended annually for children age ≥6 months with certain risk factors (including but not limited to children with asthma, cardiac disease, sickle cell disease, human immunodeficiency virus infection, and diabetes; and household members of persons in high-risk groups [see *MMWR* 2003;52(RR-8):1–36]) and can be administered to all others wishing to obtain immunity. In addition, healthy children age 6 to 23 months are encouraged to receive influenza vaccine if feasible, because children in this age group are at substantially increased risk of influenza-related hospitalizations. For healthy persons age 5 to 49 years, the intranasally administered live-attenuated influenza vaccine (LAIV) is an acceptable alternative to the intramuscular trivalent inactivated influenza vaccine (TIV). See *MMWR* 2003;52(RR-13):1–8. Children receiving TIV should be administered a dosage appropriate for their age (0.25 mL if age 6 to 35 months or 0.5 mL if age ≥3 years). Children age ≤8 years who are receiving influenza vaccine for the first time should receive 2 doses (separated by at least 4 weeks for TIV and at least 6 weeks for LAIV).

TABLE 101–2. HEPATITIS B VACCINATION SCHEDULES[1]

	Maternal Hepatitis B Surface Antigen (HbsAg) Negative	Maternal HBsAg Unknown or Positive
Single antigen	Birth, 2 months, 6 months	Birth, 1 month, 6 months
PEDIARIX	Birth, 2 months, 4 months, 6 months	Birth, 6 weeks, 4 months, 6 months
COMVAX	Birth, 2 months, 4 months, 12–15 months	Birth, 6 weeks, 4 months, 12–15 months

[1] The first dose is always given with a single-antigen vaccine, and all infants of mothers whose HBsAg is positive or unknown should also receive 0.5 cc of hepatitis B immune globulin (HBIG) injected IM at another site.

3. **Cautions.** Local pain and a mildly elevated temperature are the most common reactions. There has been a low rate of anaphylaxis (1 case in 600,000 vaccine doses) reported; thus, further HBV doses are contraindicated for those who have had anaphylaxis in response to a previous dose. There appears to be no association between HBV immunization and Guillain-Barré syndrome.

B. **Diphtheria–tetanus–pertussis (DTaP)**
   1. **Overview.** Childhood vaccination against diphtheria, tetanus, and pertussis has been routine in the United States since the 1940s. The older DTP vaccine combining diphtheria and tetanus toxoids with inactivated whole-cell pertussis has largely been replaced by the newer DTaP using an acellular preparation of pertussis toxin. Immunity to pertussis wanes, with little protection after 5–10 years, but current DTaP vaccines should not be used for immunizing adults because the dose of diphtheria toxoid is higher than recommended for those older than 7 years.
   2. **Timing and administration.** DTaP is administered by IM injection of 0.5 cc of vaccine, given at 2, 4, and 6 months. Booster doses are given at 15–18 months (or at least 6 months after the last dose), and again at 4–6 years.
   3. **Cautions.** Mild reactions such as fever or drowsiness or more severe reactions such as high temperatures >105 °F or febrile seizures may occur after DTaP administration but are much less common than with the older DTP vaccine. If encephalopathy, such as unresponsiveness or seizures, occurs within 7 days of DTaP administration and cannot be attributed to another cause, DT (diphtheria and tetanus toxoids alone) should be used for all subsequent immunizations. Stable neurologic conditions, or a family history of seizures, are not contraindications to pertussis immunization.

C. **Haemophilus influenzae type B (Hib)**
   1. **Overview.** Before development of effective vaccinations, 1 in 200 children developed invasive *Haemophilus* disease before age 5—many of these children developed meningitis with sequelae including hearing loss and mental retardation. Vaccines against *Haemophilus influenzae* type B have been 95–100% effective in preventing invasive Hib disease. Three Hib vaccines are available:
      a. *Haemophilus* b Diphtheria Protein Conjugate (HbOC).
      b. *Haemophilus* b Meningococcal Protein Conjugate (PRP-OMP).
      c. *Haemophilus* b Diphtheria Toxoid Conjugate (PRP-D).
   2. **Timing and administration.** Hib vaccines should not be given to infants younger than 6 weeks. The recommended schedule is a dose of Hib at 2, 4, and 6 months and a booster at 12–15 months. Children who have received PRP-OMP at 2 and 4 months do not require a dose at 6 months. The number of doses needed to complete an interrupted series depends on the vaccine type and the child's age.
   3. **Cautions.** Adverse effects from Hib vaccination are rare, usually occur after the third dose if at all, and are usually limited to mild fever, or local redness, swelling, or warmth.

D. **Polio**
   1. **Overview.** Introduction of polio vaccination in the 1950s led to control of polio in the Western Hemisphere. The live oral polio vaccine (OPV) carries a small but real risk of vaccine-associated paralytic polio, and so has been replaced in the United States by use of the inactivated polio vaccine (IPV) since 2000.
   2. **Timing and administration.** Children should receive four doses of IPV, at ages 2 and 4 months, between 6 and 18 months, and between 4 and 6 years. The dose is 0.5 cc of vaccine administered SC.

3. **Cautions.** There have been no serious adverse events associated with the use of IPV.
E. **Measles–Mumps–Rubella (MMR)**
   1. **Overview.** MMR vaccination has reduced the incidence of measles, mumps, rubella ("german measles") and congenital rubella syndrome by 99% over the course of the last century, although occasional outbreaks continue to occur among unimmunized persons. The MMR vaccine combines attenuated strains of all three viruses.
   2. **Timing and administration.** The first dose of MMR vaccine is given SC at 12–15 months of age, and the second dose can be administered at either 4–6 years or 11–12 years of age depending on state school immunization requirements.
   3. **Cautions.** Pain, redness, and local irritation are common side effects of all three vaccines. Rubella vaccine may rarely cause generalized lymphadenopathy in children or a transient arthralgia in young women, and mumps vaccine may rarely cause transient orchitis in young men. These side effects generally have no long-term sequelae. Egg allergy is not a contraindication to MMR vaccine, but the vaccine should not be given to persons with severe allergy to gelatin or neomycin. Patients with human immunodeficiency virus (HIV) should be given MMR if they are asymptomatic, but it should be withheld if they have low age-specific CD4 counts.
F. **Varicella-zoster virus (VZV)**
   1. **Overview.** VZV vaccine decreases the incidence and severity of childhood varicella, reduces the incidence of later adult varicella, and decreases the risk of later perinatal transmission of the virus. The vaccine contains a live attenuated virus.
   2. **Timing and administration.** Children with no history of chickenpox should be routinely vaccinated with a single 0.5-cc dose of VZV SC between 12 and 18 months of age. Serologic testing of children between 12 months and 12 years of age without a reliable history of chickenpox infection is not warranted prior to vaccination because most of these children are susceptible and because the vaccine is well tolerated by seropositive individuals.

   Varicella-zoster immune globulin (VZIG) is indicated in susceptible individuals following significant exposure and in newborns of mothers with varicella that occurred in the interval from 5 days prior to 2 days following delivery.
   3. **Cautions.** The vaccine is highly protective (97%) and appears to confer long-lasting immunity; however, about 1% of vaccinees per year develop mild, breakthrough infection that does not appear to be contagious. Studies on the duration of immunogenicity are ongoing. The vaccine is contraindicated in immunosuppressed individuals. Transient zoster in recipients and transmission to susceptible contacts of vaccinees has been reported.
G. **Pneumococcus**
   1. **Overview.** *Streptococcus pneumoniae* is a major cause of pediatric otitis media, pneumonia, meningitis, and bacteremia. Rates of disease are higher among those younger than 5 years than in older children and are highest in infants. The pneumococcal conjugate vaccine (PCV) contains antigens from seven serotypes of pneumococcus conjugated to a carrier protein. It became available in 2000 and has been found effective in reducing invasive disease and pneumonia (vaccinating 151 patients will prevent one case of pneumonia or invasive disease).
   2. **Timing and administration.** PCV should be given as 0.5 cc IM to children at 2, 4, 6, and 12–15 months of age. Since the highest risk of invasive disease is in children younger than age 2, catch-up vaccination with PCV between ages 2 and 5 is recommended only for children with increased risk of disease due to HIV, sickle-cell disease, asplenia, or chronic illness.
   3. **Cautions.** Local redness and tenderness at the injection site are the only reported adverse effects of PCV. This vaccine is not licensed for use in adults.
H. **Hepatitis A (HAV)**
   1. **Overview.** Hepatitis A virus is usually transmitted by the fecal-oral route. While acute disease is more common in adults, children generally have asymptomatic infection and so can be an important source of infection for older individuals. Hepatitis A immune globulin has been available for several years for inducing passive immunity, and since 1995 two inactivated-virus vaccines conferring active immunity against hepatitis A have been available (HAV and VAQTA).
   2. **Timing and administration.** Individuals living in communities with high rates of hepatitis A should be immunized, as should those planning international travel to

areas with high rates of hepatitis A. Vaccination may also be used in the setting of community outbreaks. Specific information on high-risk areas for hepatitis A is available from the CDC. For pediatric usage, HAVRIX is given to individuals aged 2–18 years as two doses of 0.5 cc IM separated by 6–12 months, and VAQTA is given to individuals aged 2–17 years as two doses of 0.5 cc IM separated by 6–18 months.
3. **Cautions.** The only reported adverse effects from HAV vaccination are local warmth and soreness and occasional headache.

I. **Influenza**
   1. **Overview.** Influenza virus has been found second only to respiratory syncytial virus (RSV) in causing hospitalizations among children with chronic illness, and even among healthy children in the first 2 years of life influenza hospitalization rates are as high as 187 per 100,000 children. In 2002, an initial recommendation was made to annually vaccinate all children aged 6–23 months against influenza and to continue annual influenza vaccination beyond 23 months for children with chronic disease who are at particularly high risk of influenza complications. Because the antigenic strains of influenza A and B that are prevalent change from year to year, revaccination on an annual basis is needed to maintain protection against disease.
   2. **Timing and administration.** Vaccination against influenza should ideally be done during October or November. Children aged 6–35 months receive 0.25 cc IM, and all those 3 years or older receive 0.5 cc IM. Anyone 8 years or younger receiving influenza immunization for the first time should receive two doses at least 4 weeks apart. The vaccine is not recommended for children younger than 6 months, though they may be protected from influenza by vaccination of household contacts.
   3. **Cautions.** Patients who are concerned about the influenza vaccine causing disease should be educated that the vaccine contains noninfectious killed virus, thus cannot cause disease, but will not protect against coincident infection with other viruses. Local reactions of redness and tenderness are the most common adverse reactions, though anaphylactic reactions to residual egg protein from the virus culture process have rarely been reported.

J. **Bacille Calmette-Guérin (BCG)**
   1. **Overview.** Tuberculosis (TB) incidence rates began to climb again in the mid 1980s after a steady decline over 40 years. Most persons infected with *Mycobacterium tuberculosis* have latent infection, but approximately 10% of immunocompetent persons with latent TB will progress to active disease during their lifetime, and children younger than age 2 are at especially high risk of tuberculous meningitis or disseminated miliary TB. There are a number of BCG vaccines in use worldwide, all originating from the same attenuated strain of *Mycobacterium bovis*. Recent studies have found that BCG vaccination is 80% effective at preventing serious TB (miliary or meningeal) in young children, but it does not appear effective at preventing pulmonary TB, and long-lasting protection into adolescence or adulthood is uncertain.
   2. **Timing and administration.** BCG vaccination should be considered for children with a negative tuberculin skin test result who are continually exposed to a person with TB who is untreated, ineffectively treated, or known to be resistant to isoniazid and rifampin.
   3. **Cautions.** Though BCG may cause local irritation, more severe side effects (BCG lymphadenitis, local ulceration, BCG osteitis) are quite rare. BCG may cause the subsequent purified protein derivative skin tests to react with up to 19 mm of induration, but this response declines with time and is unlikely to persist beyond 10 years after BCG vaccination.

III. **Adolescent Immunizations.** Immunization status should be reviewed at age 11 or 12, and plans made for catching up on any missed vaccination doses. Recommended adolescent immunizations are included on the annually updated childhood vaccination schedule from the CDC.
   A. **Hepatitis B (HBV).** Part of the effort to increase population immunity to hepatitis B and decrease the burden of suffering from liver disease and hepatocellular carcinoma includes ensuring that adolescents who have not previously been immunized against hepatitis B receive all doses necessary to complete the three-dose primary series. The second dose should be administered at least 1 month after the first dose, and the third dose should be administered at least 4 months after the first dose. All patients 11 years or older can be given the adult dose of 1.0 cc IM of Recombivax or Engerix-B.

B. **Tetanus–diphtheria (Td).** The tetanus-diphtheria booster should be given as 0.5 cc IM at age 11 or 12 if the last DTP, DTaP, or DT was given 5 or more years before, then routine Td boosters should be given every 10 years.

C. **Measles–mumps–rubella (MMR).** Children who did not receive the second dose of MMR at 4–6 years of age should receive their second dose at 11–12 years.

D. **Varicella-zoster virus (VZV).** The severity of varicella disease is usually worse in individuals older than age 15, and complications such as encephalitis, hepatitis, and pneumonia are more frequent. Adolescents with no documented history of chickenpox should be vaccinated against varicella, but serologic testing is not needed because a history of chickenpox is adequate assurance of immunity. Individuals older than age 13 should receive two 0.5-cc doses SC at least 4 weeks apart.

E. **Meningococcal vaccine.** See section IV,H.

F. **Other vaccines.** Adolescents with certain health conditions may require additional protection from certain diseases. In patients at increased risk of pneumococcal disease due to heart disease or cardiomyopathy, diabetes mellitus, immunosuppression, or depressed or absent spleen function (eg, due to sickle cell disease or splenectomy), a single dose of the 23-valent pneumococcal polysaccharide vaccine (PPV) is administered as 0.5 cc SC and may be repeated once after at least 5 years if the risk of infection is particularly high. Adolescents living in communities at high risk for hepatitis A should be vaccinated with two doses of HAVRIX or VAQTA as outlined above. Annual influenza vaccination should be given to adolescents with asthma, diabetes, or other chronic metabolic disease, hemoglobinopathies, or immunosuppression due to medications or illness, or those on chronic aspirin therapy (due to the increased risk of Reye's syndrome associated with taking aspirin during influenza illness).

IV. **Adult Immunizations.** While immunizations may be given at routine health maintenance, many adults seek medical care only for acute injury or illness; thus, episodes of acute care also are important times for assessing and updating immunization status. Also, many adults may not have had all recommended immunizations. Recommendations are published on the CDC web site, and the 2004 adult immunization schedule is listed in Table 101–3.

A. **Tetanus–diphtheria (Td).** Adults who have completed a primary series of Td vaccinations should continue to receive a Td booster (0.5 cc IM) every 10 years. Those who have not completed a primary series should receive three doses of Td, with the second dose 4 weeks after the first, and the third dose 6 months after the second. During routine wound management, Td administration is not required unless more than 10 years has elapsed since the last dose for clean, minor wounds. For contaminated or deep wounds, a booster is recommended if it has been longer than 5 years since the last dose or the immunization history is unclear. Tetanus immune globulin (250 IU intramuscularly) is also indicated for contaminated wounds in those with uncertain histories or with less than three primary Td doses.

B. **Influenza.** All adults 65 years or older should receive influenza vaccination (0.5 cc IM) annually in October or November. Annual influenza vaccination should also be given to residents of nursing homes or chronic-care facilities and to adults of any age with the following risk factors: asthma or other respiratory disorders, diabetes or other chronic metabolic disease, hemoglobinopathies, immunosuppression due to medications or illness, or chronic aspirin therapy. Pregnant women past 13 weeks' gestation should also be immunized. Influenza vaccine is 90% effective in preventing infection in young healthy adults, but only 30–40% effective in frail elderly or compromised adults. Health workers should be vaccinated annually to reduce the risk of transmitting influenza to susceptible individuals. Depending on vaccine availability, all adults may be offered influenza vaccination. Persons who contract influenza following immunization usually have a milder course and are less likely to have complications.

C. **Pneumococcus.** The 23-valent pneumococcal polysaccharide vaccine (PPV) should be given (0.5 cc SC) to all adults aged 65 or older due to their high risk of complications from pneumococcal disease. Anyone between ages 2 and 64 with chronic cardiovascular disease, chronic pulmonary disease (chronic obstructive pulmonary disease, but not asthma), diabetes mellitus, alcoholism, chronic liver disease, cerebrospinal fluid leaks, functional or anatomic asplenia, or immunosuppression, or anyone living in a chronic-care facility is also at risk of pneumococcal disease and should be vaccinated. One-time revaccination after an interval of 5 years is recommended for those aged 65 or older whose first dose was before age 65.

TABLE 101–3. RECOMMENDED ADULT IMMUNIZATION SCHEDULE, UNITED STATES, 2003–2004

by Age Group

Vaccine ▼ / Age Group ▶	19–49 Years	50–64 Years	65 Years and Older
Tetanus, Diphtheria (Td)*	1 dose booster every 10 years[1]		
Influenza	1 dose annually[2]	1 dose annually[2]	
Pneumococcal (polysaccharide)	1 dose[3,4]		1 dose[3,4]
Hepatitis B*	3 doses (0, 1–2, 4–6 months)[5]		
Hepatitis A	2 doses (0, 6–12 months)[6]		
Measles, Mumps, Rubella (MMR)*	1 dose if measles, mumps, or rubella vaccination history is unreliable; 2 doses for persons with occupational or other indications[7]	1 dose	
Varicella*	2 doses (0, 4–8 weeks) for persons who are susceptible[8]		
Meningococcal (polysaccharide)	1 dose[9]		

by Medical Conditions

Medical Condition ▼ / Vaccine ▶	Tetanus-Diphtheria (Td)*[1]	Influenza[2]	Pneumococcal (polysaccharide)[3,4]	Hepatitis B*[5]	Hepatitis A[6]	Measles, Mumps, Rubella (MMR)*[7]	Varicella*[8]
Pregnancy		A					
Diabetes, heart disease, chronic pulmonary disease, chronic liver disease, including chronic alcoholism		B	C		D		
Congenital immunodeficiency, leukemia, lymphoma, generalized malignancy, therapy with alkylating agents, antimetabolites, radiation or large amounts of corticosteroids			E				F
Renal failure/end stage renal disease, recipients of hemodialysis or clotting factor concentrates			E	G			
Asplenia including elective splenectomy and terminal complement component deficiencies		H	E, I, J				
HIV infection		H	E, K			L	

| For all persons in this group | Catch-up on childhood vaccinations | For persons with medical/ exposure indications | Contraindicated |

See Special Notes for Medical Conditions below—also see Footnotes for Recommended Adult Immunization Schedule, by Age Group and Medical Conditions, United States, 2003–2004.

*Covered by the Vaccine Injury Compensation Program. For information on how to file a claim call 800-338-2382. Please also visit www.hrsa.gov/osp/vicp To file a claim for vaccine injury contact: U.S. Court of Federal Claims, 717 Madison Place, N.W., Washington D.C. 20005, 202-219-9657.

This schedule indicates the recommended age groups for routine administration of currently licensed vaccines for persons 19 years of age and older. Licensed combination vaccines may be used whenever any components of the combination are indicated and the vaccine's other components are not contraindicated. Providers should consult the manufacturer's package inserts for detailed recommendations.

Report all clinically significant post-vaccination reactions to the Vaccine Adverse Event Reporting System (VAERS). Reporting forms and instructions on filing a VAERS report are available by calling 800-822-7967 or from the VAERS website at www.vaers.org

For additional information about the vaccines listed above and contraindications for immunization, visit the National Immunization Program Website at www.cdc.gov/nip/ or call the National Immunization Hotline at 800-232-2522 (English) or 800-232-0233 (Spanish).

Approved by the Advisory Committee on Immunization Practices (ACIP), and accepted by the American College of Obstetricians and Gynecologists (ACOG) and the American Academy of Family Physicians (AAFP).

From the Advisory Committee on Immunization Practices, Centers for Disease Control and Prevention. Department of Health and Human Services, 2004.

Special Notes for Medical Conditions

A. For women without chronic diseases/conditions, vaccinate if pregnancy will be at 2nd or 3rd trimester during influenza season. For women with chronic diseases/conditions, vaccinate at any time during the pregnancy.

B. Although chronic liver disease and alcoholism are not indicator conditions for influenza vaccination, give 1 dose annually if the patient is age 50 years or older, has other indications for influenza vaccine, or if the patient requests vaccination.

C. Asthma is an indicator condition for influenza but not for pneumococcal vaccination.

D. For all persons with chronic liver disease.

E. For persons <65 years, revaccinate once after 5 years or more have elapsed since initial vaccination.

F. Persons with impaired humoral immunity but intact cellular immunity may be vaccinated. MMWR 1999; 48(RR-06):1–5.

G. Hemodialysis patients: Use special formulation of vaccine (40 μg/mL) or two 1.0 mL 20 μg doses given at one site. Vaccinate early in the course of renal disease. Assess antibody titers to hep B surface antigen (anti-HBs) levels annually. Administer additional doses if anti-HBs levels decline to <10 milliinternational units (mIU)/mL.

H. There are no data specifically on risk of severe or complicated influenza infections among persons with asplenia. However, influenza is a risk factor for secondary bacterial infections that may cause severe disease in asplenics.

I. Administer meningococcal vaccine and consider Hib vaccine.

J. Elective splenectomy: vaccinate at least 2 weeks before surgery.

K. Vaccinate as close to diagnosis as possible when CD4 cell counts are highest.

L. Withhold MMR or other measles containing vaccines from HIV-infected persons with evidence of severe immunosuppression. MMWR 1998;47(RR-8):21–22; MMWR 2002; 51(RR-02):22–24.

1. **Tetanus and diphtheria (Td) toxoids**—Adults including pregnant women with uncertain histories of a complete primary vaccination series should receive a primary series of Td. A primary vaccination series for adults is 3 doses: the first 2 doses given at least 4 weeks apart and the 3rd dose, 6–12 months after the second. Administer 1 dose if the person had received the primary series and the last vaccination was 10 years ago or longer. Consult MMWR 1991;40(RR-10):1–21 for administering Td as prophylaxis is wound management. The ACP Task Force on Adult Immunization supports a second option for Td use in adults: a single Td booster at age 50 years for persons who have completed the full pediatric series, including the teenage/young adult booster. Guide for Adult Immunization. 3rd ed. ACP 1994:20.

2. **Influenza vaccination**—Medical indications: chronic disorders of the cardiovascular or pulmonary systems including asthma; chronic metabolic diseases including diabetes mellitus, renal dysfunction, hemoglobinopathies, or immunosuppression (including immunosuppression caused by medications or by human immunodeficiency virus [HIV]), requiring regular medical follow-up or hospitalization during the preceding year; women who will be in the second or third trimester of pregnancy during the influenza season. Occupational indications: health-care workers. Other indications: residents of nursing homes and other long-term care facilities; persons likely to transmit influenza to persons at high-risk (in-home care givers to persons with medical indications, household contacts and out-of-home caregivers of children from birth to 23 months of age, or children with asthma or other indicator conditions for influenza vaccination, household members and care givers of elderly and adults with high-risk conditions); and anyone who wishes to be vaccinated. For healthy persons aged 5–49 years without high risk conditions, either the inactivated vaccine or the intranasally administered influenza vaccine (Flumist) may be given. MMWR 2003;52(RR-8);1–36;MMWR 2003;53(RR-13);1–8.

3. **Pneumococcal polysaccharide vaccination**—Medical indications: chronic disorders of the pulmonary system (excluding asthma), cardiovascular diseases, diabetes mellitus, chronic renal failure or nephrotic syndrome, functional or anatomic asplenia (e.g., sickle cell disease or splenectomy), immunosuppressive conditions (e.g., congenital immunodeficiency, HIV infection, leukemia, lymphoma, multiple myeloma, Hodgkins disease, generalized malignancy, organ or bone marrow transplantation), chemotherapy with alkylating agents, anti-metabolites, or long-term systemic corticosteroids. Geographic/other indications: Alaskan Natives and certain American Indian populations. Other indications: residents of nursing homes and other long-term care facilities. MMWR 1997;46(RR-8):1–24.

4. **Revaccination with pneumococcal polysaccharide vaccine**—One time revaccination after 5 years for persons with chronic renal failure or nephrotic syndrome, functional or anatomic asplenia (e.g., sickle cell disease or splenectomy),

(continued)

TABLE 101–3. RECOMMENDED ADULT IMMUNIZATION SCHEDULE, UNITED STATES, 2003–2004 (*Continued*)

immunosuppressive conditions (e.g., congenital immunodeficiency, HIV infection, leukemia, lymphoma, multiple myeloma, Hodgkins disease, generalized malignancy, organ or bone marrow transplantation), chemotherapy with alkylating agents, anti-metabolites, or long-term systemic corticosteroids. For persons 65 and older, one-time revaccination if they were vaccinated 5 or more years previously and were aged less than 65 years at the time of primary vaccination. *MMWR* 1997;46(RR-8):1–24.

5. Hepatitis B vaccination—Medical indications: hemodialysis patients, patients who receive clotting-factor concentrates. Occupational indications: health-care workers and public-safety workers who have exposure to blood in the workplace, persons in training in schools of medicine, dentistry, nursing, laboratory technology, and other allied health professions. Behavioral indications: injecting drug users, persons with more than one sex partner in the previous 6 months, persons with a recently acquired sexually-transmitted disease (STD), all clients in STD clinics, men who have sex with men. Other indications: household contacts and sex partners of persons with chronic HBV infection, clients and staff of institutions for the developmentally disabled, international travelers who will be in countries with high or intermediate prevalence of chronic HBV infection for more than 6 months, inmates of correctional facilities. *MMWR* 1991;40(RR-13):1–19. (www.cdc.gov/travel/diseases/hbv.htm)

6. Hepatitis A vaccination—For the combined HepA-HepB vaccine use 3 doses at 0, 1, 6 months). Medical indications: persons with clotting-factor disorders or chronic liver disease. Behavioral indications: men who have sex with men, users of injecting and noninjecting illegal drugs. Occupational indications: persons working with HAV-infected primates or with HAV in a research laboratory setting. Other indications: persons traveling to or working in countries that have high or intermediate endemicity of hepatitis A. *MMWR* 1999;48(RR-12):1–37. (www.cdc.gov/travel/diseases/hav.htm)

7. Measles, Mumps, Rubella vaccination (MMR)—Measles component: Adults born before 1957 may be considered immune to measles. Adults born in or after 1957 should receive at least one dose of MMR unless they have a medical contraindication, documentation of at least one dose or other acceptable evidence of immunity. A second dose of MMR is recommended for adults who:

—are recently exposed to measles or in an outbreak setting

—were previously vaccinated with killed measles vaccine

—were vaccinated with an unknown vaccine between 1963 and 1967

—are students in post-secondary educational institutions

—work in health care facilities

—plan to travel internationally

Mumps component: 1 dose of MMR should be adequate for protection. Rubella component: Give 1 dose of MMR to women whose rubella vaccination history is unreliable and counsel women to avoid becoming pregnant for 4 weeks after vaccination. For women of child-bearing age, regardless of birth year, routinely determine rubella immunity and counsel women regarding congenital rubella syndrome. Do not vaccinate pregnant women or those planning to become pregnant in the next 4 weeks. If pregnant and susceptible, vaccinate as early in postpartum period as possible. *MMWR* 1998;47(RR-8):1–57; *MMWR* 2001;50:1117.

8. Varicella vaccination—Recommended for all persons who do not have reliable clinical history of varicella infection or serological evidence of varicella zoster virus (VZV) infection who may be at high risk for exposure or transmission. This includes, health-care workers and family contacts of immunocompromised persons, those who live or work in environments where transmission is likely (e.g., teachers of young children, day care employees, and residents and staff members in institutional settings), persons who live or work in environments where VZV transmission can occur (e.g., college students, inmates and staff members of correctional institutions, and military personnel), adolescents and adults living in households with children, women who are not pregnant but who may become pregnant in the future, international travelers who are not immune to infection. Note: Greater than 95% of U.S. born adults are immune to VZV. Do not vaccinate pregnant women or those planning to become pregnant in the next 4 weeks. If pregnant and susceptible, vaccinate as early in postpartum period as possible. *MMWR* 1996;45(RR-11):1–36; *MMWR* 1999;48(RR-6):1–5.

9. Meningococcal vaccination (quadrivalent polysaccharide vaccine for serogroups A, Y, and W-135)—Consider vaccination for persons with medical indications: adults with terminal complement component deficiencies, with anatomic or functional asplenia. Other indications: travelers to countries in which disease is hyperendemic or epidemic ("meningitis belt" of sub-Saharan Africa, Mecca, Saudi Arabia for Hajj). Revaccination at 3–5 years may be indicated for persons at high risk for infection (e.g., persons residing in areas in which disease is epidemic). Counsel college freshmen, especially those who live in dormitories, regarding meningococcal disease and the vaccine so that they can make an educated decision about receiving the vaccination. *MMWR* 2000;49(RR-7):1–20. Note: The AAFP recommends that colleges should take the lead on providing education on meningococcal infection and vaccination and offer it to those who are interested. Physicians need not initiate discussion of the meningococcal quadrivalent polysaccharide vaccine as part of routine medical care.

D. Hepatitis B (HBV). HBV should be offered to all young adults; persons with occupational risk (health care workers and public service workers); persons with lifestyle risk (homosexual or bisexual men, heterosexual persons with multiple partners or with any sexually transmitted disease, and injectable drug users); persons with hepatitis C or hemophilia and hemodialysis patients; and those with environmental risk factors (including household or sexual contacts of hepatitis B carriers, prison inmates, and immigrants from hepatitis B–endemic areas). All pregnant women should be screened prenatally for active HBV infection (HBsAg positive). HBV vaccine is administered as 1 cc IM, with a second dose given 1 month later and the third dose given at 6 months. Though not routinely recommended, booster doses of HBV vaccine and pre- and post-immunization serologic testing may be considered, based on the patient's risk factors. Postexposure prophylaxis using 0.06 cc/kg IM of HBIG, in addition to the HBV vaccine series, should be offered to persons with percutaneous or mucous-membrane exposure to blood or secretions known to be HBsAg positive, as soon as possible after exposure (within 72 hours).

E. Hepatitis A (HAV). Immunization against hepatitis A should be given to adults who live in endemic areas or travel internationally to countries with endemic hepatitis A. Other groups at risk who should be immunized are men who have sex with men, users of illegal drugs, patients with clotting factor disorders, patients with chronic liver disease, and those with occupational exposure to HAV. Adult vaccination is given with 1.0 cc HAVRIX or VAQTA IM. Immediate postexposure protection against hepatitis A can be achieved with immune serum globulin (ISG, 0.02–0.06 cc/kg IM). ISG should be given within 2 weeks of exposure to close household and sexual contacts of persons with hepatitis A and to health care workers and patients in centers with active cases of hepatitis A. ISG affords protection against hepatitis A for 3–6 months, depending on the dose given. The protective effect of HAV immunization takes 4 weeks to develop. For international travelers, it may be necessary to administer ISG at a different site, in addition to the vaccine, if travel is anticipated before 4 weeks has elapsed.

F. Measles–mumps–rubella (MMR). All persons born after in 1957 or later who lack evidence of immunity to measles, mumps, or rubella or do not have documentation of having received MMR on or after their first birthday should receive a 0.5 cc SC dose of MMR. Persons born in 1956 or before are generally assumed to be immune. MMR or other live-virus vaccines should not be given during pregnancy. Any woman who is not pregnant and who has no history of MMR vaccination or evidence of immunity to rubella should be immunized with MMR or rubella vaccine (0.5 cc SC) and agree to avoid pregnancy for 3 months. Susceptible pregnant women should be immunized in the immediate postpartum period, with the same instructions.

G. Varicella zoster (VZV). Adults with a reliable history of chickenpox are assumed to be immune and do not need vaccination or serologic testing. All adults without a history of chickenpox should be assumed susceptible and offered immunization with two 0.5-cc doses at least 4 weeks apart to decrease the risk of severe varicella, pneumonia, hepatitis, or encephalitis.

H. Meningococcal polysaccharide vaccine. Meningococcal disease occurs at a rate of about 1 case per 100,000 per population in the United States, causing a case fatality rate of 10% as well as substantial morbidity, despite continued sensitivity to many antibiotics. The quadrivalent meningococcal vaccine against serogroups A, C, Y, W-135 is over 85% protective against these groups. While most outbreaks in the United States are caused by serogroup C, sporadic outbreaks of group Y and group B (which are not covered by the vaccine) also occur. The dose for adults and children is a single 0.5-cc SC injection, and protective antibodies are present in 7–10 days. College freshmen living in dormitories are at increased risk of meningococcal disease, and it is recommended to discuss with freshmen and parents the potential risk for disease and benefits of vaccination. Individuals should also be vaccinated if they are at increased risk of disease due to anatomic or functional asplenia, terminal complement component deficiencies, occupational exposure in a research or clinical setting, or travel to an endemic area (especially the "meningitis belt" of sub-Saharan Africa from Senegal to Ethiopia). Postexposure chemoprophylaxis may be given with rifampin (600 mg twice daily for 2 days), ciprofloxacin (500-mg single dose), or ceftriaxone (250-mg single dose).

I. Rabies vaccine. The rabies virus is transmitted by the saliva of infected animals, causing an encephalitis that is nearly always fatal. Veterinarians, animal handlers, cave explorers, and hunters are at increased risk of disease and should be immunized. Seemingly insignificant contact with bats has resulted in clinical rabies even in the absence of a bite. Three vaccines are in use in the United States: Human Diploid Cell Vaccine (HDCV), Rabies Vaccine Adsorbed (RVA), and Purified Chick Embryo Cell Vaccine (PCEC). Pre-exposure prophylaxis is given with three 1.0-cc IM doses of HDCV, RVA, or PCEC on days 0, 7, and 21 or 28 or three 0.1-cc ID doses of HDCV on days 0, 7, and 21 or 28. (Only HDCV is approved for intradermal use.) If exposure continues, booster doses are indicated every 2 years or if antibody titers are found inadequate. Postexposure prophylaxis includes thorough wound washing and human rabies immune globulin (HRIG) 20 IU/kg, with half administered at the bite site and the rest administered IM. Rabies immunization should be initiated without delay following contact of an unvaccinated person with a potentially rabid animal. Postexposure immunization includes five doses on days 0, 3, 7, 14, and 28 following exposure.

V. **Combination Vaccines.** Combination vaccines allow adequate administration of recommended vaccines with fewer total injections, but only US Food and Drug Administration–licensed combination vaccines should be used. Combination vaccines covering measles, mumps, rubella, diphtheria, pertussis, and tetanus have been available for many years. More recent combinations include COMVAX (combining HBV and Hib) and Pediarix (combining HBV, DtaP, and IPV). Combination vaccines are appropriate when any component vaccine is indicated and none of the component vaccines are contraindicated. Whenever possible, a vaccine series should be completed with all doses coming from the same manufacturer.

REFERENCES

American Academy of Pediatrics (AAP): *2000 Red Book: Report of the Committee on Infectious Diseases,* 25th ed. AAP; 2000.

Centers for Disease Control and Prevention: Preventing pneumococcal disease among infants and young children: Recommendations of the Advisory Committee on Immunization Practices (ACIP). MMWR 2000;**49**(No. RR-9):1. (http://www.cdc.gov/mmwr/preview/mmwrhtml/rr4909a1.htm)

Centers for Disease Control and Prevention: Prevention and control of influenza: Recommendations of the Advisory Committee on Immunization Practices (ACIP). MMWR 2001;**50**(No. RR-4):1. (http://www.cdc.gov/mmwr/preview/mmwrhtml/rr5004a1.htm)

Centers for Disease Control and Prevention: Prevention and control of meningococcal disease and meningococcal disease and college students: Recommendations of the Advisory Committee on Immunization Practices (ACIP). MMWR 2000;**49**(No. RR-7):1. (http://www.cdc.gov/mmwr/preview/mmwrhtml/rr4907a1.htm)

Centers for Disease Control and Prevention: Use of diphtheria toxoid-tetanus toxoid-acellular pertussis vaccine as a five-dose series: Supplemental recommendations of the Advisory Committee on Immunization Practices (ACIP). MMWR 2000;**49**(No. RR-13):1. (http://www.cdc.gov/mmwr/preview/mmwrhtml/rr4913a1.htm)

General Recommendations on Immunization: Recommendations of the Advisory Committee on Immunization Practices (ACIP) and the American Academy of Family Physicians (AAFP) MMWR 2002;**51**(No. RR02):1. (http://www.cdc.gov/mmwr/preview/mmwrhtml/rr5102a1.htm)

Zimmerman RK, et al: Routine vaccines across the life span, 2003. J Fam Pract 2003;**52**(1 suppl):S1. Review. (http://www.jfponline.com/supplements/vaccine_jan03/vaccine_s1.pdf)

---

102   Screening Tests

Larry L. Dickey, MD, MPH

I. **Quick Screening Guide.** The following screening tests and examinations should be considered for children and adults. Those tests designated with an asterisk (*) have been recommended by some, but not all, major authorities.

A. **Children**
   1. Body measurement
      a. Head circumference (until age 2 years)
      b. Height and weight
      c. Blood pressure (beginning at age 3 years)*

2. Blood tests
   a. Hypothyroidism (newborns)
   b. Phenylketonuria (newborns)
   c. Hemoglobinopathies (newborns)
   d. Anemia (at 6–12 months of age and adolescent girls at risk)*
   e. Glucose (high-risk)
   f. Lead (high-risk at 12 and 24 months)
   g. Cholesterol (high-risk, after age 2 years)
3. Sensory screening
   a. Hearing* (newborns, children, and adolescents)
   b. Vision (amblyopia/strabismus until age 3–4 years, acuity* beginning at age 3–4 years)
4. Mental health screening
   a. Depression (high-risk adolescents)
5. Infectious diseases tests
   a. Hepatitis C (high-risk)
   b. Human immunodeficiency virus (HIV) (high-risk)
   c. Chlamydia/gonorrhea/syphilis (high-risk adolescents)
   d. Tuberculosis (high-risk)
6. Cancer tests
   a. Testicular examination* (boys beginning at age 15)

B. Adults
1. Body measurement
   a. Height and weight
   b. Blood pressure
   c. Bone density (women, beginning at age 60)
2. Blood tests
   a. Cholesterol (men aged 35–65 years, women aged 45–65 years)
   b. Glucose (high-risk)
   c. Thyroid (high-risk)
3. Sensory screenings
   a. Hearing (beginning at age 65)
   b. Vision (beginning at age 65)
   c. Glaucoma (high-risk)
4. Mental health screening
   a. Depression
5. Infectious diseases tests
   a. Hepatitis C (high-risk)
   b. HIV (high-risk)
   c. Chlamydia/gonorrhea/syphilis (high-risk)
   d. Tuberculosis (high-risk)
6. Cancer tests
   a. Breast examination and mammogram (women beginning at age 40)
   b. Cervical—Pap smear (women)
   c. Colorectal screening (stool guaiac cards, flexible sigmoidoscopy, barium enema, or colonoscopy beginning at age 50)
   d. Prostate examination and prostate-specific antigen (PSA* (men beginning at age 50)
   e. Skin examination*
   f. Testicular examination* (men)
   g. Thyroid examination*

II. **Body Measurement Screening**
   A. **Head circumference.** The American Academy of Pediatrics (AAP) has recommended measurement of head circumference at every visit until a child is 2 years old. Other authorities have not made recommendations for or against this.
   B. **Height and weight.** All major authorities have recommended regular measurement of height and weight at all ages. For children and adolescents, these can be plotted using age-specific growth curve charts. For adults, standard height and weight charts can be used (Table 102–1) for assessing norms. Several authorities recommend periodic calculation and charting of body mass index [BMI = weight (kg)/height^2 (m)], since BMI is believed to be more reflective of total body fat than weight for height norms. According

TABLE 102-1. WEIGHT CHART FOR ADULT MEN AND WOMEN

Height[1]

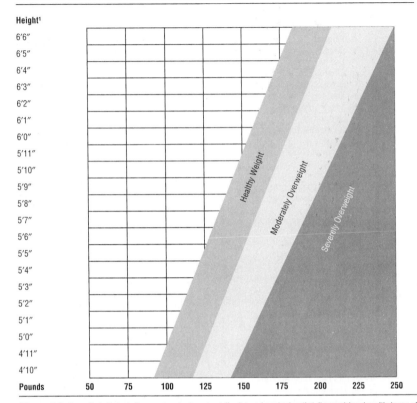

¹ The use of shading reflects the lack of consensus about exact cutoff points and emphasizes that disease risk varies with degree of overweight.

Note: To use this chart, find your height in feet and inches (without shoes) along the left side of the graph. Trace the line corresponding to your height across the figure until it intersects with the vertical line corresponding to your weight in pounds (without clothes). The point of intersection lies within a band that indicates whether your weight is healthy or is moderately or severely overweight. The higher weights apply mainly to men, who have more muscle and bone.

Reprinted from US Department of Agriculture, US Department of Health and Human Services: *Nutrition and Your Health: Dietary Guidelines for Americans.* US Government Printing Office; 1995. Home and Garden Bulletin 232.

to the US Department of Agriculture, BMI of ≥25 constitutes overweight for adults, the point at which negative health consequences begin. The AAP classifies children with BMIs >95th percentile to be obese, and children with BMIs between the 85th and 95th percentiles to be at risk of being overweight.

C. **Waist/hip measurement.** Some authorities, such as the US Department of Agriculture and the US Department of Health and Human Services, have recommended measurement of waist and hip circumferences and calculation of waist/hip ratio (WHR) for adults. By some reports, this may be a more accurate predictor of negative health consequences than height/weight or BMI values. Upper limits of healthy WHR values are usually cited as 0.8 for women and 1.0 for men. According to the National Heart, Lung, and Blood Institute, an abdominal circumference of >40 inches for men and >35 inches for women constitutes abdominal obesity and should be considered a cardiovascular disease risk factor.

D. **Blood pressure**
   1. **Children and adolescents.** The AAP and NHLBI recommend regular blood pressure screening of all children beginning at age 3 years. For children, values above

TABLE 102–2. 95TH PERCENTILE OF BLOOD PRESSURE BY SELECTED AGES IN GIRLS AND BOYS, BY THE 50TH AND 75TH HEIGHT PERCENTILES

Age (Years)	Girls' SBP/DPB		Boys' SBP/DBP	
	50th Percentile for Height	75th Percentile for Height	50th Percentile for Height	75th Percentile for Height
1	104/58	105/59	102/57	104/58
6	111/73	112/73	114/74	115/75
12	123/80	124/81	123/81	125/82
17	129/84	130/85	136/87	138/88

DBP, diastolic blood pressure; SBP, systolic blood pressure.
Reprinted from National Institutes of Health: *The Sixth Report of the Joint National Committee on Prevention, Detection, Evaluation, and Treatment of High Blood Pressure*. US Department of Health and Human Services; 1997. NIH Publication No. 98-4080.

the 95th percentile are considered elevated (Table 102–2). In 2003, the US Preventive Services Task Force (USPSTF) found insufficient evidence to recommend for or against routine screening of children and adolescents, stating that evidence is poor that routine blood pressure measurement accurately identifies children and adolescents at increased risk for cardiovascular disease and that treatment of elevated blood pressure in children or adolescents decreases the incidence of cardiovascular disease.

2. **Adults.** All authorities recommend regular routine screening of adults for elevated blood pressure. The NHLBI recommends screening every 2 years for persons with systolic blood pressure <130 mm Hg and diastolic blood pressure <85 mm Hg, with more frequent screening for adults with higher pressures. The USPSTF has found insufficient evidence to recommend an optimal screening interval. For adults, systolic pressures ≥140 mm Hg and diastolic pressures ≥90 mm Hg are considered elevated. Elevated values should be confirmed on at least one or two additional visits before hypertension is diagnosed. In 2003, the NHLBI issued guidelines that adult systolic pressures >120 mm Hg or diastolic pressures >80 mm Hg be classified as "pre-hypertension," for which lifestyle modifications should be considered.

E. **Bone density.** The USPSTF recommends routine screening for normal-risk women age 65 or older and for high-risk women age 60 or older. Although the optimal interval screening is not determined, intervals of at least 2 years may be necessary in order to detect changes. Other groups, such as the American Academy of Family Physicians, have stated that screening may be useful for high-risk women. Since July 1998, Medicare has provided coverage for bone densitometry screening of estrogen-deficient women, including postmenopausal women, as well as for persons at high risk due to receiving long-term glucocorticoid therapy, persons with primary hyperparathyroidism, and persons being monitored to assess the response to an osteoporosis drug therapy approved by the US Food and Drug Administration (FDA).

III. **Blood Test Screening**

A. **Cholesterol**

1. **Children and adolescents.** No major authority recommends routine cholesterol screening of children or adolescents. Several authorities, including the AAP, American Medical Association (AMA), and NHLBI, recommend total cholesterol screening of children older than 2 years and adolescents who have a parent with a total cholesterol level ≥240 mg/dL. These authorities also recommend lipoprotein analysis of children older than 2 years old and adolescents who have a family history of premature cardiovascular disease (before age 55) in a parent or grandparent. The National Cholesterol Education Program (NCEP) recommends screening for at-risk children and adolescents every 5 years. The AMA states that during adolescence screening is needed only once if values are normal. The NCEP has classified cholesterol levels in children and adolescents as follows: acceptable (total <170 mg/dL, low-density lipoprotein [LDL] <110 mg/dL); borderline (total 170–199 mg/dL, LDL 110–129 mg/dL); and high (total = 200 mg/dL, LDL = 130 mg/dL).

2. **Adults.** Recommendations vary regarding screening of adults. The most aggressive recommendations are those of the NCEP, which recommends screening all

adults at least once every 5 years for total cholesterol and at the same time, if accurate results are available, for high-density lipoprotein (HDL) cholesterol. The USPSTF recommends screening for total cholesterol in men aged 35–65 years and women aged 45–65 years. The USPSTF does not recommend screening younger men and women unless they are at high risk and found insufficient evidence to recommend for or against screening after age 65. The USPSTF states that the appropriate interval for screening is unknown. The NCEP has classified cholesterol level in adults without coronary artery disease as follows: desirable (total <200 mg/dL, LDL <130 mg/dL); borderline (total 200–239 mg/dL, LDL 130–159 mg/dL); and high (total ≥240 mg/dL, LDL ≥160 mg/dL). The NCEP considers HDL levels <35 mg/dL and ≥60 mg/dL to be positive and negative risk factors, respectively, for coronary artery disease.

B. Glucose
1. **Children and adolescents.** Because of the growing prevalence of type II diabetes in children and adolescents, the American Diabetes Association (ADA) recommends plasma glucose screening for overweight children and adolescents (BMI >85th percentile) with any two of the following risk factors: family history of type II diabetes in first or second-degree relatives; belonging to a high-risk race/ethnic group (Native American, African American, Hispanic American, Asian/South Pacific Islander); or having signs of insulin resistance or conditions associated with insulin resistance (acanthosis nigricans, hypertension, dyslipidemia, polycystic ovary syndrome). Other authorities have not issued recommendations for screening children and adolescents.
2. **Adults.** The USPSTF has found insufficient evidence to recommend routine plasma glucose screening of normal-risk adults and has recommended screening for adults with hypertension or hyperlipidemia. The ADA recommends that screening be considered at 3-year intervals for those 45 years or older, particularly with a BMI >25 kg/m².

C. Hemoglobin/hematocrit
1. **Children and adolescents.** The AAP recommends screening all children for anemia once between 9 and 12 months of age and annually during adolescence for menstruating teenagers. The USPSTF recommends screening infants at high risk for iron deficiency between 6 and 12 months of age. The USPSTF defines high-risk factors as poverty; race—blacks, Native Americans, and Alaskan Natives; immigrants from developing countries; preterm and low-birth-weight infants; and infants whose principal intake is unfortified cow's milk. According to the Centers for Disease Control and Prevention (CDC), the cutoff points for defining anemia in children aged 6 months to 2 years are hemoglobin ≤11.0 g/dL and hematocrit ≤33.0%.
2. **Adults.** No major authority recommends routine screening of asymptomatic, nonpregnant adults for anemia. The American College of Obstetricians and Gynecologists (ACOG) recommends periodic screening of women with a history of excessive menstrual flow and women of Caribbean, Latin American, Asian, Mediterranean, or African ancestry. In nonpregnant women and adolescent girls older than 15 years, the cutpoints for anemia are hemoglobin ≤12 g/dL and hematocrit ≤36%.

D. Lead. In 1997 the CDC recommended that state health officials develop plans for targeted blood lead level (BLL) screening of children based on assessments of the lead exposure and screening capacity in specific regions of the state. For targeted screening, the CDC recommends screening of children who reside in a zip code in which >27% of housing was built before 1950; receive services from public assistance programs for the poor, such as Medicaid or the Supplemental Food Program for Women, Infants, and Children; or whose parents answer "yes" or "don't know" to any of three question of a personal-risk questionnaire (Table 102–3). In areas where exposure to lead from older housing is unlikely, the CDC states that the personal-risk questionnaire could contain questions about other risk factors, such as parental occupation or use of lead-containing ceramic ware or traditional remedies. In the absence of a targeted screening plan or other formal guidance from state health officials, the CDC recommends universal screening of all children at age 1 and 2 years and of children 36–72 months of age not previously screened.

Diagnostic testing of venous blood should be performed for all patients with elevated BLLs >10 µg/dL at a follow-up interval based on degree of elevation of BLL (see Table 102–4). The AAP has endorsed the 1997 CDC recommendations. The USPSTF

TABLE 102–3. BASIC LEAD PERSONAL RISK PROFILE

1. Does your child live in or regularly visit a house that was built before 1950? This question could apply to a facility such as a home day-care center or the home of a babysitter or relative.
2. Does your child live in or regularly visit a house built before 1978 with recent or ongoing renovations or remodeling (within the last 6 months)?
3. Does your child have a sibling or playmate who has or did have lead poisoning?

Reprinted from Centers for Disease Control and Prevention: *Screening Young Children for Lead Poisoning: Guidance for State and Local Public Health Officials.* US Department of Health and Human Services; 1997.

recommends screening children at increased risk for lead exposure. The USPSTF states that this screening should occur at about 12 months of age and that the optimal frequency for screening or repeat testing of children with elevated BLLs is left to clinical discretion.

E. **Newborn screening.** The AAP and other authorities have recommended that newborn screening be performed according to each state's regulations. Using new tandem mass spectroscopy technology, several states have recently expanded required screening to 30 or more conditions. National authorities have made recommendations for the following important conditions:

1. **Hypothyroidism.** The AAP, American Thyroid Association (ATA), and USPSTF have recommended that all neonates be screened for congenital hypothyroidism between 2 and 6 days of life. Care should be taken to ensure that infants born at home, ill at birth, or transferred between hospitals in the first week of life are screened before 7 days of life.
2. **Phenylketonuria (PKU).** The AAFP and USPSTF have recommended that all infants be screened for PKU prior to discharge from the nursery. Premature infants and those with illnesses should be tested at or near 7 days of age. Infants tested before 24 hours of age should receive a repeat screening. According to the USP-STF, this should occur by the time the infant is 2 weeks of age.
3. **Hemoglobinopathies.** The Sickle Cell Disease Guideline Panel of the Agency for Health Care Policy and Research, US Public Health Service, has recommended universal screening of newborns for sickle cell disease. This recommendation has been endorsed by the AAP, American Nurses Association, and AMA. The USP-STF has also recommended neonatal screening for sickle hemoglobinopathies, but it has stated that whether screening should be universal or targeted to high-risk groups should depend on the proportion of high-risk persons in the screening area. All screening must be accompanied by comprehensive counseling and treatment services.

F. **Thyroid function.** No authorities recommend screening of asymptomatic adults for thyroid dysfunctions. The ACOG recommends measurement of thyroid-stimulating hormone (TSH) levels adult women with a strong family history of thyroid disease. In 1998, the American College of Physicians (ACP) stated, "It is reasonable to screen women older than age 50 for unsuspected but symptomatic thyroid disease. The preferred screening method is a sensitive TSH test." This recommendation is based on

TABLE 102–4. SCHEDULE FOR DIAGNOSTIC TESTING OF A CHILD WITH AN ELEVATED BLOOD LEAD LEVEL ON A SCREENING TEST

If result of screening test (µ/dL) is:	Perform diagnostic test on venous blood within:
10–19	3 months
20–44	1 month–1 week[1]
45–59	48 hours
60–69	24 hours
≥70	Immediately as an emergency lab test

[1] The higher the screening blood lead level, the more urgent the need for a diagnostic test.
Reprinted from Centers for Disease Control and Prevention: *Screening Young Children for Lead Poisoning: Guidance for State and Local Public Health Officials,* US Department of Health and Human Services; 1997.

the estimate that 1 of 71 women older than 50 years will have unsuspected but symptomatic overt hypothyroidism or overt hyperthyroidism that will respond to treatment. Treatment of subclinical hyperthyroidism or hypothyroidism is of uncertain benefit. Other organizations, such as the USPSTF, have found insufficient evidence for screening of this population, recommending instead that clinicians remain alert for subtle or nonspecific symptoms of thyroid dysfunction when examining older women, postpartum women, and persons with Down syndrome.

IV. **Sensory Screening**
  A. **Hearing**
    1. **Children.** The Joint Committee on Infant Hearing (composed of the AAP, American Speech-Language-Hearing Association, American Academy of Otolaryngology—Head and Neck Surgery, and American Academy of Audiology) has endorsed universal screening of all neonates. These authorities recommend screening neonates for hearing impairment prior to hospital discharge, but not later than 3 months of age. The USPSTF has found insufficient evidence to recommend for or against universal screening of neonates. The AAP has recommended routine screening of asymptomatic children with pure-tone audiometry at ages 3, 4, 5, 10, 12, 15, and 18 years. The USPSTF has recommended against routine screening of asymptomatic children. The Joint Committee on Infant Hearing has identified recurrent or persistent otitis media with effusion for at least 3 months to be a risk factor requiring screening.
    2. **Adults.** All major authorities recommend screening older adults for hearing impairment. However, the modality for screening remains poorly defined. The American Speech-Language-Hearing Association recommends using a hearing handicap questionnaire or pure-tone audiometry. The USPSTF recommends first questioning patients about hearing impairment and performing audiometry on those reporting abnormalities. Patients found to have evidence of hearing loss by screening should be considered for referral to a specialist for comprehensive audiologic evaluation, especially if they feel handicapped by the hearing loss. Because about 10% of persons with hearing loss are amenable to medical or surgical treatment and because some patients are incorrectly identified as having hearing loss by screening, patients should not be referred directly to a hearing aid dealer. The primary care clinician should make sure that appropriate follow-up management is provided to all patients referred for audiologic evaluation. Patients may need considerable support and training to use their hearing aids effectively.
  B. **Vision**
    1. **Children.** Recommendations regarding vision screening for children vary among authorities. The AAP has recommended questioning of parents regarding a child's vision at well-child visits, with the first objective test of visual acuity at age 3 years. If the child is uncooperative, this should be rescheduled 6 months later. Subsequent objective testing is recommended at 4, 5, 10, 12, 15, and 18 years of age. The USPSTF recommends that clinicians be alert for signs of ocular misalignment in examining all newborns, infants, and children. The USPSTF recommends testing for amblyopia and strabismus once before the child enters school, preferably at age 3–4 years, and states that stereotesting is more effective for this purpose than visual acuity testing. Physical examination procedures for detecting amblyopia and strabismus include the corneal light reflex, fixation, differential occlusion, and cover/uncover tests. The USPSTF has found insufficient evidence to recommend for or against routine visual acuity testing of schoolchildren, because refractive errors of consequence present symptomatically and respond to corrective lenses without lasting effects.
    2. **Adults.** Recommendations for vision screening of adults vary considerably among authorities.
      a. **Visual acuity.** All major authorities recommend routine visual acuity screening for normal-risk adults beginning at age 65.
      b. **Eye examination.** No major authority recommends routine examination by primary care physicians, including the use of tonometry to detect glaucoma. Most authorities recommend referral to an ophthalmologist for patients at risk for glaucoma, especially African Americans older than 40 years. The American Academy of Ophthalmology recommends comprehensive eye examinations by an ophthalmologist every 2–4 years from ages 40 to 64 and every 1–2 years

beginning at age 65. The National Eye Institute recommends comprehensive eye examinations every 2 years starting at age 60, with examinations beginning at age 40 for African Americans. All authorities recommend frequent, yearly, comprehensive eye examinations by eye care specialists for patients with diabetes mellitus.

V. **Mental Health and Cognition**
  A. **Depression.** The USPSTF recommends screening adults for depression in clinical practices that have systems in place to assure accurate diagnosis, effective treatment, and follow-up. The USPSTF found limited evidence on the accuracy and reliability of screening tests in children and adolescents and limited evidence on the effectiveness of therapy in children and adolescents identified in primary care settings. Although formal screening tools (such as the Beck Depression Inventory or the Zung Self-Assessment Depression Scale) are available, the USPSTF states that asking two simple questions ("Over the past 2 weeks, have you felt down, depressed, or hopeless?" and "Over the past 2 weeks, have you felt little interest or pleasure in doing things?") may be as effective as using long instruments. The AAP recommends that pediatricians ask questions about depression in history-taking with adolescents, and the AMA recommends screening for depression in treating adolescents who may be at risk due to family problems, drug or alcohol use, or other risk factors.
  B. **Dementia.** Although instruments such as the Mini-Mental State Examination are often used for screening older adults, the USPSTF has found insufficient evidence to recommend for or against routine screening of asymptomatic older adults for dementia. The AAFP recommends that physicians be alert for cognitive and functional decline in elderly patients. The USPSTF recommends that clinicians assess cognitive function whenever cognitive impairment or deterioration is suspected.

VI. **Infectious Disease**
  A. **Hepatitis C.** In recognition of the heavy burden of disease caused by hepatitis C (1.8% of the US population infected, >$600 million in medical and work-loss expenses annually), the CDC has recommended screening of high-risk populations (Table 102–5).
  B. **Human immunodeficiency virus (HIV).** All major authorities recommend that HIV screening be offered to patients at risk: those with another sexually transmitted disease (STD), homosexual and bisexual men; past or present injection drug users; persons with a history of prostitution or multiple sexual partners; persons whose past (or present) sexual partners are HIV-infected or injection drug users, or both; patients with a history of blood transfusion between 1978 and 1985; and persons born in, or with long-term residence in, a community in which HIV is prevalent. The AMA also recommends offering testing and counseling to high-risk persons receiving family planning services or undergoing surgery. The CDC recommends that health facilities with an HIV seroprevalence rate of at least 1% or an AIDS diagnosis rate of 1 or more per

---

TABLE 102–5. PERSONS WHO SHOULD BE TESTED ROUTINELY FOR HEPATITIS C VIRUS (HCV) INFECTION

Persons who should be tested routinely for hepatitis C virus (HCV) infection based on their risk for infection
- Persons who ever injected illegal drugs, including those who injected once or a few times many years ago and do not consider themselves as drug users.
- Persons with selected medical conditions, including
  - Persons who received clotting factor concentrates produced before 1987;
  - Persons who were ever on chronic (long-term) hemodialysis; and
  - Persons with persistently abnormal alanine aminotransferase levels.
- Prior recipients of transfusions or organ transplants, including
  - Persons who were notified that they received blood from a donor who later tested positive for HCV infection;
  - Persons who received a transfusion of blood or blood components before July 1992; and
  - Persons who received an organ transplant before July 1992.

Persons who should be tested routinely for HCV-infection based on a recognized exposure
- Healthcare, emergency medical, and public safety workers after needle sticks, sharps, or mucosal exposures to HCV-positive blood.
- Children born to HCV-positive women.

Reprinted from Centers for Disease Control and Prevention: Recommendations for prevention and control of Hepatitis C Virus (HCV) infection and HCV-related chronic disease. MMWR 1998;**47**(RR-19):1.

1000 discharges should consider a policy of routine counseling and voluntary HIV testing for patients aged 15–54 years. Because of the high effectiveness of prenatal antiviral treatments, the CDC and ACOG recommend universal, voluntary HIV testing of all pregnant women.

   C. Other sexually transmitted diseases

      1. Chlamydia and gonorrhea. The AAP and AMA have advocated screening all sexually active adolescents. The AAP recommends annual urine leukocyte esterase dipstick tests for all sexually active adolescents. The USPSTF recommends screening all sexually active females younger than age 25 and other high-risk adult women for chlamydia. Chlamydia risk factors include a history of prior STDs, a new partner or multiple sex partners, inconsistent barrier contraceptive use, cervical ectopy, and being unmarried. In areas of high prevalence, screening of all women for chlamydia may be justified. For gonorrhea, women at risk are commercial sex workers, those with repeated episodes of gonorrhea, and women younger than age 25 with two or more sex partners in the last year. The USPSTF has found insufficient evidence to recommend for or against screening asymptomatic males for chlamydia or gonorrhea, although in settings in which prevalence is high, such as urban adolescent clinics, broader screening, including screening of males, may be justified. Although dipstick leukocyte testing is convenient and inexpensive, its positive predictive value has been found to be as low as 11% for chlamydia and 30% for gonorrhea. Thus, confirmation with more specific tests is required for all positive results.

        Screening of urine for chlamydia with new nucleic acid amplification and antigen detection tests offers promise for rapid, accurate, noninvasive screening. However, the optimal screening technique for chlamydia has not been established. The CDC has released laboratory guidelines that outline the advantages and disadvantages of available tests (http://www.cdc.gov/STD/LabGuidelines).

      2. Syphilis. All major authorities recommend that screening be performed for persons at high risk for infection. These persons may include sexual partners of known syphilis cases, those with multiple sexual partners—especially in high-prevalence areas; prostitutes or those who trade sex for drugs, and males who engage in sex with other males. Routine screening of sexually active adolescents has not been advocated. Because the causative agent of syphilis cannot be cultured, screening relies on serology. A nontreponemal test, either the VDRL or RPR, is recommended for initial screening. Because the specificity of these tests is limited, follow-up testing with a treponemal test, such as the FTA (fluorescent treponemal antibody), is required for positive results. Because the sensitivity of nontreponemal tests may be as low as 75% in primary syphilis, patients who have had recent contact with a person with a documented case of syphilis should be treated, even if serologic tests are negative.

   D. Tuberculosis (TB). All major authorities recommend screening of persons at high risk for TB. In general, authorities have not specified how often high-risk persons should be screened, although the AAP has recommended annual screening for children at risk. Populations at risk include (1) medically underserved, low-income populations, including those of African American, Hispanic, Asian, Native American, and Alaskan Native heritage; (2) foreign-born persons from high-prevalence countries (eg, Asia, Africa, and Latin America); (3) persons in close contact with infectious TB cases (sharing accommodations as well as playing or working in the same enclosed area); (4) alcoholics and injection drug users; (5) residents of high-risk environments, including long-term care facilities, correctional institutions, and mental institutions; and (6) persons with medical conditions known to substantially increase the risk of TB, such as HIV infection, diabetes mellitus, and chronic renal failure.

      The appropriate criterion for defining a positive skin-test reaction depends on the likelihood of TB exposure and the risk of TB if exposure has occurred. For persons with HIV infection, close contacts of infectious cases, and those with fibrotic lesions on chest radiograph, a reaction of ≥5 mm is considered positive. For other at-risk persons, including all infants and children younger than 4 years, a reaction of ≥10 mm is considered positive. Persons who are not likely to be infected with *Mycobacterium tuberculosis* should generally not be skin-tested because the predictive value of a positive skin test in low-risk populations is poor. If a skin test is performed on a person who is not in a high-risk category or who is not exposed in a high-risk environment, a cutoff point of

≥15 mm is considered positive, although prophylaxis with isoniazid is not necessarily recommended for these persons.

In 2002, the FDA approved the use of a blood test, QuantiFERON-TB Test, for screening. Like skin testing, this new test should not be used to screen normal-risk persons. Children (younger than 17 years), pregnant women, or persons with suspected tuberculosis should not be tested. Positive test results should be confirmed with a skin test.

VII. Cancer Screening

A. Breast cancer

1. **Clinical breast examination (CBE).** Most major authorities recommend regular CBEs for women aged 50 years and older. The American Cancer Society and ACOG recommend annual breast examinations in this age range, while AAFP recommends them every 1–2 years until age 70. The USPSTF has found insufficient evidence to recommend for against CBE for screening at any age. The ACS recommends CBE every 3 years for women aged 20–39 years and annually thereafter. ACOG recommends CBE annually beginning at age 18. In performing the CBE, the examiner should be systematic, palpating every portion of the breast with the patient in both an upright and supine position. One of the best indicators of examiner accuracy is thought to be the amount of time spent.

2. **Mammography.** All major authorities now recommend regular mammography for women aged 40 years and older. The ACS recommends annual screening beginning at age 40. The USPSTF recommends mammography every 1–2 years for all women older than 40 years. The ACOG and the National Cancer Institute recommend mammography every 1–2 years for women aged 40–49 years and annually thereafter.

   The clinician should keep in mind that the sensitivity of a mammogram is limited— about 90%. Thus, symptoms and positive physical findings should not be dismissed strictly on the basis of a negative mammogram result. The specificity is similarly limited; thus, women should be counseled against alarm based strictly on a positive mammogram result.

B. Cervical cancer.
All major authorities recommend routine Papanicolaou (Pap) smears for sexually active adolescent and adult women. The USPSTF and ACS recommend beginning screening within 3 years of initiation of sexual activity or by age 21, depending on which comes first. The ACS and ACOG recommend annual Pap smears, stipulating that after three normal annual tests, Pap smears can be performed less frequently at the discretion of the patient and clinician. The USPSTF recommends screening at least every 3 years and found evidence that yield of screening was low in previously screened women after age 65. ACS recommendations suggest stopping cervical cancer screening at age 70 if 3 or more screenings have been normal and no screenings have been abnormal in the last 10 years. The USPSTF recommends screening in older women who have not been previously screened, when information about previous screening is unavailable, or when screening is unlikely to have occurred in the past (eg, among women from countries without screening programs).

The use of an endocervical brush and wooden spatula provides the best yield of adequate samples, defined as containing endocervical cells. Although the presence of endocervical cells has not been demonstrated to result in improved clinical outcomes, it remains the accepted standard for adequacy of Pap smears. The USPSTF recommends against screening women who are without a cervix due to hysterectomy and found insufficient evidence to recommend the use of new screening technologies, such as liquid-based cytology, human papillomavirus (HPV) testing, and computerized rescreening. The ACS states that the use of liquid-based cytology is acceptable and that with HPV testing the frequency of cervical cytology testing in women older than age 30 may be decreased to every 3 years.

C. Colorectal cancer

1. **Digital rectal examination.** Digital rectal examination is no longer recommended by major authorities as a modality for screening for colorectal cancer because of its poor sensitivity (<10%).

2. **Fecal occult blood testing.** All major authorities now recommend annual fecal occult blood testing for normal-risk persons beginning at age 50. Some authorities, such as the USPSTF and ACS, state that its use may be optional if sigmoidoscopy or colonoscopy is performed regularly. The sensitivity and specificity of fecal occult blood testing are limited, resulting in many false-negative and false-positive results.

The positive predictive value may be <10%. Those undergoing annual screening have a lifetime risk of about 40% of experiencing a false-positive result. The improved mortality attributed to screening may actually be partially due to the high rate of sigmoidoscopy and colonoscopy used to evaluate incidental false-positive fecal occult blood tests. Rehydration of samples with a few drops of water before development improves sensitivity but significantly decreases specificity. Clinicians should keep in mind that, because of limited sensitivity and the intermittent nature of colorectal cancer bleeding, cancer cannot be ruled out by repeated fecal occult blood testing after a positive result.

3. **Sigmoidoscopy.** All major authorities now recommend sigmoidoscopy every 5 years as an acceptable screening tool for persons beginning at age 50. According to the USPSTF and ACS, this screening can be performed in addition to or in conjunction with annual fecal occult blood testing. The sensitivity of sigmoidoscopy is limited by the length of the scope, with about 40% of malignancies being beyond the reach of a 60-cm flexible scope. For this reason, some authorities recommend offering procedures that are able to examine the entire colon, such as colonoscopy and barium enema.

4. **Colonoscopy.** Several authorities (ACS, American Gastroenterological Association (AGA), and USPSTF) recommend colonoscopy every 10 years—beginning at age 50 for normal-risk patients—as an alternative to fecal occult blood and sigmoidoscopy screening. The USPSTF stated that it is unclear whether the increased accuracy of colonoscopy compared with alternative screening methods offsets the procedure's additional complications, inconvenience and costs.

5. **Barium enema.** Several authorities (ACS, AGA, and USPSTF) have recommended a barium enema every 5 years—beginning at age 50 for normal-risk patients—as an alternative to other screening modalities. The USPSTF stated that there is no direct evidence that barium enema screening is effective in reducing mortality rates.

6. **Virtual colonoscopy.** The development of new radiographic techniques now enables detailed "visualization" of the colon without endoscopy. However, this technique does not allow for concomitant biopsy and both the USPSTF and ACS have stated that the evidence is insufficient to recommend its use in routine screening.

D. **Oral cancer.** The ACS recommends oral cavity examinations at least every 3 years until age 40 and yearly thereafter as part of a cancer-related check-up. The USPSTF states that there is insufficient evidence to recommend for or against screening examinations, but suggests that clinicians may wish to provide such examinations to persons at risk because of a history of chewing or smoking tobacco or regular alcohol use.

E. **Ovarian cancer**
1. **Bimanual pelvic examination.** The USPSTF and ACOG do not recommend screening for ovarian cancer with bimanual pelvic examination. The ACS continues to recommend that bimanual examination be performed as a part of the routine gynecologic examination. The main limitation of pelvic examination for screening is its limited sensitivity, with many tumors becoming large in size before becoming detectable by examination.

2. **Tumor markers.** No major authorities have recommended screening normal-risk women using tumor markers, such as CA-125. A National Institutes of Health consensus conference has recommended using annual CA-125 measurements and transvaginal ultrasonography to screen women at particularly high risk because of hereditary cancer syndrome. Because of limited specificity and low prevalence of the disease, the use of tumor makers for screening in normal-risk populations results in large numbers of false-positive results.

3. **Ultrasonography.** No major authority currently recommends the use of ultrasonography to screen normal-risk women, largely because of its poor positive predictive value. As previously described, some authorities have recommended its use in combination with tumor marker measurement to screen high-risk women.

F. **Prostate cancer.** The ACS and American Urological Association (AUA) recommend offering annual digital rectal examination (DRE) and prostate-specific antigen (PSA) testing for normal-risk men beginning at age 50, and beginning at age 45 for men at high risk due to being African American or having a first-degree relative with a history of prostate cancer. The USPSTF found insufficient evidence to recommend for or against routine screening with DRE or PSA testing and, like other authorities, recommends that men be informed of the uncertain benefits and possible harms of prostate cancer screening. The DRE has limited sensitivity (33–69%) and positive predictive value (6–33%) for detecting prostate cancer in asymptomatic men. The positive predictive value of PSA testing is estimated to be 10–35%, thus leading to many unnecessary biopsies. Efforts to refine PSA testing using age, prostate size based on ultrasound findings, and rates of change in PSA over time may lead to improvements in sensitivity and specificity. No major authority currently recommends using transrectal ultrasonography (TRUS) to screen for prostate cancer. Because TRUS cannot distinguish between benign and malignant nodules, its positive predictive value is lower than that of PSA testing.

G. Skin cancer. The ACS recommends skin examinations every 3 years from ages 20 to 40 years and yearly thereafter. The ACOG states that skin examination may be a component of the annual examination for adult women. The USPSTF has found insufficient evidence to recommend for or against routine skin examinations by primary care clinicians, while recommending that they remain alert for skin lesions with malignant features, particularly in patients at risk. Risk groups include fair-skinned men and women older than 65 years, patients with atypical moles, and those with >50 moles. Major characteristics that make a lesion suspicious for malignant melanoma may be remembered by the ABCDs: A, asymmetry; B, irregular borders; C, variation in color; and D. diameter greater than 6 mm.

H. Testicular cancer. The AUA recommends annual testicular examinations beginning at age 15. The ACS recommends examinations every 3 years starting from 20 to 40 years of age and annual examinations thereafter. The USPSTF has found insufficient evidence to recommend for or against routine screening, while stating that patients at increased risk because of history of cryptorchidism or testicular atrophy should be counseled about the risk of cancer and offered the options of physician examinations or self-examinations. A major factor against screening is the excellent prognosis of testicular cancer, regardless of how it is detected.

I. Thyroid cancer. The ACS recommends thyroid palpation every 3 years until age 40 and yearly thereafter. The ACOG states that thyroid palpation may be a component of the annual examination for adult women. The USPSTF has found inadequate evidence to recommend for or against routine screening by thyroid palpation, while stating that screening of persons at high risk because of a history of external upper body radiation in infancy and childhood may be justified on other grounds, such as patient preference or anxiety.

REFERENCES

American Academy of Family Physicians, Commission on Public Health and Scientific Affairs: *Periodic Health Examinations, Version 5.3 August 2002.* http://www.aafp.org/exam.xml

American Academy of Pediatrics, Committee on Infectious Disease: *2000 Red Book.* American Academy of Pediatrics; 2000.

American Academy of Pediatrics, Committee on Practice and Ambulatory Medicine: Recommendations for preventive pediatric health care. Pediatrics 2000;**105**:645. http://www.aap.org/policy/re9939.html

American Cancer Society: *Cancer Detection Guidelines.* American Cancer Society; 2003.

American College of Obstetricians and Gynecologists: *Routine Cancer Screening.* ACOG Committee Opinion 247, American College of Obstetricians and Gynecologists; 2000.

American College of Obstetricians and Gynecologists: *Primary and Preventive Care: Periodic Assessments.* Committee Opinion 246. American College of Obstetricians and Gynecologists; 2000.

American College of Physicians. *Screening for Thyroid Disease.* http:www.acponlin.org/sci-policy/thyralgo.htm

American Diabetes Association. Screening for type 2 diabetes. Diabetes Care 2003;**26**:S21.

Centers for Disease Control and Prevention. Screening tests to detect *Chlamydia trachomatis* and *Neisseria gonorrhoeae* infections—2002. MMWR 2002;**51**:RR-15:1. (http://www.cdc.gov/STD/LabGuidelines)

US Department of Health and Human Services: *The Seventh Report of the Joint National Committee on Prevention, Detection, Evaluation, and Treatment of High Blood Pressure (JNC 7).* http://www.nhlbi.nih.gov/guidelines/hypertension/index.htm

US Preventive Services Task Force: *Guide to Clinical Preventive Services,* 3rd ed. 2000–2003. http://www.ahrq.gov/clinic/cps3dix.htm

US Preventive Services Task Force: *Guide to Clinical Preventive Services,* 2nd ed. Williams & Wilkins; 1996.

103 Chemoprophylaxis

Shelly S. Harkins, MD

I. **Definition.** Prophylaxis is derived from the Greek (*pro phulax*), which means "to put up a guard before it is necessary." Chemoprophylaxis is the use of a chemical or medication to prevent a disease. Chemoprophylaxis is widely utilized in modern medicine from preventing infectious diseases to treating chronic disease states.

II. **Bacterial Meningitis**
   A. **Pathogens**
      1. *Haemophilus influenzae*
         a. The mortality rate is about 5%, with 20–30% of survivors having neurologic sequelae.
         b. The risk of infection in a 1996 national study was 6% in children younger than 1 year, 2.1% in those younger than 4 years, and 0% in those older than 5 years.
         c. In the United States, the incidence is greatest in Native Americans, blacks, those in lower socioeconomic groups, and those with complement or immunoglobulin deficiencies.
            (1) The near universal administration of the *H influenzae* type b vaccine has significantly reduced the incidence of this disease since 1987 and made the need for prophylaxis relatively rare.
      2. *Neisseria meningitidis*
         a. The mortality rate is about 10%, with children younger than 1 year of age having the greatest incidence.
         b. Vaccines against serotypes a and c have been developed, but just over 50% of meningococcal infections in the United States are caused by type b, for which there is no vaccine.
         c. Meningococci are carried by 15% of contacts in their throats, but only 3–4% will carry a pathogenic strain. Eradication of this pharyngeal carriage and subsequent transmission is the goal of chemoprophylaxis.
      3. *Streptococcus pneumoniae*
         a. The mortality rate is about 26%, with the greatest mortality in patients older than age 60.
         b. Most cases occur during the first 2 years of life, but a second peak occurs in the elderly.
         c. Eighty-eight percent of organisms causing bacteremic disease in the United States are represented in the 23-valent pneumococcal vaccine.
         d. In the United States, the incidence is greatest in patients who are asplenic or alcoholic and those with sickle cell disease, human immunodeficiency virus (HIV) infection, and deficiencies of immunoglobulins and complement.
   B. **Prophylaxis**
      1. *H influenzae* type b meningitis
         a. **Criteria for prophylaxis**
            (1) There is no need to for prophylaxis in families with a child with *H influenzae* meningitis if no one else in the environment is younger than 4 years.
            (2) If there is another child in the household younger than age 4, the entire family (including the infected child) should receive prophylaxis.
            (3) Personnel of day-care centers **should receive prophylaxis** when two or more cases occur within 60 days.
            (4) Prophylaxis is not needed when all children in day care are older than 4 years of age.
            (5) Prophylaxis for day-care contacts >20 hours/week should be considered in a setting where children are younger than 4 years.
         b. **Regimen.** Rifampin, administered orally at 20 mg/kg/day in one dose for 4 days (maximum dose, 600 mg/day).
      2. *N meningitidis* meningitis
         a. **Criteria for prophylaxis**
            (1) Household, day-care, and nursery school contacts if contact is prolonged, generally >20 hours/week.
            (2) Personnel who have had contact with oral secretions of the index case.

(3) Prophylaxis is not indicated if exposure to the index case is brief. This includes most health care workers unless they have been directly exposed to respiratory secretions via intubation, suctioning, or oral care.

(4) Protection is only temporary, as colonization rates rise quickly back to baseline by 6–12 months post prophylaxis.

b. Regimen

(1) Rifampin, administered orally every 12 hours at 5 mg/kg per dose in children younger than 1 year, 10 mg/kg per dose in children aged 1–12 years, and 600 mg in adults and children aged older than 12 years for a total of four doses (maximum 600 mg/day).

(2) Ciprofloxacin, administered as a single oral 500-mg dose in adults, is equally as effective if rifampin is not tolerated.

(3) Ceftriaxone, administered as a single intramuscular dose of 125 mg for children younger than 12 years and a dose of 250 mg for adults, may eliminate meningococcal carriage of serogroup a strains.

(4) Outbreaks of serogroup a strains need antibiotic prophylaxis for all persons 3 months or older and the meningococcal a vaccine.

(5) Meningococcal c vaccines are used in the United States where serotype c epidemics occur.

III. Cardiovascular Disease

A. Primary prevention

1. Large-scale meta-analysis clearly demonstrates that aspirin reduces the risk of a first myocardial infarction (MI) by at least one third.

2. Any recommendation to begin aspirin therapy should rely on the physician's clinical judgment after careful consideration of risk and patient preferences.

3. The United States Preventive Services Task Force "strongly recommends" that aspirin be considered in all patients whose Framingham 10-year risk score is 6% or greater (Tables 103–1 and 103–2). Other national organizations make very similar recommendations.

4. **Dosage recommendations in primary prevention.** The studies that have demonstrated significant impact have used aspirin at dosages from 81 mg/day to 325 mg/day with an average dose of 273 mg/day. Generally, a 325-mg dose should be given, with the lower doses reserved for those at higher risk of gastrointestinal (GI) side effects.

5. Aspirin also appears to reduce the severity of a new episode if its use had been instituted prior to the event.

B. Acute MI

1. The Second International Study of Infarct Trial (ISIS-2) randomized patients on aspirin, intravenous streptokinase, both agents, or neither drug during an acute MI. Aspirin was demonstrated to provide a significant reduction in mortality at 5 weeks (23%), which was equivalent to intravenous streptokinase. The absolute mortality reduction was 24 vascular deaths prevented per 1000 patients treated. Aspirin was also demonstrated to significantly reduce the number of nonfatal MIs and strokes. There was no increase in risk of major bleeding/hemorrhage. Aspirin was by far the most cost-effective agent.

2. **Dosage recommendations for acute MI**

   a. A loading dose of preferably 325 mg of uncoated aspirin should be administered within 24 hours of an acute MI.

   b. If the only preparation available is enteric-coated, then the tablet should be chewed or crushed.

   c. Therapy should be continued at a dose of 81–325 mg (enteric-coated) for a minimum of 30 days.

3. Several clinical trials have established the efficacy of aspirin therapy in non-ST segment elevation coronary syndromes, in non Q-wave MIs, and in unstable angina. Aspirin significantly reduced the risk of an acute MI or death at 5, 30, and 90 days and at 1 year of treatment when used in these settings.

4. **Recommendations for aspirin in non-MI coronary syndromes**

   a. Aspirin should be considered for all patients with new-onset angina, angina at rest, or crescendo angina at a dose of 325 mg/day.

   b. Patient with GI distress may tolerate a lower dose of aspirin or can take clopidogrel or ticlopidine.

TABLE 103–1. FRAMINGHAM POINT SCORES IN MEN[1,2]

Age (years)	Points
20–34	−9
35–39	−4
40–44	0
45–49	3
50–54	6
55–59	8
60–64	10
65–69	11
70–74	12
75–79	13

Total Cholesterol mg/dL (mmol/L)	Age 20–39	Age 40–49	Age 50–59	Age 60–69	Age 70–79
<160 (3.4)	0	0	0	0	0
160–199 (3.4–5.15)	4	3	2	1	0
200–239 (5.17–6.18)	7	5	3	1	0
240–279 (6.2–7.21)	9	6	4	2	1
≥280 (7.24)	11	8	5	3	1

	Age 20–39	Age 40–49	Age 50–59	Age 60–69	Age 70–79
Nonsmoker	0	0	0	0	0
Smoker	8	5	3	1	1

HDL Cholesterol mg/dL (mmol/L)	Points
≥60 (1.55)	−1
50–59 (1.29–1.53)	0
40–49 (1.03–1.27)	1
<40 (1.03)	2

Systolic Blood Pressure (mm Hg)	Untreated	Treated
<120	0	0
120–129	0	1
130–139	1	2
140–159	1	2
≥160	2	3

Point Total	10 Year Risk (%)	Point Total	10 Year Risk (%)
0	1	10	6
1	1	11	8
2	1	12	10
3	1	13	12
4	1	14	16
5	2	15	20
6	2	16	25
7	3	≥17	≥30
8	4		
9	5		

[1] The point total is determined in each category and the 10-year risk determined in the bottom row.
[2] These risk estimates for the development of coronary heart disease do not account for all important cardiovascular risk factors. Not included are diabetes mellitus, which is considered a coronary heart disease equivalent, alcohol intake, and the serum C-reactive protein concentration.
HDL, high-density lipoprotein.
Adapted from Adult Treatment Panel III at http://www.nhlbi.nih.gov/

TABLE 103–2. FRAMINGHAM POINT SCORES IN WOMEN[1,2]

Age (years)	Points
20–34	−7
35–39	−3
40–44	0
45–49	3
50–54	6
55–59	8
60–64	10
65–69	12
70–74	14
75–79	16

Total Cholesterol mg/dL (mmol/L)	Age 20–39	Age 40–49	Age 50–59	Age 60–69	Age 70–79
<160 (3.4)	0	0	0	0	0
160–199 (3.4–5.15)	4	3	2	1	1
200–239 (5.17–6.18)	8	6	4	2	1
240–279 (6.2–7.21)	11	8	5	3	2
≥280 (7.24)	13	10	7	4	2

	Age 20–39	Age 40–49	Age 50–59	Age 60–69	Age 70–79
Nonsmoker	0	0	0	0	0
Smoker	9	7	4	2	1

HDL Cholesterol mg/dL (mmol/L)	Points
≥60 (1.55)	−1
50–59 (1.29–1.53)	0
40–49 (1.03–1.27)	1
<40 (1.03)	2

Systolic Blood Pressure (mm Hg)	Untreated	Treated
<120	0	0
120–129	1	3
130–139	2	4
140–159	3	5
≥160	4	6

Point Total	10 Year Risk (%)	Point Total	10 Year Risk (%)
<9	<1	18	6
9	1	19	8
10	1	20	11
11	1	21	14
12	1	22	17
13	2	23	22
14	2	24	27
15	3	≥25	≥30
16	4		
17	5		

[1] The point total is determined in each category and the 10-year risk determined in the bottom row.
[2] These risk estimates for the development of coronary heart disease do not account for all important cardiovascular risk factors. Not included are diabetes mellitus, which is considered a coronary heart disease equivalent, alcohol intake, and the serum C-reactive protein concentration.
HDL, high-density lipoprotein.
Adapted from Adult Treatment Panel III at http://www.nhlbi.nih.gov/

C. Acute stroke
1. The International Stroke Trial (IST) demonstrated that aspirin-treated patients had significant reductions in the 14-day recurrence of ischemic stroke (2.8% vs. 3.9%) and in the combined outcome of nonfatal stroke or death (11.3% vs. 12.4%) when administered within 48 hours of the onset of symptoms compared to subcutaneous heparin or no treatment.
2. The Chinese Acute Stroke Trial (CAST) demonstrated a 14% reduction in total mortality at 4 weeks in the aspirin group compared to placebo.
3. These two trials demonstrate that aspirin therapy is crucial in the acute stroke setting, with an overall reduction of 13 deaths or significant residual impairment per 1000 patients treated at a 6-month follow up.
4. **Recommendations in acute stroke**
   a. Aspirin should be administered to all patients with acute ischemic stroke if no contraindication exists.
   b. Dosing should fall between 162.5 mg and 325 mg based on current literature. Enteric-coated preparations should be chewed or crushed initially.
   c. Therapy should continue indefinitely and the risk-benefit ratio must be examined individually.
   d. Other antiplatelet drugs including clopidogrel, ticlopidine, or the combinations of aspirin and dipyridamole may be equally effective after the acute event for those who cannot tolerate aspirin, but aspirin should be used initially. (See Chapter 86 for dosages)

D. Secondary prevention
1. The Multicenter Myocardial Ischemia Research Group evaluated the efficacy of aspirin vs. placebo as secondary prevention after an acute MI or in unstable angina. Aspirin use provided significantly lower rates of all-cause mortality (2.5% vs. 6.5%), cardiac death (1.6% vs. 5.4%), and nonfatal MI (6.5% vs. 11.4%) when compared to placebo.
2. The sixth American College of Chest Pain Physicians Consensus Conference on Antithrombotic Therapy recommends that all patients with evidence of coronary artery disease or with stable angina receive aspirin for secondary prevention indefinitely.
3. **Dosage recommendations for secondary prevention**
   a. The most universally accepted regimen used in the trials demonstrating the benefit of aspirin in secondary prevention was 75–325 mg/day.
   b. Higher aspirin dosages were not shown to be more effective.
   c. Lower doses were shown to be less beneficial.
4. There is no evidence to support that other antiplatelet drugs, such as clopidogrel, are preferable to aspirin and are far less cost-effective.
5. However, clopidogrel in addition to aspirin further decreases the risk of secondary events without increasing the risk of life-threatening bleeds.

E. Atrial fibrillation (AF)
1. **Aspirin**
   a. Several trials have attempted to demonstrate the efficacy of aspirin in the prevention of thromboembolic events in patients with AF, with conflicting results.
   b. Meta-analysis of the trials (including the AFASAK trial and the SPAF-I trial) reveals that although there is modest benefit of aspirin, this benefit varies widely with age and risk.
   c. Aspirin should be considered for primary prevention only in the patient with no other risk factors, including hypertension, diabetes mellitus, history of transient ischemic attack, and poor left ventricular function.
2. **Warfarin**
   a. Meta-analysis of five primary stroke prevention trials clearly demonstrates that anticoagulation with warfarin significantly reduces the risk of stroke in patients with AF when compared to aspirin or placebo. Overall, treating 100 patients with warfarin will prevent nearly three strokes per year.
   b. Trials evaluating the additive effect of warfarin plus aspirin therapy demonstrate that the combination is **not** beneficial.
   c. **Indications for warfarin therapy in atrial fibrillation**
      (1) Warfarin should be administered to patients with AF who are at risk to maintain the International Normalized Ratio (INR) at 2.0–3.0. Risk factors include a prior embolic event, left ventricular dysfunction, valvular heart disease, especially mitral stenosis, hypertension, age >60 years, and diabetes.

    (2) Patients with severe dilated cardiomyopathy, mitral stenosis, or prosthetic valves should be maintained at 2.0–4.5.

F. Diabetes mellitus

    1. The Antithrombotic Trialist's Collaboration analyzed nine trials evaluating aspirin as a preventive agent in diabetic patients. Based on these data, aspirin is recommended for all patients with diabetes mellitus who have one additional risk factor for cardiovascular disease.

IV. Bacterial Endocarditis

A. Pathophysiology

1. Infective endocarditis (IE) is a localized infection consisting of fibrin, platelets, and microorganisms that adhere to the cardiac valves. The pathogenesis of IE initiates with a bacteremia.

2. Procedures that result in transient bacteremia include invasive oral and dental surgery where the mucosa is penetrated or traumatized. Invasive genitourinary or GI procedures are less likely to cause a significant bacteremia.

3. Without appropriate treatment, the mortality rate approaches 100%.

4. Clinical manifestations include fever, cardiac murmurs, anemia, splenomegaly, petechiae, pyuria, and peripheral emboli.

5. The causative organisms for native valves are *Streptococcus viridans* and other streptococci (60%), *Staphylococcus aureus* (25%), enterococci (10%), and other gram-negative organisms (5%). For prosthetic valves beyond 2 months of placement, *S viridans* and other streptococci account for 30% of cases; coagulase-negative staphylococci, 20%; *S aureus,* 15%; and enterococci and gram-negative organisms, 10%.

6. Diagnosis is made by using clinical, microbiologic, and echocardiographic data (Tables 103–3 and 103–4).

B. Prophylaxis

1. Although only proved to prevent endocarditis in experimental animals, chemoprophylaxis is recommended for invasive procedures that cause bacteremia in humans having cardiac lesions highly associated with endocarditis.

    a. Those at high risk for cardiac lesions include people with prosthetic heart valves, a history of previous bacterial endocarditis, cyanotic congenital heart disease (single ventricle, transposition of the great vessels, and tetralogy of Fallot), pulmonary shunts or conduits, and advanced aortic or mitral valve disease.

    b. Those at moderate risk for lesions include people with uncorrected congenital heart conditions (patent ductus arteriosus, ventricular septal defect, primary atrial septal defect, coarctation of the aorta, and bicuspid aortic valve), acquired valvular dysfunction, and hypertrophic cardiomyopathy. Aortic or mitral

---

TABLE 103–3. MODIFIED DUKE CRITERIA FOR DIAGNOSIS OF INFECTIVE ENDOCARDITIS—I[1]

Definite IE
Pathologic criteria
Microorganism: demonstrated by culture or histology in a vegetation, or in a vegetation that has embolized, or in an intracardiac abscess **OR**
Pathologic lesions: vegetation or intracardiac abscess, confirmed by histology showing active endocarditis

Clinical criteria—using specific definitions listed in the following table
2 major criteria **OR**
1 major and 3 minor criteria **OR**
5 minor criteria

Possible IE[1]
1 major criterion and 1 minor criterion **OR** 3 minor criteria

Rejected IE
Firm alternate diagnosis for manifestations of endocarditis **OR**
Resolution of manifestations of endocarditis, with antibiotic therapy for 4 days or less **OR**
No pathologic evidence of infective endocarditis at surgery or autopsy after antibiotic therapy for 4 days or less
Does not meet criteria for possible infective endocarditis, as above

---

[1] The category of possible IE represents a modification from the previous published Duke criteria.
From Li JS, et al, Clin Infect Dis 2000;**30**:633.

TABLE 103-4. MODIFIED DUKE CRITERIA FOR DIAGNOSIS OF INFECTIVE ENDOCARDITIS—II

Major criteria

Positive blood cultures for IE

Typical microorganism for infective endocarditis from two separate blood cultures in the absence of a primary focus

    Viridans streptococci

    Streptococcus bovis, including nutritional variant strains

    HACEK group—*Haemophilus* spp, *Actinobacillus actinomycete* comitants, *Cardiobacterium hominis, Eikenella* spp, and *Kingella kingae*

    Community-acquired *Staphylococcus aureus* or enterococci

Persistently positive blood culture, defined as recovery of a microorganism consistent with IE from:

    Blood cultures drawn more than 12 hours apart **OR**

    All of three or a majority of four or more separate blood cultures, with first and last drawn at least 1 hour apart

Single positive blood culture for *Coxiella burnetii* or antiphase I IgG antibody titer >1:800[1]

Evidence of endocardial involvement

Positive echocardiogram for IE

TEE recommended in patients with prosthetic valves, rated at least "possible IE" by clinical criteria, or complicated IE [paravalvular abscess]; TTE as first test in other patients[1]

Definition of positive echocardiogram

    Oscillating intracardiac mass, on valve or supporting structures, or in the path of regurgitant jets, or on implanted material, in the absence of an alternative anatomic explanation **OR**

    Abscess **OR**

    New partial dehiscence of prosthetic valve

New valvular regurgitation

Increase in change in pre-existing murmur not sufficient

Minor criteria

Predisposition—predisposing heart condition or intravenous drug use

Fever—38.0 °C (100.4 °F)

Vascular phenomena—major arterial emboli, septic pulmonary infarcts, mycotic aneurysm, intracranial hemorrhage, conjunctival hemorrhages, Janeway lesions

Immunologic phenomena—glomerulonephritis, Osler's nodes, Roth spots, rheumatoid factor

Microbiologic evidence—positive blood culture but not meeting major criterion as noted previously (excluding single positive cultures for coagulase-negative staphylococci and organisms that do not cause endocarditis) **OR** serologic evidence of active infection with organism consistent with IE

Echocardiographic minor criteria eliminated[1]

---

[1] Modifications from the previous published Duke criteria.

TEE, transesophogeal echocardiography.

From Li JS, et al: Clin Infect Dis 2000;**30:**633.

valve diseases that do not have an associated murmur, click, or other evidence of significant leakage may be considered moderate risk. Otherwise, they are high risk.

    c. Low-risk conditions (not requiring antibiotic prophylaxis) include isolated secundum atrial septal defect, surgically corrected congenital heart lesions (atrial septal defect, ventricular septal defect, or patent ductus arteriosus without residua beyond 6 months), previous coronary artery bypass graft, previous Kawasaki disease without valvular dysfunction, and previous rheumatic fever without valvular dysfunction. Patients with cardiac pacemakers or innocent or functional murmurs are also not at risk.

    d. Specific dental and nondental procedures for which endocarditis prophylaxis is recommended or not recommended in patients with moderate- and high-risk conditions are listed in Tables 103-5 and 103-6.

2. The specific antibiotic prophylaxis guidelines in Tables 103-4, 103-7, and 103-8 and were designed to improve practitioner and patient compliance, reduce cost and potential GI adverse effects, and lessen risk of increasing bacterial resistance.

3. The importance of excellent oral hygiene for those patients at risk for IE cannot be underestimated. This includes brushing and flossing regularly, using oral antiseptics, providing atraumatic care for acneiform pustules, avoiding nail biting, and careful gum care.

TABLE 103–5. DENTAL PROCEDURES FOR WHICH ENDOCARDITIS PROPHYLAXIS IS RECOMMENDED OR NOT RECOMMENDED IN PATIENTS WITH HIGH AND MODERATE RISK CARDIAC DISEASES

Endocarditis Prophylaxis Recommended	Endocarditis Prophylaxis Not Recommended
• Dental extractions • Periodontal procedures including surgery, scaling and root planing, probing, and recall maintenance • Dental implant placement and reimplantation of avulsed teeth • Endodontic (root canal) instrumentation or surgery only beyond the apex • Subgingival placement of antibiotic fibers or strips • Initial placement of orthodontic bands but not brackets • Intraligamentary local anesthetic injections • Prophylactic cleaning of teeth of implants where bleeding is anticipated	• Restoration dentistry[1] (operative or prosthodontic with or without retraction cord)[2] • Local anesthetic injections (nonintraligamentary) • Intracanal endodontic treatment; post placement and buildup • Placement of rubber dams • Postoperative suture removal • Placement of removable prosthodontic or orthodontic appliances • Taking of oral impressions • Fluoride treatments • Taking of oral radiographs • Orthodontic appliance adjustment • Shedding of primary teeth

[1] This includes restoration of decayed teeth (filling cavities) and replacement of missing teeth.
[2] Clinical judgment may indicate antibiotic use in selected circumstances that may create significant bleeding.
Data from Dajani AS, et al: JAMA 1997;**277**:1797.

4. Although it is still considered important by many orthopedic physicians, there is no compelling evidence to support prophylaxes of patients with joint replacements prior to oral, GI, or genitourinary procedures.

V. Neural Tube Defects (NTDs)

A. Studies reveal that 20% of women whose pregnancies ended in miscarriages and up to 30% of women with recurrent miscarriages had an inadequate folate level. Several

TABLE 103–6. NONDENTAL PROCEDURES FOR WHICH ENDOCARDITIS PROPHYLAXIS IS RECOMMENDED OR NOT RECOMMENDED IN PATIENTS WITH HIGH- AND MODERATE-RISK CARDIAC DISEASES

Endocarditis Prophylaxis Recommended	Endocarditis Prophylaxis Not Recommended

Respiratory tract
• Tonsillectomy and/or adenoidectomy
• Surgical operations that involve the respiratory mucosa
• Bronchoscopy with a rigid bronchoscope
 	
Gastrointestinal tract[1]
• Sclerotherapy for esophageal varices
• Esophageal stricture dilation
• Endoscopic retrograde cholangiopancreatography with biliary obstruction
• Biliary tract surgery
• Surgical operations that involve the intestinal mucosa
 	
Genitourinary tract
• Prostatic surgery
• Cystoscopy
• Urethral dilation
	Respiratory tract
	• Endotracheal intubation
	• Bronchoscopy with a flexible bronchoscope with or without biopsy[2]
	• Tympanostomy tube insertion
	
	Gastrointestinal tract
	• Transesophageal echocardiography[2]
	• Endoscopy with or without gastrointestinal biopsy
	
	Genitourinary tract
	• Vaginal hysterectomy[2]
	• Vaginal delivery[2]
	• Cesarean section
	• In uninfected tissue:
	  Urethral catheterization
	  Uterine dilatation and curettage
	  Therapeutic abortion
	  Sterilization procedures
	  Insertion or removal of intrauterine devices
	
	Other
	• Cardiac catheterization, including balloon angioplasty
	• Implanted cardiac pacemakers, defibrillators, and coronary stents
	• Incision or biopsy of surgically scrubbed skin
	• Circumcision

[1] Prophylaxis is indicated for high-risk patients, optional for medium-risk patients.
[2] Prophylaxis is optional for high-risk patients.
Data from Dajani AS, et al: JAMA 1997;**277**:1797.

TABLE 103–7. PROPHYLACTIC REGIMENS FOR DENTAL, ORAL, RESPIRATORY TRACT, OR ESOPHAGEAL PROCEDURES

Situation	Agent	Regimen[1]
Standard general prophylaxis	Amoxicillin	Adults: 2.0 g; children: 50 mg/kg orally 1 h before procedure
Unable to take oral medications	Ampicillin	Adults: 2.0 g IM or IV; children: 50 mg/kg IM or IV within 30 min before procedure
Allergic to penicillin	Clindamycin *or*	Adults: 600 mg; children: 20 mg/kg orally 1 h before procedure
	Cephalexin[2] or cefadroxil[2] *or*	Adults: 2.0 g; children: 50 mg/kg orally 1 h before procedure
	Azithromycin or clarithomycin	Adults: 500 mg; children: 15 mg/kg orally 1 h before procedure
	Clindamycin *or*	Adults: 600 mg; children: 20 mg/kg IV within 30 min before procedure
Allergic to penicillin and unable to take oral medications	Cephazolin[2]	Adults: 1.0 g; children: 25 mg/kg IM or IV within 30 min before procedure

[1] Total children's dose should not exceed adult dose.
[2] Cephalosporins should not be used in individuals with immediate-type hypersensitivity reaction (urticaria, angioedema, or anaphylaxis) to penicillins.
IM, intramuscular; IV, intravenous.
Reprinted from Dajani et al: Prevention of bacterial endocarditis. CID 1997;**25**:1454.

TABLE 103–8. PROPHYLACTIC REGIMENS FOR GENITOURINARY OR GASTROINTESTINAL (EXCLUDING ESOPHAGEAL) PROCEDURES

Situation	Agents[1]	Regimen[2]
High-risk patients	Ampicillin plus gentamicin	Adults: ampicillin 2.0 g IM or IV plus gentamicin 1.5 mg/kg (not to exceed 120 mg) within 30 min of starting the procedure; 6 h later, ampicillin 1 g IM/IV or amoxicillin 1 g orally Children: ampicillin 50 mg/kg IM or IV (not to exceed 2.0 g) plus gentamicin 1.5 mg/kg within 30 min of starting the procedure; 6 h later, ampicillin 25 mg/kg IM/IV or amoxicillin 25 mg/kg orally
High-risk patients allergic to ampicillin/amoxicillin	Vancomycin plus gentamicin	Adults: vancomycin 1.0 g IV over 1–2 h plus gentamicin 1.5 mg/kg IV/IM (not to exceed 120 mg); complete injection/infusion within 30 min of starting the procedure Children: vancomycin 20 mg/kg IV over 1–2 h plus gentamicin 1.5 mg/kg IV/IM; complete injection/infusion within 30 min of starting the procedure
Moderate-risk patients	Amoxicillin or ampicillin	Adults: amoxicillin 2.0 g orally 1 h before procedure; or ampicillin 2.0 g IM/IV within 30 min of starting the procedure Children: amoxicillin 50 mg/kg orally 1 h before procedure, or ampicillin 50 mg/kg IM/IV within 30 min of starting the procedure
Moderate-risk patients allergic to ampicillin/amoxicillin	Vancomycin	Adults: vancomycin 1.0 g IV over 1–2 h; complete infusion within 30 min of starting the procedure Children: vancomycin 20 mg/kg IV over 1–2 h; complete infusion within 30 min of starting the procedure

[1] Total children's dose should not exceed adult dose.
[2] No second dose of vancomycin or gentamicin is recommended.
Reprinted from Dajani et al: Prevention of bacterial endocarditis. CID 1997;**25**:1455.

studies suggest that consumption of folic acid decreases the incidence of NTDs in the fetuses of pregnant women when taken during the first 6 weeks after conception. These studies include trials of folate supplementation, dietary consumption of folate, and folate concentrations in serum and red blood cells.

B. **Recommendations for folate supplementation**

1. The US Public Health Service and The Food and Nutrition Board of the Institute of Medicine recommend that all women of childbearing age capable of becoming pregnant consume 0.4 mg of folic acid per day in order to reduce their risk of having a child with NTD, since nearly half of all pregnancies are unplanned.

2. Many experts recommend doses far higher than this (800 µg/day) for women trying to conceive. All women should consume 0.6 mg of folate per day during pregnancy and 0.5 mg of folate per day during lactation.

3. Women who have delivered a child with an NTD should consume 4 mg/day of folate 1 month prior to conception and for the first 3 months of pregnancy. The minimal effective folate dose is unknown.

C. The US Food and Drug Administration decided in 1993 to fortify staple foods by adding 1.4 mg folic acid/kg of cereal grain. Folic acid consumption may mask the hematologic manifestations of pernicious anemia in the elderly. Folate doses should be kept under 1 mg/day in those with low vitamin B_{12} levels, particularly those with achlorhydria and gastric atrophy lacking intrinsic factor.

D. Moderate increases in folate supply should also lower serum homocysteine in patients heterozygous for the gene for homocystinuria. Elevated homocysteine levels appear to be a strong independent risk factor for coronary vascular disease.

VI. **Rheumatic Fever**

A. Rheumatic fever is a **complication of group A β-hemolytic streptococcal infection** of the upper respiratory tract that is most frequently observed in children aged 5–13 years.

B. Diagnosis is based on meeting the **Jones criteria:** two major criteria or one major and two minor criteria plus evidence of a preceding streptococcal infection (Table 103–5).

C. **Prophylaxis**

1. The goal of prophylaxis against group A strep is to prevent a **recurrence** of acute rheumatic fever. Recurrence rates decrease with increasing age, but recurrences have been documented as late as the fifth or sixth decade.

2. **Recommendations for treatment duration**

   a. Patients who have had rheumatic fever with carditis and residual heart disease need prophylaxis for at least 10 years beyond the last episode and until age 40 years or perhaps for life.

   b. Patients who have had rheumatic fever with carditis but without residual heart disease need prophylaxis for at least 10 years since the last episode or well into adulthood, whichever is longer.

   c. Patients who have had rheumatic fever without carditis need prophylaxis for at least 5 years since the last episode or until age 21, whichever is longer.

3. **Recommended regimen**

   a. Benzathine penicillin G (1,200,000 U intramuscularly every 3–4 weeks).

   b. Penicillin V (250 mg by mouth twice daily).

   c. Sulfadiazine (500 mg/day orally if <60 lbs; 1 g/day orally if >60 lbs).

   d. Erythromycin (250 mg by mouth twice daily).

4. A possible alternative to long-term prophylaxis in the future may be a streptococcal vaccine that would eliminate primary rheumatic fever by eliminating the causative organism.

VII. **Group B Streptococcal Disease (GBS).** GBS is a Gram-positive bacterium that colonizes the human GI tract and genitourinary tract. It is the most frequently encountered bacterial pathogen in neonates, and prevention of GBS transmission during vaginal delivery is crucial.

A. **History of intrapartum antibiotic prophylaxis (IAP)**

1. Two approaches to IAP existed prior to 2002. The first was risk factor based and the second was screening based.

2. A 1999 study raised questions about the inconsistency of these two strategies. Infants born to women whose physicians used the risk factor–based approach were 50% more likely to have early-onset GBS disease.

B. **Revised 2002 IAP Screening Guidelines**

1. All pregnant women should be screened for GBS colonization with swabs of both the lower vagina and the rectum at 35–37 weeks' gestation.

   2. Patients with GBS bacteriuria in the current pregnancy or with a positive GBS infant in a previous pregnancy should receive IAP regardless.

C. Patients recommended for IAP
   1. Pregnant women with a positive GBS screen unless a planned cesarean section is performed in the absence of labor or rupture of membranes.
   2. Pregnant women who have had a prior infant with GBS disease.
   3. Women with GBS bacteriuria during the current pregnancy.
   4. Pregnant women whose culture status is unknown and who also have delivery at <37 weeks, rupture >18 hours, or temperature spike to >100.4 °F.

D. Regimen
   1. Penicillin G (5 million units intravenously initial dose, then 2.5 million units every 4 hours)
   2. Ampicillin (2 g intravenously initial dose, then 1 g every 4 hours). Penicillin has a narrower spectrum and is preferred.
   3. Cefazolin (2 g initial dose, then 1 g every 8 hours).
   4. If a patient has an anaphylaxis risk to penicillins, the physician may give clindamycin (900 mg intravenously every 8 hours) or erythromycin (500 mg intravenously every 6 hours).

REFERENCES

American Diabetes Association. Position statement: Aspirin therapy in diabetes. Diabetes Care 2001;**24**(suppl 1):S62.

Baker CJ: Chemoprophylaxis for the prevention of Group B streptococcal disease. In: UpToDate, Rose BD (editor), UpToDate, (Wellesley, MA); 2003.

Braunwald E, et al: ACC/AHA 2002 Guideline update for the management of patients with unstable angina and non-ST segment elevation myocardial infarction summary article. A report of the American College of Cardiology/American Heart Association task force on practice guidelines. J Am Coll Cardiol 2002;**40**:1366.

CAST (Chinese Acute Stroke Trial): Randomized placebo-controlled trial of early aspirin use in 20,000 patients with acute ischemic stroke. Cast Collaborative Group. Lancet 1997;**349**:1641.

Collaborative meta-analysis of randomized trials of antiplatelet therapy for prevention of death, myocardial infarction and stroke in high risk patients. BMJ 2002;**324**:71.

Dajani A, et al: Prevention of bacterial endocarditis: Recommendations by the American Heart Association. Circulation 1997;**96**:358.

Dajani A, et al: Treatment of acute streptococcal pharyngitis and prevention of rheumatic fever: A statement for health professionals. Pediatrics 1995;**96**:758.

Goldstein RE, et al for the Multicenter Myocardial Ischemia research group: Marked reduction in long-term cardiac deaths with aspirin after a coronary event. J Am Coll Cardiol 1996;**28**:326.

Hart RG, et al: Aspirin for the primary prevention of stroke and other major vascular events: Meta-analysis and hypotheses. Arch Neurol 2000;**57**:326.

Hennekens CH, Dyken ML, Fuster V: Aspirin as a therapeutic agent in cardiovascular disease: A statement for healthcare professionals from the American Heart Association. Circulation 1997;**96**:2751.

The International Stroke Trial (IST): A randomized trial of aspirin, subcutaneous heparin, both, or neither among patients with acute ischemic stroke. International Stroke Trial Collaborative Group. Lancet 1997;**349**:1569.

Lauer MS: Clinical practice. Aspirin for the primary prevention of coronary events. N Engl J Med 2002;**346**:1468.

Pearson TA, et al: AHA guidelines for the primary prevention of cardiovascular disease and stroke: 2002 Update: consensus panel guide to comprehensive risk reduction for adult patients without coronary or other atherosclerotic vascular diseases. American Heart Association Science Advisory and Coordinating Committee. Circulation 2002;**106**:388.

---

104   Travel Medicine

Lowell G. Sensintaffar, MD, & Matthew E. Ulven, MD, MPH

I. Quick Treatment Guide
  A. Know your traveler!
   1. Age, gender.
   2. Destination, duration.

   3. Modes of travel.
   4. High-risk activities or behaviors.
   5. Comorbid illnesses or pregnancy.
   B. Nonpharmacologic measures
     1. Arthropod bite prevention. Proper coverage with 30–35% DEET on exposed areas of skin and permethrin-impregnated clothing can afford nearly 100% protection from ticks and mosquitoes.
     2. Food and water precautions. "Boil it, peel it, cook it, or forget it." Avoid unpasteurized milk and reheated foods (especially from street vendors). Food should be served and eaten piping hot. Consume seafood with caution. Drink bottled, boiled, or treated water only.
     3. Sunscreen. Sunscreen should have a Sun Protection Factor (SPF) of 15 or greater.
   C. Vaccinations. See Tables 104–1 and 104–2.
   D. Malarial chemoprophylaxis. See Table 104–3 and 104–4.
   E. Motion sickness and jet lag. See Tables 104–6 and 104–7.
   F. Staying current. Review the Centers for Disease Control and Prevention (CDC) and the World Health Organization (WHO) web sites for current information before finalizing treatment plans.
     1. CDC—http://www.cdc.gov/travel
     2. \eh6\WHO—www.who.int
II. Introduction. In 2001, 693 million people traveled internationally. Despite recent global economic downturns, a surge in global terrorism, and regional conflicts, and emerging new diseases such as Severe Acute Respiratory Syndrome, the overall trend in international travel is increasing. An 80% increase in international travel between 1995 and 2010 is predicted. Travel medicine addresses the travel-specific health concerns of these people.
   A. The pre-travel visit. The clinic visit should be at least 4–6 weeks before travel to ensure adequate time for vaccinations. Nevertheless, a clinic visit just days prior to travel, while not ideal, can be beneficial.
   B. Vaccinations (routine and travel-related)
     1. Routine vaccinations. All routine and childhood vaccinations should be current according to established guidelines. An accelerated vaccination schedule can be used to catch-up children who are delinquent prior to travel (Table 104–1). Guidelines notwithstanding, there are some important aspects of some routine vaccinations that need to be considered before embarking on travel, particularly to developing countries (Table 104–2).
       a. *Haemophilus influenza b* (Hib) vaccines. All splenectomized travelers (including functional asplenia, eg, sickle cell disease) and other individuals at

TABLE 104–1. ACCELERATED IMMUNIZATION SCHEDULE FOR TRAVELING CHILDREN

Vaccine	Minimum Age for First Dose	Minimum Interval for Second Dose	Minimum Interval for Third Dose	Minimum Interval for Fourth Dose
Hepatitis B	Birth	4 weeks	8 weeks	NA
Diphtheria–tetanus–acellular pertussis (DtaP)	6 weeks	4 weeks	4 weeks	6 mos.
Inactivated poliomyelitis vaccine (IPV)	6 weeks	4 weeks	4 weeks	4 weeks
Haemophilus influenza b (Hib)[1]	6 weeks	4 weeks	4 weeks	Booster after 12 mos. of age
Prevnar	6 weeks	4 weeks	4 weeks	8 weeks, but not earlier than 12 mos. of age
Measles–Mumps–Rubella (MMR)	6 mos.[2]	12 mos. of age	4 weeks	NA
Varicella[3]	12 mos.	4 weeks[4]	NA	NA

[1] The Hib vaccine that is conjugated to the outer membrane protein does not require a third or fourth dose.
[2] If given at 6–12 mos, a booster is required again at 12 months, at least 4 weeks after the first vaccination.
[3] Children with a reliable history of chickenpox should be considered immune and vaccination is not necessary.
[4] The second dose of varicella vaccine is only required for susceptible children older than 12 years.
From Stauffer WM, Kamat D: Traveling with infants and children. Part 2: Immunizations. J Travel Med 2002;9(2):82.

TABLE 104–2. RECOMMENDATIONS FOR THE PREVENTION OF VACCINE-PREVENTABLE DISEASES IN TRAVELERS

Vaccinations (Earliest Effective Date)	Indication	Administration	Booster?	Contraindications[1]	Miscellaneous Comments
Cholera Whole-cell-B subunit vaccine **Dukoral** (7 days after last dose) Live attenuated vaccine **Mutacol** (8 days after last dose)	Consider for long-term travel to cholera-endemic areas or areas with active cholera outbreak	Dukoral: two doses (ages >6 years) or 3 doses (age 2–6 years) at intervals of 7–42 days. Mutacol single dose (ages 2 years and older). Vaccine should not be administered within 1 week of antibiotics or chloroquine or within 8 hours of oral typhoid vaccine.	Dukoral: Every 3 months for ages >2 years to insure ETEC protection. Otherwise every 2 years for age >6 years and every 6 months for ages 2–6 years. Mutacol: Every 6 months for all age groups.	Live, attenuated vaccine is contraindicated in phenyl-ketonurics, severely immunocompromised travelers (eg, those with AIDS), and children <2 years old. Not approved in pregnancy but risk is remote and theoretical. Benefits should outweigh risk.	Dukoral vaccine effective against ETEC travelers' diarrhea after two doses. Mutacol has no effect on ETEC. Vaccines not available in the United States. Contact manufacturers for availability: www.activebiotech.com and www.berna.com
Tetanus–diphtheria (TD) and tetanus–diphtheria–acellular pertussis (DtaP)	All travelers	For those 7 years or older or who have not received the full tetanus–diphtheria series should receive a 3-dose series of Td. First 2 doses, 4–8 weeks apart and the third dose 6–12 months after the second. If last dose cannot be insured, the third dose can be administered 4–8 weeks after the second.	At ages 11–12 years if it had been at least 5 years since last pediatric dose. Every 10 years for all others.	High fevers can occur in children who receive the DTP formulations. For these children, DTaP should be used. Children with some neurologic disorders may not be able to take the pertussis component. For these individuals the DT formulation is recommended.	All children <7 years old should be vaccinated with DTaP according to routine immunization schedule
Hepatitis A[2] (1 month after first dose)	All travelers to endemic areas	2 doses, 6–24 months apart	None		
Immune globulin (Immediately effective)	Travelers to areas with high hepatitis A endemicity or who have a contraindication to hepatitis A vaccine or did not receive the vaccine prior to 1 month pre-travel	Short-term (1–2 mo) cover-age: 0.02 mg/kg IM Long-term (3–6 mo) cover-age: 0.06 mg/kg IM	Booster dependent on initial dose given and length of continued stay. Booster not needed if hepatitis A vaccine given just prior to travel.		

Vaccine (interval)	Indications	Primary schedule	Booster	Notes/Contraindications
Hepatitis B (2 weeks after second dose)	All travelers	3 doses at 0, 1 month, and 6–12 months	None	
Hib (*Haemophilus influenzae*, type b)	All travelers <5 years of age and previously unvaccinated asplenic travelers	Single dose in splenectomized people >5 years. Accelerated program available for infant travelers (Table 104–1)	NA	
Influenza[1,3] (2 weeks)	All travelers		Annually	Egg allergy. See text for tropical and opposite hemisphere considerations
Japanese encephalitis (after 2 doses)	Travelers for >1 month to endemic rural areas of eastern Asia including the Indian subcontinent	3 doses on days 0, 7, and 14–30.	Every 3 years	Hypersensitivity reactions have occurred as late as 10 days post vaccination (after any dose in series). Delay of travel recommended for at least 10 days if traveling to area with poor medical access
Meningococcal (10 days)	Hajj or umra pilgrims. Consider for travel to sub-Saharan Africa; unvaccinated asplenic patients	Single injection	Every 3 years	Meningococcal vaccine must be at least 10 days old for entry into Saudi Arabia
Measles–mumps–rubella (MMR)	All travelers over 6 mos. of age. (see notes for travelers 6–12 months of age)	Accelerated vaccination program available for infant travelers	Booster >4 weeks after first dose. See notes for immunization in 6- to 12-month age group	Known allergy to neomycin, gelatin. **Allergy to eggs is not a contraindication.** CD4+ count <200 cell/μL
Pneumococcal disease[1] (2 weeks)	Age >65 years, persons with chronic diseases, and asplenic travelers	Single injection	5-year booster in some populations	
Polio (inactivated poliomyelitis vaccine (IPV) or oral polio vaccine (OPV) (4 weeks))	All travelers		Single dose administered by injection (IPV) or orally (OPV) prior to travel to an endemic area	Known reaction to formaldehyde. OPV contraindicated in immunosuppressed individuals.

(continued)

TABLE 104–2. RECOMMENDATIONS FOR THE PREVENTION OF VACCINE-PREVENTABLE DISEASES IN TRAVELERS (Continued)

Vaccinations (Earliest Effective Date)	Indication	Administration	Booster?	Contraindications[1]	Miscellaneous Comments
Rabies[1] (1 week after final dose)	Recommended for pre-exposure prophylaxis for prolonged stays in hyper-endemic areas, or parks and game reserves in endemic areas	Series of 3 injections at 0, 7, and 21–28 days for pre-exposure prophylaxis	2–3 years depending on risk of exposure. Pre-exposure vaccination does not eliminate need for post-exposure management.		3 vaccines available: –Human Diploid Cell Vaccine (HDCV) 1-cc IM dose or 0.1-cc intradermal dose. –Purified Chick Embryo Cell (PCEC). 1 cc IM only –Rabies Vaccine Absorbed (RVA) 1 cc IM only
Tick-borne encephalitis[1] (2 weeks after second dose)	High-risk travelers to rural areas of Europe	Series of 3 IM injections at 0 days, 4–12 weeks, and 9–12 months	3 years	Sensitivity to thiomersal	Vaccine not available in the United States. Available in Canada and Europe. Disease can be acquired by tick bite and by consuming unpasteurized milk.
Tuberculosis (BCG) (4 weeks)	Consider for infants <6 mos. of age and high-risk health care workers	One dose, intradermally	None	Severely immunocompromised	
Typhoid fever[1] (1 week)	Recommended for high-risk areas.[4] Parenteral age >2 years Oral age >6 years	Parenteral, one dose IM. Oral, 4 doses on days 1, 3, 5, and 7.	Parenteral—3 years Oral—6 years. (Stop proguanil, mefloquine, and antibiotics 1 week before and after administration of oral vaccine.)	Parenteral vaccine more likely to cause a systemic reaction	
Yellow fever (10 days)	Sub-Saharan Africa and tropical South America	Single injection	10 years	Egg allergy, age <6 mos. Pregnancy is a relative contraindication.	

[1] Hypersensitivity can occur with any vaccine. Previous hypersensitivity is a contraindication to further vaccination.
[2] Immunoglobulin is recommended for children younger than 2 years of age. Hepatitis A vaccine is approved for children older than 1 year of age in Europe.
[3] Because of seasonal variations between hemispheres, may need to receive vaccination at destination. Indicated for travel at any time to tropical areas.
[4] Typhoid vaccination strongly recommended for travel to high-risk areas for more than 1 month.
ETEC, enterotoxigenic *Escherichia coli*.

increased risk for infections from encapsulated organisms should receive a single Hib vaccination if childhood vaccination cannot be confirmed.

b. **Influenza vaccine.** Although seasonal in temperate regions, in tropical regions influenza is a perennial disease. Furthermore, the peak incidence of influenza in one hemisphere is opposite that of the other hemisphere (ie, influenza season runs November through March in the Northern temperate regions and May through September in Southern temperate regions). Interhemispheric travelers should take these seasonal differences into consideration and be vaccinated, if needed, upon arrival at their destination. Influenza vaccines from the northern and southern hemispheres are not necessarily the same, so vaccination with one vaccine does not necessarily confer immunity in the opposite hemisphere. Travelers in situations where multinational groups (perhaps from the opposite hemisphere) gather in close quarters (eg, cruise vacations and international conventions) should also consider vaccination. While not a substitute for vaccination, prophylactic medications such as amantadine, zanamivir, or oseltamivir can be prescribed if influenza vaccine is unavailable.

c. **Measles–Mumps–Rubella (MMR) vaccine.** While the MMR vaccine is normally first given between ages 12–15 months, children aged 6–12 months traveling to the developing world may benefit from an early MMR or monovalent measles vaccine. Maternal antibodies and the immature immune systems of young infants can decrease the measles seroconversion rate in young infants, but morbidity and mortality studies on infants in developing, measles-endemic countries have demonstrated some benefit to earlier vaccination. If an MMR is given prior to the first birthday, the routine MMR vaccine schedule must be restarted at age 12–15 months.

d. **Poliomyelitis vaccine.** Because the risk of vaccine-associated paralytic poliomyelitis in the United States exceeds that of the infection with the wild virus, the attenuated live oral polio vaccine (OPV) is no longer recommended in the United States. A single injected inactivated poliomyelitis vaccine (IPV) booster is recommended before travel to endemic areas.

2. **Travel-related vaccinations** (Table 104–2).

a. **Bacille-Calmette-Guérin (BCG) vaccine.** This vaccine is rarely administered in the United States. Nevertheless, BCG vaccination has been shown to protect very young children from severe tuberculosis, particularly neurotuberculosis. BCG vaccine should be considered in very young children who will have prolonged contact with indigenous people in developing countries. Health care workers with prolonged exposure to populations with high tuberculosis endemicity may also benefit from BCG vaccination.

b. **Cholera vaccine.** The risk of cholera for the average western traveler to a developing nation is so remote (0.2 per 100,000 travelers) that cholera vaccination is of questionable benefit in this population. However, some long-term travelers to cholera-endemic areas or areas with an active cholera outbreak may benefit from this vaccine. Due to poor efficacy of the cholera parenteral vaccine, two oral vaccines, whole-cell-B subunit vaccine (Duracol) and a live, attenuated vaccine (Mutacol) have been developed. In addition to cholera, Duracol vaccine also affords some protection against the enterotoxigenic *Escherichia coli* (ETEC), a very common cause of traveler's diarrhea. Mutacol does not afford any protection from ETEC.

c. **Hepatitis A vaccine.** Hepatitis A vaccine is recommended for all travelers to areas endemic for hepatitis A. If the vaccine is not administered at least 1 month prior to travel, immune globulin prophylaxis prior to travel is recommended. Hepatitis A is generally a mild disease in young children, but they can shed the virus for months. For this reason, hepatitis A vaccination of young children, particularly those in diapers, may promote the health of the family and other caregivers. Although hepatitis A vaccine is approved for children older than age 2 years, data suggest that the vaccine is safe and efficacious in children as young as 1 year. Hepatitis A vaccination in Canada and Europe is approved in children older than 1 year. Use of the vaccine in children younger than 2 years old in the United States should be considered off-label. Young children who do not receive the vaccine should receive immune globulin prior to travel.

d. Japanese encephalitis vaccine. Japanese encephalitis is a mosquito-borne viral disease endemic to rural Southeast Asia. Although most travelers are at low risk for this disease, those traveling in these rural areas for more than 1 month should consider this vaccination series.

e. Meningococcal vaccine. Pilgrims entering Saudi Arabia for the Hajj, umra, or seasonal work must show proof of quadrivalent (A, C, W-135, Y) meningococcal vaccination not >3 years or <10 days prior to arrival. Travelers to sub-Saharan Africa, particularly during the dry season (December–June), or in areas of current outbreaks of these serotypes should also consider vaccination. Travelers with surgical or functional asplenia are at particular risk of meningococcal disease and should be vaccinated. Meningococcal disease tends to be more severe in the very young and very old. Unfortunately, the quadrivalent (A,C,W-135,Y) vaccine is poorly immunogenic in young children. This is particularly true of serogroups C, W-135 and Y. In spite of this short-coming, the vaccine is still recommended in children traveling to high-risk areas. A monovalent conjugate vaccine to serogroup C is available in Canada, Australia, and Europe and is highly effective in people of all ages. It should be noted, however, that the predominant serotype in sub-Saharan Africa is serogroup A and vaccines to other serogroups are not effective. It is also important to note that there is no effective vaccine for serogroup B, a common serogroup in the Western Hemisphere and Europe.

f. Rabies vaccine. Pre-exposure prophylaxis is recommended for high-risk travelers including animal handlers, trekkers, cyclists, veterinarians, spelunkers, field biologists, and missionaries. Due to their curiosity concerning animals and immaturity, children may be at particular risk for rabies. There are three vaccines available: Human Diploid Cell Vaccine (HDCV), Purified Chick Embryo Cell (PCEC) vaccine, and Rabies Vaccine Absorbed (RVA). PCEC and RVA are given at a dose of 1 cc intramuscularly. HDCV can be given intramuscularly or intradermally (ID) at a dose of 1 cc or 0.1 cc, respectively. Pre-exposure vaccines, regardless of type, should never be given in the gluteal muscle because of decreased efficacy with this route. The smaller HDCV intradermally dose can be much less expensive. Concomitant dosing of HDCV with chloroquine or mefloquine can dampen the immune response. HDCV should not be given within 1 week of mefloquine or chloroquine. Pre-exposure rabies vaccination does simplify the post-bite rabies regimen but does not eliminate the need for prompt medical care that can include an abbreviated post-exposure regimen.

g. Typhoid vaccine. Two vaccines are available—the oral TY21a and injectable Vi capsular vaccines. The injectable vaccine is more likely to cause systemic reactions, needs a booster every 2 years, and is approved for ages older than 2 years. The oral vaccine requires four doses on days 1, 3, 5, and 7, lasts 5 years, has fewer side effects, and is approved for ages 6 years and up. Breast-feeding may confer passive immunity.

h. Yellow fever vaccine. A valid International Certificate of Vaccination documenting yellow fever vaccination is required for entry into some countries. The certificate is valid 10 days after immunization and expires after 10 years. Yellow fever vaccine should never be used in infants younger than 6 months due to an increased risk of post-vaccine encephalitis and should only be used in children from 6 to 9 months of age if traveling to an area with an active yellow fever outbreak. For those individuals in whom yellow fever vaccination is contraindicated (immunocompromised persons, infants, pregnant women, or persons with an egg allergy), a waiver letter on a physician's letterhead should be given and an official stamp placed on the vaccination card. Pregnant women should receive the vaccine only when the benefit outweighs the risk. Although yellow fever vaccination is required every 10 years, evidence suggests that protective antibodies remain for 35–40 years. For this reason, pregnant women who have a history of yellow fever vaccination will likely gain no benefit from repeat vaccination and a waiver letter should be issued regardless of perceived risks.

3. Chemoprophylaxis

a. Malaria. Malarial prophylaxis is absolutely critical. Local resistance patterns should be considered prior to prescribing prophylaxis (Table 104–3). Please refer to Table 104–4 for dosage instructions. For travelers with prolonged travel

TABLE 104–3. MALARIAL RESISTANCE AND PROPHYLACTIC DRUG CHOICE

Geographic Resistance/Susceptibility	Drug Choices in Order of Preference
Chloroquine-susceptible areas	Chloroquine, doxycycline, mefloquine, atovaquone-proguanil
Chloroquine-resistant areas	Mefloquine, doxycycline, atovaquone-proguanil
Mefloquine-resistant areas	Doxycycline, atovaquone-proguanil

to areas endemic with *Plasmodium vivax* or *ovale,* terminal prophylaxis with primaquine may be needed. The most deadly malaria by far is *Plasmodium falciparum.* People traveling to areas where *P falciparum* malaria is endemic who will be unable to access medical care within 24 hours should be proactively prescribed emergency antimalarial treatment. Up-to-date recommendations for emergency antimalarial treatment can be found at the WHO web site (www.who.int/ith).

   b. **Travelers' diarrhea (TD)**
   1. **Prophylaxis.** Currently the CDC does not recommend prophylactic antibiotics for TD in most travelers. Nevertheless, some travelers may elect to take prophylactic antibiotics particularly if even a portion of a lost day to illness would be catastrophic (eg, diplomats, athletes, business people, etc). Ciprofloxacin (500 mg daily), norfloxacin (400 mg daily), ofloxacin (400 mg daily), levofloxacin (500 mg daily), and Pepto-Bismol (2 tablets four times daily) are all reasonable choices.
   2. **Treatment of TD.** Most travelers' diarrhea is self-limited. Antibiotics can hasten recovery in most cases. Dosages can be found in Table 104–5. Oral rehydration therapy is critical, particularly for children.
III. **Illness and Injury Prevention**
   A. **Arthropod bite prevention**
      1. *N,N*-diethyl-3-methylbenzamide (DEET): DEET is the most used, most effective, and best-studied insect repellent on the world market. When used as directed, its safety profile is unmatched. Plant-based repellents (Bite Blocker, Skin-so-Soft, and citronella) are much less effective than DEET-based products. DEET is available in 5–100% concentrations. The higher concentrations afford longer protection times between applications. Studies have shown that 50% DEET provides around 4 hours of protection. It should be noted that increasing the concentration to 100% increases the duration of protection by only 1 hour. Extended-release DEET preparations have made it possible to increase the duration of action while lowering the concentration. For the vast majority of travelers, including pregnant women and children, a DEET concentration of 30–35% provides adequate protection. The traveler should reapply DEET every 4 hours and more often when perspiring heavily or after swimming. When one is applying sunscreen and insect repellent together, the sunscreen should be applied first. While the *Anopheles* and *Culex* species of mosquitoes are nighttime feeders, *Aedes* species, responsible for yellow and dengue fevers, are daytime feeders. Round-the-clock protection is necessary in endemic areas.
      2. **Permethrin.** Permethrin is a contact insecticide that is applied to clothing to augment DEET protection. Combined with DEET, permethrin can afford nearly 100% protection from ticks and mosquitoes. Permethrin is sold in 0.5% sprays and 13.3% soaks. Once applied, permethrin's insecticidal effects linger through several launderings.
      3. **Other measures.** Using permethrin-impregnated mosquito netting for sleeping, having air-conditioned sleeping quarters, spraying sleeping quarters with insecticide for flying insects (eg, Raid), wearing light-colored clothing, and avoiding colognes and perfumes can further reduce the risk of arthropod bites.
      4. **Special note of caution.** Tsetse flies, the cause of African trypanosomiasis (African sleeping sickness), are not well repelled by DEET. These black flies elicit a painful bite. Onset of fever with or without a chancre at the bite site in the weeks following a painful fly bite in Eastern or Western Africa should prompt immediate medical attention.
   B. **Food and drinking water safety.** TD and other food-borne illnesses are the most common causes of morbidity among travelers to developing countries.
      1. **Water.** The traveler should avoid consuming nonbottled water in developing countries. Tap water that has been boiled for 1 minute at sea level (boil longer at higher

TABLE 104-4. MALARIA CHEMOPROPHYLAXIS DRUG DOSAGES

Drug	Adult Dosing	Pediatric Dosing/Concerns	Pregnancy/Lactation Concerns	Side Effects, Precautions, and Miscellaneous Concerns
Chloroquine (Aralen)	500 mg weekly beginning 12 weeks before travel and continuing 4 weeks after return	5 mg/kg up to adult dose. Liquid formulation available in some countries. May require pharmacy compounding.	Safe in pregnancy and lactation. Concentrations in breast milk are not protective for infant.	Usually minor: itching, skin eruptions, headache. Contraindicated in patients with severe hepatic insufficiency. The therapeutic window is fairly narrow. Fatal overdoses of young children have been reported at doses as little as 300 mg. Accurate dosing in young children is critical.
Mefloquine (Lariam)	250 mg weekly beginning 1–2 weeks before travel and continuing 4 weeks after return	**<15 kg:** 5 mg/kg weekly (will require pharmacy compounding into liquid form for accurate dosing) **15–19 kg:** ¼ tablet weekly **20–30 kg:** ½ tablet weekly **31–45 kg:** ¾ tablet weekly **>45 kg:** adult dose	Safe in second and third trimesters.	25–40% will experience mild side effects (nausea, headaches) Neuropsychiatric side effects uncommon in prophylactic dosages. Contraindicated in patients with epilepsy, serious psychiatric illness, or cardiac conduction disturbance.
Atovaquone-proguanil (Malarone)	250 mg/100 mg daily beginning 1–2 days before travel and stopping 1 week after return.	**<11 kg:** not recommended at this time **11–20 kg:** 1 pediatric tablet (62.5/25) po daily **21–30 kg:** 2 pediatric tablets po daily **31–40 kg:** 3 pediatric tablets po daily **>40 kg:** 1 adult tablet po daily	First trimester usage unstudied, but most experts feel that real risk of malaria outweighs any theoretical risk of taking medication. Concentrations in breast milk are not protective for nursing infant.	Contraindicated in patients with severe renal insufficiency (creatinine clearance <30 mL/min)
Doxycycline (Vibramycin and others)	100 mg po daily beginning 1–2 days before travel and continuing for 4 weeks after return	**>8 years:** 2 mg/kg/day up to adult dose. Contraindicated in children 8 years old and younger.	Contraindicated in pregnancy and lactation	A photo sensitizer. Increases risk for sunburn. Recommend sunscreen.
Primaquine (Palum)	26.3 mg po daily for 14 days after departure for those individuals with prolonged exposure to *Plasmodium vivax* and *Plasmodium ovale*	0.5 mg/kg up to adult dose	Contraindicated in pregnancy since the G6PD status of the newborn is unknown.	Contraindicated in G6PD deficiency.

TABLE 104–5. TREATMENT OF TRAVELERS' DIARRHEA (TD)

Drug	Adult Dosing	Pediatric Dosing/Concerns	Pregnancy/Lactation Concerns	Side Effects, Precautions, and Miscellaneous Concerns
Ciprofloxacin (Cipro)	500 mg po bid × 3 days after onset of diarrhea	15–20 mg/kg/dose bid up to adult dose. Some experts recommend for severe TD/dysentery.	Relative contraindication in pregnancy: Some experts recommend for severe TD/dysentery.	Relative contraindication in childhood and in pregnancy due to studies showing arthropathy in immature animals.
Azithromycin (Zithromax)	200 mg daily for 3 days	10 mg/kg/day × 3 days after onset of diarrhea	May use in pregnancy.	
Loperamide (Imodium)	4 mg followed by 2 mg for each unformed stool. Maximum of 16 mg/day	**30–45 kg:** ½ adult dose Maximum 6 mg/day **22–29 kg:** ¼ adult dose, Maximum 4 mg/day **<22 kg or <6 years old:** not recommended	May use in pregnancy.	Avoid use with serious illness such as fever or bloody diarrhea, as this may worsen/prolong illness.
Bismuth Subsalicylate (eg, Pepto-Bismol)	524 mg (2 tablets or 30 cc) qid	**9–12 years:** 1 tablet or 15 cc qid **6–8 years:** ⅔ tablet or 10 cc qid **3–6 years:** ⅓ tablet or 5 cc qid Not recommended for children <3 years	Should avoid during last half of pregnancy	Not recommended for travel longer than 3 weeks. Contraindicated in aspirin allergy, renal insufficiency, or gout.

altitudes) or properly treated with water purification systems or halogen additives (chlorine or iodine) may be safe. Using ice in beverages and using tap water to brush teeth are common lapses in travelers' water discipline.

2. **Vegetables and fruits.** Raw, unpeeled vegetables and salads should be avoided. Melons and other fruit should be closely inspected for puncture marks. Unscrupulous vendors will often inject fruit with water to increase the weight.
3. **Dairy products.** Unpasteurized dairy products should be avoided. Diseases transmitted via unpasteurized milk include brucellosis, *Mycobacterium bovis,* and Q fever, among others.
4. **Seafood.** Fish and shellfish can harbor pathogens and toxins.
   a. **Shellfish poisoning.** The four most common shellfish poisonings are paralytic, diarrheic, amnesic, and neurotoxic shellfish poisonings. These toxins are tasteless and odorless and can be found in fresh shellfish. Unfortunately, these toxins are heat-stable and are not neutralized by cooking. Dinoflagellate toxins released during red and brown algae blooms cause these poisonings. Many federal and regional authorities will issue shellfish warnings in response to algae blooms. Many developing countries, however, do not reliably surveil for these conditions. Contacting local officials and tour and hotel operators regarding this risk is recommended.
   b. **Ciguatera poisoning.** This biotoxin is also produced by dinoflagellates. The toxin is concentrated in large, predaceous fin and coral reef fish such as barracuda, red snapper, grouper, amberjack, and mackerel. This toxin is odorless, tasteless, and heat-stable and can be found in freshly caught fish. Symptoms of ciguatera poisoning include gastroenteritis followed by symptoms such as dysthesias, the sensation of loose teeth, temperature reversal (cold feeling hot and vice versa), and weakness. An expensive testing kit, Cigua-Check (Oceanit Test Systems, Inco, Honolulu, Hawaii) is available at http://www.cigua.com. The traveler should contact local officials and hotel and tour operators regarding local risks.
   c. **Scombroid poisoning.** Scombroid toxin is produced by a bacterial overgrowth in improperly refrigerated fish, particularly tuna, mackerel, mahi-mahi, amberjack, and bluefish, herring, among others. The bacteria metabolize histidine into histamine, resulting in a histamine-rich muscle. Consuming the fish results in "histamine poisoning" characterized by flushing, wheezing, tachycardia, hypotension, and urticaria. Fortunately, severe, life-threatening sequelae are rare. Prevention involves eating only properly refrigerated fish. Fish unrefrigerated for more than 2 hours should be avoided.
   d. **Fugu poisoning.** Puffer fish (fugu fish) is a delicacy popular in Japan. If improperly prepared, this delicacy can harbor tetrodotoxin. Tetrodotoxin poisoning has a 60% case fatality rate. It is imperative to only eat fugu prepared by specially trained, government-licensed chefs.
C. **Unintentional injuries during travel.** Nearly one quarter of overseas fatalities are due to accidents, the most common causes being motor vehicle accidents and drowning. The most common nonfatal injuries were falls and water recreation–related injuries. Alcohol consumption correlates with an increased risk of injury and death while traveling. Advise travelers to avoid drinking and driving and to buckle up if seat belts are available. Travelers should bring personal protective gear such as helmets if they intend to ride bicycles or motorbikes. They should become familiar with road conditions and laws and customs of the road. If travelers are going to be participating in water-based recreation during their travel, encourage them to know the area well before engaging in these activities, particularly higher-risk activities like scuba diving.
D. **Terrorism.** Many travelers may have concerns about terrorist threats during their travels. Statistically, travelers are at greater risk from accidents and diseases. Nevertheless, travelers should consult the State Department web site for traveler security alerts before beginning their trip at http://travel.state.gov.
E. **Deep vein thromboses.** Deep vein thromboses and pulmonary emboli associated with long airline flights are very rare, but there appears to be an increased risk in travelers, particularly those with hypercoagulable states. These travelers should stretch and walk frequently about the plane, taking into consideration flying conditions and air turbulence. Compression stockings may offer some protective benefit in these patients. Aspirin has not been shown to reduce the risk of thromboembolic events in travelers. Low-molecular-weight heparin is unstudied for this indication.

F. Motion sickness. Motion sickness (air sickness, seasickness) is thought to be caused by an asynchrony between the sight and vestibular senses. The symptoms include fatigue, headache, nausea, and vomiting. Several medications have been shown to be effective in preventing or reducing the symptoms of motion sickness (see Table 104–6).

1. The scopolamine patch is effective 6–8 hours after the patch is placed. Oral medications are effective within 1–2 hours.

2. Scopolamine patch efficacy may be enhanced and drowsiness reduced with concurrent use of sympathomimetics (ephedrine, D-amphetamine, and methylphenidate). While useful in refractory cases, abuse potential and potential legal problems in some countries limit use.

3. Nonpharmacologic methods of preventing motion sickness (acupressure bracelets, ginger) have not been shown to be effective in clinical trials.

4. Motion sickness can be reduced by sitting in the front seat of the car or over the wings in an aircraft.

G. Sun protection. Sun exposure has short- and long-term consequences, including sunburn, photo-aging, and skin cancer. Wearing protective clothing, avoiding exposure during the time of day when the sun's rays are most intense (10:00 AM to 3:00 PM), and applying sufficient sunscreen are strategies to reduce the untoward consequences of sun exposure. The Sun Protection Factor (SPF) determines a sunscreen's strength. While a sunscreen with an SPF factor of 15, when applied as directed, can afford over 90% protection, most people apply sunscreen much more sparingly and less frequently than recommended. Recommending a higher SPF can partially compensate for this deficiency.

H. Sexually transmitted disease (STD) prevention. It has been estimated that as many as 15% of international travelers will report at least one new sexual encounter during their travels. Travelers need to be aware that human immunodeficiency virus (HIV) and hepatitis B infection rates may be very high in some countries, particularly among prostitutes. Abstinence is strongly encouraged. Latex condoms, consistently and correctly used, may afford some protection to those unwilling to abstain. A post-travel examination to screen for STDs is also recommended for these travelers. Hepatitis B vaccination of these high-risk travelers prior to travel is strongly recommended.

I. Jet lag. Rapidly crossing multiple time zones disrupts a traveler's normal sleep-wake cycle. This effect increases as more time zones are crossed and is particularly troublesome for travelers traveling in an easterly direction. Adjustment to a new time zone usually requires 1 day for every time zone crossed. Strategies to reduce jet lag are summarized in Table 104–7.

TABLE 104–6. MOTION SICKNESS PROPHYLAXIS

Drug	Dosages	Side Effects	Additional Comments
Scopolamine hydrobromide (Transderm Scōp, Scopace)	1.5 mg transdermal patch behind ear q 3 days 0.4 mg tablet po, 1–2 tabs po q 8 hours	Dry mouth (66%), drowsiness (33%)	Tablets better suited for shorter outings. Patch costs 10 × more than tablets.
Promethazine (Phenergan) 25-, 12.5-mg tablets, 12.5-mg/5-cc elixir	25 mg po q 6–18 hours; 1 mg/kg/dose for children	Less dry mouth and more drowsiness compared to scopolamine	Usual dosing interval is 12 hours
Dimenhydrinate (Dramamine)	50–100 mg po q 6–8 hr (12 years and older); 25–50 mg po q 6–8 hr (6–12 years old); 12.5–25 mg q 6–8 hrs (2–6 years old)		Most effective over-the-counter medication. Chewable tablet formulations available.
Cyclizine (Marezine)	50 mg po q 4–6 hr	Less sedation compared with other antihistamines	
Meclizine (Antivert, Bonine) 12.5-, 25-, 50-mg tablets	25–50 mg po daily (12 years and older)		Pregnancy category B. Chewable tablet formulations available.

TABLE 104-7. STRATEGIES FOR LESSENING JET-LAG SYMPTOMS

Direction of Travel	Pre-Travel Bedtime Adjustments	Wakefulness During Flight	Bright Light Exposure at Destination	Vigorous Exercise at Destination
Eastward	Go to bed 1 hour earlier each night for 3 nights prior to departure	Try to sleep on plane. Avoid caffeinated beverages.	Bright light in early morning—avoid sunglasses for first few days	Mid-morning exercise
Westward	Go to bed 1 hour later each night for 3 nights prior to departure	Try to stay awake during flight. Drink caffeinated beverages.	Bright light in late afternoon—avoid sunglasses for first few days	Late afternoon exercise

Melatonin is not a regulated substance, and formulations vary considerably. While the sedative effects of melatonin are generally accepted, its ability to "re-set" the chronobiologic clock is disputed. Nevertheless, several trials have demonstrated remarkable effectiveness in reducing the symptoms of jet lag. The benefit is greater the more time zones are crossed and for eastward flights. Many pre-travel, en route, and post-travel melatonin-dosing regimens have been described—some can be quite complicated. A simplified dosing regimen is 5 mg en route taken at the destination bedtime and 5 mg orally nightly for 3–5 nights post-travel. Short-acting agents such as zolpidem (Ambien) and benzodiazepines can be used in a similar manner.

IV. **Special Travelers**
  A. **Pregnant travelers**
    1. **Air travel.** Many women will elect to travel well into their third trimester. Commercial air travel generally does not pose a significant risk to the pregnant patient or her fetus. Decreased PaO_2 present at the standard cabin altitude of 5000–8000 ft (1500–2500 m) has little, if any, effect on fetal oxygenation due to a favorable fetal hemoglobin disassociation curve. Pregnancy does confer an increased risk of thromboembolism, so it is recommended that the pregnant traveler should walk about frequently while traveling, flying conditions and turbulence permitting. Each airline has defined policies regarding the pregnant traveler. US domestic and intra-European travel is usually allowed up until the 36th week in uncomplicated pregnancies. Air travel across great distances, particularly transoceanic travel, is permitted up until the 32nd week of uncomplicated pregnancies. Many airlines require medical authorization before permitting travel by pregnant women beyond 28 weeks' gestation. Pregnant travelers should carry a copy or summary of the prenatal record. Blood type and due date are particularly important data to carry.
    2. **Vaccines in pregnancy.** Most vaccines are safe in pregnancy. MMR and varicella are the notable exceptions and should be avoided until the postpartum period. Other live viral/bacterial vaccines (oral typhoid, oral polio, Japanese encephalitis virus vaccine, yellow fever vaccine) have relative contraindications but can be given if travel to areas with active outbreaks or high levels of endemicity cannot be avoided and the vaccine's benefit outweighs any perceived risks. Indications for killed, inactivated, or split-virus vaccines are not altered by pregnancy status.
    3. **TD and food-borne illnesses in pregnancy.** While quinolones are contraindicated in pregnancy, many experts believe that these medications should not be withheld from the pregnant patient for cases of severe TD (severe enough to cause dehydration or dysentery). Azithromycin, cefixime, and furazolidone are also reasonable choices. Hepatitis E, which is not vaccine-preventable, is usually contracted from contaminated food or water. This infection carries a 17–33% case fatality rate in the pregnant patient. Strict food and water discipline is critical for the pregnant traveler.
    4. **Malaria and the pregnant traveler.** Malaria can be catastrophic to the pregnant patient and her fetus. Maternal mortality can approach 10%. Travel to malarious areas during pregnancy should be avoided if at all possible. In the event that travel to malarious areas is unavoidable, malarial prophylaxis and arthropod vector control is paramount. Chloroquine and mefloquine are safe throughout pregnancy. Travel to mefloquine-resistant areas should be avoided during pregnancy because

no proven safe prophylaxis exists at this time. While doxycycline has a relative contraindication during pregnancy, it should be noted that the fetal "side effects" attributed to doxycycline have actually been reported in tetracycline and not doxycycline. There is very little evidence that a class effect exists in this regard. Data on the safety of atovaquone-proguanil (Malarone) are incomplete at this time and cannot be formally recommended for use in the pregnant traveler. Nevertheless, if travel to a mefloquine-resistant area is unavoidable, the provider and the pregnant traveler may decide that the real risks of *P falciparum* malaria outweigh any theoretical risks of doxycycline or atovaquone-proguanil prophylaxis and prescribe one of these medications. Primaquine is contraindicated during pregnancy because the glucose-6-phospate dehydrogenase (G6PD) status of the fetus is unknown. In cases where primaquine terminal prophylaxis is necessary, chloroquine should be continued until delivery (even if it requires months of treatment after return). Primaquine can then begin in the postpartum period. DEET and permethrin, used as directed, are safe in pregnancy.

5. **Miscellaneous travel hazards in pregnancy.** Scuba diving and water skiing are contraindicated during pregnancy, as is horseback riding after the first trimester. Acetazolamide for high-altitude illness prophylaxis is not recommended during the first trimester. Nifedipine and dexamethasone are safe throughout pregnancy.

B. **The pediatric traveler**
1. **Air travel.** The CDC recommends that children younger than 6 weeks old should avoid air travel. The WHO, on the other hand, recommends that children younger than 1 week old avoid air travel. There are no prospective or case-control studies substantiating these recommendations. Most US carriers have no lower age restrictions for air travel. Nevertheless, contacting the airline well in advance of travel is recommended. Ear pain during ascent and descent has been reported in as many as 15% of pediatric air travelers. Bottle-feeding, nursing, and decongestants have been advocated to ameliorate these symptoms but multiple small studies have shown little, if any, benefit.
2. **Vaccinations in childhood.** See section II,B above and Tables 104–1 and 104–2.
3. **Malarial chemoprophylaxis in childhood.** Children are at increased risk of mortality from *P falciparum* malaria. Chloroquine and mefloquine, in appropriate doses, are safe for all ages. Overdoses of these medications can be fatal, so proper compounding of suspensions and accurate dosing are critical. In situations where a mosquito-free microenvironment can be assured (eg, permethrin-impregnated netting over a bassinet, stroller, playpen or car seat, combined with DEET), one may defer chemoprophylaxis.
4. **TD in childhood.** Quinolones are the most effective treatment for TD in all age groups, including children. Quinolone use has caused long bone arthropathy in skeletally immature experimental animals, but clinical use of long-term quinolones in children with cystic fibrosis has not demonstrated this risk. Azithromycin, cefixime, and furazolidone can also be used, but quinolones should be considered first-line treatment in cases of children with severe TD with dehydration or dysentery (bloody diarrhea with high fever). Vigorous rehydration of children with TD is absolutely critical. WHO recommends rehydration with reconstituted prepackaged WHO Oral Rehydration Salts (ORS) in the following amounts:
   a. Children under 2 years: 1/4–1/2 cup (50–100 mL) after each loose stool
   b. Children 2–10 years: 1/2–1 cup (100–200 mL) after each loose stool
   c. Older children and adults: unlimited amount (As a substitute to the prepackaged WHO ORS: 6 level tsp of sugar plus 1 level tsp of salt in 1 liter/quart of safe drinking water can be used.)

C. **Travelers with chronic diseases**
1. **General considerations.** Prescribed medications should be hand-carried and in sufficient quantity to last the duration of the trip. A reserve supply of medications should be packed in a separate, checked bag. Medications should be in their original containers and labeled with generic names. A letter on official letterhead from the physician explaining dosages and indications of medications, particularly scheduled medications and diabetic needles and syringes, may avert legal problems at some international borders and assist with replacement, if needed.
2. **Immunosuppressed travelers.** The risk of infectious disease is increased in the immunocompromised traveler, including those who are infected with HIV.

a. **TD in the immunocompromised traveler.** Antibiotics are not routinely recommended to prevent TD in HIV-positive travelers. However, certain circumstances where any time lost due to illness may be considered critical or where the risk of illness would significantly compromise the traveler's health may warrant the use of daily prophylactic antibiotics such as ciprofloxacin 500 mg a day. HIV-positive travelers on trimethoprim-sulfamethoxazole (TMP-SMX) prophylaxis may also experience some benefit in the prevention of TD. TMP-SMX should not be prescribed for TD to those not currently taking it, as it does have potential side effects and may promote resistance when it becomes needed for other reasons. Acute treatment plans as outlined in Table 104–5 are also effective in this group, but may need to be extended for 7 days.

b. **Immunizations in the immunocompromised traveler**
   (1) **HIV-positive travelers.** Vaccine immunogenicity may be decreased in HIV-positive patients with CD4$^+$ peripheral cell count <300 cells/µL. Generally, live vaccines should be avoided in the severely immunocompromised traveler. For HIV-positive persons, severely immunocompromised can be defined as the presence of opportunistic infections or a CD4$^+$ peripheral cell count <200 cells/µL. Inactivated vaccines should be used in place of live vaccines wherever possible (eg, poliomyelitis, typhoid, cholera). Measles and yellow fever vaccines should only be given to those with CD4$^+$ peripheral cell count >200 cells/µL. Killed vaccines are generally considered safe.
   (2) **Other immunocompromised travelers.** Travelers who have recently received high-dose steroids for >14 days should delay vaccination 2 weeks after the completion of high-dose steroid therapy. Similarly, many cancer patients undergoing radiation or chemotherapy may also be immunosuppressed and should avoid vaccinations during this time. Cancer patients who are not actively being treated may be vaccinated. Travelers with leukemia who have been in remission for 3 months or transplant patients no longer needing immunosuppression may also be vaccinated.

c. **Travel restrictions for the HIV-positive patient.** In most countries, travelers staying <1 month are not required to show proof of being HIV-negative. For travelers wishing to stay >1 month, many countries require HIV testing, and most foreigners who are HIV-positive will be denied entry. Many countries have policies of expelling foreigners with AIDS. Some countries will deny entry to travelers carrying antiretroviral medications. HIV-positive travelers should consult the US State Department web site (http://www.travel.state.gov/HIVtestingreq.html) for further information. Since regulations change frequently, contacting the consulate of the country in question prior to travel planning is also recommended.

3. **The diabetic traveler.** It is critical that the diabetic traveler carry adequate medications and monitoring supplies on the trip. This equipment and medication (including Glucagon) should be hand-carried during travel. Insulin can be stored at room temperature for up to 30 days without losing effectiveness. Nevertheless, exposure of insulin to sunlight and temperature extremes should be avoided.

   Travel across time zones can shorten or lengthen the "24-hour day," changing insulin and meal requirements. Travel in an easterly direction shortens the day and may decrease insulin and meal requirements. Conversely, westward travel lengthens the day and can increase insulin and meal requirements. Frequent blood glucose monitoring is essential. Having ready access to snack foods is recommended.

   Coordinating pre-meal insulin dosing with unpredictable meal times during air-travel can be simplified with short-acting insulin (eg, insulin lispro).

   Insulin concentrations may vary from the standard U100 concentration prescribed in North America. U80 and U40 concentrations with corresponding syringes can be found in other countries. Mixing syringes with different concentrations of insulin increase the chances of overdosing or underdosing. Bringing adequate diabetic supplies can minimize this risk.

   Severe TD can predispose the diabetic traveler to wildly fluctuating blood glucoses and adverse sequelae such as diabetic ketoacidosis. Emergency standby treatment for TD should be prescribed to diabetic travelers.

4. **Travelers with cardiovascular disease.** A recent report determined that approximately two thirds of in-flight fatalities on US carriers are due to cardiac disease.

Hypobaric hypoxemia (decreased partial pressure of oxygen at altitude) can increase the risk of cardiac events.

Special considerations for air travelers with cardiac disease include the following:

a. Those with compensated congestive heart failure, stable angina, or a sea-level Pao_2 <70 mm Hg should arrange for in-flight oxygen.

b. Carrying a recent copy of electrocardiogram (ECG) results is recommended, (with and without magnet ECG for pacemakers).

c. A wallet card documenting pacemaker/AICD placement can speed transit through airport security.

Cardiovascular contraindications to air travel are summarized in Table 104–8.

5. **Travelers with pulmonary disease.** As with travelers with cardiac disease, those with pulmonary disease are also susceptible to the hypobaric hypoxemia of air travel. A Pao_2 >70 mm Hg at room air does not usually require supplemental oxygen at altitude. If a pre-travel arterial blood gas measurement is not feasible, a traveler who can walk up a flight of stairs or walk 50 meters at a brisk pace without becoming severely dyspneic will usually tolerate flight without supplemental oxygen. A more sophisticated test, the High Altitude Simulation Test (HAST), in which 15% Fio_2 is inhaled to mimic the partial pressure of oxygen at altitude, can be used to assess the pulmonary status prior to air travel.

If in-flight supplemental oxygen is required, special arrangements must be made:

a. Filled personal oxygen bottles are not permitted on commercial aircraft. Personal O_2 bottles must be purged and transported as checked luggage.

b. In-flight oxygen can be arranged through each airline. It is recommended that the traveler contact the airline well in advance of travel. Most airlines will require a letter or prescription from a physician.

c. If supplemental oxygen is needed during layovers, arrangements for oxygen must be made with venders in that particular locale. The airline usually does not provide this service.

Pulmonary contraindications to air travel include severe, labile, uncontrolled asthma and individuals with a pneumothorax. For individuals at high risk of pneumothorax (eg, bullous emphysema), preflight end-expiratory chest radiographs should be performed.

V. **Accessing health care overseas.** Consular officers at embassies can assist in locating appropriate medical services, but the costs of care and, if necessary, air evacuation, are usually the traveler's financial responsibilities.

A. **Travelers' medical insurance.** If the traveler's insurance plan provides for international coverage, it is important to bring an insurance card as proof of coverage and a claim form. Many insurance plans do not provide coverage at the point of service, and the traveler may be responsible for payment even before services are rendered. Some plans will offer partial or complete reimbursement upon return, so it is critical to save all receipts. **Medicare does not cover health expenses incurred outside of the United States.** Seniors may want to contact the American Association of Retired Persons about a Medicare supplement that provides international coverage.

B. **Evacuation insurance.** Since medical care in most of the developing world is substandard by Western standards, the most prudent thing in the event of severe illness or injury

---

TABLE 104–8. CARDIOVASCULAR CONTRAINDICATIONS TO AIR TRAVEL

1. Uncomplicated myocardial infarction within 2–3 weeks
2. Complicated myocardial infarction within 6 weeks
3. Unstable angina
4. Decompensated congestive heart failure
5. Uncontrolled hypertension
6. Coronary artery bypass grafting within 10–14 days
7. Stroke within 2 weeks
8. Uncontrolled ventricular or supraventricular tachycardia
9. Eisenmenger syndrome
10. Severe symptomatic valvular heart disease

From Aerospace Medical Association MGTF: *Medical Guidelines for Airline Travel,* 2nd ed. Aviat Space Environ Med 2003;**74**(5, Section II):A1.

may be air evacuation. Evacuation can be prohibitively expensive, costing as much as $100,000 for a private air ambulance. Evacuation insurance is strongly recommended.

C. **Sources for travelers' medical and evacuation insurance.** Medical and evacuation insurance can be purchased at a reasonable cost through a travel agent or online. See the US State Department web site at www.travel.state.gov/medical.html for a list of private insurance and air evacuation companies.

D. **Accessing care overseas.** Lists of English-speaking health care providers by country can be obtained from the following sources:
   1. Office of Overseas Citizens Services, Room 4811, 2201 C Street, N.W., Washington, DC 20520. Indicate country or region of interest when you write.
   2. International Association for Medical Assistance to Travelers (IAMAT), (519) 836-0102.
   3. International Society of Travel Medicine (ISTM), www.istm.org (directory of clinics and providers).

E. Travelers should carry the name, phone number, and e-mail address of their personal physician for consultation if needed.

VI. Special Activities

A. **Travel to high-altitude destinations.** Altitude illness can occur in travelers who travel to high altitude destinations. These illnesses include acute mountain sickness (AMS), high altitude cerebral edema (HACE), and high altitude pulmonary edema (HAPE). HACE and HAPE can be life-threatening. The risk of occurrence is dependent on rate of ascent, sleeping altitude, the traveler's home altitude, and other aspects of individual physiology. AMS, the most common and least severe type of high-altitude illness, occurs in roughly one quarter of travelers to elevations of 7000–9000 ft (1850–2750 m) and >40% of travelers to elevations of 10,000 ft (3000 m). The incidence of HACE and HAPE is 0.1–4.0%. AMS and HACE are likely the same disease process at different points along a continuum—HACE being a very severe form of AMS. It is critical that travelers are aware of symptoms of high-altitude illness so immediate corrective action can be taken. Table 104–9 summarizes the symptoms, signs, prevention, and treatment of high-altitude illnesses.

B. **Freshwater activities**
   1. **Schistosomiasis prevention.** Travelers to areas endemic for schistosomiasis (Africa, tropical South America, South and Southeast Asia, the eastern Caribbean) should be cautioned against swimming in fresh water due to risk of acquiring this disease. Precise areas of endemicity can be found at the CDC and WHO web sites.
   2. **Leptospirosis prevention.** Travelers participating in activities such as kayaking, canoeing, whitewater rafting, or swimming in areas endemic or epidemic for leptospirosis are at increased risk for acquiring this potentially fatal disease. Leptospirosis, while a global disease, is particularly a problem in Latin America and Southeast Asia. Recent heavy rains and flooding increase the risk of this disease. For at-risk travelers, doxycycline prophylaxis (200 mg orally weekly beginning 1–2 days prior to activity and continuing for the duration of the activity) can be protective.
   3. **Scuba diving.** Scuba diving is generally well regulated in developed countries. Many popular dive sites in underdeveloped countries may not be as well regulated, and instruction/supervision of novice divers may be rudimentary at best. Obtaining education and certification by a reputable instructor prior to travel and diving with experienced divers are strongly recommended.
      Air travel after diving increases the risk of decompression sickness. A minimum surface interval of 12 hours prior to air travel after a single dive is recommended before flying. For repetitive dives in a single day, a longer surface interval (at least 17 hours) prior to flying is recommended.
      The Divers Alert Network (www.diversalertnetwork.org) is a reputable resource for medical concerns associated with diving.

VII. Travel After-care. Between 20% and 70% of travelers to developing countries will have an illness or injury associated with their travel. Of these travelers, 1–5% will seek medical care during travel or shortly after return. Travelers, particularly those to developing nations, are advised to seek medical attention upon return in the following situations:

A. Persistent diarrhea.
B. Jaundice.
C. Newly acquired skin disorders.

TABLE 104-9. SUMMARY OF SYMPTOMS/SIGNS, PROPHYLAXIS, AND TREATMENT
FOR HIGH-ALTITUDE ILLNESSES

	Symptoms/Signs	Prophylaxis	Treatment
Acute mountain sickness (AMS)	• Headache (most common) • Nausea • Difficulty sleeping • Fatigue • Anorexia	• Gradual ascent (<300 m/daily) at elevations >3000 m with rest day every 2–3 days. • Sleeping altitudes most critical. Climb high but sleep low. • Acetazolamide 250 mg po bid starting 1 day prior to ascent • Dexamethasone 4 mg po bid starting 1 day prior to ascent • Gingko biloba 120 mg po bid starting 5 days prior to ascent	• Rest • Avoid further ascent until symptoms resolve • Descent for severe AMS • Antiemetics • Oxygen • Acetazolamide 250 mg po bid–tid • Dexamethasone 4 mg po/IM q 6 hours
High altitude cerebral edema (HACE)	• Ataxia—inability to walk heel-to-toe (tandem walk test) • Altered level of consciousness ± • Symptoms of AMS	• Avoid hypothermia • Keep well hydrated • Avoid sedatives/narcotics that result in hypoventilation during sleep	• Immediate descent to lower altitude • Oxygen • Acetazolamide or dexamethasone in doses noted above • Portable hyperbaric chamber
High altitude pulmonary edema (HAPE)	• Dyspnea on exertion • Cough • Blood-tinged sputum • Often coexists with AMS/HACE • Crackles, especially RML early on	• Gradual ascent, avoidance of hypothermia, hydration, and avoidance of sedatives and narcotics • Nifedipine SR 20 mg po tid • Salmeterol MDI 1–2 puffs bid • Persons with prior history of HAPE are at extremely high risk of recurrence (66% recurrence in one study). Avoidance of rapid altitude increases in these individuals should be strongly encouraged.	• Immediate descent • Reduce exertion • Oxygen • Continuous positive airway pressure • Portable hyperbaric chamber • Nifedipine 10 mg po followed by 20–30 mg SR bid–qd • Inhaled β-adrenergic agonists may be helpful

From Basnyat B, Murdoch DR: High-altitude illness. Lancet (June 7) 2003;**361**:1967.

D. Persistent vomiting.

E. Possible STDs.

F. Fever. If a fever occurs more than 6 days after the first exposure to a malaria-endemic area, malaria must be ruled out. A useful web tool for determining the etiology of a fever in an otherwise healthy, nonpregnant adult traveler can be found at www.fevertravel.ch.

G. Long-term travelers/expatriates (>3 months in a developing country).

H. Travelers who are concerned that they have been exposed to a serious infectious disease.

REFERENCES

General References

Centers for Disease Control and Prevention. *Yellow Book 2003/2004;* 2003. (Has information on vaccinations (routine and travel-related), travelers' diarrhea; precautions in consuming water and dairy products abroad; and air travel for pediatric travelers).

Hargarten SW, Baker TD, Guptill K: Overseas fatalities of United States citizen travelers: An analysis of deaths related to international travel. Ann Emerg Med (June) 1991;**20**(6):622.

World Health Organization. *International Travel and Health;* 2003. (Has information on vaccinations (routine and travel-related), travelers' diarrhea; fever onset from fly bite in trypanosomiasis; precautions in consuming water and dairy products abroad; precautions in consuming food and water in pregnant patients; and air travel for pediatric travelers).

World Tourism Organization. http://www.world-tourism.org/.

High Altitude Illness & Diving
Basnyat B, Murdoch DR: High-altitude illness. Lancet (June 7) 2003;**361**:1967.
Divers Alert Network. http://www.diversalertnetwork.org

Illness & Injury Prevention
Barbier HM, Diaz JH: Prevention and treatment of toxic seafoodborne diseases in travelers. J Travel Med (January) 2003;**10**(01):29.
Fradin MS: Mosquitoes and mosquito repellents: A clinician's guide. Ann Intern Med (June 1) 1998; **128**:931.
Matteelli A, Carosi G: Sexually transmitted diseases in travelers. Clin Infect Dis (April 1) 2001;**32**:1063.
Scurr J Frequency and prevention of symptomless deep venous thrombosis in long-haul flights: A randomised trial. Lancet (May 12) 2001;**357**:1485.

Jet Lag & Motion Sickness
Herxheimer A, Petrie K: Melatonin for the prevention and treatment of jet lag (Cochrane Review). Cochrane Database Syst Rev 2003;2(CD001520).
Sherman CR: Motion sickness: Review of causes and preventive strategies. J Travel Med (September) 2002;**9**(05):251.

Travel After-care
World Health Organization. http://www.who.int travel after-care

Travelers with Special Needs
Aerospace Medical Association MGTF: *Medical Guidelines for Airline Travel,* 2nd ed. Aviat Space Environ Med 2003;**74**(5, Section II):A1.
American College of Obstetrics and Gynecology Committee on Obstetric Practice: Committee Opinion Number 282: Immunization during pregnancy. Obstet Gynecol (January) 2003;**101**(1):207.
Castelli F, Patroni A: The human immunodeficiency virus-infected traveler. Clin Infect Dis (December) 2000;**31**:1403.
Stauffer WM, Kamat D, Magill AJ: Traveling with infants and children. Part IV: Insect avoidance and malarial prevention. J Travel Med (July/August) 2003;**10**(4):225.
Stauffer WM, Konop RJ, Kamat D: Traveling with infants and young children. Part I: Anticipatory guidance: Travel preparation and preventive health advice. J Travel Med (September) 2001;**8**(5):254.
Stauffer WM, Kamat D: Traveling with infants and children. Part II: Immunizations. J Travel Med 2002;**9**(2):82.
Stauffer WM, Konop RJ, Kamat D: Traveling with infants and young children. Part III: Travelers' diarrhea. J Travel Med 2002;**9**(3):141.

Vaccinations
American Academy of Family Physicians. AAFP Clinical Recommendations for Immunizations. www.aafp.org/x10631.xml.
Cetron MS: Yellow fever vaccine: Recommendations of the Advisory Committee on Immunization Practices (ACIP), 2002. Morbid Mortal Wkly Rep (November 8) 2002;**51**(RR-17):1.
Duke T, Mgone CS: Measles: Not just another viral exanthem. Lancet (March 1) 2003;**361**:763.
Pollard AJ, Shlim DR: Epidemic meningococcal disease and travel. J Travel Med (January) 2002; **9**(01):29.
Ryan ET, Calderwood SB: Cholera vaccines. J Travel Med (March) 2001;**8**(02):82.
Watson D, Ashley R: Pretravel health advice for asplenic individuals. J Travel Med 2003;**10**(02):117.

---

105   Preoperative Evaluation

Sarah R. Edmonson, MD

I. Quick Evaluation Guide

    A. The purpose of the preoperative evaluation is to identify and manage risk, not to guarantee a problem-free surgery.

    B. The most common complications of surgery are infectious, cardiac, and pulmonary problems.

    C. Preoperative testing should be customized to the findings of the history and physical examination. No test is recommended for every patient.

D. The operative plan should include measures to decrease the patient's operative risk as much as possible. For example, patients with pulmonary disease should have incentive spirometry ordered, and patients with coronary artery disease should receive perioperative beta blockers.

E. The final important step in a preoperative evaluation is communication of your findings to both the patient and the consulting surgeon.

F. Figure 105–1 shows a suggested algorithm for approaching the preoperative evaluation.

II. Introduction

A. Role of the primary care physician

1. The primary care physician is frequently asked to perform a preoperative evaluation on surgical patients. When this consultation is made, the implicit task is to identify and quantify the patient's risk for adverse outcome from the surgical procedure. The preoperative evaluation cannot "clear" the patient for surgery, as all surgeries involve some level of risk.

2. This evaluation allows the patient to balance the need for surgery against the risk of adverse outcome, and hence to make an informed decision.

3. The consultation also allows the surgeon and primary care physician to work together to minimize the known risks before, during, and after the procedure.

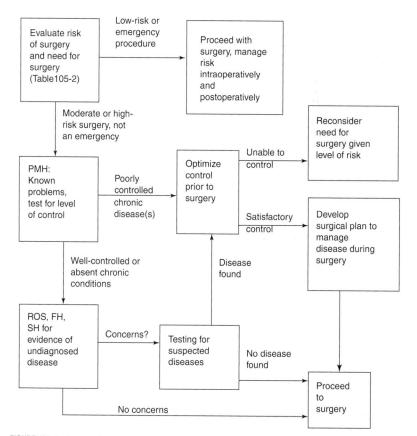

FIGURE 105–1. Preoperative evaluation algorithm. FH, Family history; PMH, previous medical history; ROS, review of systems; SH, social history.

4. Preoperative evaluation is cost-effective, because operative risks are identified and controlled in the outpatient setting, hospital stays are shorter, and fewer surgeries are cancelled or postponed.

5. The ideal timing for the preoperative assessment is several weeks before the procedure. This timing allows the provider time to evaluate problems and initiate therapy without having to postpone a scheduled surgery. The Joint Commission on Accreditation of Healthcare Organizations requires all surgical patients to have a medical history and physical examination within 30 days of surgery.

B. **Outcomes.** Overall, between 15 and 20% of surgeries cause at least one complication. Prospective studies to determine if preoperative evaluation reduces the rate of complications have not been published. However, preoperative evaluation can help the physician predict and manage these complications, whether or not they are avoidable. Surgical morbidity and mortality rates vary depending on the type of surgery, the anatomical location of the procedure, and the condition of the patient. The most common adverse outcomes of surgery are:

1. **Infectious.** The most frequent complication of surgery is bacterial infection. It may include wound infections, pneumonia, urinary tract infections, bacterial endocarditis, and frank systemic sepsis.

2. **Cardiac.** Myocardial infarction, cardiac arrest, pulmonary edema, and complications of congestive heart failure are among the most frequent problems occurring during and immediately after surgery. In addition, these are the most commonly lethal complications.

3. **Pulmonary.** Pneumonia, atelectasis, bronchitis, respiratory failure with unplanned intubation, inability to wean from the respirator, and pulmonary embolus make up the third significant category of common and highly dangerous perioperative events. Pulmonary complications are most common for abdominal or thoracic surgery, and among obese patients.

4. **Thrombosis.** In addition to thrombotic events leading to pulmonary or cardiac complications, surgical procedures increase the chances of venous thromboses in the peripheral veins. In addition, arterial disease affecting the kidneys, mesentery, or extremities may present in the perioperative period. Diagnosis of postoperative venous thromboembolism can be difficult as more than half of cases are asymptomatic.

5. **Adverse reaction to anesthesia.** While rare, anesthesia reactions present a highly dangerous intraoperative and postoperative risk. Malignant hyperthermia stands out as a particularly toxic example. Other medications or surgical equipment, such as latex gloves, can trigger life-threatening allergic reactions.

6. **Gastrointestinal.** The combination of disrupted alimentation, emotional and physical stress, and sometimes direct disturbance of the abdominal cavity presents a unique challenge for the digestive system. Gastritis and ulcers can be triggered, as well as postoperative constipation or ileus.

7. **Psychosocial.** Surgical procedures can be extremely disruptive to both psychological and social stability. The patient misses work, will require increased assistance with ordinary functions of life, and will undergo a physical invasion that leaves his or her body permanently altered. Even with medical management, the patient is likely to experience pain and other unpleasant symptoms such as nausea. Postoperative delirium can occur, leading to distress for both the patient and family. Visible scarring may undermine the patient's self-confidence, and changes in bodily function—even positive changes—may startle the patient and disrupt assumptions about body image. Patients with known psychiatric disease are prone to increased symptoms in the perioperative period, and patients without a prior history of mental health problems may also need evaluation and support during this time.

III. **Preoperative Assessment**

A. **Urgency of surgery.** If the risk of delaying surgery outweighs the benefits of preoperative evaluation, then the patient must obviously proceed to surgery. Such situations are innately high-risk for the patient, regardless of underlying medical condition. Surgery for acute trauma often falls into this category, as do surgeries for rupture of intraperitoneal organs such as spleen, bowel or bladder.

B. **Previous surgical experience.** Patients who have had bleeding complications, anesthesia reactions (such as malignant hyperthermia), or other adverse responses to surgery should have their previous history investigated carefully. This history should strongly influence the perioperative care plan. For example, work-up of a patient with prior bleeding complications may show a clotting disorder, which can be treated with preoperative supplementation of clotting factor or fresh frozen plasma immediately before surgery.

C. **Cardiac evaluation.** Because of the high morbidity and mortality associated with perioperative cardiac problems, every patient should have a careful cardiac evaluation.

1. Well-known **preoperative algorithms** can be used to evaluate cardiac risk. These include Goldman's risk index, Detsky's risk index, the American Society of Anesthesiology's preoperative guideline, the Lee Risk Index, the American College of Physicians guideline, and the American College of Cardiology/American Heart Association (ACC/AHA) guideline. Comparative studies have not established the superiority of any one of these guidelines, and all may be cumbersome in the clinical setting. A summary of the ACC/AHA guideline is shown in Figure 105–2.

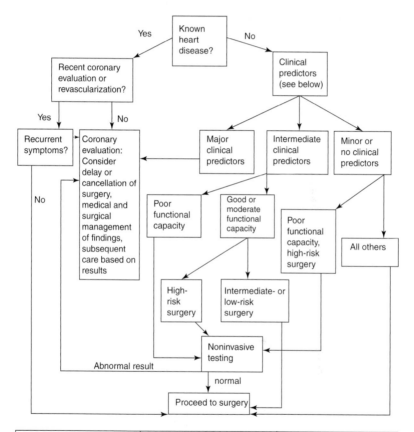

Major Clinical Predictors	Intermediate Clinical Predictors	Minor Clinical Predictors
Unstable coronary syndromes	Mild angina pectoris	Advanced age
Decompensated CHF	Prior myocardial infarction	Abnormal electrocardiogram
Significant arrhythmias	Compensated CHF	Rhythm other than sinus
Severe valvular disease	Diabetes mellitus	Low functional capacity
	Renal insufficiency	History of stroke
		Uncontrolled hypertension

FIGURE 105–2. American College of Cardiology/American Heart Association guidelines for preoperative cardiac evaluation (summarized). CHF, congestive heart failure.

2. The initial evaluation should divide the patients into the following groups:
   a. Patients with clearly established, uncontrolled disease should defer surgery until better control is achieved. People with clinically important coronary artery disease should defer noncardiac procedures until 6 months after revascularization, when possible. See section III,C,3 below for more information on this group.
   b. Patients with intermediate risk should receive additional testing to better define their level of disease. These patients may have signs and symptoms consistent with previously undiagnosed heart disease, such as exertional chest pain, dyspnea, and poor functional status (see section III,C,5,c). Patients who have multiple cardiac risk factors (Table 105–1) should also be evaluated for cardiac disease.
   c. Patients who have no concerning history or symptoms and who have fewer than two risk factors are at low risk for heart disease and can proceed to surgery.
3. **Patients with known heart disease or anginal symptoms**
   a. Even under optimal medical management, patients with congestive heart failure, previous myocardial infarction, or coronary artery obstruction that is not amenable to repair are at higher risk of perioperative cardiac events. This risk has to be balanced against the benefits of surgery on a case-by-case basis.
   b. In known or suspected coronary artery disease, perioperative beta-blocker therapy reduces risk. Administer an initial dose of atenolol intravenously 30 minutes before the procedure. After the procedure, order either atenolol 5 mg intravenously every 12 hours, or 50–100 mg orally once daily up to a maximum of 7 days. This therapy is contraindicated in patients with hypotension, active congestive heart failure, bronchospasm, bradycardia, or third degree heart block.
   c. Patients with ongoing or recurrent symptoms that have been previously established to be angina should have evaluation of their coronary arteries (catheterization or angiography) prior to surgery. Often revascularization should be performed before elective surgery is scheduled.
   d. Asymptomatic patients who have had a normal stress test in the past 2 years, bypass surgery in the past 5 years, or angioplasty in the past 5 years are unlikely to have developed significant new disease. These patients may proceed to surgery without further cardiac work-up.
   e. Patients who have undergone cardiac revascularization in the past 6 months should defer surgery or have repeat evaluation of their coronary arteries prior to surgery.
   f. If the patient has had a recent myocardial infarction, he or she is at high risk for another attack during or after surgery, and the operation should be deferred whenever possible. As the risk for recurrent myocardial infarction decreases after 6 weeks, the patient should be re-evaluated at that time.
   g. Patients with congestive heart failure (CHF) should be stabilized to optimal function before surgery and should consider avoiding surgery when possible. Decompensated CHF puts the patient at high risk for perioperative cardiac arrest. Assessment of left ventricular function (such as echocardiogram) does not change the management of these patients and is not recommended.
   h. Arrhythmias generally indicate some level of underlying cardiac damage. Preoperative assessment of the arrhythmia involves investigation for the under-

TABLE 105–1. PATIENT RISK FACTORS FOR CARDIOVASCULAR DISEASE

Hypertension, particularly uncontrolled
History of stroke
Diabetes mellitus
Advanced age
Previous abnormal electrocardiogram
Non-sinus cardiac rhythm (asymptomatic)
Tobacco use
Hyperlipidemia
Obesity
Family history of heart disease, particularly in male first-degree relatives who develop heart disease when younger than 50 years and female first-degree relatives younger than 60 years

lying problem, addressing any hemodynamic instability caused by the arrhythmia, and managing any thrombogenic potential generated by the arrhythmia. For arrhythmias that increase the risk of thrombosis (such as atrial fibrillation), postoperative prophylaxis against pulmonary embolus or deep venous thrombosis can be used. See section III,F,5 for details.

  i. Valvular disease can cause both hemodynamic instability and increased risk for bacterial endocarditis. All patients with valvular disease should receive antibiotic prophylaxis before and during the procedure (see Chapter 103 for more information).

4. If the review of systems reveals symptoms consistent with angina or anginal equivalent, the patient should undergo noninvasive (stress) testing to clarify the likelihood of coronary artery disease.

5. Asymptomatic patients with no known history of heart disease should be evaluated for cardiac risk factors and functional capacity.

  a. The use and weighting of risk factors for cardiac disease varies depending on the guideline used. Overall, factors that have been shown to predispose a patient to coronary artery disease are summarized in Table 105–1.

  b. The presence of three or more risk factors indicates a need for additional cardiac evaluation. Noninvasive stress testing is generally used for such patients.

  c. Functional capacity refers to the intensity of physical effort that the patient is capable of regularly performing.

  (1) Typically functional capacity is measured in METs (metabolic equivalents of oxygen consumption) according to the Duke Activity Status Index, Table 105–2.

  (2) A patient who is able to perform moderate intensity activity (>4 MET equivalent) is unlikely to have significant coronary artery disease.

  (3) Poor functional capacity correlates highly with coronary artery disease and may require further preoperative work-up. Intermediate functional capacity should be considered for evaluation, particularly if one or more risk factors are also present.

  (4) Functional capacity cannot be evaluated in a number of patients because of noncardiac factors that limit exercise. For example, a patient with mobility impairment due to osteoarthritis cannot run, but may have intact coronary vasculature. When functional capacity is unknown, it is advisable to err on the side of caution.

  d. Certain surgical procedures are associated with a higher risk of perioperative myocardial infarction (Table 105–3). The physician threshold for cardiac testing should be lower for the patient preparing to undergo a high-risk surgery.

D. Pulmonary evaluation

1. Pulmonary complications of surgery are most common in surgeries that are anatomically close to the diaphragm.

TABLE 105–2. DUKE ACTIVITY STATUS INDEX

Functional Class	METs	Activity
I	7.5–8	Heavy housework
		Strenuous sports
		Can run a short distance
II	4.5–5.5	Climb one flight of stairs
		Sexual relations
		Light yardwork
III	2.5–3.5	Light housework
		Walk two level blocks
		Self-care (dressing, bathing)
IV	1.75	Walk short distances indoors

METs, metabolic equivalents of oxygen consumption.
From Hlatky MA, et al: A brief self-administered questionnaire to determine functional capacity (the Duke Activity Status Index). Am J Cardiol 1989;**64**:651.

TABLE 105–3. RISK OF CERTAIN SURGERIES

High-risk surgeries	High anticipated blood loss
	Aortic or peripheral vascular surgery
Moderate-risk surgeries	Abdominal or thoracic surgery
	Head and neck surgery
	Carotid endarterectomy
	Orthopedic surgery
	Prostate surgery
Low-risk surgeries	Breast surgery
	Cataract surgery
	Superficial dermatologic surgery
	Endoscopy

   2. Pre-existing respiratory disease such as asthma, chronic obstructive pulmonary disease (COPD), pulmonary fibrotic diseases such as sarcoidosis, pneumonia, tuberculosis, or other pulmonary conditions increase the chance of bad outcomes.
   3. Smoking, obesity, dyspnea, and a history of cough are risk factors for pulmonary problems after surgery.
   4. Evaluation
      a. Chest X-ray is indicated for evaluation of physical examination abnormalities or reported symptoms of dyspnea or cough. Radiography may also be helpful for clarifying the status of previously diagnosed problems. Routine baseline chest x-rays in all patients undergoing surgery has been shown to be unhelpful.
      b. Pulmonary function testing is useful for evaluation of patients with suspected asthma or COPD. This testing may also be useful for demonstrating the status of these problems prior to surgery.
      c. Arterial blood gases are rarely useful in the preoperative patient. Patients whose pulmonary function is diminished enough to affect blood oxygenation are at inherently high surgical risk; these patients should be easily identifiable from the history and physical alone.
   5. Pulmonary medication, including steroids, should be continued perioperatively. Patients with severe COPD or asthma may benefit from a course of prophylactic steroid therapy prior to surgery.
   6. High-risk patients can be taught to perform incentive spirometry before, during, and after the procedure to minimize the chances of pulmonary complications.
E. Diabetes mellitus may increase the risk of cardiac events as well as perioperative infection.
   1. Patients with previously diagnosed diabetes should be evaluated for current diabetic control and presence of secondary organ damage. If not recently done, testing including hemoglobin A_{1C}, urine microalbumin levels, and renal function testing should be performed. In addition, diabetic patients should be considered high risk for cardiac disease and evaluated as such.
   2. All patients undergoing surgery should be screened for the signs and symptoms of diabetes mellitus, including polyuria, thirst, weight loss, blurring vision, acanthosis nigricans, and truncal obesity. All patients older than age 50, patients with a family history of diabetes, or patients whose history or physical suggests any possibility of diabetes mellitus should have a fasting blood glucose test performed.
   3. New or uncontrolled diabetes mellitus should be brought into good glycemic control prior to surgery.
F. Additional conditions that affect perioperative risk
   1. Immunocompromise. Certain patients are at high risk for infectious complications, including patients with genetic immune deficiencies, rheumatologic disease requiring immunosuppressive therapy, HIV, and diabetes mellitus, as well as chemotherapy recipients. In addition, patients with asplenia and valvular heart disease are at increased risk of catastrophic bacterial infection. These patients should be considered for prophylactic antibiotic therapy during the procedure and should be closely monitored throughout the operative period.
   2. Anemia. Anemia may result from a number of causes and can be particularly dangerous when the proposed surgery is likely to result in significant blood loss. Re-

view of systems may reveal fatigue, syncope, or cold intolerance, and examination may reveal pallor, pale mucus membranes, rapid pulse, or a functional heart murmur. A hemoglobin level should be checked in any patient with a history of anemia or a suggestive history or physical examination; hemoglobin may also be a useful test prior to surgeries that often cause significant bleeding. Any finding of anemia warrants work-up to determine the cause prior to surgery. Transfusion may be necessary prior to any surgery that cannot be deferred.

3. **Malnutrition.** Individuals with protein-calorie malnutrition or specific vitamin or mineral deficiencies have a much higher rate of postoperative complications. Weight loss, edema, fatigue, syncope, pallor, dental disease, financial or social deprivation, anemia, or frequent illness can be warning signs of malnutrition. Laboratory tests to evaluate malnutrition should include a blood count, albumin level, and specific vitamin assays. Supplements and hyperalimentation prior to and immediately after the procedure are helpful. For surgeries that require a fasting patient, parenteral nutrition may be chosen to sustain the malnourished patient.

4. **Peripheral vascular disease.** In general, the risk of peripheral vascular disease closely parallels that of ischemic cardiac disease. Thus, the presence of one should promote evaluation for both, and all patients with claudication symptoms or abnormal peripheral pulses should receive both peripheral vascular and cardiac evaluation. Noninvasive peripheral arterial evaluation may include Doppler or Duplex scanning, high-resolution computerized tomography, or magnetic resonance angiography (MRA). If the testing shows evidence of peripheral vascular disease, the postoperative plan should include prevention of pressure ulcers.

5. **Hypercoagulable state.** The patient should be questioned about a personal or family history of hypercoagulable conditions as well as rheumatologic disease. At-risk patients should receive perioperative prophylaxis against venous thromboembolism including subcutaneous heparin (5000 U subcutaneously every 8 hours) or low-molecular-weight heparin (such as enoxaparin, 40 mg subcutaneously once daily), and intermittent limb compression.

6. **Peptic ulcer disease.** Most postoperative gastrointestinal complications are new-onset, so all patients should be monitored closely. However, patients who have a prior history of peptic ulcer, or who are experiencing symptoms of dyspepsia or reflux, should receive prophylactic therapy in the pre operative and perioperative periods.

7. **Renal or hepatic failure.** Patients with end-stage liver or kidney disease face unique surgical challenges. Maintenance of blood pressure and fluid balance is more difficult in such patients, and many medications are metabolized at different rates in these patients. In addition, patients with renal failure often have disrupted hematopoiesis and concurrent anemia. Liver failure leads to decreased synthesis of important proteins including clotting factors. Prior to end-stage disease, the physiologic stress of surgery may worsen the organ's function either temporarily or permanently. Patients with significant renal disease should consider preparation for dialysis prior to surgery, including placement of long-term or permanent venous access. Patients with significant liver failure should not undergo surgery except in life-threatening situations.

8. **Psychiatric disease.** Symptomatic control should be evaluated in all patients with known psychiatric disease. In addition, all patients should be monitored for signs of active psychiatric disease, and their social support system assessed. Patients with evidence of or predisposition for psychiatric disturbance should delay surgery until acute problems are controlled and should be monitored during and after surgery for exacerbation.

9. **Lifestyle risks**
   a. **Drug or alcohol use/abuse.** Patients who abuse alcohol or drugs must be evaluated for use-associated organ damage such as alcoholic hepatitis. In addition, the perioperative period presents risks for withdrawal symptoms. Ideally, the addicted patient should undergo medically monitored detoxification prior to surgery (see Chapter 88). If a history of intravenous drug use is elicited, testing for HIV and hepatitis C is warranted.
   b. **Cigarette smoking.** Smokers have a higher risk of cardiovascular and pulmonary disease and should be evaluated carefully for those problems. In addition, smokers should be advised that smoking cessation at least 8 weeks before surgery can improve their mucociliary capacity considerably and thus decrease their chances of postoperative pneumonia. Fewer than 8 weeks of

smoking cessation has not been associated with an improvement in operative morbidity or mortality.

   c. Sexual behavior. Brief questioning about sexual behavior will uncover female patients at risk for pregnancy and will help identify patients at risk for HIV. A urine pregnancy test should be performed in all sexually active, premenopausal women.

  10. Medications. Certain medications can increase the patient's perioperative risk. Anticoagulant therapy such as warfarin or platelet aggregation inhibitors should be stopped 1 week before surgery. For some patients, the risk of even short-term discontinuation of anticoagulants exceeds the risk of surgery. These patients can be started on intravenous unfractionated heparin, titrated to maintain an activated partial thromboplastin time level of 55–85 seconds, or given a low-molecular-weight heparin subcutaneously, at a typical dose of 1 mg/kg body weight. Heparin can be discontinued several hours before the procedure to minimize intraoperative bleeding complications. Over-the-counter anti-inflammatories or some herbal remedies also cause a predisposition for excess bleeding, and the patient may not think to mention these products without specific prompting.

IV. Special Cases

  A. Children. Children are far less likely to have coronary artery disease but are at higher risk of having undiagnosed pulmonary, immunologic, anatomic, or genetic abnormalities. The preoperative history should include the prenatal and birth history and a history of recent infections. Upper respiratory infections or pneumonia should be allowed to completely resolve prior to surgery.

  B. Patients who are unable to give a history. Evaluation of functional capacity and current symptoms is impossible if a patient is unconscious or incapable of communicating with the physician. In this case, a careful physical examination becomes the only tool the primary care doctor has to identify risks. In this situation, a lower threshold for ordering predictive tests should be employed.

  C. Pregnancy. Except in life-threatening situations, surgery should be avoided in all pregnant women.

  D. Elderly patients. The likelihood of serious medical problems increases with age, and thus the perception arises that older patients are at higher risk during surgery. In fact, healthy geriatric patients do not have a higher surgical morbidity. These patients should be carefully evaluated for medical problems or social support issues, but can expect to undergo surgery quite successfully. Because of the high prevalence of dementia, the primary care examiner should perform a mental status examination on every geriatric patient.

V. The Perioperative Plan

  A. Communication of results to surgeon. The primary care consultation to the surgeon should include the following:

    1. A listing of the patient's known risk factors and medical conditions.

    2. Appraisal of how these factors will affect the patient's overall surgical risk.

    3. Suggestions for controlling, minimizing, or eliminating risks discovered in the preoperative evaluation.

  B. Patient counseling. The primary care doctor should discuss the risks and benefits of surgery clearly with the patient. The patient should understand:

    1. That all surgery may include unanticipated complications.

    2. Any factors that create particularly high risk for this patient.

    3. Your suggestions to the patient for minimizing risk.

    4. Your suggestion for long-term follow-up of any medical problems found in the examination.

REFERENCES

Eagle KA, et al: ACC/AHA Guideline Update on Perioperative Cardiovascular Evaluation for Noncardiac Surgery: A report of the American College of Cardiology/American Heart Association Task Force on Practice Guidelines (Committee to Update the 1996 Guidelines on Perioperative Cardiovascular Evaluation for Noncardiac Surgery). 2002; American College of Cardiology web site. http://www.acc.org/clinical/guidelines/perio/dirIndex.htm.

Karnath BM: Preoperative cardiac risk assessment. Am Fam Physician 2002;**66:**1889.

King MS: Problem-oriented diagnosis: Preoperative evaluation. Am Fam Physician 2000;**62:**387.

Michota FA, Frost SD: Perioperative management of the hospitalized patient. Med Clin North Am 2002;**86:**731.

Index